Acute
Coronary
Care

Acute
Coronary
Care

Second Edition

ROBERT M. CALIFF

Associate Professor, Division of Cardiology
Department of Medicine
Director, Cardiac Care Unit
Duke University Medical Center
Durham, North Carolina

DANIEL B. MARK

Associate Professor, Division of Cardiology
Department of Medicine
Co-Director, Cardiac Care Unit
Director, Outcomes Research and
    Assessment Group
Duke University Medical Center
Durham, North Carolina

GALEN S. WAGNER

Associate Professor, Division of Cardiology
Department of Medicine
Duke University Medical Center
Durham, North Carolina

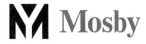 Mosby

St. Louis Baltimore Berlin Boston Carlsbad Chicago London Madrid
Naples New York Philadelphia Sydney Tokyo Toronto

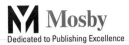

Mosby
Dedicated to Publishing Excellence

Editor: Laura DeYoung
Developmental Editor: Carolyn Malik
Project Manager: John Rogers
Production Editor: Lavon Wirch Peters
Cover Designer: Eleanor Safe

The authors and publisher have made every effort to ensure that the patient care recommendations herein, including the choice of drugs and drug dosages, are in accord with accepted standards and practices at the time of publication. However, because research and regulations constantly change clinical standards, the reader is urged to check the product information sheet included in the package of each drug, which includes recommended doses, warnings, and contraindications. This is particularly important with new and infrequently used drugs.

Second Edition

Printed in the United States of America

Mosby–Year Book, Inc.
11830 Westline Industrial Drive
St. Louis, Missouri 63146

Library of Congress Cataloging-in-Publication Data

Acute coronary care / [edited by] Robert M. Califf, Daniel B. Mark, Galen S. Wagner. — 2nd ed.
    p. cm.
    Rev. ed. of: Acute coronary care in the thrombolytic era. c1988.
    Includes bibliographical references and index.
    ISBN 0-8016-6753-4
    1. Coronary heart disease.   2. Coronary heart disease — Chemotherapy.
3. Fibrinolytic agents. I. Califf, Robert M. II. Mark, Daniel B. III. Wagner, Galen S. IV. Acute coronary care in the thrombolytic era.
    [DNLM: 1. Coronary Disease. 2. Critical Care. 3. Fibrinolytic Agents — therapeutic use. 4. Myocardial Infarction. WG 300 A1854 1994]
RC685.C6A285 1994
616.1'23 — dc20
DNLM/DLC
for Library of Congress
          94-4498
          CIP

94 95 96 97 98 / 9 8 7 6 5 4 3 2 1

CONTRIBUTORS

R. WAYNE ALEXANDER, M.D.
R. Bruce Logue Professor of Medicine, Director, Division of Cardiology, Emory University School of Medicine, Atlanta, Georgia

JOHN A. AMBROSE, M.D.
Professor of Medicine, Mount Sinai School of Medicine; Director, Cardiac Catheterization Laboratory, Mount Sinai Hospital, New York, New York

BRADI BARTRUG, R.N.
Clinical Nurse Specialist, Office of the Director of Nursing, Duke University Medical Center, Durham, North Carolina

THOMAS M. BASHORE, M.D.
Professor of Medicine, Division of Cardiology, Director, Cardiac Catheterization Laboratory, Duke University Medical Center, Durham, North Carolina

ERIC R. BATES, M.D.
Associate Professor of Internal Medicine, Director, Cardiac Catheterization Laboratory, The University of Michigan Medical Center, Department of Internal Medicine, Division of Cardiology, Ann Arbor, Michigan

ROBERT P. BAUMAN, M.D.
Research Associate, Durham Veterans Affairs Medical Center; Assistant Professor, Department of Medicine, Division of Cardiology, Duke University Medical Center, Durham, North Carolina

JAMES R. BENGTSON, M.D., M.P.H.
Director of Research, Michigan Heart and Vascular Institute, Ann Arbor, Michigan

DONALD A. BERKOW, M.D.
Emergency Room Department, Lancaster General Hospital, Lancaster, Pennsylvania

JONI R. BESHANSKY, R.N., M.P.H.
Research Coordinator, Division of Clinical Care Research, Center for Cardiovascular Health Services Research, Department of Medicine, New England Medical Center; Instructor of Medicine, Tufts University School of Medicine, Boston, Massachusetts

EDWIN G. BOVILL, M.D.
Professor and Chairman, Department of Pathology, University of Vermont, Burlington, Vermont

DAMIAN A. BREZINSKI, M.D.
Fellow, Division of Cardiology, Duke University Medical Center, Durham, North Carolina

WANDA BRIDE, R.N.
Head Nurse, Cardiac Intensive Care Unit, Duke University Medical Center, Durham, North Carolina

ROBERT M. CALIFF, M.D.
Associate Professor, Department of Medicine, Division of Cardiology, Director, Cardiac Care Unit, Duke University Medical Center, Durham, North Carolina

RONALD W.F. CAMPBELL, M.B., CH.B.
Professor of Cardiology, University of Newcastle-Upon-Tyne, Freeman Hospital, Newcastle-Upon-Tyne, United Kingdom

BERNARD R. CHAITMAN, M.D.
Professor of Medicine, Division of Cardiology, Department of Internal Medicine, Chief of Cardiology, Saint Louis University School of Medicine, St. Louis, Missouri

M. LEE CHENEY
Young, Moore, Henderson & Alvis, P.A., Raleigh, North Carolina

ROBERT CHRISTENSEN, PH.D.
Director, Clinical Chemistry Laboratory, University of Maryland, Baltimore, Maryland

FREDERICK R. COBB, M.D.
Professor, Department of Medicine, Division of Cardiology, Duke University Medical Center, Durham, North Carolina

DÉSIRÉ COLLEN, M.D., PH.D.
Professor of Medicine, Department of Molecular and Cardiovascular Research, Katholieke Universiteit Leuven, Center for Molecular and Vascular Biology, Leuven, Belgium

CHARLES J. DAVIDSON, M.D., F.A.C.C.
Associate Professor of Medicine, Northwestern University Medical School, Director, Cardiac Catheterization Laboratory, Northwestern Memorial Hospital, Chicago, Illinois

ANTHONY C. DeFRANCO, M.D.
Staff Physician, Interventional and Critical Care Cardiology, The Cleveland Clinic Foundation, Cleveland, Ohio

LESLIE DOMALIK, M.D.
Associate, Division of Endocrinology, Department of Medicine, Duke University Medical Center, Durham, North Carolina

JAMES M. DOUGLAS, JR., M.D., F.C.C.P.
Assistant Professor, Department of Surgery, Duke University Medical Center; Attending Physician, Department of Surgery, Durham Veterans Administration Medical Center, Durham, North Carolina

KATHLEEN DRACUP, R.N., D.N.S.C.
Professor, School of Nursing, University of California, Los Angeles, Los Angeles, California

GARY DUNHAM, B.S. PHARM.
Clinical Pharmacy Specialist on Cardiology, Department of Pharmacy, Clinical Instructor and Director—S.D.L.T. Lab, Department of Medicine, Duke Medical Center, Durham, North Carolina; Clinical Assistant Professor, University of North Carolina School of Pharmacy, Chapel Hill, North Carolina

DEBRA A. ECKART, R.N., M.S.N.
Nurse Clinician, Clinical Cardiac Electrophysiology, Duke University Medical Center; Clinical Associate, School of Nursing, Duke University, Durham, North Carolina

CAROLA C. EKELUND, L.P.T.
Exercise Physiologist, Duke University Center for Living, Durham, North Carolina

LARS G. EKELUND, M.D., PH.D., F.A.C.C.
Instructor, Duke University Diet and Fitness Center, Durham, North Carolina

STEPHEN G. ELLIS, M.D.
Director, Sones Cardiac Catheterization Laboratory, Department of Cardiology, The Cleveland Clinic Foundation, Cleveland, Ohio; Professor of Medicine, Ohio State University, Columbus, Ohio

ERLING FALK, M.D., PH.D.
Pathologist, Cardiac Unit, Massachusetts General Hospital; Visiting Associate Professor, Harvard University, Boston, Massachusetts

MICHAEL E. FARKOUH, M.D., F.R.C.P.C.
HGH McMaster Clinic, Hamilton General Hospital, Hamilton, Ontario, Canada

FREDERICK FEIT, M.D.
Director, Cardiac Catheterization, Tisch and Bellevue Hospitals; Associate Professor of Medicine, New York University School of Medicine, New York, New York

WENDY S. FITTS, R.N., B.S.N.
Nurse Manager, Emergency Department, Lancaster General Hospital, Lancaster, Pennsylvania

KEVIN FITZPATRICK, P.A.-C.
Health System User Analyst, Medical Center Information Systems, Duke University Medical Center, Durham, North Carolina

MARCUS D. FLATHER, M.D.
Senior Research Fellow, Division of Cardiology, McMaster University, HGH McMaster Clinic, Hamilton General Hospital, Hamilton, Ontario, Canada

WALTER L. FLOYD, M.D.
Professor of Medicine, Department of Medicine, Division of Cardiology, Duke University Medical Center, Durham, North Carolina

MATTHEW FLYNN, B.S.
Research Analyst, Duke University Medical Center, Durham, North Carolina

VICTOR F. FROELICHER, M.D.
Professor of Medicine, Stanford University School of Medicine, Cardiology Section, Veterans Administration Medical Center, Palo Alto, California

VALENTIN FUSTER, M.D., PH.D.
Director, Cardiovascular Institute, Arthur M. and Hilda A. Master Professor, The Mount Sinai Medical Center, New York, New York

KIRK N. GARRATT, M.D.
Assistant Professor of Medicine, Division of Cardiovascular Diseases and Internal Medicine, Mayo Clinic, Rochester, Minnesota

JEAN-MICHEL GASPOZ, M.D., M.SC.
Premier Chef-de-Clinique, Clinique de Medecine, Department of Medicine, University Hospital of Geneva, Geneva Medical School, University of Geneva, Geneva, Switzerland

BERNARD J. GERSH, M.B., CH.B., D.PHIL.
Chief, Division of Cardiology, Georgetown University Hospital, Washington, DC

DONALD D. GLOWER, M.D.
Associate Professor, Division of General and Thoracic Surgery, Duke University Medical Center, Durham, North Carolina

HERMAN K. GOLD, M.D.
Associate Professor of Medicine, Harvard Medical School, Massachusetts General Hospital, Boston, Massachusetts

ROBERT J. GOLDBERG, PH.D.
Professor of Medicine in Epidemiology, University of Massachusetts Medical Center, Worcester, Massachusetts

LEE GOLDMAN, M.D., M.P.H.
Chief Medical Officer, Brigham and Women's Hospital; Professor of Medicine, Harvard Medical School, Boston, Massachusetts

CHRISTOPHER B. GRANGER, M.D.
Assistant Professor of Medicine, Department of Medicine, Division of Cardiology, Co-Director, Cardiac Care Unit, Duke University Medical Center, Durham, North Carolina

JOSEPH C. GREENFIELD, JR., M.D.
Chairman and James B. Duke Professor, Department of Medicine, Durham Veterans Affairs Medical Center, Duke University Medical Center, Durham, North Carolina

RUTH ANN GREENFIELD, M.D.
Assistant Professor, Division of Cardiology, Department of Medicine, Duke University Medical Center, Durham, North Carolina

JOHN L. GRIFFITH, PH.D.
Statistician, Center for Cardiovascular Health Services Research, Division of Clinical Care Research, Department of Medicine, New England Medical Center; Assistant Professor of Medicine, Tufts University School of Medicine, Boston, Massachusetts

CINDY L. GRINES, M.D.
Director, Cardiac Catheterization Laboratories, Department of Cardiology, William Beaumont Hospital, Royal Oak, Michigan

ROBERT A. HARRINGTON, M.D.
Associate in Medicine, Department of Medicine, Division of Cardiology, Duke University Medical Center, Durham, North Carolina

J. KEVIN HARRISON, M.D.
Assistant Professor of Medicine, Department of Medicine, Division of Cardiology, Duke University Medical Center, Durham, North Carolina

WILLIAM R. HATHAWAY, M.D.
Fellow in Cardiology, Department of Medicine, Division of Cardiology, Duke University Medical Center, Durham, North Carolina

STEVEN E. HEARNE, M.D.
Fellow, Division of Cardiology, Department of Medicine, Duke University Medical Center, Durham, North Carolina

WILLIAM R. HERZOG, M.D.
Assistant Professor of Medicine, Director, VA Cath Lab, University of Maryland Hospital, Division of Cardiology, Baltimore, Maryland

MICHAEL B. HIGGINBOTHAM, M.B.
Director, Heart Failure Program, Director, Cardiopulmonary Exercise Laboratory, Medical Director, Heart Transplant Program, Associate Professor of Medicine, Department of Medicine, Division of Cardiology, Duke University Medical Center, Durham, North Carolina

JACK HIRSH, M.D.
Director, Hamilton Civic Hospitals Research Centre, Henderson General Hospital; Professor, Department of Medicine, McMaster University, Hamilton, Ontario, Canada

CRAIG E. HJEMDAHL-MONSEN, M.D., F.A.C.C.
Assistant Professor of Medicine, Department of Medicine, Division of Cardiology, New York Medical College, Westchester County Medical Center, Valhalla, New York

MARK HLATKY, M.D.
Associate Professor of Health Research and Policy and of Medicine (Cardiovascular Medicine), Stanford University School of Medicine, Stanford, California

DAVID R. HOLMES, JR., M.D.
Professor of Medicine, Department of Cardiovascular Diseases and Internal Medicine, Mayo Clinic, Rochester, Minnesota

JODIE L. HURWITZ, M.D.
Assistant Professor of Medicine, North Texas Heart Center, Dallas, Texas

IK-KYUNG JANG, M.D.
Assistant Professor of Medicine, Harvard University Medical School, Massachusetts General Hospital, Boston, Massachusetts

ROBERT H. JONES, M.D.
Mary and Deryl Hart Professor of Surgery, Department of Surgery, Duke University Medical Center, Durham, North Carolina

ANDREW J. KAPLAN, M.D.
Cardiology Fellow in Electrophysiology, Emory University School of Medicine, Atlanta, Georgia

DEAN J. KEREIAKES, M.D., F.A.C.C.
Director, Division of Coronary Intervention, The Christ Hospital Cardiovascular Research Center, The Christ Hospital, Cincinnati, Ohio

JOSEPH KISSLO, M.D.
Professor of Medicine, Department of Medicine, Division of Cardiology, Director, Adult and Pediatric Echocardiography, Duke University Medical Center, Durham, North Carolina

NEAL S. KLEIMAN, M.D.
Assistant Director, Cardiac Catheterization Laboratory, Department of Medicine, The Methodist Hospital; Assistant Professor, Department of Medicine, Baylor College of Medicine, Houston, Texas

EVA KLINE, R.N., M.S.
Clinical Nurse Specialist, Division of Cardiology, University of Michigan Medical Center, Ann Arbor, Michigan

EUGENE KOVALIK, M.D., F.R.C.P.(C.)
Director of Dialysis Unit, Division of Nephrology, Duke University Medical Center, Durham, North Carolina

MITCHELL W. KRUCOFF, M.D.
Assistant Professor of Medicine, Division of Cardiology, Department of Medicine, Duke University Medical Center, Durham, North Carolina

MARINO LABINAZ, M.D.
Fellow, Interventional Cardiology, Duke University Medical Center, Durham, North Carolina; Research Fellow of the Heart and Stroke Foundation of Canada, Ottawa, Ontario, Canada

THOMAS H. LEE, M.D.
Associate Professor of Medicine, Chief, Section of Clinical Epidemiology, Brigham and Women's Hospital and Harvard Medical School, Boston, Massachusetts

HENRI ROGER LIJNEN, PH.D.
Associate Professor, Department of Molecular and Cardiovascular Research, Katholieke Universiteit Leuven, Center for Molecular and Vascular Biology, Leuven, Belgium

B. GAIL MACIK, M.D.
Assistant Professor, Departments of Medicine and Pathology, Duke University Medical Center, Durham, North Carolina

VICTOR J. MARDER, M.D.
Professor of Medicine, Hematology Unit/Department of Medicine, Strong Memorial Hospital; Attending Physician, University of Rochester School of Medicine and Dentistry, Rochester, New York

DANIEL B. MARK, M.D., M.P.H.
Associate Professor of Medicine, Department of Medicine, Division of Cardiology, Co-Director, Cardiac Care Unit, Director, Outcomes Research and Assessment Group, Duke University Medical Center, Durham, North Carolina

JENNY MARTIN, R.N.
Research Coordinator, M.I.T.I. Coordinating Center, Division of Cardiology, University of Washington, Seattle, Washington

RICHARD L. McCANN, M.D.
Professor of Surgery, Chief, Department of Vascular Surgery, Duke University Medical Center, Durham, North Carolina

JAMES J. MERRILL, M.D.
Associate, Division of Cardiology, Department of Medicine, Duke University Medical Center, Durham, North Carolina

MEG MOLLOY, M.P.H., R.D., L.D.N.
Dietician Clinician, Duke University Center for Living, Durham, North Carolina

KENNETH G. MORRIS, M.D.
Assistant Clinical Professor, Department of Medicine, Division of Cardiology, Duke University Medical Center; Chief, Cardiology Section, Department of Cardiology, Veterans Administration Medical Center, Durham, North Carolina

MITCHELL MROZ, M.S.
Medical Student, Duke University Medical Center, Durham, North Carolina

JAMES E. MULLER, M.D.
Chief, Cardiology Division, New England Deaconess Hospital; Associate Professor of Medicine, Harvard Medical School, Boston, Massachusetts

MARGARET B. MUNSTER, R.N., M.S.N.
Patient Advice Nurse, Scott and White Clinic, College Station, Texas

PAUL E. NATHAN, M.D.
Cardiologist, Long Island College Hospital, Brooklyn, New York

C. DAVID NAYLOR, M.D., D.PHIL.
Director, Clinical Epidemiology Program, Sunnybrook Health Science Centre; Associate Professor of Medicine, University of Toronto; Chief Executive Officer, The Institute for Clinical Evaluative Sciences in Ontario (Inc.), Toronto, Ontario, Canada

CHRISTOPHER M. O'CONNOR, M.D.
Assistant Professor of Medicine, Department of Medicine, Division of Cardiology, Duke University Medical Center, Durham, North Carolina

E. MAGNUS OHMAN, M.D., F.R.C.P.I.
Assistant Professor of Medicine, Department of Medicine, Division of Cardiology, Coordinator, Clinical Trials, Interventional Cardiology, Duke University Medical Center, Durham, North Carolina

SUMITA D. PAUL, M.D., M.P.H.
Clinical/Research Fellow in Cardiology, Cardiac Unit, Massachusetts General Hospital; Clinical/Research Fellow in Cardiology, Harvard Medical School, Boston, Massachusetts

HARRY R. PHILLIPS, M.D.
Associate Professor of Medicine, Director, Interventional Cardiac Catheterization Laboratory, Department of Medicine, Division of Cardiology, Duke University Medical Center, Durham, North Carolina

JAMES E. POPE, M.D.
Consulting Associate, Division of Cardiology, Department of Medicine, Duke University Medical Center, Durham, North Carolina

ERIC N. PRYSTOWSKY, M.D.
Director, Clinical Electrophysiology Laboratory, St. Vincent Hospital, Indianapolis, Indiana; Consulting Professor of Medicine, Duke University Medical Center, Durham, North Carolina

JOSEPH A. PUMA, D.O.
Consulting Associate, Division of Cardiology, Department of Medicine, Duke University Medical Center, Durham, North Carolina

JUDITH C. REMBERT, PH.D.
Physiologist, Durham Veterans Affairs Medical Center; Associate Medical Research Professor of Medicine, Department of Medicine, Duke University Medical Center, Durham, North Carolina

JOSEPH G. REVES, M.D.
Professor and Chairman, Department of Anesthesiology, Director, The Heart Center, Duke University Medical Center, Durham, North Carolina

LEIGH ANN ROGERS, R.N., B.S.N.
Cardiology Nurse Clinician, Cardiac Care Unit, Duke University Medical Center, Durham, North Carolina

MARK C. ROGERS, M.D.
Vice Chancellor for Health Affairs, Executive Director and CEO, Duke University Hospital and Health Network, Durham, North Carolina

ALLAN M. ROSS, M.D.
Professor and Associate Chairman, Department of Medicine, Director, Cardiovascular Research Institute, George Washington University Medical Center, Washington, D.C.

DEBORAH A. ROTH, M.S.
Administrative Director, Duke Heart Center, Duke University Medical Center, Durham, North Carolina

JOHN A. RUMBERGER, M.D., PH.D.
Associate Professor of Medicine, Department of Cardiovascular Diseases, Mayo Medical School, Rochester, Minnesota

DAVID C. SANE, M.D.
Assistant Professor of Internal Medicine, The Bowman Gray School of Medicine, Winston-Salem, North Carolina

SHARON T. SAWCHAK
Clinical Research Nurse, Division of Cardiology, Department of Medicine, Duke University Medical Center, Durham, North Carolina

STEVEN J. SCHWAB, M.D.
Professor of Medicine, Department of Medicine, Division of Nephrology, Duke University Medical Center, Durham, North Carolina

LEWIS B. SCHWARTZ, M.D.
Chief Resident, Department of Surgery, Duke University Medical Center, Durham, North Carolina

HARRY P. SELKER, M.D., M.S.PH.
Chief, Division of Clinical Care Research, Director, Center for Cardiovascular Health Services Research, Department of Medicine, New England Medical Center; Associate Professor of Medicine, Tufts University School of Medicine, Boston, Massachusetts

RONALD H. SELVESTER, M.D.
Professor of Medicine, Retired, LAC-USC Medical Center, Los Angeles, California

AKBAR SHAH, M.D.
Research Fellow in Cardiology, Duke University Medical Center, Durham, North Carolina

ROBERT D. SIMARI, M.D.
Assistant Professor of Medicine, Department of Internal Medicine, Division of Cardiovascular Diseases, Mayo Clinic, Rochester, Minnesota

MICHAEL H. SKETCH, JR., M.D.
Assistant Professor, Department of Medicine, Division of Cardiology, Director, Interventional Cardiac Catheterization Laboratory, Duke University Medical Center, Durham, North Carolina

DEBORAH D. SMITH, R.N.
Regional Coordinator, GUSTO Trial, Duke Databank for Cardiovascular Disease, Duke University Medical Center, Durham, North Carolina

ROBERT A. SORRENTINO, M.D.
Assistant Professor, Division of Cardiology, Department of Medicine, Duke University Medical Center, Durham, North Carolina

JAMES L. SPIRA, PH.D., M.P.H.
Assistant Clinical Professor, Division of Medical Psychology, Department of Psychiatry, Duke University Medical Center, Durham, North Carolina

RICHARD S. STACK, M.D.
Associate Professor, Department of Medicine, Division of Cardiology, Director, Interventional Cardiac Catheterization Program, Duke University Medical Center, Durham, North Carolina

MARTIN J. SULLIVAN, M.D.
Assistant Professor, Department of Medicine, Division of Cardiology, Duke University Medical Center, Durham, North Carolina

JOSEPH M. SUTTON, M.D.
Director, Acute Coronary Intervention, Department of Cardiology, The Cleveland Clinic Foundation, Cleveland, Ohio

JAMES E. TCHENG, M.D.
Assistant Professor of Medicine, Division of Cardiology, Duke University Medical Center, Durham, North Carolina

ALAN N. TENAGLIA, M.D.
Assistant Professor, Division of Cardiology, Tulane University Medical Center, New Orleans, Louisiana

KOON K. TEO, M.B.B.CH., PH.D., M.R.C.P.I., F.R.C.P.C.
Assistant Professor of Medicine, Director, Cardiac Clinical Trials, Division of Cardiology, University of Alberta, Edmonton, Alberta, Canada

FRANK D. TICE, M.D.
Assistant Professor of Clinical Medicine, The Ohio State University Medical Center, Columbus, Ohio

GEOFFREY H. TOFLER, M.B.
Co-Director, Institute for Prevention of Cardiovascular Disease, New England Deaconess Hospital; Instructor in Medicine, Harvard Medical School, Boston, Massachusetts

ERIC J. TOPOL, M.D.
Chairman, Department of Cardiology, Director, Center for Thrombosis and Arterial Biology, The Cleveland Clinic Foundation, Cleveland, Ohio

RUSSELL P. TRACY, PH.D.
Associate Professor of Pathology and Biochemistry, Department of Pathology, University of Vermont, Burlington, Vermont

CHARLES B. TREASURE, M.D.
Assistant Professor of Medicine, Emory University School of Medicine, Atlanta, Georgia

KATHLEEN M. TROLLINGER
Clinical Research Nurse, Division of Cardiology, Department of Medicine, Duke University Medical Center, Durham, North Carolina

FRANS VAN DE WERF, M.D., PH.D.
Professor of Medicine, Department of Cardiology, University Hospital Gasthuisberg, Leuven, Belgium

MARC VERSTRAETE, M.D., PH.D.
Professor of Medicine, Center for Molecular and Vascular Biology, Katholieke Universiteit Leuven, Leuven, Belgium

GALEN S. WAGNER, M.D.
Associate Professor of Medicine, Department of Medicine, Division of Cardiology, Duke University Medical Center, Durham, North Carolina

NANCY B. WAGNER, B.A. (DECEASED)
Clinical Research Coordinator, Department of Medicine, Division of Cardiology, Duke University Medical Center, Durham, North Carolina

THOMAS C. WALL, M.D., F.A.C.C.
Division of Cardiology, Drs. LeBauer, Weintraub, Brodie, Patterson & Associates, P.A., Greensboro, North Carolina

W. DOUGLAS WEAVER, M.D.
Professor of Medicine in Cardiology, Director of Cardiovascular Care, University of Washington, Seattle, Washington

J. MARCUS WHARTON, M.D.
Associate Professor of Medicine, Director, Clinical Cardiac Electrophysiology, Duke University Medical Center, Durham, North Carolina

HARVEY D. WHITE, M.B., F.A.C.C.
Director, Coronary Care and Cardiovascular Research, Green Lane Hospital, Auckland, New Zealand

RICHARD D. WHITE, M.D.
Head, Section of Cardiac Imaging, Division of Radiology, The Cleveland Clinic Foundation, Cleveland, Ohio

REDFORD B. WILLIAMS, M.D.
Professor of Psychiatry and Psychology, Associate Professor of Medicine, Director, Behavioral Medicine Research Center, Duke University Medical Center, Duke University, Durham, North Carolina

VANCE E. WILSON, M.D.
Lecturer, Internal Medicine, Division of Cardiology, Department of Internal Medicine, University of Michigan, Ann Arbor, Michigan

LYNN H. WOODLIEF, M.S.
Research Analyst, Duke University Medical Center, Durham, North Carolina

SETH JOSEPH WORLEY, M.D.
Director of Electrophysiology and Clinical Research, Department of Cardiology, Lancaster General Hospital, Lancaster, Pennsylvania

SALIM YUSUF, M.B.B.S., D.PHIL., F.R.C.P.(U.K.), F.R.C.P.C., F.A.C.C.
Professor of Medicine, Director, Division of Cardiology, McMaster University, Hamilton, Ontario, Canada

K. MICHAEL ZABEL, M.D.
Fellow in Cardiology, Department of Medicine, Division of Cardiology, Duke University Medical Center, Durham, North Carolina

DEDICATION

More than any other edition of the coronary care texts we have edited, this edition has tested the mettle of our loved ones, friends and colleagues. As we have been swept up in the frenzy of health care reform, the reshaping of academic medical centers, and the revolution in knowledge about cardiovascular medicine, we have often felt like sailors trying to sail out of the Golden Gate against the tide, catching the wind at full sail, yet moving backwards nevertheless. Just as a chapter was considered almost complete, a new clinical trial or observation would become available. In this complex environment we have relied on pillars of stability for inspiration and support.

Most importantly, this book is dedicated to our families, who continually remind us of the reason we are driven to improve our understanding of cardiovascular disease and how to treat it: the net of love and support that leads to the desire to help mankind and individuals in a tangible way.

Professionally, the editors share a common bond of friendship with and admiration for a mentor, Dr. Joseph C. Greenfield, Jr. As Dr. Greenfield prepares to move from being our Department Chairman but remains our most trusted advisor, we wish to recognize the critical nature of his selfless support of our efforts and to express our appreciation for his willingness to listen to us and to provide us with pithy and memorable direction.

The flavor of this book reflects the collaborative spirit that has been our heritage in the Cardiology Division at Duke Medical Center and that has in many ways overtaken the field of cardiovascular medicine. We have personally collaborated with the authors of this book either in patient care or in research and sometimes in both, and thus the book in many ways represents a collective wisdom developed over years of working together. Many of our colleagues have contributed to the book without being authors, either by reviewing the chapters through the DUCCS organization or through collegial interactions at the bedside.

Finally, without the constant prodding and encouragement of Carolyn Malik at Mosby–Year Book and our editorial staffs, including Serena Smith, Lisa Breslau, Penny Hodgson and Patricia Williams, we would never have completed this constantly evolving task.

PREFACE

Acute coronary care is being swept up in the revolution of changes in medical practice. Simultaneous with a virtual explosion in the understanding of the biology of atherosclerosis and acute cardiac events, tremendous economic pressure is being applied to health care providers, resulting in increased demand for knowledge about what is effective in the practice of cardiology. For these reasons the number of clinical investigations and reports on clinical investigations has increased dramatically during the writing of this book. Thus the material presented in the book represents an attempt to hit a moving target.

This edition of *Acute Coronary Care* is meant to follow in the tradition of its predecessors. We have tried throughout to avoid the traditional textbook style; instead we have sought to provide the reader with a series of concepts that can be applied to an understanding of acute cardiac care, both at the bedside and in the research arena. Authors of the chapters have all been collaborators in research or clinical care. We have asked them to provide broad concepts as much as possible so that a framework will be established for the many

advances on the horizon. Where specifics are critical for clinical practice, we have sought to include the needed detail also.

After a first draft of each chapter was received, it was forwarded to a member of the Duke University Clinical Cardiology Society (DUCCS) for review. This special step enabled us to evaluate whether the chapters would be received as intended, and these reviews resulted in substantial useful modifications.

As the hype about the "information highway" is progressively transformed into reality, we have a vision that scientific and medical advances will be rapidly transmitted to appropriate audiences for consideration and feedback. In a way this book reflects a precursor to an eventual electronic, interactive environment. Much of the material represents original information developed in a collaborative fashion and shaped into a presentation through the interaction of scientists and clinicians over a broad geographic range. The ability to achieve this collaboration "in real time" will make future editions of *Acute Coronary Care* even more challenging, but we believe that the rewards will also be greater.

CONTENTS

Acute
Coronary
Care

Part I

BASIC CONCEPTS

Chapter 1

ATHEROGENESIS AND THROMBOSIS

Erling Falk

Very different pathologic processes underlie the slow progression of atherosclerotic plaques over decades, as opposed to the sudden, rapid progression responsible for acute heart attacks.[1] *Time-dependent, slow progression* is caused by cell proliferation, matrix production, and lipid accumulation. The individual significance of and interplay between cells (endothelium, macrophages, smooth muscle cells, and lymphocytes) and lipids during atherogenesis in humans are poorly understood. However, the complicating *time-independent, rapid progression* is clearly related to the extracellular lipids that soften plaques, making them vulnerable to rupture; ruptured plaques with superimposed thrombosis underlie the great majority of acute heart attacks.[1,2] Because soft extracellular lipid and thrombus are the key components of the lesion responsible for life-threatening clinical disease, this chapter will focus primarily on the soft atherothrombotic plaques responsible for acute unstable angina (pain at rest), acute myocardial infarction, and many cases of sudden coronary death.

ATHEROSCLEROSIS

Atherosclerotic plaques differ in composition, consistency, and vulnerability. As the name "atherosclerosis" implies, *atheromatous gruel* (lipid-rich, soft) and *sclerotic tissue* (collagen-rich, hard) are the main plaque components (Fig. 1-1 and 1-2). Interplaque and intraplaque composition vary greatly, but the hard, sclerotic component is usually much more voluminous than the soft atheromatous one.[3] Some patients have only hard or soft plaques, but most patients have plaques containing variable amounts of both hard and soft components.

Although these two plaque components are usually considered to represent different stages of atherosclerosis, their pathogenesis and relationship—with each other and with age-related adaptive intimal thickening[4]—are poorly understood.[3]

PLAQUE VULNERABILITY

Although hard, collagenous tissue usually constitutes the most voluminous component of coronary plaques, it is stable and rather innocuous. Soft atheromatous gruel, on the other hand, is definitely dangerous because it determines plaque vulnerability and rupture risk. Typically a vulnerable plaque consists of a pool of soft extracellular lipid (gruel) separated from the vascular lumen by a cap of fibrous tissue (see Figs. 1-1, *B*, and 1-2, *B*). The cap varies greatly in thickness (thick in 1-1 *B*, very thin in 1-2, *B*), cellularity, strength, and stiffness. It is often thinnest and most heavily infiltrated by macrophage foam cells at its junction with the adjacent, more normal intima (shoulders of the plaque).

Importantly, vulnerability is not a simple function of *plaque size* (i.e. severity of stenosis). The crucial factor is *plaque type* (i.e. the composition of the lesion).[5] Clinically, nonstenotic lesions appear more dangerous than stenotic ones,[1] probably because collaterals do not protect the nonstenotic lesions in case of sudden thrombotic occlusion.[6]

CAP RUPTURE: VULNERABILITY VS. TRIGGERS

Most ruptures are tiny, occurring at the shoulder regions of the plaque.[7] At the rupture site, the cap is often thin and foam cell infiltrated (Fig. 1-3), indicating

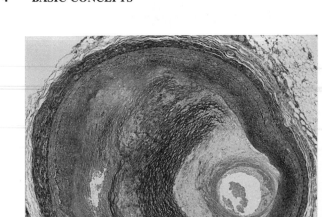

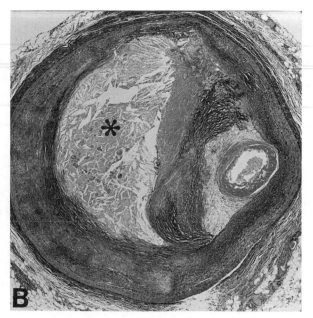

Fig. 1-1. The two main plaque components. **A,** Hard, collagen-rich, and innocuous plaque. **B,** Soft, lipid-rich, and potentially dangerous plaque. *Lipid-rich, atheromatous gruel with cholesterol crystals.

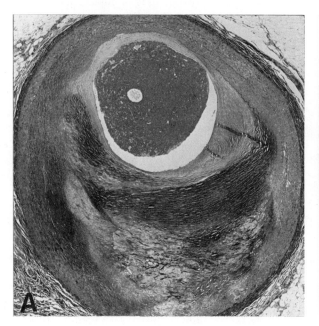

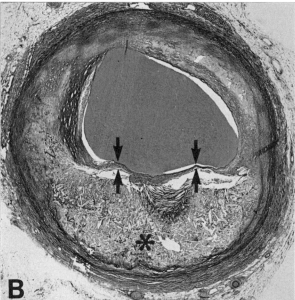

Fig. 1-2. Plaque vulnerability. **A,** Stable sclerotic (collagen-rich) plaque. **B,** Vulnerable plaque, consisting of a pool of soft, lipid-rich, atheromatous gruel (*) separated from the vascular lumen only by a very thin cap of fibrous tissue (between *arrows*). Although plaque **A** is more voluminous/stenotic than plaque **B,** the latter is the most dangerous.

ongoing disease activity, at least locally.[7,8] Progressive extracellular lipid accumulation (gruel formation) and cap weakening, possibly because of ongoing macrophage activity within the cap,[9,10] may determine the plaque's vulnerability, which may change with time.

The shoulder regions are, however, not only "weak points" but probably also points of "maximal stress."[7] Therefore, the questions arise: Is plaque rupture caused solely by ongoing disease activity within the plaque, causing progressive weakening *(vulnerability),* or do factors external to the plaque *(triggers)* also contribute?

Muller et al.[11,12] considered these possibilities in the

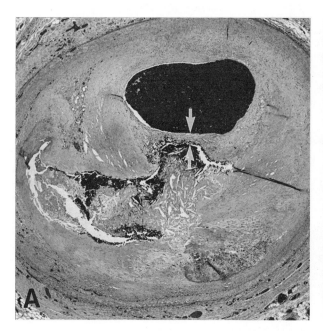
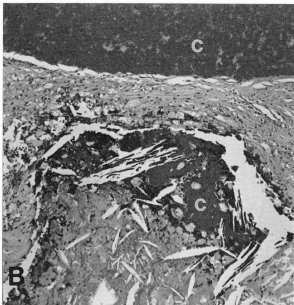

Fig. 1-3. Cap weakening. **A** and **B,** The contrast medium *(c)* injected postmortem has found its way into the plaque, indicating that the plaque surface is ruptured nearby. In this section, the fibrous cap is intact but very thin (between *arrows* in **A**) and heavily foam cell infiltrated **(B),** indicating ongoing disease activity that may have weakened the cap, predisposing it to rupture.

"circadian-triggering" concept: a plaque becomes vulnerable because of internal changes. Then, even a minor stress may trigger onset, most frequently between 6 A.M. and noon.[11,12] As possible rupture triggers, most attention has been paid to hemodynamic and mechanical stresses. In particular, "surges in sympathetic activity" increasing the blood pressure, heart rate, myocardial contractility, coronary flow, and coronary tone might physically stress and disrupt a vulnerable plaque. I believe, however, that vulnerability plays a more important role in rupture than triggers, because only vulnerable plaques are rupture prone, and the majority of rupture/thrombus-related acute heart attacks occur during *normal* daily activities without an obvious precipitator. In addition, exercise stress testing (usually associated with much greater hemodynamic changes than the morning "surge") of patients with advanced coronary artery disease rarely "triggers" a rupture/thrombus-related acute heart attack.[13] The circadian rhythm in clinical disease could be caused by a parallel variation in thrombogenic factors superimposed, as the thrombus, on ruptured plaques.[11,12]

PLAQUE RUPTURE CAUSING UNSTABLE LESION

Rupture of a vulnerable plaque may cause rapid plaque progression because of hemorrhage into the plaque or luminal thrombosis (or both) (Figs. 1-4 and 1-5). Autopsy studies suggest that acute coronary events occur frequently during plaque evolution.[3,8,14] However, the majority of such events are probably clinically silent,

because most ruptures involve progression from a nonstenotic to a more severe, still nonstenotic lesion. *Most ruptured plaques are sealed by a small mural thrombus and become dangerous only if a major, flow-limiting thrombus evolves at the rupture site.*

Three major factors seem to determine the outcome of a plaque rupture (mural vs. occlusive thrombosis)[1,15]: (1) the amount and character of exposed thrombogenic material at the rupture site (thrombogenic substrates), (2) local flow disturbances caused by preexisting atherosclerotic stenosis (stenosis/flow), and (3) the actual thrombotic-thrombolytic equilibrium (thrombotic propensity).

Thrombogenic substrates

Experimentally, the amount and character of exposed thrombogenic material after intimal injury dominantly affect the outcome (thrombotic response), often via local thrombin generation with platelet activation.[1] *However, factors other than thrombin may dominate at high shear stress (i.e., thrombus formation within severely stenotic lesions).*[16] A recent coronary angioscopic study indicated a similar substrate-thrombosis relation in humans: *mild intimal irregularities with mural thrombosis were found in unstable angina, whereas more extensive injuries with occlusive thrombus were present in acute myocardial infarction.*[17] Collagen and lipids, including lipoprotein (a),[18] could be key substrates in human thrombus formation. Special attention has recently been focused on tissue factor.[19]

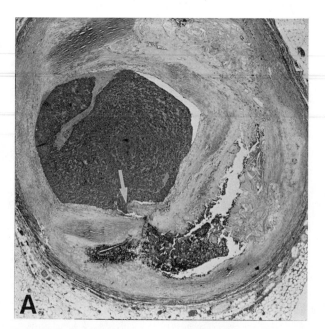

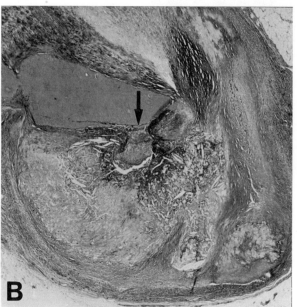
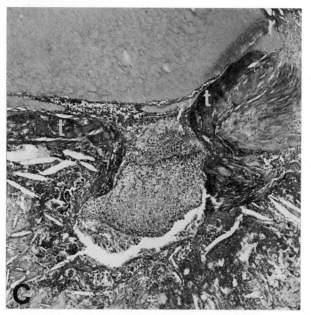

Fig. 1-4. Unstable plaques. **A,** Ruptured plaque surface (at *arrow*) with hemorrhage into the plaque. No luminal thrombus is seen. **B** and **C,** Ruptured plaque surface (at *arrow*) with hemorrhage into the plaque and missing (embolized) plaque material. A small mural thrombus *(t)* has evolved over the exposed collagen-rich cap at the rupture site.

Stenosis/flow

Postmortem and clinical observations indicate that, to some extent, the degree of preexisting atherosclerotic stenosis determines the outcome of a plaque rupture: as the degree of atherosclerotic stenosis increases, *the risk of major thrombus formation also increases.*[15,20] Thus, a stenosis seems to promote arterial thrombosis, probably via *shear-induced platelet activation.*[21] Experimentally, a platelet thrombus may form and grow within a severe stenosis, predominantly at the apex where the blood

velocity and shear forces are highest.[22,23] Unlike venous thrombosis, arterial thrombosis is not primarily associated with blood stagnation; many atherosclerotic stenoses underlying infarct-related thrombi are hemodynamically insignificant.[24,25] Although mild or moderate stenoses most frequently progress to infarct-related occlusion,[1,5] severe stenoses most frequently occlude,[20,21, 26-29] but such events are often clinically silent because of well-developed collateral vessels.

Thrombus formation may also extend poststenoti-

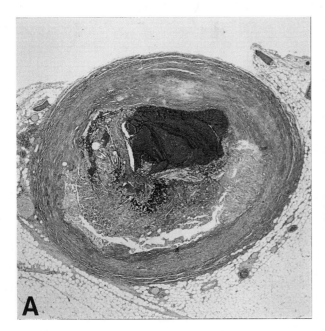
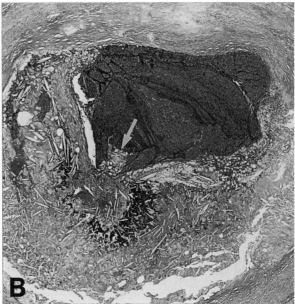

Fig. 1-5. Occlusive thrombosis. **A** and **B,** Ruptured plaque with hemorrhage into the soft gruel and luminal thrombus. The cap is heavily foam cell infiltrated. It is totally disintegrated with soft plaque material displaced through the ruptured surface into the lumen (at *arrow*), where it is buried within the thrombus.

cally, where flow separation, recirculation, and turbulence probably offer ideal fluid dynamic conditions for progressive growth. This free-floating thrombus "tail" extends downstream, often growing much larger than the mural thrombus within the stenosis and exhibiting a high potential to embolize.[24] Accordingly, angiographic filling defects thought to represent nonoccluding thrombi are typically poststenotic.[30]

Thrombotic propensity

Platelet aggregation, plasma fibrinogen, and fibrinolytic activity are associated with the development of acute myocardial infarction. People at risk of plaque rupture (stable angina) or thought to have ruptured coronary plaques (unstable angina) may benefit from antithrombotic therapy with antiplatelet agents or anticoagulants.[1] Aspirin may postpone the complication of progressing atherosclerosis with life-threatening thrombosis.[31] Thus, in cases of plaque rupture, the actual thrombotic-thrombolytic equilibrium may play a decisive role.

Experimentally, some plasma lipoproteins, epinephrine, cigarette smoke, and exercise promote platelet aggregation and arterial thrombosis.[1]

CORONARY THROMBOSIS

Most fatal and nonfatal coronary thrombi ($>75\%$) are precipitated by the sudden rupture of a plaque surface, which exposes thrombogenic material to the flowing blood (see Fig. 1-5).[3,15] Only minor and super-

ficial intimal irregularities (i.e., no deep injury) are found beneath the rest of the thrombi, usually in combination with a severe atherosclerotic stenosis. The microstructure of the luminal thrombus may illuminate the significance of the individual components, particularly platelets and fibrin, and their temporal, dynamic interplay.

Early platelet-rich thrombus

In fatal, acute heart attack victims, the most recent thrombus growth causing the final symptoms consists predominantly of aggregated platelets (Fig. 1-6), often admixed with displaced atheromatous plaque material.[8,32] The latter or intimal flaps may project into the narrowed lumen and form a predominantly nonthrombotic, vascular occlusion (Fig. 1-7). In addition, evidence strongly suggests that rethrombosis (reinfarction) is platelet mediated like the initial thrombotic occlusion at the site.[33]

Consolidated platelet-rich thrombus

The early platelet-rich thrombus is soon infiltrated by fibrin, which eventually enmeshes the platelets, giving rise to a homogeneous, structureless mass (when viewed under light microscope) (see Fig. 1-6). However, the primary platelet structure is still apparent under electron microscope, where platelets appear "concealed" in a fibrin network.[34] Although the platelet thrombus may now appear "transformed" into a fibrinous thrombus, the early platelet thrombus is merely stabilized by fibrin.

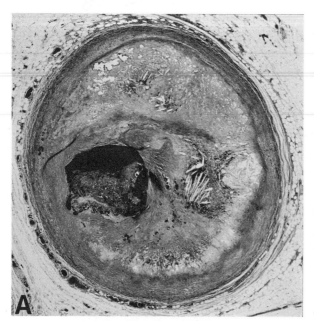
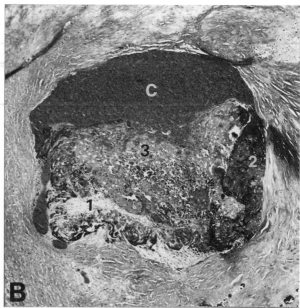

Fig. 1-6. Coronary thrombosis: episodic growth. **A** and **B,** Nonocclusive luminal thrombus formed in at least three stages. The most recent part, located centrally *(3),* consists predominantly of aggregated platelets. The older part of the thrombus *(2)* is homogeneous (fibrin stabilized), whereas the oldest part *(1)* is being incorporated into the plaque. *c,* contrast medium injected postmortem. (From Falk E: Coronary thrombosis: pathogenesis and clinical manifestations. Am J Cardiol 68:28B-35B, 1991. Used by permission.)

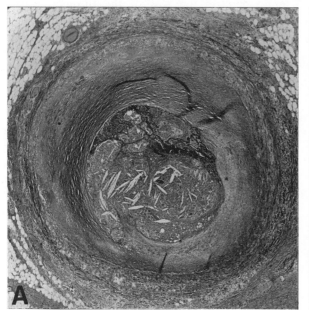
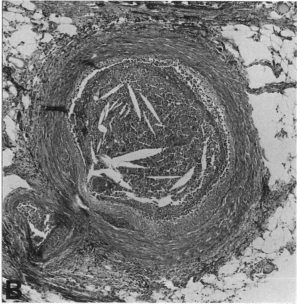

Fig. 1-7. Nonthrombotic vascular occlusion. Coronary artery **(A)** and a distal side branch **(B)** occluded by atheromatous gruel with cholesterol crystals. A huge, soft, atheromatous plaque was ruptured just proximal to section **A,** with extrusion of the occluding plaque material into the vascular lumen.

Thus, both platelets and fibrin play a role in the evolution of a coronary thrombus. The primary flow obstruction is usually caused by platelet aggregation. However, the flowing blood may easily sweep away an unstable platelet thrombus unless fibrin subsequently enmeshes the platelets and stabilizes the thrombus. Such a temporal interplay between platelets and fibrin, also found in experimental studies, explains why both anti-platelet agents and anticoagulants may benefit patients at risk of coronary thrombosis[1] and also why fresh

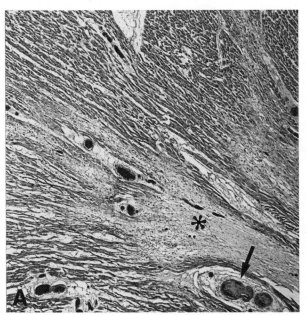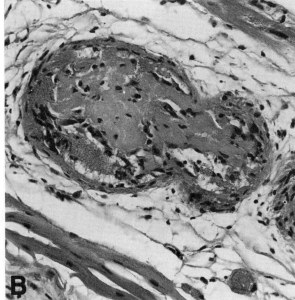

Fig. 1-8. Coronary thrombosis: embolization. **A,** Small thromboemboli *(arrow)* and microinfarcts (*) are frequently found in the myocardium downstream from evolving coronary thrombi. **B,** thromboembolus at arrow in **A.**

thrombi are more easiy lysed than older, consolidated thrombi.[15,35]

Dynamic thrombosis

More than 80% of coronary thrombi have a *layered* structure indicating repeated mural deposits (Fig. 1-6).[32] Episodic growth apparently alternates with thrombus fragmentation and peripheral embolization, evidenced by the frequently found, small thrombus fragments impacted in intramyocardial arteries downstream from evolving coronary thrombi. These fragments are often associated with microinfarcts (Fig. 1-8).[32,36,37] In total, coronary thrombosis is a dynamic process in which the thrombus waxes and wanes, causing intermittent coronary obstruction. Also, clinical observations indicate that thrombosis and thrombolysis occur simultaneously.[38] Thus, the goal of rapid and sustained reperfusion may be reached most effectively by targeting both processes: inhibiting thrombosis and enhancing thrombolysis.

Thrombosis and vasospasm often coexist; the former may give rise to the latter.[39] Although spasm often contributes to the dynamic flow obstruction in patients suffering an acute heart attack, thrombosis is most important to initial reperfusion and survival.[40]

Thrombus propagation

If the white, platelet-rich thrombus at the rupture site evolves into an occlusive thrombus, the blood proximal and distal to the occlusion may stagnate and coagulate (clot). The red stagnation thrombosis, similar to a venous thrombus found in stagnant blood, is composed primarily of fibrin-bound erythrocytes (Fig. 1-9). Depending

on side branches and collateral flow, the extent of thrombus propagation varies greatly both downstream and upstream. Particularly in coronary vein grafts (lacking side branches)[41] and in the right coronary artery (with few major side branches), this secondarily formed clot may contribute significantly to the "thrombotic burden." If not too huge, the clot is probably more easily lysed than the primary platelet-rich thrombus at the rupture site.[42]

CLINICAL MANIFESTATIONS

Most hemodynamically insignificant lesions are likely to rupture asymptomatically. Unstable angina likely is caused by rapid plaque progression as a result of plaque rupture. The natural history of acute unstable angina probably mirrors that of the underlying ruptured plaque: stabilization (sealing the rupture), symptom accentuation (mural thrombosis), or infarction (occlusive thrombosis). The collateral flow's magnitude would naturally modify the history.

As previously mentioned, a great proportion of total occlusions result from severe stenoses' silent progression, in which collateral vessels probably protect the myocardium when thrombotic occlusion supervenes.[26-29] Typically, coronary angiography and angioscopy performed during acute heart attacks have revealed transient, nonocclusive thrombi in unstable angina with pain at rest. These procedures have also revealed severe stenoses probably representing mural thrombosis or early spontaneous recanalized thrombi that may progress to total occlusion in non–Q-wave infarction. Occlusive thrombi that may persist or lyse spontaneously

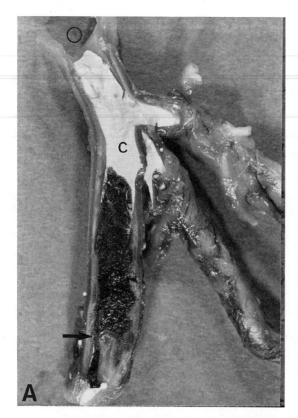
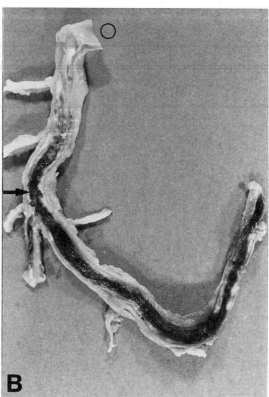

Fig. 1-9. Thrombus propagation. **A,** Left anterior descending coronary artery cut open longitudinally, showing a dark (red) stagnation thrombosis propagating upstream from the initiating rupture/platelet-rich thrombus at the arrow. In this case, the thrombus has propagated proximally up to the nearest major side branch (the first diagonal branch). **B,** The right coronary artery cut open longitudinally, showing a huge stagnation thrombosis propagating downstream from the initiating rupture/platelet-rich thrombus at the arrow. Unlike upstream thrombus propagation, downstream propagation may, like here, occlude major side branches. *O,* coronary ostium; *c,* contrast medium injected postmortem. (From Falk E: Coronary thrombosis: pathogenesis and clinical manifestations. Am J Cardiol 68:28B-35B, 1991. Used by permission.)

(but too late for significant myocardial salvage) seem to characterize Q-wave infarction.[17,43-46] Apparently the culprit lesion responsible for out of hospital cardiac arrest or sudden death often resembles that of unstable angina: plaque rupture with mural thrombosis.[47,48]

Thus, a ruptured plaque with a superimposed dynamic thrombosis (with or without concomitant vasospasm) seems to underlie the majority of acute coronary syndromes. Clinical presentation and outcome depend on the severity and duration of ischemia. The degree of vascular obstruction and the persistence of flow limitation are important, as is the magnitude of collateral flow.

INTERVENTION

An acute heart attack usually results from the following chain of events: plaque, leading to vulnerability (and trigger?), leading to rupture, leading to thrombosis. Preventing just one of these "processes" will eliminate the life-threatening potential of coronary atherosclerosis.

Vulnerability and rupture risk

The dynamic interplay between the plaque's vulnerability and external triggers probably determines the likelihood, time, and point of rupture. Vulnerability predisposes the plaque to rupture; triggers may precipitate it. The plaque components responsible for vulnerability (soft extracellular lipid and maybe macrophages) usually constitute only a small fraction of plaque volume. However, these plaque components are most likely to regress with treatment. Therefore, lipid lowering may stabilize the plaque, reducing vulnerability and rupture risk (clinical disease) without causing a dramatic change in plaque volume (i.e., stenosis severity).[49]

Currently we cannot differentiate angiographically between stable and vulnerable plaques. In particular, plaque size (degree of stenosis) does not predict vulnerability and rupture risk. Therefore, to prevent rupture/thrombus-related acute heart attacks, therapy must address the entire coronary tree (systemic) and not just obstructive lesions.[5] The primary aim should be to arrest disease progression. However, it might be possible to postpone rupture of a progressing, vulnerable plaque by reducing trigger activity (*acute* risk factor reduction)[12] with β-blockers and heart rate–decreasing calcium antagonists. In the future, new imaging techniques may help identify soft, rupture-prone lesions, guiding choice of treatment.[50]

Evolving, dynamic thrombosis

The *actual* thrombotic-thrombolytic equilibrium (thrombotic propensity) is very important to the outcome of plaque rupture. Thrombosis and thrombolysis occur simultaneously in patients with acute coronary syndromes; both processes are enhanced by current pharmacologic thrombolysis.[38] Therefore, the efficacy of thrombolysis may depend crucially on effective, conjunctive antithrombotic therapy. Its importance was first indicated clearly by the results of the ISIS-2 trial: aspirin alone reduced mortality to the same extent as streptokinase alone. Combined, their effects were additive.[33] Heparin may be just as good.[51]

Generally, effective antithrombotic therapy (plus endogenous thrombolysis) usually prevents occlusion of the culprit lesions in acute unstable angina (mural thrombus).[52] On the other hand, pharmacologic thrombolysis and conjunctive antithrombotic therapy are needed for rapid and sustained reperfusion of occluded, infarct-related arteries.[53] In weeks or months, endogenous thrombolysis alone will gradually reopen most thrombosed arteries, but unaided it works slowly, and a severe stenosis usually persists.[54] Pharmacologic thrombolysis works faster, but the ultimate coronary result is probably not much better than that achieved by effective antithrombotic therapy.[55,56]

Failed thrombolysis

Current thrombolytic regimens fail to reperfuse a substantial proportion (20%?) of infarct-related arteries. Persistent occlusion (i.e., unsuccessful thrombolysis) remains a problem. In fatal cases, an occluding thrombus will nearly always be found at autopsy.[57-60] Clinical studies also indicate the presence of an occluding thrombus, despite the failure of standard intravenous thrombolytic treatment to reperfuse.[61] The reason for the partly age-dependent, apparently intrinsic thrombolytic resistance of some thrombi is unknown, but experimental data indicate that not all thrombi are equally susceptible to thrombolysis. Thus, thrombi formed within arterial stenoses[62] and other platelet-rich thrombi appear particularly resistant to lysis, unlike erythrocyte-rich clots formed in stagnant blood.[42] Accordingly, clinical data indicate that the relatively small but probably platelet-rich thrombus within the atherosclerotic stenosis disappears only slowly during thrombolysis; it may resist even prolonged intracoronary

streptokinase infusion. On the other hand, the thrombus "tail" extending downstream usually dissolves rapidly and completely.[24] The difficulty of lysing thrombi formed within severe stenoses is consistent with the lower patency rate after infarction in patients with preceding chronic angina (compared with patients without preceding angina[63]), indicating an underlying severe atherosclerotic stenosis.

Thus, the presence of a strong thrombogenic stimulus in the form of a tight atherosclerotic stenosis or extensive plaque disruption[64] seems to be associated with lytic failure, maybe because thrombi formed under such conditions are particularly rich in platelets.[16,42] Other causes of unsuccessful thrombolysis could be extensive stagnation thrombosis (see Fig. 1-9, *B*)[41] or nonthrombotic obstructions: major plaque "disasters" with dissecting plaque hemorrhages, intimal flaps, or extruded atheromatous plaque material (see Fig. 1-7). Vasospasm probably does not play a role in the occlusion's persistence.[65]

Importantly, the character of the infarct-related lesions usually treated by "rescue" angioplasty (persistent occlusions despite thrombolysis), "adjunctive" angioplasty (residual stenoses after thrombolytic reperfusion), and "primary" angioplasty (all infarct-related lesions without antecedent thrombolytic therapy) probably differs significantly, which may explain the different complication rates.[66]

ACKNOWLEDGMENTS

Thanks to Pam Atanasoff for editorial assistance and to Doris Petersen for preparation of the figures.

REFERENCES
1. Fuster V, Badimon L, Badimon JJ, et al: The pathogenesis of coronary artery disease and the acute coronary syndromes, *N Engl J Med* 326:242-250, 310-318, 1992.
2. Falk E: Morphologic features of unstable atherothrombotic plaques underlying acute coronary syndromes, *Am J Cardiol* 63:114E-120E, 1989.
3. Davies MJ: A macro and micro view of coronary vascular insult in ischemic heart disease, *Circulation* 82(suppl II):II38-II46, 1990.
4. Stary HC, Blankenhorn DH, Chandler AB, et al: A definition of the intima of human arteries and of its atherosclerosis-prone regions, *Circulation* 85:391-405, 1992.
5. Little WC: Angiographic assessment of the culprit coronary artery lesion before acute myocardial infarction, *Am J Cardiol* 66:44G-47G, 1990.
6. Cohen M, Sherman W, Rentrop KP, et al: Determinants of collateral filling observed during sudden controlled coronary artery occlusion in human subjects, *J Am Coll Cardiol* 13:297-303, 1989.
7. Richardson PD, Davies MJ, Born GVR: Influence of plaque configuration and stress distribution on fissuring of coronary atherosclerotic plaques, *Lancet* 2:941-944, 1989.
8. Falk E: Plaque rupture with severe pre-existing stenosis precipitating coronary thrombosis. Characteristics of coronary atherosclerotic plaques underlying fatal occlusive thrombi, *Br Heart J* 50:127-134, 1983.

9. Lendon CL, Davies MJ, Born GVR, et al: Atherosclerotic plaque caps are locally weakened when macrophages density is increased, *Atherosclerosis* 87:87-90, 1991.

10. Falk E: Why do plaques rupture? *Circulation* 86(suppl III): 30-42, 1992.

11. Muller JE, Tofler GH, Stone PH: Circadian variation and triggers of onset of acute cardiovascular disease, *Circulation* 79:733-743, 1989.

12. Muller JE, Abela GS, Nesto RW, et al: Triggers, acute risk factors and vulnerable plaques: the lexicon of a new frontier, *J Am Coll Cardiol* 23:809-813, 1994.

13. Rochmis P, Blackburn H: Exercise tests. A survey of procedures, safety and litigation experience in approximately 170,000 tests, *JAMA* 217:1061-1069, 1971.

14. Davies MJ, Bland JM, Hangartner JRW, et al: Factors influencing the presence or absence of acute coronary artery thrombi in sudden ischaemic death, *Eur Heart J* 10:203-208, 1989.

15. Falk E: Coronary thrombosis: Pathogenesis and clinical manifestations, *Am J Cardiol* 68:28B-35B, 1991.

16. Folts J: An in vivo model of experimental arterial stenosis, intimal damage, and periodic thrombosis, *Circulation* 83 (suppl IV):IV3-IV14, 1991.

17. Mizuno K, Miyamoto A, Satomura K, et al: Angioscopic coronary macromorphology in patients with acute coronary disorders, *Lancet* 337:809-812, 1991.

18. Smith E, Cochran S: Factors influencing the accumulation in fibrous plaques of lipid derived from low density lipoprotein: II. Preferential immobilization of lipoprotein (a) (Lp(a)), *Atherosclerosis* 84:173-181, 1990.

19. Wilcox JN, Smith KM, Schwartz SM, et al: Localization of tissue factor in the normal vessel wall and in the atherosclerotic plaque, *Proc Natl Acad Sci USA* 86:2839-2843, 1989.

20. Haft JI, Al-Zarka AM: The origin and fate of complex coronary lesions, *Am Heart J* 121:1050-1061, 1991.

21. Taeymans Y, Theroux P, Lesperance J, et al: Quantitative angiographic morphology of the coronary artery lesions at risk of thrombotic occlusion, *Circulation* 85:78-85, 1992.

22. Badimon L, Badimon JJ: Mechanisms of arterial thrombosis in nonparallel streamlines: platelet thrombi grow on the apex of stenotic severely injured vessel wall. Experimental study in the pig model, *J Clin Invest* 84:1134-1144, 1989.

23. Lassila R, Badimon JJ, Vallabhajosula S, et al: Dynamic monitoring of platelet deposition on severely damaged vessel wall in flowing blood. Effects of different stenoses on thrombus growth, *Arteriosclerosis* 10:306-315, 1990.

24. Brown BG, Gallery CA, Badger RS, et al: Incomplete lysis of thrombus in the moderate underlying atherosclerotic lesion during intracoronary infusion of streptokinase for acute myocardial infarction: quantitative angiographic observations, *Circulation* 73:653-661, 1986.

25. Hackett D, Davies G, Maseri A: Pre-existing coronary stenoses in patients with first myocardial infarction are not necessarily severe, *Eur Heart J* 9:1317-1323, 1988.

26. Danchin N, Oswald T, Voiriot P, et al: Significance of spontaneous obstruction of high degree coronary artery stenoses between diagnostic angiography and later percutaneous transluminal coronary angioplasty, *Am J Cardiol* 63:660-662, 1989.

27. Bissett JK, Ngo WL, Wyeth RP, et al: Angiographic progression to total coronary occlusion in hyperlipidemic patients after acute myocardial infarction, *Am J Cardiol* 66:1293-1297, 1990.

28. Webster MW, Chesebro JH, Smith HC, et al: Myocardial infarction and coronary artery occlusion: a prospective 5-year angiographic study [abstract], *J Am Coll Cardiol* 15:218A, 1990.

29. Berder V, Danchin N, Juilliere Y, et al: Angiographic study of spontaneous obstruction of coronary artery stenoses: do the tightest stenoses have the most benign clinical course [abstract]? *Eur Heart J* 12(suppl):231, 1991.

30. Ambrose JA, Hjemdahl-Monsen CE: Arteriographic anatomy and mechanisms of myocardial ischemia in unstable angina [editorial], *J Am Coll Cardiol* 9:1397-1402, 1987.

31. Schreiber TL, Macina G, Bunnell P, et al: Unstable angina or non-Q wave infarction despite long-term aspirin: response to thrombolytic therapy with implications on mechanisms, *Am Heart J* 120:248-255, 1990.

32. Falk E: Unstable angina with fatal outcome: dynamic coronary thrombosis leading to infarction and/or sudden death. Autopsy evidence of recurrent mural thrombosis with peripheral embolization culminating in total vascular occlusion, *Circulation* 71:699-708, 1985.

33. ISIS-2: Randomised trial of intravenous streptokinase, oral aspirin, both, or neither among 17 187 cases of suspected acute myocardial infarction, *Lancet* 13:349-360, 1988.

34. Jørgensen L, Rowsell HC, Hovig T, et al: Resolution and organization of platelet-rich mural thrombi in carotid arteries of swine, *Acta Pathol Microbiol Scand* 51:681-719, 1967.

35. Kanamasa K, Watanabe I, Cercek B, et al: Selective decrease in lysis of old thrombi after rapid administration of tissue-type plasminogen activator, *J Am Coll Cardiol* 14:1359-1364, 1989.

36. Davies MJ, Thomas AC, Knapman PA, et al: Intramyocardial platelet aggregation in patients with unstable angina suffering sudden ischemic cardiac death, *Circulation* 73:418-427, 1986.

37. Frink RJ, Rooney PA, Trowbridge JO, et al: Coronary thrombosis and platelet/fibrin microemboli in death associated with acute myocardial infarction. *Br Heart J* 59:196-200, 1988.

38. Chesebro JH, Fuster V: Dynamic thrombosis and thrombolysis. Role of antithrombins [editorial], *Circulation* 83:1815-1817, 1991.

39. Zeiher AM, Schachinger V, Weitzel SH, et al: Intracoronary thrombus formation causes focal vasoconstriction of epicardial arteries in patients with coronary artery disease, *Circulation* 83:1519-1525, 1991.

40. Kaski JC: Mechanisms of coronary artery spasm, *TCM* 1:289-294, 1991.

41. Grines CL, Booth DC, Nissen SE, et al: Mechanism of acute myocardial infarction in patients with prior coronary artery bypass grafting and therapeutic implications, *Am J Cardiol* 65:1292-1296, 1990.

42. Jang I-K, Gold HK, Ziskind AA, et al: Differential sensitivity of erythrocyte-rich and platelet-rich arterial thrombi to lysis with recombinant tissue-type plasminogen activator. A possible explation for resistance to coronary thrombolysis, *Circulation* 79:920-928, 1989.

43. DeWood MA, Spores J, Notske R, et al: Prevalence of total coronary occlusion during the early hours of transmural myocardial infarction, *N Engl J Med* 303:897-902, 1980.

44. DeWood MA, Stifter WF, Simpson CS, et al: Coronary arteriographic findings soon after non-Q-wave myocardial infarction, *N Engl J Med* 315:417-423, 1986.

45. Freeman MR, Williams AE, Chisholm RJ, et al: Intracoronary thrombus and complex morphology in unstable angina. Relation to timing of angiography and in-hospital cardiac events, *Circulation* 80:17-23, 1989.

46. Forrester J: Intimal disruption and coronary thrombosis: its role in the pathogenesis of human coronary disease, *Am J Cardiol* 68:69B-77B, 1991.

47. Lo Y-SA, Cutler JE, Blake K, et al: Angiographic coronary morphology in survivors of cardiac arrest, *Am Heart J* 115:781-785, 1988.

48. Davies MJ: Anatomic features in victims of sudden coronary death. Coronary artery pathology, *Circulation* 85(suppl I):I19-I24, 1992.

49. Brown G, Albers JJ, Fisher LD, et al: Regression of coronary artery disease as a result of intensive lipid-lowering therapy in men with high levels of apolipoprotein B, *N Engl J Med* 323:1289-1298, 1990.

50. Honye J, Mahon DJ, Tobis JM: Intravascular ultrasound imaging, *TCM* 1:305-311, 1991.

51. MacMahon S, Collins R, Knight C, et al: Reduction in major morbidity and mortality by heparin in acute myocardial infarction, *Circulation* 78(suppl II):II98, 1988.

52. Ambrose JA, Israel DH: Angiography in unstable angina, *Am J Cardiol* 68:78B-84B, 1991.

53. Sobel BE, Hirsh J: Principles and practice of coronary thrombolysis and conjunctive treatment, *Am J Cardiol* 68:382-388, 1991.

54. Pichard AD, Ziff C, Rentrop P, et al: Angiographic study of the infarct-related coronary artery in the chronic stage of acute myocardial infarction, *Am Heart J* 106:687-692, 1983.

55. Van Lierde J, De Geest H, Verstraete M, et al: Angiographic assessment of the infarct-related residual coronary stenosis after spontaneous or therapeutic thrombolysis, *J Am Coll Cardiol* 16:1545-1549, 1990.

56. Braunwald E: Coronary artery patency in patients with myocardial infarction [editorial], *J Am Coll Cardiol* 16:1550-1552, 1990.

57. Mattfeldt T, Schwarz F, Schuler G, et al: Necropsy evaluation in seven patients with evolving acute myocardial infarction treated with thrombolytic therapy, *Am J Cardiol* 54:530-534, 1984.

58. Schroder S, Schofer J, Kloppel G, et al: Myocardial haemorrhage after intracoronary thrombolysis, *Eur Heart J* 6(suppl E):155-162, 1985.

59. Onodera T, Fujiwara H, Tanaka M, et al: Cineangiographic and pathological features of the infarct related vessel in successful and unsuccessful thrombolysis, *Br Heart J* 61:385-389, 1989.

60. Gertz SD, Kalan JM, Kragel AH, et al: Cardiac morphologic findings in patients with acute myocardial infarction treated with recombinant tissue plasminogen activator, *Am J Cardiol* 65:953-961, 1990.

61. Verstraete M, Arnold AER, Brower RW, et al: Acute coronary thrombolysis with recombinant human tissue-type plasminogen activator: initial patency and influence of maintained infusion on reocclusion rate, *Am J Cardiol* 60:231-237, 1987.

62. Bush LR, Shebuski RJ: In vivo models of arterial thrombosis and thrombolysis, *FASEB* 4:3087-3098, 1990.

63. Riccitelli MA, Nul DR, Sarubbi AL, et al: The clinical presentation of acute myocardial infarction predicts the severity of the lesion in the infarct-related artery, *Eur Heart J* 12:210-213, 1991.

64. Davies MJ: Successful and unsuccessful coronary thrombolysis, *Br Heart J* 61:381-384, 1989.

65. Rentrop KP, Feit F, Sherman W, et al: Serial angiographic assessment of coronary artery obstruction and collateral flow in acute myocardial infarction. Report from the Second Mount Sinai–New York University Reperfusion Trial, *Circulation* 80:1166-1175, 1989.

66. Topol EJ, Gacioch GM: Discordance in results of right coronary intervention [letter], *Circulation* 84:955, 1991.

Chapter 2

TRIGGERING OF THE ACUTE CORONARY ARTERY SYNDROMES

Sumita D. Paul
Geoffrey H. Tofler
James E. Muller

New insight into triggering of acute coronary artery syndromes is emerging. This information describes *acute* risk factors and provides a needed supplement to our knowledge of the role of chronic risk factors for several reasons. First, the traditional chronic risk factors do not explain a substantial portion of the variance in the occurrence of heart disease in a population.[1] Second, they do not explain why some patients with little obstructive coronary artery disease develop myocardial infarction (MI), whereas others with severe coronary obstructive disease remain asymptomatic or experience only stable angina.[2] Third, they do not explain why onset occurs on a particular day at a particular moment. Increased knowledge about acute risk and potential triggering activities may help overcome these significant limitations.

Knowledge about the triggering process also provides an opportunity to extend recent progress in the treatment of the acute coronary syndromes to include prevention. This is an essential step, because most cardiac deaths occur before treatment can be given.

Fig. 2-1 shows the limitations of thrombolytic therapy and emphasizes the need for improved prevention that might be obtained through improved knowledge of acute coronary risk factors. Of the 675,000 patients hospitalized with MI in the United States in 1988, only 124,000 (18%) received thrombolysis.[3] Although short-term mortality may have been reduced by 25% (from 12% to 9%, a 3% absolute reduction),[4] the number of lives saved (3720) was less than 1% of the 500,000 deaths attributed to "heart attack,"[5] the combined term for MI and sudden cardiac death. The extremely low percentage of deaths prevented occurs because approximately 300,000 heart attack deaths occur before the patient reaches the hospital,[5] thereby limiting the potential value of thrombolysis and preventing access of these patients to the major improvements in the care of hospitalized patients. Although the number of patients treated with thrombolytics and the speed with which they are treated must be increased, even a fourfold increase in lives saved by thrombolysis would prevent only 4% of heart attack deaths. This intrinsic limitation of treatment once the infarction has begun is the strongest argument for intensive investigation of the events occurring in the crucial minutes before the onset of the disease.

HISTORY OF THE CONCEPT OF TRIGGERING OF CORONARY ARTERY DISEASE

History provides numerous anecdotes of stress triggering the death of prominent individuals. In 1746, King Philip V of Spain died suddenly after being told that the Franco-Spanish fleet had been defeated by the Austro-Sardinians in the battle of Piacenza.[6,7] John Hunter, the renowned eighteenth century English surgeon, suffered

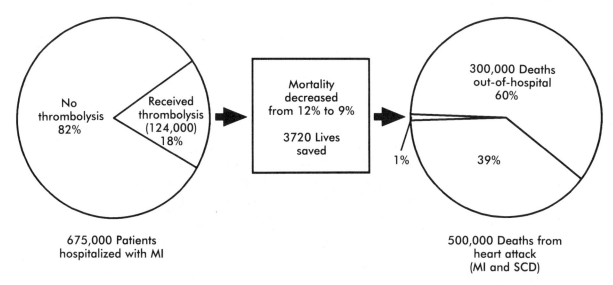

Fig. 2-1. Theoretical analysis of the contribution of thrombolytic therapy to reduction of the total number of deaths due to "heart attack." The circle on the left represents the proportion of hospitalized patients with myocardial infarction *(MI)* who receive thrombolysis.[3] The circle on the right shows the resulting decrease in mortality expressed as a percentage reduction of all deaths from heart attacks.[4,5] In 1988, it is estimated that only 1% of the 500,000 deaths from heart attacks were saved by thrombolysis. *SCD,* sudden cardiac death.

from angina pectoris for 20 years and appeared to have a reactive personality type that left him especially susceptible to triggering. He often said that his life was in the hands of "any rascal who chose to annoy and tease him." Indeed, on Oct. 16, 1793, after an argument with his colleagues at a medical board meeting, Hunter was said to have "immediately ceased speaking, struggled to suppress the tumult of his passion, hurried to an adjoining room, and fell over lifeless."[8]

In the original description of the clinical features of acute MI in 1910, Obraztsov and Strazhesko stated that infarction was frequently triggered and presented graphic examples of stressful activities preceding its onset: "The infarct began in one case on climbing a high staircase, in another during an unpleasant conversation, and in a third during emotional distress associated with a heated card game."[9] In 1933, Fitzhugh and Hamilton collected a series of 100 cases of coronary thrombosis and found that the attacks were frequently precipitated by some unusual event.[10] Fifty five of these cases had coronary occlusion or fatal angina directly after unaccustomed exertion and 13 after unusual emotional strain.

The view that cardiac events were frequently triggered was challenged in 1937 by Master et al.,[11] who analyzed the events preceding 530 cases of coronary thrombosis. They found that unusual exertion preceded only 2% of cases, excitement preceded 5%, and mild activity 37%. No significant trigger was found in the remainder. Subsequently, a debate ensued between investigators for and against the hypothesis of triggering. The debate ended with the widespread acceptance of the

conclusion of Master[12] that "coronary occlusion takes place irrespective of the physical activity being performed or the type of rest taken."

The concept of triggering has now gained renewed attention because of support from an unexpected source, the recognition of the circadian variation of onset of MI.

EPIDEMIOLOGIC EVIDENCE OF CIRCADIAN VARIATION IN THE ONSET OF MI

In subsequent years, a number of authors reported an increase in the frequency of infarction during the late morning hours.[13-16] Unfortunately, these claims received limited attention because of their reliance on subjective reporting of pain onset. It was believed that certain infarcts could begin during sleep but that the symptoms were not experienced by the patients until they awakened. The distribution of MI based on the onset of pain would therefore be skewed toward the hours after awakening. The recall and the differential misclassification biases complicating these reports were sufficient to block acceptance of the observation of morning increase in onset of acute ischemic events.

Advances in quantitative methods of timing the onset of ischemic events enabled investigators to overcome the biases inherent in subjective recall studies. In 1985, the Multicenter Investigation of Limitation of Infarct Size (MILIS) used the initial appearance of creatine kinase in the plasma to objectively measure time of infarct onset.[17] Infarct onset was considered to have begun 4 hours before the first appearance of creatine kinase (CK) in the plasma. Use of this method provided the first objective evidence that MI is three times more likely to

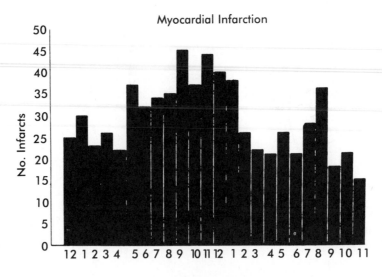

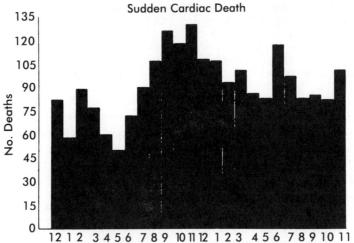

Fig. 2-2. Time of day of onset of myocardial infarction, sudden death, stroke, and transient myocardial ischemia in four different groups of patients.[17,24,29,40] The number of events is shown on the y axis and the hour of the day on the x axis. Each of the disorders exhibits a prominent increase in frequency of onset in the period from 6:00 A.M. to noon. (From Muller JE, et al: *Circulation* 79:733, 1989. Used by permission.)

begin in the morning than in the late evening (Fig. 2-2). The findings of the MILIS study were subsequently confirmed by those of the Intravenous Streptokinase in Acute Myocardial Infarction (ISAM) study, which also used CK timing of onset.[18] Because both of these studies were randomized multicenter clinical trials with restrictive inclusion criteria, the generalizability of these results to the general population could be questioned. However, in both MILIS and ISAM, a relatively strong correlation was found between CK-determined onset and pain-determined onset, indicating that pain-determined onset was not associated with its suspected biases, and could be used to determine timing in less selected populations.

Such studies have now allowed others to extend the analysis of timing of onset. Hjalmarson et al.[15] found the circadian pattern blunted or abolished in subgroups of

patients who were advanced in age or who had diabetes, a history of smoking, or a prior history of infarction.[15] Further, Goldberg et al.[16] have demonstrated that the morning increase results from an increase in events in the first 4 hours after awakening.[16] This observation suggests that events associated with awakening and initiation of morning activities trigger onset of MI.

EPIDEMIOLOGIC EVIDENCE ON TRIGGERING OF MI

Sumiyoshi et al.[19] performed a systematic study of the activities before the onset of MI in 416 patients admitted to the National Heart Center of Japan from 1977 to 1985. They used the frequency of emotional and physical stress during the same month 1 year before infarction as their control data. This approach permitted comparison of the frequency of stress in the month immediately before MI

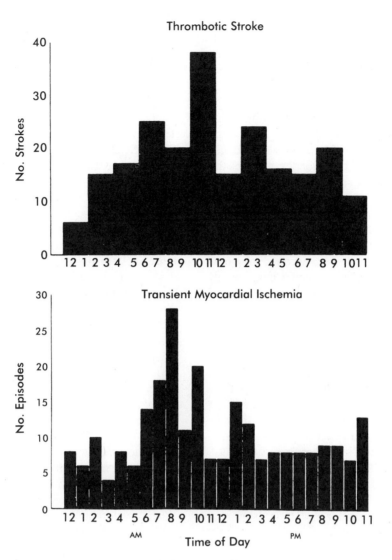

Fig. 2-2. —cont'd

with that in the same month 1 year earlier. Fifty-eight percent of patients reported stress (moderate to heavy exercise, emotional stress, or excitation) in the month immediately before their MI vs. only 34% during the control period 1 year earlier (P < 0.01). However, recall bias favoring reporting of recent events vs. those more than 1 year old complicates interpretation of these results.

Our group investigated the frequency of possible triggering of MI as reported by patients enrolled in the MILIS study. Almost half (48.5%) of the patients reported a possible trigger.[20] The most common possible triggers reported were emotional upset (18.4%), moderate physical activity (14.1%), multiple possible triggers (13%), heavy physical activity (8.7%), lack of sleep (8.0%), overeating (6.9%), sexual activity (1.2%), surgery (0.4%), and miscellaneous triggers (6.6%). Younger patients, those without diabetes, and men were more likely to report a possible trigger. The size of the infarct

had no effect on the likelihood that the patient would report a trigger.

Although the previously mentioned studies suggest that potentially identifiable triggers may play an important role in the onset of acute MI, progress in this area is limited by a lack of information regarding the exact nature, duration, and time relation of possible triggers to onset of acute MI. In addition, there is limited information about effect modifiers, and most important, there is an absence of appropriate control data.

These limitations are being addressed by the ongoing Myocardial Infarction Onset study (ONSET), supported by the National Heart Lung and Blood Institute. More than 1000 patients admitted to the 50 participating hospitals have now completed an hour-long interview on the events before their MI. This study uses the novel case-crossover design.[21] With this method, the frequency of a potential trigger occurring during a designated hazard period (the 2 hours before the onset of MI) is compared with the frequency of the trigger during the identical 2-hour period 24 to 26 hours before the MI. This design is analogous to a retrospective crossover experiment in which each subject serves as his or her own control.

In ONSET, the relative risk for MI onset in the subsequent hour after heavy physical exertion (estimated by history to be $\geq$ 6 METS) was 2.4 among regular exercisers but 10.7 among those who did not exercise regularly.[22] The case-crossover design solves the problem of selection bias for controls (each patient is well matched as his or her own control) and between person confounding (by matched pair analysis). The potential for information bias still exists for two reasons. First, the subjects may be less likely to remember the events of the day before their MI. Second, they may overreport potential triggers in the hours immediately before the MI in a search for a cause of the onset of their disease.

These problems of information bias are being addressed in ONSET by the use of a traditional case-control study in addition to the case-crossover study that will permit consistency checks between the two methods. An age- and gender-matched neighbor of the MI patient is identified and asked to serve as a control. The subject is given a beeper that is set off at the time of day that the matched patient experienced the MI. The control is then interviewed about the activity levels occurring before the beeper activation.

In January 1991, the Iraqi missile war provided an opportunity to methodically study the effects of psychologic stress on cardiovascular events in Israeli civilians.[23] During the initial week of missile attacks on Israel (Jan. 17-25, 1991), 20 people developed an acute MI in the area served by the Sapir Medical Center, 24 km northeast of Tel Aviv, compared with an average of 8 MIs in each of 5 control periods before the war. In addition, there were 41 out of hospital sudden deaths during January 1991, compared with only 22 during the same period in 1990. Although these results suggest that psychologic stress triggered the onset of MI and sudden death, the absolute number of events was small, and the possibility exists of confounding by such factors as the use of gas masks, changes in diet, and exertion patterns.

CIRCADIAN VARIATION OF SUDDEN CARDIAC DEATH

Data revealing that sudden cardiac death has a prominent circadian variation similar to that of MI have been obtained from two large studies: the mortality records for Massachusetts for 1983[24] and the Framingham Heart Study.[25] The time of day of sudden cardiac death as indicated by death certificates was determined for the 2203 individuals dying out of the hospital in Massachusetts in 1983. Sudden cardiac death was found to have a peak incidence between 7:00 and 11:00 A.M., with a low incidence during the night (see Fig. 2-2), a pattern similar to that for the onset of nonfatal MI and episodes of transient myocardial ischemia.

Subsequently, the time of day of sudden cardiac death (SCD) in the Framingham Heart Study was analyzed. There was a peak incidence from 7:00 to 9:00 A.M. The risk of SCD was at least 70% higher during this period than the average risk during other times of the day. A recent study from Berlin has used electrocardiography (ECG) findings at the time of out of hospital cardiopulmonary resuscitation to determine the type of preterminal arrhythmia present.[26] Patients with ventricular tachycardia leading to ventricular fibrillation were the most likely to show a morning increase in onset.

A possible physiologic mechanism for increased SCD in the morning may be the well-documented increase in sympathetic activity after assumption of the upright posture.[27] The increase in plasma catecholamines could contribute in two ways to the morning increase of SCD. First, it could increase the likelihood of plaque rupture and occlusive thrombosis. Second, it may result in an increased electrical instability of the myocardium. A morning increase in electrical instability has recently been demonstrated by Siegel et al.[28] in their study involving 199 hypertensive men between 35 to 70 years old, who were withdrawn from diuretic treatment and received 1 month of oral electrolyte repletion.[28] As assessed by 24-hour Holter monitoring, there was a higher prevalence of ventricular arrhythmias per hour in the interval from 6 A.M. to noon than in the interval from midnight to 6 A.M. ($P < 0.01$).

CIRCADIAN VARIATION IN THE ONSET OF TRANSIENT MYOCARDIAL ISCHEMIA

The technique of ambulatory ECG monitoring has enabled the timing of transient myocardial ischemia to be determined without a potential bias arising from lack of monitoring during periods of sleep. The pattern of transient ischemic episodes has been found to closely parallel the circadian variation of acute MI and sudden cardiac death.[29] Adjustment of the timing of ischemic episodes for variable wake time indicates that the peak number of ischemic events occurs in the first 1 to 2 hours after awakening, as does the risk for infarction.

The relative contribution of increased myocardial oxygen demand[29-33] vs. decreased oxygen supply[29,34-37] in causing transient ischemia may vary during the day. Hausmann et al.[38] have shown that the heart rate at the onset of ischemic episodes and the maximal heart rate during ischemic episodes are lower between midnight and 6 A.M. compared with the remaining hours of the day.[38] In patients with stable coronary disease who undergo exercise treadmill testing, the time to onset of

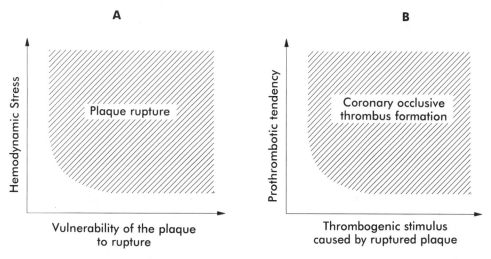

Fig. 2-3. A, Proposed inverse relation between the vulnerability of a plaque to rupture and the hemodynamic stress required to produce plaque rupture. **B,** Proposed inverse relation between the thrombogenic stimulus caused by the ruptured plaque and the prothrombotic tendency of the blood required to produce coronary occlusive thrombus formation.

ST-segment depression is shorter in the morning compared with other times of the day.[39]

EVIDENCE FOR TRIGGERING OF TRANSIENT MYOCARDIAL ISCHEMIA

The role of external activities in triggering the occurrence of transient ischemic episodes has been closely examined by numerous investigators. Barry et al.[34] have shown that when potential mental, as well as physical, causes of ischemia are considered, more than half of transient ischemic episodes are preceded by possible triggering activities.[34] Further, an analysis that adjusted for the time spent engaged in the activity revealed a high likelihood of occurrence during increased physical or mental stress.

CIRCADIAN VARIATION IN THE ONSET OF STROKE

The timing of stroke onset shows a remarkable similarity to that of MI and sudden cardiac death (see Fig. 2-2). The methodologic problem of determining the time of onset of events detected on patient awakening has been overcome by considering these events to have occurred randomly during the 8 hours before awakening. Even with this assumption against the hypothesis of a morning increase, there still remains a prominent increase from 6:00 A.M. to noon.[40] Tsementzis et al.[40] examined the diurnal variation in the onset of stroke in 194 patients with subarachnoid hemorrhage, 118 with intracerebral hemorrhage, and 245 with thromboembolic cerebral infarction.[40] All three types of strokes exhibited a peak incidence between 10 A.M. and noon. There was no difference in the time of onset of stroke between normotensive and treated or untreated hypertensive patients.

MORNING INCREASE IN PHYSIOLOGIC PROCESSES LIKELY TO TRIGGER AN EVENT

Several systemic physiologic processes have been identified that increase in intensity in the morning and may trigger disease onset in an individual with an atherosclerotic plaque that is vulnerable to rupture. The processes may exert their effects either by causing plaque rupture or by promoting formation of an occlusive thrombus (Fig. 2-3). For example, the morning arterial pressure surge,[30] accompanied by a heart rate increase, may cause plaque rupture. An increase in vascular resistance[41] may worsen the flow reduction produced by a fixed stenosis. Increased blood viscosity[42] and platelet aggregability,[43] resulting from assumption of the upright posture[44] and associated with low circulating tissue plasminogen (t-PA) activity,[45,46] may produce a thrombotic tendency.

The variation during a 24-hour period of eight physiologic processes possibly contributing to the increased morning frequency of disease onset is shown in Fig. 2-4. Recently, Panza et al.[47] have demonstrated that forearm vascular resistance is higher in the morning than at other times of the day. They provided evidence that the increase in resistance was caused by a morning peak in α-adrenergic activity, because the increase could be abolished by the intraarterial infusion of the α-blocking agent, phentolamine.

The morning increase in the onset of cardiovascular events serves as a model for investigation into the onset of cardiovascular events throughout the day, because the physiologic changes that are present in the morning can also occur at other times of the day in response to activities such as physical exertion, emotional stress, or exposure to cold.

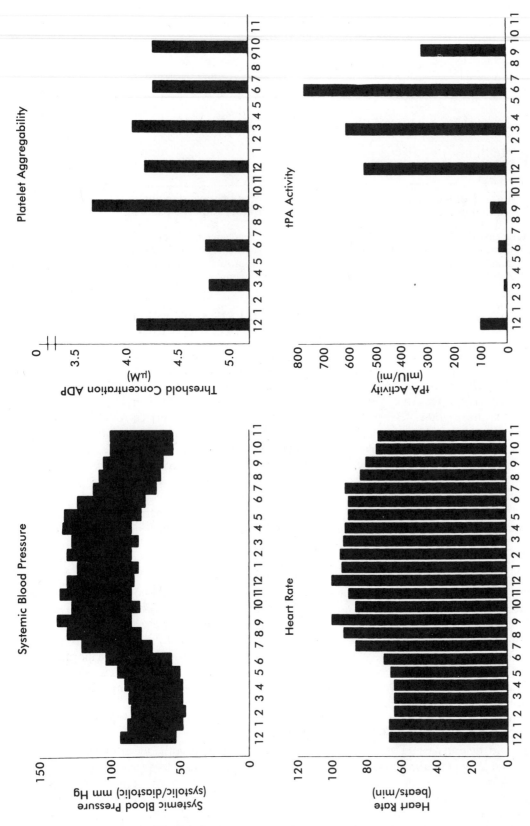

Fig. 2-4. Variation during a 24-hour period of eight physiologic processes possibly contributing to the increased morning frequency of disease onset.[30,41-43,46,89] *t-PA*, tissue plasminogen activator. (From Muller JE, et al: *Circulation* 79:733, 1989. Used by permission.)

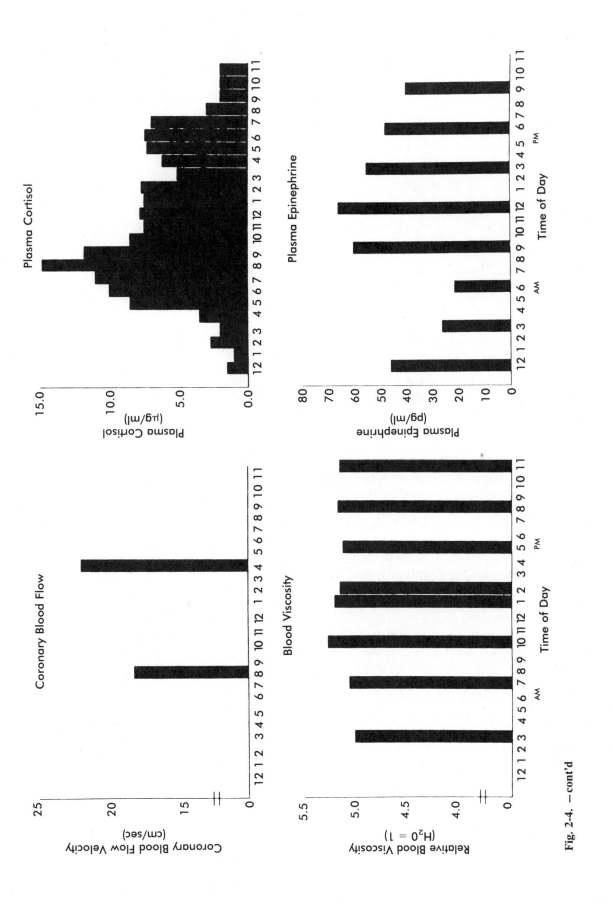

Fig. 2-4. —cont'd

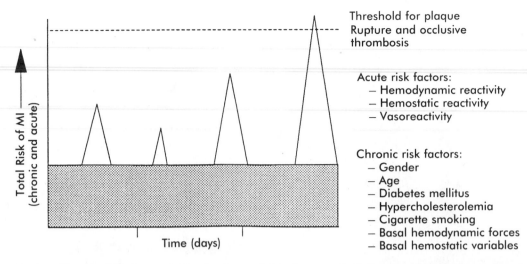

Fig. 2-5. Hypothetical diagram indicating the total risk of myocardial infarction *(MI)*, which consists of the sum of the traditional chronic risk factors and acute risk factors. Disease onset occurs when the total risk exceeds the threshold for plaque rupture and occlusive thrombus formation.

PHYSIOLOGIC PROCESSES THAT MIGHT LEAD TO TRIGGERING OF ONSET OF MI

Although a 24-hour periodicity of disease onset is well established, the degree to which the periodicity results from a true, endogenous circadian rhythm or from the daily rest-activity cycle is only partially characterized. Cortisol secretion, for example, is an endogenous circadian process not dependent on daily activity, whereas the increase in morning platelet aggregability is abolished if the subject remains at bedrest. The rest/activity cycle seems to be a major determinant of disease onset because adjustment for time of awakening shows that infarction onset, sudden cardiac death, and increases of transient ischemia follow awakening, but such adjustment could also align the population for their endogenous circadian rhythms. Also, an interaction between circadian and rest/activity cycles may exist; for example, assumption of the upright posture leading to sympathetic activation may be more likely to cause intense vasoconstriction when endogenously controlled cortisol levels are high.

Plaque rupture and occlusive thrombosis probably occur at a critical moment when a combination of hemodynamic, prothrombotic, and vasoconstricting forces interact with a vulnerable plaque. Using an atherosclerotic rabbit model, Constantinides[48] has demonstrated that a sudden increase in systemic arterial pressure plus infusion of a prothrombotic agent result in plaque fissuring and subsequent thrombosis. The vascular injury determines the site of thrombus location in the animal model. This animal model could be used to examine the newly generated hypothesis concerning triggering of cardiovascular disease in patients.

Fuster et al.[49] have proposed a three-stage patho-

physiologic classification of vascular injury: type 1 consists of functional alterations of endothelial cells without substantial morphologic changes, type 2 represents endothelial denudation and intimal damage with intact internal elastic lamina, and type 3 represents endothelial denudation with damage to both the intima and media. Richardson et al.[50] have described that a plaque with a high lipid content and surrounded by a thin capsule is particularly prone to rupture leading to endothelial denudation and damage to both the intima and media (type 3 damage), with subsequent thrombus formation. It has also been demonstrated by Little et al.[2] that plaque rupture followed by occlusive thrombosis often occurs in the absence of a preexisting critical stenosis.

A summary of the physiologic changes likely to occur during several potential triggering activities is presented in Table 2-1.[51-69] This table describes the overall responses to stressors and indicates the significant differences in coronary artery reactivity that occur in patients with coronary disease. Because of abnormal endothelial function, such patients frequently exhibit paradoxical vasoconstriction in response to stimuli that produce coronary vasodilation in individuals with normal arteries.[70-73]

Angiographic studies in patients have shown that in the presence of coronary atherosclerosis, dynamic exercise,[70] handgrip,[71] exposure to cold,[72] and infusion of acetylcholine[73] produce coronary vasoconstriction when vasodilation would be the normal response. These findings are supported by in vitro observations that an atherosclerotic artery shows exaggerated constriction to a number of normally occurring vasoconstrictors such as norepinephrine and serotonin[74-76] and a paradoxical vasoconstrictive response to acetylcholine.[77]

Table 2-1. Physiologic changes during possible triggering activities*

Possible triggers	Systemic arterial pressure	Heart rate	Coronary vascular resistance or narrowing†	Plasma catechols	Platelet activity	Fibrinolytic activity
Exercise	↑	↑	↑	↑	↑ ↔	↑
Assumption of upright posture	↓ ↔	↑	?	↑	↑	↑
Handgrip	↑	↑	↑	↑	?	?
Cold exposure	↑	↑	↑ ↔	↑	↑ ↔	↑
Cigarette smoking	↑	↑	↑	↑	↑ ↔	↑ Acute ↓ Chronic
Mental stress	↑	↑	↑	↑	↑	↑

From Muller JE, et al: Circulation 79:733, 1989. Used by permission.

* ↑, increased; ↓, decreased; ↔, no change; ?, limited information. Multiple responses reflect either variability within subject populations, or conflicting results.

†Response observed with coronary atherosclerosis. Normal response is a resistance decrease, or dilatation.

Exaggerated systemic hemodynamic reactivity has also been observed in certain individuals. Eliot[78] has used the term "hot reactors" to describe subjects with marked blood pressure and heart rate increases after mental stress.[78] Although the prognostic significance of this classification is not fully clarified, hypertensive patients who are hot reactors have a predisposition to the development of left ventricular hypertrophy.[79]

The conflicting data regarding type A behavior and coronary heart disease could perhaps be clarified if anger and hostile behavior were studied as *acute* rather than chronic risk factors. Additional data on anger before acute disease onset and during appropriate control intervals are needed.

In addition to marked subgroup differences in *hemodynamic* responses, there are also significant subgroup differences in *hemostatic* responses to stressors. These reactivity differences are often more marked than basal differences between the subgroups. For example, patients with coronary artery disease, advanced diabetes mellitus, and hypercholesterolemia have a diminished fibrinolytic response to physical exercise compared with healthy subjects.[80-82] The ratio of plasma thromboxane A_2 to plasma 6-keto-prostaglandin $F_{1\alpha}$ released with exercise was also greater (i.e., the response was more prothrombotic) in patients with coronary artery disease than in normal subjects (1.9 vs. 0.1).[83]

Although the severity of atherosclerosis increases slowly with time, hemodynamic, hemostatic, and vasoconstricting forces may increase rapidly after external stresses and act as acute risk factors. We propose that MI is most likely to occur when a combination of chronic and acute risk factors reaches a critical threshold. In Fig. 2-5, the total risk for an MI is portrayed as the sum of acute plus chronic risk. Chronic risk is a summation of factors such as age, total cholesterol levels, high-density lipoprotein, basal systolic blood pressure, current smoker status, the presence of diabetes mellitus, and the presence of left ventricular hypertrophy by ECG,[84] whereas the acute risk for MI depends on the exposure to a triggering activity and the instantaneous hemodynamic, hemostatic, and vasoconstrictive reactivity to that trigger.

PHARMACOLOGIC PREVENTION OF MI

The triggering hypothesis can provide insight into the ability of aspirin and β-blockade to prevent MI. The beneficial effects of aspirin in the secondary prevention of cardiovascular events have been well documented in subjects with unstable angina and with acute MI. Further, the Physician's Health Study has demonstrated the ability of aspirin to provide primary protection against MI.[85] In this randomized, double-blind, placebo-controlled study, there were 342 cases of nonfatal MI, and time of onset was available in 211 (62%). The placebo-treated group demonstrated a prominent morning increase in onset of MI as expected from prior studies. However, in the aspirin-treated physicians, there was a marked reduction in the morning peak of infarction, which was maximal during the 3-hour period immediately after awakening. Aspirin produced a 59.3% reduction in the incidence of MI during the period from 6 A.M. to noon compared with a 34.1% reduction for the remaining hours of the day. These findings support the hypothesis that increased platelet aggregability in the morning contributes to the occurrence of nonfatal MI.

In both the MILIS and ISAM studies, the morning increase in the risk of infarction was blunted in those subjects receiving β-blockers before their MI. A reduction in the morning occurrence of sudden deaths in patients after MI was also demonstrated in the randomized Beta-Blocker Heart Attack Trial.[86] In this study, propranolol-treated patients had a 44% lower occurrence of death during the morning period than the placebo-treated group, whereas there was no significant benefit of β-blockers during the 2 P.M. to 2 A.M. period.

Because most β-blockers have only minimal antiplatelet activity, it is likely that β-blockers exert their protective effect by blunting the response to the morning increase in sympathetic activity associated with awakening and activity.

Coy et al.[87] have reported that β-adrenergic blockade, which exerts its effect on myocardial ischemia predominantly by lowering myocardial oxygen demand, markedly blunts the morning increase in heart rate and ischemia.[87] This suggests that increases in heart rate and blood pressure secondary to the increased catecholamine levels play a significant role in the pathogenesis of the morning peak in occurrence of transient myocardial ischemia.

CLINICAL IMPLICATIONS

The presence of a morning peak in the onset of the acute coronary artery syndromes suggests that for patients already receiving antiischemic and antihypertensive therapy, pharmacologic protection should be provided during the morning hours. Although no scientific studies have been performed to test the hypothesis, it seems reasonable that long-acting antiischemic agents would have an advantage over short-acting agents in providing protection against cardiovascular events in the morning when the effects of short-acting agents taken the night before may attenuate. Pharmacologic therapy (aspirin and β-blockers), which blunts the physiologic changes that occur in the morning, has been shown to be of particular benefit against morning onset of disease.

Questions have arisen as to the timing of nitrate-free intervals and the morning increase in cardiovascular events. It is difficult to provide a complete answer to this issue because the exact role of coronary and systemic vasoconstriction in causing disease onset at various times of the day is not understood; although events are more frequent in the hours after awakening, it is possible that the events caused by vasoconstriction are actually more frequent at some other time of day, possibly during the sleeping hours. Therefore, further research is required before the optimal timing of nitrate-free intervals is known.

Clinical implications for morning exercise

Because of the widespread awareness of the morning peak in MI, both physicians and patients have questioned whether exercise in the morning is more dangerous than exercise at other times of the day. Murray et al.[88] compared the incidence of ischemic events in patients who underwent cardiac rehabilitation in the morning vs. the event rate in those who attended an afternoon program. There were 3 ischemic events per 100,000 patient hours of exercise in the morning and 2.3 events per 100,000 patient hours of exercise in the afternoon

($P = NS$). Although the power of detecting a difference in the timing of the events was low because there were so few events, the absolute risk of having such an event was extremely low. Because exercise is beneficial and the absolute risk of an event is quite low, exercising in the morning appears to be preferable to not exercising. Determination as to whether the timing of exercise influences the relative risk of cardiovascular events requires further study.

The recognition of the circadian patterns of physiologic processes and cardiovascular events has helped in the understanding of the mechanism of disease onset. With improved understanding of the triggering mechanism, it may be possible to design therapy to sever the link between a potential triggering process and its pathologic consequences.

REFERENCES

1. Marmot MG, Shipley MJ, Rose G: Inequalities in death-specific explanations of a general pattern? *Lancet* 1:1003-1006, 1984.
2. Little WC, et al: Can coronary angiography predict the site of a subsequent myocardial infarction in patients with mild to moderate coronary artery disease? *Circulation* 78:1157-1166, 1988.
3. Muller DWM, Topol EJ: Selection of patients with acute myocardial infarction for thrombolytic therapy, *Ann Intern Med* 113:949-960, 1990.
4. Yusuf S, et al: Routine medical management of acute myocardial infarction: lessons from overviews of recent randomized controlled trials, *Circulation* 82(suppl II):II117-II134, 1990.
5. American Heart Association: *Heart and stroke facts 1991,* Dallas, 1990, American Heart Association National Center.
6. Zimmerman, JG: *A treatise on experience in physic,* London, 1782, vol II, p 274.
7. War of the Austrian succession. In *Encyclopedia Americana.* 1959, Americana Corporation, vol XXV, p 795.
8. Palmer JF (ed): *The works of John Hunter, with notes,* 1835, Longman, Rees, Orme, Brown, Green, Longman, vol I, p 131.
9. Obraztsov VP, Strazhesko ND: The symptomatology and diagnosis of coronary thrombosis. In Vorobeva VA, Konchalovski MP (eds): *Works of the First Congress of Russian Therapists,* 1910, Comradeship Typography of AE Mamontov, pp 26-43.
10. Fitzhugh G, Hamilton BE: Coronary occlusion and fatal angina pectoris. Study of the immediate causes and their prevention, *JAMA* 100:475-480, 1933.
11. Master AM, et al: Factors and events associated with onset of coronary artery thrombosis, *JAMA* 109:546, 1937.
12. Master AM: The role of effort and occupation (including physicians) in coronary occlusion, *JAMA* 174:942-948, 1960.
13. Pell S, D'Alonzo CA: Acute myocardial infarction in a large industrial population: report of a 6-year study of 1,356 cases, *JAMA* 185:831-838, 1963.
14. Thompson DR, et al: Time of onset of chest pain in acute myocardial infarction, *Int J Cardiol* 7:139-146, 1985.
15. Hjalmarson A, et al: Differing circadian pattern of symptom onset in subgroups of patients with acute myocardial infarction, *Circulation* 80:267-275, 1989.
16. Goldberg R, et al: Time of onset of acute myocardial infarction, *Am J Cardiol* 66:140-144, 1990.
17. Muller JE, et al: Circadian variation in the frequency of onset of acute myocardial infarction, *N Engl J Med* 313:1315-1322, 1985.
18. Willich SN, et al: Increased morning incidence of myocardial

infarction in the ISAM Study: absence with prior beta-adrenergic blockade, *Circulation* 80:853-858, 1989.

19. Sumiyoshi T, et al: Evaluation of clinical factors involved in onset of myocardial infarction, *Jpn Circ J* 50:164-173, 1986.

20. Tofler GH, et al: Analysis of possible triggers of acute myocardial infarction (MILIS Study), *Am J Cardiol* 66:28-30, 1990.

21. Maclure M: The case-crossover design: A method for studying transient effects on the risk of acute events, *Am J Epidemiol* 133:144-153, 1991.

22. Mittleman M, et al: Triggering the acute myocardial infarction by heavy physical exertion—protection against triggering by regular exertion, *N Engl J Med* 329:1677-1683, 1993.

23. Meisel SR, et al: Effect of Iraqi missile war on incidence of acute myocardial infarction and sudden death in Israeli civilians, *Lancet* 338:660-661, 1991.

24. Muller JE, et al: Circadian variation in the frequency of sudden cardiac death, *Circulation* 75:131-138, 1987.

25. Willich SN, et al: Circadian variation in the incidence of sudden cardiac death in the Framingham Heart Study Population, *Am J Cardiol* 60:801-806, 1987.

26. Arntz R, et al: Circadian variability of sudden cardiac death is caused by age dependent variations in the incidence of ventricular fibrillation, *J Am Coll Cardiol* 19:105A, 1992.

27. Muller JE, et al: Circadian variation of cardiovascular disease and sympathetic activity, *J Cardiovasc Pharmacol* 10(suppl 2):S104-S109, 1987.

28. Seigel D, et al: Circadian variation in ventricular arrhythmias in hypertensive men, *Am J Cardiol* 69:344-347, 1992.

29. Rocco MB, et al: Circadian variation of transient myocardial ischemia in patients with coronary artery disease, *Circulation* 75:395-400, 1987.

30. Millar-Craig MW, Bishop CN, Raftery EB: Circadian variation of blood pressure, *Lancet* 1:795-797, 1978.

31. Davies AB, et al: Simultaneous recording of continuous arterial pressure, heart rate, and ST segment in ambulant patients with stable angina pectoris, *Br Heart J* 50:85-91, 1983.

32. Quyyumi AA, et al: Nocturnal angina: precipitating factors in patients with coronary artery disease and those with variant angina, *Br Heart J* 56:346-352, 1986.

33. Hinderliter, et al: Myocardial ischemia during daily activities: the importance of increased myocardial oxygen demand, *J Am Coll Cardiol* 18:405-412, 1991.

34. Barry J, et al: Frequency of ST segment depression produced by mental stress in stable angina pectoris from coronary artery disease, *Am J Cardiol* 61:989-993, 1988.

35. Singh BN, et al: Hemodynamic and electrocardiographic correlates of symptomatic and silent myocardial ischemia: pathophysiologic and therapeutic implications, *Am J Cardiol* 58:3B-10B, 1986.

36. Freeman LJ, et al: Psychological stress and silent myocardial ischemia, *Am Heart J* 114:477-482, 1987.

37. Moncada S, Vane JR: Arachidonic acid metabolites and the interactions between platelets and blood-vessel walls, *N Engl J Med* 300:1142-1147, 1979.

38. Hausmann D, et al: Circadian distribution of the characteristics of ischemic episodes in patients with stable coronary artery disease, *Am J Cardiol* 66:668-672, 1990.

39. Henkels U, Blumchen G, Ebner F: Zur Problematick vone Belastungsprufungen in Abhangigkeit von der Tageszeit bei Patienten mit Koronarinsuffizienz, *Herz* 9:343-347, 1977.

40. Tsementzis SA, et al: Diurnal variation of and activity during the onset of stroke, *Neurosurgery* 17:901-904, 1985.

41. Fujita M, Franklin D: Diurnal changes in coronary blood flow in conscious dogs, *Circulation* 76:488-491, 1987.

42. Ehrly AM, Jung G: Circadian rhythm of human blood viscosity, *Biorheology* 10:577-583, 1973.

43. Tofler GH, et al: Concurrent morning increase in platelet aggregability and the risk of myocardial infarction and sudden cardiac death, *N Engl J Med* 316:1514-1518, 1987.

44. Brezinski DA, et al: Morning increase in platelet aggregability: association with assumption of the upright posture, *Circulation* 78:35-40, 1988.

45. Rosing DR, et al: Blood fibrinolytic activity in man: diurnal variation and the response to varying intensities of exercise, *Circ Res* 27:171-184, 1970.

46. Andreotti F, et al: Major circadian fluctuations in fibrinolytic factors and possible relevance to time of onset of myocardial infarction, sudden cardiac death, and stroke, *Am J Cardiol* 62:635-637, 1988.

47. Panza JA, Epstein SE, Quyyumi AA: Circadian variation in vascular tone and its relation to α-sympathetic vasoconstrictor activity, *N Engl J Med* 325:986-990, 1991.

48. Constantinides P: Plaque fissure in human coronary thrombosis, *Atherosclerosis* 1:1-17, 1966.

49. Fuster V, et al: The pathogenesis of coronary artery disease and the acute coronary syndromes, *N Engl J Med* 326:242-249, 1992.

50. Richardson PD, Davies MJ, Born GVR: Influence of plaque configuration and stress distribution on fissuring of coronary atherosclerotic plaques, *Lancet* 2:941-944, 1989.

51. Robertson D, et al: Comparative assessment of stimuli that release neuronal and adrenomedullary catecholamines in man, *Circulation* 59:637-643, 1979.

52. Green LH, Seroppian E, Handin RI: Platelet activation during exercise-induced myocardial ischemia, *N Engl J Med* 302:193-197, 1980.

53. Mathis PC, et al: Lack of release of platelet factor 4 during exercise-induced myocardial ischemia, *N Engl J Med* 304:1275-1278, 1981.

54. Estelles A, et al: Reduced fibrinolytic activity in coronary heart disease in basal conditions and after exercise, *Thromb Res* 40:373-383, 1985.

55. Speiser W, et al: Increased blood fibrinolytic activity after physical exercise: comparative study in individuals with different sporting activities and in patients after myocardial infarction taking part in a rehabilitation sports program, *Thromb Res* 51:543-555, 1988.

56. Shannon RP, et al: The effect of age and sodium depletion on cardiovascular response to orthostasis, *Hypertension* 8:438-443, 1986.

57. Nabel EG, et al: Dilation of normal and constriction of atherosclerotic coronary arteries caused by the cold pressor test, *Circulation* 77:43-52, 1988.

58. De Servi S, et al: Coronary vasoconstrictor response to cold pressor test in variant angina: lack of relation to intracoronary thromboxane concentrations, *Am Heart J* 114:511-515, 1987.

59. Fitchett D, et al: Platelet release of beta-thromboglobulin within the coronary circulation during cold pressor stress, *Am J Cardiol* 52:727-730, 1983.

60. Mangue M, Haynes EM, Lipner H: Coagulation and fibrinolytic responses to exercise and cold exposure, *Aviat Space Environ Med* 55:291-295, 1984.

61. Cryer PE, et al: Norepinephrine and epinephrine release and adrenergic mediation of smoking-associated hemodynamic and metabolic events, *N Engl J Med* 295:573-577, 1976.

62. Maouad J, et al: Diffuse or segmental narrowing (spasm) of the coronary arteries during smoking demonstrated on angiography, *Am J Cardiol* 53:354-555, 1984.

63. Belch JJF, et al: The effects of acute smoking on platelet behavior, fibrinolysis, and haemorheology in habitual smokers, *Thromb Haemost* 51:6-8, 1984.

64. Siess W, et al: Plasma catecholamines, platelet aggregation and associated thromboxane formation after physical exercise, smoking or norepinephrine infusion, *Circulation* 66:44-48, 1982.

65. Allen RA, Kluft C, Brommer EJP: Acute effect of smoking on fibrinolysis: increase in the level of circulating extrinsic (tissue-type) plasminogen activator, *Eur J Clin Invest* 14:354-361, 1984.

66. Allen RA, Kluft C, Brommer EJP: Effect of chronic smoking on fibrinolysis, *Arteriosclerosis* 5:443-450, 1985.

67. Rebecca G, et al: Pathogenetic mechanisms causing transient myocardial ischemia with mental arousal in patients with coronary artery disease [abstract], *Clin Res* 34:338A, 1986.

68. Levine SP, et al: Platelet activation and secretion associated with emotional stress, *Circulation* 71:1129-1134, 1985.

69. Ogston D: Fibrinolytic activity and anxiety and its relation to coronary artery disease, *J Psychosom Med* 8:219-222, 1964.

70. Gage JE, et al: Vasoconstriction of stenotic coronary arteries during dynamic exercise in patients with classic angina pectoris: reversibility by nitroglycerin, *Circulation* 73:865-876, 1986.

71. Brown BG, et al: Reflex constriction of significant coronary stenoses as a mechanism contributing to ischemic left ventricular dysfunction during isometric exercise, *Circulation* 70:18-24, 1984.

72. Mudge Jr GH, et al: Reflex increase in coronary vascular resistance in patients with ischemic heart disease, *N Engl J Med* 295:1333-1337, 1976.

73. Ludmer PL, et al: Paradoxical vasoconstriction induced by acetylcholine in atherosclerotic coronary arteries, *N Engl J Med* 315:1046-1051, 1986.

74. Ginsburg R, et al: Quantitative pharmacologic responses of normal and atherosclerotic isolated human epicardial coronary arteries, *Circulation* 69:430-440, 1984.

75. Ganz P, Alexander RW: New insights into the cellular mechanisms of vasospasm, *Am J Cardiol* 56:11E-15E, 1985.

76. Ganz W: Coronary spasm in myocardial infarction: fact or fiction? *Circulation* 63:487-488, 1981.

77. Furchgott RF, Zawadzki JV: The obligatory role of endothelial cells in the relaxation of arterial smooth muscle by acetylcholine, *Nature* 288:373-376, 1980.

78. Eliot RS: Stress and the heart. Contemporary problems in cardiology. 1974;1.

79. Devereaux RB, et al: Left ventricular hypertrophy in patients with hypertension: importance of blood pressure response to regularly occurring stress, *Circulation* 68:470-476, 1983.

80. Khann PK, et al: Effect of submaximal exercise on fibrinolytic activity in ischemic heart disease, *Br Med J (Clin Res)* 2:910-912, 1975.

81. Almer LO, Pandolfi M: Fibrinolysis and diabetic retinopathy, *Diabetes* 25(suppl 2):807-810, 1976.

82. Epstein SE, et al: Impaired fibrinolytic response to exercise in patients with type-IV hyperlipoproteinemia, *Lancet* 2:631-634, 1970.

83. Mehta J, Mehta P, Horalek C: The significance of platelet-vessel wall prostaglandin equilibrium during exercise-induced stress, *Am Heart J* 105:895-900, 1983.

84. Anderson KM, et al: An updated coronary risk profile. A statement for health professionals. American Heart Association/Scientific Statement, *Circulation* 83:356-362, 1991.

85. Ridker PM, et al: Circadian variation of acute myocardial infarction and the effect of low-dose aspirin in a randomized trial of physicians, *Circulation* 82:897-902, 1990.

86. Peters RW: Propranolol and the morning increase in sudden cardiac death: the Beta-Blocker Heart Attack Trial Experience, *Am J Cardiol* 66:57G-59G, 1990.

87. Coy KM, et al: Application of time series analysis to circadian rhythms: effect of beta-adrenergic blockade upon heart rate and transient myocardial ischemia, *Am J Cardiol* 66:22G-24G, 1990.

88. Murray PM, et al: Should patients with coronary artery disease exercise in the morning or afternoon [abstract]? *J Am Coll Cardiol* 17:296A, 1991.

89. Weitzman ED, et al: Twenty-four hour pattern of the episodic secretion of cortisol in normal subjects, *J Clin Endocrinol Metab* 20:446-456, 1960.

Chapter 3

HEMOSTASIS AND RISK OF ISCHEMIC DISEASE

Epidemiologic evidence with emphasis on the elderly

Russell P. Tracy
Edwin G. Bovill

COAGULATION, FIBRINOLYSIS, AND THROMBOSIS

Over the last 20 years, it has become increasingly clear that thrombosis is involved in most ischemic cardiovascular events.[1] Although it is not yet a certainty, it appears likely that variations in the plasma levels of coagulation factors, possibly even variations within the "normal" ranges, may be important in determining an individual's response to a vascular insult such as plaque ulceration. Some individuals with deficiencies of the anticoagulant proteins antithrombin III, protein C, and protein S and others with abnormalities of fibrinolysis factors such as plasminogen activator inhibitor-1 (PAI-1) experience thrombotic diatheses.[2] It seems reasonable, therefore, to hypothesize that relatively minor deviations from normal, identified by test values in the "low-" or "high-normal" range, might also be associated with disease. The first part of this chapter presents an overview of the coagulation and fibrinolytic systems, identifying specific measurable factors and the manner in which they interact. Following this, we explore the evidence that relates to the previously mentioned hypothesis and attempt to put the findings in the context of the overall pathophysiology of ischemic heart disease.

Finally, it is evident that ischemic heart disease, to a large extent, may be considered a disease of the elderly, in that the majority of clinical events occur in people over

the age of 65.[3] The last part of this chapter examines what is known about changes in coagulation, thrombosis, and fibrinolysis in the elderly and how these changes might affect the relationships between coagulation, fibrinolysis, and thrombosis.

GENERAL REVIEW OF COAGULATION AND FIBRINOLYSIS

The coagulation system is responsible for halting blood loss through ruptures in the vasculature; after the opening is sealed, the fibrinolytic system is responsible for the gradual removal of the initial blood clot. However, both of these systems are involved in a variety of other functions, some physiologic and some pathophysiologic, such as the thrombotic response to atherosclerotic plaque rupture. The two systems are complimentary and interactive, and both interact with a third system, comprised primarily of platelets. The coagulation system may be considered as two subsystems: the procoagulant and anticoagulant systems. In the same manner the fibrinolytic system may be broken down into the profibrinolytic and antifibrinolytic systems. Normally the procoagulant and anticoagulant systems may be considered to be in balance or dynamic equilibrium; the same may be said of the profibrinolytic and antifibrinolytic systems. In addition, the coagulant and fibrinolytic systems may also be considered to be in balance.

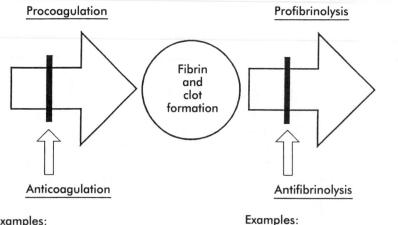

Examples:
   factor VII
   fibrinogen
   activated platelet surface

Examples:
   plasminogen activators
   cellular plasminogen receptors
   fibrin surface

Procoagulation

Profibrinolysis

Fibrin
and
clot
formation

Anticoagulation

Antifibrinolysis

Examples:
   protein c
   antithrombin III
   endothelial cell thrombomodulin

Examples:
   plasminogen activator inhibitor-1
   alpha-2 antiplasmin
   lp (a)?

Fig. 3-1. Schematic representation of "coagulant balance." This figure describes the dynamic relationships between the factors that control clot formation (procoagulant and anticoagulant factors) and those that control clot removal (profi-brinolytic and antifibrinolytic factors). As part of this scheme we hypothesize that a decrease in anticoagulation potential may have a similar overall effect as an increase in antifibrinolysis, both resulting in an increase in clot formation. (Modified from Tracy R, Mann K, and Bovill E: Mechanisms of thrombosis. In Esekowitz M: *Cardiac sources of systemic embolization,* New York, 1992, Marcel Dekker.)

Evidence is presented to support the position that there are a low level of coagulation and reactive fibrinolysis going on at all times. This level may be higher in some individuals and lower in others. The "coagulant balance" is disrupted in times of stress, as when a blood vessel is injured or an atherosclerotic plaque is ruptured. This overall scheme of "coagulant balance" is shown in Fig. 3-1. Fig. 3-2 provides an overview of the important coagulation and fibrinolysis factors.

Procoagulation occurs when inactive zymogen forms of circulating coagulation factors are proteolytically activated to enzymic forms. For example, factor X is not an enzyme, whereas the proteolytically activated form, factor Xa, is an enzyme. This ongoing procoagulation is limited by an active anticoagulant system and balanced by a low level of ongoing fibrinolysis. There is much experimental and observational support for this position, gathered from measurements of circulating levels of the products of these activities, such as prothrombin fragment 1·2 and fibrinopeptide A.[4,5] It remains speculative whether or not this low-level activity is some sort of "priming" activity, allowing the full response to be expressed rapidly on demand, or simply a response to a constant series of slight provocative events, such as small vascular lesions or unavoidable brief blood stasis occurring in certain vascular locations. It is also unclear whether or not this slight activity is directly associated with a platelet response; however, because platelet activation markers such as plasma β-thromboglobulin[6] and thromboxane A_2[7] reach measurable levels in "normal" individuals, it seems likely that it is.

At some point in time, this low-level procoagulant activity is dramatically amplified by a precipitating event such as the rupture of an atherosclerotic plaque. At least briefly, the procoagulant activity exceeds both the anticoagulant activity and the fibrinolytic response. These reactions occur almost entirely on surfaces through the assembly of the relevant macromolecular enzyme complexes. It is possible that platelet activation after adherence is the initial event, with activated platelets then expressing procoagulant sites on their surfaces. However, thrombin generation may precede platelet activation if tissue factor is expressed on cells such as circulating monocytes. In some cases of myocardial infarction, the occlusion appears to be formed primarily by platelets, whereas in other cases there is a major fibrin component. The factors that regulate the type of hemostatic plug are not well understood.

The formation of specialized "sites" on the surface of cells is a key step in propagating the coagulant response. Such sites might serve to generate thrombin from prothrombin, or factor Xa from factor X. These sites use factors from within the cells, as well as from the blood plasma, and may be expressed on platelets,[8]

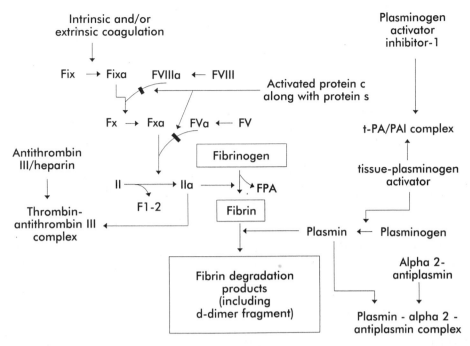

Fig. 3-2. Schematic overview of coagulation and fibrinolysis. This diagram is meant to put several key factors in the context of the overall process of clot formation and resolution. Several factors mentioned in the text are shown, including the fibrin D-dimer fragment, prothrombin fragment 1·2 (*F1-2*), and fibrinopeptide A (*FPA*). The coagulation factors factor V, factor VII, factor VIII, factor IX, and factor X are abbreviated as *FV, FVII, FVIII, FIX,* and *FX,* respectively. Prothrombin is shown as *II.* Active forms of the coagulation zymogens include the suffix *a.*

monocytes,[9] and possibly endothelial cells.[10] Cells also provide for the ultimate limitation of coagulation by expressing sites for the generation of anticoagulants such as activated protein C (endothelial cell thrombomodulin expression[11]) and profibrinolytics such as plasmin (the plasminogen-binding site[12,13]). Fibrin itself acts as a profibrinolytic agent by facilitating the conversion of plasminogen to plasmin through the catalytic activity of tissue-type plasminogen activator (t-PA). The processes of coagulation and fibrinolysis are not separate but interactive. The interaction of various key elements is shown in Fig. 3-3.

MEASUREMENTS OF COAGULATION AND FIBRINOLYSIS

Although we can measure circulating factors and activation products, currently we have no way to accurately assess the actual and potential cellular "sites" that might exist at any point in time in an individual. Because of this lack of information concerning specific microenvironments (e.g., those surrounding a ruptured atherosclerotic plaque), our measurements can only help estimate the true status of an individual. Nonetheless, we believe that much useful information can be obtained from the available analytes.

Concerning soluble coagulation and fibrinolytic factors, three types of measurement might be considered.

The first type concerns the factors in the "passive" state, that is, the circulating levels of unactivated zymogen forms of enzymes, and unprocessed forms of structural proteins such as fibrinogen. This includes not only immunoassays of specific factors but also the measurement of factors after the deliberate activation of the zymogen present in the sample, as is done in one-stage clotting assays.

The second type of assay concerns measurement of products of in situ enzymatic activity. Such assays include activation peptides (e.g., prothrombin fragment 1·2 as an indication of thrombin generation) and enzyme-inhibitor complexes (e.g., thrombin-antithrombin III complex).[14] Although these assays reflect the ongoing activity of interest, the interpretation of the results should take into account several possible confounding factors: artifact caused by venipuncture and blood collection, alterations in endogenous elimination rates, and the potential for differential reactivity of the assay reagents (commonly antibodies) with different forms of the protein of interest.

The third type of measurement involves the direct assay of circulating active enzymatic forms such as thrombin[15] and activated protein C.[16] This type of measurement has the advantage of directly assessing the key enzymes of coagulation and fibrinolysis. However, this has proved difficult for a variety of reasons, not the

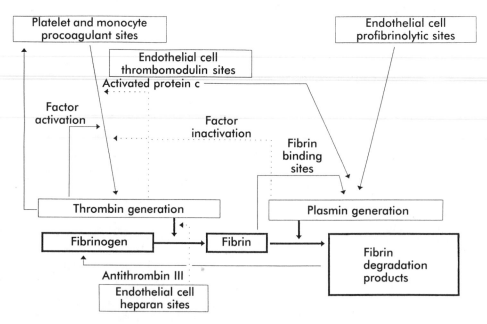

Fig. 3-3. Interrelationships between coagulation and fibrinolysis. The thick, solid lines indicate major processes. The thin, solid lines indicate positive influences, whereas the thin, dotted lines indicate negative influences. The cellular components and the interactions between systems are stressed in this schematic.

least of which is sample collection. Because many enzymes have circulating inhibitors, this is another factor that has made direct assay of plasma enzymes difficult. Table 3-1 describes the three types of assays and emphasize measurements that have proved useful to date.

KEY INTERACTIVE ROLES OF THROMBIN AND PLASMIN

Although virtually all identified coagulation and fibrinolytic enzymes appear to be important, two enzymes hold special places in the overall process, thrombin and plasmin (Table 3-2; see Fig. 3-3). As the ultimate coagulation enzyme, thrombin is responsible for the conversion of fibrinogen to fibrin. However, thrombin appears to play many other roles as well. Thrombin is capable of enzymatic activity toward several of the coagulation factors and cofactors (e.g., factor V[17]), causing an acceleration of procoagulation. Even in the face of antiplatelet agents such as aspirin, thrombin is a powerful platelet agonist.[18,19] However, if thrombin is completely inhibited by a small, fast-acting inhibitor such as D-Phe-Pro-Arg chloromethyl ketone (PPACK), platelet aggregation is virtually completely eliminated under conditions where thrombus formation has been stimulated.[20]

After the expression of thrombomodulin, thrombin acts as an *anticoagulant* by activating protein C to activated protein C,[21] which, along with protein S, acts to inactivate the factor Xa cofactor, factor Va. Not only does activated protein C inactivate factor Va, but it also appears to play a role in promoting fibrinolysis, through

a mechanism that is as yet unclear.[22] Thrombin also appears to have growth factor activity[23] and vasoactive properties.[24] Thrombin is inhibited in situ by antithrombin III when either therapeutic heparin or naturally occurring heparans are present.[25] Antithrombin III also acts to inhibit factor Xa[25] and factor VIIa,[26] enzymes that lead to the generation of thrombin from prothrombin, thereby limiting not only thrombin activity but also thrombin generation. Interestingly, antithrombin III can also inactivate plasmin, although this reaction is considerably weaker than the reaction to inhibit thrombin.[25]

Plasmin is the ultimate profibrinolytic enzyme, effecting the conversion of insoluble fibrin to soluble fibrin degradation products (FDPs). FDPs may affect the "coagulant balance" by inhibiting the fibrinogen-mediated cross-linking of platelets[27] and stimulating the production of fibrinogen.[28] Plasmin is responsible for the elimination of fibrin in physiologic clots and the maintenance of "coagulant balance" under the low-level conditions discussed earlier. Plasmin is also capable of moving the "balance" toward clot dissolution by degrading fibrinogen (thereby eliminating the substrate for fibrin formation and producing FDPs, which can inhibit platelet cross-linking), as well as by activating and subsequently inactivating factor V (and probably factor VIII),[29] thereby acting as an anticoagulant. It is likely that these latter activities are at least partly responsible for some hemorrhagic events seen with thrombolytic therapy.

Plasmin is a particularly nonspecific enzyme capable of cleaving a wide variety of proteins, with many

Table 3-1. Measurements of coagulation and fibrinolysis

Type of assay	Screening	Type 1	Type 2	Type 3
Description	Integrative assays that cover entire systems	Assays that estimate the circulating concentration of individual zymogen and inhibitor concentrations	Assays that measure molecular species formed as a result of in vivo enzyme activity	Assays that directly measure plasma enzymes
Methods	Clot-based or clot lysis-based assays	Clot-based, immunologic, or chromogenic assays	Immunoassays	Specialized assays, often using components from chromogen and/or immunologic assay systems
Examples	Activated partial thromboplastin time; prothrombin time; euglobulin clot lysis assay	Fibrinogen; factor V, VII, VIII, etc.; plasminogen activator inhibitor-1	Prothrombin fragment 1 · 2; fibrin fragment D-dimer; fibrinopeptide A; thrombin-antithrombin complex	Activated protein C; factor VIIa; thrombin
Advantages	Detects major abnormalities Easy to perform No special blood collection	Relatively easy to perform Reproducible and sensitive Usually no special blood collection is required	Results reflect in vivo enzymatic activity Reproducible and sensitive	Results reflect in vivo enzymatic activity
Disadvantages	No information on specific factors Difficult to standardize Not sensitive	Some assays require special collection Minor changes are difficult to interpret	Most require special collection or processing; collection artifacts are difficult to avoid Difficult to standardize Effect of endogenous enzyme inhibitors and clearance rates complicate results	Research-level assays Effect of endogenous enzyme inhibitors and clearance rates complicate results Most require special collection or processing; collection artifacts are difficult to avoid

important physiologic activities of plasmin being unrelated to fibrinolysis.[30-32] Plasmin itself is inhibited by α_2-antiplasmin, an inhibitor that does not require a cofactor.[33] α_2-Antiplasmin is a particularly fast-acting inhibitor but acts only when plasmin is free in solution.[34] Plasmin bound to insoluble fibrin is poorly inhibited by α_2-antiplasmin. Plasmin is produced from plasminogen by the action of the circulating enzyme t-PA, most effectively in the presence of fibrin.[35] The most effective way to inhibit plasmin is to inhibit its generation, which is done physiologically primarily by PAI-1[36] and, to a lesser extent, by two similar proteins PAI-2[37] and PAI-3.[38] PAI-3 is also an inhibitor of activated protein C,[39] thereby affecting coagulant balance by two mechanisms: the inhibition of plasminogen activation and the inhibition of factor Va inactivation.

Table 3-2. Thrombin and plasmin: key enzymes in coagulant balance

	Thrombin	Plasmin
Principal role	Cleave fibrinogen to yield fibrin I and fibrin II	Cleave fibrin to yield soluble FDPs*
	Form blood clots	Resolve blood clots
Complementary roles	Cleave other pro-coagulant factors to yield active components (e.g., factor V, factor VIII)	Soluble FDPs act to enhance plasmin formation from plasminogen
	Activate platelets	Inactivate factors V and VIII
Antagonistic roles	Cleave protein C to yield activated protein C	Activate factor V
Other roles	Vasoconstriction	Broad specificity for tissue proteins
	Chemoattraction	

*FDPs, Fibrin degradation products.

CURRENT MODEL FOR THE RELATIONSHIP OF THROMBOSIS AND ATHEROSCLEROSIS TO ISCHEMIC HEART DISEASE

The work of DeWood et al.[1] made it clear that the majority of the clinical events associated with ischemic heart disease have thrombosis as their proximal cause. Thrombolytic therapy makes use of this understanding, and the rapid lysis of occlusive blood clots, with the attendant reperfusion, has significant clinical benefit. It is believed that the formation of thrombi is stimulated by a procoagulant surface, such as the surface associated with an ulcerated atherosclerotic plaque. The active components of a surface may be several: exposed subendothelial collagen and von Willebrand factor (platelet adherence), adenosine diphosphate liberated from damaged cells and activated platelets (platelet adherence and aggregation), and tissue factor elaboration by damaged cells (thrombin generation).

Recently, investigators Ross,[40] Fuster,[41-43] Davies,[44] and Chandler[45] have emphasized that thrombosis may also be involved with atherosclerotic development, not just with precipitating the clinical event. This position was originally championed by von Rokitansky,[46] Mallory,[47] Clark,[48] and Duguid[49] (see Chandler[45] for brief review). The possible role of growth factors and cytokines in even the earliest atherosclerotic development has been postulated, and one of the key candidates is platelet-derived growth factor (PDGF). It appears likely that platelet and monocyte adherence, as a response to "damaged" endothelium, may be an early event in atherogenesis,[40,50,51] possibly mediated by the same adherence events that play a role in thrombosis and coagulation. True thrombosis probably comes later, in response to the ulceration of lipid-rich plaque,[43] although there is evidence that fibrinogen and FDPs are present within even very early atherosclerotic lesions.[52,53] The fragile, lipid-rich plaque, most likely resulting primarily from the play of "atherogenic risk factors," is characterized by a fluid center and a thin, fragile cap. Ultimately, when this plaque ruptures, "thrombotic risk factors" come into play (Fig. 3-4), determining the extent and duration of thrombus formation, as well as the time to lysis.[43] It is believed that occlusive thrombi of this type are often clinically more serious, because there has not been a "gradual" development of stenosis, with attendant collateral development.[43] Nonocclusive thrombi are most likely incorporated into the plaque, and "reorganization" occurs, with the size and composition of the resulting thrombus, along with other thrombotic risk factors, determining the frequency of recurrent thrombosis at this site. If cyclical nonocclusive events occur, there may be time for the development of extensive collateral circulation so that the ultimate occlusive event may be clinically silent. The general scheme is depicted in Fig. 3-4.

One interesting area of investigation that has not been fully developed concerns the possible role of inflammation in atherogenesis and thrombosis. In a recent discussion, Esmon et al.[54] suggest that disseminated intravascular coagulation (DIC) after *Escherichia coli* challenge in baboons may be mediated through the complement pathway. C_4B-binding protein, which functions as an inhibitor of anticoagulation, through its properties to bind the anticoagulant factor protein S,[55] is elevated during inflammation, possibly causing a deficiency in protein S–mediated anticoagulation. Although this acute change is interesting, presumably longer time scales are at play in the development of atherosclerosis. Recent data suggest that inflammatory mediators such as the interleukins, tissue necrosis factor, and other cytokines may play a role if chronically elevated,[56] and certain plasma protein changes that have been identified as cardiovascular disease risk factors (e.g., elevated fibrinogen[57] or decreased albumin[58]) are also associated with chronic inflammation. Research is needed in this intriguing area to determine if acute and chronic inflammation play roles in the development of atherosclerosis or thrombosis.

THROMBOSIS AFTER PHARMACOLOGIC FIBRINOLYSIS

Recurrent ischemic events following closely behind thrombolytic therapy for myocardial infarction continue to be a major cause for concern. Ongoing thrombin activity is probably associated with these events, a

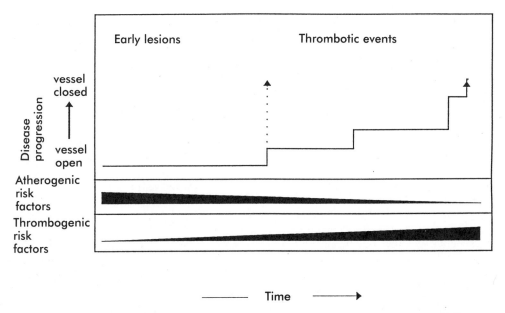

Fig. 3-4. Schematic representation of the natural history of ischemic heart disease.[41-43] The time-dependent progression of disease (i.e., "vessel open" → "vessel closed") may be relatively gradual *(solid line)* or precipitous *(dotted line),* depending on the interplay of thrombotic and atherogenic risk factors. It seems likely that atherogenic risk factors (e.g., plasma lipids) may play a dominant role early in the process, whereas thrombogenic risk factors (e.g., fibrinogen) may be dominant at later stages. It seems equally likely, however, that both atherogenic and thrombotic risk factors are important to some degree at all stages of disease. (Modified from Fuster V, Badimon L, Badimon J, et al: *N Engl J Med* 326:242-250, 310-318, 1992; Fuster V, Stein B, Ambrose J, et al: *Circulation* 82:II47-II59, 1990.)

position strengthened by the finding that fibrinopeptide A, a product of the action of thrombin on fibrinogen, is present during the administration of thrombolytic therapy such as streptokinase,[59] urokinase, and t-PA.[60] In one study of 19 patients with myocardial infarction treated with streptokinase, recanalization was associated with a fall in the level of fibrinopeptide A,[59] whereas in another study of 34 patients receiving t-PA, there was increased risk of reocclusion when fibrinopeptide A levels remained high after therapy.[61] In a third study of 55 patients receiving either urokinase or t-PA, persistent patency was associated with decreasing values of thrombin–antithrombin III complex formation (indicating decreased thrombin activity), whereas an unfavorable course was associated with increased complex formation.[60] These three studies indicate that thrombin formation during and after thrombolytic therapy may be an important risk factor for recurrent events.

Although t-PA is capable of generating fibrinopeptide A from fibrinogen itself, the rate is slow and could not account for the amount of fibrinopeptide A observed.[62] There are two possibilities for the origin of this thrombin. First, thrombin could come from the fibrin clot that is being dissolved, because it has been demonstrated that thrombin is bound to the fibrin as it is formed, and a significant pool of thrombin exists in fibrin deposits.[63] The size of the clot that precipitated

the ischemic event is in all likelihood too small to provide the amount of thrombin observed, but there is the possibility that other regions of the vasculature contain fibrin deposits, which would be affected by systemic fibrinolysis. The second possibility is that there is newly generated thrombin present during and after thrombolytic therapy, a concept supported by the finding that there is increased prothrombin fragment 1·2 present at this time, indicating ongoing prothrombin activation.[64] There are many possible mechanisms for such procoagulant activity, including the continued exposure of the damaged endothelium that precipitated the initial event in the first place and a possible direct effect of plasminogen activation,[60] the mechanism for which remains unclear but may include the activation of factors V and VIII.[29] It seems likely that, in fact, both mechanisms are contributing thrombin after thrombolytic therapy, even in the face of systemic heparinization.

At this time it is unclear whether or not there is significant interindividual variation in the overall capacity to respond to the events of thrombolytic therapy with thrombin generation. That is, we have little evidence that an individual's genetic and environmental makeup is such that one person may respond to a given set of physiologic conditions with greater thrombin production than another. Studies addressing this issue from an

Table 3-3. Prospective epidemiologic evidence that fibrinogen is a cardiovascular disease risk factor

Study	No. of participants (Gender)	Follow-up (yr)	Endpoints*
Northwick Park Heart Study[57]	1511 (men)	10	Fatal or nonfatal CHD
Wilhelmsen et al.[69]	792 (men)	13.5	Myocardial infarction
PROCAM (Munster)[74]	1674 (men)	2.5	Myocardial infarction or sudden cardiac death
Leigh[72]	297 (men)	7.3	Myocardial infarction
Framingham[70]	541 (men), 733 (women)	18	Fatal and nonfatal CHD or CVD
Caerphilly & Speedwell[73]	4860 (men)	5.1 (Caerphilly); 3.2 (Speedwell)	Fatal and nonfatal CHD

*CHD, Coronary heart disease; CVD, cardiovascular disease.

epidemiologic perspective are just beginning and are discussed more fully later on.

THROMBOTIC RISK FACTORS

Thrombotic risk factors may be defined as those factors that control the initiation, propagation, termination, and elimination of thrombus formation.[65] Such risk factors may include procoagulant, anticoagulant, profibrinolytic, and antifibrinolytic factors as described earlier, as well as factors influencing platelet, monocyte, and endothelial cell activation. Plasma lipids may also be thrombotic risk factors, because there is some evidence that certain plasma lipids may be associated with the expression of activity by procoagulant factors such as factor VII.[66] At this time, only a few of the soluble coagulation factors have been examined as risk factors using epidemiologic techniques. Only measurements of circulating factors have been made, although several studies are currently underway exploring measurements of activation peptides such as prothrombin fragment 1·2.

Fibrinogen

In several studies, fibrinogen has been shown to be an independent risk factor for cardiovascular disease, with an importance similar to that of total serum cholesterol. The initial findings of Meade et al.[57,67,68] in the Northwick Park Heart Study and Wilhelmsen et al.[69] in the Gotenborg study established this firmly, and this relationship has been confirmed in several studies since that time, including the Framingham study,[70,71] Leigh[72] study, and Caerphilly and Speedwell[73] studies. These all are prospective studies, and for the most part, when multivariate analysis has been done, fibrinogen has remained a significant predictor of incident disease, both coronary heart disease and stroke. Generally methods that measure either the amount of fibrinogen that can form a clot or the rate of clot formation have been used to estimate fibrinogen concentrations. Table 3-3 lists the principal findings from these studies.

The nature of the association between fibrinogen and cardiovascular risk remains speculative. Certainly it is possible that increased fibrinogen values may directly contribute to increased risk through several mechanisms. First, kinetic modeling has demonstrated that higher fibrinogen concentrations, even within the "normal" range, most likely cause higher rates of fibrin formation, all other factors being equal.[75] In these models, fibrinogen is a substrate for thrombin, and increased substrate concentration results in increased reaction rate. If true in situ, fibrinogen would be a procoagulant risk factor.

Second, because fibrinogen acts as a cross-linker for platelet aggregation,[76] increased fibrinogen concentration might result in an increased propensity toward platelet aggregation. There are data in the literature that both support and refute this position. Meade et al.[77] have performed in vitro platelet aggregation studies using different fibrinogen concentrations and have seen a dose response with respect to certain measures of aggregation but not with respect to others. However, the dissociation constant for the fibrinogen–fibrinogen receptor (GPIIb-IIIa) interaction has been estimated as between 0.05 and 0.5 μM, considerably lower than the plasma fibrinogen concentration of 10 μM, indicating that variation with the twofold to threefold "normal" range is unlikely to affect fibrinogen binding to the receptor.[8] This possibility awaits further study for resolution.

Third, because fibrinogen is a major component of plasma viscosity,[78] increased fibrinogen concentration may result in increased risk through viscosity. Several studies have indicated that plasma viscosity may be related to cardiovascular disease, with the most recent being a prospective study indicating an independent association of viscosity with risk.[73] Interestingly, in a multivariate analysis, both fibrinogen and viscosity remained significant, suggesting that both may have effects independent of each other.

Fourth, fibrinogen may not be a causative agent in cardiovascular disease but may reflect the inflammatory nature of atherosclerotic disease. It has been shown in vitro that fibrinogen elaboration by cultured hepatoma cells, like that of other "acute phase" proteins, is responsive to inflammation mediating cytokines such as interleukin-6 (IL-6).[79] Because it is likely that atherosclerosis, especially advanced atherosclerosis, is an inflammatory process,[54,56,58,80-83] fibrinogen concentration may reflect circulating or localized cytokine concentrations. Possible cytokine regulation of fibrinogen concentration is most likely only one aspect of overall regulation, because there is some evidence that there is a significant genetic component that contributes to fibrinogen plasma concentration as well.[84,85] Little is known about other forms of regulation, such as dietary influences; however, it is clear that smoking exerts a strong influence on circulating fibrinogen concentration.[86-88]

It is important to consider that these four possibilities are not necessarily exclusive, and all may be acting in concert. Fibrinogen concentrations may well be initially regulated by genetic, environmental (diet, smoking, etc.), and pathobiologic (inflammation) processes, reflecting cardiovascular risk. At the same time, elevated fibrinogen concentrations may increase the likelihood of recurrent thrombotic episodes and the development of significant disease. Further atherosclerotic progression, with its attendant inflammation, may then result in further increases in fibrinogen concentrations.

Factor VII

The only other coagulation factor that has been studied extensively as a risk factor is factor VII, the zymogen/enzyme responsible for the conversion of factor X to factor Xa and factor IX to factor IXa during procoagulation. It is likely that the tissue factor–factor VIIa complex is the initiating enzymatic complex for procoagulation in many circumstances.

Only one study, the Northwick Park Heart Study,[57,67] has reported on the status of factor VII as an independent, prospective risk factor for cardiovascular disease. In this study, factor VII was a risk factor with importance similar to that of cholesterol and fibrinogen. To date there have been no confirming prospective studies. Preliminary results from the Munster study (PROCAM) seemed to indicate that factor VII was an independent risk factor,[74] but more recent results indicate that although factor VII baseline values were higher in those who went on to have ischemic events than in those that did not, this difference did not reach statistical significance.[89] Several cross-sectional studies have established a relationship between factor VII plasma concentration and prevalent cardiovascular disease. Elevated factor VII levels have been demonstrated in men at risk for coronary heart disease, with risk based on smoking, cholesterol level, and family history,[90-92] previous myocardial infarction[93]; peripheral vascular disease; and hyperlipidemia of various types.[94,95] In all cases factor

VII was estimated either by clot rate assay (i.e., one-stage factor assay using factor VII–deficient plasma) or immunoassay.

Factor VII levels have been correlated to plasma lipids in several studies. In particular, factor VII, as measured in a one-stage factor assay, appears to be associated with plasma triglyceride and plasma total cholesterol values in a positive manner.[87,91-93,95-97] Interestingly, factor VII also demonstrates a positive correlation with plasma high-density lipoprotein (HDL)–cholesterol.[87,98] The mechanism behind these factor VII–lipid associations remains unknown. It may concern the biochemistry of factor VII activation or may reflect a dependence of the factor VII assay on plasma lipids.[66]

Recently a study of plasma from pregnant women has revealed that the elevated factor VII levels seen in pregnancy may be reduced when the plasma is pretreated with phospholipase C, a lipid-cleaving enzyme.[99] Men at risk for cardiovascular disease also exhibit this phenomenon.[90] The initial explanation for this finding was that there were "factor VII–phospholipid complexes" having factor VIIa–like activity, which could be inactivated by the action of phospholipase C. At this time, however, the most likely explanation is the presence in these plasma samples of a form of plasma lipid (probably VLDL) particularly susceptible to phospholipase C, which exhibits a factor VII–binding region or regions after enzymatic activity. We hypothesize that the binding of factor VII by this modified lipid inactivates the factor VII, causing the decrease in plasma factor VII activity seen after phospholipase C treatment.[100] Recent work by Hubbard and Parr[101] supports this position; they have demonstrated a strong dependence of phospholipase C–dependent factor VII activity on the plasma triglyceride level.

Several studies, but not all, have demonstrated a relationship between factor VII plasma levels and dietary fat intake. The original study of Miller et al.[102] indicated that a change in total dietary fat was accompanied by a change in factor VII levels in a one-stage clotting assay. This was supported by a study showing that factor VII levels decreased after a change to a diet characterized as low fat and high fiber.[103] However, a recent study that purported to alter the subjects' diet concerning fat but not in any other way failed to result in altered factor VII levels.[104] Although the question remains open, it has been suggested that to decrease factor VII levels significantly, it may require altering more than a single component of the diet.[104]

Because there is no evidence that factor VII is an "acute phase" protein, its status as a prospective risk factor, if confirmed, would most likely relate to its role as a procoagulant factor. It will be necessary to confirm the independence of factor VII, because, as mentioned earlier, several studies have demonstrated a strong association between factor VII and plasma lipids, which are risk factors in their own right.

Other procoagulant and anticoagulant factors

Deficiency states of virtually all the procoagulant factors have been associated with hemorrhagic complications, but it does not necessarily hold that high circulating concentrations of these procoagulants are associated with a tendency toward thrombosis. A single report has discussed the association of factor X levels with hyperlipidemia,[105] but no prospective information has been presented for this factor or for other factors or cofactors. Much research is needed in this area.

The evidence for the association of other anticoagulant factors comes primarily from studies of individuals with deficiencies and not from studies of "normal" populations or populations at risk. Deficiency states of the anticoagulant factors protein C, protein S, and antithrombin III all have been associated with thrombosis,[106-108] and protein C deficiency has been firmly established not only through many studies in the world literature but also through detailed study of a large New England kindred characterized by a high frequency of protein C deficiency.[109] These deficiency states have been established by examining the levels of the anticoagulant protein themselves in relationship to prevalent thrombotic disease and by demonstrating that prothrombin activation to thrombin occurs at an accelerated rate in deficient individuals by analysis of prothrombin fragment 1·2.

Prospective studies will be forthcoming concerning these anticoagulant factors and other procoagulant and anticoagulant factors in the near future. In particular, two large, multicenter NIH-funded prospective epidemiologic studies are making careful and comprehensive examinations of thrombotic risk factors. These are the Atherosclerosis Risk in Communities Study, which is concentrating of middle-aged individuals,[110] and the Cardiovascular Health Study, which is emphasizing elderly participants.[111] These studies have many features in common, including the use of carotid ultrasonography to assess carotid atherosclerosis and careful longitudinal assessment of incident myocardial infarction, unstable angina, stroke, and peripheral vascular disease. We anticipate learning much about thrombosis risk factors from studies such as these.

t-PA and PAI-1

Concerning the relationship of fibrinolysis to cardiovascular risk, it has been pointed out in the Northwick Park Heart Study,[57,68] and in several other studies as well,[112,113] that cardiovascular disease is associated with decreased fibrinolytic potential. The association identified in the Northwick Park results, although relatively weak, concerned prospective data, whereas much of the other information concerns cross-sectional data.

Work from Hamsten et al.[113] has identified elevated PAI-1 levels and decreased t-PA activity in individuals with a previous myocardial infarction compared with those without. Moreover, these workers have determined that in individuals with previous infarction, those with higher PAI-1 levels were more likely to have a second infarction compared with those with lower levels.[112] These data may be interpreted as indicating that increased PAI-1 causes a decreased fibrinolytic response, which is, in turn, associated with increased thrombosis. However, because PAI-1 is an acute phase reactant, care must be taken in making such an interpretation. The possibility that PAI-1 simply reflects more severe coronary disease, through an inflammatory mechanism, cannot be ruled out at this time.

PAI-1, like factor VII, has been associated with plasma lipids, especially plasma triglyceride.[114-118] Elevations of PAI-1 have been described in non-insulin-dependent diabetics,[119] and PAI-1 levels have been shown to correlate to insulin levels in normals,[116,120] nondiabetic obese persons,[116-118,120] non-insulin-dependent diabetics,[119] and persons with angina pectoris.[121] Efforts at lowering insulin levels through diet[116,120,122,123] and pharmacologic intervention[121] have been associated with increased fibrinolytic capacity and with decreased PAI-1, and PAI-1 secretion is sensitive to insulin in tissue culture.[124-126] However, an increase in PAI-1 after an acute increase in insulin has not been observed in humans in clinical studies.[127,128] Therefore, it remains unclear whether or not PAI-1 in vivo is responsive to plasma insulin or is more closely linked to other diabetes-associated changes such as plasma triglyceride levels.

Other profibrinolytic and antifibrinolytic factors

Very little research has been done to examine other fibrinolytic factors, such as plasminogen and α_2-antiplasmin, and plasminogen activator inhibitors other than PAI-1, such as PAI-2, and PAI-3. Existing data would indicate that these are most likely not involved in the ongoing regulation of fibrinolysis, but this remains to be demonstrated in clinical studies under conditions where thrombosis is likely. Assays are available for the study of ongoing fibrinolytic activity, including PAI-1–t-PA complex,[129-131] α_2-antiplasmin-plasmin complex[132] and markers of plasmin activity such as the fibrin D-dimer fragment.[133,134] Concerning this latter analyte, it has been shown in small studies that D-dimer values are elevated in individuals with prevalent disease,[135] but whether or not this finding may be substantiated in larger studies or whether or not D-dimer is predictive of recurrent disease is unknown.

There is considerable effort underway to examine the

relationship of a relatively new lipoprotein particle, Lp(a), to cardiovascular risk. Several studies have suggested an association, with most of these studies[136-141] but not all[142] being cross-sectional. Lp(a) has been found to be incorporated into atherosclerotic plaque, which implies it might function as an atherogenic risk factor.[143] However, another proposed mechanism of action for Lp(a) concerns fibrinolysis. Lp(a) is similar to the low-density lipoprotein (LDL) particle in general structure, with the addition of the apolipoprotein (a) moiety, a polypeptide chain characterized by multiple copies of a particular amino acid sequence. This sequence is highly analogous to one of the so-called Kringle domains in plasminogen,[144] a region of the plasminogen molecule at least partly responsible for the binding of plasminogen to fibrin. Lp(a) exhibits considerable genotypic variation in the actual number of Kringle-like structures present per Lp(a) molecule,[145] and Lp(a) structure and plasma concentration appear to be under considerable genetic regulation.[146] It has been proposed that Lp(a) might interrupt the association of fibrin with plasminogen (and possibly other important fibrin-binding factors such as t-PA) and thereby limit fibrinolysis.[147] Although isolated Lp(a) can clearly do this in vitro,[147-149] it remains to be established that this is an important pathophysiologic mechanism in vivo.[150]

Role of genetics

For three of the factors mentioned earlier (fibrinogen, factor VII, and PAI-1), there are at least preliminary data indicating that genotype plays a significant role in regulating the plasma concentration.

Concerning fibrinogen, it has been estimated that 51% of the plasma fibrinogen variance may be explained genetically,[85] a figure, however, that has been questioned by us[151] and others.[84] Whatever the exact number, it appears that at least a fraction of the fibrinogen variance may be heritable. Humphries et al.[152] have identified a restriction fragment length polymorphism (RFLP) that is associated with elevated fibrinogen levels. This polymorphism appears to explain approximately 3% of the plasma fibrinogen variance. The frequency of the allele associated with higher fibrinogen (H2) values is approximately 0.2, similar in smokers and nonsmokers. The effect of the H2 allele is the same in smokers and nonsmokers. In multivariate analysis, the presence of the H2 allele was the strongest predictor of fibrinogen levels after smoking. A single factor explaining this fraction of plasma variance may play an important role defining the cardiovascular disease risk associated with fibrinogen.

For factor VII, a common polymorphism (gene frequency of approximately 0.1) has been identified that is located in the gene itself, coding for a G $\rightarrow$ A substitution in the second position of the codon for amino acid 353.[153] This leads to a change at this position from argi-

nine to glutamine ($Arg_{353} \rightarrow Gln_{353}$). The Gln_{353} allele is consistently associated with decreased factor VII activity levels and factor VII antigen levels, with heterozygotes expressing factor VII levels decreased by 20% to 30% and homozygotes expressing levels approximately 30% to 60% of normal.[154] As mentioned earlier, factor VII is known to exhibit relatively tight correlation to levels of plasma triglycerides and cholesterol. In one small study, when this correlation was explored in people in whom factor VII genotypes were also known, this correlation was only in the Arg/Arg individuals and not in those with the Gln_{353} allele, suggesting that this structural change may have profound implications concerning the putative physical association of plasma lipids and factor VII.[154] These results support the hypothesis that the presence of Gln_{353} may be associated with lower prevalence and incidence rates of cardiovascular disease. This hypothesis is being pursued at this time.

Finally, for the fibrinolytic control protein PAI-1, two different (but tightly correlated) polymorphisms have been reported that are associated with what appears to be an increase in PAI-1 levels of approximately 30%.[155] The HindIII RFLP has been studied the most, and because neither it nor the other polymorphism is in a coding region of the PAI-1 gene, it has been postulated that these polymorphisms are in linkage disequilibrium with another polymorphism in a response element associated with the PAI-1 gene, such as the glucocorticoid responsive element.[152] The frequency of these polymorphisms is approximately 0.5. PAI-1 is known to correlate with plasma triglyceride levels,[115] and this correlation was examined in individuals who were also typed for the HindIII polymorphism.[152] Different associations between PAI-1 and triglycerides were observed in the three possible HindIII genotypes (i.e., 1-1, 1-2, 2-2), indicating that this polymorphism may be related to a functional property of PAI-1 through the linkage disequilibrium mechanism mentioned earlier. Recently, Humphries et al.[152] have reported on another polymorphism in the PAI-1 gene, coding for either a 4G or 5G repeat sequence at position -675. Interestingly this polymorphism may be associated with the responsiveness of the PAI-1 gene to acute phase mediators, possibly cytokines such as IL-2 and IL-6.

THROMBOTIC RISK FACTORS IN THE ELDERLY

It is clear that risk of myocardial infarction increases with age, and greater than 80% of the individuals affected by cardiovascular disease in the United States are more than age 65.[3] None of the studies examining thrombotic risk factors has contained large numbers of elderly participants, however, so it is uncertain at this time whether or not elevated levels of these factors confer added risk in older individuals. Fibrinogen has received the most attention, and it has been demonstrated that fibrinogen goes up with age, both in middle-aged individuals[86,87] and, recently, in the elderly.[156,157] There appears to be little difference in fibrinogen values between elderly men and women, which is similar to the situation in middle-aged persons.

Concerning cardiovascular risk and age, the little information that is available concerning fibrinogen is inconsistent. In the Northwick Park Heart Study, Meade[67] reported that the value of fibrinogen as a predictive risk factor in men declined with age (women were not included in this study). However, in the Framingham study, fibrinogen was observed to be a predictive risk factor independent of the age of the men at entry.[71] In Framingham women, the association between plasma fibrinogen concentration and cardiovascular risk declined with age. The reason for these inconsistent results is unknown. Possibly differences in the study populations, the assay methodologies, as well as the relatively small numbers of older participants may account for the discrepant results. The Cardiovascular Health Study,[98] a prospective epidemiologic study of cardiovascular risk in elderly individuals, is currently underway and should provide definitive answers to these questions.

A preliminary report has appeared concerning the fibrinogen-associated variables in the elderly using a multivariate analysis of data from the Cardiovascular Health Study.[98] Fibrinogen plasma concentrations are positively associated with age, smoking, obesity, total cholesterol level, and black race and negatively associated with levels of HDL-cholesterol and triglyceride and

alcohol consumption. However, even with considerable knowledge about associated variables, a multivariate model can explain only approximately 10% of the plasma variation. Further research is needed to identify the other environmental factors, as well as the genetic factors, which are responsible for regulation of fibrinogen.

Several research groups have reported that factor VII values increase with age in the middle aged,[86,87] and data from the Cardiovascular Health Study[157] indicate that values in the elderly, although no longer increasing, are higher than in the middle aged. In two different studies of factor VII in middle-aged populations, it has been reported that factor VII values are the same in men and women and higher in women than in men, respectively. In the elderly it appears that factor VII values are significantly higher in women than in men by approximately 18%. There are no prospective studies of factor VII as a cardiovascular risk factor that include significant numbers of elderly persons, but, as just mentioned, the Cardiovascular Health Study will soon address this issue.

Concerning associated variables, plasma factor VII levels in the elderly have been shown to be positively associated with gender, plasma lipid levels (total cholesterol, triglyceride, and HDL-cholesterol), obesity, postmenopausal estrogen levels, and smoking and negatively associated with alcohol consumption.[157] As for fibrinogen, this list is very similar to published associations for factor VII in middle-aged individuals. Approximately 26% of the plasma factor VII variation can be explained by such associations.

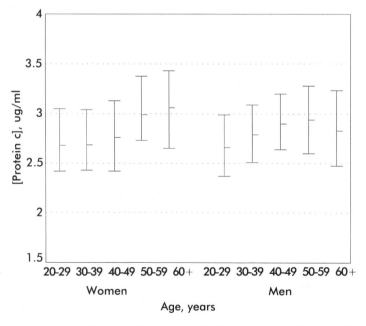

Fig. 3-5. Age distribution of protein C antigen in 2743 blood donors. Plasma collected at time of donation was frozen at −70° C and later thawed and assayed for protein C antigen. The results are expressed as the median value for each age-gender group, plus the 25th and 75th percentile. Note that the Y-axis is truncated. (Modified from Howard P, Bovill E, Mann K, et al: *Clin Chem* 34:324-330, 1988.)

There is not much known about the effect of aging on other thrombotic risk factors. Even when there is information on age-associated changes, the mechanisms directing such changes are unknown. Age-related changes in measurements for several other coagulation factors have been identified, such as an increase in factor VIII[158] and a decrease in prothrombin.[5] Also, age-related decreases have been noted for anticoagulant factors such as antithrombin III and protein C.[5,158] In fact, protein C appears to exhibit a complex relationship with age, with mean values in cross-sectional population studies rising through the first five decades and decreasing thereafter. Fig. 3-5 illustrates this finding, with data from 2743 donors from the Vermont/New Hampshire Red Cross.

In the measurement of activation peptides, although only a few studies have been done, the data suggest that in general coagulation activity increases with age. The thrombin activation peptide prothrombin fragment 1·2, as well as the protein C activation peptide, the factor IX activation peptide, and fibrinopeptide A, all exhibit elevated mean values with aging in normal population cross-sectional studies.[5,159] Age-related elevations in D-dimer have also been observed.[160] These results imply a generalized increase in procoagulant activity. Whether or not this increase is related to the decrease in anticoagulant proteins noted earlier, however, remains speculative at this time.

Table 3-4. Age-associated changes in coagulation and fibrinolytic factors

Factor	Changes in middle age (approximately 20-60 yr)	Changes in older age (approximately > 60 yr)
Fibrinogen*	Increases	Increases
Prothrombin†	Decreases	Decreases
Factor VII*	Increases	Stays the same
Factor VIII*	Increases	Increases
von Willebrand factor*	Increases	?
Protein C*	Increases	Decreases
Antithrombin III†	Stays the same	Stays the same
Protein C activation peptide†	Increases	Increases
Factor IX activation peptide†	Increases	Increases
Prothrombin fragment 1·2†	Increases	Increases
Fibrinopeptide A†	Increases	Increases
Tissue plasminogen activator†	Increases	?
Plasminogen activator inhibitor-1†	Increases	?

*Information from large population-based cross-sectional studies (n, several hundred to several thousand).
†Information from smaller cross-sectional studies.

Finally, concerning fibrinolysis, the data that have been gathered to date suggest that there are age-associated increases in both t-PA and PAI-1 antigens. However, it is unclear as to the relative magnitude of these increases. Some data indicate that the increase in PAI-1 antigen exceeds that in t-PA, with measurements of t-PA activity decreasing with age.[161,162] Other studies have shown that the ratio of PAI-1 antigen to t-PA antigen is stable with age, resulting in not decreased fibrinolysis but either unchanged or increased fibrinolytic activity.[163] There are indications that although t-PA may go up with age in both men and women, PAI-1 may go up only in women.[163] This issue remains unresolved.

Consistent with our general hypothesis (i.e., coagulation and fibrinolysis are in a state of dynamic balance), in the healthy elderly person an increase in procoagulant activity should be accompanied by an increase in either anticoagulant potential or fibrinolytic capacity or both. Whether or not this is true, however, remains to be demonstrated.

Although there is some inconsistency in the data currently available, it appears most likely that the age-associated changes in plasma levels of thrombotic risk factors, as illustrated in Table 3-4, all tend toward increasing the possibility for a thrombotic event. It remains to be proved whether or not these changes truly contribute to the increased thrombosis observed in the elderly and, if they do, whether or not they can be modified to reduce cardiovascular risk. There is clear evidence that inhibition of the cyclooxygenase-associated pathway of platelet activation can help reduce the risk of thrombotic episodes, especially in patients with atrial fibrillation.[164] Warfarin, which downregulates procoagulant factor production, can also help reduce risk of stroke in this latter group.[164] However, at this time it is unclear whether or not procoagulant factor modification would be useful, neutral, or detrimental in a "normal" population, because there would almost certainly be increased risk of bleeding.

In a speculative vein, we believe that there are compelling data to support the positions that (1) individuals vary in their capacity to respond to a vascular "insult" from a coagulation standpoint and that (2) this variation is important is determining when a severe thrombotic event will take place, how extensive that event will be, and how rapidly it will be resolved. The systems that are involved (i.e., procoagulation and anticoagulation and profibrinolysis and antifibrinolysis), however, are quite complex and interactive, not only among themselves but most likely with other systems as well, such as the lipoprotein metabolism system. Much work is needed to tease out those measurements that can effectively summarize ongoing thrombotic status and report clinically useful information. This is an exciting challenge that will require an integrated approach involving basic scientists, clinicians, and epidemiologists over the next 5 to 10 years.

REFERENCES

1. DeWood M, Spores J, Notske R, et al: Prevalence of total coronary occlusion during the early hours of transmural myocardial infarction, *N Engl J Med* 303:897-902, 1980.
2. Colman R, Hirsh J, Marder V, et al (eds): *Hemostasis and thrombosis: basic principles and clinical practice,* Philadelphia, 1987, JB Lippincott.
3. National Center for Health Statistics: *Advance report of final mortality statistics, 1987,* Hyattsville, Md, Public Health Service 1989.
4. Bauer K, Rosenberg R: The pathophysiology of the prethrombotic state in humans: insights gained from studies using markers of hemostatic system activation, *Blood* 70:343-350, 1987.
5. Bauer K, Weiss L, Sparrow D, et al: Aging-associated changes in indices of thrombin generation and protein C activation in humans, *J Clin Invest* 80:1527-1534, 1987.
6. Kaplan K, Owen J: Plasma levels of beta-thromboglobulin and platelet factor 4 as indices of platelet activation in vivo, *Blood* 57:199-202, 1981.
7. Granstrom E, Diczfalusy U, Hamberg M, et al: Thromboxane A2: biosynthesis and effect on platelets, *Adv Prostaglandin Thromboxane Leukotriene Res* 10:15-57, 1982.
8. Plow E, Ginsberg M: Cellular adhesion: GPIIb-IIIa as a prototypic adhesion receptor. In Coller B: *Progress in hemostasis and thrombosis,* Philadelphia, 1989, WB Saunders, pp 117-156.
9. Rapaport S: Inhibition of factor VIIa/tissue factor-induced blood coagulation: with particular emphasis upon a factor Xa-dependent inhibitory mechanism, *Blood* 73:359-365, 1989.
10. Tijburg P, de Groot P: Endothelial cell-mediated thrombin formation, *Semin Thromb Hemost* 18:256-260, 1992.
11. Esmon C: The roles of protein C and thrombomodulin in the regulation of blood coagulation, *J Biol Chem* 264:4743-4753, 1987.
12. Hajjar K, Harpel P, Jaffe E, et al: Binding of plasminogen to cultured human endothelial cells, *J Biol Chem* 261:11656-11662, 1986.
13. Miles L, Plow E: Plasminogen receptors: ubiquitous sites for cellular regulation of fibrinolysis, *Fibrinolysis* 2:61-71, 1988.
14. Teitel J, Bauer K, Lau H, et al: Studies of the prothrombin activation pathway utilizing radioimmunoassays for the F2/F1 + 2 fragment and thrombin-antithrombin complex, *Blood* 59:1086-1095, 1982.
15. Mann K, Williams E, Krishnaswamy S, et al: Active site-specific immunoassays, *Blood* 76:755-766, 1990.
16. Gruber A, Griffin J: Direct detection of activated protein C in blood from human subjects, *Blood* 79:2340-2348, 1992.
17. Nesheim M, Mann K: Thrombin-catalyzed activation of single-chain bovine factor V, *J Biol Chem* 254:1326-1338, 1979.
18. Coller B: Platelets and thrombolytic therapy, *N Engl J Med* 322:33-42, 1990.
19. Friedman F, Detwiler T: Stimulus secretion coupling in platelets: effects of drugs on secretion of adenosine 5'-triphosphate, *Biochemistry* 14:1315-1318, 1975.
20. Krupski W, Bass A, Kelly A, et al: Heparin-resistant thrombus formation by endovascular stents in baboons: interruption by a synthetic antithrombin, *Circulation* 81:570-577, 1990.
21. Esmon C, Owen W: Identification of an endothelial cell co-factor for thrombin-catalyzed activation of protein C, *Proc Nat Acad Sci USA* 1578:2249-2252, 1981.
22. Bajzar L, Fredenburgh J, Nesheim M: The activated protein C–mediated enhancement of tissue-type plasminogen activator-induced fibrinolysis in a cell-free system, *J Biol Chem* 265:16948-16954, 1990.
23. Gospodarowicz D, Brown C, Birdwell C, et al: Control of proliferation of human vascular endothelial cells, *J Cell Biol* 77:774-788, 1978.
24. Malik A, Fenton J: Thrombin-mediated increase in vascular endothelial permeability, *Semin Thromb Hemost* 18:193-199, 1992.
25. Rosenberg R: Chemistry of the hemostatic mechanism and its relationship to the action of heparin, *Fed Proc* 36:10-18, 1977.
26. Lawson J, Butenas S, Ribarik N, et al: Complex-dependent inhibition of factor VIIa by antithrombin III and heparin, *Circulation* 86 (suppl I): I680, 1992.
27. Gouin I, Lecompte T, Morel M-C, et al: In vitro effect of plasmin on human platelet function in plasma: inhibition of aggregation caused by fibrinogenolysis, *Circulation* 85:935-941, 1992.
28. Ritchie D, Levy B, Adams M, et al: Regulation of fibrinogen synthesis by plasmin-derived fragments of fibrinogen and fibrin: an indirect feedback pathway, *Proc Natl Acad Sci USA* 79:1530-1534, 1982.
29. Lee C, Mann K: Activation/inactivation of human factor V by plasmin, *Blood* 73:185-190, 1989.
30. Gurewich V: Importance of fibrin specificity in therapeutic thrombolysis and the rationale of using sequential and synergistic combinations of tissue plasminogen activator and pro-urokinase, *Semin Thromb Hemost* 15:123-128, 1989.
31. Robbins K: The plasminogen-plasmin enzyme system. In Colman R, Hirsh J, Marder V, et al: *Hemostasis and thrombosis: basic principles and clinical practice,* ed 2, Philadelphia, 1987, JB Lippincott, pp 318-339.
32. Saksela O: Plasminogen activation and regulation of proteolysis, *Biochim Biophys Acta* 823:35-65, 1985.
33. Wiman B, Collen D: On the mechanism of the reaction between human alpha-2 antiplasmin and plasmin, *J Biol Chem* 254:9291-9301, 1979.
34. Wiman B, Lijnen H, Collen D: On the specific interaction between the lysine-binding sites in plasmin and complementary sites in alpha-2-antiplasmin and in fibrinogen, *Biochim Biophys Acta* 579:142-154, 1979.
35. Collen D: Tissue-type plasminogen activator (t-PA) and single chain urokinase-type plasminogen activator (scu-PA): potential for fibrin-specific thrombolytic therapy. In Coller B: *Progress in hemostasis and thrombosis,* Orlando, Fla, 1986, Grune & Stratton, pp 1-18.
36. Kruithof E, Tran-Thang C, Ransijn A, et al: Demonstration of a fast-acting inhibitor of plasminogen activators in human plasma, *Blood* 64:907-913, 1984.
37. Astedt B, Lecander I, Ny T: The placental type plasminogen activator inhibitor, PAI-2, *Fibrinolysis* 1:203-208, 1987.
38. Stump D, Thienpont M, Collen D: Purification and characterization of a novel inhibitor of urokinase from human urine, *J Biol Chem* 261:12759-12766, 1986.
39. Heeb M, Espana F, Geiger M, et al: Immunologic identity of heparin-dependent plasma and urinary protein C inhibitor and plasminogen activator inhibitor-3, *J Biol Chem* 262:15813-15816, 1987.
40. Ross R: The pathogenesis of atherosclerosis—an update, *N Engl J Med* 314:488-500, 1986.
41. Fuster V, Badimon L, Badimon J, et al: Pathogenesis of coronary artery disease and the acute coronary syndromes: part 1, *N Engl J Med* 326:242-250, 1992.
42. Fuster V, Badimon L, Badimon J, et al: The pathogenesis of coronary artery disease and the acute coronary syndromes: Part 2, *N Engl J Med* 326:310-318, 1992.
43. Fuster V, Stein B, Ambrose J, et al: Atherosclerotic plaque rupture and thrombosis: evolving concepts, *Circulation* 82:II47-II59, 1990.
44. Woolf N, Davies M: Interrelationship between atherosclerosis and thrombosis. In Fuster V, Verstraete M: *Thrombosis in*

cardiovascular disorders, Philadelphia, 1992, WB Saunders, pp 41-77.

45. Chandler A: An overview of thrombosis and platelet involvement in the development of the human atherosclerotic plaque. In Glagov S, W Newman, S Schaffer: *Pathobiology of the human atherosclerotic plaque,* New York, 1990, Springer-Verlag New York, pp 359-378.

46. Rokitansky C: *A manual of pathological anatomy,* Philadelphia, Blanchard & Lee, 1855.

47. Mallory F: *The infectious lesions of blood vessels,* Philadelphia, 1913, JB Lippincott, pp 150-166.

48. Clark E, Graef I, Chasis H: Thrombosis of the aorta and coronary arteries with special reference to "fibrinoid" lesions, *Arch Pathol* 22:183-212, 1936.

49. Duguid J: Thrombosis as a factor in the pathogenesis of coronary atherosclerosis, *J Pathol* 58:207-212, 1946.

50. Gerrity R: The role of the monocyte in atherogenesis: I. Transition of blood-borne monocytes into the foam cells in fatty lesions, *Am J Pathol* 103:181-190, 1981.

51. Gerrity R: The role of the monocyte in atherogenesis: II. Migration of foam cells from atherosclerotic lesions, *Am J Pathol* 103:191-200, 1981.

52. Bini A, Fenoglio J, Mesa-Tejada R, et al: Identification and distribution of fibrinogen, fibrin, and fibrin(ogen) degradation products in atherosclerosis: use of monoclonal antibodies, *Arteriosclerosis* 9:109-121, 1989.

53. Smith E, Keen G, Grant A, et al: Fate of fibrinogen in human arterial intima, *Arteriosclerosis* 10:263-275, 1990.

54. Esmon C, Taylor F, Snow T: Inflammation and coagulation: linked processes potentially regulated through a common pathway mediated by protein C, *Thromb Haemost* 66:160-165, 1991.

55. Dahlback B, Stenflo J: High molecular weight complex in human plasma between vitamin K–dependent protein S and complement component C4b-binding protein, *Proc Natl Acad Sci USA* 78:2512-2516, 1981.

56. Libby P, Clinton S: Possible roles for cytokines in atherogenesis, *J Cellular Biochem* 16(suppl A):2, 1992.

57. Meade T, Brozovic M, Chakrabarti R, et al: Haemostatic function and ischaemic heart disease: principal results of the Northwick Park Heart Study, *Lancet* 2:533-537, 1986.

58. Kuller L, Eichner J, Orchard T, et al: The relation between serum albumin levels and risk of coronary heart disease in the Multiple Risk Factor Intervention Trial, *Am J Epidemiol* 134:1266-1277, 1991.

59. Eisenberg P, Sherman L, Rich M, et al: Importance of continued activation of thrombin reflected by fibrinopeptide A to the efficacy of thrombolysis, *J Am Coll Cardiol* 7:1986.

60. Gulba P, Barthels M, Westhoff-Bleck M, et al: Increased thrombin levels during thrombolytic therapy in acute myocardial infarction: relevance for the success of therapy, *Circulation* 83:937-944, 1991.

61. Rapold H, Kuemmerli H, Weiss M, et al: Monitoring of fibrin generation during thrombolytic therapy of acute myocardial infarction with recombinant tissue-type plasminogen activator, *Circulation* 79:980-989, 1989.

62. Weitz J, Cruickshank M, Thong B, et al: Human tissue-type plasminogen activator releases fibrinopeptides A and B from fibrinogen, *J Clin Invest* 82:1700-1707, 1988.

63. Francis C, Markham R, Barlow G, et al: Thrombin activity of fibrin thrombi and soluble plasmic derivatives, *J Lab Clin Med* 102:220-230, 1983.

64. Eisenberg P, Sobel B, Jaffe A: Activation of prothrombin accompanying thrombolysis with recombinant tissue–type plasminogen activator, *J Am Coll Cardiol* 19:1065-1069, 1992.

65. Mann K: Normal hemostasis. In Kelley W: *Textbook of internal medicine,* New York, 1992, JB Lippincott, pp 1240-1245.

66. Mann K: Factor VII assays, plasma triglyceride levels and cardiovascular disease risk, *Arteriosclerosis* 9:783-784, 1989.

67. Meade T: The epidemiology of haemostatic and other variables in coronary artery disease. In Verstraete M, Vermylen J, Lijnen H, et al: *Thrombosis and haemostasis 1987,* Leuven, Belgium, 1987, International Society on Thrombosis and Haemostasis and Leuven University Press, pp 37-59.

68. Meade T, Chakrabarti R, Haines A, et al: Haemostatic function and cardiovascular death: early results of a prospective study, *Lancet* 1:1050-1054, 1980.

69. Wilhelmsen L, Svardsudd K, Korsan-Bengtsen K, et al: Fibrinogen as a risk factor for stroke and myocardial infarction, *N Engl J Med* 311:501-505, 1984.

70. Kannel W, D'Agostino R, Belanger A: Update on fibrinogen as a cardiovascular risk factor, *Ann Epidemiol* 2:457-466, 1992.

71. Kannel W, Wolf P, Castelli W, et al: Fibrinogen and risk of cardiovascular disease: the Framingham study, *JAMA* 258:1183-1186, 1987.

72. Stone M, Thorp J: Plasma fibrinogen—a major coronary risk factor, *J R Coll Gen Pract* 35:565-569, 1985.

73. Yarnell J, Baker I, Sweetnam P, et al: Fibrinogen, viscosity, and white blood cell count are major risk factors for ischemic heart disease, *Circulation* 83:836-844, 1991.

74. Balleisen L, Schulte H, Assmann G, et al: Coagulation factors and the progress of coronary heart disease, *Lancet* 2:461, 1987.

75. Naski M, Shafer J: A kinetic model for the alpha-thrombin-catalyzed conversion of plasma levels of fibrinogen to fibrin in the presence of antithrombin III, *J Biol Chem* 266:13003-13010, 1991.

76. Marguerie G, Plow E, Edgington T: Human platelets possess an inducible and saturable receptor specific for fibrinogen, *J Biol Chem* 254:5357-5363, 1979.

77. Meade T, Vickers M, Thompson S, et al: The effect of physiological levels of fibrinogen on platelet aggregation, *Thromb Res* 38:527-534, 1985.

78. Letcher R, Chien S, Pickering T, et al: Direct relationship between blood pressure and blood viscosity in normal and hypertensive subjects: role of fibrinogen and concentration, *Am J Med* 70:1195-1202, 1981.

79. Baumann H, Isseroff H, Latimer J, et al: Phorbol ester modulates Interleukin-6 and Interleukin-1–regulated expression of acute phase plasma proteins in hepatoma cells, *J Biol Chem* 263:1530-1534, 1988.

80. Marcus A: Thrombosis and inflammation as multicellular processes: pathophysiologic significance of transcellular metabolism, *Blood* 76:1903-1907, 1990.

81. Munro J, Cotran R: Biology of disease: the pathogenesis of atherosclerosis: atherogenesis and inflammation, *Lab Invest* 58:249-261, 1988.

82. Schwartz C, Sprague E, Valente A, et al: Inflammatory components of the human atherosclerotic plaque. In Glagov S, W Newman, S Schaffer: *Pathobiology of the human atherosclerotic plaque,* New York, 1990, Springer-Verlag, New York, pp 107-120.

83. Schwartz C, Valente A, Sprague E, et al: Atherosclerosis as an inflammatory process: the roles of the monocyte-macrophage, *NY Acad Sci* 454:115-120, 1985.

84. Berg K, Kierulf P: DNA polymorphisms at the fibrinogen loci and plasma fibrinogen concentration, *Clin Genet* 36:229-235, 1989.

85. Hamsten A, Iselius L, DeFaire U, et al: Genetic and cultural inheritance of plasma fibrinogen concentration, *Lancet* 2:988-991, 1987.

86. Balleisen L, Bailey J, Epping P-H, et al: Epidemiological study on factor VII, factor VIII and fibrinogen in an industrial population: I. Baseline data on the relation to age, gender, body-weight, smoking, alcohol, pill-using, and menopause, *Thromb Haemost* 54:475-479, 1985.

87. Folsom A, Wu K, Davis C, et al: Population correlates of plasma

fibrinogen and factor VII, putative cardiovascular risk factors, *Atherosclerosis* 91:191-205, 1991.

88. Meade T, Chakrabarti R, Haines A, et al: Characteristics affecting fibrinolytic activity and plasma fibrinogen concentrations, *Br Med J (Clin Res)* 1:153-156, 1979.

89. van de Loo J: Paper presented at the American Heart Association 65th Scientific Sessions, New Orleans, November 1992.

90. Dalaker K, Hjermann I, Prydz H: A novel form of factor VII in plasma from men at risk for cardiovascular disease, *Br J Haematol* 61:315-322, 1985.

91. Hoffman C, Miller R, Lawson W, et al: Elevation of factor VII activity and mass in young adults at risk of ischaemic heart disease *J Am Coll Cardiol* 14:941-946, 1989.

92. Hoffman C, Shah A, Sodums M, et al: Factor VII activity state in coronary artery disease, *J Lab Clin Med* 111:475-481, 1988.

93. Dalaker K, Smith P, Arnesen H, et al: Factor VII–phospholipid complex in male survivors of acute myocardial infarction, *Acta Med Scand* 222:111-116, 1987.

94. Bruckert E, Carvalho de Sousa J, Giral P, et al: Interrelationship of plasma triglyceride and coagulant factor VII levels in normotriglyceridemic hypercholesterolemia, *Atherosclerosis* 75:129-134, 1989.

95. Carvalho de Sousa J, Bruckert E, Giral P, et al: Plasma factor VII, triglyceride concentration and fibrin degradation products in primary hyperlipidemia: a clinical and laboratory study, *Haemostasis* 19:83-90, 1989.

96. Miller G, Walter S, Stirling Y, et al: Assay of factor VII activity by two techniques: evidence for increased conversion of VII to VIIa in hyperlipidaemia, with possible implications for ischaemic heart disease, *Br J Haematol* 59:249-258, 1985.

97. Skartlien A, Lyberg-Beckmann S, Holme I, et al: Effect of alteration in triglyceride levels on factor VII–phospholipid complexes in plasma, *Arteriosclerosis* 9:798-801, 1989.

98. Tracy R, Psaty B, Bovill E, et al: Fibrinogen and factor VIII, but not factor VII, are positively associated with prevalent cardiovascular disease in older adults: analyses from the Cardiovascular Health Study. In *32nd Annual Conference on Cardiovascular Disease Epidemiology,* Abstract P31, 1992.

99. Dalaker K, Prydz H: Coagulation factor VII in pregnancy, *Br J Haematol* 56:233-241, 1984.

100. Hayes T, Pike J, Tracy R: Factor VII assays: a review, *Arch Pathol Lab Med* 117:52-57, 1993.

101. Hubbard A, Parr L: Phospholipase C mediated inhibition of factor VII requires triglyceride-rich lipoproteins, *Thromb Res* 62:335-344, 1991.

102. Miller G, Martin J, Webster J, et al: Association between dietary fat intake and plasma factor VII coagulant activity—a predictor of cardiovascular mortality, *Atherosclerosis* 60:269-277, 1986.

103. Marckmann P, Sandstrom B, Jespersen J: Effect of total fat content and fatty acid composition in diet on factor VII coagulant activity and blood lipids, *Atherosclerosis* 80:227-233, 1990.

104. Marckmann P, Sandstrom B, Jespersen J: Fasting blood coagulation and fibrinolysis of young adults unchanged by reduction in dietary fat content, *Arterioscler Thromb* 12:201-205, 1992.

105. Simpson H, Meade T, Stirling Y, et al: Hypertriglyceridaemia and hypercoagulability *Lancet* 1:786-790, 1983.

106. Bertina R: Hereditary protein S deficiency, *Haemostasis* 15:241-246, 1985.

107. Hirsh J, Piovella F, Pini M: Congenital antithrombin III deficiency: incidence and clinical features, *Am J Med* 87(suppl 3B):34S-38S, 1989.

108. Miletich J: Laboratory diagnosis of protein C deficiency, *Semin Thromb Hemost* 16:169-176, 1990.

109. Bovill E, Bauer K, Dickerman J, et al: The clinical spectrum of heterozygous protein C deficiency in a large New England kindred, *Blood* 73:712-717, 1989.

110. Sharrett A, and ARIC Investigators: The Atherosclerosis Risk in Communities Study: introduction and objectives of the hemostasis component, *Ann Epidemiol* 2:467-469, 1992.

111. Fried L, Borhani N, Enright P, et al: The Cardiovascular Health Study: design and rationale, *Ann Epidemiol* 1:263-276, 1991.

112. Hamsten A, de Faire U, Walldius G, et al: Plasminogen activator inhibitor in plasma: risk factor for recurrent myocardial infarction, *Lancet* 2:3-9, 1987.

113. Hamsten A, Wiman B, de Faire U, et al: Increased plasma levels of a rapid inhibitor of tissue plasminogen activator in young survivors of myocardial infarction, *N Engl J Med* 313:1557-1563, 1985.

114. Donders S, Lustermans F, van Wersch J: Fibrinolysis factors and lipid composition of the blood in treated and untreated hypertensive patients, *Blood Coag Fibrinolysis* 3:61-67, 1992.

115. Juhan-Vague I, Alessi M, Vague P: Increased plasma plasminogen activator inhibitor 1 levels: a possible link between insulin resistance and atherothrombosis, *Diabetologia* 34:457-462, 1991.

116. Juhan-Vague I, Vague P, Alessi M, et al: Relationships between plasma insulin, triglyceride, body mass index, and plasminogen activator inhibitor 1, *Diabete Metab* 13:331-336, 1987.

117. Vague P, Juhan-Vague I, Alessi M, et al: Metformin decreases the high plasminogen activator capacity, plasma insulin and triglyceride levels in non-diabetic obese subjects, *Thromb Haemost* 57:326-328, 1987.

118. Vague P, Juhan-Vague I, Chabert V, et al: Fat distribution and plasminogen activator inhibitor activity in nondiabetic obese women, *Metabolism* 38:913-915, 1989.

119. Juhan-Vague I, Roul C, Alessi M, et al: Increased plasminogen activator inhibitor activity in non-insulin dependent diabetic patients—relationship with plasma insulin *Thromb Haemost* 61:370-373, 1989.

120. Vague P, Juhan-Vague I, Aillaud M, et al: Correlation between blood fibrinolytic activity, plasminogen activator inhibitor level, plasma insulin level, and relative body weight in normal and obese subjects, *Metabolism* 35:250-253, 1986.

121. Juhan-Vague I, Alessi M, Joly P, et al: Plasma plasminogen activator inhibitor-1 in angina pectoris: influence of plasma insulin and acute-phase response, *Arteriosclerosis* 9:362-367, 1989.

122. Geiger M, Binder B: Plasminogen activation in diabetes mellitus: normalization of blood sugar levels improves impaired enzyme kinetics in vitro, *Thromb Haemost* 54:413-414, 1985.

123. Juhan-Vague I, Vague P, Poisson C, et al: Effect of 24 hours of normoglycaemia on tissue-type plasminogen activator plasma levels in insulin-dependent diabetes, *Thromb Haemost* 51:97-98, 1984.

124. Alessi M, Juhan-Vague I, Kooistra T, et al: Insulin stimulates the synthesis of plasminogen activator inhibitor 1 by the human hepatocellular cell line HepG2, *Thromb Haemost* 60:491-494, 1988.

125. Kooistra T, Bosma P, Tons H, et al: Plasminogen activator inhibitor 1: biosynthesis and mRNA level are increased by insulin in cultured human hepatocytes, *Thromb Haemost* 62:723-728, 1989.

126. Schneider D: Augmentation of synthesis of plasminogen activator inhibitor type 1 by insulin and insulin-like growth factor type I: implications for vascular disease in hyperinsulinemic states, *Proc Natl Acad Sci USA* 88:9959-9963, 1991.

127. Grant P, Kruithof E, Felley C, et al: Short-term infusions of insulin, triacylglycerol and glucose do not cause acute increases in plasminogen activator inhibitor-1 concentrations in man, *Clin Sci* 79:513-516, 1990.

128. Landin K, Tengborn L, Chmielewska J, et al: The acute effect of insulin on tissue plasminogen activator and plasminogen activator inhibitor in man, *Thromb Haemost* 65:130-133, 1991.

129. Alessi M, Juhan-Vague I, Declerck P, et al: Correlations between

t-PA and PAI-1 antigen and activity and t-PA/PAI-1 complexes in plasma of control subjects and of patients with increased t-PA or PAI-1 levels, *Thromb Res* 60:509-516, 1990.

130. Chandler W, Trimble S, Loo S-C, et al: Effect of PAI-1 levels on the molar concentrations of active plasminogen activator (t-PA) and t-PA/PAI-1 complex in plasma, *Blood* 76:930-937, 1990.

131. Declerck P, Collen D: Measurement of plasminogen activator inhibitor 1 (PAI-1) in plasma with various monoclonal antibody-based enzyme-linked immunosorbent assays, *Thromb Res* (suppl X):3-9, 1990.

132. Holvoet P, de Boer A, Verstreken M, et al: An enzyme-linked immunosorbent assay (ELISA) for the measurement of plasmin-alpha-2-antiplasmin complex in human plasma — application to the detection of in vivo activation of the fibrinolytic system, *Thromb Haemost* 56:124-127, 1986.

133. Declerck P, Mombaerts P, Holvoet P, et al: Fibrinolytic response and fibrin fragment D-dimer levels in patients with deep vein thrombosis, *Thromb Haemost* 58:1024-1029, 1987.

134. Elms M, Bunce H, Bundesen P, et al: Measurement of cross-linked fibrin degradation products. An immunoassay using monoclonal antibodies, *Thromb Haemost* 50:591-594, 1983.

135. Kruskal J, Commerford P, Franks J, et al: Fibrin and fibrinogen-related antigens in patients with stable and unstable coronary artery disease, *N Engl J Med* 317:1362-1365, 1987.

136. Armstrong V, Cremer P, Eberle E, et al: The association between Lp(a) concentrations and angiographically assessed coronary atherosclerosis: dependence on serum LDL levels, *Atherosclerosis* 62:249-257, 1986.

137. Dahlen G, Guyton J, Attar M, et al: Association of levels of lipoprotein (a), plasma lipids, and other lipoproteins with coronary artery disease documented by angiography, *Circulation* 74:758-765, 1986.

138. Kostner G, Avogaro P, Cazzolato G, et al: Lipoprotein Lp(a) and the risk for myocardial infarction, *Atherosclerosis* 38:51-61, 1981.

139. Murai A, Miyahara T, Fujimoto N, et al: Lp(a) lipoprotein as a risk factor for coronary heart disease and cerebral infarction, *Atherosclerosis* 59:199-204, 1986.

140. Rhoads G, Dahlen G, Berg K, et al: Lp(a) lipoprotein as a risk factor for myocardial infarction, *JAMA* 256:2540-2544, 1986.

141. Sandkamp M, Funke H, Schulte H, et al: Lipoprotein (a) is an independent risk factor for myocardial infarction at a young age, *Clin Chem* 36:20-23, 1990.

142. Rosengren A, Wilhelmsen L, Eriksson E, et al: Lipoprotein (a) and coronary heart disease: a prospective case-control study in a general population sample of middle aged men, *Br Med J (Clin Res)* 301:1248-1251, 1990.

143. Rath M, Niendorf A, Reblin T, et al: Detection and quantitation of lipoprotein (a) in the arterial wall of 107 coronary bypass patients, *Atheriosclerosis* 9:579-592, 1989.

144. Eaton D, Fless G, Kohr W, et al: Partial amino acid sequence of apolipoprotein (a) shows that it is homologous to plasminogen, *Proc Natl Acad Sci USA* 84:3224-3228, 1987.

145. Scanu A, Fless G: Lipoprotein (a): heterogeneity and biological relevance, *J Clin Invest* 85:1709-1715, 1990.

146. Kraft H, Sandholzer C, Menzel H, et al: Apolipoprotein (a) alleles determine lipoprotein (a) particle density and concentration in plasma, *Arterioscler Thromb* 12:302-306, 1992.

147. Miles L, Fless G, Levin E, et al: A potential basis for the thrombotic risks associated with lipoprotein(a), *Nature* 339:301-303, 1989.

148. Loscalzo J, Weinfeld M, Fless G, et al: Lipoprotein (a), fibrin binding, and plasminogen activation, *Arteriosclerosis* 10:240-245, 1990.

149. Rouy D, Laplaud P, Saboureau M, et al: Hedgehog lipoprotein (a) is a modulator of activation of plasminogen at the fibrin surface: an in vitro study, *Arterioscler Thromb* 12:146-154, 1992.

150. Alessi M, Parra H, Joly P, et al: The increased plasma Lp(a):B lipoprotein particle concentration in angina pectoris is not associated with hypofibrinolysis, *Clin Chem Acta* 188:119-128, 1990.

151. Reed T, Tracy RP, Fabsitz RR: Minimal genetic influences on plasma fibrinogen level in adult males in the NHLBI twin study, *Clin Genet* 45:71-77, 1994.

152. Humphries S, Lane A, Dawson S, et al: The study of gene-environment interactions that influence thrombosis and fibrinolysis: genetic variation at the loci for factor VII and plasminogen activator inhibitor-1, *Arch Pathol Lab Med* 116:1322-1329, 1992.

153. Green F, Kelleher C, Wilkes H, et al: A common genetic polymorphism associated with low coagulation factor VII levels in healthy individuals, *Arterioscler Thromb* 11:540-546, 1991.

154. Lane A, Cruickshank J, Stewart J, et al: Genetic and environmental determinants of factor VII coagulant activity in different ethnic groups at differing risk of coronary heart disease, *Atherosclerosis* 94:43-50, 1992.

155. Dawson S, Hamsten A, Wiman B, et al: Genetic variation at the plasminogen activator inhibitor-1 locus is associated with altered levels of plasminogen activator inhibitor-1 activity, *Arterioscler Thromb* 11:183-190, 1991.

156. Tracy R, Bovill E: Thrombosis and cardiovascular risk in the elderly, *Arch Pathol Lab Med* 116:1307-1312, 1992.

157. Tracy R, Bovill E, Fried L, et al: The distribution of coagulation factors VII, VIII and fibrinogen in adults over the age of 65 years: results from the Cardiovascular Health Study, *Ann Epidemiol* 2:509-519, 1992.

158. Folsom A, Conlan M, Davis C, et al: Relations between hemostasis variables and cardiovascular risk factors in middle-aged adults, *Ann Epidemiol* 2:481-494, 1992.

159. Bauer K, Kass B, ten Cate H, et al: Factor IX is activated in vivo by the tissue factor mechanism, *Blood* 76:731-736, 1990.

160. Currie M, Vala M, Pisetsky D, et al: Correlation between erythrocyte CR1 reduction and other blood proteinase markers in patients with malignant and inflammatory disorders, *Blood* 75:1699-1704, 1990.

161. Hashimoto Y, Kobayashi A, Yamazaki N, et al: Relationship between age and plasma t-PA, PA-inhibitor, and PA activity, *Thromb Res* 46:625-633, 1987.

162. Krishnamurti C, Tang D, Barr C, et al: Plasminogen activator and plasminogen activator inhibitor activities in a reference population, *Am J Clin Pathol* 89:747-752, 1988.

163. Sundell I, Nilsson T, Ranby M, et al: Fibrinolytic variables are related to age, sex, blood pressure, and body build measurements: a cross-sectional study in Norsjo, Sweden, *J Clin Epidemiol* 42:719-723, 1989.

164. Stroke Prevention in Atrial Fibrillation Study Group (SPAF): Preliminary report of the stroke prevention in atrial fibrillation study, *N Engl J Med* 322:863-868, 1990.

Chapter 4

THE ROLE OF THE COLLATERAL CIRCULATION IN MAINTAINING CELLULAR VIABILITY DURING CORONARY OCCLUSION

Robert P. Bauman
Judith C. Rembert
Joseph C. Greenfield, Jr.

In this chapter, the salient features of the anatomy of the coronary circulation and the pathophysiology of myocardial blood flow regulation are delineated briefly. These data provide a background for a better understanding of the processes that occur during the two major events secondary to the development of coronary atherosclerosis: gradual occlusion of the lumen of a major coronary artery by atherosclerotic disease or acute occlusion of a major coronary artery secondary to thrombus formation on an arteriosclerotic plaque. The primary thrust of this chapter is to outline the factors that initiate the development of the coronary collateral circulation and explore the extent to which collateral vessels may function to perfuse the myocardium at risk during coronary artery occlusion, thereby maintaining cellular viability. This description cannot be exhaustive; therefore, the reader is referred to two excellent extensive reviews on myocardial blood flow.[1,2]

The coronary arterial supply consists of two large coronary arteries (right and left) that originate at the coronary ostia in the sinus of Valsalva of the aorta. The left main coronary artery divides almost immediately into the left anterior descending and circumflex arteries. The arteries branch to form a network of large vessels that traverse the surface of the heart and, in turn, give off branches that penetrate into the ventricular myocardium. These penetrating arteries branch to form a network within the transmural myocardium as schematically illustrated in Fig. 4-1. The atria receive their arterial supply from branches originating from the right and circumflex coronary arteries. This system of large arteries, collectively referred to as capacitance vessels, branch further to form the arterioles (resistance vessels) and finally the capillary bed. The capillary bed is drained by a series of venules and veins that connect to surface veins and empty into the coronary sinus. The primary drainage from the heart is through the coronary sinus, although a significant fraction may drain directly into the right ventricle.

The purpose of this complex circulatory system is to

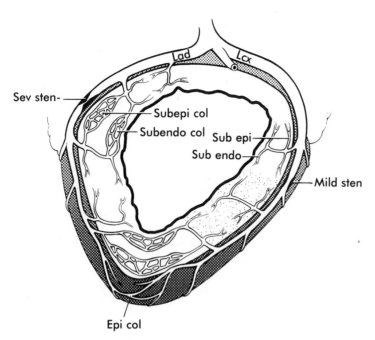

Fig. 4-1. Various components of the coronary arterial circulation perfusing a section of the left ventricle are illustrated schematically. The left anterior descending artery *(LAD)* is depicted as having severe stenosis *(Sev Sten)* and the left circumflex artery *(LCX)* a mild stenosis *(Mild Sten)*. Both arteries are shown to have branches that penetrate the myocardium and perfuse the subepicardial *(Sub Epi)* and subendocardial *(Sub Endo)* transmural layers. In the region distal to the mild stenosis, no collateral vessels are shown. Well-developed collateral vessels are illustrated distal to the severe stenosis in both the transmural layers *(SubEpi Col* and *SubEndo Col)* and on the epicardial surface *(Epi Col)*. The potential area at risk for myocardial infarction to occur after total occlusion at the site of the mild stenosis is illustrated by the stippled area. On the other hand, the absence of a stippled region distal to the severe stenosis assumes that collateral blood flow is adequate to prevent myocardial infarction when this vessel is occluded.

supply each cardiac myocyte with sufficient blood to maintain normal contractile function over a wide range of metabolic needs. Three mechanisms are responsible for maintaining myocardial blood flow: the degree of vasomotor tone primarily of the resistance vessels, the magnitude of the perfusion pressure, and diastolic perfusion time. Vasomotor tone is regulated via a complex synergistic interaction of metabolic, neurogenic, and myogenic mechanisms coupled closely to myocyte metabolism. Recent studies have shown that myocardial blood flow can be regulated rapidly, responding to beat-to-beat variations in myocyte metabolism. The coronary circulation has a marked capacity to autoregulate through changes in vasomotor tone; for example, myocardial perfusion is maintained at a constant level during variations in perfusion pressure ranging from 60 to 150 mm Hg.

Perfusion pressure is defined as the "driving pressure" (mean aortic pressure) minus the "back pressure." Although right atrial pressure is the back pressure for the entire coronary circulation, both left ventricular end diastolic pressure and transmural tissue pressure contribute significantly and variably to the back pressure. In

the left ventricle there is a transmural gradient in these components of the back pressure, with the highest values found in the subendocardial layers. During systole the tissue pressure impedes flow completely to the subendocardial layer. As blood is conducted to the distal segments of the surface capacitance vessels, perfusion pressure decreases by only 3 to 4 mm Hg. There is an unmeasurable further drop in perfusion pressure as blood is conducted from epicardial to endocardial layers of the ventricle (see Fig. 4-1). This reduction in perfusion pressure, coupled with the aforementioned gradient in back pressure, makes the subendocardial layer very vulnerable to reduced perfusion, especially during pathologic conditions. For example, patients with severe aortic stenosis commonly experience angina pectoris during exercise. In these patients the aortic outflow obstruction reduces the driving pressure, and the increased tissue pressure associated with pressure overload hypertrophy increases the back pressure, which results in a critical reduction in perfusion pressure.

Because myocardial perfusion to the inner layers of the left ventricle occurs only during diastole, significant increases in heart rate, which primarily shortens diastolic perfusion time theoretically, may result in inadequate perfusion. However, if the coronary anatomy is normal, the other regulatory mechanisms are sufficient so that marked increases in heart rate are only rarely associated with ischemia of the endocardium.

Studies in dogs have shown that flow requirements vary considerably across the four chambers of the heart during basal conditions: right atria (0.27 ± 0.04), left atria (0.35 ± 0.04), right ventricle (0.47 ± 0.05), and left ventricle (0.90 ± 0.09) ml/min/g, respectively.[3] Thus, the atria receive approximately 4% of the coronary flow. In addition, a differential in flow occurs across the wall of the left ventricle such that subendocardial flow is 10% to 20% greater than subepicardial flow. Because arterial oxygen extraction by myocytes in the ventricles has been found to be constant and quite high, differences in regional myocardial blood flows are generally assumed to represent differences in regional oxygen consumption (i.e., metabolic requirements). During maximum or near maximum levels of exercise, myocardial blood flow increases 300% to 400% from resting levels. It is important to note that although the increase in flow during physiologic stress is substantial, it is significantly less than the maximum flow potential of the coronary vasculature as measured during either infusion of a potent coronary vasodilator or the reactive hyperemic response after transient occlusion of the coronary artery. The capacity to further vasodilate during any given metabolic state is defined as coronary flow reserve. In general, myocardial blood flow is considered to be adequate if coronary flow reserve can be demonstrated.

Gradual occlusion of a major coronary artery is associated with two pathophysiologic responses that attempt to maintain adequate myocardial perfusion: a reduction in coronary flow reserve and development of the collateral vasculature. When the encroachment of the lumen becomes hemodynamically significant (i.e., approximately a 50% reduction in cross-sectional area under resting conditions), a pressure gradient develops across the stenosis, resulting in a reduction of the distal perfusion pressure. To compensate for this fall in perfusion pressure, the resistance vessels dilate to maintain adequate blood flow to the capillary bed; thus, coronary flow reserve decreases. As the atherosclerotic process further reduces the luminal cross-sectional area, coronary flow reserve is exhausted. At this juncture the stenosis is termed critical, implying that an obligatory reduction in myocardial perfusion will occur. Under resting conditions a 90% decrease in luminal area usually will be associated with a complete loss of coronary flow reserve. In patients, perfusion pressures in the range of 20 to 30 mm Hg have been measured distal to stenoses of this magnitude. Obviously conditions that require enhanced blood flow in the large coronary arteries such as exercise or myocardial hypertrophy will

be associated with an exhaustion of coronary flow reserve with lesser degrees of coronary stenosis. As noted in the preceding discussion, perfusion of the subendocardial myocardial layer is especially vulnerable to reductions in perfusion pressure. Thus, the presence of a critical coronary stenosis leads to the clinical manifestation of subendocardial ischemia (e.g., angina pectoris).

The second response to maintain adequate myocardial perfusion is the development of the collateral vasculature as the vascular lumen is reduced by the atherosclerotic process. Although two different mechanisms may be employed to enhance collateral flow, namely, neovascularization and enlargement of existing vessels, the latter mechanism appears to be predominant in the noninfarcted myocardium. Collateral vessel enlargement occurs in humans at both the epicardial and intramyocardial locations, as illustrated schematically in Fig. 4-1. In stimulating collateral development, two interrelated mechanisms seem to be operative: the development of a pressure gradient across the stenotic lesion and the presence of myocardial ischemia. It is unclear which of these mechanisms is paramount because it is difficult experimentally to produce one without the other. As noted earlier, as the degree of stenosis increases, a decrease in distal perfusion pressure occurs, resulting in a pressure gradient that forces blood through small existing collateral channels. The hemodynamic stresses secondary to blood flow tend to disrupt the intimal surface of these channels, leading to a reparative process that enlarges the vascular lumen.[4] Ischemia initiates the release of growth factors, which accelerate or may even initiate the process of collateral development. Several studies support ischemia as the sole mechanism; microembolization has been shown to induce ischemia and collateral vessel enlargement without altering the pressure gradient,[5] and radiolabeled DNA demonstrates proliferation among both venules and arterioles, supporting a generalized response of vascular cells to growth factors.[6] Other models that have been used to stimulate collateral vessel development are associated with both a pressure gradient and ischemia. Studies in dogs whereby transient episodes of ischemia were produced by a 2-minute occlusion of the circumflex coronary artery and repeated at hourly intervals have been effective in inducing marked collateral formation in approximately 14 days such that a sustained total occlusion did not produce ischemia.[7] Similar findings regarding both the rapidity and the magnitude of collateral development have been observed in both dogs and pigs using either gradual occlusion or a fixed stenosis of a major coronary artery to stimulate collateral development. Collateral vessels developing for approximately 21 days have been found to perfuse the myocardium adequately during exercise. Although it has been impossible to carry out similar studies in humans, it seems quite likely that the same general principles are present. Certainly patients found by angiography to have two of the major coronary arteries occluded but a normal ejection fraction is irrefutable evidence that collateral development has kept pace with the occlusive process. This anatomic finding is especially interesting when noted in patients who have never had symptomatic ischemia (i.e., angina). The role of episodic silent ischemia in this scenario is unknown but may well play an important role in stimulating collateral development.

Another feature of collateral vessels is that they do not become fully operative immediately after total coronary occlusion but may take several minutes or even longer for maximum perfusion to occur through collateral channels. Regression studies have shown that collateral vessels gradually lose a significant component of perfusion capacity, as well as take longer to open fully. However, they do maintain the ability to perfuse significantly the ischemic myocardium. It should be noted that blood flow through collateral vessels is subject to the same hemodynamic conditions that apply to native coronary arteries. Thus, if the capacity for collateral flow is inadequate for any given state, the blood will preferentially perfuse the epicardial layer, resulting in ischemia of the subendocardium.

Developing methods to stimulate collateral vessel growth might be an interesting new approach to the treatment of patients with coronary disease. These strategies must take into account whether or not a hemodynamically significant stenosis is present. If this is the case, either exercise or another modality that intermittently increases the magnitude of the transstenotic pressure gradient, especially if accompanied by ischemia either silent or symptomatic, might prove to be effective. Because it seems fairly certain that several specific growth factors are involved in vascular development, techniques to augment these effects on collateral development might prove to be a useful therapeutic approach to hasten this process. If hemodynamically significant stenoses are not present, the task to enhance collateral capacity becomes more difficult. Repetitive, frequent occlusions of coronary vessels as used experimentally will have little clinical applicability. However, if the molecular mechanisms that initiate and control collateral vessel development can be precisely defined, a potentially valuable therapeutic modality may be formulated.

In the event of a sudden total occlusion of a major coronary artery, the extent of the resulting myocardial necrosis depends on four interrelated factors: the amount of myocardium normally perfused by the occluded vessel or "the area at risk," the magnitude of the residual or collateral blood flow, the duration of the ischemia, and the transmural location of the ischemic area. As depicted in Fig. 4-1, the myocardium is perfused

through a series of arteries and arterioles that do not overlap significantly so that the lateral border in which the flow changes from ischemic to normal is narrow (1 to 2 mm). The amount of residual blood flow in the ischemic region, when collateral blood vessels have not been stimulated to develop, is species dependent. For example, the porcine myocardium is densely ischemic (approximately 0.05 ml/min/g) with little transmural gradient, whereas in the canine heart the blood flow is higher, and a significant transmural gradient favoring the epicardial layer is present. In humans, precise measurements are unavailable, but in the primate, blood flow during coronary occlusion has been found to be between those of the pig and the dog. As described earlier, if collateral vessels have been stimulated to develop, acute interruption of coronary arteries, as illustrated in Fig. 4-1, may result in an amount of collateral blood flow that will range from dense ischemia to essentially normal perfusion. If the former is the case, myocardial necrosis may occur but may be delayed. Unfortunately, it is impossible at the present state of knowledge to precisely define the level of blood flow necessary to maintain myocardial viability as a function of the duration of the ischemia. It is clear that a low level of blood flow in the range of 20% to 30% of normal flow can significantly retard the necrotic process. For example, Reimer and Jennings[8] have shown in the papillary muscle of the dog that interruption of the blood supply results in a "wavefront" phenomenon in which cell death is initiated within 20 minutes of ischemia at the endocardial layers and progresses as a function of time to the epicardial region so that the process is essentially completed in the epicardial layer within approximately 4 to 6 hours. This phenomenon parallels distribution of the low level of innate collateral flow. Another factor not well understood is that the endocardial layers seem to be more vulnerable to cell death when compared with epicardial layers experiencing similar degrees of ischemia. The important conclusion from this discussion is that if significant collateral flow is available, the myocardium may in fact cease contracting but may remain viable for a considerable period. Thus, it is incorrect to conclude that reperfusion occurring after 4 to 6 hours cannot reduce the degree of myocardial necrosis in acute myocardial infarction.

From the foregoing discussion, it seems reasonable to conclude that in patients in whom the collateral vasculature remains in the native or unstimulated state, blood flow through these channels will be insufficient to prevent myocardial necrosis in the event of a catastrophic occlusion of one of the primary coronary arteries. In this scenario the magnitude of the resulting myocardial infarction will be delineated to a major extent within 4 hours. However, if collaterals have been stimulated to develop, these channels may well provide alternative sources of blood flow so that the magnitude of the resulting myocardial infarction may be remarkably reduced or even eliminated. In addition, collateral perfusion may markedly lengthen the time that the myocardium remains viable so that reperfusion may result in normal function. This issue has been evaluated in patients using two different approaches to estimate collateral perfusion. Studies in 87 patients with acute myocardial infarction undergoing reperfusion at 0.5 to 21.5 hours using sestamibi labeled with technetium 99m to estimate the presence of collateral flow indicated that the final infarct size showed a strong and independent correlation with the degree of collateral perfusion when the duration of the occlusion was taken into account.[9] In another study, contrast echocardiography was used to estimate collateral perfusion in patients with acute myocardial infarction. If significant collateral blood flow was demonstrated, reperfusion occurring even after a prolonged period (12 ± 2 days) was associated with improvement in wall motion in the ischemic region.[10] Thus, it seems obvious that treatment strategies cannot be based solely on the premise that myocardial salvage will not occur if reperfusion is effected 4, 6, or more hours after the onset of the ischemic event. The obvious question facing a clinician attempting to develop an appropriate therapeutic strategy for a patient having an acute coronary ischemic event with clear evidence for an evolving myocardial infarction is to ask, "What is the potential for significant myocardial salvage?" Unfortunately, there are no precise methods to rapidly determine myocardial viability in this setting. Electrocardiographic evidence of injury as defined by the degree of ST-segment elevation, as well as continual chest pain, has been of some utility but clearly is not of sufficient discriminatory value to be reliable. Because now it has been clearly demonstrated by the GUSTO trial that short-term survival in patients with acute myocardial infarction is related to the size of the myocardial infarction, it would seem logical that every effort should be made to develop an aggressive strategy to open the occluded vessel if any evidence of continued myocardial viability is suspected. In addition, an aggressive research effort should be mounted to develop methodologies to determine the presence of collateral vessels and associated viable myocardium within the ischemic area to stratify patients into treatment groups in which myocardial salvage can be anticipated when reperfusion occurs. A second reason for employing an aggressive strategy is that data indicate an improved long-term survival in patients in which the coronary artery is opened early during the course of myocardial infarction in the absence of obvious myocardial salvage.[11,12]

In summary, the primary function of this chapter has been to define briefly the pathophysiology of the consequences of coronary artery occlusion. From this discussion, it seems reasonable to conclude that in humans, a significant collateral circulation can develop that, if present, may markedly reduce the extent of myocardial infarction after a total catastrophic occlusion of a coronary artery. If this is the case, an arbitrary time to initiate reperfusion based on studies of myocardial infarction without significant collateral vasculature is not warranted. Because at the present time it is impossible to determine the magnitude of collateral flow during the ischemic process, an aggressive approach that includes longer periods to initiate reperfusion would seem to be justified in some patients.

ACKNOWLEDGMENTS

We would like to express our appreciation to Carole A. Gunter for continuous secretarial support, Marie B. Anderson for library searches, Larry D. Moy for technical and search assistance, and Medical Media at Duke Medical Center for the illustration.

REFERENCES

1. Marcus ML: *The coronary circulation in health and disease,* New York, 1983, McGraw-Hill.
2. Feigl E: Coronary physiology, *Physiol Rev* 63:1-205, 1983.
3. Bauman, RP, Rembert JC, Greenfield Jr JC: Regional blood flow in canine atria during exercise, *Am J Physiol* 265:H629-H632, 1993.
4. Schaper W, Schaper J, Xhonneux R, et al: The morphology of intercoronary anastomoses in chronic coronary artery occlusion, *Cardiovasc Res* 3:315-323, 1969.
5. Chillian WM, Mass HJ, Williams SE, et al: Microvascular occlusions promote coronary collateral growth, *Heart Circ Physiol* 27:H1103-H1111, 1990.
6. Görge G, Schmidt T, Ito BR, et al: Microvascular and collateral adaptation in swine hearts following progressive coronary artery stenosis, *Basic Res Cardiol* 84:524-535, 1989.
7. Fujita M, McKown DP, McKown MD, et al: Evaluation of coronary collateral development by regional myocardial function and reactive hyperaemia, *Cardiovasc Res* 21:377-384, 1987.
8. Reimer KA, Jennings RB: The "wavefront" phenomenon of myocardial ischemic cell death, *Lab Invest* 40:633-644, 1979.
9. Christian TF, Schwartz RS, Gibbons RJ: Determinants of infarct size in reperfusion therapy for acute myocardial infarction, *Circulation* 86:81-90, 1992.
10. Sabia PJ, Powers ER, Ragosta M, et al: An association between collateral blood flow and myocardial viability in patients with recent myocardial infarction, *N Engl J Med* 327:1825-1831, 1992.
11. Stadius ML, Davis K, Maynard C, et al: Risk stratification for 1 year survival based on characteristics identified in the early hours of acute myocardial infarction: the Western Washington Intracoronary Streptokinase Trial, *Circulation* 74:703-711, 1986.
12. Stack RS, Califf RM, Hinohara T, et al: Survival and cardiac event rates in the first year after emergency coronary angioplasty for acute myocardial infarction, *J Am Coll Cardiol* 11:1141-1149, 1988.

Chapter 5

PSYCHOSOCIAL FACTORS

Redford B. Williams

Psychosocial factors contribute to the pathogenesis of acute ischemic events in two ways. First, psychosocial stressors acting over extended periods appear to play a role in the formation of the atherosclerotic plaque, thereby acting *indirectly* to help set the stage for acute events. Second, once atherosclerosis is present, psychosocial stressors appear capable of playing a more *direct* role in the precipitation of acute ischemic events.

The strongest evidence for a role of psychosocial factors in both plaque formation and the triggering of acute events comes from research that began by focusing on the type A behavior pattern as a potential coronary risk factor. More recently this research has identified hostility and anger as the only "toxic" part of the overall type A complex. Besides the epidemiologic evidence that points to hostility and anger as causal factors in coronary artery disease (CAD), laboratory and field research have identified acute physiologic responses to stress in hostile persons that are biologically plausible contributors to the formation of atherosclerotic plaques, as well as to the precipitation of acute events in the setting of clinically significant CAD.

Once coronary heart disease (CHD) has become clinically manifest, considerable evidence has accumulated showing that patients who are socially isolated or depressed are two to four times more likely to suffer a recurrent ischemic event as those patients who are not depressed and who have higher levels of social support.

In this chapter we review the epidemiologic and biologic evidence documenting the role of hostility, social isolation, and depression in the pathogenesis of acute ischemic events. We take some care to note the implications of this evidence for the efforts of the practicing physician to help patients reduce their risk of acute ischemic events in the first place, as well as after clinical coronary disease is present.

PSYCHOSOCIAL FACTORS AND ISCHEMIC EVENTS
Epidemiologic evidence

Type A behavior and hostility. The earliest recorded instance of an acute (probably ischemic) cardiac event brought on by psychosocial stress can be found in the Acts of the Apostles in the *New Testament.* Ananias and his wife Sapphira had sold some land and given what they said were all the proceeds to Peter to support the work of the early church. This was not true, however, because they held back some of the money for their own use. Peter discovered this deceit and called Ananias in and chastised him so severely that he dropped dead on the spot. Soon after, Sapphira underwent the same confrontation, with a similar fatal outcome.

Such anecdotal evidence as this makes a strong case that, at least for some people caught in the wrong circumstances, acute psychosocial stress can indeed precipitate acute coronary events. More modern research has shown that most persons who die acutely under conditions that appear similar to the one that killed Ananias and Sapphira already are suffering from subclinical coronary atherosclerosis (or CAD). A complete understanding of the role of psychosocial factors in causing acute ischemic events must include, therefore, consideration of how psychosocial factors contribute to the development of CAD, thereby providing the substrate for acute ischemic events.

It was not until nearly 2000 years after Peter scared Ananias and Sapphira to death that two San Francisco cardiologists, Meyer Friedman and Ray Rosenman, provided the first convincing epidemiologic evidence that a psychosocial factor (in this case, the type A behavior pattern consisting of time urgency, ambitious achievement, striving, and hostility) predicts increased risk of all manifestations of CHD. In the study by

Rosenman et al.,[1] over an 8½ year follow-up period, the type A men experienced twice as many ischemic events of all types when compared with their less hurried, competitive, and hostile type B counterparts.

These results, along with other studies showing type A behavior to be more prevalent among patients with angiographically documented CAD,[2] led in the late 1980s to the conclusion that type A behavior is probably a coronary risk factor of similar magnitude to smoking, hyperlipidemia, and hypertension.[3]

At about the same time, however, the picture was clouded by the publication of several studies that failed to find type A predicting coronary risk.[4] Two studies even found that once clinically significant coronary disease was present, type A patients actually survived longer.[5,6] Despite type A's early promise to become the first psychosocial stressor to be accepted as a coronary risk factor, these later studies rekindled skepticism in the cardiologic and medical community about the real potency of psychosocial stress in the pathogenesis of acute ischemic events.

The negative studies led many working in the field of behavioral medicine to evaluate the separate components of type A behavior, namely, time urgency, ambition, and hostility, with the goal of seeing whether, just as with the "good" and "bad" cholesterol, some aspects of type A are toxic, whereas others are benign. For various reasons, not the least of which was its intuitive appeal, the hypothesis that hostility is the toxic component (the "bad" cholesterol) of type A behavior received considerable attention.

Initially we[7] found that scores on a hostility scale (the Ho scale) derived from the Minnesota Multiphasic Personality Inventory (MMPI), a long used standard psychodiagnostic test, correlated positively with severity of angiographically documented atherosclerotic coronary lesions. Because archival MMPI data were available for various groups that had been studied in the past, it has been possible for several investigative teams to rescore the old MMPIs to derive Ho scores that could be evaluated for prediction of ischemic events. An analogy with lipid research would be the discovery of carefully preserved frozen sera from 25 years earlier on a sample of people whose coronary event rate over the interval is known.

Two studies found that in both a group of physicians who had taken the MMPI in medical school and a group of factory workers who took the MMPI as part of a prospective coronary risk factor study, those with higher Ho scores experienced, over follow-up periods of 10 to 25 years, higher rates of ischemic coronary events and death from all causes than those with lower Ho scores.[8,9] Another study in which there were too few coronary events to provide adequate statistical power nevertheless did document a nearly fivefold higher all-cause mortality

rate among attorneys with higher Ho scores in law school 25 years earlier compared with those with lower Ho scores.[10] In this same study, analysis of the individual items on the Ho scale suggested that only those reflecting a cynical mistrust of others, frequent experience of angry emotions, and frequent overt aggressive behaviors were accounting for the prediction of increased mortality by the overall Ho score.

Three other studies applied a similar approach (reevaluating archival MMPI data in samples being followed up in the present) and failed to find Ho scores predicting either acute ischemic events or all-cause mortality. One of these studies was methodologically flawed[11]; applicants to medical school were asked to complete the MMPI while visiting the school for their admission interviews, and it therefore need not be considered further. The other two studies had no such obvious flaws and weaken the case that hostility as measured by the Ho scale predicts either acute ischemic events or all-cause mortality.[12,13]

In contrast to these negative studies using the Ho scale, a self-report instrument, results have been more consistent when the method of assessing hostility was behavioral observation of the study subjects during a structured interview to assess type A behavior. Dembroski et al.[14] found that potential for hostility ratings based on behaviors displayed during the structured interview correlated positively with severity of angiographically documented lesions.

In prospective studies, too, hostility ratings from the structured interview predicted increased risk of ischemic events. Whereas Shekelle et al.[4] found no prediction of ischemic events by structured interview assessments of the global type A behavior pattern in the Multiple Risk Factor Intervention Trial (MRFIT) Study, Dembroski et al.[15] performed behavioral assessments on the same MRFIT tape-recorded interviews and found that of all the components scored, including overall type A behavior, only hostility was an independent predictor of increased coronary risk. A similar result was obtained when Hecker et al.[16] evaluated interview-based hostility assessments as predictors of ischemic events in the Western Collaborative Group Study.

In research focusing on the effects of psychosocial stressors on ischemic events in clinical coronary samples, we have already noted that type A predicts not shorter but longer survival. In contrast, in the same study Barefoot et al.[5] found that Ho scores were not significantly related to survival.

Taken altogether, the available epidemiologic evidence makes a strong case that high levels of hostility, especially aspects of hostility reflecting cynicism, anger, and aggression, place persons at high risk of being exposed to psychosocial stress that, over time, accelerates the initiation and growth of the atherosclerotic plaque, thereby setting the stage for the precipitation of acute ischemic events.

As for the type A concept, it now appears likely that type A does increase risk of ischemic events but only because type A persons have high levels of hostility. Type A is a multifaceted construct, with some aspects, namely, hostility, that have been shown to predict increased CHD risk, whereas other aspects (i.e., time urgency) have been evaluated and found to add no further prognostic information.

Social isolation and depression. Although we did not find Ho predictive of survival in our patients with significant CAD at Duke, we did find a related psychosocial variable, social isolation, to be a strong independent prognostic factor. In a follow-up study of 1369 patients, those who were not married and reported they lacked a confidant experienced a 50% 5-year mortality.[17] In contrast, those with a spouse, confidant, or both experienced only a 17% 5-year mortality. When the study controlled for such strong physical prognostic factors as ejection fraction and coronary anatomy, those who were socially isolated were more than three times more likely to die within 5 years than those with a spouse or confidant.

Other studies have confirmed the strong and clinically significant impact of social isolation on prognosis in established CAD, with socially isolated patients experiencing twofold to fivefold higher rates of ischemic and arrhythmic events than patients with higher levels of social support.[18,19] Social isolation also appears to increase the risk of developing CHD in healthy populations, though the evidence is stronger for all-cause mortality than for CHD-specific events.[20]

Because studies in normal samples have frequently found low levels of reported social support among persons scoring high on hostility,[21] hostility may contribute to the social isolation that was associated with reduced survival in clinical CHD samples.

In addition to social isolation, there is mounting evidence that depression increases the risk of ischemic events in patients with CHD. In a very recent study, Frasure-Smith et al.[22] found a fivefold higher mortality rate among post–myocardial infarction (MI) patients with major depression than in those who were not depressed. This strong impact of depression on mortality was only slightly decreased (to fourfold) when physical prognostic factors like ejection fraction, Killip class, and prior MI were controlled for.

Prior studies of depression and prognosis in CHD using retrospective designs and self-report measures of depression had also found increased ischemic/arrhythmic event rates in post-MI patients who were depressed. By confirming these earlier findings in a well-designed prospective study using a state of the art clinical interview to diagnose depression, Frasure-Smith et al.[22]

enable us to add depression to social isolation as psychosocial factors that are clearly increasing the risk of ischemic/arrhythmic events in established CHD.

Besides the epidemiologic evidence that psychosocial factors increase the risk of ischemic/arrhythmic events, research into the biologic mechanisms whereby hostility might contribute to the development of atherosclerotic plaques and the precipitation of acute events adds further evidence for the pathogenic potential of hostility. Although not as extensive, there is also some evidence as to mechanisms whereby social isolation and depression affect prognosis in CHD.

Biologic evidence

Type A behavior and hostility. The case for the biologic plausibility of type A behavior as a risk factor for ischemic events was strengthened by studies (see Krantz and Manuck[23] for review) showing larger physiologic responses to standardized laboratory stressors (e.g., mental arithmetic) in type As. When these same cognitive stressors were used in analogous studies of subjects selected for high vs. low hostility levels, however, no association was found between hostility and physiologic reactivity.

Investigators studying this issue soon realized that cognitive stressors like mental arithmetic might not be relevant to hostility; stressors that induce anger would be required. When such stressors as role playing interpersonal conflicts,[24] receiving misleading instructions about unsolvable anagrams,[25] and being harassed during task performance[26] were used, it quickly became apparent that subjects with higher scores on the Ho scale were indeed physiologically hyperreactive. Harassment during task performance had no effect, for example, on the forearm blood flow and blood pressure responses of low Ho-scoring subjects to an anagram task; in contrast, harassment caused markedly larger forearm blood flow and blood pressure responses in high Ho-scoring subjects.[26]

A recent study using ambulatory blood pressure monitoring found that high hostile subjects exhibited higher blood pressure when experiencing angry emotions[27]; in contrast, angry emotions had no effect on blood pressure in low hostile subjects. Thus, the cardiovascular hyperactivity observed during anger-inducing laboratory situations in hostile persons appears to generalize to real world settings.

Another study has extended our understanding of the relationship between hostility and acute reactivity to stress by showing a differential association between blood cholesterol levels and catecholamine reactivity as a function of hostility levels.[28] Among middle-aged men with high scores on the Ho scale, there was a *positive* association between serum cholesterol levels and plasma catecholamine responses to a mental task; in contrast, among low Ho-scoring men this association was *negative.*

This combination of a high cholesterol level with a larger catecholamine response to stress only in hostile men would be expected to accelerate the development of CAD. This hypothesis was supported in a study using implanted osmotic minipumps to maintain chronically high norepinephrine levels in Egyptian sand rats consuming a high cholesterol diet.[29] Although diet alone caused only moderate intimal hyperplasia and lipid accumulation in the aortic wall after 2 months, the animals receiving norepinephrine infusions developed marked intimal hyperplasia and lipid accumulation after the same interval.

In addition to the biologic plausibility of these excessive *sympathetically* mediated responses to anger-inducing stimuli as contributors to processes involved in atherogenesis and the precipitation of acute events, a recent study suggests that hostile persons may also be placed at higher risk of acute ischemic and arrhythmic events by virtue of weaker *parasympathetic* antagonism of sympathetic effects on the heart.[30] Because weaker parasympathetic function is becoming increasingly recognized as a risk factor for acute ischemic events in CAD patients,[31] this finding adds a new dimension of evidence in support of the biologic plausibility of hostility as a cause of acute ischemic events.

The reader is also referred to Chapter 2 for a consideration of the role of acute stressors in precipitating ischemic events.

A final, still newer dimension to our understanding of how hostility might speed the development of CAD comes from a follow-up study of nearly 5000 university graduates who took the MMPI as part of freshman orientation 25 years ago.[32] Those who scored higher on the MMPI Ho scale in college at age 18 or 19 are found now, at age 43, to have a higher body mass index and worse cholesterol/HDL ratio, to be more likely to smoke, and to consume more alcohol than their low Ho-scoring counterparts. Thus, it appears that hostile persons eat more (as reflected in their increased body mass index and lipid ratio), smoke more, and drink more.

To summarize the biologic evidence supporting the pathogenic potential of hostility, the following characteristics have been documented in studies of hostile persons: (1) increased sympathetic nervous system reactivity to anger-inducing social situations (especially if a high cholesterol level is present), (2) decreased parasympathetic antagonism of sympathetic effects on the heart, (3) increased eating, and (4) increased smoking. Increased alcohol consumption has also been found among hostile people and may contribute to pathogenesis via effects to raise blood pressure.

Elsewhere I have reviewed evidence suggesting that all these pathogenic characteristics of hostile persons could be the result of a single "lesion": deficient function of the neurotransmitter serotonin in the central nervous system.[33] The effect of weak brain serotonin function on autonomic balance, for example, has been documented in studies (reviewed by Saxena and Villalon[34]) showing that stimulation of a specific class of brain serotonin receptor (designated $5HT_{1A}$) causes a reduction in sympathetic outflow and an increase in vagal outflow — just the pattern found when low hostile subjects are compared with those with high hostility levels.

If confirmed in further research, this "serotonin deficiency" hypothesis has specific implications for prevention and treatment of the cardiovascular problems associated with high hostility levels. Verrier[35] has noted, for example, the effect of increased brain serotonin function to reduce sympathetic outflow and has documented the protective potential of this effect in studies showing that increasing brain serotonin via tryptophan loading confers protection against ventricular fibrillation during acute coronary occlusion in an animal model.

Social isolation and depression. In contrast to type A behavior and hostility, where there has been considerable research aimed at identifying pathogenic mechanisms, the major effort in research on social isolation and depression in CHD has been directed toward demonstrating an effect on prognosis, with little attention having been given to mechanisms.

Among the potential mechanisms that have been proposed to account for the increased rate of ischemic events in CHD patients who are depressed or socially isolated are (1) increased sympathetic nervous system reactivity to the stress of daily life, (2) decreased parasympathetic protection of the myocardium against sympathetic effects, (3) decreased adherence to medical regimens, and (4) increased risk behaviors.[17,22] Research efforts are currently under way to increase our understanding of how these mechanisms are acting in patients with established CHD.

Implications for prevention and treatment

Of what practical importance to the practicing physician are the findings just reviewed that socially isolated, depressed, and hostile persons are at higher risk for ischemic events and that this risk appears to be mediated by a variety of biobehavioral mechanisms, including stronger sympathetic reactivity, weaker parasympathetic function, and increased indulgence in such risky behaviors as overeating, alcohol consumption, and smoking? What would it imply for prevention and treatment if the neurobiologic substrate for the biologic mediators of increased risk in hostile persons (as well, perhaps, as those who are socially isolated and depressed) were proved to be weak brain serotonin function?

The first and most obvious implication is that interventions that help reduce depression and hostility and increase social support would be helpful in both prevention and treatment of coronary disease. One such intervention is behavior modification training that provides for cognitive restructuring of hostile (i.e., cynical) attitudes, reduction of angry feelings, and curbing of aggressive behaviors. In the Recurrent Coronary Prevention Project, such an approach was employed to reduce all aspects of type A behavior, with considerable emphasis on hostility and anger, in a randomized clinical trial of male post-MI patients.[36] Compared with those men randomized to usual care, those receiving behavior modification training experienced fewer recurrent ischemic events.

Clearly such a result in a single well-designed study calls out for an intensification of research efforts aimed at evaluating the use of behavior modification approaches to hostility and anger reduction in both primary and secondary prevention. Meanwhile, most cardiologists appear to accept at least the potential benefits of stress reduction techniques as a component of any comprehensive cardiac rehabilitation program. It would appear prudent, because it may help and is unlikely to do harm, to include as a part of such stress management training specific skills designed to help patients reduce their hostility and anger.

A self-help approach that patients (and healthy folks trying to avoid becoming patients) can use to gain better control over their hostile impulses is described in a recent book *Anger Kills: Seventeen Strategies for Controlling the Hostility that Can Harm Your Health.*[37] To know when to advise their patients to seek training in hostility control, physicians can use the hostility assessment questionnaire in the box on p. 54, which is adapted from a longer instrument in *Anger Kills.* People who score in the high hostile range need to learn when to act (assertively, not aggressively) on their anger, how to deflect their anger when action is not appropriate, how to improve their relationships with others, and how to adopt more positive attitudes.

Considering that one pathway whereby hostility may increase risk of ischemic events is via the harmful effects of reduced social support,[17] physicians might also begin to seek ways of helping their patients increase their social support resources. This help could take the form of advice to seek out and cultivate friendships, become more active in civic or religious groups, and the like. It could also involve an actual intervention to increase social support by having, for example, a nurse call the patient regularly to learn of any problems and offer assistance for any that are reported. Just such an approach was used in a Canadian study, and it significantly improved survival in post-MI patients.[38]

Patient support groups are another vehicle whereby

psychosocial interventions to reduce hostility and increase social support can be effectively delivered, especially as part of comprehensive cardiac rehabilitation programs. The content presented in such support groups varies but usually consists of training to control hostility and anxiety, to increase social support, and to convert negative attitudes into more positive attitudes.*

While interventions to reduce hostility or increase social support have the potential to directly reduce ischemic event rates, they are just as likely to prove beneficial indirectly, e.g., via improved risk factor reduction.[39]

Aerobic exercise training has effects, such as increased vagal tone and decreased sympathetic responses to stress,[40] that could help to ameliorate the harmful potential of the altered sympathetic-parasympathetic balance observed in hostile persons. Therefore, the time-honored recommendation to engage in regular aerobic exercise could have the added benefit of reducing risk of ischemic and arrhythmic events especially well in hostile persons.

Looking further into the future, if ongoing research confirms the hypothesis that brain serotonin deficiency is responsible for at least some of the harmful biologic effects associated with hostility and anger, it could guide the development of pharmacologic approaches to prevention and treatment. A growing number of drugs that enhance brain serotonin function by either direct agonist action (e.g., the $5HT_{1A}$ agonist buspirone) or selective serotonin reuptake inhibition (e.g., fluoxetine, sertraline, and fluvoxamine) are already available.

These latter agents are effective antidepressants, with a favorable cardiovascular side effect profile. In fact, in addition to their antidepressant actions, they have other effects, such as decreased anger and aggression, decreased craving for tobacco and alcohol, and decreased sympathetic reactivity,[41] with potential to directly reduce the risk of ischemic and arrhythmic events.

In conclusion, the time has come when our knowledge of the impact of psychosocial factors in risk of ischemic and arrhythmic events, particularly once CHD is clinically manifest,[42] has advanced far enough to call for interventions aimed at ameliorating this impact. Among the interventions that should now be evaluated in controlled clinical trials are (1) psychosocial interventions training patients to control hostility, increase social support, reduce depression, and manage stress; (2) pharmacologic interventions to reduce depression and perhaps at the same time interdict the biobehavioral mechanisms whereby both hostility and depression increase CHD

---

*For a workshop leader's manual showing how to present the strategies described in *Anger Kills,*[37] in a support group format, write to Redford Williams, M.D., Box 3926, Duke University Medical Center, Durham, NC 27710. Include $2.50 for handling and postage.

Hostility assessment questionnaire to determine whether efforts to reduce hostility are needed

How hostile are you?

Find out how hostile you are on the road, in a supermarket line, and at the office by answering these questions. Choose the answer that most closely describes your response to the situation described.

1. I am in the express checkout line at the supermarket, where a sign reads: "No more than 10 items, please!"
   A. I pick up a magazine to pass the time.
   B. I glance ahead to see if anyone has more than 10 items.
2. My spouse, boyfriend, or girlfriend is going to get me a birthday present.
   A. I prefer to pick it out myself.
   B. I prefer to be surprised.
3. Someone is speaking very slowly during a conversation.
   A. I am apt to finish his or her sentences.
   B. I am apt to listen until he or she finishes.
4. Someone treats me unfairly.
   A. I usually forget it rather quickly.
   B. I am apt to keep thinking about it for hours.
5. The person who cuts my hair trims off more than I wanted.
   A. I tell him or her what a lousy job he or she did.
   B. I figure it'll grow back, and resolve to give my instructions more forcefully next time.
6. I am riding as a passenger in the front seat of a car.
   A. I take the opportunity to enjoy the scenery.
   B. I try to stay alert for obstacles ahead.
7. At times, I have to work with incompetent people.
   A. I concentrate on my part of the job.
   B. Having to put up with them ticks me off.
8. Someone bumps into me in a store.
   A. I pass it off as an accident.
   B. I feel irritated at the person's clumsiness.
9. Someone is hogging the conversation at a party.
   A. I look for an opportunity to put him or her down.
   B. I soon move to another group.
10. There is a really important job to be done.
    A. I prefer to do it myself.
    B. I am apt to call on my friends or coworkers for help.

11. Someone criticizes something I have done.
    A. I feel annoyed.
    B. I try to decide whether the criticism is justified.
12. Another driver butts ahead of me in traffic.
    A. I usually flash my lights or honk my horn.
    B. I stay farther behind such a driver.
13. I see a very overweight person walking down the street.
    A. I wonder why these people have such little self-control.
    B. I think that he or she might have a metabolic defect or a psychological problem.
14. There have been times when I was very angry with someone.
    A. I have always been able to stop short of hitting them.
    B. I have, on occasion, hit or shoved them.
15. I recall something that angered me previously.
    A. I feel angry all over again.
    B. The memory doesn't bother me nearly as much as the actual event did.

Rating your hostility

Responses to 15 questions will not determine whether your hostility level is a health risk, but they can suggest whether you would benefit from defusing hostile thoughts.

Questions 1, 2, 6, 10, and 13 are designed to measure cynicism, a "mistrusting attitude" toward people's motives and a tendency to be "constantly on guard" against others' misbehavior. If you answered two or more with the responses in parentheses—1(B), 2(A), 6(B), 10(A), 13(A)—your cynicism level is high.

Questions 4, 7, 8, 11, and 15 measure anger, the tendency to respond with "anger, irritation, or annoyance when faced with life's frustrations." If your answers match two or more of the responses in parentheses—4(B), 7(B), 8(B), 11(A), 15(A)—your anger level is probably quite high.

Questions 3, 5, 9, 12, and 14 measure aggression, the tendency to express your anger, either physically or verbally. A highly aggressive person would most likely choose the responses in parentheses two or more times—3(A), 5(A), 9(A), 12(A), 14(B).

Modified from Williams RB, Williams VP: *Anger kills: seventeen strategies for controlling the hostility that can harm your health,* New York, 1993, Time Books. Used by permission.

risk; and (3) combination therapies, such as a selective serotonin reuptake inhibitor combined with a support group focusing on hostility control.

Pursuing this course can lead to major breakthroughs in our understanding of the pathogenesis of acute ischemic events and their prevention. Moreover, because the psychosocial and pharmacologic interventions that are likely to be helpful are far less costly than such high-tech interventions as angioplasty and coronary bypass surgery, application of interventions aimed at psychosocial factors can also help our national efforts to control spiraling medical costs.

REFERENCES

1. Rosenman RH, et al: Coronary heart disease in the Western Collaborative Group Study: final follow-up experience of 8½ years, *JAMA* 233:872, 1975.
2. Blumenthal JA, et al: Type A behavior pattern and coronary atherosclerosis, *Circulation* 58:634, 1978.
3. Review Panel on Coronary-prone Behavior: Coronary-prone behavior pattern and coronary disease risk, *Circulation* 63:1199, 1981.

4. Shekelle RB, et al: The MRFIT behavior pattern study: II. Type A behavior and incidence of coronary heart disease, *Am J Epidemiol* 122:559, 1985.

5. Barefoot JC, et al: Type A behavior and survival: a follow up study of 1,467 patients with coronary artery disease, *Am J Cardiol* 64:427, 1989.

6. Ragland DR, Brand RJ: Type A behavior and mortality from coronary heart disease, *N Engl J Med* 313:65, 1988.

7. Williams RB, et al: Type A behavior, hostility, and coronary heart disease, *Psychosom Med* 42:539, 1980.

8. Barefoot JC, et al: Hostility, CHD incidence, and total mortality: a 25-year follow-up study of 255 physicians, *Psychosom Med* 45:219, 1983.

9. Shekelle RB, et al: Hostility, risk of coronary disease, and mortality, *Psychosom Med* 45:219, 1983.

10. Barefoot JC, et al: The Cook-Medley Hostility scale: item content and ability to predict survival, *Psychosom Med* 51:46, 1989.

11. McCranie E, et al: Hostility, coronary heart disease (CHD) incidence and total mortality: lack of association in a 25-year follow-up study of 478 physicians, *J Behav Med* 9:119, 1986.

12. Hearn MD, Murray DM, Luepker RV: Hostility, coronary heart disease, and total mortality: a 33-year follow-up study of university students, *J Behav Med* 12:105, 1989.

13. Leon GR, et al: Inability to predict cardiovascular disease from hostility scores or MMPI items related to Type A behavior, *J Consult Clin Psychol* 56:597, 1988.

14. Dembroski TM, et al: Components of Type A, hostility, and anger-in: relationship to angiographic findings, *Psychosom Med* 47:219, 1985.

15. Dembroski TM, et al: Components of hostility as predictors of sudden death and myocardial infarction in the Multiple Risk Factor Intervention Trial, *Psychosom Med* 51:514, 1989.

16. Hecker MHL, et al: Coronary-prone behaviors in the Western Collaborative Group Study, *Psychosom Med* 50:153, 1988.

17. Williams RB, et al: Prognostic importance of social and economic resources among medically treated patients with angiographically documented coronary artery disease, *JAMA* 267:520, 1992.

18. Ruberman W, et al: Psychosocial influences on mortality after myocardial infarction, *N Engl J Med* 311:552, 1984.

19. Case RB, et al: Living alone after myocardial infarction: impact on prognosis, *JAMA* 267:515, 1992.

20. House JS, et al: The association of social relationships and activities with mortality: prospective evidence from the Tecumseh Community Health Study, *Am J Epidemiol* 116:123, 1982.

21. Smith TW: Hostility and health: current status of a psychosomatic hypothesis, *Health Psychol* 11:139, 1992.

22. Frasure-Smith N, et al: Depression following myocardial infarction: impact on 6-month survival, *JAMA* 270:1819, 1993.

23. Krantz DS, Manuck SB: Acute psychophysiologic reactivity and risk of cardiovascular disease: a review and methodological critique, *Psychol Bull* 96:435, 1984.

24. Hardy JH, Smith TW: Cynical hostility and vulnerability to disease: social support, life stress, and physiological response to conflict, *Health Psychol* 7:447, 1988.

25. Weidner G, et al: Hostility and cardiovascular reactivity to stress in women and men, *Psychosom Med* 51:36, 1989.

26. Suarez EC, Williams RB: Situational determinants of cardiovascular and emotional reactivity in high and low hostile men, *Psychosom Med* 51:404, 1989.

27. Suarez EC, Blumenthal JA: Ambulatory blood responses during daily life in high and low hostile patients with a recent myocardial infarction, *J Cardiopulmonary Rehab* (in press).

28. Suarez EC, et al: Biobehavioral basis of coronary-prone behavior in middle-aged men: II. Serum cholesterol, the Type A behavior pattern, and hostility as interactive modulators of physiological reactivity, *Psychosom Med* 53:528, 1991.

29. Mikat EM, et al: Chronic norepinephrine infusion accelerates atherosclerotic lesion development in sand rats maintained on a high cholesterol diet [abstract], *Psychosom Med* 53:211, 1991.

30. Fukudo S, et al: Accentuated vagal antagonism of β-adrenergic effects on ventricular repolarization: evidence of weaker antagonism in hostile Type A men, *Circulation* 85:2045, 1992.

31. Schwartz P, LaRovere MT, Vanoli E: Autonomic nervous system and sudden cardiac death. Experimental basis and clinical observations for post-myocardial infarction risk stratification, *Circulation* 85(suppl 1):I77, 1988.

32. Siegler IC, et al: Hostility during late adolescence predicts coronary risk factors at midlife, *Am J Epidemiol* 136:146-154, 1992.

33. Williams RB: A relook at personality types and coronary heart disease. In Zipes D, Rowlands D (ed): *Progress in Cardiology 4.2,* Philadelphia, 1991, Lea & Febiger.

34. Saxena PR, Villalon CM: Cardiovascular effects of serotonin agonists and antagonists, *J Cardiovasc Pharmacol* 7:S17, 1990.

35. Verrier RL: Neurochemical approaches to the prevention of ventricular fibrillation, *Fed Proc* 45:2191, 1986.

36. Friedman M, et al: Alteration of Type A behavior and its effect on cardiac recurrences in post-myocardial infarction patients: summary results of the Recurrent Coronary Prevention Project, *Am Heart J* 112:653, 1986.

37. Williams RB, Williams VP: *Anger kills: seventeen strategies for controlling the hostility that can harm your health,* New York, 1993, Times Books.

38. Frasure-Smith N, Prince R: The Ischemic Heart Disease Life Stress Monitoring Program: impact on mortality, *Psychosom Med* 47:431, 1985.

39. Taylor CB, et al: Smoking cessation after acute myocardial infarction: effects of a nurse managed intervention, *Ann Intern Med* 113:118, 1990.

40. Blumenthal JA, et al: Exercise training in healthy type A middle-aged men: effects on behavioral and cardiovascular response, *Psychosom Med* 50:418, 1988.

41. Williams RB: Neurobiology, molecular biology, and psychosomatic medicine, *Psychosom Med* (in press).

42. Williams RB, Chesney MA: Psychosocial factors and prognosis in established coronary artery disease: interventions are needed to reduce suffering and save lives and money, *JAMA* 270:1860, 1993.

Chapter 6

ANGINA PECTORIS, MYOCARDIAL INFARCTION, AND THE BIOLOGY OF ATHEROSCLEROSIS

Charles B. Treasure
R. Wayne Alexander

Clinical and pathologic studies have taught us much about the pathophysiologic basis for stable and unstable angina and myocardial infarction. Several distinct mechanisms contribute to produce ischemia in these syndromes. Vasoconstriction, thrombosis, and increases in oxygen demand in the setting of flow-limiting obstruction appear to be the primary pathophysiologic mechanisms. Vasoconstriction and thrombosis are particularly important in unstable angina and myocardial infarction.

Only recently have we begun to understand these clinical syndromes in the context of biologic processes within the vessel wall. This understanding is the subject of intense clinical and research interest for two reasons. First, from a knowledge of vessel wall biology, we have a better understanding of the episodic nature of plaque rupture and alterations in coronary tone in unstable and stable coronary syndromes, leading to improved mechanistically directed therapies. Second, the clinical cardiologist's view of the acute and episodic nature of coronary atherosclerotic disease, previously difficult to marry with the traditional pathologic view of slow linear progression of atherosclerosis, is becoming reconciled through this understanding of vessel wall pathobiology.

Classically, the pathologist's view of coronary atherosclerosis has been quite different from that of the clinician. The pathologist sees a chronic illness with years of progressive and gradual plaque deposition leading to lumen encroachment. The clinician sees episodic and cyclic punctuations of this progressive course with catastrophic bursts of activity manifested as myocardial infarction and unstable angina. Although we have made great strides in recent years in our understanding of atherosclerotic plaque pathobiology, the basic biologic processes that transform the stable atherosclerotic plaque into an unstable, fissured, thrombus-forming, "active" plaque are unknown. This "activated" atherosclerotic lesion is the cornerstone for myocardial infarction and unstable angina. Understanding the initiating event or events and the cellular cascade leading to atherosclerotic lesion activation are prerequisites for developing a strategy to prevent these two most unfortunate manifestations of coronary atherosclerosis.

This chapter reviews the current state of knowledge of the cell biology of atherosclerosis in the context of angina pectoris and myocardial infarction. It will provide a better understanding of the spectrum of ischemic coronary syndromes based on what is currently known of the underlying cellular pathobiology of atherosclerosis.

BIOLOGY OF ATHEROSCLEROSIS

Atherosclerotic lesion formation is confined to the epicardial coronary arteries. Typically atherosclerotic lesions form at flow dividers in areas of low shear stress.

The lesion is composed of smooth muscle cells and monocytes all migrating into the intima. These smooth muscle cells have been transformed into a growth phenotype referred as the "modulated state."[1] Monocyte adherence to and migration through the endothelium lead to transformation into a tissue macrophage-like cell called the "foam" cell. Foam cells are a principal component of the atherosclerotic plaque. These lipid-laden cells are formed from the uptake of oxidized low-density lipoprotein (LDL) via a "scavenger" receptor that does not recognize native LDL. Other inflammatory cells such as T lymphocytes also reside in the atherosclerotic plaque.[2] These T cells express late-activation antigens, suggesting that they have been immunologically activated.[3] Plaque neovascularization from the adventitial surface also occurs.[4] The presence of inflammatory cells and mediators within the atherosclerotic lesion has led to conceptualization of the atherosclerotic process as an inflammatory response to vascular injury.

Risk factors for coronary atherosclerosis (including hyperlipidemia, hypertension, and other as yet unappreciated factors) and balloon angioplasty damage the coronary vessel wall. These metabolic and physical insults appear to stimulate an inflammatory response within the wall, resulting in a final common outcome, the atherosclerotic plaque. This concept of atherosclerosis has led to an enhanced understanding of the pathogenesis of atherosclerosis and to a framework for understanding the episodic nature of the disease.[5]

Recent work by Steinberg et al.[6] has contributed greatly to our understanding of the basic biology of atherosclerosis. These investigators noted that native LDL could not be taken up by monocytes or macrophages in vitro. However, when modified by endothelial cells, LDL was readily taken up, forming foam cells.[7] Subsequent studies have demonstrated that oxidation of LDL with an increase in lysophosphatidylcholine (LPC) content were the critical modifications for LDL uptake.[8]

Modified (oxidized) LDL and LPC can stimulate endothelial monocyte and lymphocyte adhesion molecules,[9] monocyte chemotactic protein expression,[10] and endothelial growth factor production.[11] Thus, oxidative alterations in plasma lipoproteins may be of central importance in the initiation of an inflammatory cascade leading to atherosclerosis. Indeed, animal studies suggesting that lesion formation can be inhibited by antioxidants have indirectly confirmed this concept.[12]

IMPORTANCE OF THE ENDOTHELIUM

The endothelium actively mediates blood vessel wall interactions. It is of central importance in preventing intraluminal thrombus formation. The discovery of leukocyte adhesion molecules on the endothelial surface illustrates its importance as a mediator of the inflammatory response. Through release of a variety of mediators, the endothelium also exerts profound influence on the contractile and growth state of underlying vascular smooth muscle. Damage to the endothelium could alter any or all of these functions, predisposing the artery to inflammation, thrombosis, vasoconstriction, and vascular smooth muscle growth, the key components in the pathogenesis of the ischemic coronary syndromes.

For a time, we believed that loss of endothelial cells was an early step in the development of atherosclerosis. Exposure of the subendothelium permitted platelet adhesion, clot formation, and growth factor release.[13] As a corollary, a healthy, structurally intact endothelium was presumed essential for prevention of atherosclerosis. However, morphologic studies demonstrated that the endothelium overlying atherosclerotic plaque was structurally intact,[14] leading to the concept of endothelial "dysfunction" in atherosclerosis. This perception that the endothelium can be phenotypically modified to a dysfunctional state is an important element of our current view of the pathogenesis of atherosclerosis. Table 6-1 summarizes the consequences of endothelial dysfunction in atherosclerosis.

Table 6-1. Endothelial function in normal and atherosclerotic arteries

Normal endothelium	Dysfunctional endothelium in atherosclerosis	Biologic mechanisms of dysfunction	Consequences of dysfunction
Maintenance of nonthrombogenic surface	Potential promotion of thrombus formation	Cytokines and free radical production	Mural thrombus and plaque progression
Arterial dilation	Diminished dilation; enhanced constriction (?)	Free radical–mediated inactivation of NO	Vasospasm
Inhibition of vascular smooth muscle growth	Vascular smooth muscle growth stimulation	Accelerated growth factor production; diminished release of growth inhibitors (?)	Lesion progression
Inhibition of inflammatory activity	Promotion of inflammatory response	Leukocyte adhesion molecule and chemotactic protein expression on endothelial surface	Possible plaque destabilization

Endothelium-dependent vasodilation

The pioneering work of Furchgott and Zawadzki[15] led to the idea of a vasorelaxant compound intrinsic to the endothelium called endothelium-derived relaxing factor (EDRF). It is now known that EDRF is predominantly nitric oxide.[16] Many agents called endothelium-dependent vasodilators bind to receptors on the endothelial surface and stimulate nitric oxide production and release. Such agents include bradykinin, acetylcholine, serotonin, and substance P. Once stimulated, the endothelial cell produces nitric oxide from L-arginine using the enzyme nitric oxide synthase. By stimulating cytosolic guanylate cyclase within the smooth muscle cell (leading to a rise in intracellular levels of cyclic guanosine monophosphate [cGMP]), nitric oxide leads to dilation of vascular smooth muscle. Nitric oxide is rapidly degraded by oxygen-derived free radicals,[17] a fact that may have particular relevance in the oxidative environment of atherosclerosis.

Inflammation

The endothelium can regulate monocyte and lymphocyte localization within the vasculature. Leukocyte adhesion molecules such as vascular cell adhesion molecule-1 (VCAM-1) are expressed on the luminal surface of the endothelial cell in lesion-prone areas.[18] The endothelium may also express chemotactic proteins (e.g., monocyte chemotactic protein-1) in response to metabolic stresses.[10] Inflammatory cytokines (tumor necrosis factor [TNF], interleukin-1 [IL-1], interferon-γ [IFN-γ]) produced in the vessel wall can target the endothelium-stimulating adhesion molecule and chemotactic protein expression, further amplifying the inflammatory response.[20] Thus, the endothelium may be the focal point for initiation and propagation of the inflammatory response associated with atherosclerosis. The clinical activity of ischemic heart disease may relate directly to the self-perpetuating nature of the inflammatory response orchestrated by the endothelium.

Thrombosis

The normal endothelium produces substances such as prostacyclin, nitric oxide, and tissue-type plasminogen activator that inhibit platelet aggregation and clot formation. Endothelial injury leading to an inflammatory response could hinder this function of the endothelium. The endothelium can become prothrombogenic or less antithrombogenic when exposed to inflammatory mediators.[21,22] This may have particular relevance in the more acute coronary syndromes of unstable angina and myocardial infarction.

Growth regulation

A normal healthy endothelium inhibits vascular smooth muscle growth.[23] The diseased dysfunctional endothelium appears to shift from this growth-inhibitory mode to a growth-promoting mode. The mechanism of growth inhibition by the endothelium is poorly understood. Growth promotion is probably accomplished via endothelial production of growth factors such as platelet-derived growth factor, insulin-like growth factor-1, and fibroblast growth factor.

STABLE ANGINA PECTORIS

Stable angina has been classically characterized as a consistent, exertional chest pain pattern. The threshold and duration of pain are predictable. Stimuli that increase myocardial oxygen demand such as exercise or emotional stress typically induce symptoms. The classic teaching has been that obstructive coronary atherosclerotic lesions that are not hemodynamically important at rest become flow limiting with any increase in myocardial oxygen demand. This fixed obstruction accounts for the reproducibility of time to onset of ischemia with provocative testing.

This view of stable angina should be amended. Anginal thresholds are not entirely fixed in most "stable angina" patients. Ambulatory monitoring has suggested that patients with stable angina develop symptoms at different heart rates, suggesting that myocardial oxygen demand is not the only determinant of ischemia.[24] This inconsistency in angina threshold is related to alterations in coronary vasomotor tone rather than alterations in myocardial oxygen demand. The pathophysiology of ischemia in stable angina not only is a "fixed stenosis-increased demand" problem but also involves a "dynamic stenosis-decreased supply" problem in most patients. In 1978, Maseri et al.[25] first demonstrated the dynamic nature of coronary atherosclerotic disease in patients with unstable angina. Local regulators of vessel tone are the primary contributors to this vasoconstrictor response affecting the production of ischemia not only in patients with stable angina but also in patients with unstable angina and infarction.

PATHOPHYSIOLOGY OF VASOSPASM

In the early 1980s, as we began to appreciate the importance of vasospasm as a contributor to myocardial ischemia, Furchgott and Zawadzki[15] discovered the importance of the endothelium as a local mediator of vessel tone. Subsequent experimental studies demonstrated abnormalities of endothelium-mediated relaxation in hypercholesterolemia and atherosclerosis, extending the theory that impaired endothelium-dependent vasodilation contributes greatly to coronary vasospasm in atherosclerosis.

Subsequent studies have proved this theory in the intact human coronary circulation. Ludmer et al.[26] demonstrated dramatic paradoxical vasoconstriction to the endothelium-dependent vasodilator acetylcholine in minimally and severely atherosclerotic arteries. Others have demonstrated abnormal endothelium-dependent responses in atherosclerotic arteries to more physiologically relevant stimuli such as serotonin,[27] exercise,[28] blood flow,[29] and cold pressor testing[30] (Figs. 6-1 to 6-3).

At least three important points can be gleaned from these clinical studies. First, the degree of endothelial dysfunction correlates with the degree of vascular injury (as measured by the number of risk factors for coronary atherosclerosis),[31] providing evidence for a cause-effect association of the initiating events in atherosclerosis and endothelial dysfunction. Second, endothelium-mediated dilator responses are impaired before significant atherosclerosis has become apparent angiographically, suggesting that endothelial dysfunction is an early step in the pathogenesis of atherosclerosis[31] and the substrate on which more advanced coronary artery disease develops. Third, this functional abnormality extends into the coronary microvessels where morphologic evidence of atherosclerosis does not exist.[32] Abnormalities of tone regulation by the microvascular endothelium may contribute to vasospasm-induced myocardial ischemia. Thus, endothelium-dependent vasodilation in large and small coronary arteries is impaired early in atherosclerosis and undoubtedly contributes to vasospastic phenomena in this disease.

The role of increased vascular smooth muscle sensitivity to circulating vasoconstrictors or augmented local concentrations of vasoconstricting agonists in atherosclerosis continues to be debated.[33] The observed enhancement in vasoconstriction to the nonspecific constrictor ergonovine supports the argument for increased vascular smooth muscle sensitivity in atherosclerosis. However, the fact that atherosclerotic and normal coronary arteries dilate similarly to nitroglycerin and calcium channel antagonists would not support this contention. Currently no convincing data exist suggesting that local concentrations of constricting agonists are increased in the ischemic coronary syndromes.

Cellular mechanisms of impaired vasodilation and enhanced vasoconstriction in atherosclerosis

Experimental and clinical data agree that nitric oxide activity is decreased in atherosclerosis. There are two explanations for this: (1) nitric oxide production is diminished, or (2) nitric oxide is rapidly degraded to inactive metabolites before eliciting any effect on vascular smooth muscle. Experimental studies have suggested that the substrate for nitric oxide production, the amino acid L-arginine, may be deficient in atherosclerosis. Endothelium-dependent vasodilation can be restored by administration of L-arginine in hypercholesterolemic models.[34] Others have suggested that endothelial cell surface receptors or signal transduction pathways are altered by atherosclerosis so that proper signaling for nitric oxide production does not occur.[35]

Evidence is accumulating, however, suggesting that nitric oxide production is normal or increased in atherosclerosis. This is consistent with the hypothesis that nitric oxide degradation is augmented, leading to decreased vasodilator activity.[36] Recent experimental work has supported this contention. In situ hybridization and immunohistochemistry techniques in human atherosclerotic plaques have demonstrated increased expression of the enzyme nitric oxide synthase.[37] Nitric oxide vasodilator activity is diminished in the setting of increased nitric oxide metabolite production in the hypercholesterolemic rabbit. In this same model, production of the nitric oxide degrader superoxide anion is dramatically increased after only 1 month of cholesterol feeding.[38] Scavenging this oxygen-derived free radical with superoxide dismutase restores endothelium-mediated relaxation to near normal.[39] These important findings are consistent with the theory that free radical–mediated destruction of nitric oxide accounts for diminished nitric oxide activity, leading to the clinical observation of impaired vasodilation and enhanced vasoconstriction in atherosclerosis.

These findings are particularly interesting in light of previously discussed information on the redox state in the vessel wall. In atherosclerosis, this redox state is altered favoring oxidation. The oxidative state is essential for propagation of the atherosclerotic process. Therefore, any by-products of oxidative metabolism (e.g., free radicals) are good candidates for important contributors to the molecular pathobiology of atherosclerosis.

Clinical implications of vasospasm

The endothelium's intrinsic vasodilating ability appears to be diminished in virtually all patients with coronary atherosclerosis, regardless of the clinical activity of the disease. Less intrinsic vasodilation (or more relative vasoconstriction) could explain the efficacy of vasodilators such as nitrates and calcium channel antagonists in the ischemic coronary syndromes. Free radical degradation of nitric oxide may be the molecular link accounting for this dysfunctional state of the endothelium. This is in accordance with the developing concept that an enhanced oxidative state is the fundamental metabolic defect in the pathobiology of atherosclerosis.

Understanding the molecular mechanisms of vasospasm in atherosclerosis should lead to better therapies directed at the primary biologic abnormalities. Although unproved in humans, hypercholesterolemia-induced endothelial dysfunction in monkeys can be reversed by simply withdrawing the high-cholesterol diet and allowing cholesterol levels to return to normal.[40] Accordingly, aggressive lipid lowering (with diet and medication) may

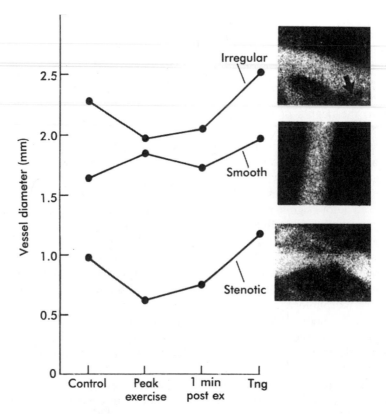

Fig. 6-1. Exercise-induced changes in vasomotion in diseased and normal coronary arteries. The effects are shown of exercise and nitroglycerin on vessel diameter as determined by quantitative coronary arteriography in a normal coronary segment and in segments with minimal obstruction and advanced stenosis. Exercise induced on the catheter table caused constriction of both the irregular segment (*upper panel*) and the segment with the high-grade stenosis (*lower panel*). In contrast, the segment that is angiographically smooth (*middle panel*) dilated in response to exercise. Endothelial dysfunction was implicated in these responses because simultaneous studies showed that segments constricting with exercise also constricted in response to acetylcholine, an endothelial-dependent vasodilator. In contrast, segments dilating to exercise dilated in response to acetylcholine. β-Blockade only partially attenuated the vasodilator response to exercise, thus invoking other mechanisms, presumably endothelium-dependent dilation stimulated by flow. Note that all three segments dilate in response to nitroglycerin, an NO donor, which bypasses the defective endothelial control mechanism and directly dilates the smooth muscle. (From Gordon JB, Ganz P, Nabel EG, et al: *Circulation* 83:1946-1952, 1989. Used by permission.)

become part of our armamentarium for treatment of vasospasm associated with the ischemic coronary syndromes. Antioxidant therapy (vitamins A and E, probucol) may also prove to be effective. Clinical assessment of the integrity of endothelial tone regulation may become a starting point for directing preventive approaches and an endpoint for evaluation of therapeutic efficacy in coronary atherosclerosis.

UNSTABLE ANGINA AND MYOCARDIAL INFARCTION

Unstable angina and myocardial infarction are considered together for two reasons. First, within the vessel wall, the underlying cellular mechanisms responsible for these two clinical syndromes are probably identical. Second, the pathologic features of plaque rupture and mural thrombus are central characteristics to both

syndromes. Partial or transient vessel occlusion with mural thrombus creates unstable angina. Prolonged complete vessel occlusion produces myocardial infarction. Unstable angina frequently precedes myocardial infarction, providing further evidence of the molecular and pathologic similarities of these two manifestations of coronary atherosclerosis.

These two unstable coronary syndromes frequently punctuate the course of chronic stable angina. An abrupt change in the pattern of chest pain is typical. The exercise threshold may be lowered. Rest angina may also occur. This conversion from a stable to an unstable syndrome is caused by a primary reduction in blood flow. As has been demonstrated in humans,[41] this alteration in blood flow is most often directly related to atherosclerotic plaque rupture and intraarterial thrombosis. The degree and duration of thrombotic vessel obstruction

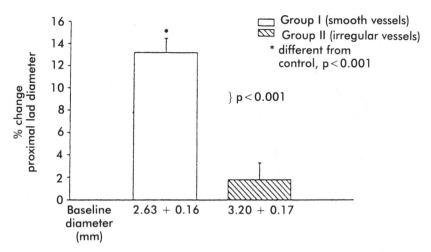

Fig. 6-2. Effects of atherosclerosis on flow-mediated vasodilation, an endothelium-dependent function. At cardiac catheterization, maximal coronary flow was stimulated by intracoronary infusion of adenosine (2.2 mg/min). Coronary artery diameter changes proximal to the tip of the infusion catheter (exposed to only increased flow) were compared in patients with mildly atherosclerotic coronary arteries and patients with smooth coronary arteries. This graph shows changes in proximal left anterior descending diameter in response to this increase in blood flow. The smooth left anterior descending segments in group 1 dilate significantly from control when coronary blood flow is increased by infusing adenosine, whereas segments with angiographic evidence of atherosclerosis in group 2 fail to dilate significantly. Thus, flow-mediated dilation, an endothelium-dependent function, is impaired in patients with atherosclerosis. (From Cox DA, Vita JA, Treasure CB, et al: *Circulation* 80:458-465, 1989. Used by permission.)

determine the clinical outcome. Complete occlusion for several hours in the absence of substantial collateral flow produces necrosis (infarction). Short-term or incomplete obstruction may produce only episodic or rest angina.

Usually thrombosis occurs when the plaque is disrupted or endothelial cells are removed,[42] exposing tissue thromboplastins and thrombogenic surfaces. Although it has not been demonstrated convincingly in vivo, thrombus could form on intact endothelium because inflammatory mediators such as IL-1 and TNF (present in active lesions) can stimulate the procoagulant tissue factor expression in cultured endothelial cells.[21] These and other inflammatory mediators could contribute to plaque destabilization by destroying connective tissue structural support and predisposing to fracture and fissuring.

In addition to plaque rupture and mural thrombus formation, vasospasm is an important contributor to the pathophysiology of unstable angina.[25] Vessel wall sensitivity to circulating vasoconstrictors may be enhanced. Thrombin and platelet aggregates (which release serotonin and thromboxane A_2), present at the site of vessel disruption, further augment vasoconstriction locally.[43]

Cellular mechanisms of unstable angina and myocardial infarction

Understanding the biologic mystery of conversion from a stable atherosclerotic plaque to an "active" unstable lesion is one of the central questions in cardiovascular medicine today. Enhanced inflammatory activity within the lesion is likely to contribute to plaque instability. Several studies have supported this hypothesis. In 1958, an autopsy study noted increased inflammatory cell infiltration in the infarct vessel adventitia of patients experiencing myocardial infarction and sudden death.[44] It is unlikely that this adventitial inflammation is secondary inflammation from infarction. Presumably the adventitial inflammation contributed to the unstable picture. Others have reproduced this finding[45] and have reported an increased number of monocytes and macrophages in the coronary arteries of autopsied patients who had had unstable angina.[46] Pultaceous plaques are frequent at sites of thrombosis and ulceration. T cells and macrophages are prominent in these active sites,[47] and TNF and IL-2 are also expressed in these plaques.

Altered plaque structural integrity

The evidence suggests that activation of the inflammatory response within the atherosclerotic plaque directly contributes to plaque instability. The interactions of macrophages and T cells are of particular importance. Both cell types are present in most atherosclerotic lesions.[2] Activation of the inflammatory response could stimulate these cells to express factors recruiting additional leukocytes into the lesion in unstable angina.[45,46] IL-1 or TNF (from T cells, macrophages, or the endothelium) can increase expression of endothelial adhesion molecules. Via attachment to these adhesion molecules, additional mononuclear cells can find their

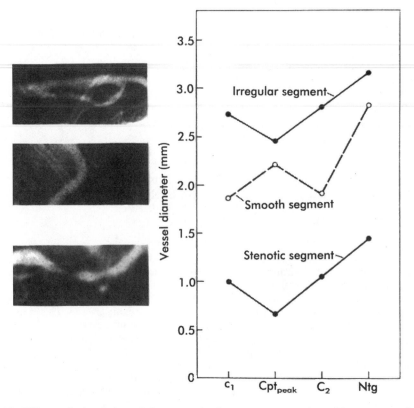

Fig. 6-3. Effects of stimulation of the sympathetic nervous system by cold pressor testing on coronary artery diameter. At catheterization the sympathetic nervous system was stimulated by the immersion of a hand in an ice slurry for 90 seconds. The middle panel shows a normal adaptive response to increased diameter at a time when myocardial oxygen consumption is increased, thus contributing to increased flow. This response in a perfectly smooth segment is contrasted with the response in a minimally diseased segment (*upper panel*) and a segment with advanced stenosis (*lower panel*). In both of these instances there was constriction of the artery. In the case of the stenotic segment, this extent of constriction contributed importantly to a decrease in blood flow and might precipitate ischemia. The mechanisms mediating the dilator response undoubtedly include endothelium-dependent stimulation to dilation caused by an increase in blood flow. The constrictor responses reflect, at least in part, the loss of endothelium-dependent dilation. As in the case of exercise depicted in Fig. 6-1, nitroglycerin dilates both diseased and normal vessels by delivering nitric oxide directly to the smooth muscle. (Nabel EG, Ganz P, Gordon JB, et al: *Circulation* 77:43-52, 1988. Used by permission.)

way into the intima and amplify the inflammatory response. In addition, cytokine-stimulated production of chemotactic factors such as monocyte chemotactic protein-1 (MCP-1) may lead to further monocyte recruitment.[10]

Many other substances released from activated lymphocytes and macrophages could contribute to plaque destabilization. Oxygen-derived free radical release and hydrogen peroxide formation in conjunction with the degradative enzymes collagenase and hyaluronidase can erode the connective tissue skeleton in the lesion, compromising plaque stability. Indeed, plaque fissuring and fracture seem to occur at sites of increased macrophage and foam cell concentration.[48] Clotting factors derived from macrophages and the lipid core of the atherosclerotic lesion contribute to luminal clot formation after plaque rupture.

In addition, plaque stability may be compromised by neovascularization from the adventitia. These thin-walled new vessels penetrate into the core of the lesion and are prone to rupture. The resulting intramural hemorrhage could contribute to destabilization and plaque rupture. The postulated cellular events leading to plaque destabilization are depicted in Fig. 6-4.

Episodic thrombosis

From postmortem studies of unstable angina patients,[49] we know that luminal clot formation is episodic. In patients dying after one or more episodes of unstable angina, histologic sections of the active epicardial coronary lesion showed a layering of thrombi of differing ages. In the vascular bed distal to this active lesion, changes ranging from old fibrotic areas of healed microinfarction to fresh platelet-rich isoemboli were

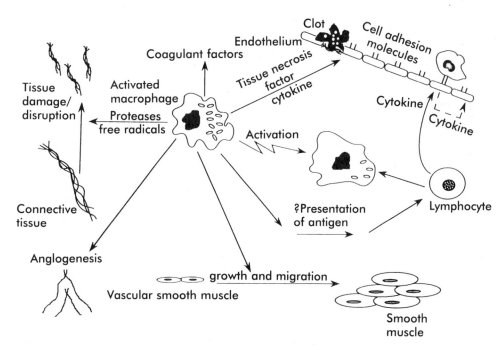

Fig. 6-4. Postulated cellular mechanism in an "active" atherosclerotic lesion leading to mononuclear cell recruitment, lesion disruption, and clot formation. Activation of the lesion is thought to be associated with enhanced production of cytokines such as tumor necrosis factor and interleukin-1, as well as enhanced production of growth factors contributing to lesion growth, smooth muscle cell migration, and proliferation. It is very likely that there is interaction between resident T cells and macrophages, and this may perhaps involve antigen presentation or processing that contributes to activation of the cells. Cytokine production will result in increased adhesion molecule expression and further recruitment of mononuclear cells and lymphocytes. The activated macrophage will produce procoagulant factors and growth factors. Importantly, the activated macrophage is likely to produce proteolytic agents such as collagenase, elastase, and free radicals that will lead to tissue damage and disruption. Fracture of the connective tissue can interfere with structural integrity of the plaque, leading to plaque fissuring and mural thrombus formation. The macrophages may also contribute angiogenic factors that increase the neovascularization of the plaque. This may be a source of intramural hemorrhage that can also compromise the structural integrity of the plaque. Decreasing inflammatory response in the plaque will, in the future, be a therapeutic objective and possibly is a major contributor to the decrease in cardiac event rates that have been reported in lipid-lowering trials.

observed, providing further evidence of episodic lesion activation. These pathologic data supporting episodic thrombosis in conjunction with the observed cyclic clinical activation of the disease would suggest that within the atherosclerotic lesion, cyclic changes in biologic activity are occurring, leading to recurrent thrombosis. Thus, according to this theory, the propensity toward unstable angina and myocardial infarction would be a function of lesion inflammatory activity rather than stenosis severity. The clinical implications of this assertion are substantial.

Clinical implications

This conceptualization of the pathogenesis of the unstable coronary syndromes in an inflammatory context is based on the premise that resident or newly recruited monocytes or macrophages and T cells, activated within the lesion, produce an aggressive inflammatory response, converting a stable lesion to an unstable one. Thus, the

episodic nature of these syndromes may represent periodic activation of a chronic inflammatory focus analagous to other chronic inflammatory diseases such as rheumatoid arthritis. Although initiating factors for inflammatory activation are unknown and details of the biologic events need further study, this postulated pathobiologic process within the vessel wall is in agreement with available evidence about the pathogenesis of atherosclerosis and clinical observations of the episodic nature of the disease.

PRECIPITATORS OF LESION ACTIVATION

The mechanisms of lesion activation remain unknown. Among the possibilities are (1) as yet unappreciated local factors in the vessel wall that initiate inflammatory cell activation or (2) antigen generation within the lesion leading to T-cell activation of the inflammatory response via macrophage-antigen-T-cell interactions (Fig. 6-4). Interestingly, oxidized LDL is a potent immunogen. It generates antibodies in some patients with atherosclerosis, making it a potential candidate for an inflammatory stimulus.[50,51]

It is possible that the trigger for lesion activation is systemic. Although systemic infection and inflammation and coronary lesion activation are difficult to link, several investigators have suggested such a relationship. Febrile illness frequently precedes myocardial infarction.[52] Some reports have suggested that patients with acute coronary syndromes have increased antibody titers against *Chlamydia pneumoniae*[53] and that chronic *C. pneumoniae* infection may be a risk factor for coronary artery disease.[54]

It is well established that an acute infectious illness may trigger activation of other chronic inflammatory diseases. It has been suggested that the unstable coronary syndromes may also be activated by an infectious process triggering systemic inflammatory responses.[55] Acute-phase reactants such as C-reactive protein are increased in patients with unstable angina,[56] providing direct evidence of systemic inflammatory activation. Tissue factor production is augmented in the coincubated macrophages and T cells of patients with unstable angina,[57] and this is lost 6 weeks later when the lesion has stabilized. Although the evidence suggests a relationship of systemic inflammation with atherosclerotic lesion activation, a cause and effect relationship has not been established.

SUMMARY AND FUTURE CLINICAL IMPORTANCE

From this merging of clinical and experimental data, two fundamental concepts in our understanding of the ischemic coronary syndromes emerge. First, cyclic changes in the cell biology of the atherosclerotic plaque are responsible for the clinically manifest episodic nature of coronary atherosclerosis (Fig. 6-5). Second, these biologic processes within the plaque are an inflammatory response to metabolic or physical injury initially to the endothelium. From this paradigm, clinical thinking regarding the therapy of coronary atherosclerosis is being refined. The "high-risk," life-threatening coronary lesion is not necessarily the most severely stenotic lesion but the lesion having the most active state of inflammation.

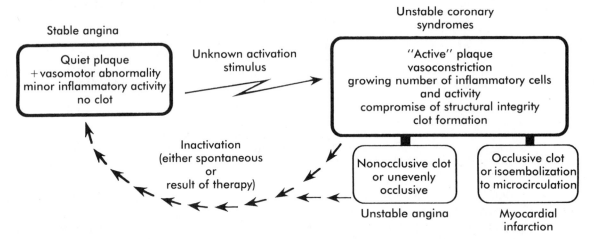

Fig. 6-5. Cyclic nature of the coronary ischemic syndromes. Stable angina is associated with plaque that has intact structural integrity and probably minimal inflammatory activity. Resident inflammatory cells are not in an active state. Effort angina is a result of the hemodynamic consequences of lumen narrowing, as well as the loss of endothelium-dependent vasodilator mechanisms that may be chronic. An activation stimulus, the nature of which is not yet understood, likely causes increased inflammatory activity. There is increased recruitment of inflammatory cells, and there is activation of these cells. As a result of the activation, the tendencies for enhanced vasoconstriction become even more prominent. Because of the inflammatory response, there may be compromise of the structural integrity of the plaque that may be associated with fissuring or fracture with thrombosis formation. A mural nonocclusive thrombus (or one that is only transiently occlusive) would be associated with unstable angina, whereas prolonged occlusion or isoembolization and microvascular occlusion would manifest as myocardial infarction. Inactivation of the plaque inflammatory activity would result in termination of the unstable state. The mechanisms for termination of lesion activity are also unknown but may be analogous to spontaneous inactivation or quiescence of inflammatory responses elsewhere. Plaque inactivation may account for the dramatic lowering of cardiac event rates in lipid-lowering regression trials.

Clinical data support this formulation. Residual lesions after thrombolysis are often minimally stenotic.[58,59] One cannot predict the anatomic location of plaque rupture based on the angiographic location and severity of coronary stenoses.[60] The results of coronary atherosclerosis regression trials also support this position. In the Familial Atherosclerosis Treatment Study, aggressive lipid-lowering therapy was associated with a dramatic reduction in cardiac events (death, myocardial infarction, or need for intervention) despite very little change in angiographic lumenal diameter (2% to 3% improvement).[61] In the St. Thomas Atherosclerosis Regression Study, low-cholesterol diet or diet plus cholestyramine was associated with a similar outcome.[62] Apparently aggressive lipid lowering alters the biology of the atherosclerotic lesion, favoring an inactive state. These data all support the notion that *the biologic state of an atherosclerotic lesion is a more important determinant of clinical course than is extent of stenosis.*

These observations may have considerable impact on our management of coronary atherosclerosis in the future. If this formulation, that coronary atherosclerosis progression is not one of linear plaque growth and progressive luminal compromise but rather cyclic lesion growth dependent on the state of inflammatory activation is correct, future therapy will focus on prevention of lesion activation or, conversely, inactivation of unstable lesions. A treatment strategy focusing strictly on the hemodynamic consequences of coronary stenoses may become passé. Treatment would focus on converting active to inactive lesions (i.e., lesions with minimal numbers of inflammatory cells, a solid connective tissue framework, and a healthy endothelium). Indeed, when hypercholesterolemic monkeys with active coronary atherosclerosis are placed on a low-cholesterol diet for 1 year, coronary artery morphology and function return to this inactive state.[63]

Return to this inactive state may directly relate to diminished oxidation of LDL-cholesterol.[6] Other studies indirectly support antioxidant therapy as a mode of lesion inactivation. In a recent trial, dietary supplementation with the antioxidant vitamin E was associated with a reduced risk of ischemic coronary events (relative risk of 0.63 in men, 0.59 in women).[64,65] Thus, antioxidants may, in the future, prove to be therapeutically effective by the prevention of plaque activation. This possibility is supported by the observation that at least one of the mechanisms involved in recruiting monocytes to attach to the endothelium involves an oxidation-sensitive pathway.[66] Other antiinflammatory strategies that prevent leukocyte incorporation into atherosclerotic lesions may be developed to prevent or reverse plaque activation.

Thus, inactive quiescent coronary atherosclerotic lesions could be associated with stable angina pectoris but have little potential for causing devastating clinical events. This interpretation would explain the dramatic clinical improvements seen in the atherosclerosis regression trials despite minimal angiographic change. Such a formulation provides a strong argument against intervening on less than severely stenotic lesions simply because of their presence.

With the current state of knowledge of vascular injury, the evidence provides a rationale for aggressive risk factor modification (hypertension, smoking, hyperlipidemia) as a treatment for active atherosclerosis in most patients with clinical evidence of vascular disease. As our understanding of the pathogenesis of atherosclerosis evolves, even more effective and specific therapeutic approaches (e.g., antioxidants, antiinflammatory agents) will become available. New technologies capable of reliably diagnosing early coronary atherosclerosis and new effective therapies to combat the disease could significantly diminish its catastrophic clinical consequences.

REFERENCES

1. Ross R, Masuda J, Raines EW: Cellular interactions, growth factors, and smooth muscle proliferation in atherogenesis, *Ann NY Acad Sci* 598:102-112, 1990.
2. Hansson GK, Jonasson L, Seifert PS, et al: Immune mechanisms in atherosclerosis, *Arteriosclerosis* 9:567-578, 1989.
3. Stemme S, Holm J, Hansson GK: T lymphocytes in human atherosclerotic plaques are memory cells expressing CD45RO and the integrin VLA-1, *Arterioscler Thromb* 12:206-211, 1992.
4. Kamat BR, Galli SJ, Barger AC, et al: Neovascularization and coronary atherosclerotic plaque: cinematographic localization and quantitative histologic analysis, *Hum Pathol* 18:1036-1042, 1987.
5. Munro JM, Cotran RS: The pathogenesis of atherosclerosis: atherogenesis and inflammation, *Lab Invest* 58:249-261, 1988.
6. Steinberg D, Parthasarathy S, Carew TE, et al: Beyond cholesterol. Modifications of low-density lipoprotein that increase its atherogenicity, *N Engl J Med* 320:915-924, 1989.
7. Henriksen T, Mahoney EM, Steinberg D: Enhanced macrophage degradation of low density lipoprotein previously incubated with cultured endothelial cells: recognition by receptor for acetylated low density lipoprotein, *Proc Natl Acad Sci USA* 78:6499-6503, 1981.
8. Steinbrecher UP, Parthasarathy S, Leake DS, et al: Modification of low density lipoprotein by endothelial cells involves lipid peroxidation and degradation of low density lipoprotein phospholipids, *Proc Natl Acad Sci USA* 81:3883-3887, 1984.
9. Fostegard J, Haegerstrand A, Gidlund M, et al: Biologically modified LDL increases the adhesive properties of endothelial cells, *Atherosclerosis* 90:112-126, 1991.
10. Cushing SD, Berliner JA, Valente AJ, et al: Minimally modified low density lipoprotein induces monocyte chemotactic protein-1 in human endothelial cells and smooth muscle cells, *Proc Natl Acad Sci USA* 87:5134-5138, 1990.
11. Rajavashirth TB, Andalibi A, Territo MC, et al: Induction of endothelial cell expression of granulocyte and macrophage colony stimulating factor by modified low-density lipoproteins, *Nature* 344:254-257, 1990.
12. Carew TE, Schwenke DC, Steinberg D: Antiatherogenic effect of probucol unrelated to its hypocholesterolemic effect; evidence that antioxidants in vivo can selectively inhibit low density lipoprotein

degradation in macrophage-rich fatty streaks and slow the progression of atherosclerosis in the Watanabe heritable hyperlipidemic rabbit, *Proc Natl Acad Sci USA* 84:7725-7729, 1987.

13. Ross R, Glomset J, Harker L: Response to injury and atherogenesis, *Am J Pathol* 86:675-684, 1977.

14. Gimbrone Jr MA: Endothelial dysfunction and the pathogenesis of atherosclerosis. In Gotto A, Smith LC, Allen B (eds): *Atherosclerosis-V. Proceedings of the Vth international symposium on atherosclerosis.* New York, 1980, Springer-Verlag, New York, pp 415-425.

15. Furchgott RF, Zawadzki JV: The obligatory role of endothelial cells in the relaxation of arterial smooth muscle by acetylcholine, *Nature* 288:373-376, 1980.

16. Palmer RM, Ferrige AG, Moncada S: Nitric oxide release accounts for the biological activity of endothelium-derived relaxing factor, *Nature* 327:524-526, 1987.

17. Gryglewski RJ, Palmer RM, Moncada S: Superoxide anion is involved in the breakdown of endothelium-derived vascular relaxing factor, *Nature* 320:454-456, 1986.

18. Kume N, Cybulsky MI, Gimbrone Jr MA: Lysophosphatidylcholine, a component of atherogenic lipoproteins, induces mononuclear leukocyte adhesion molecules in cultured human and rabbit arterial endothelial cells, *J Clin Invest* 90:1138-1144, 1992.

19. Reference deleted in proofs.

20. Libby P, Hansson GK: Involvement of the immune system in human atherogenesis: current knowledge and unanswered questions, *Lab Invest* 64:5-15, 1991.

21. Bevilacqua MP, Gimbrone Jr MA: Inducible endothelial functions in inflammation and coagulation, *Semin Thromb Hemost* 13:425-433, 1987.

22. Bevilacqua MP, Schleff RR, Gimbrone Jr MA, et al: Regulation of the fibrinolytic system of cultured human vascular endothelium by interleukin 1, *J Clin Invest* 78:587-591, 1986.

23. Edelman ER, Nugent MA, Smith LT, et al: Basic fibroblast growth factor enhances the coupling of intimal hyperplasia and proliferation of vaso vasorum in injured rat arteries, *J Clin Invest* 89:465-473, 1992.

24. Deanfield JE, Maseri A, Selwyn AP, et al: Myocardial ischaemia during daily life in patients with stable angina: its relation to symptoms and heart rate changes, *Lancet* 2:753-758, 1983.

25. Maseri A, Labbate A, Baroldi G, et al: Coronary vasospasm as a possible cause of myocardial infarction. A conclusion derived from the study of "preinfarction" angina, *N Engl J Med* 299:1271-1277, 1978.

26. Ludmer PL, Selwyn AP, Shook TL, et al: Paradoxical vasoconstriction induced by acetylcholine in atherosclerotic coronary arteries, *N Engl J Med* 315:1046-1051, 1986.

27. Golino P, Piscione F, Willerson JT, et al: Divergent effects of serotonin on coronary artery dimensions and blood flow in patients with coronary atherosclerosis and control patients, *N Engl J Med* 324:641-648, 1991.

28. Gordon JB, Ganz P, Nabel EG, et al: Atherosclerosis influences the vasomotor response of epicardial coronary arteries to exercise, *J Clin Invest* 83:1946-1952, 1989.

29. Cox DA, Vita JA, Treasure CB, et al: Atherosclerosis impairs flow-mediated dilation of coronary arteries in humans, *Circulation* 80:458-465, 1989.

30. Nabel EG, Ganz P, Gordon JB, et al: Dilation of normal and constriction of atherosclerotic coronary arteries caused by the cold pressor test, *Circulation* 77:43-52, 1988.

31. Vita JA, Treasure CB, Nabel EG, et al: Coronary vasomotor response to acetylcholine relates to risk factors for coronary artery disease, *Circulation* 81:491-497, 1990.

32. Ryan Jr TJ, Treasure CB, Yeung AC, et al: Impaired endothelium-dependent dilation of the coronary microvasculature in patients with atherosclerosis, *Circulation* 84:II624, 1991.

33. Ganz, P, Alexander RW: New insights into the cellular mechanisms of vasospasm, *Am J Cardiol* 56:11E-15E, 1985.

34. Cooke JP, Singer AH, Tsao P, et al: Antiatherogenic effects of L-arginine in the hypercholesterolemic rabbit, *J Clin Invest* 90:1168-1172, 1992.

35. DeMeyer GRY, Bult H, Van Hoydonck AE, et al: Neointima formation impairs endothelial muscarinic receptors while enhancing prostacyclin-mediated responses in the rabbit carotid artery, *Circ Res* 68:1669-1680, 1991.

36. Minor Jr RL, Myers P, Guerra Jr R, et al: Diet-induced atherosclerosis increases the release of nitrogen oxides from rabbit aorta, *J Clin Invest* 86:2109-2116, 1990.

37. Sundell CL, Marsden PA, Subramanian RR, et al: Nitric oxide synthase is expressed by endothelial cells overlying human atherosclerotic plaques, *Circulation* 86:I473, 1992.

38. Ohara Y, Peterson TE, Harrison DG: Hypercholesterolemia increases endothelial superoxide anion production, *J Clin Invest* 91:2546-2551, 1993.

39. Mugge A, Elwell JH, Peterson TE, et al: Chronic treatment with polyethylene-glycolated superoxide dismutase partially restores endothelium-dependent vascular relaxations in cholesterol-fed rabbits, *Circ Res* 69:1293-1300, 1991.

40. Freiman PC, Mitchell GG, Heistad DD, et al: Atherosclerosis impairs endothelium-dependent vascular relaxation to acetylcholine and thrombin in primates, *Circ Res* 58:783-789, 1986.

41. Mizuno K, Satomura K, Miyamoto A, et al: Angioscopic evaluation of coronary-artery thrombi in acute coronary syndromes, *N Engl J Med* 326:287-291, 1992.

42. Sherman CT, Litvack F, Grundfest W, et al: Coronary angioscopy in patients with unstable angina pectoris, *N Engl J Med* 315:913-919, 1986.

43. Willerson JT, Yao SK, McNatt J, et al: Frequency and severity of cyclic flow alternations and platelet aggregation predict the severity of neointimal proliferation following experimental coronary stenosis and endothelial injury, *Proc Natl Acad Sci USA* 88:10624-10628, 1991.

44. Pomerance A: Periarterial mast cells in coronary atheroma and thrombosis, *Pathol Bacteriol* 76:55-70, 1958.

45. Sato T, Takebayashi S, Kohchi K: Increased subendothelial infiltration of the coronary arteries with monocytes/macrophages in patients with unstable angina, *Atherosclerosis* 68:191-197, 1987.

46. Kohchi K, Takebayashi S, Hiroki T, et al: Significance of adventitial inflammation of the coronary artery in patients with unstable angina: results at autopsy, *Circulation* 71:709-716, 1985.

47. Arbustini E, Grasso M, Diegoli M, et al: Coronary atherosclerotic plaques with and without thrombus in ischemic heart syndromes: a morphologic, immunohistochemical, and biochemical study, *Am J Cardiol* 68:36B-50B, 1991.

48. Richardson PD, Davies MJ, Born GV: Influence of plaque configuration and stress distribution on fissuring of coronary atherosclerotic plaques, *Lancet* 2:941-944, 1989.

49. Falk E: Unstable angina with fatal outcome: dynamic coronary thrombosis leading to infarction and/or sudden death. Autopsy evidence of recurrent mural thrombosis with peripheral embolization culminating in total vascular occlusion, *Circulation* 71:699-708, 1985.

50. Palinski W, Yla-Herttuala S, Rosenfeld ME, et al: Antisera and monoclonal antibodies specific for epitopes generated during oxidative modification of low density lipoprotein, *Arteriosclerosis* 10:325-335, 1990.

51. Salonen JT, Yla-Herttuala S, Yamamoto R, et al: Autoantibody against oxidised LDL and progression of carotid atherosclerosis, *Lancet* 339:883-887, 1992.

52. Spodick DH: Infection and infarction. Acute viral (and other) infection in the onset, pathogenesis and mimicry of acute myocardial infarction, *Am J Med* 81:661-668, 1986.

53. Thom DH, Wang SP, Grayston JT, et al: *Chlamydia pneumoniae* strain TWAR antibody and angiographically demonstrated coronary heart disease, *Arterioscler Thromb* 11:547-551, 1991.

54. Saikku P, Leinonen M, Tenkanen L, et al: Chronic *Chlamydia pneumoniae* infections as a risk factor for coronary heart disease in the Helsinki Heart Study, *Ann Intern Med* 116:273-278, 1992.

55. Valtonen VV: Infection as a risk factor for infarction and atherosclerosis, *Ann Med* 23:539-543, 1991.

56. Berk BC, Weintraub WS, Alexander RW: Elevation of C-reactive protein in "active" coronary artery disease, *Am J Cardiol* 65:168-172, 1990.

57. Serveri GG, Abbate R, Gori AM, et al: Transient intermittent lymphocyte activation is responsible for the instability of angina, *Circulation* 86:790-797, 1992.

58. Ganz W, Buchbinder N, Marcus H, et al: Intracoronary thrombolysis in evolving myocardial infarction, *Am Heart J* 101:4-13, 1981.

59. Hackett D, Davies G, Maseri A: Pre-existing coronary stenoses in patients with first myocardial infarction are not necessarily severe, *Eur Heart J* 9:1317-1323, 1988.

60. Little WC, Constantinescu M, Applegate RJ, et al: Can coronary angiography predict the site of a subsequent myocardial infarction in patients with mild to moderate coronary artery disease? *Circulation* 78:1157-1166, 1988.

61. Brown G, Albers JJ, Fisher LD, et al: Regression of coronary artery disease as a result of intensive lipid-lowering therapy in men with high levels of apolipoprotein B, *N Engl J Med* 323:1289-1298, 1990.

62. Watts GF, Lewis B, Brunt JNH, et al: Effects on coronary artery disease of lipid-lowering diet, or diet plus cholestyramine, in the St. Thomas' Atherosclerosis Regression Study (STARS), *Lancet* 339:563-569, 1992.

63. Harrison DG, Armstrong ML, Freiman PC, et al: Restoration of endothelium-dependent relaxation by dietary treatment of atherosclerosis, *J Clin Invest* 80:1808-1811, 1987.

64. Rimm EB, Stampfer MJ, Ascherio A, et al: Vitamin E consumption and the risk of coronary artery disease in men, *N Engl J Med* 328:1450-1456, 1993.

65. Stampfer MJ, Hennekens CH, Manson JE, et al: Vitamin E consumption and the risk of coronary disease in women, *N Engl J Med* 328:1444-1449, 1993.

66. Marui N, Offerman M, Swerlick R, et al: Vascular cell adhesion molecule-1 (VCAM-1) gene transcription and expression are regulated through an antioxidant sensitive mechanism in human vascular endothelial cells, *J Clin Invest* 92:1866-1874, 1993.

Chapter 7

THE PARADIGM OF ACUTE REPERFUSION AND THE GUSTO-I TRIAL

Robert M. Califf
Eric J. Topol

The concept of reperfusion therapy for acute myocardial infarction (AMI) has been one of the most intensively studied issues in the history of medicine. Following a series of pathologic observations suggesting that thrombus was an important component of the pathophysiology of AMI, initial clinical studies with intravenous thrombolysis were largely disregarded despite promising clinical results. Seminal studies in animal models demonstrating that early reperfusion was associated with substantial myocardial salvage and reduction in infarct size caused a resurgence of interest in this field, but it was not until the powerful visual image of coronary artery occlusion and reperfusion was produced in the angiographic laboratory that the imagination of the cardiovascular community became fully involved in the pursuit of reperfusion. This chapter will review the pathophysiologic and clinical basis for the practice of reperfusion, with an emphasis on the role of the GUSTO-I trial in solidifying the concepts of early reperfusion—salvage of myocardium to preserve left ventricular function and survival.

Animal models of reperfusion

The critical work on the fundamental basis of reperfusion was conducted in a series of experiments by Reimer et al.,[1] which have been solidified and expanded by multiple collaborators over the past 20 years. In essence, by occluding an epicardial coronary vessel in a canine model and releasing that occlusion

at various points in time, these investigators demonstrated that myocardial necrosis begins developing within 15 to 45 minutes after occlusion. The necrosis progresses in a "wavefront" fashion from the endocardium to the epicardium. Other than the duration of the occlusion, the only other modifier of the extent of necrosis that has been observed consistently is the collateral circulation. The fact that collateral vessels are predominantly confined to the epicardium, and the higher metabolic demands and downstream loss of "pressure-head" in the endocardium probably account for the wavefront. Although the concept of a lateral "border zone" or reversibly injured myocardium in an MI is attractive to the clinician, it has yet to be borne out as constituting anything more than wishful thinking. Fundamentally, restoration of blood flow is the only therapy that has been demonstrated to be markedly effective in reducing infarct size.

For years investigators have evaluated promising agents designed to assist reperfusion in reducing infarct size, but when put to the test in humans, these experiments have been negative. The reasons for the failure of the animal model to accurately identify promising agents that may affect infarct size are complex and unclear. The one exception is the effect of ischemic "preconditioning" on future infarct size: repetitive bouts of ischemia before total vessel occlusion will reduce the size of the subsequent infarction. Unfortunately, a clinical approach to adopting this

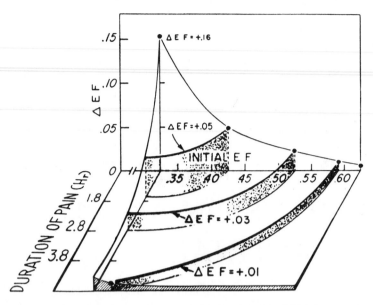

Fig. 7-1. A conceptual model relating changes of ejection fraction (ΔEF) from preintervention to chronic angiography, duration of infarct symptoms (hours), and preintervention EF (initial EF). The two key factors are the duration of symptoms before reperfusion and the size of the infarction. (From Rentrop P, Smith H, Painter L, et al: Changes in left ventricular ejection fraction after intracoronary thrombolytic therapy: results of the Registry of the European Society of Cardiology, *Circulation* 68 (suppl I):I-55-I-60, 1983.)

phenomenon to improve patient outcome is not intuitively apparent.

The species variability in the time course of the wavefront of necrosis appears to be secondary to heterogeneity in collateral blood flow. In pigs, which have almost no collateral flow, a fully transmural infarction develops within 45 minutes after coronary occlusion. In comparison, rats rarely develop a transmural infarction if the occlusion is sustained because they have excellent collateral flow. Humans apparently can fall anywhere within this spectrum, depending upon such vicissitudes as the development of an acute plaque rupture in the presence of poorly developed collateral flow.

Historical developments

From the early use of intracoronary thrombolytic therapy it was believed that reperfusion would reduce mortality and favorably affect other clinical endpoints by reducing MI size in exactly the same manner as the canine experiments demonstrated. In a classic review in 1983, Rentrop et al. displayed a theoretic model (Fig. 7-1) indicating that the benefit of thrombolytic therapy would be a function of time from coronary occlusion, the amount of myocardium at risk, and the presence of collaterals.[2] Although the path has not been clear throughout the entire course, our thesis is that the observational studies and clinical trials since that time have been consistent with Rentrop's model. We believe that the key to understanding the seeming inconsisten-

cies is to realize that the model is dependent upon both the duration of occlusion and the maintenance of perfusion, and that the physiological and clinical results are "noisy" because of the wavefront phenomenon itself and the multiple confounding factors in the human situation, including variable collaterals, fallibility of the human memory regarding onset of symptoms, inconsistent administration of therapy, concomitant administration of other effective therapies, difficulty measuring surrogate endpoints, and random chance.

Mortality trials

Until the seminal overview by Yusuf et al.[3] using the creative insight of the Oxford group, the field was confused by multiple small trials, none of which convincingly demonstrated a mortality benefit of thrombolytic therapy. Yusuf demonstrated that when the results of all these trials were systematically combined, the best estimate was a 27% reduction in mortality with thrombolysis. After arguing persuasively that large trials were essential to answer this question and many others confronting practicing cardiologists, both the ISIS group[4] and the GISSI group[5] performed convincing individual trials demonstrating a 25% to 30% reduction in mortality with streptokinase compared with placebo. In 1994 the Fibrinolysis Trialists' (FTT) Collaborative Group[6] combined individual patient data from over 70,000 patients treated with thrombolytic therapy versus conventional care and essentially confirmed these results (Fig. 7-2).

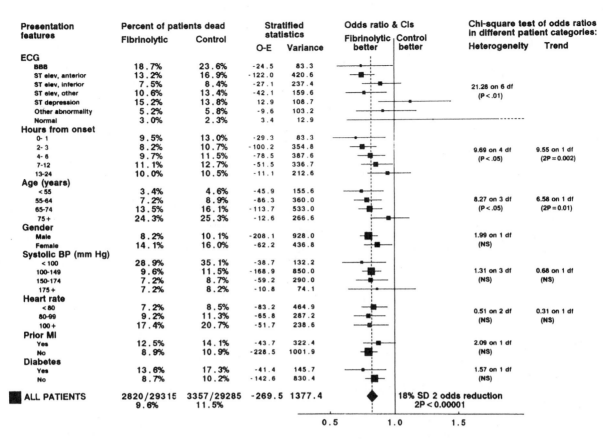

Presentation features	Percent of patients dead		Stratified statistics		Odds ratio & CIs		Chi-square test of odds ratios in different patient categories:	
	Fibrinolytic	Control	O-E	Variance	Fibrinolytic better	Control better	Heterogeneity	Trend
ECG								
BBB	18.7%	23.6%	-24.5	83.3				
ST elev, anterior	13.2%	16.9%	-122.0	420.6			21.28 on 6 df	
ST elev, inferior	7.5%	8.4%	-27.1	237.4			(P<.01)	
ST elev, other	10.6%	13.4%	-42.1	159.6				
ST depression	15.2%	13.8%	12.9	108.7				
Other abnormality	5.2%	5.8%	-9.6	103.2				
Normal	3.0%	2.3%	3.4	12.9				
Hours from onset								
0-1	9.5%	13.0%	-29.3	83.3				
2-3	8.2%	10.7%	-100.2	354.8			9.69 on 4 df	9.55 on 1 df
4-6	9.7%	11.5%	-78.5	387.6			(P<.05)	(2P=0.002)
7-12	11.1%	12.7%	-51.6	336.7				
13-24	10.0%	10.5%	-11.1	212.6				
Age (years)								
<55	3.4%	4.6%	-45.9	155.6				
55-64	7.2%	8.9%	-86.3	360.0			8.27 on 3 df	6.58 on 1 df
65-74	13.5%	16.1%	-113.7	533.0			(P<.05)	(2P=0.01)
75+	24.3%	25.3%	-12.6	266.6				
Gender								
Male	8.2%	10.1%	-208.1	928.0			1.99 on 1 df	
Female	14.1%	16.0%	-62.2	436.8			(NS)	
Systolic BP (mm Hg)								
<100	28.9%	35.1%	-38.7	132.2				
100-149	9.6%	11.5%	-168.9	850.0			1.31 on 3 df	0.68 on 1 df
150-174	7.2%	8.7%	-59.2	290.0			(NS)	(NS)
175+	7.2%	8.2%	-10.8	74.1				
Heart rate								
<80	7.2%	8.5%	-83.2	464.9				
80-99	9.2%	11.3%	-65.8	287.2			0.51 on 2 df	0.31 on 1 df
100+	17.4%	20.7%	-51.7	238.6			(NS)	(NS)
Prior MI								
Yes	12.5%	14.1%	-43.7	322.4			2.09 on 1 df	
No	8.9%	10.9%	-228.5	1001.9			(NS)	
Diabetes								
Yes	13.6%	17.3%	-41.4	145.7			1.57 on 1 df	
No	8.7%	10.2%	-142.6	830.4			(NS)	
■ **ALL PATIENTS**	2820/29315	3357/29285	-269.5	1377.4			18% SD 2 odds reduction	
	9.6%	11.5%					2P < 0.00001	

0.5   1.0   1.5

Fig. 7-2. Proportional effects of fibrinolytic therapy on mortality during days 0 to 35, subdivided by presentation features. "Observed minus expected" (O − E) number of events among fibrinolytic-allocated patients (and its variance) is given for subdivisions of presentation features, stratified by trial. This is used to calculate odds ratios (ORs) of death among patients allocated to fibrinolytic therapy vs. that among those allocated control. ORs (black squares with areas proportional to amount of "statistical information" contributed by the trials) are plotted with their 99% CIs (horizontal lines). Squares to the left of the solid vertical line indicate benefit (significant at $2P < 0.01$ only where entire CI is to left of vertical line). Overall result and 95% CI is represented by the diamond, with overall proportional reduction in the odds of death and statistical significance given alongside. Chi-square tests for evidence of heterogeneity of, or trends in, size of ORs in subdivisions of each presentation feature are also given. (From Fibrinolytic Therapy Trialists' (FTT) Collaborative Group: Indications for fibrinolytic therapy in suspected acute myocardial infarction: collaborative overview of early mortality and major morbidity results from all randomised trials of more than 1000 patients, *Lancet* 343:311-322, 1994.)

Relative and absolute benefit

A review of subgroup data from the FTT effort reveals three consistent themes: the benefit is time-related, sicker patients by and large receive the most benefit, and the very elderly have a reduction in the estimate of relative benefit. Although thrombolytic therapy is beneficial even up to 12 hours from the onset of symptoms, the most dramatic benefit is in the first hour, with a substantially greater proportional reduction in mortality in this time frame (Figs. 7-3 and 7-4). Other than time, no other consistent modifier of the relative mortality reduction is observed. In general, given the same 25% to 30% reduction in the risk of death, patients with the greatest risk of death without thrombolytic

therapy derive the greatest benefit from it. The outcomes in elderly patients are especially important and complex (Fig. 7-5). The best estimate of relative treatment effect is a slight reduction of benefit in the elderly, but because of their excessive risk of dying without reperfusion the absolute reduction in mortality is equivalent.

The large mortality trials comparing thrombolytic agents before GUSTO-I[7,8] showed a convincing lack of difference in mortality (Fig. 7-6). The sizable study population effectively ruled out chance as a cause of the lack of mortality difference, suggesting either that the earlier perfusion rates observed with t-PA were irrelevant or that the dosing and/or adjunctive therapy were canceling the benefit of this earlier therapy.

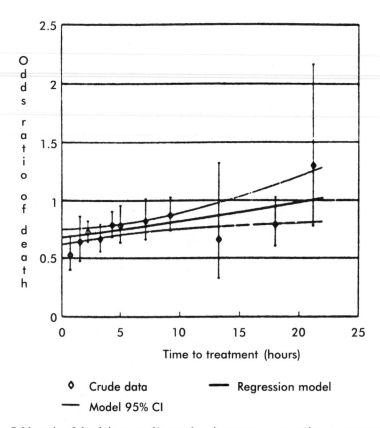

Fig. 7-3. Odds ratio of death in treated/control patients versus mean time to treatment. Error bars shows odds ratios and 95% confidence intervals (CI) for the 65 trials as combined by Mantel-Haenszel statistics to form 11 subgroups by time to treatment. The logistic regression model estimates of this association ($\chi^2 = 7.6, P = 0.006$) and its 95% confidence intervals are displayed. (Reprinted with permission from Honan et al: Cardiac rupture and thrombolytic therapy, J Am Coll Cardiol 16:359-367, 1990.)

Perfusion data

Studies of coronary perfusion after thrombolysis have also shown a consistent pattern of the most rapid perfusion with t-PA, followed by anistreplase, and then streptokinase[9] (Fig. 7-7). Following the administration of "accelerated" t-PA, the perfusion rates were even higher than with standard t-PA in the first 90 minutes, particularly the rates of TIMI grade 3 flow (Fig. 7-8). Within the first several hours after treatment the perfusion rates seem similar, regardless of thrombolytic agent.

Before accelerated dosing of t-PA, the reocclusion rate was twice as high with t-PA as with streptokinase. Aggregated reocclusion data with "front-loaded" t-PA show a substantially lower rate of reocclusion than with standard dose t-PA (Fig. 7-9).

LV function data

Comparative studies of left ventricular function have been somewhat disappointing, with a small difference in left ventricular ejection fraction when thrombolytic-treated patients were compared with control patients (Fig. 7-10). This has been attributed partly to the fact that patients who survived the infarction in the treated group were likely to include a higher proportion of patients with compromised left ventricular function, whereas many patients with low ejection fractions would not have survived in the control group, leaving a group of patients with better left ventricular function. Multivariable analyses have consistently demonstrated that baseline left ventricular dysfunction[10,11] is the most potent predictor of improvement in follow-up, although achievement of TIMI grade 3 flow by 90 minutes after treatment is also a significant predictor.

Stroke

The details of the stroke information are discussed in Chapter 52, but the aggregated data now demonstrate an increase in overall risk of stroke with thrombolytic therapy, consisting of a combination of a dramatic increase in the risk of hemorrhagic stroke and a modest decrease in the risk of nonhemorrhagic stroke.[6] t-PA exaggerates the increase in the risk of hemorrhagic stroke.

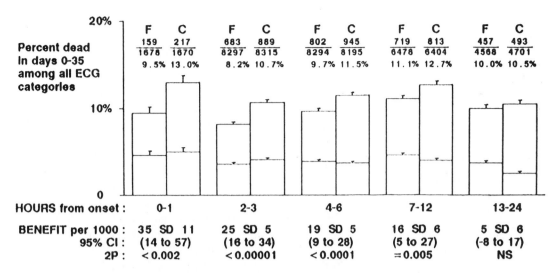

Fig. 7-4. Absolute effects of fibrinolytic therapy on mortality during days 0 to 35, subdivided by delay from symptom onset. Unstratified percentages dead during days 0 to 35 among all those allocated fibrinolytic therapy *(F)* and all those allocated control *(C)* in these trials are plotted (± SD), subdivided by time from symptom onset. The portion below the horizontal line within each column represents deaths during days 0 to 1; the portion above the line represents deaths during days 2 to 35. (From Fibrinolytic Therapy Trialists' (FTT) Collaborative Group: Indications for fibrinolytic therapy in suspected acute myocardial infarction: collaborative overview of early mortality and major morbidity results from all randomised trials of more than 1000 patients, *Lancet* 343:311-322, 1994.)

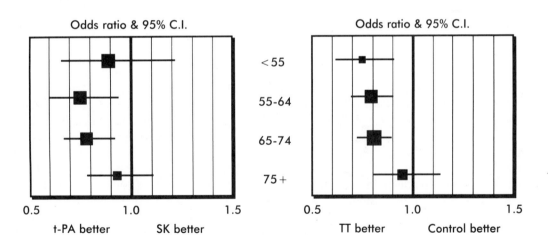

Fig. 7-5. The figure demonstrates that thrombolysis is superior to no thrombolysis in all age groups and that the "booster" effect of the benefit of accelerated t-PA compared with streptokinase has a similar distributional effect. The relative benefit in the elderly is less, and the confidence limits cross unity. However, because of the extremely high mortality rate in elderly patients regardless of treatment, the *absolute* benefits of thrombolysis vs. no thrombolysis and for accelerated t-PA versus streptokinase are similar in the elderly and in younger patients.

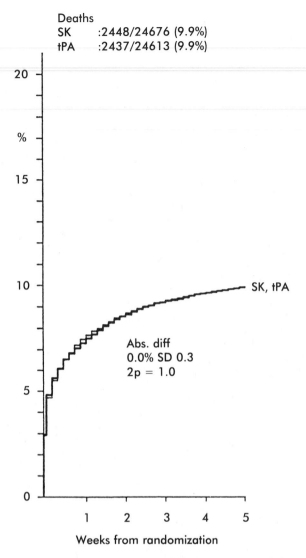

Deaths
SK   :2448/24676 (9.9%)
tPA   :2437/24613 (9.9%)

Abs. diff
0.0% SD 0.3
2p = 1.0

SK, tPA

Fig. 7-6. Cumulative percentage of deaths in days 0 to 35 shows no difference between patients treated with streptokinase (SK) and those treated with t-PA in the ISIS-3 and GISSI-2 trials.

GUSTO-I
Planning considerations

The GUSTO-I trial was planned in an effort to reconcile the difference between the pathophysiological model indicating the critical importance of rapid, complete, and sustained reperfusion and the absence of a mortality benefit of t-PA in the large clinical trials. One possibility was that the standard dosing regimen of t-PA did not translate into a mortality benefit because the previous mortality trials did not use concomitant intravenous, carefully monitored heparin. Multiple previous trials[12-14] had shown a modest increase in late coronary perfusion (48 hours to 1 week) when heparin was compared with placebo after standard-dose t-PA. A second possibility was that standard-dose t-PA simply did not achieve enough of a difference in early perfusion to lead to a mortality benefit, especially after considering the impact of the additional strokes on the subsequent mortality rate after t-PA.

Study design (Fig. 7-11)

In order to address the issue a trial was designed, initially having three treatment arms. The standard treatment arm was designed to include streptokinase, given as 1.5 million units over 1 hour, and intravenous heparin, given as a 5000-unit bolus followed by 1000 units per hour with adjustment according to the aPTT. A treatment arm consisting of "accelerated" t-PA was designed, based on the results of angiographic pilot studies, to achieve rapid perfusion with a 10-mg bolus followed by 0.75 mg per kg over 30 minutes, then 0.50 mg per kg over 60 minutes in addition to the same heparin regimen as the streptokinase-treated patients. A very aggressive experimental treatment arm consisting of t-PA in a dose of 1 mg per kg over 60 minutes (up to 90 mg maximum) in combination with 1 million units of streptokinase and the same heparin regimen was included in an effort both to achieve early perfusion and to prevent the higher reocclusion rate that had been observed with standard dosing of t-PA.

Shortly after the study began enrolling patients the ISIS-3 investigators reported that streptokinase with subcutaneous heparin was the superior treatment because it had equivalent mortality to t-PA and fewer strokes at a much lower cost. Consequently a fourth treatment arm was added to the GUSTO-I trial, consisting of 1.5 million units of streptokinase given over 1 hour with subcutaneous heparin. When the results of ISIS-3 were published 1 year after this arm was added, it became known that streptokinase with no heparin did as well as streptokinase with subcutaneous heparin.

The consensus before the GUSTO-I trial started was that the sample size should be large enough to allow for detection of a 1% absolute difference in mortality or a 15% relative difference, whichever was smaller. This approach led to the construction of a sample size of 30,000 patients for three arms and of 41,000 patients for four arms. Another point of considerable discussion was whether the study should be blinded. Because of the complexity of the treatment regimens and because the key endpoints (stroke and death) were objective, the decision was made to proceed without blinding.

Substudies

Concomitant with the mortality trial a decision was made to proceed with several key substudies to provide the pathophysiological and economic underpinnings for the mortality results. An angiographic substudy called for the performance of angiograms on 2400 patients in a randomly allocated sequence to provide a "snapshot" of coronary perfusion and left ventricular function with

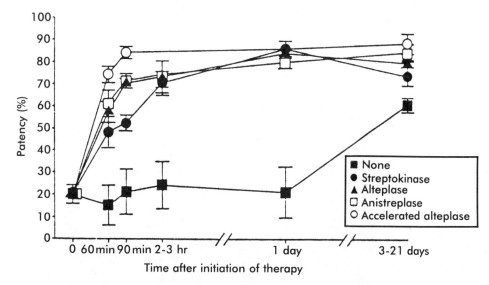

Fig. 7-7. Pooled analysis of angiographic patency rates over time after various thrombolytic agents: patency rates are highest following accelerated t-PA, early rates with conventional t-PA and anistreplase are strikingly similar, and the patency rate following streptokinase has "caught up" to conventional t-PA and anistreplase within 2 to 3 hours; includes 13,728 angiographic observations. (From Granger CB, Califf RM, Topol EJ: Thrombolytic therapy for acute myocardial infarction: a review, *Drugs* 44:293-325, 1992.)

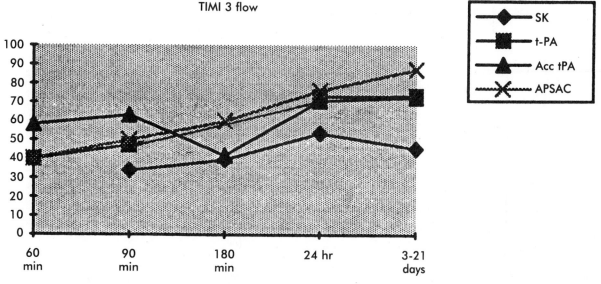

Fig. 7-8. Pooled analysis of TIMI grade 3 flow determined in several time periods following thrombolysis demonstrates the early advantage of accelerated t-PA at 60 and 90 minutes.

each thrombolytic strategy at 90 minutes, 3 hours, 24 hours, and 7 days. A detailed economic and quality-of-life study focused on the United States and Canada to allow for both the comparison of outcomes as a function of for both treatment and an analysis of outcomes of patients with AMI in the two health care systems. A major substudy organized by the study coordinators evaluated time to treatment, and the results of this substudy are discussed in Chapter 22. Specific substudies evaluated the details of prognosis and outcome in pa-

tients with stroke, cardiogenic shock, and reinfarction. In particular, an effort to obtain a brain imaging study on every patient with suspected stroke had 93% success, and quality of life was directly measured via a structured questionnaire in all patients with stroke in North America.

Mortality results

The mortality results indicated that t-PA was associated with a 14% relative reduction in risk of death and a

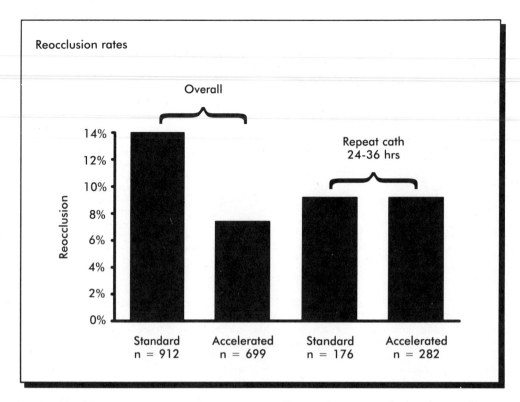

Fig. 7-9. Patients given accelerated t-PA are less likely to have a reocclusion than patients given standard t-PA.

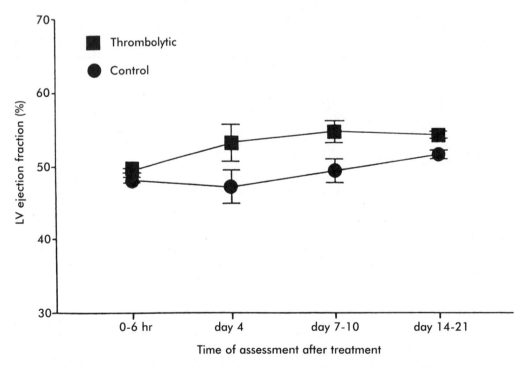

Fig. 7-10. Pooled analysis of left ventricular ejection fraction from randomized trials of thrombolytic therapy versus control: thrombolytic therapy results in significantly higher ejection fraction ($P \leq 0.001$ for each time point), and the difference between thrombolytic and control does not increase after day 4; includes 3066 ventriculographic observations.   (From Granger CB, Califf RM, Topol EJ: Thrombolytic therapy for acute myocardial infarction: a review, *Drugs* 44:293-325, 1992.)

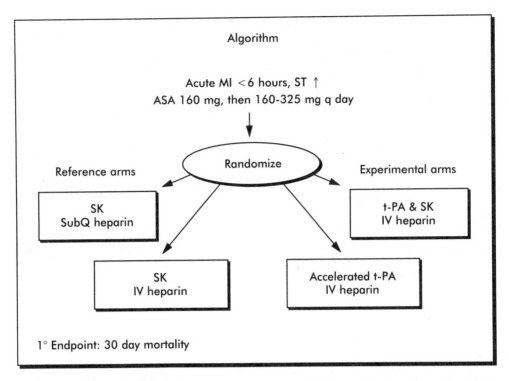

Fig. 7-11. The GUSTO-I trial originally included the two experimental arms and one reference arm in which patients would receive streptokinase and intravenous heparin. The second reference arm, streptokinase and subcutaneous heparin, was added several months after the trial began because of the results of the ISIS-3 investigation.

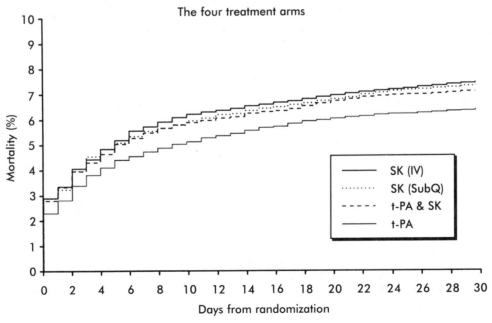

Fig. 7-12. After 30 days the mortality rate among patients who received t-PA was significantly lower than among patients who received one of the other three strategies.

Prior MI

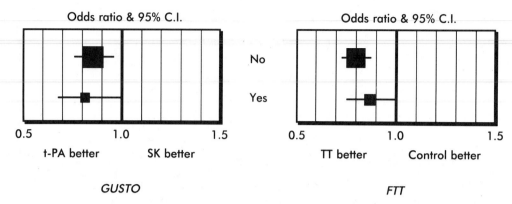

GUSTO

FTT

Fig. 7-13. The following six figures present data from the GUSTO-I and FTT trials, showing odds ratios and 95% confidence intervals (C.I.) for accelerated tissue-plasminogen activator (t-PA) vs. streptokinase (SK) in GUSTO-I and for thrombolytic therapy (TT) vs. control in the FTT data. Thrombolytic therapy is clearly better than control for patients with and without a previous MI, as is accelerated t-PA over SK.

Diabetes

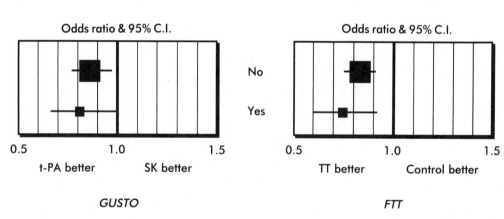

GUSTO

FTT

Fig. 7-14. Among patients with and without diabetes, thrombolytic therapy is better than none and accelerated t-PA is superior to SK.

MI location

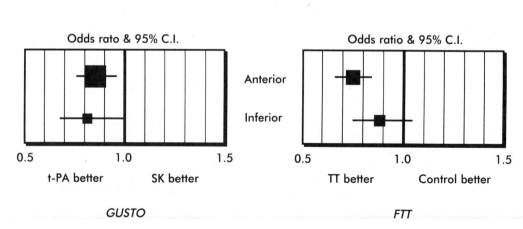

GUSTO

FTT

Fig. 7-15. Patients with anterior or inferior myocardial infarctions (MI) benefit more from thrombolytic therapy and from t-PA among thrombolytics.

Systolic blood pressure

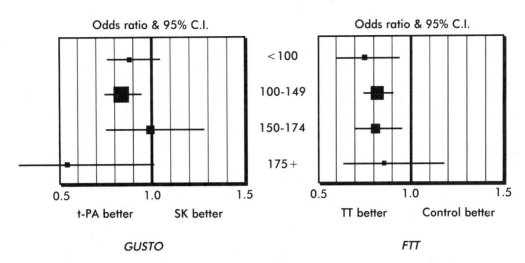

Fig. 7-16. From the FTT data patients within all ranges of systolic blood pressure do best with thrombolytic therapy. The same is true for GUSTO-I patients who received accelerated t-PA, although those in the 150 to 174 mm Hg range were equivocal, probably representing the "play of chance."

Heart rate

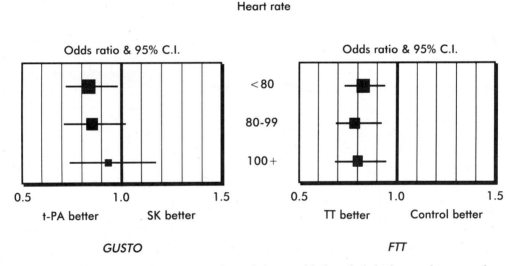

Fig. 7-17. Regardless of heart rate, patients do better with thrombolytic therapy than control, and the patterns for accelerated t-PA versus SK are similar.

1% absolute reduction (Fig. 7-12).[15] This difference was already highly significant within 24 hours of randomization, with a 0.5% mortality difference, suggesting that the "early hazard" of dying may be accentuated by streptokinase. As demonstrated in Figures 7-13 to 7-18 these results were remarkably consistent across subgroups, indicating that t-PA for the most part extended the beneficial results of streptokinase compared with placebo.

Angiographic substudy

The design of the angiographic substudy (Fig. 7-19) called for randomization at the time of angiography to allow estimation of coronary perfusion throughout the course of angiography.[16] The only major difference was observed at the 90-minute angiogram, at which time 57% of patients treated with accelerated t-PA had TIMI grade 3 flow compared with close to 30% in the streptokinase group (Fig. 7-20). At all other time points no significant differences were seen. When reocclusion was directly measured, to our surprise no differences were found among the regimens. The differences in early perfusion translated into measurable differences in left ventricular function with better ejection fraction, regional wall motion, and smaller ventricular volumes in the accelerated t-PA group. Interestingly, these differ-

Time to treatment (hours)

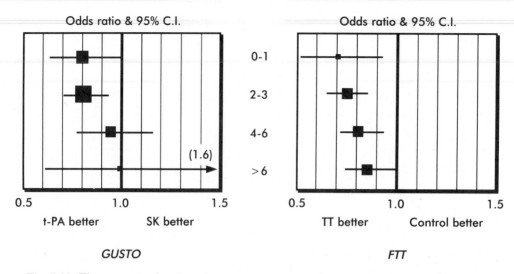

Fig. 7-18. The sooner patients receive thrombolytic therapy the better their odds, although thrombolytic therapy up to 6 hours after onset of symptoms is better than control. Patients receiving t-PA do better than patients receiving SK up to 6 hours, at which point the results appear equivalent with SK.

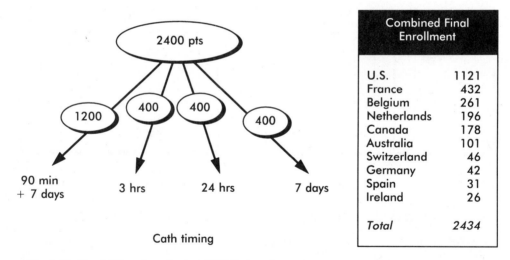

Combined Final Enrollment	
U.S.	1121
France	432
Belgium	261
Netherlands	196
Canada	178
Australia	101
Switzerland	46
Germany	42
Spain	31
Ireland	26
Total	2434

Fig. 7-19. The 2400 patients in the GUSTO-I angiographic substudy were randomized to one of four arms.

ences were present within the first 90 minutes, perhaps indicating that reperfusion arrests the wavefront rather than restores the function of stunned myocardium.

When the angiographic results were correlated with clinical outcome the most striking finding was the strong relationship between initial TIMI grade flow at 90 minutes and the risk of death. The major predictor of survival was TIMI grade 3 flow at 90 minutes. Additionally, as expected, impaired left ventricular function was closely correlated with an increased risk of death.

Net clinical benefit

The previous large studies had led the Steering Committee to expect that if the more aggressive regimens reduced mortality, the trade-off would be an excess risk of strokes. Because stroke after AMI often leads to death, adding the strokes and deaths together would give an exaggerated picture of negative endpoints, so the endpoint of net clinical benefit was defined as freedom from death or nonfatal, disabling stroke. The endpoint of disabling stroke was validated through quality-of-life

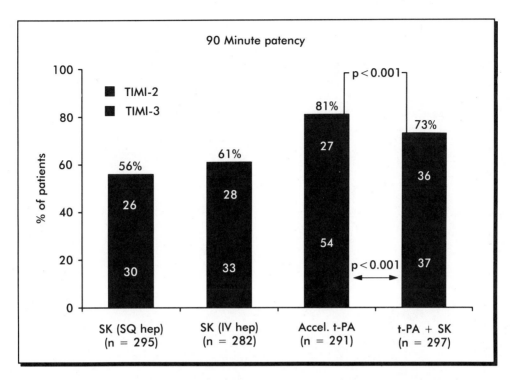

Fig. 7-20. Patients randomized to accelerated t-PA who underwent angiography after 90 minutes had significantly higher rates of patency (TIMI grade 2 and 3 flow) than patients in the other three arms of the GUSTO-I trial, and the difference in TIMI grade 3 flow was significant.

Mortality or stroke

	SK (SubQ)	SK (IV)	t-PA	t-PA & SK
Treated	1000	1000	1000	1000
Deaths	72	74	63	70
Fatal strokes	5 ⎫	6 ⎫	7 ⎫	7 ⎫
Disabling strokes	5 ⎬ 12	5 ⎬ 14	6 ⎬ 16	6 ⎬ 16
Recovered strokes	2 ⎭	3 ⎭	3 ⎭	3 ⎭
Death or stroke	79	82	72	79
Death or disabling stroke	77	79	69	76

Fig. 7-21. The net clinical benefit of t-PA is evident in the bottom line of this figure, where the number of patients who died or suffered a disabling stroke is 8 to 10 fewer per 1000 patients treated than in either SK arm.

Table 7-1. Secondary endpoints in the GUSTO-I trial[1]

Complication	SK and SC heparin (N = 8669)	SK and IV heparin (N = 9260)	Accelerated t-PA and IV heparin (N = 9235)	t-PA + SK and IV heparin (N = 9193)	P value, accelerated t-PA vs. both SK groups
Percentage of patients with:					
Allergic reaction	5.7	5.8	1.6	5.4	<0.001
Anaphylaxis	0.7	0.6	0.2	0.6	<0.001
Congestive heart failure	17.5	16.8	15.2	16.8	<0.001
Cardiogenic shock	6.9	6.3	5.1	6.1	<0.001
Sustained hypotension	13.3	12.5	10.1	12.4	<0.001
Atrioventricular block*	9.5	8.7	7.3	8.4	<0.001
Sustained ventricular tachycardia	6.8	6.5	5.6	6.1	0.001
Ventricular fibrillation	7.1	6.9	6.3	6.9	0.02
Asystole	6	6.4	5.3	6.4	0.003
Atrial fibrillation or flutter	9.9	9.8	8.6	9.1	0.001
Reinfarction	3.4	4	4	4	0.26
Recurrent ischemia	19.9	19.6	19	18.8	0.14
Acute mitral regurgitation	1.6	2.6	1.3	1.4	0.11
Acute VSD	0.5	0.4	0.4	0.6	0.59

*Refers to second- or third-degree block.

measurements. Although t-PA was associated with a significant excess of intracranial hemorrhage, the total stroke rate was only marginally greater and the net clinical benefit was in favor of accelerated t-PA, with 8 to 10 lives saved free of disabling stroke per 1000 patients treated (Fig. 7-21).

Other endpoints

The accelerated t-PA treatment group had fewer arrhythmias, less evidence of left ventricular dysfunction, less systemic bleeding, and fewer allergic manifestations (Table 7-1). As expected, no difference in recurrent ischemia was observed. In essence the secondary clinical endpoints reinforced the congruence among earlier reperfusion, better left ventricular function, and lower mortality.

Economics

The consumption of resources did not differ appreciably in the four treatment arms. A slight excess of bypass surgery in the accelerated t-PA group was offset by the greater need for other procedures in the streptokinase groups. This simplified the cost analysis because the only difference in cost between the treatments was the cost of the drug. Because accelerated t-PA saved 1 life per 100 patients treated and the difference in cost was $2400 per patient in the United States, the cost per life saved is approximately $240,000. The life expectancy of the average GUSTO-I hospital survivor is 10 to 11 years based on previous studies, so the cost per

year of life saved for the average GUSTO-I patient is $20,000 to $25,000. These figures compare favorably with other therapies that have been evaluated and found to be acceptable for practice.

Patient-specific information

Although the subgroup information suggests that the clinical value and cost effectiveness may be somewhat unevenly distributed as a function of individual characteristics, the GUSTO-I database allows for a much more sophisticated evaluation of the degree of treatment benefit. Using the general relationship between baseline characteristics and survival and factoring in the specific effect of time to treatment on the degree of benefit, the expected survival benefit and cost effectiveness for the use of accelerated t-PA in the individual patient can be calculated. With this information the physician, health care system, or society can make a decision about the value of the more expensive but more effective treatment in the individual patient.

Summary

The GUSTO-I trial has solidified the concept that early reperfusion is associated with enhanced survival and better left ventricular function, which also results in fewer complications reflecting arrhythmias and pump dysfunction. This fundamental paradigm is far more important than the specific issue of which drug achieved the desired effect in this trial. In essence the effect of accelerated t-PA may be viewed as a "booster" effect compared with streptokinase. The same relationship is observed with accelerated t-PA and streptokinase in GUSTO-I as with streptokinase and conservative treatment in the FTT. Especially with the clear superiority of TIMI grade 3 flow the goal of current and future therapies is to achieve normal perfusion as quickly as possible in as many patients as possible. As described elsewhere in this book, this goal may be achieved by more rapid administration of t-PA, use of more efficient thrombolytics, efficient use of direct coronary angioplasty, or the development of more effective antithrombin or antiplatelet agents. The most important effort, however, should be the widespread adoption of effective and efficient strategies to identify and treat patients as rapidly as possible.

REFERENCES

1. Reimer KA, Lowe JE, Rasmussen MM, et al: The wave-front phenomenon of ischemic cell death: myocardial infarct size versus duration of coronary occlusion in dogs, *Circulation* 56:786-794, 1977.
2. Rentrop P, Smith H, Painter L, et al: Changes in left ventricular ejection fraction after intracoronary thrombolytic therapy: results of the Registry of the European Society of Cardiology, *Circulation.* 68(suppl I):I-55-I-60, 1983.
3. Yusuf S, Collins R, Peto R, et al: Intravenous and intracoronary fibrinolytic therapy in acute myocardial infarction: overview of results on mortality, reinfarction and side-effects from 33 randomized controlled trials, *Eur Heart J* 6:556-585, 1985.
4. ISIS-2: Randomised trial of intravenous streptokinase, oral aspirin, both, or neither among 17,187 cases of suspected acute myocardial infarction: ISIS-2, *Lancet* 2:349-360, 1988.
5. Gruppo Italiano per lo Studio della Streptochinasi nell'Infarto Miocardico (GISSI): Effectiveness of intravenous thrombolytic treatment in acute myocardial infarction, *Lancet* 1:397-402, 1986.
6. Fibrinolytic Therapy Trialists' (FTT) Collaborative Group: Indications for fibrinolytic therapy in suspected acute myocardial infarction: collaborative overview of early mortality and major morbidity results from all randomised trials of more than 1000 patients, *Lancet* 343:311-322, 1994.
7. ISIS-3 Collaborative Group: ISIS-3: a randomised comparison of streptokinase vs tissue plasminogen activator vs anistreplase and of aspirin plus heparin vs aspirin alone among 41,299 cases of suspected acute myocardial infarction. ISIS-3 (Third International Study of Infarct Survival) Collaborative Group, *Lancet* 339:753-770, 1992.
8. GISSI-2 (Gruppo Italiano per lo Studio della Sopravvivenza nell'Infarto Miocardico): GISSI-2: a factorial randomised trial of alteplase versus streptokinase and heparin versus no heparin among 12,490 patients with acute myocardial infarction, *Lancet* 336:65-71, 1990.
9. Granger CB, Califf RM, Topol EJ: Thrombolytic therapy for acute myocardial infarction. A review, *Drugs* 44:293-325, 1992.
10. Harrison JK, Califf RM, Woodlief LH, et al. and the TAMI Study Group: Systolic left ventricular function after reperfusion therapy for acute myocardial infarction: an analysis of determinants of improvement, *Circulation* 87:1531-1541, 1993.
11. Verani MS, Lacy JL, Guidry GW, et al: Quantification of left ventricular performance during transient coronary occlusion at various anatomic sites in humans: a study using tantalum-178 and a multiwire gamma camera, *J Am Coll Cardiol* 19:297-306, 1992.
12. de Bono DP, Simoons ML, Tijssen J, et al: Effect of early intravenous heparin on coronary patency, infarct size, and bleeding complications after alteplase thrombolysis: results of a randomised double-blind European Cooperative Study Group trial, *Br Heart J* 67:122-128, 1992.
13. Hsia J, Hamilton WP, Kleiman N, et al: A comparison between heparin and low-dose aspirin as adjunctive therapy with tissue plasminogen activator for acute myocardial infarction. Heparin-Aspirin Reperfusion Trial (HART) Investigators, *New Engl J Med* 323:1433-1437, 1990.
14. Bleich SD, Nichols TC, Schumacher RR, et al: Effect of heparin on coronary arterial patency after thrombolysis with tissue plasminogen activator in acute myocardial infarction, *Am J Cardiol* 66:1412-1417, 1990.
15. The GUSTO Investigators: An international randomized trial comparing four thrombolytic strategies for acute myocardial infarction, *New Engl J Med* 329:673-682, 1993.
16. The GUSTO Angiographic Investigators: The effects of tissue plasminogen activator, streptokinase, or both on coronary-artery patency, ventricular function, and survival after acute myocardial infarction, *New Engl J Med* 329:1615-1622, 1993.

Chapter 8

FIBRINOLYTIC SYSTEM: IMPLICATIONS FOR THROMBOLYTIC THERAPY

Désiré Collen
H.R. Lijnen

Mammalian blood contains an enzymatic system, the blood coagulation system, that is responsible for the formation of fibrin, the solid noncellular component of the thrombus. Sequential activation of proteins in the clotting cascade occurs on the surface of various types of blood cells, especially platelets and monocytes, and is counterbalanced by inhibitors. Activation and inhibition of the blood coagulation system occur continuously under physiologic conditions to maintain vascular integrity. Disturbance of the balance of these events may lead to bleeding, in the case of coagulation factor deficiencies, or to thrombosis, in the case of coagulation inhibitor deficiencies.[1]

Human plasma also contains an enzymatic system for the dissolution of fibrin, known as the fibrinolytic system, which is responsible for restoring and maintaining vascular patency after fibrin formation. Although fibrinolysis plays an important role in several biologic processes, such as tissue repair, malignant transformation, macrophage function,[2] and fertility,[3] this chapter focuses on its role in removal of fibrin from the bloodstream.

COMPONENTS OF THE FIBRINOLYTIC SYSTEM

The fibrinolytic system (Fig. 8-1) contains a proenzyme, plasminogen, which, by the action of plasminogen activators, is converted to the active enzyme plasmin, which in turn digests fibrin to soluble degradation products. Inhibition of the fibrinolytic system occurs both at the level of the plasminogen activators, by

plasminogen activator inhibitors (plasminogen activator inhibitor-1 [PAI-1] and plasminogen activator inhibitor-2 [PAI-2]) and at the level of plasmin, mainly by α_2-antiplasmin. The physiologic plasminogen activators, tissue-type plasminogen activator (t-PA) and single-chain urokinase-type plasminogen activator (scu-PA), activate plasminogen preferentially at the fibrin surface. Plasmin, associated with the fibrin surface, is protected from rapid inhibition by α_2-antiplasmin and may thus efficiently degrade the fibrin of a thrombus.[4] These molecular interactions determining the fibrin specificity of fibrinolysis are illustrated in Fig. 8-2 and are discussed further later on in the chapter.

Plasminogen

Human plasminogen is a single-chain glycoprotein with a molecular weight of 92 kD, present in plasma at a concentration of 1.5 to 2 μM. It was reported to consist of 790 amino acids with 24 disulfide bridges, and it contains 5 homologous triple-loop structures, or "kringles."[5] Subsequently, the cDNA sequence revealed the presence of an extra isoleucine at position 85, yielding a total of 791 amino acids in human plasminogen.[6]

Native plasminogen has NH$_2$-terminal glutamic acid ("Glu-plasminogen") but is easily converted by limited plasmic digestion to modified forms with NH$_2$-terminal lysine, valine, or methionine, commonly designated "Lys-plasminogen." This conversion occurs by hydrolysis of the Arg[67]-Met[68], Lys[76]-Lys[77], or Lys[77]-Val[78] peptide

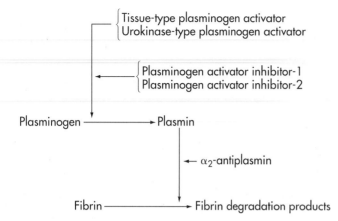

Fig. 8-1. Schematic representation of the fibrinolytic system. The proenzyme plasminogen is activated to the active enzyme plasmin by tissue or urokinase plasminogen activator. Plasmin degrades fibrin into soluble fibrin degradation products. Inhibition of the fibrinolytic system may occur at the level of the plasminogen activators, by plasminogen activator inhibitors, or at the level of plasmin, mainly by α_2-antiplasmin.

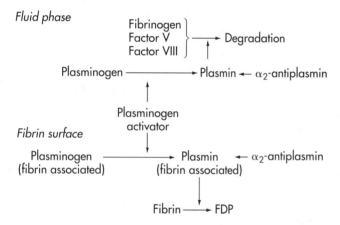

Fig. 8-2. Molecular interactions determining the fibrin specificity of plasminogen activators. Non–fibrin-specific plasminogen activators (streptokinase, urokinase, anisoylated plasminogen–streptokinase activator complex) activate both plasminogen in the fluid phase and fibrin-associated plasminogen. Fibrin-specific plasminogen activators (tissue-type or single-chain urokinase-type plasminogen activator) preferentially activate fibrin-associated plasminogen. *FDP,* Fibrin degradation product.

bonds. Plasminogen is converted to plasmin by cleavage of the Arg[560]-Val[561] peptide bond. The plasmin molecule is a two-chain trypsinlike serine proteinase with an active site composed of His[602], Asp[645], and Ser[740]. The plasminogen molecule contains structures, called lysine-binding sites, that interact specifically with amino acids such as lysine and 6-aminohexanoic acid. These lysine-binding sites mediate the specific binding of plasminogen to fibrin and the interaction of plasmin with α_2-antiplasmin and play a crucial role in the regulation of fibrinolysis.[4]

Plasminogen activators

t-PA. Human t-PA is a serine proteinase with relative molecular mass (M_r) about 70 kD, composed of one polypeptide chain containing 527 amino acids with Ser as the NH$_2$-terminal amino acid[7]; its primary structure is schematically represented in Fig. 8-3. It was subsequently shown that native t-PA contains an NH$_2$-terminal extension of three amino acids, but in general the initial numbering system has been maintained. Limited plasmic hydrolysis of the Arg[275]-Ile[276] peptide bond converts the molecule to a two-chain activator held together by one interchain disulfide bond. The t-PA molecule contains four domains: (1) a 47-residue-long (residues 4-50) amino-terminal region (F domain), which is homologous with the finger domains mediating the fibrin-affinity of fibronectin; (2) residues 50 to 87 (E domain), which are homologous with human epidermal growth factor; (3) two regions comprising residues 87 to 176 and 176 to 262 (K$_1$ and K$_2$ domains), which share a high degree of homology with the five kringles of plasminogen; and (4) a serine proteinase domain (residues 276-527) with the active site residues His[322], Asp[371], and Ser[478].

t-PA is a poor enzyme in the absence of fibrin, but fibrin enhances the activation rate of plasminogen by t-PA by at least two orders of magnitude.[8]

u-PA. scu-PA (prourokinase) is a single-chain glycoprotein with a relative molecular mass (M_r) 54 kD containing 411 amino acids[9]; its primary structure is schematically represented in Fig. 8-4. On limited hydrolysis by plasmin or kallikrein of the Lys[158]-Ile[159] peptide bond, the molecule is converted to a two-chain derivative (tcu-PA, or urokinase).[10] The NH$_2$-terminal chain contains a region homologous to human epidermal growth factor (E; residues 9-45) and one kringle region (K; residues 45-134). The catalytic center is located in the proteinase domain (residues 159-411) and is composed of His[204], Asp[255], and Ser[356]. A low-M_r, two-chain urokinase (M_r 33 kD) can be generated by hydrolysis of the Lys[135]-Lys[136] peptide bond with plasmin. A low-M_r scu-PA with M_r 32 kD (scu-PA-32k) can be obtained by specific hydrolysis of the Glu[143]-Leu[144] peptide bond in scu-PA by an unidentified protease.[11]

scu-PA has a very low reactivity toward low-molecular-weight synthetic substrates or active site inhibitors that are very reactive toward tcu-PA. In mixtures of purified scu-PA and plasminogen, both tcu-PA and plasmin are quickly generated, suggesting that scu-PA has intrinsic plasminogen activating activity. The magnitude of this intrinsic activity is, however, still controversial.[12-14]

Streptokinase and anisoylated plasminogen–streptokinase activator complex. Streptokinase is produced by several strains of hemolytic streptococci; it consists of a single polypeptide chain with M_r 47 to 50 kD and

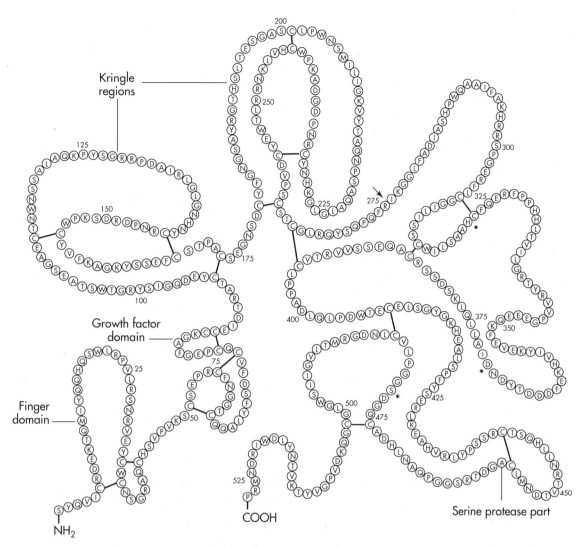

Fig. 8-3. Schematic representation of the primary structure of tissue-type plasminogen activator (t-PA). The amino acids are represented by their single letter symbols, and black bars indicate disulfide bonds. The active site residues His[322], Asp[371], and Ser[478] are indicated with asterisks. The arrow indicates the plasmin cleavage site for conversion of single-chain t-PA to two-chain t-PA.

contains 414 amino acids.[15] Streptokinase cannot directly cleave peptide bonds, but it activates plasminogen to plasmin indirectly, following a three-step mechanism.[16] In the first step, streptokinase forms an equimolar complex with plasminogen. This complex undergoes a conformational change, resulting in the exposure of an active site in the plasminogen moiety. In the second step, this active site catalyzes the activation of plasminogen to plasmin. In a third step, plasminogen-streptokinase molecules are converted to plasmin-streptokinase complex. The active site residues in the plasmin-streptokinase complex are the same as those in the plasmin molecule. However, plasmin is unable to activate plasminogen, whereas the plasmin(ogen)-streptokinase complex is not inhibited by α_2-antiplasmin.

Most individuals have measurable circulating streptokinase-neutralizing antibodies, which may result from previous infections with β-hemolytic streptococci. Therefore, during thrombolytic therapy, sufficient streptokinase must be infused to neutralize those antibodies. A few days after streptokinase administration, the antistreptokinase titer rises rapidly to 50 to 100 times the preinfusion value and remains high for 4 to 6 months, during which period renewed treatment is impracticable.

Anisoylated plasminogen–streptokinase activator complex (APSAC) was constructed with the aim to control the enzymatic activity of the plasmin(ogen)-streptokinase complex by a specific reversible chemical protection of its catalytic center (i.e., by titration with a *p*-anisoyl group).[17] APSAC is an equimolar noncovalent

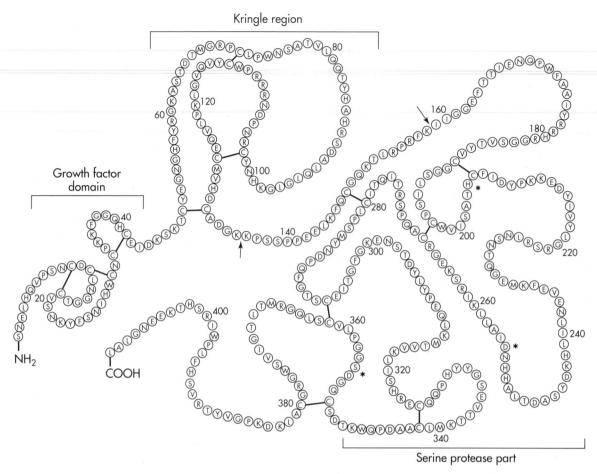

Fig. 8-4. Schematic representation of the primary structure of single-chain urokinase plasminogen activator (scu-PA). The amino acids are represented by their single letter symbols, and black bars indicate disulfide bonds. The active site residues His[204], Asp[255], and Ser[356] are indicated with asterisks. The arrows indicate the plasmin cleavage sites for conversion of relative molecular mass (M_r) 54 kD scu-PA to M_r 54 kD two-chain urokinase-type plasminogen activator (tcu-PA) and of M_r 54 kD tcu-PA to M_r 33 kD tcu-PA.

complex between human Lys-plasminogen and streptokinase, containing the titrated catalytic center and the lysine-binding sites of plasminogen. Reversible acylation of the catalytic center would thus not affect the weak fibrin-binding capacity of Lys-plasminogen in the complex. Deacylation of APSAC, which regenerates the catalytic center, occurs both in the circulation and at the fibrin surface. A plasma half-life of 70 minutes was found for APSAC compared with 25 minutes for the plasminogen-streptokinase complex formed in vivo after administration of streptokinase.[18] Patients with high streptokinase antibody titers do not respond to APSAC, and APSAC causes a marked increase in the streptokinase antibody titer within 2 to 3 weeks, which persists for months.

Staphylokinase. Staphylokinase, an M_r-15.5 kD protein produced by *Staphylococcus aureus,* was shown to have profibrinolytic properties more than 40 years ago.[19]

The gene coding for the bacterial protein has now been cloned and expressed in *Escherichia coli*[20] and *Bacillus subtilis.*[21] Staphylokinase, like streptokinase, forms a stoichiometric complex with plasminogen[22] that activates other plasminogen molecules. Streptokinase and plasminogen produce a complex that exposes the active site in the plasminogen molecule without proteolytic cleavage,[23] whereas the generation of plasmin is required for the exposure of the active site in the complex with staphylokinase.[24] In purified systems, α_2-antiplasmin rapidly inhibits the plasmin-staphylokinase complex, whereas addition of 6-aminohexanoic acid or of fibrin fragments induces a concentration-dependent reduction of the inhibition rate.[25]

Inhibitors of the fibrinolytic system

Inhibition of the fibrinolytic system may occur at the level of plasmin or at the level of the plasminogen activators. α_2-Antiplasmin is the main physiologic plasmin inhibitor in human plasma, whereas inhibition of the physiologic plasminogen activators t-PA and u-PA occurs primarily by PAI-1 and PAI-2.

α_2-Antiplasmin

α_2-Antiplasmin is a single-chain glycoprotein with a molecular weight of 70 kD consisting of 452 amino acids.[26] α_2-Antiplasmin belongs to the *serine proteinase inhibitor* protein family (serpins). Its P_1-P_1' reactive site peptide bond consists of Arg[364]-Met[365]. The concentration of the inhibitor in plasma is about 1 μM. In the presence of calcium ions and activated coagulation factor XIII, α_2-antiplasmin is cross-linked to the fibrin α-chain.[27] This fibrin cross-linking site involves the Gln residue in the second NH_2-terminal position of the inhibitor.

α_2-Antiplasmin forms a 1:1 stoichiometric complex with plasmin that is devoid of protease or esterase activity. The inhibition of plasmin (P) by α_2-antiplasmin (A) can be represented by two consecutive reactions: a fast, second-order reaction producing a reversible inactive complex (PA), which is followed by a slower first-order transition resulting in an irreversible complex (PA'). This model can be represented by

$$P + A \underset{K_{-1}}{\overset{K_1}{\rightleftharpoons}} PA \overset{K_2}{\rightarrow} PA'.$$

The second-order rate constant of the inhibition of plasmin by α_2-antiplasmin ($K_1 = 2$ to $4 \times 10^7 \text{ M}^{-1}\text{s}^{-1}$) is among the fastest protein-protein reactions described.[28] This high inhibition rate constant is dependent on the presence of a free lysine-binding site and active site in the plasmin molecule and of the plasminogen-binding site and the reactive site in the inhibitor.

PAI-1

PAI-1 was first identified in conditioned media of cultured human endothelial cells and rat hepatoma cells and subsequently in plasma, platelets, placenta, and conditioned media of fibrosarcoma cells and hepatocytes (for references see Kruithof[29]). It is a single-chain glycoprotein with M_r about 52 kD consisting of 379 amino acids. The cDNA has been sequenced, revealing that PAI-1 is a member of the serine protease inhibitor (serpin) family. Its reactive site consists of Arg[346]-Met[347].[30,31]

PAI-1 is stabilized by binding to a PAI-binding protein identified as S protein or vitronectin[32]. PAI-1 is the primary inhibitor of both t-PA and u-PA in human plasma.[33,34]

The synthesis or release of PAI-1 from various cells is regulated by several stimuli, including thrombin, dexamethasone, endotoxin, interleukin-1, transforming growth factor-β, and tumor necrosis factor (for references, see Kruithof[29]). PAI-1 levels are elevated in several disease states, including venous thromboembolism, obesity, sepsis, and coronary artery disease.[35]

PAI-2

PAI-2 in plasma occurs most frequently in association with pregnancy, although it has occasionally been identified in men and nonpregnant women[36]; it is also secreted by leukocytes and fibrosarcoma cells. PAI-2 exists in two different forms with comparable inhibition properties: an intracellular nonglycosylated form with M_r 47 kD and isoelectric point (pI) 5.0 and a secreted glycosylated form with M_r 60 kD and pI 4.4 (for references, see Kruithof[29]). The cDNA has been sequenced[37]; PAI-2 is a serpin, containing 393 amino acids with reactive site peptide bond Arg[358]-Thr[359].

PAI-2 inhibits tcu-PA with a second-order rate constant, which is about tenfold slower than that of PAI-1. PAI-2 also efficiently inhibits two-chain t-PA, less efficiently single-chain t-PA, and it does not inhibit scu-PA. Secretion of PAI-2 is regulated by endotoxin and phorbol esters, which stimulate the gene transcription of PAI-2 more than 50-fold (for references, see Kruithof[29]).

MECHANISMS OF FIBRIN-SPECIFIC FIBRINOLYSIS

The physiologic plasminogen activators t-PA and scu-PA dissolve fibrin in a plasma milieu with a high degree of fibrin specificity. The mechanism of fibrin specificity, as detailed later on, is different for both activators. The elucidation of these molecular interactions has triggered great interest in the use of t-PA and scu-PA as thrombolytic agents. The availability of sufficient quantities of both t-PA[38] and scu-PA[39] has aided in their biologic characterization. These properties, summarized in Table 8-1, illustrate that although biochemically and pathophysiologically they are quite distinct, pharmacologically and thrombolytically definite similarities exist. Both have demonstrated absolutely fibrin-specific thrombolysis in numerous animal models and relative clot selectivity in clinical studies.[40-42] Both appear to be cleared rapidly from the circulation via a hepatic route.[43-45]

t-PA

t-PA is a poor enzyme in the absence of fibrin, but the presence of fibrin strikingly enhances the activation rate of plasminogen.[8] In the presence of fibrin, the Michaelis constant equals 0.16 μM compared with 65 μM in the absence of fibrin. The kinetic data of Hoylaerts et al.[8] support a mechanism in which fibrin provides a surface to which t-PA and plasminogen adsorb in a sequential

Table 8-1. Comparative properties of tissue-type plasminogen activator (t-PA) and single-chain urokinase-type plasminogen activator (scu-PA)

Property	t-PA	scu-PA
Fibrin-specific thrombolysis	Relative	Relative
Affinity for fibrin	High	Low
Affinity for plasminogen	Low	High
Stability in plasma	Low	High
Inhibition by plasma	Irreversible	Reversible by fibrin
Function in two-chain form	Similar	Different
Plasma half-life (in vivo)	Biexponential (90% <5 min)	Biexponential (90% <5 min)
Major organ of clearance	Liver	Liver
Role in physiologic fibrinolysis	Responsive	Static

and ordered way, yielding a cyclic ternary complex. Fibrin essentially increases the local plasminogen concentration by creating an additional interaction between t-PA and its substrate. The high affinity of t-PA for plasminogen in the presence of fibrin thus allows efficient activation on the fibrin clot, whereas plasminogen activation by t-PA in plasma is a comparatively inefficient process. Plasmin formed on the fibrin surface has both its lysine-binding sites and active site occupied and is thus only slowly inactivated by α_2-antiplasmin (half-life of about 10 to 100 seconds); in contrast, free plasmin, when formed, is rapidly inhibited by α_2-antiplasmin (half-life of about 0.1 second).[28] However, others have claimed that fibrin influences both the K_m and k_{cat} of the activation of plasminogen by t-PA.[46]

It was proposed that initial binding of t-PA to fibrin would be governed by the finger domain and that partial degradation of fibrin would result in enhanced binding of t-PA via kringle 2 to newly exposed COOH-terminal lysine residues.[47] Early fibrin digestion by plasmin may accelerate fibrinolysis by increasing the binding of both t-PA and plasminogen. The fibrinolytic process thus seems to be triggered by and confined to fibrin.

u-PA

Two-chain urokinase-type plasminogen activator (tcu-PA) has no fibrin specificity and activates fibrin-bound and circulating plasminogen relatively indiscriminately. Extensive plasminogen activation and depletion of α_2-antiplasmin may occur after treatment of patients with thromboembolic disease with tcu-PA, leading to degradation of several plasma proteins, including fibrinogen, factor V, and factor VIII (see Fig. 8-2).

scu-PA, in contrast to tcu-PA, has a significant fibrin specificity. Several hypotheses for the mechanism of plasminogen activation and fibrin specificity of clot lysis with scu-PA in a plasma milieu have been proposed. One hypothesis claims that scu-PA is inactive toward circulating native plasminogen (Glu-plasminogen) but active toward conformationally altered plasminogen (Lys-plasminogen) bound to partially digested fibrin.[48] Second, scu-PA has been proposed to be a genuine proenzyme with negligible activity toward plasminogen,[13] and fibrinolysis with scu-PA would thus depend entirely on generation of tcu-PA. Alternatively, scu-PA was claimed to have some intrinsic plasminogen-activating potential counteracted by a competitive inhibitory mechanism in plasma, that is, reversed by fibrin.[12] Studies in human plasma in vitro have suggested that conversion of scu-PA to tcu-PA during clot lysis constitutes a primary positive feedback system, whereas binding of plasminogen to fibrin or predigestion of fibrin by plasmin was found to result in relatively minor additional acceleration of fibrinolysis.[12] The observation that plasmin-resistant mutants of scu-PA (i.e., scu-PA K158E) have only a threefold to fivefold lower in vivo thrombolytic potency compared with wild-type scu-PA[49] suggests that for in vivo thrombolysis conversion of scu-PA to tcu-PA may play a less important role.

Staphylokinase

In contrast to streptokinase, the bacterial protein staphylokinase induces clot lysis in a citrated human plasma milieu without associated fibrinogen breakdown.[25,50] In animal models of venous thrombosis, staphylokinase was shown to be an efficient thrombolytic agent, with a potency comparable with that of streptokinase.[51]

The following mechanism for the relatively fibrin-specific clot lysis with staphylokinase in a plasma milieu has been proposed.[25,50] In plasma in the absence of fibrin, the plasminogen-staphylokinase complex is rapidly neutralized by α_2-antiplasmin, thus preventing systemic plasminogen activation. In the presence of fibrin, the plasminogen-staphylokinase complex binds via the lysine-binding sites of the plasminogen moiety to the clot. Thereby its inhibition rate by α_2-antiplasmin is reduced 130-fold (t½ prolonged from 0.26 to 35 seconds), allowing preferential plasminogen activation at the fibrin surface.[25] However, staphylokinase also dissociates in active form from the plasmin-staphylokinase complex after neutralization by α_2-antiplasmin and may be recycled.[52] In the absence of fibrin, no significant amounts of active plasmin-staphylokinase complex in plasma are formed, which contributes to the absence of extensive systemic plasminogen activation in plasma. Fibrin both facilitates generation of the plasmin-staphylokinase complex and delays its inhibition at the clot surface.[53]

IMPLICATIONS FOR THROMBOLYSIS
IN ACUTE MYOCARDIAL INFARCTION

The recognition that thrombosis within the infarct-related coronary artery plays a major role in the pathogenesis of acute myocardial infarction[54] and the observation that early administration of thrombolytic agents results in recanalization of occluded coronary arteries[55] have provided the basis for the development of thrombolytic therapy in acute myocardial infarction. The hypothesis underlying this form of treatment is that coronary artery occlusion leads to ischemia and cell death, resulting in ventricular dysfunction and reduced life expectancy, and that timely recanalization prevents cell death, reduces infarct size, preserves myocardial function, and reduces early and late mortality. The most rational treatment of patients with acute myocardial infarction is therefore likely to be thrombolytic therapy with agents or combinations that produce stable coronary artery recanalization as frequently and as rapidly as possible with an acceptable safety. Several observations suggest that late opening of an occluded coronary artery may still have some beneficial effect. Indeed, late reperfusion may limit left ventricular remodeling, improve the electrical stability of the heart, or provide collateral vessels to viable myocardium.[56] Furthermore, adjunctive therapy with anticoagulant or antiplatelet agents may contribute to the efficacy of thrombolysis.[57]

The elucidation of the mechanism of fibrin-specific plasminogen activation has fueled the hope that more specific and efficacious thrombolysis might be achieved. The use of non-fibrin-specific agents, such as streptokinase or urokinase, has indeed required doses high enough to generate free plasmin in the circulation, which is possible only after exhaustive plasminogen activation, leading to α_2-antiplasmin depletion and fibrinogen breakdown, the so-called lytic state. The major concerns with this mode of therapy have been a lower efficacy of coronary arterial thrombolysis as a result of plasminogen "steal" at the fibrin surface[58,59] and the potential predisposition toward bleeding associated with breakdown of the hemostatic system.[60,61]

Implications of fibrin specificity
for efficacy of coronary thrombolysis

Comparative studies between the non-fibrin-selective streptokinase and fibrin-selective rt-PA have indeed shown a difference in efficacy for early coronary artery recanalization,[62] and this conclusion has been supported by results of several noncomparative studies with similar design and endpoints (for references see Collen[63]). Coronary artery patency is present in approximately 22% of patients within 90 minutes after the start of placebo infusion (usually heparin and occasionally aspirin), probably around 35% after 24 to 48 hours and around 65% after 1 to 3 weeks. Streptokinase adminis-

tration is associated with around 53% patency at 90 minutes and 75% after 1 to 3 weeks, whereas rt-PA given as a "standard" 100-mg infusion over 3 hours in combination with intravenous heparin is associated with 75% patency at 90 minutes, 85% at 24 to 48 hours, and 81% at 1 to 3 weeks.[64] Thus, early patency, measured around 90 minutes after the start of therapy, is significantly increased over placebo (22%) with both streptokinase (53%) and "standard" rt-PA (75%), whereas the efficacy for coronary recanalization with rt-PA is about 50% higher than with streptokinase. This difference between rt-PA and streptokinase is observed in patients with both early (<3 hours) and later (3 to 6 hours) initiation of thrombolytic therapy.[62,64]

Two megatrials directly comparing streptokinase and rt-PA, the International t-PA/SK Mortality Trial (GISSI/Int)[65] and the ISIS-3 study,[66] have not shown a difference in survival. This lack of correlation between initial efficacy and clinical outcome may have several explanations: (1) the simplified protocols with delayed subcutaneous administration of heparin, as used in the megatrials, may have blunted the differences in efficacy between thrombolytic agents[67-70] and thereby the demonstration of potential differences in mortality; (2) delayed recanalization, which after a catch-up phenomenon over several hours occurs to a comparable extent with both streptokinase and rt-PA, may be a major contributor to clinical benefit; or (3) there may be no direct correlation between early recanalization and clinical benefit, but other (unknown) mechanisms may be major contributors.

Because of the uncertainties about the design and monitoring of the GISSI/Int[65] and the ISIS-3[66] trials, the recently reported GUSTO trial (Global Utilization of Streptokinase and rt-PA for the treatment of occluded coronary arteries) was undertaken.[71] In the GUSTO trial, 4 randomized groups of approximately 10,000 patients each were studied: treatment with streptokinase plus either subcutaneous or intravenous heparin, accelerated rt-PA[72] plus intravenous heparin, and a combination of streptokinase and rt-PA plus intravenous heparin. To define the correlation between early patency and clinical outcome, an angiographic substudy was performed in approximately 2400 patients.

The primary endpoint of the study, 30-day mortality, was lower with accelerated rt-PA and intravenous heparin than with streptokinase plus either intravenous or subcutaneous heparin. Because there were no significant differences in outcome between the two groups receiving streptokinase plus intravenous or subcutaneous heparin, these data are pooled in Table 8-2. Thus, 30-day mortality was 6.3% in 10,344 patients treated with rt-PA compared with 7.3% in 20,172 patients receiving streptokinase ($P = 0.001$). The combination of streptokinase and rt-PA did not result in improved 30-day mortality rate (7.0% in 10,327 patients) compared with streptokinase. The relative mortality reduction with accelerated rt-PA and intravenous heparin was 14% for the trial as a whole and was even more pronounced in patients randomized within 2 hours of the onset of symptoms (mortality of 5.4% in 5350 patients receiving rt-PA compared with 6.5% in 10,644 patients treated with streptokinase). The incidence of stroke was higher in the rt-PA group compared with both streptokinase groups combined (see Table 8-2).

However, the net clinical benefit was greater with accelerated rt-PA plus intravenous heparin than with streptokinase: death or stroke in 7.2% of patients treated with rt-PA compared with 8.1% in both streptokinase groups combined (see Table 8-2). Preliminary data from the angiographic substudy demonstrated that induction of patency within 90 minutes (TIMI flow grade 2 or 3) was more frequent in the rt-PA group (81% of 291 patients) than in both streptokinase groups combined (58% of 577 patients; $P < 0.001$ vs. the rt-PA group) (see Table 8-2). Induction of patency (TIMI flow grade 2 or 3) within 90 minutes was correlated with survival in all the treatment groups.

The relative risk of dying after streptokinase vs. rt-PA in the GUSTO trial was 1.17 (95% confidence interval: 1.06 to 1.28). In the combined GISSI/International and ISIS-3 studies, this relative risk was 1.00 (95% confidence interval 0.94 to 1.06) (Table 8-3). The lack of overlap between these confidence intervals suggests that accelerated rt-PA plus intravenous heparin in the GUSTO trial had a significantly greater effect on 30- to 35-day mortality than standard rt-PA with delayed subcutaneous heparin, as used in these two previous megatrials. Furthermore, homogeneity testing of the relative risk in GISSI/International vs. ISIS-3 vs. GUSTO yields a P value of 0.012, which precludes metaanalysis of the combined data of the three studies.

The data of the GUSTO trial thus establish that clinical benefit in patients with acute myocardial infarction is correlated with the rapidity and frequency of sustained recanalization and that effective thrombolysis requires adequate anticoagulation. The hypothesis that early recanalization is a major determinant of clinical outcome, which was challenged in the previous megatrials, thus seems to be conclusively validated by the results of the GUSTO trial.

Implications of fibrin specificity for bleeding complications

The implications of fibrin-specific thrombolytic therapy for bleeding complications are less clear. Theoretically the ability to promote efficient plasminogen activation while sparing degradation of circulating blood coagulation components might afford protection against hemorrhagic events. In line with this hypothesis most major trials have found that the risk of systemic bleeding

Table 8-2. Comparative data obtained in the GUSTO trial with accelerated recombinant tissue-type plasminogen activator (rt-PA) plus intravenous heparin or with streptokinase plus either subcutaneous or intravenous heparin

	Streptokinase		rt-PA		
	%	No.	%	No.	P
Mortality (30 days)	7.3	20,172	6.3	10,344	0.001
Stroke	1.31	20,023	1.55	10,268	0.0091
ICB	0.52	20,023	0.72	10,268	0.03
Death or stroke	8.1	20,173	7.2	10,344	0.006
Coronary patency					
TIMI 2 + 3 (90 minutes)	58	577	71	291	<0.001
(180 minutes)	75	198	77	95	NS
TIMI 3 (90 minutes)	31	577	54	291	<0.001

Data presented at the AFCR meeting, Washington DC, April 30, 1993.

Table 8-3. Thirty- to 35-day mortality in GISSI/Int, ISIS-3, and GUSTO*

	SK	t-PA	RR (95% CI)
GISSI/Int	958 (10,067)	993 (10,028)	0.96 (0.87-1.05)
ISIS-3	1455 (13,780)	1418 (13,746)	1.03 (0.95-1.11)
Combined			1.00 (0.94-1.06)
GUSTO	1471 (20,172)	652 (10,344)	1.17 (1.06-1.28)

*Homogeneity test: GISSI/Int vs. ISIS-3: p = 0.26; GISSI/Int vs. ISIS-3 vs. GUSTO: p = 0.012.

with fibrin-specific t-PA has been significantly although not dramatically lower than with non–fibrin-specific streptokinase. However, the causes of bleeding are multiple and complex. Moreover, the lysis of fibrin will occur, even during fibrin specific therapy, at all vascular sites where thrombus formation is ongoing. Thus, it can be anticipated that lysis of the pathologic thrombus will not necessarily be achieved in the absence of lysis of the physiologic thrombus as would occur at a vascular access site.

The frequency of intracranial bleeding in the International t-PA/SK Mortality Study[65] and ISIS-3[66] deserves some comment. Indeed, the frequency of cerebral bleeding, as defined in these studies, was identical at 0.3% in both streptokinase groups. The frequency of intracerebral bleeding with 100 mg of alteplase in the International t-PA/SK mortality trial was 0.4% ($P = \mathrm{NS}$) and with 0.6M clot lysis units of duteplase/kg of body weight in ISIS-3 was 0.7% ($P < 0.001$). The difference in cerebral bleeding rates between these studies thus appears to be due primarily to a difference between duteplase and alteplase and not between alteplase and streptokinase.

A dose of 0.6M clot lysis units of duteplase/kg of body weight corresponds to 2 mg/kg of body weight. For the average 75-kg patient, this would correspond to a total dose of 45 megaunits, or 150 mg. Based on the activity of both preparations in the standard clot lysis assay, the 45-megaunit dose of duteplase, given to the 75-kg patient in ISIS-3, would appear to be somewhat underdosed relative to the 58 megaunits contained in 100 mg of alteplase. However, based on the gravimetric amount of material given in ISIS-3, the average dose of 150 mg of duteplase would be clearly overdosed relative to the 100-mg alteplase dose. In the absence of directly comparative studies between alteplase and duteplase, their equivalence in either clot lysis units or amount remains enigmatic.

The TIMI-2 trial showed that 150 mg of alteplase, given in combination with intravenous heparin, was associated with an intracerebral bleeding rate of 1.6%.[73] This observation caused cessation of the testing of the 150-mg dose after several hundred patients and a worldwide reduction of the dose to a maximum 100 mg. In view of these earlier events, it is most surprising that the ISIS-3 trial, which was initially planned to enter 30,000 patients, was extended to 45,000 patients without a protocol change.

In the GUSTO trial,[71] the incidence of intracerebral bleeding was somewhat higher in the patients treated with t-PA (0.72% of 10,268 patients) compared with patients receiving streptokinase (0.52% of 20,023 patients; $P = 0.03$), suggesting that the combination of accelerated alteplase with aspirin and intravenous heparin may be associated with a modestly higher degree of

intracranial hemorrhage (or conversion of ischemic to hemorrhagic stroke) than the combination of streptokinase and aspirin with subcutaneous or intravenous heparin (see Table 8-2).

CONCLUSIONS

The clinical benefit of thrombolytic therapy in patients with acute myocardial infarction is well established, and the GUSTO trial has documented a close correlation between early coronary artery recanalization and clinical outcome. Further studies at both the basic mechanistic and the clinical outcome level will help define the optimal thrombolytic regimen in terms of thrombolytic agent and conjunctive anticoagulant or antiplatelet agents. Indeed, thrombolytic therapy can no longer be considered as a monotherapy with a single thrombolytic agent but must consist of conjunctive use of thrombolytic, anticoagulant, and antiplatelet agents.

REFERENCES

1. Mann KG, Fass DN: The molecular biology of blood coagulation. In Fairbanks VF (ed): *Current hematology II,* Somerset, NJ, 1983, John Wiley & Sons, p 347.
2. Reich E: Plasminogen activator: secretion by neoplastic cells and macrophages. In Reich E, Rifkin DB, Shaw E (eds): *Proteases and biological control,* Cold Spring Harbor, NY, 1975, Cold Spring Harbor Laboratory, p 333.
3. Strickland S: Studies on the role of plasminogen activator in ovulation and early embryogenesis. In Magnusson S, Ottesen M, Foltman B, et al (eds): *Regulatory proteolytic enzymes and their inhibitors,* New York, Pergamon Press, 1978, pp 181-185.
4. Collen D: On the regulation and control of fibrinolysis, *Thromb Haemost* 43:77-89, 1980.
5. Dayhoff MO (ed): *Atlas of protein sequence and structure,* Washington DC, 1978, National Biomedical Research Foundation, vol 5, supplement 3, p 91.
6. Forsgren M, Raden B, Israelsson M, et al: Molecular cloning and characterization of a full-length cDNA clone for human plasminogen, *FEBS Lett* 213:254-260, 1987.
7. Pennica D, Holmes WE, Kohr WJ, et al: Cloning and expression of human tissue-type plasminogen activator cDNA in *E. coli, Nature* 301:214-221, 1983.
8. Hoylaerts M, Rijken DC, Lijnen HR, et al: Kinetics of the activation of plasminogen by human tissue plasminogen activator. Role of fibrin, *J Biol Chem* 257:2912-2919, 1982.
9. Holmes WE, Pennica D, Blaber M, et al: Cloning and expression of the gene for prourokinase in *Escherichia coli, Biotechnology* 3:923-929, 1985.
10. Günzler WA, Steffens GJ, Ötting F, et al: Structural relationship between human high and low molecular mass urokinase, Hoppe-Seyler's Z. *Physiol Chem* 363:133-141, 1982.
11. Stump DC, Lijnen HR, Collen D: Purification and characterization of a novel low molecular weight form of single-chain urokinase-type plasminogen activator, *J Biol Chem* 261:17120-17126, 1986.
12. Lijnen HR, Van Hoef B, De Cock F, et al: The mechanism of plasminogen activation and fibrin dissolution by single chain urokinase-type plasminogen activator in a plasma milieu in vitro, *Blood* 73:1864-1872, 1989.
13. Husain SS: Single-chain urokinase-type plasminogen activator does not possess measurable intrinsic amidolytic or plasminogen activator activities, *Biochemistry* 30:5797-5805, 1991.
14. Manchanda N, Schwartz BS: Single chain urokinase. Augmenta-

tion of enzymatic activity upon binding to monocytes, *J Biol Chem* 266:14580-14584, 1991.

15. Jackson KW, Tang J: Complete amino acid sequence of streptokinase and its homology with serine proteases, *Biochemistry* 21:6620-6625, 1982.

16. Reddy KNN: Mechanism of activation of human plasminogen by streptokinase. In Kline DL, Reddy KNN (eds.): *Fibrinolysis,* Boca Raton, Fla, 1980, CRC Press, pp 71-94.

17. Smith RAG, Dupe RJ, English PD, et al: Fibrinolysis with acyl-enzymes: a new approach to thrombolytic therapy, *Nature* 290:505-508, 1981.

18. Staniforth DH, Smith RAG, Hibbs M: Streptokinase and anisoylated streptokinase plasminogen complex. Their action on haemostasis in human volunteers, *Eur J Clin Pharmacol* 24:751-756, 1983.

19. Lack CH: Staphylokinase: an activator of plasma protease, *Nature* 161:559-560, 1948.

20. Sako T: Overproduction of staphylokinase in *Escherichia coli* and its characterization, *Eur J Biochem* 149:557-563, 1985.

21. Behnke D, Gerlach D: Cloning and expression in *Escherichia coli, Bacillus subtilis* and *Streptococcus sanguis* of a gene for staphylokinase—a bacterial plasminogen activator, *Molec Gen Genet* 210:528-534, 1987.

22. Kowalska-Loth B, Zakrzewski K: The activation by staphylokinase of human plasminogen, *Acta Biochim Pol* 22:327-339, 1975.

23. Collen D, Schlott B, Engelborghs Y, et al: On the mechanism of the activation of human plasminogen by recombinant staphylokinase, *J Biol Chem* 268:8284-8289, 1993.

24. McClintock DK, Bell PH: The mechanisms of activation of human plasminogen by streptokinase, *Biochem Biophys Res Commun* 43:694-702, 1971.

25. Lijnen HR, Van Hoef B, De Cock F, et al: On the mechanism of fibrin-specific plasminogen activation by staphylokinase, *J Biol Chem* 266:11826-11832 1991.

26. Holmes WE, Nelles L, Lijnen HR, et al: Primary structure of human α_2-antiplasmin, a serine protease inhibitor (serpin), *J Biol Chem* 262:1659-1664, 1987.

27. Ichinose A, Tamaki T, Aoki N: Factor XIII-mediated cross-linking of NH$_2$-terminal peptide of α_2-plasmin inhibitor to fibrin, *FEBS Lett* 153:369-371, 1983.

28. Wiman B, Collen D: On the kinetics of the reaction between human antiplasmin and plasmin, *Eur J Biochem* 84:573-578, 1978.

29. Kruithof EKO: Plasminogen activator inhibitors—a review, *Enzyme* 40:113-121, 1988.

30. Ny T, Sawdey M, Lawrence D, et al: Cloning and sequence of a cDNA coding for the human β-migrating endothelial-cell-type plasminogen activator inhibitor, *Proc Natl Acad Sci USA* 83:6776-6780, 1986.

31. Pannekoek H, Veerman H, Lambers H, et al: Endothelial plasminogen activator inhibitor (PAI): a new member of the serpin gene family, *EMBO J* 5:2539-2544, 1986.

32. Declerck PJ, De Mol M, Alessi MC, et al: Purification and characterization of a plasminogen activator inhibitor-1 binding protein from human plasma. Identification as a multimeric form of S protein (Vitronectin), *J Biol Chem* 263:15454-15461, 1988.

33. Kruithof EKO, Tran-Thang C, Ransijn A, et al: Demonstration of a fast-acting inhibitor of plasminogen activators in human plasma, *Blood* 64:907-913, 1984.

34. Juhan-Vague I, Moerman B, De Cock F, et al: Plasma levels of a specific inhibitor of tissue-type plasminogen activator (and urokinase) in normal and pathological conditions, *Thromb Res* 33:523-530, 1984.

35. Wiman B, Hamsten A: The fibrinolytic enzyme system and its role in the etiology of thromboembolic disease, *Semin Thromb Haemost* 16:207-216, 1990.

36. Lecander I, Astedt B: Occurrence of a specific plasminogen

activator inhibitor of placental type, PAI-2, in men and non-pregnant women, *Fibrinolysis* 3:27-30, 1989.

37. Ye RD, Wun TC, Sadler JE: cDNA cloning and expression in *Escherichia coli* of a plasminogen activator inhibitor from human placenta, *J Biol Chem* 262:3718-3725, 1987.

38. Rijken DC, Collen D: Purification and characterization of the plasminogen activator secreted by human melanoma cells in culture, *J Biol Chem* 256:7035-7041, 1981.

39. Stump DC, Lijnen HR, Collen D: Purification and characterization of single-chain urokinase-type plasminogen activator from human cell cultures, *J Biol Chem* 261:1274-1278, 1986.

40. Collen D: Human tissue-type plasminogen activator: from the laboratory to the bedside, *Circulation* 72:18-20, 1985.

41. Stump DC, Lijnen HR, Collen D: Biochemical and biological properties of single-chain urokinase-type plasminogen activator, *Cold Spring Harbor Symp Quant Biol* 51:563-569, 1986.

42. Collen D, Lijnen HR, Todd PA, et al: Tissue-type plasminogen activator. A review of its pharmacology and therapeutic use as a thrombolytic agent, *Drugs* 38:346-388, 1989.

43. Korninger C, Stassen JM, Collen D: Turnover of human extrinsic (tissue-type) plasminogen activator in rabbits, *Thromb Haemost* 46:658-661, 1981.

44. Collen D, De Cock F, Lijnen HR: Biological and thrombolytic properties of proenzyme and active forms of human urokinase: II. Turnover of natural and recombinant urokinase in rabbits and squirrel monkeys, *Thromb Haemost* 24:24-26, 1984.

45. Stump DC, Kieckens L, De Cock F, et al: Pharmacokinetics of single-chain forms of urokinase-type plasminogen activator, *J Pharmacol Exp Ther* 242:245-250, 1987.

46. Nieuwenhuizen W, Voskuilen M, Vermond A, et al: The influence of fibrin(ogen) fragments on the kinetic parameters of the tissue-type plasminogen-activator-mediated activation of different forms of plasminogen, *Eur J Biochem* 174:163-169, 1988.

47. van Zonneveld AJ, Veerman H, Pannekoek H: On the interaction of the finger and kringle-2 domain of tissue-type plasminogen activator with fibrin, *J Biol Chem* 261:14214-14218, 1986.

48. Pannell R, Gurewich V: Pro-urokinase: a study of its stability in plasma and of a mechanism for its selective fibrinolytic effect, *Blood* 67:1215-1223, 1986.

49. Collen D, Mao J, Stassen JM, et al: Thrombolytic properties of Lys-158 mutants of recombinant single chain urokinase-type plasminogen activator (scu-PA) in rabbits with jugular vein thrombosis, *J Vasc Med Biol* 1:46-49, 1989.

50. Matsuo O, Okada K, Fukao H, et al: Thrombolytic properties of staphylokinase, *Blood* 76:925-929, 1990.

51. Lijnen HR, Stassen JM, Vanlinthout I, et al: Comparative fibrinolytic properties of staphylokinase and streptokinase in animal models of venous thrombosis, *Thromb Haemost* 66:468-473, 1991.

52. Silence K, Collen D, Lijnen HR: Interaction between staphylokinase, plasmin(ogen) and α_2-antiplasmin. Recycling of staphylokinase after neutralization of the plasmin-staphylokinase complex by α_2-antiplasmin, *J Biol Chem* 268:9811-9816, 1993.

53. Silence K, Collen D, Lijnen HR: Regulation by α_2-antiplasmin and fibrin of the activation of plasminogen with recombinant staphylokinase in plasma, *Blood* 82:AA75-AA83, 1993.

54. De Wood MA, Spores J, Notske R, et al: Prevalence of total coronary occlusion during the early hours of transmural myocardial infarction, *N Engl J Med* 303:897-902, 1980.

55. Rentrop KP: Thrombolytic therapy in patients with acute myocardial infarction, *Circulation* 71:627-631, 1985.

56. Braunwald E: Myocardial reperfusion, limitation of infarct size, reduction of left ventricular dysfunction, and improved survival. Should the paradigm be expanded? *Circulation* 79:441-444, 1989

57. Gold HK: Conjunctive antithrombotic and thrombolytic therapy for coronary-artery occlusion, *N Engl J Med* 323:1483-1485, 1990.

58. Sabovic M, Lijnen HR, Keber D, et al: Effect of retraction on the lysis of human clots with fibrin specific and non-fibrin specific plasminogen activators, *Thromb Haemost* 62:1083-1087, 1989.

59. Sobel BE, Nachowiak DA, Fry ETA, et al: Paradoxical attenuation of fibrinolysis attributable to "plasminogen steal" and its implications for coronary thrombolysis, *Coron Art Dis* 1:111-119, 1990.

60. Verstraete M: A far-reaching program: rapid, safe and predictable thrombolysis in man. In Kline DL, Reddy KNN (eds): *Fibrinolysis,* Boca Raton, Fla, 1980, CRC Press, p 129.

61. Duckert F: Urokinase. In Markwardt F (ed): *Fibrinolytics and antifibrinolytics,* New York, 1978, Springer-Verlag New York, p 209.

62. Chesebro JH, Knatterud G, Braunwald E: Thrombolytic therapy [correspondence], *N Engl J Med* 319:1544-1545, 1988.

63. Collen D: Coronary thrombolysis: streptokinase or recombinant tissue-type plasminogen activator? *Ann Intern Med* 112:529-538, 1990.

64. Collen D: On the future of thrombolytic therapy in acute myocardial infarction. In Haber E, Braunwald E (eds): *Thrombolysis: basic contributions and clinical progress,* St Louis, 1991, Mosby, pp 315-331.

65. International Study Group: In-hospital mortality and clinical course of 20,891 patients with suspected acute myocardial infarction randomised between alteplase and streptokinase with or without heparin, *Lancet* 336:71-75, 1990.

66. ISIS-3 (Third International Study of Infarct Survival) Collaborative Group: A randomised comparison of streptokinase vs tissue plasminogen activator vs anistreplase and of aspirin plus heparin vs aspirin alone among 41,299 cases of suspected acute myocardial infarction, *Lancet* 339:753-770, 1992.

67. Topol EJ, George BS, Kereiakes DJ, et al: A randomized controlled trial of intravenous tissue plasminogen activator and early intravenous heparin in acute myocardial infarction, *Circulation* 79:281-286, 1989.

68. Hsia J, Hamilton WP, Kleiman N, et al: A comparison between heparin and low-dose aspirin as adjunctive therapy with tissue plasminogen activator for acute myocardial infarction, *N Engl J Med* 323:1433-1437 1990.

69. Bleich SD, Nichols TC, Schumacher RR, et al: Effect of heparin on coronary arterial patency after thrombolysis with tissue plasminogen activator in acute myocardial infarction, *Am J Cardiol* 66:1412-1417, 1990.

70. de Bono DP, Simoons ML, Tijssen J, et al: Effect of early intravenous heparin on coronary patency, infarct size, and bleeding complications after alteplase thrombolysis: results of a randomised double blind European Cooperative Study Group trial, *Br Heart J* 67:122-128, 1992.

71. The GUSTO Investigators: An international randomized trial comparing four thrombolytic strategies for acute myocardial infarction, *N Engl J Med* 329:673-682, 1993.

72. Neuhaus KL, von Essen R, Tebbe U, et al: Improved thrombolysis in acute myocardial infarction with front-loaded administration of alteplase: results of the rt-PA-APSAC patency study (TAPS), *J Am Coll Cardiol* 19:885-891, 1992.

73. The TIMI Study Group: The Thrombolysis in Myocardial Infarction (TIMI) trial: phase I findings, *N Engl J Med* 312:932-936, 1985.

Chapter 9

ROLE OF PLATELET AND CLOTTING FACTORS

IK-Kyung Jang
Herman K. Gold
Valentin Fuster

Acute ischemic coronary syndromes (acute myocardial infarction, unstable angina pectoris, and sudden ischemic death) have as their common underlying pathologic condition rupture of atherosclerotic plaque with intraluminal thrombus formation.[1-6] This thrombus may embolize and cause sudden ischemic death[7-10] or progressively encroach the coronary arterial lumen to cause unstable angina pectoris[3,10,11] or acute myocardial infarction[12-14] (Fig. 9-1). The rupture is caused by a tear of the thin fibrous "cap" separating the fatty material of a soft atheromatous plaque, or "abscess," from the arterial lumen. The exact mechanism of plaque rupture is unknown: it may include ulceration by shear forces engendered by hypertension, changes in coronary tone or turbulent flow at the stenosis, or disruption of ingrown vasa vasorum, causing intraplaque hemorrhage and plaque expansion.[5] It may just be an incidental event in the evolution and growth of the atherosclerotic plaque, which occurs when the cap has become thinned to the extent that normal hemodynamic stresses may fragment it.[3] Another explanation for plaque rupture has been the belief that macrophages release enzymes, which digest collagen and elastin, and thereby weaken the cap. Then, several events may occur: (1) the contents of the atheromatous abscess may discharge into the lumen and embolize distally; (2) blood from the lumen may enter into the plaque and cause intraplaque hemorrhage; (3) platelet aggregation may occur at the site of the rupture, leading to peripheral embolization of platelet clumps or progression toward luminal occlusion; and (4) the occlusive thrombus may propagate both proximally and distally.[3,5,13] The composition of the intraluminal thrombus formed in association with plaque rupture depends to a significant extent on whether plaque material extends into the lumen or whether blood leaks into the abscess cavity.[13] In the latter case, the thrombi usually appear to be homogeneous in structure and consist of red blood cells with a few atheromatous elements, platelets, and fibrin strands. In the former case the thrombus usually consists of distinct zones, a "head" and "body" and frequently also a "tail." The body, which is contiguous to the area of plaque rupture, consists predominantly of aggregated platelets with scattered red blood cells, components derived from the atheroma and strands of fibrin. The head, which occupies the lumen proximal to the area of wall fracture, and the distally extending tail are composed almost entirely of red blood cells and fibrin (Fig. 9-2).

Intravenous thrombolysis has become a standard therapy for acute myocardial infarction.[15-19] However, this thrombolytic therapy has several problems: failure rate of 20% to 25%, delay in time to reperfusion (averaging 45 minutes), and high reocclusion rate.[20-25] This is not surprising in view of the heterogeneous composition of the coronary thrombus, which comprises zones of platelet-rich material, which may be more resistant to dissolution than erythrocyte-rich zones. Moreover, platelets play a crucial role in mediating acute reocclusion after initial successful thrombolysis. Indeed, platelet aggregates formed in plasma are much more

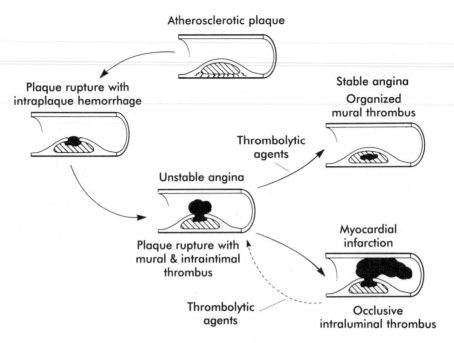

Fig. 9-1. Diagram of the pathogenesis of ischemic syndromes. (From Gold HK, Johns JA, Leinbach RC, et al: *J Am Coll Cardiol* 10:91B-95B, 1987. Used by permission.)

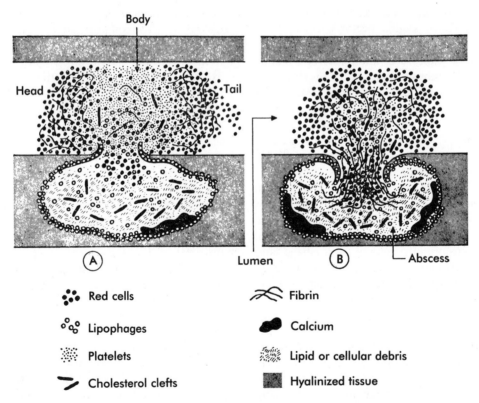

Fig. 9-2. Mechanism of platelet-rich and fibrin-rich thrombus. **A,** exposure of atheromatous abscess contents into the lumen leads a platelet-rich thrombus in the body with fibrin and erythrocyte components in the head and tail portions of the thrombus. **B,** collapse of atheromatous capsule into the abscess predisposes the homogenous fibrin- and erythrocyte-rich thrombus. (From Friedman M, Van den Bovenkamp GJ: *Am J Pathol* 48:19-44, 1966. Used by permission.)

resistant to dispersion than whole blood clots by activation of the fibrinolytic system.[26,27] Similar phenomenon was observed in in vivo experiments.[28] These observations suggest that these problems might be able to be overcome by the addition of platelet-blocking agents or thrombin inhibitors.

This chapter is divided into three sections: pathophysiology of acute thrombotic occlusion of coronary artery and reocclusion after reperfusion, thrombin inhibitors in thrombolysis, and other platelet and clotting blocking agents in thrombolysis.

PATHOPHYSIOLOGY OF ACUTE THROMBOTIC OCCLUSION OF CORONARY ARTERY AND REOCCLUSION AFTER REPERFUSION
Activation of platelets

Platelets are activated by three different pathways (Fig. 9-3). First, after plaque rupture, collagen, exposed on the subendothelium, and thrombin, generated by activation of the extrinsic and intrinsic coagulation systems, are strong agonists for platelet aggregation. Adenosine diphosphate released from red blood cells constitutes another pathway for platelet activation. Secretory granules in platelets are dense granules, α-granules, lysosomes, and peroxisomes. Dense granules contain adenosine diphosphate, serotonin, calcium, and phosphate. α-Granules can release fibrinogen, von Willebrand factor, fibronectin, albumin, thrombospon-

din, platelet factors 4 and 5, β-thromboglobulin, and platelet-derived growth factor. Activated platelets release calcium from the dense granules into the cytoplasm by the action of phospholipase on platelet membrane phosphatidylinositol. Calcium causes platelet contraction, with a further release of serotonin, adenosine diphosphate, and arachidonate. Adenosine diphosphate, a strong platelet agonist in the presence of calcium and fibrinogen, constitutes the second pathway. It induces platelet-platelet interaction by exposure of binding receptors such as IIb/IIIa to fibrinogen and von Willebrand's factor, resulting in platelet aggregation.[29] Third, arachidonate from platelet membrane is converted to thromboxane A$_2$ by cyclooxygenase and thromboxane synthetase. Thromboxane A$_2$ is not only a strong agonist for platelet aggregation but also a strong vasoconstrictor. It exposes occult fibrinogen and von Willebrand's factor–binding site in glycoprotein IIb/IIIa complex by mobilizing intracellular calcium.[30,31]

Activated platelets expose membrane receptors such as glycoprotein Ib, Ia, and IIb/IIIa (Fig. 9-4). Glycoprotein IIb/IIIa binds to fibrinogen, von Willebrand's factor, and fibronectin and plays an important role for platelet-platelet interaction. von Willebrand's factor binds to glycoprotein Ib[32] and is important for platelet adhesion to subendothelium at high shear rates.[33,34] Glycoprotein Ib binds to exposed collagen. There has been a debate about roles of fibrinogen and von Willebrand's factor

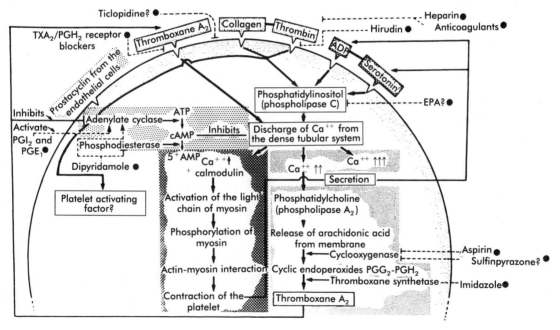

Fig. 9-3. Three different pathways of platelet activation. Collagen and thrombin constitute a major pathway after plaque rupture. Adenosine diphosphate *(ADP)* and arachidonate initiate other two pathways. Calcium causes platelet contraction with a further release of serotonin, ADP, and arachidonate. *ATP,* Adenosine triphosphate; *PGG$_2$* and *PGH$_2$,* prostaglandin G$_2$ and H$_2$. (From Stein B, Fuster V, Israel DH, et al: *J Am Coll Cardiol* 14:813-836, 1989. Used by permission.)

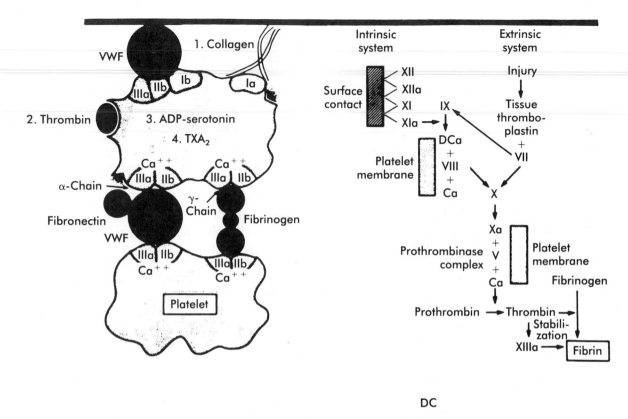

Fig. 9-4. *Left,* Platelet membrane receptor (glycoprotein Ia, Ib, and IIb/IIIa) and adhesive macromolecules on the disrupted vessel wall. *Right,* Intrinsic and extrinsic pathways of the coagulation system. Factor VII activates not only factor X but also factor IX. *Ca,* Calcium; *VWF,* von Willebrand's factor. (From Fuster V, Badimon L, Cohen M, et al: *Circulation* 77:1213-1220, 1988. Used by permission.)

in platelet-platelet interaction. Fibrinogen has been thought to be a key factor for this interaction because of defective aggregation in thrombasthenia patients. However, recent studies showed that platelet adhesion to subendothelium and platelet aggregation were preserved in afibrinogenemia.[33,35,36] A peptide-specific monoclonal antibody that blocks the binding of von Willebrand's factor to glycoprotein IIb/IIIa [152B6] without affecting the binding of other Arg-Gly-Asp [RGD]–dependent glycoproteins has been shown to reduce the platelet deposition to human atherosclerotic vessel wall.[37] Moreover, pigs with von Willebrand's disease but with normal fibrinogen levels showed much less platelet deposition in subendothelium[38] and collagen type I bundle[39] at different shear rates.[40] All these evidences suggest that von Willebrand's factor rather than fibrinogen plays a crucial role in platelet adhesion to vessel walls.

Activation of the coagulation system

When the plaque ruptures, both intrinsic and extrinsic coagulation cascades become activated by the exposure of collagen and tissue factor in the subendothelium (Fig. 9-4). Factors IX and VIII and factors X and V are activated on platelet membrane. Tissue factor binds factors VII and VIIa in the presence of calcium, and this complex activates factors IX and X[41,42] and thereby plays a major role in the activation of both the "intrinsic" and "extrinsic" pathways of blood coagulation. The final product, thrombin, produces fibrin by catalizing fibrinogen, induces the cross-linking of fibrin by activating factor XIII, and stimulates new thrombin generation by stimulating factors V and VIII. Polymerized fibrin protects the thrombus from embolization by the high shear rate. At the same time, thrombin is a strong agonist for platelet aggregation.[43-45] Activated platelets increase prothrombinase activity,[46,47] which promotes further thrombin production from prothrombin. Thrombin is readily inhibited by antithrombin III in the circulation, but fibrin-bound thrombin is partially protected from circulating antithrombin. Thus, thrombin in the thrombus continues to produce fibrin and activate platelets.

Reocclusion of coronary artery after reperfusion

The surface of residual thrombus after partial thrombolysis constitutes a strong thrombogenic stimulus for both platelet aggregation and fibrin formation.[48] Thrombin, incorporated into the thrombus during initial clot formation, is exposed on the surface during thrombolysis and continues to activate both the coagulation system and platelets.[49] Tissue factor and collagen in the atheromatous plaque or subendothelium are exposed after thrombolysis and initiate the extrinsic and intrinsic pathways of the coagulation system, resulting in the generation of new thrombin. It has also been shown that platelets are activated during thrombolytic therapy with both streptokinase and recombinant tissue-type plasminogen activator (rt-PA),[50-53] possibly by plasmin generation.[54] Platelet activation, again, augments thrombin formation and causes a vicious cycle.

SELECTIVE THROMBIN INHIBITORS FOR THE ACCELERATION OF REPERFUSION AND PREVENTION OF REOCCLUSION

As mentioned before, although thrombolytic therapy has become a standard therapy for acute myocardial infarction, it has several problems to be solved, such as resistance to therapy, delayed time to reperfusion, and reocclusion after initial successful reperfusion. To overcome these shortcomings, researchers have tested a number of pharmacologic approaches. These include the use of aspirin,[55] prostaglandin E1,[56] selective thromboxane A_2 synthase inhibitors,[57,58] selective thromboxane A_2 receptor antagonists in combination with serotonin receptor antagonists,[59,60] and combined thromboxane A_2 synthase inhibitors/prostaglandin endoperoxide receptor antagonists.[58,61]

Since the study of Hanson and Harker[43] showing that thrombin is the principal mediator of platelet-rich thrombus formation, several studies have been published about the effect of selective thrombin inhibitors on the enhancement of thrombolysis.[62-64] Fitzgerald and FitzGerald[62] showed that Argatroban, ([2R, 4R]-4-methyl-1-[N2-(3-methyl-1,2,3,4-tetrahydro-8-quinoline-sulfonyl)-1-arginyl]-2-piperidinecarboxylic acid monohydrate), a synthetic specific thrombin inhibitor, shortens the time to reperfusion with rt-PA from 59 to 28 minutes in the dog platelet–rich coronary thrombus model. However, Argatroban itself was not potent enough to prevent reocclusion after thrombolysis. Addition of thromboxane A_2 antagonist GR 32191 to Argatroban was required to abolish cyclic changes of reflow and reocclusion. Jang et al.[63] also showed that Argatroban, compared with heparin, increases the reperfusion rate, shortens the time to reperfusion (from 37 to 12 minutes), and prevents reocclusion (0/5 in the Argatroban group vs. 3/5 in the heparin group) in rabbits with erythrocyte-rich thrombus. In this study, addition of aspirin to Argatroban further decreased the residual thrombus after reperfusion when analyzed by scanning electron and light microscopy. These results were confirmed in the similar dog coronary artery thrombosis model by the same group.[64] Hirudin also shortens the

time to reperfusion with t-PA (from around 43 to 19 minutes) compared with heparin in the platelet-rich coronary artery thrombosis model in conscious dogs.[65] In this study reocclusion was completely prevented during a 90-minute follow-up period by hirudin alone without an additional platelet-blocking agent, whereas in the heparin group, five of six dogs showed reocclusion after an average of 37 minutes.

Selective thrombin inhibitors have been more widely tested for the prevention of platelet deposition or platelet-mediated arterial occlusion. Hanson and Harker[43] showed that the synthetic covalent antithrombin D-phenylalanyl-L-prolyl-L-arginyl chloromethyl ketone (FPRCH2Cl) effectively prevented platelet-rich thrombosis in a nonhuman primate vascular graft model. In rabbit models with platelet-rich thrombus, Jang et al.[45] showed that 1-hour intraarterial infusion of Argatroban was effective for the prevention of acute thrombotic occlusion up to 3 hours after the end of infusion. Although this study was not designed to address the occurrence and mechanism of reduced thrombogenicity of the vessel wall, the results suggested that an apparent "passivation" of the thrombogenic surface seemed to occur after a short-term local infusion of a selective thrombin inhibitor. In the other study,[66] chloromethyl ketone (FPRCH2CL) prevented platelet deposition in a stainless steel endovascular stent model in baboons, whereas heparin was totally ineffective.

OTHER PLATELET AND CLOTTING BLOCKING AGENTS FOR THE ACCELERATION OF REPERFUSION AND PREVENTION OF REOCCLUSION

Gold et al.[67] reported that F(ab′)2 fragment of a murine monoclonal antibody (7E3) against human platelet GP IIb/IIIa receptor [7E3-F(ab′)2] enhanced rt-PA–induced thrombolysis and prevented the reocclusion in the dog coronary artery thrombosis model with fibrin-rich clot and superimposed high-grade stenosis. The reperfusion time was shortened from 33 minutes in the heparin group to 6 minutes in the antibody group, and reocclusion did not occur during the follow-up period. The same group showed that the arterial surface after antibody treatment was covered with a monolayer of platelets without clumps.[68] Mickelson et al.[69] studied the effect of this antibody [7E3 F(ab′)2] on the prevention of rethrombosis after rt-PA–induced reperfusion in the dog circumflex coronary artery thrombosis model. Whereas rethrombosis occurred in all animals in the control group receiving the saline diluent, rethrombosis occurred in only one of nine dogs in the antibody-treated group. The thrombus mass at the end of the experiment was also significantly less in the antibody group (1.5 vs. 7.0 mg) than in the control group. The same antibody was tested for the lysis of thrombolysis-resistant platelet-rich coronary thrombus in the dog with rt-PA.[70] This resistance was overcome by the combined use of a reduced dose of rt-PA and the antibody. In this model antibody combined with rt-PA induced reperfusion in all five animals, whereas heparin with rt-PA reperfused only one of five dogs. Other antiplatelet GP IIb/IIIa receptor antibodies, such as AP-2 and LJ-CP8, showed a reduction in platelet deposition in Dacron vascular grafts in the baboon.[71] The shortcomings of these antibodies are protracted inhibition of platelet aggregation, prolongation of the bleeding time, and risk of immunogenicity. The platelet glycoprotein IIb/IIIa receptor may also be inhibited by peptides containing the Arg-Gly-Asp (RGD) recognition sequence.[72,73] These peptides compete with fibrinogen in binding to the GP IIb/IIIa receptor. RGD-containing peptides include low-molecular-weight linear synthetic peptides,[74,75] snake venom polypeptides such as trigramin,[76] echistatin,[77] bitistatin,[78] and kistrin,[79] or high-affinity cyclic derivatives.[80] Shebuski et al.[75] reported that Ac-Arg-Gly-Asp-Ser-NH2 abolished intracoronary cyclic platelet aggregation when given locally at high concentrations. Haskel et al.[75] also showed arginine-glycine-aspartate-o-methyltyrosine amide (RGDY) could prevent reocclusion after reperfusion with rt-PA in dogs. However, in this model RGDY, even at high doses (4 mg/kg/min), was not more efficient than intravenous aspirin. Because of their weak potency, their future clinical use is obscure. On the other hand, RGD-containing viper venom peptides are 100 to 1000 times more potent than linear GRGDS peptides for the inhibition of both fibrinogen binding to platelets and platelet aggregation. Among these peptides, bitistatin and kistrin have been tested in the animal model for the prevention of reocclusion. Bitistatin in conjunction with heparin prevented reocclusion after reperfusion with rt-PA in the dog coronary artery thrombosis model.[81] The reocclusion rate of the combined treatment of bitistatin and heparin was 22%, whereas heparin alone or bitistatin alone showed reocclusion in more than 80% of the animals.

In the dog coronary artery thrombosis model, kistrin shortened the rt-PA–induced reperfusion time to 6 minutes compared with 37 minutes in the control group receiving heparin, with a transient prolongation of bleeding time.[82] Reocclusion was prevented in the kistrin group even after the bleeding time returned to normal.

Recently recombinant tick anticoagulant peptide (rTAP), a selective factor Xa inhibitor, was tested in conjunction with rt-PA for the acceleration of thrombolysis in a canine model with platelet-rich thrombosis and a superimposed stenosis.[83] In this study rTAP induced reperfusion in all 8 animals, whereas in the control group reperfusion was achieved in 5 of 12 dogs ($P < 0.05$). The time to reperfusion was also shortened from 68 minutes in the control group to 23 minutes in the rTAP group. Reocclusion was, however, not completely abolished with rTAP.

Another important recent finding is the role of lipoprotein-associated coagulation inhibitor (LACI), which is a physiologic inhibitor of tissue factor–induced coagulation.[84] In the dog femoral artery thrombosis model, induced by extensive vascular injury, LACI prevented reocclusion and nearly abolished cyclic flow changes. This suggests that reocclusion after thrombolysis is mediated mainly by the activation of the extrinsic pathway of the coagulation system, and the inhibition of this pathway by LACI may be a highly targeted approach to maintaining patency. Another study supporting this hypothesis was done in rabbits with platelet-rich femoral artery thrombosis, where a monoclonal antibody to tissue factor was shown to be effective for the prevention of platelet-mediated arterial thrombosis.[85]

FUTURE ANTITHROMBOTIC THERAPY

Among various antithrombotic agents, aspirin has been shown to be effective in the prevention and treatment of acute coronary syndromes. However, because aspirin blocks only one pathway of platelet activation, its effect is limited. Therefore, the combination of aspirin and an anticoagulant with or without thrombolytic therapy is required for the treatment of acute coronary syndromes in conjunction with vasodilators and β-blockers. Heparin, however, is also a nonselective thrombin inhibitor and requires antithrombin III to be effective. Clot-bound thrombin is inaccessible to the heparin–antithrombin III complex, and therefore heparin has limited value in the treatment of acute coronary syndromes. The key issue in the clinical application of the specific therapies outlined in this chapter is whether a more potent approach to preventing ischemic events can be employed without increasing bleeding risk.

Other antiplatelet agents that block enzymes or receptors in the thromboxane or serotonin pathway have been widely tested in animal models. However, their role in patients with acute coronary syndromes is not yet clear. Agents that block tissue factor may be very effective in the prevention of activation of the coagulation system and platelets and may have a promising therapeutic future.

The most promising antithrombotic agent at the present time is the selective thrombin inhibitor hirudin, which does not require antithrombin III and can inhibit clot-bound thrombin. Future therapy for unstable angina pectoris may be the combination of hirudin and aspirin with standard medical therapy, although the dose and duration of the therapy remains undetermined. For acute myocardial infarction, a combination of a thrombolytic agent, hirudin, and aspirin could be the preferred choice. Hirudin is currently in the midst of large-scale clinical trials in both acute myocardial infarction and unstable angina. Another possibility is the combination of a thrombolytic agent, a potent platelet glycoprotein IIb/IIIa blocker, such as a monoclonal antibody or peptide, and heparin. Whether the combination of a thrombolytic agent, hirudin, and a potent platelet glycoprotein IIb/IIIa–blocking agent at lower doses would be better than the current therapy remains to be investigated.

REFERENCES

1. Friedman M: The coronary thrombus: its origin and fate, *Hum Pathol* 2:81-128, 1971.
2. Ridolfi RL, Hutchins GM: The relationship between coronary artery lesions and myocardial infarct: ulceration of atherosclerotic plaques precipitating coronary thrombosis, *Am Heart J* 93:468-486, 1977.
3. Falk E: Plaque rupture with severe pre-existing stenosis precipitating coronary thrombosis: characteristics of coronary atherosclerotic plaques underlying fatal occlusive thrombi, *Br Heart J* 50:127-134, 1983.
4. Falk E: Unstable angina with fatal outcome: dynamic coronary thrombosis leading to infarction and/or sudden death. Autopsy evidence of recurrent mural thrombosis with peripheral embolization culminating in total vascular occlusion, *Circulation* 71:699-708, 1985.
5. Davies MJ, Thomas AC: Plaque fissuring: the cause of acute myocardial infarction, sudden ischemic death, and crescendo angina, *Br Heart J* 53:363-373, 1985.
6. Fuster V, Badimon L, Badimon JJ, et al: The pathogenesis of coronary artery disease and the acute coronary syndrome, *N Engl J Med* 326:242-250, 1992.
7. Haerem JW: Platelet aggregates in intramyocardial vessels of patients dying suddenly and unexpectedly of coronary artery disease, *Atherosclerosis* 5:199-213, 1972.
8. El-Maraghi N, Genton E: The relevance of platelet and fibrin thromboembolism of the coronary microcirculation with special reference to sudden cardiac death, *Circulation* 62:936-944, 1980.
9. Davies MJ, Thomas A: Thrombosis and acute coronary artery lesions in sudden cardiac ischemic death, *N Engl J Med* 310:1137-1140, 1984.
10. Davies MJ, Thomas AC, Knapman PA, et al: Intramyocardial platelet aggregation in patients with unstable angina suffering sudden ischemic cardiac death, *Circulation* 73:418-427, 1986.
11. Levin DC, Fallon JT: Significance of the angiographic morphology of localized coronary stenoses: histopathologic correlations, *Circulation* 66:316-320, 1982.
12. Davies MJ, Woolf N, Robertson WB: Pathology of acute myocardial infarction with particular reference to occlusive coronary thrombi, *Br Heart J* 38:659-664, 1976.
13. Friedman M, Van den Bovenkamp GJ: The pathogenesis of a coronary thrombus, *Am J Pathol* 48:19-44, 1966.
14. Erhardt LR, Lundman T, Mellstedt H: Incorporation of 125I-labelled fibrinogen into coronary arterial thrombi in acute myocardial infarction in man, *Lancet* 1:387-390, 1973.
15. Rentrop KP, Blanke H, Karsch KR, et al: Initial experience with transmural recanalization of the recently occluded infarct-related coronary artery in acute myocardial infarction—comparison with conventionally treated patients, *Clin Cardiol* 2:92-105, 1979.
16. TIMI Study Group: The thrombolysis in myocardial infarction (TIMI) trial. Phase I findings, *N Engl J Med* 312:932-936, 1985.
17. Gruppo Italiano per lo Studio della Streptochinasi nell'Infarto Miocardico (GISSI): Effectiveness of intravenous thrombolytic treatment in acute myocardial infarction, *Lancet* 1:397-402, 1986.
18. ISIS-2 (Second International Study of Infarct Survival) Collaborative Group: Randomised trial of intravenous streptokinase, oral aspirin, both, or neither among 17,189 cases of suspected acute myocardial infarction: ISIS 2, *Lancet* 2:349-360, 1988.
19. AIMS Trial Study Group: Effect of intravenous APSAC on mortality after acute myocardial infarction: preliminary report of a placebo-controlled clinical trial, *Lancet* 1:545-549, 1988.
20. Schaer DH, Ross AM, Wasserman AG: Reinfarction, recurrent angina, and reocclusion after thrombolytic therapy, *Circulation* 72(suppl II):II57-II62, 1987.
21. Kennedy JW, Martin GV, Davies KB, et al: The Western Washington Intravenous Streptokinase in Acute Myocardial Infarction Randomized Trial, *Circulation* 77:345-352, 1988.
22. Ohman EM, Califf RM, Topol EJ, et al: Consequences of reocclusion after successful reperfusion therapy in acute myocardial infarction, *Circulation* 82:781-791, 1990.
23. Van de Werf F, Arnold AER, European Cooperative Study Group for recombinant tissue-type plasminogen activator (rt-PA): Intravenous tissue plasminogen activator and size of infarct, left ventricular function, and survival in acute myocardial infarction, *Br Heart J* 297:1374-1379, 1988.
24. Jang IK, Vanhaecke J, De Geest H, et al: Coronary thrombolysis with recombinant tissue-type plasminogen activator: patency rate and regional wall motion after 3 months, *J Am Coll Cardiol* 8:1455-1460, 1986.
25. Neuhaus KL, von Essen R, Tebbe U, et al: Improved thrombolysis in acute myocardial infarction with front-loaded administration of alteplase: Results of the rt-PA-APSAC patency study (TAPS), *J Am Coll Cardiol* 19:885-891, 1992.
26. Matsuo O, Rijken DC, Collen D: Comparison of the relative fibrinogenolytic, fibrinolytic and thrombolytic properties of tissue plasminogen activator and urokinase in vitro, *Thromb Haemost* 45:225-229, 1981.
27. Loscalzo J, Vaughan DE: Tissue plasminogen activator promotes platelet disaggregation in plasma, *J Clin Invest* 79:1749-1755, 1987.
28. Jang IK, Gold HK, Ziskind AA, et al: Differential sensitivity of erythrocyte-rich and platelet-rich arterial thrombi to lysis with recombinant tissue-type plasminogen activator. A possible explanation for resistance to coronary thrombolysis, *Circulation* 79:920-928, 1989.
29. Peerschke EIB: The platelet fibrinogen receptor, *Semin Hematol* 22:241-259, 1985.
30. Shattil SJ, Brass LP: Induction of the fibrinogen receptor on human platelets by intracellular mediators, *J Biol Chem* 262:992-1000, 1987.
31. Coller BS: Activation affects access to the platelet receptor for adhesive glycoproteins, *J Cell Biol* 103:451-456, 1986.
32. Sakariassen KS, Nievelstein FF, Coller BS, et al: The role of platelet membrane glycoproteins, Ib and IIb/IIIa in platelet adherence to human artery subendothelium, *Br J Haematol* 63:681-191, 1986.
33. Weiss HJ, Turitto VT, Baumgartner HR: Effect of shear rate on platelet interaction with subendothelium in citrated and native blood: I. Shear rate-dependent decrease of adhesion in von Willebrand's disease and the Bernard-Soulier syndrome, *J Lab Clin Med* 92:750-754, 1978.
34. Turitto VT, Baumgartner HR: Platelet surface interactions. In *Hemostasis and thrombosis, basic principles and clinical practice,* ed 2, New York, 1987, JB Lippincott.
35. Turitto VT, Weiss JH, Baumgartner HR: Platelet interaction with rabbit subendothelium in von Willebrand's disease: altered thrombus formation distinct from defective platelet adhesion, *J Clin Invest* 74:1730-1741, 1984.
36. Weiss HJ, Turitto VT, Vicic WJ, et al: Fibrin formation, fibrinopeptide A release, and platelet thrombus dimensions on subendothelium exposed to flowing native blood: greater in

Factor XII and XI than in Factor VIII and VIII and IX deficiency, *Blood* 63:1004-1014, 1984.

37. Badimon L, Badimon J, Ruggeri Z, et al: A peptide-specific monoclonal antibody that inhibits von Willebrand factor binding to GP IIb/IIIa [152B6] inhibits platelet deposition to human atherosclerotic vessel wall [abstract], *Circulation* 82:III370, 1990.

38. Badimon L, Badimon JJ, Rand J, et al: Platelet deposition on von Willebrand factor-deficient vessels. Extracorporeal perfusion studies in swine with von Willebrand's disease using native and heparinized blood, *J Lab Clin Med* 110:634-647, 1987.

39. Badimon L, Badimon JJ, Turitto VT, et al: Platelet thrombus formation on collagen type I. Influence of blood rheology, von Willebrand Factor and blood coagulation, *Circulation* 78:1431-1442, 1988.

40. Badimon L, Badimon JJ, Turitto VT, et al: Role of von Willebrand factor in mediating platelet-vessel wall interaction at low shear rate; the importance of perfusion condition, *Blood* 73:961-967, 1989.

41. Nemerson T: The reaction between bovine brain tissue factor and factors VII and X, *Biochemistry* 5:601-608, 1966.

42. Osterud B, Rapaport SI: Activation of factor IX by the reaction product of tissue factor and factor VII: additional pathway for initiating blood coagulation, *Proc Natl Acad Sci USA* 74:5260-5264, 1977.

43. Hanson SR, Harker LA: Interruption of acute platelet-dependent thrombosis by the synthetic antithrombin D-phenylalanyl-L-prolyl-L-arginyl chloromethyl ketone, *Proc Natl Acad Sci USA* 85:3184-3188, 1988.

44. Heras M, Chesbro JH, Penny WJ, et al: Effects of thrombin inhibition on the development of acute platelet-thrombus deposit during angioplasty in pigs. Heparin vs. recombinant hirudin, a specific thrombin inhibitor, *Circulation* 79:657-665, 1989.

45. Jang IK, Gold HK, Ziskind AA, et al: Prevention of platelet-rich arterial thrombosis by selective thrombin inhibition, *Circulation* 81:219-225, 1990.

46. Rosing J, van Rijn JL, Bevers EM, et al: The role of activated human platelets in prothrombin and factor X activation, *Blood* 65:319-332, 1985.

47. Miletich JP, Jackson CM, Majerus PW: Interaction of coagulation factor Xa with human platelets, *Proc Natl Acad Sci USA* 74:4033-4036, 1977.

48. Badimon L, Lassila R, Badimon J, et al: Residual thrombus is more thrombogenic than severely damaged vessel walls [abstract], *Circulation* 78:II119, 1988.

49. Eisenberg PR, Sherman LA, Jaffe AS: Paradoxic elevation of fibrinopeptide A after streptokinase: evidence for continued thrombosis despite intense fibrinolysis, *J Am Coll Cardiol* 10:527-529, 1987.

50. Fitzgerald DJ, Catella F, Roy L, et al: Marked platelet activation in vivo after intravenous streptokinase in patients with acute myocardial infarction, *Circulation* 77:142-150, 1988.

51. Fitzgerald DJ, Wright F, FitzGerald GA: Increased thromboxane biosynthesis during coronary thrombolysis. Evidence that platelet activation and thromboxane A2 modulate the response to tissue-type plasminogen activator in vivo, *Circ Res* 65:83-94, 1989.

52. Vaughan DE, Van Houtte E, Declerck PJ, et al: Streptokinase-induced platelet aggregation. Prevalence and mechanism, *Circulation* 84:84-91, 1991.

53. Ohlstein EH, Storer B, Fujita T, et al: Tissue-type plasminogen activator and streptokinase induce platelet hyper-aggregability in the rabbit, *Thromb Res* 46:575-585, 1987.

54. Niewiarowski S, Senyi AF, Gillies P: Plasmin-induced platelet aggregation and platelet release reaction. Effects on hemostasis, *J Clin Invest* 52:1647-1659, 1973.

55. Folts JD, Crowell EB, Rowe GG: Platelet aggregation in partially obstructed vessels and its elimination with aspirin, *Circulation* 54:365-370, 1976.

56. Sharma B, Wyeth RP, Gimenes HJ, et al: Intracoronary prostaglandin E1 plus streptokinase in acute myocardial infarction, *Am J Cardiol* 58:1161-1166, 1986.

57. Aiken JW, Shebuski RJ, Miller OV, et al: Endogenous prostacyclin contributes to the efficacy of a thromboxane synthetase inhibitor for preventing coronary artery thrombosis, *J Pharmacol Exp Ther* 219:299-308, 1981.

58. Golino P, Rosolowsky M, Yao S-K, et al: Endogenous prostaglandin endoperoxides and prostacyclin modulate the thrombolytic activity of tissue plasminogen activator: effects of simultaneous inhibition of thromboxane A2 synthase and blockade of thromboxane A2/prostaglandin H2 receptors in a canine model of coronary thrombosis, *J Clin Invest* 86:1095-1102, 1990.

59. Golino P, Ashton JH, McNatt J, et al: Simultaneous administration of thromboxane A2- and serotonin S2-receptor antagonists markedly enhances thrombolysis and prevents or delays reocclusion after tissue-type plasminogen activator in a canine model of coronary thrombosis, *Circulation* 79:911-919, 1989.

60. De Clerk FB, Xhonneux L, Van Gorp L: S2-serotonergic receptor inhibition (ketanserin), combined with thromboxane A2/prostaglandin H2 receptor blockade (BM 13,177): enhanced anti-platelet effect [letter]. *Thromb Haemost* 56:236, 1986.

61. De Clerck F, Beetens J, Van der Water A, et al: R68070: thromboxane A2 synthetase inhibition and thromboxane A2/prostaglandin endoperoxide receptor blockade combined in one molecule: II. Pharmacological effects in vivo and ex vivo, *Thromb Haemost* 61:43-49, 1989.

62. Fitzgerald DJ, FitzGerald GA: Role of thrombin and thromboxane A2 in reocclusion following coronary thrombolysis with tissue-type plasminogen activator, *Proc Natl Acad Sci USA* 86:7585-7589, 1989.

63. Jang IK, Gold HK, Leinbach RC, et al: In vivo thrombin inhibition enhances and sustains arterial recanalization with recombinant tissue-type plasminogen activator, *Circ Res* 67:1552-1561, 1990.

64. Yasuda T, Gold HK, Yaoita H, et al: Comparative effects of aspirin, a synthetic thrombin inhibitor and a monoclonal antiplatelet glycoprotein IIb/IIIa antibody on coronary artery reperfusion, reocclusion and bleeding with recombinant tissue-type plasminogen activator in a canine preparation, *J Am Coll Cardiol* 16:714-722, 1990.

65. Haskel EJ, Preger NA, Sobel BE, et al: Relative efficacy of antithrombin compared with antiplatelet agents in accelerating coronary thrombolysis and preventing early reocclusion, *Circulation* 83:1048-1056, 1991.

66. Krupski WC, Bass A, Kelly AB, et al: Heparin-resistant thrombus formation by endovascular stents in baboons. Interruption by a synthetic antithrombin, *Circulation* 81:570-577, 1990.

67. Gold HK, Coller BS, Yasuda T, et al: Rapid and sustained coronary artery recanalization with combined bolus injection of recombinant tissue-type plasminogen activator and monoclonal antiplatelet GP IIb/IIIa antibody in a canine preparation, *Circulation* 77:670-677, 1988.

68. Yasuda T, Gold HK, Fallon JT, et al: Monoclonal antibody against the platelet glycoprotein (GP) IIb/IIIa receptor prevents coronary artery reocclusion after reperfusion with recombinant tissue-type plasminogen activator in dogs, *J Clin Invest* 81:1284-1291, 1988.

69. Mickelson JK, Simpson PJ, Cronin M, et al: Antiplatelet antibody [7E3 F(ab')2] prevents rethrombosis after recombinant tissue-type plasminogen activator-induced coronary artery thrombolysis in a canine model, *Circulation* 81:617-627, 1990.

70. Yasuda T, Gold HK, Leinbach RC, et al: Lysis of plasminogen activator-resistant platelet-rich coronary artery thrombus with combined bolus injection of recombinant tissue-type plasminogen activator and antiplatelet GP IIb/IIIa antibody, *J Am Coll Cardiol* 16:1728-1735, 1990.

71. Hanson SR, Pareti FI, Ruggeri ZM, et al: Effects of monoclonal antibodies against the platelet glycoprotein IIb/IIIa complex on

thrombosis and hemostasis in the baboon, *J Clin Invest* 81:149-158, 1988.

72. Ruoslahti E, Pierschbacher MD: Arg-Gly-Asp: a versatile cell recognition signal, *Cell* 44:517-518, 1986.

73. Plow EF, Pierschbacher MD, Ruoslahti E, et al: The effect of Arg-Gly-Asp containing peptides on fibrinogen and von Willebrand factor binding to platelets, *Proc Natl Acad Sci USA* 82:8057-8061, 1985.

74. Shebuski RJ, Berry DE, Bennett DB, et al: Demonstration of Ac-Arg-Gly-Asp-Ser-Nh2 as an antiaggregatory agent in the dog by intracoronary administration, *Thromb Haemost* 61:183-188, 1989.

75. Haskel EJ, Adams SP, Feigen LP, et al: Prevention of reoccluding platelet-rich thrombi in canine femoral arteries with a novel peptide antagonist of platelet glycoprotein IIb/IIIa receptors, *Circulation* 80:1775-1782, 1989.

76. Huang T-F, Holt JC, Lukasiewicz H, et al: Trigramin: A low molecular weight peptide inhibiting fibrinogen interaction with platelet receptors expressed in glycoprotein IIb/IIIa complex, *J Biol Chem* 262:16157-16163, 1987.

77. Gan Z-R, Gould RJ, Jacobs JW, et al: Echistatin: A potent platelet aggregation inhibitor from the venom of the vipor, *Echis carinatus, J Biol Chem* 263:19827-19832, 1988.

78. Shebuski RJ, Ramjit DR, Bencen GH, et al: Characterization and platelet inhibitory activity of bitistatin, a potent RGD-containing peptide from the venom of the viper, *Bitis arietans, J Biol Chem* 264:21550-21556, 1991.

79. Dennis MS, Henzel WJ, Pitti RM, et al: Platelet GP IIb/IIIa protein antagonists from snake venom: evidence for a family of platelet aggregation inhibitors, *Proc Natl Acad Sci USA* 87:2471-2475, 1990.

80. Nichols A, Vasko J, Koster P, et al: SK&F 106760, a novel GPIIb/IIIa antagonist: antithrombotic activity and potentiation of streptokinase-mediated thrombolysis [abstract], *Eur J Pharmacol* 183:2019, 1990.

81. Shebuski RJ, Stabilito IJ, Sitko GR, et al: Acceleration of recombinant tissue-type plasminogen activator-induced thrombolysis and prevention of reocclusion by the combination of heparin and the Arg-Gly-Asp-containing peptide bitistatin in a canine model of coronary thrombolysis, *Circulation* 82:169-177, 1990.

82. Yasuda T, Gold HK, Leinbach RC, et al: Kistrin, a polypeptide platelet GP IIb/IIIa receptor antagonist, enhances and sustains coronary arterial thrombolysis with recombinant tissue-type plasminogen activator in a canine preparation, *Circulation* 83:1038-1047, 1991.

83. Sitko GR, Ramjit DR, Stabilito II, et al: Conjunctive enhancement of enzymatic thrombolysis and prevention of thrombotic reocclusion with the selective factor Xa inhibitor, tick anticoagulant peptide, *Circulation* 85:805-815, 1992.

84. Haskel EJ, Torr SR, Day KC, et al: Prevention of arterial reocclusion after thrombolysis with recombinant lipoprotein-associated coagulation inhibitor, *Circulation* 84:821-827, 1991.

85. Jang IK, Gold HK, Leinbach RC, et al: Antithrombotic effect of a monoclonal antibody against tissue factor in a rabbit model of platelet-mediated arterial thrombosis, *Arterioscler Thromb* 12:948-954, 1992.

Chapter 10

MECHANISMS OF MECHANICAL REPERFUSION AND CORONARY REVASCULARIZATION

Alan N. Tenaglia
Charles J. Davidson

Reperfusion of an occluded coronary artery during acute myocardial infarction (AMI) may be achieved pharmacologically with thrombolytic therapy; mechanically with balloon angioplasty or other interventional devices; or by a combination of these methods. Revascularization of patients with coronary artery disease may be achieved by balloon angioplasty or other percutaneous interventional devices or by coronary artery bypass surgery. An understanding of the basic mechanisms of mechanical reperfusion and percutaneous revascularization could assist in the selection of the most effective option for an individual patient.

POTENTIAL MECHANISMS OF ANGIOPLASTY

There are several potential mechanisms of coronary artery interventions.[1] Plaque compression may occur, presumably with extrusion of liquid elements. Plaque fracture and vessel wall dissection may contribute to enlarging the lumen area. Vessel stretch may occur, either concentrically or, in lesions with eccentric plaque, only over the disease-free wall. Finally, plaque may be extracted, ablated, or distally embolized.

It must be emphasized that in most cases the actual in vivo mechanical effects in humans can only be inferred. Studies performed in experimental animal models have intrinsic limitations when extrapolated to humans because of differences in atherosclerotic plaque composition and other species-specific factors. For instance, in the atherosclerotic rabbit model most of the plaque is highly lipid-laden. This contrasts to the fibrous, often calcified lesions that are more typical of human coronary artery plaque. Other differences between animal models and human disease include the rapidity and means of disease induction, activity of the coagulation system, and the presence or absence of collateral blood flow. Currently the choice of animal model appears to be the pig coronary artery.[2] The most similar animal model would be the primate, although this is not routinely used because of its cost.

Human research often involves performing interventions in cadaveric arteries, which lack normal vascular tone and intact coagulation systems. Pathologic findings in patients dying soon after interventions are biased to those with adverse outcomes and may not reflect mechanisms in those with successful procedures. In addition, some pathologic findings, such as plaque splitting, may be found in specimens on which no prior intervention has been performed and therefore may represent artifact rather than effect.[3]

A distinction should be made between mechanical effects occurring during elective angioplasty and those seen with angioplasty during AMI. For example, acute interventions are more likely to be performed in cases of thrombus and soft plaque as opposed to hard and calcified plaque in chronic lesions. Thus, mechanisms are likely to differ in these two circumstances. In addition, pathologic findings such as plaque disruption may be part of the process of MI and may not be caused by the intervention itself, thus making assessment of mechanisms more difficult. Finally, the influence of concomitant thrombolytic therapy on mechanisms must also be explored.

Because contrast angiography only provides silhouette images of the vessel lumen, information on the mechanical effects on the vessel wall are poorly delineated. New imaging technologies such as intravascular ultrasound and angioscopy may overcome some of these limitations. These methods may offer new insight into the human in vivo mechanisms of mechanical reperfusion or revascularization and will be discussed further.

MECHANISMS OF BALLOON ANGIOPLASTY
Animal studies

Initial studies of balloon angioplasty mechanisms were performed in aortoiliac lesions induced in rabbits by balloon injury and feeding of a high-cholesterol diet.[4-6] These studies found that the mechanisms of successful balloon angioplasty were primarily plaque fracture and dissection of the vessel wall, usually occurring at the internal elastic lamina. In addition, Faxon et al.[5] and Sanborn et al.[6] noted stretching of nondiseased segments of vessel wall. There was no evidence of either embolization of plaque[7] or compression of plaque being significant contributors to luminal enlargement.

Cadaver studies

Given the limitations of extrapolating animal results to humans, further studies examined pathologic effects of balloon angioplasty performed in human cadaveric arteries. The earliest report by Lee et al. concluded that angioplasty caused plaque compression and minimal vascular tears.[8]

This conclusion has been contradicted by all subsequent reports. Other studies have found intimal disruption and separation of intima from media.[9,10] In another study angiographic evidence of dissection was noted in 7 of 17 vessels, although at pathology, dissections were seen in all 17 (intimal 17, medial 11, adventitial 1).[11] This illustrates the insensitivity of angiography in detecting

dissection. Finally, Lyon et al. found stretching of the media and adventitia in addition to splitting of the intima near the edge of the plaque and separation of the edges of plaque from the media.[12] No evidence of plaque compression, deformation, or remodeling was noted in any of these later studies.

Autopsy findings

An initial series of three patients dying soon after angioplasty revealed splitting of the atherosclerotic plaque and intimal dissection.[13] Further autopsy studies[14,15] have confirmed the conclusion that plaque fracture and vessel stretching play the major roles in improvement in luminal dimensions, although these reports are inherently biased towards unsuccessful cases. However, in one case report in which accidental death occurred by inadvertent intracoronary lidocaine injection following successful angioplasty, similar results were noted.[16]

Mechanisms of balloon angioplasty as assessed by newer diagnostic devices

The development of both intracoronary ultrasound and angioscopy has allowed in vivo assessment of the mechanisms of interventions in humans and can overcome some of the inherent limitations noted in the pathologic studies just discussed. The two new techniques appear to be complementary. Intracoronary ultrasound provides a 360-degree cross-sectional tomographic image of the artery, revealing details of the various layers as well as measurements of lumen, plaque, and artery sizes. It is well suited to detect dissections. On the other hand, angioscopy provides detailed imaging of the luminal surface and is therefore more sensitive in detecting processes such as thrombus.

To evaluate human in vivo mechanisms of coronary balloon angioplasty, 30 patients were imaged with intracoronary ultrasound immediately following successful balloon angioplasty.[17] Ultrasound images were analyzed quantitatively for luminal area and area within the media at both the treatment site and the adjacent angiographically-normal reference site. Qualitative analysis included presence or absence of dissection. The area within the media was significantly larger at the treated site compared with the adjacent untreated reference site, suggesting that vessel stretching had occurred (Fig. 10-1). In addition, vessel dissection was noted in 50% of lesions (Fig. 10-2). These data support a role for stretching and dissection as the major mechanisms of successful balloon angioplasty.

Angioscopy following angioplasty has revealed endothelial exfoliation. Scattered thrombi were found in 10 of 10 segments, plaque rupture in two segments, and intimal dissection in two segments.[18]

Thus, information obtained using new imaging mo-

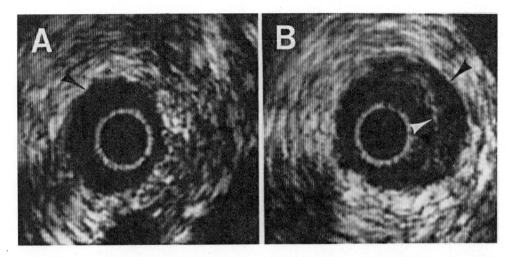

Fig. 10-1. Ultrasound appearance at reference site (**A**) and at site of balloon angioplasty (**B**). *Black arrowhead* = media; *white arrowhead* = border between lumen and plaque. Note that the area within the media is larger at the angioplasty-treated site compared with the reference site, indicating vessel stretching. (From Tenaglia et al.[17] with permission.)

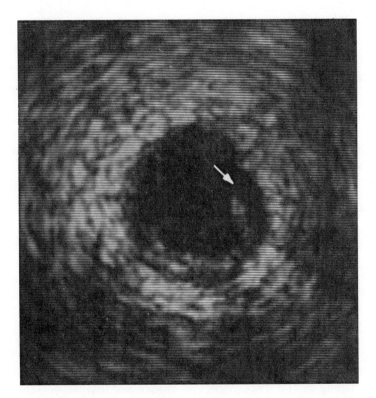

Fig. 10-2. Ultrasound appearance of dissection *(arrow)* in artery following balloon angioplasty. (From Tenaglia et al.[17] with permission.)

dalities after balloon angioplasty appear to confirm the earlier pathologic findings.

Mechanisms of balloon angioplasty in AMI

In the setting of AMI, which may be associated with preexisting plaque fracture and thrombus formation, mechanisms of balloon angioplasty may differ from those noted for treatment of chronic atherosclerosis. Colavita

et al.[19] presented pathological findings on four patients who died 6 hours to 4 days after AMI. Death was caused by ventricular arrhythmia or cardiogenic shock, so that the morphology of the dilated artery did not appear related to the cause of death. All the patients had received thrombolytic therapy in addition to balloon angioplasty. Residual stenosis, intimal hemorrhage, and plaque disruption were found in all four patients; distal embolization of plaque was noted in two patients. There were no medial dissections.

Another study examined pathologic findings in nine patients who died soon after balloon angioplasty for AMI.[20] Four of these patients also received thrombolytic therapy. In these four patients severe adventitial hemorrhage surrounded the angioplasty site, compressing and compromising the lumen in one case. Areas of plaque fracture and vessel wall dissection also contained hemorrhage in these patients. In contrast, there was no hemorrhage noted in the five patients treated with angioplasty without thrombolytic therapy.

These two small series suggest that angioplasty during AMI results in plaque fracture and vessel dissection similar to that seen after elective angioplasty. However, compared with elective angioplasty, plaque embolization may occur more frequently in this setting. Finally, the addition of thrombolytic therapy to balloon angioplasty results in vessel wall hemorrhage, which may have implications for successful outcome. For instance, hemorrhage behind a dissection plane may extend the dissection or increase the degree of luminal obstruction.

Influence of plaque composition on mechanisms of balloon angioplasty

The mechanism of balloon angioplasty probably differs depending upon the composition and morphology of the plaque. For instance, eccentric lesions potentially allow more stretching to occur because the arc of normal vessel wall is more pliable.[21]

Farb et al.[22] examined pathological findings in 28 patients in whom 40 coronary arteries were subjected to balloon angioplasty. The time from angioplasty to death ranged from less than 1 day to 3.5 years. Arteries with satisfactory luminal area (area stenosis at pathology < 75%) had evidence of medial disruption and stretching. A satisfactory lumen was more often noted for eccentric plaque compared with concentric plaque and for fibropultaceous plaque compared with primarily fibrous plaque. They hypothesized that the necrotic fibropultaceous core allowed more successful plaque and medial disruption and that the presence of eccentric plaque allowed stretching of the disease-free vessel wall.

Potkin and Roberts[23] examined 29 PTCA sites in 27 patients who died up to 960 days after the procedure (4 unsuccessful angioplasty, 25 successful). Ninety-seven percent of sites had plaque tear, which extended to the internal elastic membrane in 17% and into the media in 10%. Plaque calcium content was higher in the unsuccessful angioplasty lesions.

Finally, a study using intracoronary ultrasound imaging following successful angioplasty of 66 lesions found calcified plaque in 83%.[24] Plaque fracture was found significantly more frequently after angioplasty in the presence of calcified plaque.

Venous bypass graft stenoses

None of the prior studies specifically looked at the mechanisms of balloon angioplasty in vein bypass grafts compared with native coronary arteries. Indirect evidence has been provided by a study of angioplasty in hemodialysis fistula stenoses.[25] These "arterialized" veins are probably very similar to saphenous vein bypass grafts, thus allowing extrapolation to coronary anatomy. Intravascular ultrasound imaging was performed in 38 consecutive patients following angioplasty of hemodialysis fistula stenoses. Plaque composition was predominately soft (88%) and eccentric (94%). Vessel dissection occurred in 42% and vessel stretching in 50%. Elastic recoil was common and occurred in 50%. Thus, similar mechanisms as those noted for native coronary artery angioplasty are probably involved in angioplasty of venous bypass grafts. However, elastic recoil appears to be a more important factor.

MECHANISMS OF NEWER INTERVENTIONAL DEVICES

Newer techniques are increasingly being used for percutaneous revascularization. Although presumably different from balloon angioplasty, the mechanisms are less well studied. Currently, directional coronary atherectomy, rotational atherectomy, transluminal extraction atherectomy, excimer laser angioplasty, and coronary stenting have been approved for use by the Food and Drug Administration.

Directional coronary atherectomy

Directional coronary atherectomy is designed to shave plaque. The plaque is pressed through a window into the central housing of the catheter by means of low-pressure inflation of a balloon on the contralateral side. Although plaque is usually retrieved after successful procedures, controversy exists as to whether plaque extraction is the sole mechanism of successful atherectomy.

In cadaver coronary arteries treated with atherectomy it was noted that the procedure successfully removes plaque and that the degree of luminal enlargement is a function of the quantity of tissue removed.[26] Smooth defects were found in the plaque, with occasional extension into the media or the inner portion of the adventitia. Small cracks in the plaque were occasionally noted but this was believed to represent artifact.

An autopsy study demonstrated discrete cuts that extended variably into atheroma, media, or adventitia.[27] Otherwise there were no disruptions such as have been reported after balloon angioplasty.

Careful angiographic analysis of 78 lesions treated with directional atherectomy was performed to evaluate

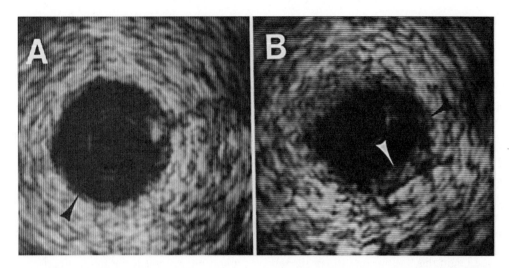

Fig. 10-3. Ultrasound appearance at reference site (**A**) and at site of directional atherectomy (**B**). *Black arrowhead* = media; *white arrowhead* = plaque. Note that the area within the media is similar at reference and treated sites. (From Tenaglia et al.[17] with permission.)

the mechanisms of the procedure.[28,29] In contrast to the prior studies it was calculated that the amount of tissue removed was not enough to account for the angiographic improvement noted. The conclusion was that part of the improvement in luminal diameter must be the result of mechanical dilation rather than tissue removal alone. This conclusion is limited somewhat by angiography's inability to assess luminal dimensions accurately, even when using quantitative techniques. This has been demonstrated by studies comparing angiography with intravascular ultrasound[30] and seems especially true for eccentric diseased and treated arteries with irregular luminal borders. Another angiographic study found dissections of 0 of 18 patients after atherectomy, compared with 6 of 18 after angioplasty ($P < 0.01$).[31]

Human in vivo intracoronary ultrasound findings provide further information. Ultrasound imaging was performed in 15 patients following successful atherectomy.[17] Smooth cuts into plaque could be seen (Fig. 10-3). The area within the media was not significantly different at treated sites compared with adjacent untreated reference sites in the same artery. In addition, in a subset of 5 patients imaging before and after atherectomy was obtained and showed no difference in the area within the media. Thus, the results suggest that significant stretching did not occur. Dissection was noted in only 1 patient. Another study using ultrasound imaging before and after directional atherectomy also demonstrated significant reduction in plaque and limited vessel expansion.[32]

Directional coronary atherectomy appears to result in increased luminal dimensions by plaque extraction, with much less evidence for plaque fracture and vessel dissection compared with balloon angioplasty. The role

of additional mechanical effects, because of either the necessary low-pressure balloon inflation or plaque displacement (Dotter effect), is still unclear. Any differences in the mechanism of the procedure in patients treated during AMI are still unexplored. For example, the relatively large profile of the device might result in more plaque and thrombus embolization in this setting.

Rotational atherectomy

Rotational atherectomy uses high-speed rotation of a diamond-tipped burr to abrade tissue and improve luminal size. In theory the device should result in a smooth lumen, with minimal damage to the underlying vessel wall. Initial studies in diseased rabbit iliac arteries demonstrated that the procedure effectively removed diseased intima.[33] Particles produced were less than 10 μm in size.

Mechanisms of action in humans have been examined by both angiography and intracoronary ultrasound. In a study using quantitative angiography after rotational atherectomy, the luminal diameter was, on average, 91% of the burr diameter, suggesting effective plaque ablation and little recoil.[34] However, dissections were noted in 30%, indicating that the smooth lumen originally hoped for with this device was not always achieved. In addition, in the majority of cases adjunctive balloon angioplasty was necessary to achieve adequate luminal size.

Intracoronary ultrasound imaging after rotational atherectomy revealed luminal enlargement by plaque ablation, especially of calcified plaque.[35] Dissections were noted in 26% of cases. Adjunctive balloon angioplasty further increased luminal size by a combination of vessel stretching and dissection.

Transluminal extraction catheter

The transluminal extraction catheter is a low-speed rotational device that cuts and removes plaque.[36] It has a particular role in treating degenerated vein grafts and lesions with thrombus, suggesting a possible role in reperfusion during AMI.[37] There are no studies using intracoronary ultrasound or angioscopy that carefully delineate its mechanism of action in human coronary arteries.

Excimer laser

Initial work with laser therapy involved continuous wave Nd:YAG or argon lasers, which destroy tissue by vaporization and pyrolysis, resulting in imprecise tissue cutting and thermal and blast damage.[38] As a result, more precise, pulsed, ultraviolet irradiation by excimer laser was developed, and this has become the preferred mode for laser treatment of coronary arteries.

It has been shown in atherosclerotic rabbit iliac arteries treated with excimer laser that a sharp vessel wall-lumen interface is created without evidence of thermal injury. Light and electron microscopy of cadaver arteries following treatment with excimer laser have also demonstrated clean cuts with histologically-normal edges.[39-41] No evidence of thermal or acoustic damage was noted.[38,41] These findings were thought to indicate photodissociation or photodisruption of tissue by excimer laser irradiation. One recent study using cadaveric arteries suggests that the mechanism of successful excimer laser angioplasty may depend on plaque composition.[42] With little calcification the primary mechanism was thought to be photoablative decomposition. As calcification increased, the mechanism shifted to more laser-induced plasma shock wave disruption.

Human in vivo mechanisms were evaluated with intracoronary ultrasound imaging, which was performed in 11 patients following successful laser angioplasty.[43] In 10 patients adjunctive balloon angioplasty was required. Compared with results following conventional balloon angioplasty alone, the images following laser treatment revealed similar postprocedural luminal dimensions, less residual plaque mass, and less evidence of vessel stretching. Dissection was noted in 1 of 5 lesions imaged after laser alone and 7 of 10 lesions imaged after laser and adjunctive balloon angioplasty. These results provide in vivo support for plaque ablation without significant stretching as the mechanism of action of lasers. In addition, the frequent occurrence of dissection appears to be the result of the adjunctive balloon treatment often required for success and not the result of the excimer laser itself.

There has been limited analysis of laser treatment by angioscopy. A single patient imaged by angioscopy following successful excimer laser did show "tissue remnants" on the vessel wall and some plaque fracture.[44] It was unclear whether adjunctive balloon angioplasty had been performed before imaging. There was no evidence of thermal damage.

The use of excimer laser in the setting of AMI has been limited by a high incidence of thrombosis. There are no data on whether the mechanism is different in this setting.

Thus, excimer laser appears to enlarge the vascular lumen by ablation of tissue without significant mechanical stretching or plaque fracture and vessel dissection. The current need for adjunctive balloon angioplasty in most cases probably results in a large proportion of cases ultimately developing dissection. Whether the development of larger laser catheters, which might obviate the need for adjunctive balloon angioplasty, will lower the rate of dissection, and what the clinical impact of this might be, are yet to be determined.

Coronary stenting

Currently the only widely available stents are the Gianturco-Roubin stent, which has been approved by the Food and Drug Administration for use in treating abrupt vessel closure, and the Palmaz-Schatz stent, which has been approved to prevent restenosis.[45,46] In arteries examined at autopsy of patients dying soon after stent implantation, the stent coils were noted to be imbedded in the vessel wall.[47] There was no evidence of thrombosis or tissue reaction to the stent wires. Thus, the stents appeared to be effectively functioning as scaffolding devices to maintain vessel patency.

REFERENCES

1. Waller BF: "Crackers, breakers, stretchers, drillers, scrapers, shavers, burners, welders and melters" — the future treatment of atherosclerotic coronary artery disease? A clinical-morphologic assessment, *J Am Coll Cardiol* 13:969-987, 1989.
2. Schwartz RS, Murphy JG, Edwards WD, et al: Restenosis after balloon angioplasty: a practical proliferative model in porcine coronary arteries, *Circulation* 82:2190-2200, 1990.
3. Isner JM, Fortin FV: Frequency in nonangioplasty patients of morphologic findings reported in coronary arteries treated with transluminal angioplasty, *Am J Cardiol* 51:689-693, 1983.
4. Block PC, Baughman KL, Pasternak RC, et al: Transluminal angioplasty: correlation of morphologic and angiographic findings in an experimental model, *Circulation* 61:778-785, 1980.
5. Faxon DP, Weber VJ, Haudenschild C, et al: Acute effects of transluminal angioplasty in three experimental models of atherosclerosis, *Arteriosclerosis* 2:125-133, 1982.
6. Sanborn TA, Faxon DP, Haudenschild C, et al: The mechanism of transluminal angioplasty: evidence for formation of aneurysms in experimental atherosclerosis, *Circulation* 68:1136-1140, 1983.
7. Sanborn TA, Faxon DP, Waush D, et al: Transluminal angioplasty in experimental atherosclerosis: analysis for embolization using an in vivo perfusion system, *Circulation* 66:917-922, 1982.
8. Lee GL, Ikeda RM, Joye JA, et al: Evaluation of transluminal angioplasty of chronic coronary artery stenosis. Value and limitations assessed in fresh human cadaver hearts, *Circulation* 61:77-83, 1980.
9. Baughman KL, Pasternak RC, Fallon JT, et al: Transluminal coronary angioplasty of postmortem human hearts, *Am J Cardiol* 48:1044-1047, 1981.

10. Castaneda-Zuniga WR, Formanek A, Tadavarthy M, et al: The mechanisms of balloon angioplasty, *Radiology* 135:565-571, 1980.

11. Hoshina T, Yoshida H, Takayama S, et al: Significance of intimal tears in the mechanism of luminal enlargement in percutaneous transluminal coronary angioplasty: correlation of pathologic and angiographic findings in postmortem human hearts, *Am Heart J* 114:503-510, 1987.

12. Lyon RT, Zarins CK, Lu CT, et al: Vessel, plaque, and lumen morphology after transluminal balloon angioplasty, *Arteriosclerosis* 7:306-314, 1987.

13. Block PC, Myler RK, Stertzer S, et al: Morphology after transluminal angioplasty in human beings, *N Engl J Med* 305:382-385, 1981.

14. Kohchi K, Takebayashi S, Block PC, et al: Arterial changes after percutaneous transluminal coronary angioplasty: results of autopsy, *J Am Coll Cardiol* 10:592-599, 1987.

15. Mizuno K, Kurita A, Imazeki N: Pathological findings after percutaneous transluminal coronary angioplasty, *Br Heart J* 52:588-590, 1984.

16. Soward AL, Essed CE, Serruys PW: Coronary arterial findings after accidental death immediately after successful percutaneous transluminal coronary angioplasty, *Am J Cardiol* 56:794-795, 1985.

17. Tenaglia AN, Buller CE, Kisslo KB, et al: Mechanisms of balloon angioplasty and directional coronary atherectomy as assessed by intracoronary ultrasound, *J Am Coll Cardiol* 20:685-691, 1992.

18. Uchida Y, Hasegawa K, Kawamura K, et al: Angioscopic observation of the coronary luminal changes induced by percutaneous transluminal coronary angioplasty, *Am Heart J* 117:769-776, 1989.

19. Colavita PG, Ideker RE, Reimer KA, et al: The spectrum of pathology associated with percutaneous transluminal coronary angioplasty during acute myocardial infarction, *J Am Coll Cardiol* 8:855-860, 1986.

20. Waller BF, Rothbaum DA, Pinkerton CA, et al: Status of the myocardium and infarct-related coronary artery in 19 necropsy patients with acute recanalization using pharmacologic (streptokinase, r-tissue plasminogen activator), mechanical (percutaneous transluminal coronary angioplasty), or combined types of reperfusion therapy, *J Am Coll Cardiol* 9:785-801, 1987.

21. Waller BF: Coronary luminal shape and the arc of disease-free wall: morphologic observations and clinical relevance, *J Am Coll Cardiol* 6:1100-1101, 1985.

22. Farb A, Virmani R, Atkinson JB, et al: Plaque morphology and pathologic changes in arteries from patients dying after coronary balloon angioplasty, *J Am J Coll Cardiol* 16:1421-1429, 1990.

23. Potkin BN, Roberts W: Effects of percutaneous transluminal coronary angioplasty on atherosclerotic plaques and relation of plaque composition and arterial size to outcome, *Am J Cardiol* 62:41-50, 1988.

24. Honye J, Mahon DJ, Jain A, et al: Morphological effects of coronary balloon angioplasty in vivo assessed by intravascular ultrasound imaging, *Circulation* 85:1012-1025, 1992.

25. Davidson CJ, Newman GE, Sheikh KH, et al: Mechanisms of angioplasty in hemodialysis fistula stenoses evaluated by intravascular ultrasound, *Kidney Int* 40:91-95, 1991.

26. Johnson DE, Braden L, Simpson JB: Mechanism of directed transluminal atherectomy, *Am J Cardiol* 65:389-391, 1990.

27. Garratt KN, Edwards WD, Vlietstra RE, et al: Coronary morphology after percutaneous directional coronary atherectomy in humans: autopsy analysis of three patients, *J Am Coll Cardiol* 16:1432-1436, 1990.

28. Penny WF, Schmidt DA, Safian RD, et al: Insights into the mechanism of luminal improvement after directional coronary atherectomy, *Am J Cardiol* 67:435-437, 1991.

29. Safian RD, Gelbfish JS, Erny RE, et al: Coronary atherectomy: clinical, angiographic, and histological findings and observations regarding potential mechanism, *Circulation* 82:69-79, 1990.

30. Nissen SE, Gurley JC, Grines CL, et al: Intravascular ultrasound assessment of lumen size and wall morphology in normal subjects and patients with coronary artery disease, *Circulation* 84:1087-1099, 1991.

31. Muller DW, Ellis SC, Debowey DL, et al: Quantitative angiographic comparison of the immediate success of coronary angioplasty, coronary atherectomy and endoluminal stenting, *Am J Cardiol* 66:938-942, 1990.

32. Suneja R, Nair RH, Reddy KG, et al: Mechanisms of angiographically successful directional coronary atherectomy: evaluation by intracoronary ultrasound and comparison with transluminal coronary angioplasty, *Am Heart J* 126:507-514, 1993.

33. Hansen DD, Auth DC, Vracko R, et al: Rotational atherectomy in atherosclerotic rabbit iliac arteries, *Am Heart J* 115:160-165, 1988.

34. Safian RD, Niazi KA, Stezelecki M, et al: Detailed angiographic analysis of high speed mechanical rotational atherectomy in human coronary arteries, *Circulation* 88:961-968, 1993.

35. Kovach JA, Mintz GS, Pichard AD, et al: Sequential intravascular ultrasound characterization of the mechanisms of rotational atherectomy and adjunct balloon angioplasty, *J Am Coll Cardiol* 22:1024-1032, 1993.

36. Sketch MH, Phillips HR, Lee M, et al: Coronary transluminal extraction endarterectomy, *J Invasive Cardiol* 3:13-18, 1991.

37. Larkin TJ, Niemyski PR, Parker MA, et al: Primary and rescue extraction atherectomy in patients with acute myocardial infarction (abstract), *Circulation* 82:II537, 1991.

38. Grundfest WS, Litvack F, Forrester JS, et al: Laser ablation of human atherosclerotic plaque without adjacent tissue injury, *J Am Coll Cardiol* 5:929-933, 1985.

39. Farrell EM, Higginson LA, Nips WS, et al: Pulsed excimer laser angioplasty of human cadaveric arteries, *J Vasc Surg* 3:284-287, 1986.

40. Isner JM, Donaldson RF, Deckelbaum LI, et al: The excimer laser: gross, light microscopic and ultrastructural analysis of potential advantages for use in laser therapy of cardiovascular disease, *J Am Coll Cardiol* 6:1102-1109, 1985.

41. Marmur JD, Sanborn TA, Kahn H, et al: Acute biologic response to excimer versus thermal laser angioplasty in experimental atherosclerosis, *J Am Coll Cardiol* 17:978-984, 1991.

42. Taylor RS, Higginson LA, Leopold KE: Dependence of the XeCl laser cut rate of plaque on the degree of calcification, laser fluence, and optical pulse duration, *Lasers Surg Med* 10:414-419, 1990.

43. Tenaglia AN, Tcheng JE, Kisslo KB, et al: Intracoronary ultrasound evaluation of excimer laser angioplasty (abstract), *Circulation* 86:I-516, 1992.

44. Diethrich EB, Santiago OJ, Hanafy HM, et al: Angioscopy after coronary excimer laser angioplasty, *J Am Coll Cardiol* 18:643, 1991.

45. Serruys PW, DeJaeger P, Kiemeneij F, et al: A comparison of balloon-expandable-stent implantation with balloon angioplasty in patients with coronary artery disease, *N Engl J Med* 331:489, 1994.

46. Fischman DL, Leon MB, Baim DS, et al: A randomized comparison of coronary-stent placement and balloon angioplasty in the treatment of coronary artery disease, *N Engl J Med* 331:496, 1994.

47. Anderson PG, Bajas RK, Baxley WA, et al: Vascular pathology of balloon-expandable flexible coil stents in humans, *J Am Coll Cardiol* 19:372-381, 1992.

Chapter 11

CORONARY ARTERY PATENCY AND LEFT VENTRICULAR REMODELING AFTER MYOCARDIAL INFARCTION: MECHANISMS AND MECHANICS

John A. Rumberger
Bernard J. Gersh

DeWood et al.[1] were the first to demonstrate total coronary artery occlusion secondary to in situ thrombosis as a prominent factor in the early phase of an evolving acute myocardial infarction. The prevalence of acute coronary thrombosis in acute myocardial infarction has subsequently been established in numerous studies and returns full circle to the studies of Herrick[2] from the early part of this century in which it was proposed to play a pivotal role. Rentrop et al.[3] in 1979 demonstrated the potential application of intracoronary streptokinase to lyse coronary thromboses and thus paved the way for the "thrombolytic era." Many studies have followed that have clearly demonstrated that establishment of coronary artery patency in the early hours after acute myocardial infarction salvages myocardium and reduces early and late cardiac mortality.

However, the clear salutary effects of early interventions such as thrombolysis and direct coronary angioplasty have not universally translated into clear advantages to preservation of resting left ventricular function. The differences between left ventricular ejection fraction at hospital discharge after coronary reperfusion and conventional therapy are mild to modest at best and are contrasted with substantial differences in mortality figures between individuals with documented early coronary patency after infarction and individuals with documented persistent coronary artery occlusion. From these data the "open artery" hypothesis has evolved. It suggests that coronary artery patency after myocardial infarction lowers short- and long-term mortality via mechanisms independent of myocardial salvage and its impact on conventional measures of left ventricular systolic function.

Numerous studies, with and without establishment of early coronary artery patency, have confirmed the pathologic and physiologic consequences of acute myocardial infarction on left ventricular size, shape, and function. Early expansion of the ventricle in the infarct

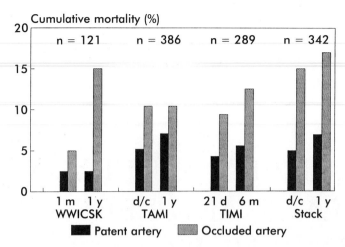

Fig. 11-1. Comparison of four angiographic studies in which early and late cumulative (all-cause) mortality was determined in individuals with documented coronary artery patency or coronary artery occlusion after acute myocardial infarction. Note that the presence of a patent infarct-related coronary artery was associated with a lowered mortality.

region results in ventricular dilation; as a continuum, changes also occur in the noninfarcted myocardium that may lead to further cavity dilation and hypertrophy. The consequences of these changes in left ventricular volumes and muscle mass, which have been termed "postinfarction left ventricular remodeling," also clearly influence postinfarct mortality and morbidity.

Recent studies have suggested that among the potential beneficial roles of the "open artery" after infarction, modulation of the extent of postinfarction ventricular remodeling, which is not well reflected by short- or long-term alterations in ejection fraction, may be one of the most prominent. This chapter explores the role of coronary artery patency after infarction through a variety of mechanisms through which the open artery may influence, in a salutary fashion, the architectural changes in the heart resulting in postinfarction left ventricular remodeling. Other mechanisms regarding the impact of a patent infarct-related artery on the electrical milieu after infarction are discussed in Chapter 66.

OPEN ARTERY HYPOTHESIS: CONTROVERSIES
Mortality vs. ejection fraction

Fig. 11-1 shows a comparison of cumulative mortality for an "open" or "closed" infarct–related coronary artery in four clinical trials of relatively early thrombolytic therapy of acute myocardial infarction. In each study, the early and late cardiac mortality was significantly reduced in patients with angiographically documented patency of the infarct-related artery.[4-7] This enhanced survival after restoration of anterograde flow using thrombolysis alone or in combination with direct angioplasty appears to be sustained long-term; Mathey et al.[8] reported a 4-year survival after myocardial infarction of 84% for individuals who had early resto-

ration of coronary flow compared with 63% in those with partial or no reperfusion.

Data from several clinical studies had previously demonstrated that the most powerful determinant of survival after myocardial infarction was left ventricular ejection fraction.[9,10] Thus, the majority of thrombolysis trials have defined left ventricular ejection fraction as an endpoint: ejection fraction functioning as both a surrogate for measurement of infarct size[11,12] and an important predictor of short- and long-term mortality.

Fig. 11-2 shows mean left ventricular ejection fractions after infarction from ten placebo-controlled randomized trials of relatively early thrombolytic therapy for acute myocardial infarction and three trials comparing the two most commonly employed thrombolytic agents, recombinant tissue-type plasminogen activator (t-PA) and streptokinase.[13] Mean left ventricular ejection fraction is, in general, well preserved after infarction (range 46%-61% for studies included in Fig. 11-2) regardless of therapy. Perhaps most curious, when comparisons were made within a given investigation, there was also little or no difference in left ventricular function between thrombolysis- and placebo-treated patients or between patients treated with different biologically active thrombolytic agents. In the study previously quoted by Mathey et al.[8] demonstrating significant reduction in mortality at 4 years after infarction for an open artery, the hospital discharge ejection fraction was identical in patients with patent and occluded infarct related coronary arteries (53% and 52%, respectively).

The controversy surrounding the apparent dissociation between reestablishment of coronary artery patency and blood flow on cardiac mortality and left ventricular function after myocardial infarction has raised the possibility that restoration of anterograde coronary flow

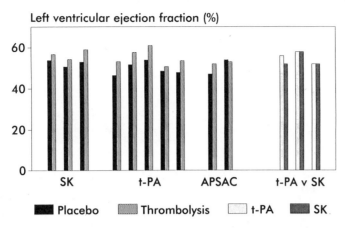

Fig. 11-2. Comparison of discharge or predischarge left ventricular ejection fraction from ten placebo-controlled trials of thrombolysis early after myocardial infarction and three trials comparing tissue-type plasminogen activator *(t-PA)* vs. streptokinase *(SK)*. In each instance, there were little or no interstudy differences in left ventricular ejection fraction.   (Adapted from Topol EJ, Wilson VE: *Heart Lung* 19:583, 1990.)

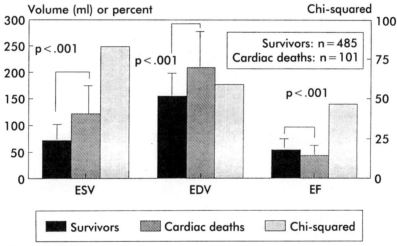

*Angiography 4-8 wks. post-MI, follow up 78 ± 32 mos.

Fig. 11-3. Survival after myocardial infarction as determined by measurements of left ventricular end-systolic volume *(ESV)*, end-diastolic volume *(EDV)*, and ejection fraction *(EF)*. Note that although each measurement was contributory, the chi-squared values indicate that end-systolic volume was the most powerful predictor of long-term survival after infarction. (Adapted from White HD, Norris RM, Brown MA, et al: *Circulation* 76:44, 1987.)

may reduce mortality through mechanisms independent of its influence on left ventricular function. Simply stated, the *open artery hypothesis* is as follows: Patency of the infarct-related coronary artery (either "early" or "late") after myocardial infarction is a major determinant of short- and long-term mortality independent of ventricular function.

Van de Werf[14] recanted these observations by suggesting that "the low ejection fractions of these early reperfused patients [who would have died without reperfusion therapy] will mask the gain in ejection fraction obtained in other reperfused patients and therefore distort the comparison with surviving controls...." Although this explanation is plausible, there

have been no definitive studies to substantiate the "time to treatment paradox." Studies by White et al.,[15] on the other hand, which confirm earlier studies by Hammermeister et al.,[16] have underscored that the absolute magnitude of left ventricular end-systolic and end-diastolic volumes are far more powerful predictors of mortality after myocardial infarction than left ventricular ejection fraction alone (Fig. 11-3).

Ejection fraction as a surrogate for mortality and infarct size after myocardial infarction

There are three caveats to the use of left ventricular ejection fraction as a surrogate for infarct size and postinfarction mortality that add to the confusion in

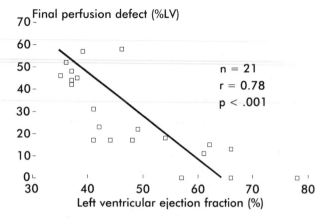

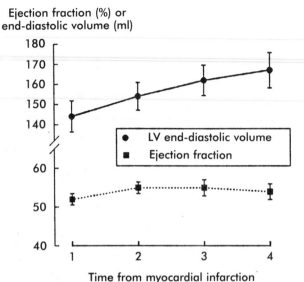

Fig. 11-4. Left ventricular ejection fraction vs. final infarct size (percent of total left ventricular perfusion defect) in patients 1 year after myocardial infarction. Note that there is an inverse correlation but that the datum scatter is broad. (From Christian TF, Behrenbeck T, Gersh BJ, et al: *Am J Cardiol* 68:21, 1991. Used by permission.)

Fig. 11-5. Absolute left ventricular end-diastolic volume (ml) and left ventricular ejection fraction in 18 patients during the first year after an index transmural myocardial infarction. Each patient had an ultrafast (cine) computed tomography study at hospital discharge (Time 1) and at 6 weeks (Time 2), 6 months (Time 3) and 1 year (Time 4) after infarction. Despite a significant (17%) increase in end-diastolic volume by 1 year after infarction, ejection fraction remains the same as that determined at hospital discharge. Data are mean ± SEM.

resolving the open-artery controversy: use of ejection fraction as a measure of infarct size, and thus a measure of myocardial salvage, is of limited value; measurement of ejection fraction in the aforementioned trials has been inaccurate; and changes in left ventricular volumes after myocardial infarction (as perhaps the best predictors of cardiac mortality) are not necessarily adequately reflected by calculation of changes in ejection fraction.

Ejection fraction as a measure of infarct size

Christian et al.[12] have demonstrated an inverse relationship between left ventricular ejection fraction and infarct size (determined as percent of final ventricular perfusion defect by technetium 99m–sestamibi) (Fig. 11-4). These results are similar to those shown by Pfeffer and Braunwald[11] comparing ejection fraction and histologic infarct size in the rate with healed infarction.

In the individual clinical situation, however, direct correlative relationships between ejection fraction determined sometime after infarction and acute infarct size must be reviewed critically because of the number of uncontrolled variables (e.g., variable preload and afterload, absence or presence of collaterals, prior infarction). The standard error of the estimate in Fig. 11-4 is on the order of 12% of the left ventricular myocardium, and the scatter of the data about the regression line is large. Thus, determinations of left ventricular ejection fraction may not be the best indicators of the degree of myocardial damage in the acute or semiacute situation; in fact, in some circumstances, recovery of regional left ventricular function can be demonstrated during the weeks to months after infarction[17] and may be dramatic in those cases of hibernating myocardium after mechanical or surgical revascularization. Although ejection

fraction appears to correlate with infarct size over a broad range of values, it is not a sufficiently reliable surrogate for infarct size when the latter is an endpoint of a large clinical trial.

Accuracy of clinical ejection fraction determinations

Consideration need be given to the overall accuracy of ejection fraction determinations made in the previously published clinical trials of thrombolysis in acute myocardial infarction. In the 13 studies that make up Fig. 11-2, 10 used contrast ventriculography and 1 used echocardiography to define left ventricular ejection fraction. For both of these commonly used clinical imaging techniques, calculation of ejection fraction is highly dependent on assumptions as to left ventricular geometry[18,19]; both have less precision in the presence of regional wall motion abnormalities. Radionuclide angiography, by determining counts per ventricular volume, requires no assumptions regarding ventricular geometry[20] but was used in only two of the aforementioned studies.

Ejection fraction as a measure of ventricular volumes

Third, ejection fraction is a measure of relative *changes* in ventricular volumes during the cardiac cycle and not a measure of volumes per se. Fig. 11-5 shows average left ventricular end-diastolic volume and ejection fraction in 18 patients who had serial ultrafast computed tomography (cine CT) examinations during the first year after an index transmural myocardial infarction. Ultrafast CT has been shown to provide quantitative data on ventricular volumes and systolic function, regardless of the clinical or experimental situation.[21-23] Overall ventricular end-diastolic volume increased 17% from hospital discharge to 1 year after infarction ($P < 0.05$); however, during this same period there was little or no change in global ejection fraction. This occurred because concomitant increases in cavitary stroke volume paralleled the changes in ventricular end-diastolic volumes.

Thus, a combination of errors in clinical calculation of ejection fraction because of the method chosen for measurement, limitations in the use of ejection fraction to define infarct size, and the limited applicability of left ventricular ejection fraction to describe progressive changes in ventricular volumes after infarction all add to difficulties in resolving the open artery controversy. Accumulating data suggest, however, that an important mechanism is modulation of the magnitude and extent of postinfarction left ventricular remodeling.

POSTINFARCTION LEFT VENTRICULAR REMODELING
Postinfarction infarct expansion and ventricular remodeling

Investigations during the 1970s and early 1980s after transmural myocardial infarction described the phenomenon of infarct expansion, defined as progressive increases in ventricular diastolic volume and myocardial segment length in the infarct region.[24-26] Pathologically such changes have been characterized largely by myocyte bundle rearrangement ("myocyte slippage") with minimal to moderate myocyte lengthening ("myocyte stretch") along individual cell bundles.[27,28] However, extensions to the early clinical studies have described relatively characteristic changes in the *non*-infarcted myocardium that appear to be in direct proportion to the degree of initial infarct expansion. Moreover, infarct expansion may be completed by 3 weeks[29] and certainly by at least 6 weeks[30] after infarction, but changes in the noninfarcted myocardium, which are also characterized by increases in segment length and cavity volume, may be observed early after infarction and persist or become progressive for weeks, months, and possibly years after the acute event (see Fig. 11-5).[31,32] The more generic term "postinfarction left ventricular remodeling" is now used to describe the scope of changes in regional and global cavity volumes, ventricular shape, and myocardial mass after an acute, transmural myocardial infarction. The extent of remodeling may well be an independent measure of cardiac exercise performance.[33]

From studies of the Framingham cohort, the prevalence of congestive heart failure increases progressively after myocardial infarction to approximately 14% by 5 years and 23% by 10 years.[34] This is likely a consequence of postinfarction remodeling and ventricular dilation. Unchecked ventricular dilation is certainly a precursor to chronic heart failure. Recent studies from the Studies of Left Ventricular Dysfunction (SOLVD) investigation have clearly shown an altered neurohormonal profile in asymptomatic patients with only mild reduction in global ejection fraction.[35] This, in turn, could predispose to further deterioration and subsequent congestive heart failure. Pfeffer et al.[36] have convincingly demonstrated that the angiotensin-converting enzyme inhibitor captopril can significantly limit postinfarction mortality in the rat model of infarction and attenuate left ventricular dilation in humans after anterior infarction.[37] In addition, reports from the Survival and Ventricular Enlargement (SAVE) protocol[38] have shown that initiation of treatment within 10 days of myocardial infarction with oral captopril can limit long-term postinfarction mortality in patients without congestive heart failure and moderately depressed ejection fraction. The CONSENSUS II trial studied the effects of intravenous enalaprilat followed by oral enalapril vs. placebo commenced within 24 hours of infarction.[39] This investigation, in contradistinction to SAVE, has suggested that there is no difference in 3- and 6-month mortality after infarction with enalaprilat/enalapril compared with placebo. Although additional studies are necessary, there are there major differences between CONSENSUS II and SAVE. In particular, CONSENSUS II commenced therapy during the throes of an acute infarction where hypotension associated with afterload reduction may be detrimental, used intravenous therapy initially rather than oral therapy, and involved limited postinfarction follow-up. If one carefully examines the SAVE data, the apparent advantage of oral captopril on all-cause mortality, cardiac mortality, and even recurrent infarction was not apparent until at least 1 year after the acute event.

The process of postinfarction left ventricular remodeling, whether a truly adaptive or pathologic mechanism, is clinically important. An objective of many therapeutic interventions for cardiac disease is to prevent or limit ventricular dilation and preserve systolic function. Because measured ventricular volumes are the most powerful predictor of late mortality after infarction, modification of dilation and remodeling is an appropriate therapeutic objective.

Coronary patency and infarct remodeling
Animal studies. Although the degree of infarct expansion is directly influenced by infarct size, coronary artery patency may also have a profound effect on

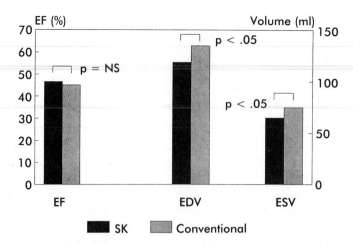

Fig. 11-6. Comparison of left ventricular ejection fraction *(EF)*, end-diastolic volume *(EDV)*, and end-systolic volume *(ESV)* in survivors of acute myocardial infarction between conventional therapy and intravenous streptokinase. Results are from GISSI-I. (Modified from Marino P, Zanolla L, Zardine P: Effect of streptokinase on left ventricular modeling and function after myocardial infarction: the GISSI Trial, *J Am Coll Cardiol* 14:1149-1158, 1989.)

remodeling. The presence of coronary artery patency during the first few hours after infarction appears to influence the remodeling process in animals at a time when any contribution to myocardial salvage is minimal. In one study performed in rats, infarct size and its extension through the ventricular wall (i.e., its transmurality) were not affected when an occluded artery was reopened after about 2 hours, allowing the muscle to reperfuse.[40] Restoring perfusion after this 2-hour period of occlusion, however, significantly inhibited subsequent infarct expansion. Thus, the degree of left ventricular remodeling was modulated by coronary artery patency when compared with a companion group of rats with persistent coronary occlusion.

Clinical studies. Efforts have been made to correlate the extent of postinfarction ventricular remodeling in humans with patency of the infarct-related coronary artery. An early report from GISSI I compared ejection fraction and left ventricular volumes at hospital discharge in patients receiving streptokinase vs. conventional therapy for an acute myocardial infarction. Between these two groups, ejection fraction was similar, but both left ventricular end-diastolic and end-systolic volumes were larger in the control subjects (Fig. 11-6).[41]

However, controversy continues in the clinical arena. For instance, Jeremy et al.[42] studied a group of patients who did not receive thrombolytic therapy for an acute Q-wave myocardial infarction. They found that the presence of infarct-related coronary patency on a discharge coronary angiogram correlated with a postinfarct reduction in overall ventricular dilation as compared with a group that had occluded coronary arteries. Remodeling in this study was defined by increases in left ventricular end-diastolic and end-systolic volume iden-

tified by radionuclide angiography. In contrast, Warren et al.[43] reported on patients given successful late thrombolysis at 5 ± 1 hours after myocardial infarction. Infarct-related coronary artery patency, as demonstrated on angiography at discharge, seemed to have no effect on limiting ventricular dilation after infarction. These findings suggested that opening the occluded vessel about 5 hours after infarction did not prove beneficial to limiting early ventricular remodeling. Finally, Villari et al.[44] found a clear inverse relationship between coronary artery patency and left ventricular volumes, as determined by angiography 8 to 10 days after infarction (Fig. 11-7). There was also a direct correlation between left ventricular volumes and the extent of regional hypokinesis or akinesis, however, suggesting that infarct extent (indexed by the magnitude of regional wall motion abnormalities[31,32]) may have been different between the two patient groups.

MECHANISMS IN WHICH PATENCY OF THE INFARCT RELATED ARTERY MAY LIMIT POST-INFARCTION REMODELING
Early vs. late patency

The general course of postinfarction left ventricular remodeling during the first few hours to days after infarction is determined largely by the initial infarct size; however, a number of mechanisms result in both early and late changes in left ventricular architecture after infarction, which may be modulated or influenced by resumption of coronary patency and flow. These mechanisms are subsequently noted and discussed later in the chapter as they pertain to the open artery controversy and are listed in Table 11-1.

However, another unresolved query that arises in the

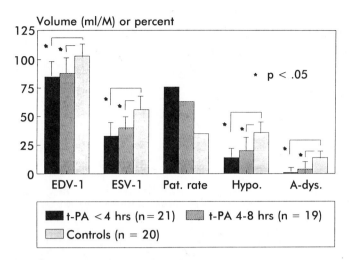

Fig. 11-7. End-diastolic volume index *(EDV-I)*, end-systolic volume index *(ESV-I)*, patency rate *(Pat. Rate)*, percent of left ventricular hypokinesis *(Hypo.)*, and percent of left ventricular akinesis or dyskinesis *(A-Dys.)* in patients given intravenous tissue-type plasminogen activator less than 4 hours after myocardial infarction, within 4 to 8 hours after myocardial infarction, and in controls given conventional therapy. Note that the ventricular volumes are inversely related to the frequency of coronary patency achieved (assessed 8 to 10 days after infarction). However, the ventricular volumes are also directly related to the extent of regional wall motion abnormalities, suggesting that differences in ventricular volumes are dependent on both patency rate and infarct size. (Adapted from Villari B, Piscione F, Bonaduce D, et al: Usefulness of late coronary thrombolysis [recombinant tissue-type plasminogen activator] in preserving left ventricular function in acute myocardial infarction, *Am J Cardiol* 66:1281-1286, 1990.)

same context is as follows: If coronary artery patency has a salutary effect on postinfarction remodeling, when during the course of acute infarction or periinfarct time period are the effects most evident? Whereas it is clear that establishment of coronary artery patency within the first few hours of an acute myocardial infarction preserves myocardium at risk and limits infarct size, the issue often is one of maintaining patency long term. In fact, although coronary artery patency with thrombolytics allow for a greater patency rate early on, there actually is little difference in coronary artery patency between early thrombolysis and "conservative" therapy when judged by direct angiography performed at several weeks to months after infarction.

Fig. 11-8 shows studies of angiographic coronary artery patency rates from ten separate angiographic studies of acute myocardial infarction, with or without

Table 11-1. Methods whereby a patent infarct-related artery may limit ventricular expansion and remodeling after myocardial infarction

---

Reduction in overall infarct size or extent
Limitation of transmurality of infarction
Resumption of antegrade collateral blood flow
Acceleration of infarct healing
"Garden hose" effect

---

thrombolysis. DeWood et al.[1] found a spontaneous coronary artery patency of 13% at 4 hours after infarction; by this time 80% of the coronary arteries may be patent in patients receiving thrombolytics.[45] (The issues of which agent may be more beneficial in a given situation or the use of adjuvant therapy with heparin are discussed in Chapters 24 and 25). Thrombolysis in Myocardial Infarction I[46] (TIMI-I) demonstrated a 17% spontaneous patency at 6 hours, and Rentrop et al.[47] showed a 27% spontaneous patency by 12 hours. However, the differences in coronary patency between early intervention and conventional therapy become diminishingly small with time from the acute event.[4,48-51] By 3 weeks after infarction, roughly 65% to 75% of infarct-related arteries are patent[52] regardless of the initial acute infarction treatment protocol. Topol et al.,[53] reporting results from TAMI-6, have shown an identical 59% coronary artery patency rate at 6 months after infarction for individuals given t-PA "late" (6-24 hours) after infarction vs. placebo. The eventual establishment of coronary patency in patients treated in a conservative manner reflects the extent of thrombus resolution occurring naturally through spontaneous in situ thrombolysis.

For the effects of coronary artery patency regarding ventricular remodeling (and by inference on short- and long-term mortality) to be so different between early

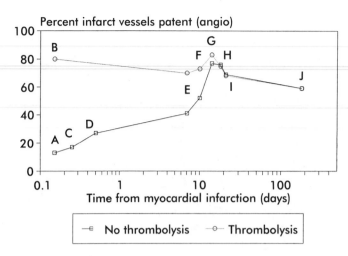

Fig. 11-8. Comparison of angiographically documented infarct-related coronary artery patency rates in ten separate clinical studies and time from myocardial infarction as modulated by early administration of a thrombolytic agent vs. nonthrombolytic (conventional) therapy. The x-axis is a semilogarithmic scale of time in days from myocardial infarction. Note that the difference in patency rates becomes diminishingly small within the first 2 to 3 weeks after infarction.

intervention (thrombolysis or angioplasty) and conservative therapy, it stands to reason that the beneficial effects of coronary patency must be influential during the postinfarction time period when coronary patency rates are significantly different. This would then narrow the time period for establishment of coronary patency and its beneficial effect on postinfarction remodeling to within the first few days after infarction and, most probably, within the first 12 hours after clinical manifestation.

The discussion that follows presents a variety of mechanisms that may limit the long-term consequences of postinfarction remodeling as modulated by reestablishment of coronary artery patency, some influential within the first hours and some within the first days after infarction.

Mechanisms

Reduction in overall infarct size or extent. The magnitude of infarct expansion and ventricular cavity dilation after infarction is directly related to infarct size.[24-31] Therefore, the smaller the infarction, the smaller the extent of postinfarct remodeling. Studies done in unanesthetized canines under well-controlled conditions have shown that little "salvage" of the myocardium occurs after 6 hours of coronary occlusion (Fig. 11-9).[54] However, because humans, unlike dogs, have a poorly developed natural coronary collateral system,[55] it is generally assumed that the time course for appreciable salvage of myocardium in the clinical situation must be much shorter than 6 hours.[56] However, studies such as ISIS-2[57] have shown a reduction in short- and long-term mortality in patients receiving thrombolysis 8 or more hours after infarction. These observations

have added to the speculation that even establishment of "late" coronary artery patency (i.e., >5 to 8 hours after infarction), although not clearly providing for additional myocardial salvage, is beneficial.

Although such considerations regarding the time window for myocardial salvage have a basis in fact, it is often most difficult to determine the exact timing of the onset of infarction in humans. Patients will frequently have waxing and waning clinical courses. The timing of angina onset is very subjective and may not be particularly predictive of the timing of coronary occlusion.

Fig. 11-10 shows results from a clinical study in which definite myocardial salvage occurred in some patients after "late" reperfusion. Here Behrenbeck et al.,[58] using [99m]Te-sestamibi scanning on clinical presentation and at 3 days after acute myocardial infarction, examined myocardial salvage in a group of patients who underwent direct coronary angioplasty after presentation. Although these data represent a select group of individuals in whom angiography was performed soon after hospital admission, clear myocardial salvage (i.e., difference between acute infarct area at risk and final infarct size) is evident in patients treated both less than and greater than 5 hours after infarction. Data such as these emphasize the heterogeneity of clinical presentations of patients with acute myocardial infarction and provide evidence that clear salvage of myocardium can occur at variable times after the onset of angina. With such data in mind one cannot eliminate entirely a degree of myocardial salvage occurring in some individuals treated "late" after myocardial infarction. However, as pointed out recently by White,[59] it is unlikely that such patients

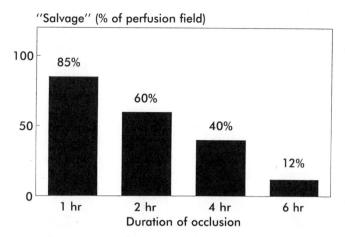

Fig. 11-9. Percent of infarct-related coronary artery perfusion field salvage vs. time of coronary artery occlusion. This study was done in conscious dogs. (From Becker LC, Ambrosio G: Myocardial consequences of reperfusion, *Prog Cardiovasc Dis* 30:23-49, 1987.)

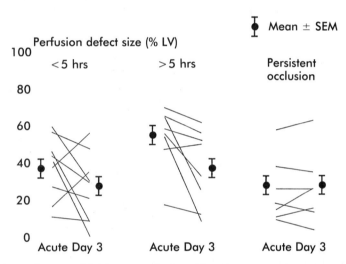

Fig. 11-10. Acute "area at risk" (presentation) and final infarct size (day 3) as determined by technetium 99m–sestamibi in patients receiving direct coronary angioplasty less than 5 hours after infarction *(far left panel)* vs. therapy 5 or more hours after infarction *(middle panel)*. The far right panel shows results from patients with chronic myocardial infarction determined 3 days apart for controls. Note that appreciable "myocardial salvage" can be seen in patients with both early and late interventions for acute myocardial infarction. (Adapted from Behrenbeck T, Pellikka P, Huber KC, et al: Primary angioplasty in myocardial infarction: assessment of improved myocardial perfusion with technetium-99m isonitrile, *J Am Coll Cardiol* 17:365-372, 1991.)

make up a large proportion of individuals entered into randomized trials.

The greatest benefits of reperfusion to myocardial salvage are most probably confined to individuals receiving therapy within 1 to 2 hours of clinical manifestation. Simoons et al.,[60] estimating infarct extent by total 72-hour myocardial enzyme release, found an overall reduction in infarct size of 30% comparing thrombolysis (N = 269) with conventional therapy (N = 264); however, in patients admitted within 1 hour, between 1 and 2 hours, and greater than 2 hours after the onset of symp-

toms, the reductions in infarct size were 51%, 31%, and 13%, respectively.

Establishment of coronary artery patency, particularly if the patient continues to have angina or persistent changes consistent with additional myocardial injury on the electrocardiogram within the first 24 hours after onset of infarction, may have an effect on infarct size and, by inference, the extent of postinfarction left ventricular remodeling.

Limitation of infarct transmurality. The experimental studies of postinfarction left ventricular remodeling have clearly shown that a full-thickness (i.e., fully trans-mural) myocardial infarction is a prerequisite to ven-tricular remodeling.[61] Preservation of an epicardial rim of myocardium by resumption of coronary artery patency early after infarction, before completion of the transmu-ral progression of necrosis, may be an additional mecha-nism by which infarct expansion and global postinfarc-tion ventricular remodeling can be limited or prevented.

The "wavefront" of myocardial infarction was first described by Reimer and Jennings.[62] Basically, myocar-dial necrosis commences at the endocardial surface and with time proceeds toward the epicardial rim. By 40 minutes in dogs with permanent coronary occlusion, the percent of necrotic myocardium is approximately 35% of the full thickness. By 6 hours infarction extends through 75% of the myocardial wall. Full-thickness, transmural necrosis is established by 24 hours after infarction. Reestablishment of coronary flow, at least during the first hours after infarction, limits not only infarct size but probably limits infarct transmurality in humans. Preser-vation of a rim of viable epicardium may be sufficient to form a buttress that resists the early expansion within the infarct zone, thus limiting early and late manifestations of infarct remodeling.

After myocardial infarction, preservation and return of regional systolic wall thickening can occur only if the majority of the thickness of the myocardium has been preserved in the infarct zone. Roughly only about 20% of the myocardial thickness needs to be necrotic before wall thickening is severely or permanently limited.[63] Touchstone et al.[64] used two-dimensional echocardiog-raphy to characterize serial changes in regional left ventricular function in the infarct region of 24 patients who received intravenous streptokinase within 4 hours of chest pain for acute myocardial infarction. Eight (45%) of the 18 patients with a patent coronary artery documented within 2 hours of the streptokinase therapy at angiography had improvement in regional left ven-tricular function; however, the improvement was not seen until 3 to 10 days after infarction, suggesting, albeit indirectly, that the ultimate improvement in regional function was secondary to nontransmural extent of necrosis. Of the five patients with evidence of infarct expansion during the 10-day follow-up, four had docu-mented coronary occlusion at angiography. Broad inter-pretation of this study, however, must be done with caution; Choong et al.[65] have suggested that late return of functional recovery in the infarct region in canines as assessed by echocardiography may result not from nontransmural infarction but from progressive reduction of infarct segment length or scar contraction.

Collateral blood flow. The existence of collateral-dependent flow to the infarct zone can have profound effects on infarct size and preservation of islands of functional myocardium. The early studies by Shaper[66] in

canines demonstrated significant variability in the time course and extent of necrosis, depending on preexisting collateral development, modulated by the myocardial oxygen demand.

Collateral flow to an infarct zone from preexisting channels can influence the magnitude of ventricular re-modeling, even in the presence of persistent coronary oc-clusion of the infarct vessel. These are commonly seen on angiography as intracoronary right-to-left/or left-to-right collaterals. The presence of such conduits has been shown by Tadakazu et al.[67] to limit the development of postinfarction left ventricular aneurysm after anterior wall infarction. Shen et al.[68] demonstrated a clear limita-tion in subsequent left ventricular volumes after infarc-tion in patients with total coronary occlusion but with preexisting collaterals compared with individuals with occlusion but no collaterals. However, it is difficult to as-certain whether these beneficial effects were as a result of return of blood flow to the perimeters of the infarct or an independent effect of reducing actual infarct size.

Patency of the infarct-related coronary artery, by itself, can be an important contributor to collateral flow to the infarct zone. For instance, a distal occlusion of the left anterior descending (LAD) coronary artery, remote from an acute and proximal LAD occlusion, could have provided for the development of left-to-left or LAD-to-LAD collaterals. Restoration of antegrade flow through the proximal LAD would be of significant benefit to the perfusion field of the anterior wall. Most probably, however, the overall effect would be in limitation of infarct size or possibly in limiting infarct transmurality by preservation of islands of viable myocardium.

Alterations in infarct healing. A key to limiting the extend of postinfarction left ventricular remodeling is to limit the initial extent of infarct expansion. Resistance to distention from alterations in preload and afterload and changes in regional wall tension after infarction must be countered by the inherent tensile strength of the myocardium. The status of regional ventricular compli-ance can have profound consequences on the magnitude of infarct expansion.

The seminal work by Hochman and Choo[40] in the rat model of anterior wall infarction has demonstrated that the extent of infarct expansion can be modulated by late reperfusion of the infarct coronary artery independent of myocardial salvage. They examined the effects of delayed coronary artery reperfusion on the extent of infarct expansion 2 weeks after anterior infarction. Rats are excellent models of human infarction because this species has very poorly developed preexisting coronary collateral channels. Here, infarct size and transmural extent of infarction were not different comparing late reperfusion with permanent occlusion. However, the extent of dilation in the infarct region was significantly attenuated by delayed coronary reperfusion (Fig. 11-11).

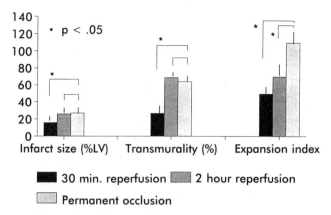

Fig. 11-11. Infarct size (percent of left ventricular muscle mass), transmurality (percent of transmural necrosis from endocardium to epicardium), and expansion index as a function of timing of reperfusion vs. permanent occlusion. Despite similar infarct size and transmurality of infarction between 2-hour reperfusion and permanent occlusion, the expansion index was significantly reduced after delayed resumption of coronary flow. (Adapted from Hochman JS, Choo H: Limitation of myocardial infarct expansion by reperfusion independent of myocardial salvage, *Circulation* 75:299, 1987.)

The primary pathologic differences were between the bland infarct seen with permanent coronary artery occlusion and the hemorrhagic infarct seen with reestablishment of coronary artery patency and delayed reperfusion. Along with hemorrhagic infarction in the reperfused hearts, they noted increased myocyte swelling, edema formation, and acceleration of contraction band necrosis; reperfusion thus hastened the overall infarct healing process. Hockman and Choo[40] speculated that the limited infarct expansion in the hemorrhagic infarction was associated with some preservation of normal compliance in the region, thus resisting the initial distending forces.

Hale and Kloner[69] examined histologic changes in the infarct region 6 weeks (presumed completion of healing[30]) after both early and late reperfusion in the rat infarction model. As would be expected and consistent with a previous discussion, early reperfusion (30 minutes) limited both infarct size and the extent of cavity dilation. Late reperfusion (90 minutes) was associated with no myocardial salvage and, in this model, no appreciable limitation of left ventricular cavity dilation compared with controls with permanent occlusion. However, infarct thickness was significantly greater in the late reperfusion group than in infarct controls. Thus, overall infarct expansion (thinning and lengthening of the infarcted myocardium) was limited by late reperfusion. Hale and Kloner[69] speculated that this would equate with an overall benefit in reducing so-called negative work (i.e., systolic bulging) during systole. This could allow for a more equitable distribution of left ventricular wall stresses between the infarct and noninfarct regions because wall stress is inversely proportional to wall thickness.

However, one must weigh the potential benefit of late coronary artery reperfusion and coronary patency, ostensibly changing from a "bland" to "hemorrhagic" infarction, against the report by Honan et al.[70] This metaanalysis suggested that aggressive attempts to reestablish coronary artery patency by 11 to 12 hours after infarction (when presumably there is little to gain with respect to myocardial salvage) may be deleterious by increasing the frequency of myocardial rupture.

Changes in myocardial compliance secondary to filled coronary vasculature (garden hose effect). Increases in regional myocardial "stiffness" by resumption of coronary blood flow in the overlying epicardial conduit may translate into beneficial effects of coronary artery patency regarding attenuation of infarct expansion. The epicardial coronary arteries are filled with blood at all times during the cardiac cycle, especially during the diastolic phase of the cardiac cycle, where two thirds or more of coronary flow occurs. In addition, intramyocardial vascular blood volume (consisting largely of blood-filled vasculature in the 100-µm or smaller arterioles and capillaries) can account for as much as 10% to 20% of the total in vivo myocardial volume,[71] especially during the peripheral vasodilation and reactive hyperemia associated with coronary reperfusion.

The presence of a fluid-filled conduit on the perimeter of the heart may influence the extent to which the heart dilates or distends during diastole. This has often been referred to as the "erectile" function of the coronary arteries but is more colloquially referred to as the garden hose effect.

No studies to date have specifically examined this effect in relation to postinfarction left ventricular remodeling. However, Vogel et al.,[72] using intravenous adenosine to produce maximum coronary vasodilation, measured the effect of increases in coronary blood flow on diastolic wall thickness and diastolic chamber compliance under normal oxygenated conditions. Under normal conditions, adenosine caused a 50% increase in blood flow but only a 4% increase in diastolic wall thickness from control; however, the diastolic pressure-volume compliance curve was significantly shifted to the left, consistent with a decrease in cardiac chamber compliance (or, alternatively, an increase in diastolic stiffness).

Brown et al.[73] examined the acute effects of delayed reperfusion on myocardial infarct shape and associated changes in left ventricular volume in dogs. Circumferentially placed myocardial ultrasonic distance crystals were used to examine dogs at control and after 5.5 hours of occlusion of the LAD, followed by 1 hour of reperfusion. Infarct size was similar in both groups. During coronary artery occlusion, left ventricular volume acutely increased by $42 \pm 6\%$ over baseline; however, within minutes after reperfusion, infarct stiffening occurred and the left volume decreased to $16 \pm 11\%$ over the baseline value. The magnitude of myocardial reperfusion blood flow was not assessed; however, this acute change in regional left ventricular compliance was temporally related to the resumption of coronary artery patency and anterograde flow.

SUMMARY AND CONCLUSIONS

Use of thrombolytics or direct coronary angioplasty has significantly reduced early and late postmyocardial infarction mortality, presumably by limiting infarct size. However, additional beneficial effects of the "open artery" after infarction have been noted regarding the extent of post–myocardial infarction left ventricular remodeling.

Post–myocardial infarction remodeling is the composite of changes in left ventricular volumes, muscle mass, and shape that occur after transmural infarction. These changes occur initially in the infarct region ("infarct expansion") but later develop in the noninfarcted myocardium. Ventricular dilation after infarction has been clinically recognized for a number of years and is believed to be primarily an adaptive response to maintenance of stroke volume via a Starling mechanism. The development of left ventricular hypertrophy appears to be delayed beyond the occurrence of ventricular dilation and is teleologically believed to occur in response to increases in regional ventricular wall stress. The extent of ventricular dilation (and as a prerequisite to the development of hypertrophy) after infarction may adversely affect prognosis. Recent studies have demonstrated the left ventricular end-systolic and end-diastolic volumes to be powerful predictors of subsequent mortality and morbidity over and above that provided from assessment of ejection fraction. In addition, the subsequent development of ventricular hypertrophy may limit flow reserve and vasodilatory capacity of the noninfarcted myocardium,[74] thus leading to a greater impairment in functional reserve and overall cardiac performance, with or without additional ischemia.

There are five mechanisms that may explain the benefits of late reperfusion on limiting post–myocardial infarction remodeling. First, there is clinical evidence that additional myocardium is preserved even if reperfusion commences more than 6 hours after infarction, thus limiting the overall extent of myocardial damage. The "wave front" of infarction has been shown to proceed from the subendocardium to the subepicardium. Thus, a second mechanism may be that late reperfusion allows preservation of a rim of myocardium in the subepicardium. Collateral blood flow to portions of the infarcted myocardium, preserving islands of viable tissue in the vascular distribution of the occluded artery, is a third possible mechanism. Reperfusion into an area of infarction results in hemorrhage, contraction band necrosis, cell swelling, and edema, thus reducing regional wall compliance and acting as a buttress to distending forces. The subsequent resistance to dilation may be a fourth mechanism. Finally, the presence of an open, blood-filled, infarct-related artery and vascular bed (the garden hose effect) may provide a scaffolding to limit "infarct expansion."

All of these mechanisms, which either increase the stiffness of the infarct region early after infarction or limit its transmural extent, possibly contribute to limitation of subsequent postnecrotic infarct expansion and left ventricular dilation after reperfusion of the infarct-related coronary artery (Fig. 11-12).

The discussions presented here emphasize the fact that the earlier the occurrence of reperfusion after myocardial infarction, the more beneficial the circumstances. In addition, there are some caveats to "late" reperfusion, as noted in the metaanalysis by Honan et al.[70] However, results from the ISIS-2 trial have suggested that late reperfusion may also be beneficial, and several of the mechanisms presented here may be contributory.

TAMI-6 was designed to evaluate benefits of administration of intravenous t-PA to patients presenting 6 to 24 hours after infarction.[53] Preliminary results do show that ventricular dilation 6 months after infarction was less in patients given thrombolysis (24-hour coronary patency rate of 63%) than in patients given placebo (24-hour patency rate of 27%). Two large randomized studies have been organized and conducted to confirm the potential benefits of late reperfusion. These are the Estudio Multicentrico Estreptoquinasa Republica Argentina (EMERA) trial (N = 4000, placebo-controlled, intravenous streptokinase given 6 to 24 hours after infarction) and the Late Assessment of Thrombolytic Efficacy (LATE) trial (similar to EMERA but using alteplase [recombinant t-PA], N = 5000). Preliminary analyses and results of these trials have been presented at several international meetings. In particular, the LATE trial showed that treatment with alteplase, initiated between 6 and 12 hours after symptom onset, reduced 35-day mortality by 27% compared with placebo.[75] This benefit apparently was sustained to at least 1 year. However, there was apparently no reduction in mortality evident among patients treated beyond 12 hours from onset of symptoms. Critical review of these data await final publication of these large clinical studies. Until that time these important issues remain incompletely resolved.

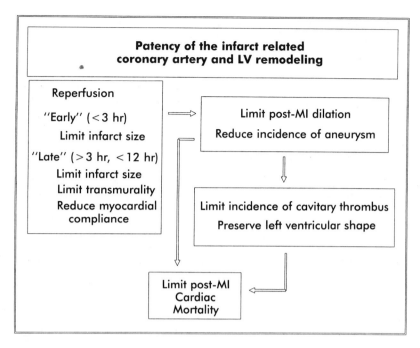

Fig. 11-12. Flow diagram indicating the salutary effects of establishment of coronary artery patency after infarction on the extent of postinfarction remodeling and mortality.

REFERENCES

1. DeWood MA, Spores J, Notske R, et al: Prevalence of total coronary occlusion during the early hours of transmural myocardial infarction, *N Engl J Med* 303:897-902, 1980.
2. Herrick JB: Clinical features of sudden obstruction of the coronary arteries, *JAMA* 59:2012-2020, 1912.
3. Rentrop P, Blanke H, Karsch KR, et al: Acute myocardial infarction: intracoronary nitroglycerin and streptokinase in combination with transluminal recanalization, *Clin Cardiol* 2:345-363, 1979.
4. Kennedy JW, Ritchie JL, Davis KB, et al: The Western Washington randomized trial of intravenous streptokinase in acute myocardial infarction: a 12 month follow up report, *N Eng J Med* 312-1073-1078, 1985.
5. Topol EJ, George BS, Kereiakes DJ, et al: A randomized controlled trial of intravenous tissue plasminogen activator and early intravenous heparin in acute myocardial infarction, *Circulation* 79:281-286, 1989.
6. Chesebro JH, Knatterud G, Roberts R, et al: Thrombolysis in myocardial infarction (TIMI) trial, phase I: a comparison between intravenous tissue plasminogen activator and intravenous streptokinase, *Circulation* 76:142-154, 1987.
7. Stack RS, O'Connor CM, Mark DB, et al: Coronary perfusion during acute myocardial infarction with a combined therapy of coronary angioplasty and high-dose streptokinase, *Circulation* 77:151-61, 1988.
8. Mathey DG, Schofer J, Sherla FH, et al: Improved survival up to four years after early coronary thrombolysis, *Am J Cardiol* 61:524-529, 1988.
9. Multicenter Postinfarction Research Group: Risk stratification and survival after myocardial infarction, *N Engl J Med* 309:331-336, 1983.
10. Norris RM, White HD: Therapeutic trials in coronary thrombosis should measure left ventricular function as primary end-point of treatment, *Lancet* 1:104-106, 1988.
11. Pfeffer MA, Braunwald E: Ventricular remodeling after myocardial infarction, *Circulation* 81:1161-1172, 1990.
12. Christian TF, Behrenbeck T, Gersh BJ, et al: Relation of left ventricular volume and function over one year after acute myocardial infarction to infarct size determined by technetium-99m sestamibi, *Am J Cardiol* 68:21-26, 1991.
13. Topol EJ, Wilson VE: Pivotal role of early and sustained infarct vessel patency in patients with acute myocardial infarction, *Heart Lung* 19:583-595, 1990.
14. Van de Werf F: Discrepancies between the effects of coronary reperfusion on survival and left ventricular functions, *Lancet* 1:1367-1368, 1989.
15. White HD, Norris RM, Brown MA, et al: Left ventricular end-systolic volume as the major determinant of survival after recovery from myocardial infarction, *Circulation* 76:44-51, 1987.
16. Hammermeister KE, DeRouen TA, Dodge HT: Variables predictive of survival with coronary disease: selection by univariate and multivariate analyses from the clinical, electrocardiographic, exercise, arteriographic and quantitative angiographic evaluations, *Circulation* 59:421-450, 1979.
17. Tamaki N, Yasuda T, Leinbach RC, et al: Spontaneous changes in regional wall motion abnormalities in acute myocardial infarction, *Am J Cardiol* 58:406, 1985.
18. Sheehan FH: Cardiac angiography. In Marcus ML, Skorton DJ, Shelbert HJ, et al (eds): *Cardiac imaging,* Philadelphia, 1991. WB Saunders, pp 109-148.
19. Force TL, Folland ED, Aebescher N, et al: Echocardiographic assessment of ventricular function. In Marcus ML, Skorton DJ, Shelbert HJ, et al (eds): *Cardiac imaging,* Philadelphia, 1991, WB Saunders, pp 374-401.
20. Gibbons RJ: Equilibrium radionuclide angiography. In Marcus ML, Skorton DJ, Shelbert HR, et al (eds): *Cardiac imaging,* Philadelphia, 1991, WB Saunders, pp 1027-1046.
21. Reiter SJ, Rumberger JA, Feiring AJ, et al: Precision of right and

left ventricular stroke volume measurements by rapid acquisition cine computed tomography, *Circulation* 74:890-900, 1986.

22. Feiring AJ, Rumberger JA, Reiter SJ, et al: Sectional and segmental variability of left ventricular function: experimental and clinical studies using ultrafast computed tomography, *J Am Coll Cardiol* 12:415-425, 1988.

23. Rumberger JA: Quantifying left ventricular regional and global systolic function using ultrafast computed tomography, *Am J Cardiac Imaging* 5:29-37, 1991.

24. Hutchins GM, Bulkley BH: Infarct expansion versus extension: two different complications of acute myocardial infarction, *Am J Cardiol* 41:1127, 1978.

25. Eaton LW, Weiss JF, Bulkley BH, et al: Regional cardiac dilatation after acute myocardial infarction, *N Engl J Med* 300:57, 1979.

26. Erlebacher JA, Weiss JL, Weisfeldt ML, et al: Early dilation of the infarcted segment in acute transmural myocardial infarction: role of infarct expansion in acute left ventricular enlargement, *J Am Coll Cardiol* 4:201, 1984.

27. Weisman HF, Bush DE, Mannisi JA, et al: Cellular mechanisms of myocardial infarct expansion, *Circulation* 78:186, 1988.

28. Olivetti G, Capasso JM, Sonnenblick EH, et al: Side-to-side slippage of myocytes participates in ventricular wall remodeling acutely after myocardial infarction in rats, *Circ Res* 67:23-34, 1990.

29. Mitchell GF, Lamas GA, Vaughan DE, et al: Left ventricular remodeling in the year after first anterior myocardial infarction: a quantitative analysis of contractile segment lengths and ventricular shape, *J Am Coll Cardiol* 19:1136-44, 1992.

30. Reimer KA, Jennings RB: The changing anatomic reference base of evolving myocardial infarction: underestimation of myocardial collateral blood flow and overestimation of experimental anatomic infarct size due to tissue edema, hemorrhage and inflammation, *Circulation* 60:866-876, 1979.

31. Lamas GA, Pfeffer MA: Increased left ventricular volumes following myocardial infarction in man, *Am Heart J* 111:30, 1986.

32. Rumberger JA, Behrenbeck T, Breen JR, et al: Non-parallel changes in global chamber volume and muscle mass during the first year following transmural myocardial infarction in man, *J Am Coll Cardiol* 21:673-682, 1993.

33. Lamas GA, Vaughan DE, Parisi AF, et al: Effects of left ventricular shape and captopril therapy on exercise capacity after anterior wall acute myocardial infarction, *Am J Cardiol* 63:1167, 1989.

34. Kannel WB, Sorlie P, McNamara PM: Prognosis after initial myocardial infarction: the Framingham study, *Am J Cardiol* 44:53, 1979.

35. Francis GS, Benedict C, Johnstone DE, et al: Comparison of neuroendocrine activation in patients with left ventricular dysfunction with and without congestive heart failure: a substudy of the studies of left ventricular dysfunction (SOLVD), *Circulation* 82:1724-1729, 1990.

36. Pfeffer MA, Pfeffer JM, Steinberg C, et al: Survival after an experimental myocardial infarction: beneficial effect of long-term therapy with captopril, *Circulation* 72:406, 1985.

37. Pfeffer MA, Lamas GA, Vaughan DE, et al: Effect of captopril on progressive ventricular dilatation after anterior myocardial infarction, *N Engl J Med* 319:80, 1988.

38. Pfeffer MA, Braunwald E, Moye LA, et al: Effect of captopril on mortality and morbidity in patients with left ventricular dysfunction after myocardial infarction: results of the Survival and Ventricular Enlargement Trial, *N Engl J Med* 327:669-677, 1992.

39. Swedberg K, Held P, Kjekshus J, et al: Effects of the early administration of enalapril on mortality in patients with acute myocardial infarction: results of the Cooperative New Scandinavian Enalapril Survival Study II (CONSENSUS II), *N Engl J Med* 327:678-684, 1992.

40. Hochman JS, Choo H: Limitation of myocardial infarct expansion by reperfusion independent of myocardial salvage, *Circulation* 75:299, 1987.

41. Marino P, Zanolla L, Zardine P: Effect of streptokinase on left ventricular modeling and function after myocardial infarction: the GISSI Trial, *J Am Coll Cardiol* 14:1149-1158, 1989.

42. Jeremy RW, Hackworthy RA, Bautovich G, et al: Infarct artery perfusion and changes in left ventricular volume in the month after acute myocardial infarction, *J Am Coll Cardiol* 9:989, 1987.

43. Warren SE, Royal HD, Markis JE, et al: Time course of left ventricular dilation after myocardial infarction: Influence of infarct-related artery and success of coronary thrombolysis, *J Am Coll Cardiol* 11:12, 1988.

44. Villari B, Piscione F, Bonaduce D, et al: Usefulness of late coronary thrombolysis (recombinant tissue-type plasminogen activator) in preserving left ventricular function in acute myocardial infarction, *Am J Cardiol* 66:1281-1286, 1990.

45. Topol EJ, Califf RM, George BS, et al: A randomized trial of immediate versus delayed elective angioplasty after intravenous tissue plasminogen activator in acute myocardial infarction, *N Engl J Med* 317:581-588, 1987.

46. TIMI Study Group: The thrombolysis in myocardial infarction (TIMI) trial, *N Engl J Med* 312:932-936, 1985.

47. Rentrop KP, Feit F, Blanke H, et al: Serial angiographic assessment of coronary artery obstruction and collateral flow in acute myocardial infarction, *Circulation* 80:1166-1175, 1989.

48. National Heart Foundation of Australia Coronary Thrombolysis Group: Coronary thrombolysis and myocardial salvage of tissue plasminogen activator given up to 4 hours after onset of myocardial infarction, *Lancet* 1:203-208, 1988.

49. Kennedy JW, Maring GV, Davis KB et al: The Western Washington intravenous streptokinase in acute myocardial infarction randomized trial, *Circulation* 77:345-352, 1988.

50. Van de Werf F, Armonl AER, European Cooperative Study Group for Recombinant Tissue-Type Plasminogen Activator (rt-PA): Effect of intravenous tissue plasminogen activator on infarct size, left ventricular function and survival in patients with acute myocardial infarction, *Br Med J (Clin Res)* 297:1374-1379, 1988.

51. Meinertz T, Kasper W, Schumacher M, et al: The German multicenter trial of anisoylated plasminogen streptokinase activator complex versus heparin for acute myocardial infarction, *Am J Cardiol* 62:347-351, 1988.

52. Bassand JP, Faivre R, Becque O, et al: Effects of early high-dose streptokinase intravenously on left ventricular function in acute myocardial infarction, *Am J Cardiol* 60:435-439, 1987.

53. Topol EJ, Califf RM, Vandormael M, et al: A randomized trial of late reperfusion therapy after acute myocardial infarction, *Circulation* 85:2090-2099, 1992.

54. Becker LC, Ambrosio G: Myocardial consequences of reperfusion, *Prog Cardiovasc Dis* 30:23-49, 1987.

55. Marcus ML: The Coronary Collateral Circulation. In Marcus ML (ed): *The coronary circulation in health and disease,* New York, 1983, McGraw-Hill, pp 221-241.

56. Tiefenbrunn AJ, Sobel BE: Timing of coronary recanalization: paradigms, paradoxes and pertinence, *Circulation* 85:2311-2315, 1992.

57. ISIS-2 Collaborative Group: Randomized trial of intravenous streptokinase, oral aspirin, both, or neither among 17,187 cases of suspected acute myocardial infarction: ISIS-2, *Lancet* 2:349-360, 1988.

58. Behrenbeck T, Pellikka P, Huber KC, et al: Primary angioplasty in myocardial infarction: assessment of improved myocardial perfusion with technetium-99m isonitrile, *J Am Coll Cardiol* 17:365-372, 1991.

59. White HD: Thrombolytic therapy for patients with myocardial infarction presenting after six hours, *Lancet* 340:221-222, 1992.

60. Simoons ML, Serruys PW, Van Den Brand M, et al: Early thrombolysis in acute myocardial infarction: limitation of infarct size and improved survival, *J Am Coll Cardiol* 7:717-728, 1986.

61. Weisman HF, Healy B: Myocardial infarct expansion, infarct extension, and reinfarction: pathophysiologic concepts, *Prog Cardiovasc Dis* 30:73-110, 1987.

62. Reimer KA, Jennings RB: The "wavefront phenomenon" of myocardial ischemic cell death: II. Transmural progression of necrosis within the framework of ischemic bed size (myocardium at risk). *Lab Invest* 40:633-644, 1979.

63. Leiberman AN, Weiss JL, Jugdutt BI, et al: Two-dimensional echocardiography and infarct size: relationship of regional wall motion and thickening to the extent of myocardial infarction in the dog, *Circulation* 63:739-746, 1981.

64. Touchstone DA, Beller BA, Nygaard TW, et al: Effects of successful intravenous reperfusion therapy on regional myocardial function and geometry in humans: A tomographic assessment using two-dimensional echocardiography, *J Am Coll Cardiol* 13:1506-1513, 1989.

65. Choong CY, Gibbons EF, Hogan RD, et al: Relationship of function recovery to scar contraction after myocardial infarction in the canine left ventricle, *Am Heart J* 117:819-829, 1989.

66. Schaper W: Residual perfusion of acutely ischemic heart muscle. In Schaper W (ed): *The pathophysiology of myocardial perfusion,* New York, 1979, North-Holland Biomedical Press.

67. Tadakazu H, Fujita M, Nakajima H, et al: Importance of collateral circulation for prevention of left ventricular aneurysm formation in acute myocardial infarction, *Circulation* 79:791-796, 1989.

68. Shen WF, Lian QC, Gong LS, et al: Beneficial effect of residual flow to the infarct region on left ventricular volume changes after acute myocardial infarction, *Am Heart J* 119:525-529, 1990.

69. Hale SL, Kloner RA: Left ventricular topographic alterations in the completely healed rat infarct caused by early and late coronary artery reperfusion, *Am Heart J* 116:1508-1513, 1988.

70. Honan MB, Harrell FE, Reimer RA, et al: Cardiac rupture and timing of thrombolytic therapy: a meta-analysis, *J Am Coll Cardiol* 16:359-367, 1990.

71. Wu XS, Ewert DL, Liu YH, et al: In-vivo relation of intramyocardial blood volume to myocardial perfusion: evidence supporting microvascular site of autoregulation, *Circulation* 85:730-737, 1992.

72. Vogel WM, Apstein CS, Briggs LL, et al: Acute alterations in left ventricular diastolic chamber stiffness: role of the "erectile" effect of coronary arterial pressure and flow in normal and damaged hearts, *Circ Res* 51:465-478, 1982.

73. Brown DJ, Swinford RD, Gadde P, et al: Acute effects of delayed reperfusion on myocardial infarct shape and left ventricular volume: a potential mechanism of additional benefits from thrombolytic therapy, *J Am Coll Cardiol* 17:1641-1650, 1991.

74. Karan R, Healy BP, Wecher P: Coronary reserve is depressed in post myocardial infarct reactive cardiac hypertrophy, *Circulation* 81:238-246, 1990.

75. LATE Trial Results: Thrombolysis with alteplase (rt-PA) provides survival benefit in 6- to 12-hour time window. In Roberts R (ed): *Clinical challenges in acute myocardial infarction,* Gardiner-Caldwell SynerMed, 1993.

Chapter 12

LARGE SIMPLE TRIALS IN CARDIOVASCULAR DISEASE: THEIR IMPACT ON MEDICAL PRACTICE

Marcus D. Flather
Michael E. Farkouh
Salim Yusuf

In the last decade science has witnessed the evolution and development of a powerful tool in medical research for the assessment of therapeutic strategies. This tool is the large simple trial (also known as the megatrial) that has helped to guide and improve therapeutic practice, particularly in cardiovascular medicine. A large simple trial can be loosely defined as a randomized controlled trial that minimizes the extra work involved and uses mortality as the main outcome measure. The underlying principles of the large simple trial have directly addressed the most challenging aspects of any therapeutic research: first to ask an important question and then to answer it reliably.

The first part of this chapter discusses the principles and design of large simple trials, and the second part gives examples and discusses the implications of these trials and future perspectives.

PRINCIPLES OF DESIGN AND ANALYSIS OF LARGE SIMPLE TRIALS[1,2]
Moderate mortality reductions are worthwhile

An important aspect of the development of the large simple trial concept was the acceptance of the hypothesis that for common, high-risk diseases (e.g., myocardial infarction, heart failure, or breast cancer) moderate reductions in mortality (on the order of 10%, 15%, or at most 25%) were all that was plausible but would still be humanly worthwhile. Furthermore, if the treatments studied were simple to use, widely applicable, and relatively inexpensive, the impact of such a moderate reduction in mortality could be substantial. The potential number of lives that could be saved by such a strategy, if a moderate reduction in mortality was demonstrated, is shown in Table 12-1. It can be seen that the "reward" for reliably demonstrating these treatment effects is the saving of many thousands of lives each year. Conversely, if a treatment increased mortality by even a small proportion, it would unnecessarily shorten the lives of many thousands of individuals. The goal of distinguishing between moderate benefit or harm or no effect has been the major driving force of investigators involved in the development and conduct of large trials.

A complementary principle that among populations chosen for a trial (i.e., those with no clear indication or contraindication), the direction of treatment effect is likely to be the same has led to substantial simplification of data collection and study procedures. Simplification can, therefore, make large trials feasible at a reasonable cost.

Table 12-1. Potential public health benefit if a large simple trial demonstrated risk reductions of 10%, 20%, or 33%*

Absolute treatment effect	Risk reduction (%)	Lives saved/year
15% down to 13.5%	10%	15,000
15% down to 12%	20%	30,000
15% down to 10%	33%	50,000

*Number of lives saved per 1 million patients (with an average mortality of 15%) treated.

Table 12-2. Total sample size estimates of a large simple trial*

Estimated risk reduction (%)	Expected event rates		
	10%	15%	20%
10	36,000	22,700	16,000
20	8600	5300	3900
30	3600	2300	1650

*Assumes 2-sided $\alpha = 0.05$, 90% power (1-B), and two arms.

IDENTIFYING AN IMPORTANT QUESTION

There are many promising treatments in medical practice, particularly in cardiovascular therapeutics, and it is a primary concern of practicing physicians to identify and use those treatments that really do benefit their patients. Treatments that appear promising by having both a sound biologic rationale and a favorable therapeutic profile but about which many physicians are ultimately uncertain (whether the treatment will influence mortality) may be considered for evaluation in a large simple trial. A rigorous review of all the available evidence is essential in planning the possible treatment strategies to be examined in a large simple trial, including pooling available data from previous randomized controlled trials of the relevant intervention using acceptable statistical methodology such as that used in systematic overviews (or meta-analyses).[3-5] These latter methods can provide a very useful guide to the overall direction of the treatment effect (benefit, little or no effect, or harm) but usually provide only a crude estimate of the size of the effect. Once the treatment or strategy has been identified by using these methods of comprehensive review, the main question of a large simple trial usually is, "Does this treatment reduce mortality or major morbidity when used for the treatment of the high-risk condition of interest?" Although this may be the main question of the trial, a number of subsidiary questions may be proposed *a priori*, but it should be made clear that these are subsidiary and should not be allowed to interfere with the assessment of the main question.

WHY IS MORTALITY AN IMPORTANT ENDPOINT?

It can be demonstrated in experimental or clinical studies that many promising treatments favorably modify important mechanisms involved in the disease process of interest. For example, a number of therapeutic agents have been shown to reduce infarct size and arrhythmias in acute myocardial infarction (MI); other agents have been shown to prevent complications of atheromatous disease, and in the treatment of cancers, various agents have been shown to reduce tumor size. However, these indirect markers of efficacy do not necessarily provide physicians with the most reliable data on which to assess overall therapeutic efficacy. The reliable demonstration of a mortality reduction would, however, be expected to be a clear indication of the balance of benefit and risks associated with a therapeutic agent that would be less open to misinterpretation and would provide physicians with a rational basis for treatment. Hence, large simple trials have often used mortality as the main outcome measure because both the method of measurement is generally undisputed and the demonstration of a mortality reduction is taken by most physicians to be a clear indication of efficacy.

DETECTING MODERATE DIFFERENCES IN MORTALITY[6,7]

The detection of the sorts of moderate differences that have been discussed (relative risk reductions of 10%, 15%, or 20%) require the reduction or elimination of biases and random errors that may obscure these moderate treatment effects. Systematic errors (or bias) can be avoided by using rigorous randomization procedures to enter patients into the large simple trial, followed by an unbiased statistical analysis of the results by using an intention-to-treat approach. This method analyzes outcomes by allocated rather than actual treatment and bases any inferences on the results of the entire trial rather than on subsidiary groups or analysis. The reduction of random error (background "noise") is also essential if moderate treatment effects are to be demonstrated. In practice this is achieved by designing and implementing trials of sufficient size to give a good chance of showing these effects. The practical implication of reducing random errors where moderate differences are expected is demonstrated in Table 12-2, which shows sample size estimates for trials expecting relative risk reductions of 10%, 15%, or 20%. These sample sizes are much larger than is generally believed to be necessary for the demonstration of therapeutic effects.

These principles should not be taken to imply that the

large randomized controlled trial is the only method for scientific advancement in medicine but that without them, moderate biases can easily obscure any real effect, and promising treatments may not be adequately assessed. Of course, treatments that have a very large beneficial (or possibly harmful) effect would still probably be discovered through clinical observation and other methods of assessment. However, even in such circumstances, a randomized trial would still be the preferred method of evaluation but the sample size required may be much smaller.

POTENTIAL INTERACTIONS IN LARGE SIMPLE TRIALS[8]

The inherent heterogeneity of biologic systems usually means that responses to a particular treatment may differ in degree or size among different patients, and these are usually termed quantitative interactions. In contrast, it is generally much less common for a treatment to have an effect that differs in direction, (i.e., a qualitative interaction) among different individuals in a particular trial. Any observed qualitative interactions are even less likely to be real if they are unanticipated, and a priori should be disbelieved unless repeatedly confirmed. Thus, when treatment effects are assessed, it is not surprising to observe differences in the amount of the effect (quantitative interactions) that are real, but it would be much more surprising (and rare) to observe different directions of effect (e.g., benefit in men, harm in women, benefit in the young, harm in the old). Therefore, in all clinical trials, including large simple trials, it is essential to emphasize the results of the primary analysis from the whole study group and reserve subgroup analyses as exercises to explore or generate predetermined hypotheses.[9]

OPERATIONAL ASPECTS OF LARGE SIMPLE TRIALS
Wide entry criteria, simple procedures, and follow-up

Table 12-2 demonstrates that the sample sizes required to detect moderate mortality differences have to be considerably larger than is commonly expected. The randomization of large numbers of patients can be achieved only through a strong collaborative network that links many hospitals and institutions that treat the disease process under investigation. If a disease is common, it follows that it will be treated in a wide range of medical facilities, most of which will not have specialized research capabilities. Therefore, it is essential for the success of large simple trials to minimize any extra work by making the entry criteria for randomization clear and broad (without too many prespecified exclusion criteria), which also allows any results of the study to be widely generalizable. The method of ran-

domization should also be reliable and efficient (e.g., by telephoning a toll-free central randomization service). After randomization there should be minimal extra investigations that are specifically study-related and simple follow-up procedures that include compliance checks and ascertainment of relevant clinical events, especially mortality. By streamlining the trial procedures in this way, one can minimize the extra work involved in randomizing and following-up patients, and busy centers can collaborate. The ultimate goal of this exercise is to make it almost as easy to treat patients within large simple trials as outside them as part of "routine" clinical practice.

ORGANIZATION OF A LARGE SIMPLE TRIAL STUDY GROUP

The most important components of a study group involved in large simple trials are the patients and the collaborating physicians, nurses, and other health professionals from the clinical centers, because this is where most of the work of a large simple trial is carried out. However, before the study starts, there needs to be careful consideration of the design and methodologic aspects, and this is usually carried out by a preappointed steering committee consisting of members with a broad range of expertise, including clinicians, trial methodologists, and biostatisticians. This committee is responsible for ensuring that the trial is properly designed and that the protocol is adhered to during the course of the study. Within the steering committee there are often a number of subcommittees that deal with particular aspects of the trial, including an operations committee that handles the day-to-day running of the trial, substudy committees, and committees that review the important outcome events on which the results of the study are based. However, to reduce any potential bias that may be introduced, the steering committee should remain blinded to any of the interim results during the course of a large simple trial. To ensure that patients and investigators are fully protected during the course of the trial if clear evidence of benefit or harm emerges, a separate group called the data monitoring committee (also known as the data and safety monitoring committee, or the external safety and efficacy committee) is appointed before the start of the study. Data monitoring committees are usually made up of a few experienced investigators and biostatisticians who periodically review the unblinded interim data from the trial to ensure that no clear evidence of benefit or harm emerges during the course of the trial and also that there is adequate quality control of the data.[10] The exact terms of reference and guidelines for recommending any modification or cessation of a particular trial varies from study to study, but if clear treatment effects do emerge, the data monitoring committee is required to recommend the appropriate course of action to the steering committee.

ETHICAL CONSIDERATIONS IN LARGE SIMPLE TRIALS

The fundamental ethics of a large simple trial are no different than of any other therapeutic clinical trial.[11] There is a prerequisite for an important scientific question, which requires that among participating physicians, there is an element of uncertainty as to the benefit of a particular treatment. In any clinical trial patient safety is clearly paramount and is ensured by proper study design (e.g., appropriate dosing), collection of adverse effects, and periodic scrutiny by the data monitoring committee during the course of the trial. Ethical responsibility for clinical trials has to be taken by the local ethical review committee and by the physician and health professionals responsible for a particular patient, especially in trials of acute MI or other conditions where patients may be too drowsy or frightened to give acceptable informed consent. Physicians are required to make the decision for each individual patient in the light of their current clinical knowledge, available research data, and the protocol requirements of the trial. The fundamental principle is that if physicians are substantially uncertain whether the treatment under investigation will benefit their patient but believe it may be beneficial, the patient may be randomized into the trial. An important ethical consideration is that having undertaken a large simple trial, it is very important to obtain a reliable answer to the question being asked, and this can be done only by continuing the trial until a clear answer is obtained or the null hypothesis has been adequately supported. The premature stopping of a trial when results are not clear can be considered to be ethically imprudent and is currently the cause of much debate. Many investigators involved in large simple trials consider that a different "standard" of ethics should not be applied to therapeutic randomized trials compared with "normal" clinical practice but that both should conform to the highest medical and ethical standards.

DETECTION OF MAJOR BUT RARE ADVERSE OUTCOMES

In recent years it has become clear that many agents that appear to have promising effects may also increase the risks of a major adverse outcome (e.g., stroke), so that the balance of benefits (e.g., mortality reduction) and risks have to be carefully weighed. However, in several instances, trials have indicated that promising interventions may actually increase mortality. Examples of these include the class I antiarrhythmic agents after myocardial infarction,[12] nondigitalis inotropic agents, or new vasodilators in heart failure. These data emphasize that large trials are needed not only to establish benefit but also to confirm safety. When the "event" is relatively uncommon (e.g., intracranial bleeds or death), only large trials can reassure clinicians of the safety of most interventions.

CAN LARGE SIMPLE TRIALS STUDY MECHANISMS?

The overall aim of large simple trials is to distinguish reliably between two plausible hypotheses: either treatment confers no material benefit, or it has a worthwhile but moderate effect on mortality. In its simplest form the large simple trial does not collect information that may answer questions related to how a particular treatment works. However, there are many examples where large simple trials have generated important hypotheses as to the mechanisms of treatment effect or disease process (e.g., that thrombolytic therapy may have a beneficial action among patients presenting beyond 6 hours from pain onset). Some large simple trials have incorporated well-designed subsidiary studies to make up for this apparent inability to examine mechanistic hypotheses. Substudies, if designed properly, can be very helpful in building up a more complete picture not only of the amount of benefit but also how the treatment may exert its action.[13] However, it must be borne in mind that subsidiary studies add a substantial burden of cost and effort to large simple trials, and this must be weighed very carefully against the overall aim of the trial and the resources available.[14]

FACTORIAL DESIGN IN LARGE SIMPLE TRIALS[2]

The effort of designing and implementing large simple trials can have greater rewards if more than one treatment can be examined in a single trial. One method of doing this efficiently is with the use of the factorial design, in which two or more treatments with a different mechanism of action may be randomized separately within the same trial. If a 2×2 factorial design is used, randomization occurs four ways (treatment A and B, treatment A only, treatment B only, or neither), and at the end of the study a retrospectively stratified analysis can be used to compare all those allocated treatment A vs. all those not allocated A and all those allocated treatment B vs. not allocated treatment B. The perceived disadvantages of these designs are their apparent complexity interfering with the conduct of the trial. Alternatively, if the combination of treatments either worked in essentially the same way or had additive adverse effects, a factorial design may not be the best strategy for detecting the effect of an individual treatment. However, the advantages are not only that two or more treatments can be effectively evaluated for the price of one study but also that generic treatments (e.g., aspirin or magnesium) that would not otherwise have enough "funding" potential to be evaluated separately can be studied in large simple trials. The factorial design can of course be extended from 2×2 designs to $2 \times 2 \times 2$ or more (but this almost always increases complexity), and in this way more than two treatments could be evaluated. Factorial designs are appropriate, particularly in the absence of interactions. On the other hand, if interactions do occur, it is clear that the factorial design may well be the only way to demonstrate this interaction. Examples of factorial designs used in large simple trials are given in the next section.

FUNDING ISSUES IN LARGE SIMPLE TRIALS

Much of the funding in biomedical research today comes from government sources and the pharmaceutical industry, either separately or jointly, and funding for large simple trials is not an exception to this generalization. Independent peer-reviewed grants from government or charitable institutions are also available, but except for a few circumstances, these grants are in themselves usually not of sufficient magnitude to completely fund a large simple trial. Wholehearted collaboration in large simple trials is clearly essential for the success of these projects, and it is strongly believed that scientific participation and the quest for improving therapy for sick patients should be the underlying rationale for collaboration. However, clearly extra effort and sometimes identifiable expense are involved in randomizing patients even in large simple trials that use streamlined protocols, and it is therefore reasonable to expect some reimbursements of any extra financial expenditure and some support for the administrative aspects (e.g., secretarial support). Financial incentives, including specific monetary payments, or allocation of free drugs, which otherwise might be quite expensive, are also gradually becoming part of the large simple trial scenario. This is a sensitive area, and there is much debate about the ethics of whether financial reimbursement should be wholeheartedly accepted or generally discouraged except to cover specific expenses.

EXAMPLES OF LARGE SIMPLE TRIALS
Noncardiovascular disease

Polio vaccine trial.[15] The largest randomized trial ever conducted was the U.S. National Polio Vaccine Trial in the United States. The trial included more than 400,000 children recruited within 1 year, ascertained outcomes by screening hospitals for polio cases (not by following each child), and demonstrated a convincing and highly significant reduction in cases of poliomyelitis. The costs of this "unfunded" trial have never been documented, but it is clear that this major public health advance was the result of the generous efforts of committed volunteers nationwide. Subsequent to the polio vaccine trial, several prevention trials in tubercu-

losis (BCG vaccines) and prevention of childhood mortality utilizing vitamin A have been conducted involving tens of thousands of subjects.

Large simple trials in acute MI (Table 12-3)

ISIS-1.[16] The first large simple trial in cardiology was conducted by the International Study of Infarct Survival (ISIS) Collaborative Group and randomized about 16,000 patients with suspected acute MI to either intravenous atenolol followed by oral atenolol for 7 days or control. Such a large sample size had been unheard of previously in the context of randomized controlled treatment trials, and although this study showed a modest benefit of the atenolol regimen used (see Table 12-3), it also clearly demonstrated that it was possible to achieve really large sample sizes through a genuine collaborative effort. Preparatory work for ISIS-1 had commenced several years previously with a thorough evaluation of the previous randomized controlled trials of β-blockers in a meta-analysis[17] and carefully conducted pilot studies of feasibility, safety, and mechanisms. Thus, the principles discussed earlier in the chapter were demonstrated very clearly in this first large simple trial.

Large simple trials of thrombolytic therapy vs. control. During the course of ISIS-1 there was renewed interest in the possibility that intravenous thrombolytic therapy could be beneficial in acute myocardial infarction. The results of a meta-analysis of 33 randomized controlled trials of streptokinase[18] suggested a risk reduction in mortality of the order of 20%, and a pilot study indicated that it was feasible to use intravenous streptokinase among a wide range of acute MI patients.[19] Members of the Italian section of the ISIS-1 Collaborative Group formed a new collaboration of 176 coronary care units (CCUs) in Italy (about 80% of all CCUs in Italy) and performed the first large simple trial of streptokinase vs. open control among 11,806 patients. This study, now known as GISSI (Gruppo Italiano per lo Studio della Streptochinasi nell'Infarto Miocardico),[20] demonstrated very clearly that streptokinase reduced mortality when given to a wide range of acute MI patients presenting within 12 hours from the onset of pain. Apart from the clear result on mortality ($P < 0.0002$), this study validated the findings of the meta-analysis of the previous streptokinase trials and also supported the hypothesis generated from experimental studies and clinical observation that those treated earlier with thrombolytic therapy benefited most. However, in spite of these clear results, the use of streptokinase for the treatment of acute MI patients increased only slowly, and the reasons for this are still somewhat unclear.[21] The second study performed by the ISIS Collaborative Group (ISIS-2) examined the same question as the GISSI study but extended the time window for entry up to 24 hours from pain onset and also looked at the randomized comparison of aspirin vs. placebo in a 2×2 factorial design.[22] ISIS-2 randomized about 17,000 patients, and the results of the streptokinase vs. placebo comparison were almost identical to those of the GISSI study. The surprising result was that aspirin alone appeared to be almost as effective as thrombolytic therapy and that the combination of both streptokinase and aspirin yielded a far greater benefit than was achieved by either agent alone (i.e., for every 1000 patients treated with the combination of streptokinase plus aspirin, about 50 deaths were prevented in the first 5 weeks without an overall excess of strokes or reinfarction.) This study not only vindicated the results of the GISSI study but also provided a strong practical validation of the factorial design and upheld the concept that this could be a very efficient way of assessing therapies that worked in different ways but were directed toward the same disease process. The presentation of the ISIS-2 results publicly, and the subsequent publication in August 1988, did cause a profound change in medical practice, with a rapid and substantial increase in the use of both streptokinase and aspirin as part of the routine treatment for acute MI patients.[21,23] It seemed, therefore, that to have a profound impact on medical practice there was a requirement for not one but two or more large simple randomized trials with very clear mortality results. This fact is still surprising to some but would appear to reinforce the general philosophy that for a scientific observation to be believed, it should at least be repeated, particularly if that observation is profound. Clearly medical practice is not just guided by the principles of science, but it does appear that physicians are more comfortable with changing their practice based on the results of two or more studies with clear results and were not at all influenced by the previous meta-analysis that showed a clear beneficial effect in the smaller trials.[18]

The EMERAS Study[24] and the LATE Study[25] have randomized patients presenting beyond 6 hours to streptokinase vs. control or tissue-type plasminogen activator (t-PA) vs. control, respectively. These two studies (which essentially tested the hypothesis generated by ISIS-2) and a meta-analysis of the large trials of thrombolytic therapy vs. control[26] have clearly demonstrated a benefit for patients with acute MI presenting up to 12 hours after symptom onset.

Trials of one thrombolytic agent vs. another: GISSI-2, ISIS-3, and GUSTO-I. The renewed interest in thrombolytic agents that became apparent during the late 1970s and early 1980s, particularly with studies of intravenous streptokinase, highlighted the need for agents that might be even more effective without the allergic side effects and hypotension that occur with streptokinase. Several new agents were developed using either

genetic engineering techniques or by biochemically modifying existing agents, and the publication of the ASSET Study confirmed that one of these newer agents, recombinant t-PA (rt-PA), was indeed effective in its own right in reducing mortality after MI.[27] Another agent called anisoylated plasminogen–streptokinase activator complex (APSAC) was also shown to be effective in a moderate-sized study.[28] t-PA had been shown to be more clot-specific and to achieve a more rapid rate of coronary patency after MI.[29] It was generally believed that these properties would make it a superior agent to streptokinase for the treatment of MI. However, despite these theoretical considerations, there were concerns about an increased risk of intracranial bleeds with t-PA. Similarly, the point estimate for the risk reduction for APSAC in the AIMS Study was about 40%, and this also made it an attractive alternative to streptokinase.[28] However, the side effect profile for APSAC was very similar to streptokinase in terms of allergic reactions because it is essentially a modified form of streptokinase, which then releases the APSAC.

The economic implications of the widespread use of the newer generation of thrombolytic agents was of substantial concern because the market cost of these agents was estimated at between five and ten times the cost of streptokinase. This powerful combination of both human health and resource implications stimulated the second generation of large simple trials of thrombolytic therapy in acute MI, where one agent was compared with one or more other agents or strategies. The GISSI-2 study and its International Extension randomized about 20,000 patients between rt-PA (alteplase) and streptokinase and found that the overall mortality between the two groups was almost exactly the same (t-PA 9.0% vs. SK 8.6%).[30,31] GISSI-2 also examined the question of whether a regimen of subcutaneous heparin vs. control would influence the outcome of acute MI in a 2×2 factorial design. There was no evidence of any difference between the groups randomized between subcutaneous heparin vs. control with or without the addition of the thrombolytic agent under investigation. There was evidence from this study, however, although the mortality outcome was the same for the two agents, there was an excess of strokes in the t-PA group, primarily because of an excess of hemorrhagic strokes.

The ISIS-3 study, which concluded shortly after GISSI-2, randomized more than 41,000 patients with suspected acute MI to streptokinase, t-PA (duteplase), or APSAC and to either subcutaneous heparin or no heparin in a 3×2 factorial design.[32] This trial reinforced the GISSI-2 results that (1) there was no apparent difference between streptokinase and t-PA on mortality after MI; (2) subcutaneous heparin, in the presence of aspirin, did not have a beneficial effect; and (3) the incidence of cerebral hemorrhage was higher in the t-PA group than the streptokinase group. In addition, there was no apparent advantage of APSAC compared with streptokinase. The conclusion of the ISIS-3 investigators was that if there was a difference in efficacy between t-PA and streptokinase, it was likely to be small.

The GUSTO-I Trial was the third large simple trial to compare different thrombolytic agents,[33] following on from GISSI-2 and ISIS-3. The main questions addressed by GUSTO-I were whether (1) accelerated t-PA with intravenous heparin was more effective than standard streptokinase with either subcutaneous heparin or intravenous heparin, (2) there was any difference in outcome between streptokinase plus subcutaneous heparin compared with streptokinase plus intravenous heparin, and (3) there was any role for the combination of streptokinase and t-PA plus intravenous heparin compared with the other thrombolytic agents studied. In summary, the trial showed that (1) for patients manifesting early with acute MI, giving t-PA in an accelerated regimen was moderately more effective than streptokinase; (2) there was no apparent difference if streptokinase was given with either subcutaneous or intravenous heparin; (3) and the combination of streptokinase and t-PA did not really provide any advantage over each agent alone. The study did confirm the previous observations that t-PA caused more cerebral hemorrhage than streptokinase and provided important information from the angiographic substudy, which supports the hypothesis that establishing early coronary artery patency in acute MI is associated with a better outcome. Apart from the therapeutic implications of these results that are discussed elsewhere, GUSTO-I is an important study because it was the first large simple trial in acute MI to be conducted outside Europe. The planning and implementation of GUSTO-I also represents an integral approach to clinically relevant questions that attempt to not only answer the therapeutic question (i.e., the safety and efficacy of different thrombolytic strategies) but also provide more information about the pathophysiology of the disease process and the mechanism of action of the agent studied through carefully-designed substudies.[13] As discussed earlier, such substudies do add complexity and expense to a large simple trial, but if undertaken in appropriate centers, they may also provide valuable information. The integration of substudies within the large simple trial is still an evolving concept, but it has been undertaken with success in the GUSTO-I Study and also in the SOLVD studies in heart failure, which are described later.

Vasodilators and magnesium in acute MI: CONSENSUS-II, GISSI-3, and ISIS-4. By the end of the 1980s, there was growing evidence that vasodilators, such as angiotensin-converting enzyme (ACE) inhibitors[34] and nitrates,[35,36] could reduce mortality after MI by attenuating ventricular enlargement and improving remodeling. Studies among high-risk populations with reduced ejection fractions or clinical heart failure after MI showed improved survival with captopril[37] or ramipril[38] when started about 3 to 10 days after the MI. The CONSENSUS-II Study was the first large simple trial to address this question among unselected patients when enalapril was started in the acute phase of MI.[39] This study was stopped prematurely when about 6000 patients had been randomized (target about 9000) because no evidence of clinical efficacy of enalapril was emerging. Two other large simple trials addressing a similar question completed their recruitment phase in 1993: GISSI-3, assessing the effects of lisinopril and nitrates starting at the acute phase of MI using a 2 × 2 factorial design,[40] and ISIS-4, assessing captopril, oral isosorbide mononitrate, and intravenous magnesium in a 2 × 2 × 2 factorial design in a similar population.[41] ISIS-4 has randomized about 58,000 patients, making it the largest randomized controlled trial of acute intervention in MI. Several studies and a meta-analysis[42,43] had shown very promising mortality results for magnesium infusions in acute MI, hence the inclusion of magnesium as a study agent in ISIS-4. These latter two trials (Table 12-3) were presented at the end of 1993.

Large simple trials in heart failure (see Table 12-4)
SOLVD and DIG trials. In the previous sections we have described the use of large simple trials in acute MI. In these studies treatments have usually been given as a bolus, a short infusion, or at most for a few days. Furthermore, randomization of patients is usually done in-hospital from a single location (e.g., CCU) and patients are acutely ill and therefore more easily recruited into trials. By contrast, patients with heart failure have diverse etiologies, have multiple complications and are older, and trials have generally required therapy for some years. Because the patients are symptomatic, this has also meant substantial problems related to noncompliance and co-interventions with other therapies. Therefore, some modifications needed to be made in applying the concept of large simple trials in heart failure. Two large trials have been conducted utilizing this concept. The first of these were the two-part SOLVD Trials, which evaluated the effects of ACE inhibitors vs. placebo and in total randomized just under 7000 patients with ejection fractions of 35% or less.[44,45] Specific features of the trial from a design point of view included utilization of many different methods (echocardiography, radionuclide or contrast angiography) for measuring ejection fraction to maximize recruitment; consent for patients to be on multiple therapies; utilization of a clinical definition of heart failure (i.e., whatever the clinic physician called heart failure, with documentation of the signs and symptoms); lack of

Table 12-3. Large simple randomized trials: acute myocardial infarction*

Trial	Publication year	Design	Eligibility criteria	Agent(s) under investigation and regimen
ISIS-1[16]	1986	Open control	Suspected acute AMI within 12 hr from symptom onset No clear contraindications to β-blockers	Atenolol 5-10 mg IV, followed by 100 mg PO daily for 7 days
GISSI-1[20]	1986	Open control	Clinical acute AMI with ECG changes < 12 hr from symptom onset No clear contraindications	SK 1.5 million units over 1 hr
ISIS-2[22]	1988	Placebo control 2 × 2 factorial	Suspected AMI Manifesting within 24 hr from symptom onset No clear contraindications to streptokinase or aspirin	(1) SK 1.5 million units over 1 hr (2) Aspirin 160 mg PO daily for 1 mo
GISSI-2[30] and International Study Group[31]	1990	Open 2 × 2 factorial	Chest pain with ST elevation on ECG Symptom onset within 6 hr No clear contraindications to thrombolytic therapy	(1) SK 1.5 million units IV over 30-60 min (2) t-PA 100 mg IV over 3 hr (10 mg bolus, 50 mg in first hr, 20 mg in second and third hr) (3) Heparin SC 12,500 units bid until discharge (first dose 12 hr after start of SK or t-PA)
ISIS-3[32]	1992	Blinded comparison of SK, t-PA, and APSAC Heparin vs. open control 3 × 2 factorial	Suspected acute MI up to 24 hr from symptom onset No clear contraindications to thrombolytic therapy	(1) SK 1.5 million units IV over 1 hr (2) t-PA 0.04 million units/kg bolus, 0.36 million units/kg in first hr, then 0.067 million units/kg for 3 hr (3) APSAC 30-unit bolus over 3 min (4) Heparin SC 12,500 units bid for 7 days (first dose 4 hr after randomization)
EMERAS[24]	1993	Placebo control	Suspected acute MI < 24 hr from symptom onset 85% > 6 hr from symptom onset	SK 1.5 million units IV over 1 hr
GUSTO-I[33]	1993	Open study 4-way randomization	Onset of symptoms of acute MI < 6 hr ECG criteria for MI	(1) SK (1.5 million units IV over 60 min) (2) SK (as in 1 above) plus intravenous heparin (bolus of 5,000 units, followed by 1000-1200 units/hr; target aPTT 60-85 sec) (3) t-PA (accelerated regimen) bolus of 15 mg, then 0.75 mg/kg over 30 min (total dose ≤ 100 mg); plus IV heparin (as in 2 above) (4) t-PA (1 mg/kg over 60 min with 10% as bolus) plus SK 1 million units over 60 min plus IV heparin (as in 2 and 3 above)
CONSENSUS-II[39]	1992	Placebo control	Acute MI BP > 100/60 mm Hg < 24 hr from symptom onset	IV enalapril at 1 mg over 2 hr then oral enalapril 2.5 mg titrating up to target of 20 mg over 4 days
GISSI-3[40]	1994	Open control 2 × 2 factorial design	Suspected acute MI < 24 hr from symptom onset Systolic BP > 100 mm Hg	(1) IV nitroglycerin for 24 hr followed by transdermal nitroglycerin 10 mg daily for 6 wk (removed at night) (2) Oral lisinopril 5 mg daily increasing to 10 mg daily after 48 hr for 6 wk
ISIS-4[41]	1994	Placebo control for captopril and isosorbide mononitrate Open control for magnesium 2 × 2 × 2 factorial	Suspected acute MI < 24 hr from symptom onset Systolic BP > 90 mm Hg	(1) Oral captopril 6.25 mg initial dose titrated up to 50 mg twice daily over 48 hr (2) Oral controlled-release isosorbide mononitrate 30 mg initial dose, increased to 60 mg daily after 24 hr (3) IV magnesium sulfate initial infusion of 8 mmol over 15 min, then 72 mmol over 24 hr

Preliminary results presented at American Heart Association meeting, November 1993.
*RRR, Relative risk reduction (proportional in events in treatment group compared with control); CI, 95% confidence intervals (%); NNT, numbers needed to treat (estimated number of patients needed to be treated to prevent one adverse event; 1/absolute risk reduction); ISIS, International Study of Infarct Survival; MI, myocardial infarction; GISSI, Gruppo Italiano per lo Studio della Streptochinasi nell'Infarto Miocardico; ECG, electrocardiographic; SK, streptokinase; t-PA, tissue-type plasminogen activator; APSAC, anisoylated plasminogen streptokinase activator complex; EMERAS, Estudio Multicentrico Estreptoquinasa Republicas de America del Sur; GUSTO-I, Global Utilization of Streptokinase and t-PA for Occluded Coronary Arteries; aPTT, activated partial thromboplastin time; CONSENSUS, Cooperative New Scandinavian Enalapril Survival Study; BP, blood pressure.

No. of centers	Total sample size	Endpoints and follow-up	Main results-deaths		RRR (%) (CI)	NNT
			Treatment	Comparison		
245	16,027	Vascular death during 7 days after acute MI	Atenolol 313/8037 (3.9%)	Control 365/7990 (4.6%)	15% (1%-27%)	143
176	11,806	21-day overall mortality	SK 628/5860 10.7%	Control 758/5852 13.0%	19% (10%-28%)	43
417	17,187	35-day mortality	SK 791/8592 9.2%	Placebo 1029/8595 12.0%	25% (18%-32%)	36
			Aspirin 804/8587 9.4%	Placebo 1016/8600 11.8%	23% (15%-30%)	40
			SK and aspirin 343/4292 8.0%	Placebo 568/4300 13.2%	42% (34%-50%)	19
	20,891	In-hospital mortality	SK 887/10,396 8.5%	t-PA 929/10,372 8.9%	NS	–
			Heparin 884/10,361 8.5%	Control 932/10,407 8.9%	NS	–
914	41,299	In-hospital mortality (up to day 35)	SK 1455/13,780 10.6%	APSAC 1448/13,773 10.5%	NS	–
			SK 1455/13,780 10.6%	t-PA 1418/13,746 10.3%	NS	–
			Heparin 2132/20,400 10.3%	Control 2189/20,375 10.6%	NS	–
236	4534	In-hospital mortality	SK 269/2257 11.9%	Placebo 282/2277 12.4%	NS	–
1081	41,021	30-day mortality	t-PA 652/103,446 0.3%	All SK 1473/20,173 7.3%	14% (6%-21%)	100
			t-PA and SK 723/10,328 7.0%	All SK 1473/20,173 7.3%	NS	–
			SK and SC heparin 705/9796 7.2%	SK and IV heparin 768/10,377 7.4%	NS	–
103	6090	Mortality up to 6 mo	312/3044 10.2%	286/3046 9.4%	NS	–
200	19,000 (approx)	Mortality and left ventricular dysfunction at 6 wk	Nitrate 617/9453 6.5%	Control 653/9442 6.9%	NS	–
			Lisinopril 597/9435 6.3%	Control 673/9460 7.1%	11% (1%-21%)	125
1086	58,000 (approx)	Mortality at 5 wk and 6 mo	Capropril 1886/27,442 6.9%	Placebo 2008/27,382 7.3%	5%	250
			Nitrate 1913/27,396 7.0%	Placebo 1981/27,428 7.2%	NS	–
			Magnesium 1997/27,413 7.3%	Control 1897/27,411 6.9%	NS	–

Table 12-4. Large simple randomized trials: heart failure*

Trial	Publication year	Design	Eligibility criteria	Agents under investigation and regimen
SOLVD Treatment[44]	1991	Placebo control	Patients with CHF Ejection fraction ≤35% Not on ACE inhibitor	Enalapril 2.5 or 5 mg twice daily initial dose titrating up to 10 mg twice daily PO
SOLVD Prevention[45]	1992	Placebo control	Ejection fraction ≤35% Known heart disease No obvious symptoms of heart failure	Enalapril 2.5 mg twice daily initial dose titrating up to 10 mg twice daily PO

*RRR, Relative risk reduction (proportional in events in treatment group compared with control); CI, 95% confidence intervals (%); NNT, numbers needed to treat (estimated number of patients needed to be treated to prevent one adverse event; 1/absolute risk reduction); SOLVD, Studies Of Left Ventricular Dysfunction; CHF, congestive heart failure; ACE, acute coronary event.

requirement of any specialized test for entry other than ejection fraction that was commonly available in North America; a run-in phase to eliminate individuals who are either unstable or noncompliant; and substantial flexibility in dosing and patient scheduling. In the main trials there were no requirements for special tests other than creatinine levels at annual visits for safety reasons. The data collection forms were simple and the outcomes easily documented. These trials have shown that treatment with an ACE inhibitor, enalapril, reduced mortality, reduced the incidence of hospitalization for heart failure, and prevented the development of overt heart failure in patients with left ventricular dysfunction.

The DIG Study (Table 12-5) was designed to be even more representative of the heart failure population than the SOLVD trials. In particular, it did not have a restriction of including only patients with ejection fractions of less than 35%. This has therefore led to inclusion of a substantial proportion of patients with ejection fractions between 35% and 45% (about 2000 patients) and a further 1000 patients with ejection fractions greater than 45%. This will be the first large trial that has included the whole spectrum of patients with congestive heart failure regardless of the level of systolic dysfunction. This trial was designed to be even simpler than the SOLVD Trials and has been conducted in approximately 300 centers in the United States and Canada. The trial completed recruitment of 7750 patients 6 months ahead of schedule and included a wide variety of centers ranging from university hospitals, Veterans Administration hospitals, community hospitals, physicians' offices, and family practices. This trial is due to report at the end of 1996 and should provide a very reliable assessment of the effects of digitalis in patients with sinus rhythm and heart failure with regard to its effects on mortality and major morbidity.

By being simple, both trials could be large and conducted at a reasonable cost. However, this has also led to lack of information on a number of pathophysiologic mechanisms. Therefore, in both trials a number of focused substudies were designed to evaluate the effects of treatment on many physiologic endpoints. In particular, in the SOLVD Trials there were eight such studies that evaluated the effects of ACE inhibitors on neurohormonal measurements, echocardiographic measurements, radionuclide measurements of ventricular volumes and function, invasive hemodynamic studies of contractility, arrhythmias, quality of life, and exercise tolerance. In the DIG Study there have been a few focused substudies that evaluated the effects of digitalis on quality of life, exercise tolerance, ventricular arrhythmias, 24-hour heart rate variability, and neurohormones. This complementary approach of having a large simple trial with nested smaller but more detailed substudies provides an opportunity to obtain reliable information on mortality and morbidity in the main trial and yet learn about the effects of the drug on various pathophysiologic mechanisms. This is a useful approach for most diseases and something that is likely to be increasingly accepted.

Large simple trials of prevention of cardiovascular disease

Healthy populations: physicians' studies (Table 12-6). Two complementary large simple trials were set up to assess whether aspirin had a role in preventing the incidence of cardiovascular disease (MI, stroke, or vascular death) in an otherwise apparently healthy population. In the United Kingdom, the British Doctors Study randomized about 5000 male physicians to either aspirin or control and did not show any clear evidence of benefit for aspirin.[46] The U.S. Physicians Study randomized about 22,000 male physicians to either aspirin or placebo or to β-carotene or placebo in a 2 × 2 factorial design.[47] The aspirin arm of the study was reported after a mean follow-up of 5 years and showed a clear reduction in the incidence of MI although, as would be expected,

No. of centers	Total sample size	Endpoints and follow-up	Main results		RRR (%) (CI)	NNT
			Treatment	Comparison		
83	2,569	Mortality (mean follow-up 41 mo)	Enalapril 452/1285 35.2%	Placebo 510/1284 39.7%	16% (5%-26%)	22
83	4,228	Mortality (mean follow-up 37 mo)	Enalapril 313/2111 14.8%	Placebo 334/2117 15.8%	NS	—

Table 12-5. Ongoing or planned large simple randomized trials in cardiovascular disease*

Trial	Start date	Design	Eligibility criteria	Agent(s) under investigation and regimen	Planned total sample size	Main endpoints and follow-up	Expected report date
DIG	1991	Placebo control	Congestive heart failure patients Ejection fraction ≤45% Sinus rhythm	Digoxin 0.125-0.5 mg daily to achieve serum levels of 0.8-2.5 ng/mL	7000	Total mortality Mean follow-up of 3 yr	1995
LIPID	1990	Placebo control	Prior MI or unstable angina	Pravastatin 40 mg daily PO	9000	Mortality from coronary heart disease	1997
HOPE	1993	Placebo control 2 × 2 factorial	History of cardiovascular disease or diabetes with at least one risk factor for cardiovascular disease >55 yr of age	(1) Ramipril target dose 10 mg daily PO (2) Vitamin E 400 IU daily PO	8000	MI Stroke or cardiovascular death 4-yr follow-up	1997
Heart Protection Study	1994	Placebo control 2 × 2 factorial	History of cardiovascular disease or diabetes	(1) Simvastatin 40 mg daily PO (2) Vitamin E (600 mg), vitamin C (250 mg), and β-carotene (20 mg) daily in a single capsule PO	20,000	Total mortality 5-yr follow-up	1998
GISSI Prevenzione	1993	Open control 2 × 2 factorial	Prior MI First randomization	(1) Fish oil (n-3 ethylester) 1 g daily PO (2) Vitamin E 300 mg daily PO	12,000	Total mortality MI Stroke	1997
			Second randomization (if cholesterol 200-300 mg/dL [5.2-7.7 mmol/L] and not being treated with cholesterol lowering therapy)	Pravastatin 20-40 mg daily PO	6000	Total mortality MI Stroke	

*DIG, Digitalis Investigation Group; LIPID, Long-term Intervention with Pravastatin in Ischemic Disease; HOPE, Heart Outcome Prevention Evaluation; MI, myocardial infarction; GISSI, Gruppo Italiano per lo Studio della Streptochinasi nell'Infarto Miocardico.

Table 12-6. Large simple randomized trials: prevention of cardiovascular events

Trial	Publication year	Design	Eligibility criteria	Agent(s) under investigation and regimen
U.K. physicians[46]	1988	Open control 2:1 random- ization	Male British physicians Not on aspirin and without a contraindication	Aspirin 500 mg daily PO
U.S. physicians[47]	1989	Placebo control 2 × 2 factorial (with β-carotene)	Male U.S. physicians Healthy	Aspirin 325 mg alternate days PO

*MI, Myocardial infarction; RRR, relative risk reduction (proportional in events in treatment group compared with control); CI, 95% confidence intervals (%); NNT, numbers needed to treat (estimated number of patients needed to be treated to prevent one adverse event; 1/absolute risk reduction).

the overall incidence was low in this otherwise healthy population (1.26% in the aspirin group vs. 2.17% in the control group). Follow-up for the β-carotene component of the U.S. Physicians Study is continuing.

Prevention in populations at risk: HOPE, Heart Protection Study, and GISSI Prevenzione (see Table 12-5). Some of the focus of large simple trials in cardiovascular disease has shifted away from acute intervention, and a number of studies have been set up to assess treatment strategies designed to prevent the progression of cardiovascular disease and events (MI, stroke, and vascular death) in populations who are at high risk of these events, (i.e, those with existing coronary disease [before MI or angina] or other established vascular disease [prior stroke or peripheral vascular disease] or others at high risk [e.g., those with diabetes]). Treatments being assessed in these studies include cholesterol-lowering agents, (e.g., simvastatin), ACE inhibitors (ramipril), vitamin E, and fish oils. These exciting and important studies will report in the latter half of this decade.

Large simple trials: future perspectives

The principles on which large simple trials have been based have now been widely accepted among the medical, research, and clinical communities, and a number of coordinating centers in different continents have the necessary expertise to conduct large simple trials. Therefore, given the necessary resources, the assessment of therapeutic strategies, both medical and surgical, has now become reasonably straightforward using the totality of the evidence from randomized controlled trials (e.g., using properly conducted meta-analyses). The ongoing prevention studies will have profound implications for the long-term treatment of patients who are at high risk of cardiovascular events and may also have major economic repercussions. The real challenge, therefore, for those involved in health care delivery is how resources will be managed. Large simple

trials can and should play an important role in the evaluation of medical and surgical therapies and in this way provide reliable information on which economic and resource decisions can be based. They may therefore provide an important method of resource management and should be placed high on the agenda of decision-makers and politicians for determining the overall cost effectiveness of different components of health care.

REFERENCES

1. Yusuf S, Collins R, Peto R: Why do we need some large, simple randomized trials? *Stat Med* 3:409-420, 1984.
2. Peto R: Clinical trial methodology, *Biomedicine* 28:24-36, 1978.
3. Peto R: Why do we need some systematic overviews of randomized trials? *Stat Med* 6:233-240, 1987.
4. Collins R, Gray R, Godwin J, et al: Avoidance of large biases and large random errors in the assessment of moderate treatment effects: the need for systemic overviews, *Stat Med* 6:245-250, 1987.
5. Yusuf S: Obtaining medically meaningful answers from an overview of randomized clinical trials, *Stat Med* 6:281-286, 1987.
6. Peto R, Pike C, Armitage P, et al: Design and analysis of randomized clinical trials requiring prolonged observation of each patient: I. Introduction and design, *Br J Cancer* 34:585, 1976.
7. Peto R, Pike C, Armitage P, et al: Design and analysis of randomized clinical trials requiring prolonged observation of each patient: II. Analysis and examples, *Br J Cancer* 35:1-27, 1977.
8. Peto R: Statistical aspects of cancer trials. In Halnan KE (ed): *Treatment of Cancer,* London, 1982, Chapman and Hall.
9. Yusuf S, Wittes J, Probstfield J, et al: Analysis and interpretation of treatment effects in subgroups of patients in randomized clinical trials, *JAMA* 266:93-98, 1991.
10. Pocock SJ: When to stop a clinical trial, *Br Med J* 305:235-240, 1992.
11. Wald N: Ethical issues in randomised prevention trials, *Br Med J* 306:563-565, 1993.
12. Cardiac Arrhythmia Suppression Trial (CAST) Investigators, Preliminary report: effect of encainide and flecainide on mortality in a randomized trial of arrhythmia suppression after myocardial infarction, *N Engl J Med* 321:406-412, 1989.
13. Topol EJ, Califf RM. Answers to complex questions cannot be derived from "simple" trials, *Br Heart J* 68:348-351, 1992.
14. Hampton JR, Skene AM: Beyond the mega-trial: certainty and uncertainty, *Br Heart J* 68:352-355, 1992.
15. Francis J Jr, et al: *Evaluation of the 1954 Field Trial of Poliomyelitis Vaccine,* Ann Arbor, Mich, 1957, Edward Bros.

Total sample size	Follow-up and endpoints	Main results		RRR (%) (CI)	NNT
		Treatment	Comparison		
5139	MI* (fatal plus nonfatal) 6-yr follow-up	79/3429 2.3%	41/1710 2.4%	NS	–
22,071	MI Mean follow-up 5 yr	139/11,037 1.26%	239/11,034 2.17%	44% (30-55)	–

16. ISIS-1 Collaborative Group: Randomized trial of intravenous atenolol among 16,027 cases of suspected acute myocardial infarction: ISIS-1, *Lancet* 2:57-66, 1986.
17. Yusuf S, Peto R, Lewis J, et al: Beta-blockade during and after myocardial infarction: an overview of the randomized trials, *Prog Cardiovasc Dis* 27:335-371, 1985.
18. Yusuf S, Collins R, Peto R, et al: Intravenous and intracoronary fibrinolytic therapy in acute myocardial inarction: overview of results on mortality, reinfarction and side-effects from 33 randomized controlled trials, *Eur Heart J* 6:556-585, 1985.
19. ISIS Pilot Study Investigators: Randomized factorial trial of high-dose intravenous streptokinase, or oral aspirin and of intravenous heparin in acute myocardial infarction, *Eur Heart J* 8:634-642, 1987.
20. GISSI (Gruppo Italiano per lo Studio della Streptochinasi nell' Infarto Miocardico): Effectiveness of intravenous thrombolytic treatment in acute myocardial infarction, *Lancet* 1:397-401, 1986.
21. Collins R, Julian D: British Heart Foundation Surveys (1987 & 1989) of United Kingdom policies for acute myocardial infarction, *Br Heart J* 66:250-255, 1991.
22. ISIS-2 (Second International Study of Infarct Survival) Collaborative Group: Randomised trial of intravenous streptokinase, oral aspirin, both, or neither among 17,187 cases of suspected acute myocardial infarction: ISIS-2, *Lancet* 2:349-360, 1988.
23. Hlatky MA, Cotugno H, O'Connor C, et al: Adoption of thrombolytic therapy in the management of acute myocardial infarction, *Am J Cardiol* 61:510-514.
24. EMERAS (Estudio Multicentrico Estreptoquinasa Republicas de America del Sur) Investigators: Randomized trial of late thrombolysis in acute myocardial infarction: EMERAS, *Lancet* 342:767-772, 1993.
25. LATE (Late Assessment of Thrombolytic Efficacy) Study Group: *Lancet* 342:759-766, 1993.
26. Fibrinolytic Therapy Trialists' (FTT) Collaborative Group: Indications for fibrinolytic therapy in suspected acute myocardial infarction: collaborative overview of mortality and major morbidity results from all randomised trials of more than 1000 patients, *Lancet* 343:311-322, 1994.
27. ASSET (Anglo-Scandinavian Study of Early Thrombolysis) Study Group: Trial of tissue plasminogen activator for mortality reduction in acute myocardial infarction, *Lancet* 2:525-530, 1988.
28. AIMS Trial Study Group: Effect of intravenous APSAC on mortality after acute myocardial infarction: Preliminary report of a placebo-controlled clinical trial, *Lancet* 1:545-549, 1988.
29. Chesebro JH, Knatterud G, Roberts R, et al: Thrombolysis in Myocardial Infarction (TIMI) Trial, Phase I: a comparison between intravenous tissue plasminogen activator and intravenous streptokinase, *Circulation* 76:142-154, 1987.
30. Gruppo Italiano per lo Studio della Sopravvivenza nell'Infarto Miocardico (GISSI). GISSI-2: a factorial randomised trial of alteplase versus streptokinase and heparin versus no heparin among 12,490 patients with acute myocardial infarction, *Lancet* 336:65-71, 1990.
31. International Study Group: In-hospital mortality and clinical course of 20,891 patients with suspected acute myocardial infarction randomised between alteplase and streptokinase with or without heparin, *Lancet* 336:71-75, 1990.
32. ISIS-3 (Third International Study of Infarct Survival) Collaborative Group: ISIS-3: A randomised trial of streptokinase vs tissue plasminogen activator vs anistreplase and of aspirin plus heparin vs aspirin alone among 41,299 cases of suspected acute myocardial infarction, *Lancet* 339:753-770, 1992.
33. GUSTO Investigators: An international randomized trial comparing four thrombolytic strategies for acute myocardial infarction, *N Engl J Med* 329:673-682, 1993.
34. Pfeffer MA, Braunwald E: Ventricular remodeling after myocardial infarction. Experimental observations and clinical implications, *Circulation* 81:1161-1172, 1990.
35. Jugdutt BI, Warnica JW: Intravenous nitroglycerin therapy to limit myocardial infarct size, expansion and complications. Effect of timing, dosage, and infarct location, *Circulation* 78:906-909, 1988.
36. Yusuf S, Collins R, MacMahon S, et al: Effects of intravenous nitrates on mortality in acute myocardial infarction: an overview of the randomised trials, *Lancet* 1:1088-1092, 1988.
37. Pfeffer MA, Braunwald E, Moyé LA, et al: Effect of captopril on mortality and morbidity in patients with left ventricular dysfunction after myocardial infarction (Survival and Ventricular Enlargement: SAVE Study), *N Engl J Med* 327:669-677, 1992.
38. The Acute Infarction Ramipril Efficacy (AIRE) study investigators: Effect of ramipril on mortality and morbidity of survivors of acute myocardial infarction with clinical evidence of heart failure, *Lancet* 342:821-828, 1993.
39. Swedberg K, Held P, Kjekshus J, et al: Effects of the early administration of enalapril on mortality in patients with acute myocardial infarction. Results of the Cooperative New Scandinavian Enalapril Survival Study II (CONSENSUS II), *N Engl J Med* 327:678-684, 1992.
40. GISSI-3-Gruppo Italiano per lo Studio della Sopravvivenza nell'Infarto Miocardico: GISSI-3 Study protocol on the effects of lisinopril, of nitrates, and of their association in patients with acute myocardial infarction, *Am J Cardiol* 70:62C-69C, 1992.
41. ISIS-4 Collaborative Group: Fourth International Study of Infarct Survival: protocol for a large simple study of the effects of oral mononitrate, of oral captopril, and of intravenous magnesium, *Am J Cardiol* 68:87D-100D, 1991.
42. Woods KL, Fletcher S, Roffe C, et al: Intravenous magnesium

sulphate in suspected acute myocardial infarction: results of the second Leicester Intravenous Magnesium Intervention Trial (LIMIT-2), *Lancet* 339:1553-1558, 1992.

43. Teo KT, Yusuf S, Collins R, et al: Effects of intravenous magnesium in suspected acute myocardial infarction: overview of randomised trials, *Br Med J (Clin Res)* 303:1499-1503, 1991.

44. SOLVD Investigators: Effect of enalapril on mortality and the development of heart failure in asymptomatic patients with reduced left ventricular ejection fractions, *N Engl J Med* 327:685-691, 1992.

45. SOLVD Investigators: Effect of enalapril on survival in patients with reduced left ventricular ejection fractions and congestive heart failure, *N Engl J Med* 325:293-302, 1991.

46. Peto R, Gray R, Collins R, et al: Randomised trial of prophylactic daily aspirin in British male doctors, *Br Med J* 296:313-316, 1988.

47. Steering Committee of the Physicians' Health Study Research Group: Final report on the aspirin component of the ongoing Physicians' Health Study, *N Engl J Med* 321:129-135, 1989.

Chapter 13

OBSERVATIONAL DATABASES

Mark Hlatky

Clinical research uses a variety of designs, from case reports to randomized clinical trials (Table 13-1). There is a general gradation in the scientific rigor of these designs in rough parallel to the quality of the control groups used. No one would seriously dispute that the randomized clinical trial is the most rigorous and reliable method of comparing therapeutic alternatives. Randomized studies, especially the large simple "megatrials," have shifted the entire paradigm for treatment of acute myocardial infarction (AMI) toward the goal of early, sustained reperfusion of ischemic myocardium. Now that the therapeutic principle of early reperfusion has been firmly established by randomized studies, considerable investigative effort is being focused on the optimal treatment regimen, including agent, dose, timing, and adjunctive therapy.

The primacy of randomized trials in the hierarchy of clinical design does not mean, however, that the other research designs lack value.[1-3] Randomized studies are difficult, time consuming, and expensive to perform, and it is simply not feasible to perform a randomized study to answer every question of therapeutic interest. Other designs may be helpful in filling the gaps in knowledge left by randomized studies. More important, many scientific questions are not amenable to study in a randomized trial but are nevertheless worthy of investigation. Examples of such questions include establishing prognostic factors or risk factors; providing information about the spectrum of disease, incidence and prevalence, and time trends in outcome; elucidating practice patterns and how they may vary between different geographic locations and over time; and evaluating quality

of care. Observational databases are well-suited to address many questions that either cannot or will not be assessed by randomized studies.

Databases can be classified according to their intended purpose into (1) administrative databases, (2) clinical databases, and (3) research databases (Table 13-2). An administrative database is assembled for purposes of organizing or financing the delivery of health services. The Health Care Finance Administration (HCFA) administers the Medicare and Medicaid programs and processes millions of claims every year to pay for the services of hospitals, physicians, and other health care providers. HCFA databases include some clinical data on diagnoses and procedures and can therefore be used in the study of a broad sample of patients. Clinical databases are assembled for use by health care professionals in the delivery of care, examples of which are coronary care unit logs and cardiac catheterization records. Research databases are distinguished from other clinical databases in that they are designed specifically for research purposes and have more rigorous attention to standard data definitions and quality control of data elements. The research database may even be derived from a clinical trial, blurring the distinction between these two designs. For example, when a randomized trial of thrombolytic therapy analyzes the correlates and outcomes of complete heart block complicating AMI, randomization assignment may not be relevant.

The different types of databases have different strengths and weaknesses. Administrative databases include unselected patients from many institutions and

Table 13-1. Clinical research designs in increasing order of rigor

---

No controls (case reports, case series)
Literature controls
Historic controls
Concurrent controls
Concurrent controls with multivariable analysis
Randomized controlled clinical trials

Table 13-2. Databases relevant to acute myocardial infarction

---

Administrative databases
  Medicare claims
  Department of Veterans Affairs files
  Hospital discharge databases (e.g., California, New York, Pennsylvania)
Clinical databases
  Coronary care unit logs
  Coronary angiography databases
Research databases
  Observational
    Duke University cardiovascular disease database
    University of California–San Diego acute myocardial infarction database
  Randomized*
    TAMI trials
    TIMI trials
    GISSI trials
    ISIS trials

---

*TAMI, Thrombolysis and Angioplasty in Acute Myocardial Infarction; TIMI, thrombolysis in myocardial infarction; GISSI, Gruppo Italian per lo Studio della Streptochinasi nell' Infarto Miocardico; ISIS, International Studies of Infarct Survival.

may therefore provide information on practice patterns and outcomes in the community instead of the academic centers that usually provide data in medical journals. The operative mortality of a surgical procedure in a typical hospital can, for example, be better established by an administrative database than by published articles from the leading referral centers. Administrative data suffer, however, from lack of clinical detail, making it difficult to study all but the simplest prognostic factors or to evaluate outcomes other than mortality. Clinical databases also provide "unselected" patient data but are limited in scope by being from one institution and often lack the rigorous quality control of research databases. Research databases have the most clinical detail and contain the most reliable data, making them best suited for multivariable prognostic studies and treatment evaluations. They are limited, however, by the selection criteria used to control patient entry into the study. The multicenter research databases overcome the limitations of using only a single institution, but institutions in research studies may have been selected for their particularly high volumes or good outcomes and there-

fore may not be representative of the community at large. The different types of databases therefore have complementary strengths in their breadth of patient selection and their depth of clinical detail.

The remainder of the chapter discusses how observational studies can address several questions of interest to clinicians.

PROGNOSIS

A rational approach to therapy rests on an evaluation of the patient's prognosis. Simply put, the high-risk patient has more to gain from an intervention than a low-risk patient. If, for example, thrombolytic therapy reduces by half the risk of death during AMI, a patient who has a risk of dying of 10% without treatment would be a more appropriate candidate for aggressive therapy than a patient with a 1% risk of dying.

The observational database is well suited for analysis of prognostic factors in AMI. Studies have been performed using research databases, clinical databases, and even administrative databases. The clinical value of such analyses depends mostly on the type and quality of data collected. Databases from the prethrombolytic era usually lack key elements such as duration of symptoms, precise electrocardiographic (ECG) findings, and thrombolytic contraindications. For some variables the database can be augmented by retrospective data collection (e.g., rereading the ECG), but for other variables (e.g., duration of symptoms) retrospective review of medical records is unlikely to be productive. Selker et al.[4] have combined data from several databases to devise prognostic index for patients with AMI. These investigators plan to incorporate the prognostic algorithm into an ECG machine to provide a real-time decision aid to physicians considering thrombolytic therapy. Prognostic studies are fundamental and by their nature derive from observations of large cohorts of unselected patients. Databases are well-suited for evaluation of prognosis.

DISEASE EPIDEMIOLOGY

Observational databases can be useful in documenting the clinical features and natural history of disease. The proportion of patients with anterior vs. inferior MI or Q-wave MI vs. non-Q-wave MI, or the age distribution of MI patients all can be established by observational data. Similarly, the incidence and clinical predictors of various complications (e.g., ventricular septal defect, myocardial rupture, complete heart block) are best appreciated from large, unselected groups of patients. The data from such series must always be analyzed with recognition of the potential biases and limitations, as with all epidemiologic data. Nevertheless, descriptive and analytic studies of the predictors, correlates, and consequences of AMI provide the essential context for all clinical decision-making.

PRACTICE PATTERNS

In the 1990s there has been increasing emphasis on the cost and outcomes of medical care. Physicians are under pressure to provide cost-effective care, and database analyses have contributed to the new focus on clinical decision-making. Temporal and geographic variations in practice patterns can provide valuable information.

Time trend data come from clinical and administrative datasets. These data may reveal that the incidence of disease is changing or that its prognosis is changing. The well-known decline in coronary artery disease mortality is an excellent example of the value of temporal analysis. The clinical research database at Duke University has been used to document the changing pattern of use for coronary bypass surgery, as well as the steadily improving outcomes of surgery.[5,6] These database analyses provide the context in which clinical trials must be interpreted.

The wide variation in physician practice among different geographic locations is a relatively recent observation. Rates of procedures such as bypass surgery may vary by a factor of 5 or more between areas with seemingly similar patient populations. These variations have highlighted the uncertainties of medical practice and led to critical self-evaluation by the medical profession. They have also catalyzed the development of "outcomes research," a field devoted to analysis of practice and outcomes, with the goal of improving care. A patient outcome research team (PORT) has been founded by the Agency for Health Care Policy and Research to examine care of AMI, and a second PORT is examining the care of patients with chronic ischemic heart disease. The PORTs plan to synthesize data from a variety of sources, including databases and randomized studies, and develop guidelines to improve patient care.[7,8]

QUALITY OF CARE

Databases have a valuable role in quality assurance in medical care. Mortality statistics can be generated from either administrative or clinical databases to examine the outcomes of care in different institutions. Medicare data have been used to screen hospitals for quality of care problems. Although these data are far from perfect (and open to abuse in a competitive environment), they can cause institutions to critically examine the care they provide. Units with excessive mortality from MI should examine their practices carefully to determine if they can be improved. The California Office of Statewide Health Planning and Development has been required by state law to develop risk-adjustment methods to compare hospitals in the outcome of patients with AMI.[9]

CONCLUSIONS

Databases derived from administrative, clinical, or research activities remain very useful tools, even in the era of large randomized trials. Databases can provide information on topics as diverse as prognosis, disease epidemiology, health care practice patterns, and quality of care. Databases and randomized trials provide complementary information valuable to clinical care.

REFERENCES

1. Hlatky MA, Lee KL, Harrell FE Jr, et al: Tying clinical research to patient care by use of an observational database, *Stat Med* 3:375-384, 1984.
2. Hlatky MA, Califf RM, Harrell FE Jr, et al: Comparisons of predictions based on observational data with the results of randomized controlled trials of coronary artery bypass surgery, *J Am Coll Cardiol* 11:237-245, 1988.
3. Hlatky MA, Califf RM, Harrell FE Jr, et al: Clinical judgment and therapeutic decision making, *J Am Coll Cardiol* 15:1-14, 1990.
4. Selker HP, Griffith JL, Beshansky JR, et al: The thrombolytic predictive instrument project: combining clinical study data bases to take medical effectiveness research to the streets. In Grady ML, Schwartz HA (ed): *Medical effectiveness research data methods,* Rockville Md, 1992, Agency for Health Care Policy and Research, pp 9-36.
5. Pryor DB, Harrell FE Jr, Rankin JS, et al: The changing survival benefits of coronary revascularization over time, *Circulation* 76(suppl V):13-21, 1987.
6. Califf RM, Harrell FE Jr, Lee KL, et al: Changing efficacy of coronary revascularization: implications for patient selection, *Circulation* 78(suppl I):185-191, 1988.
7. DeFriese GH: Measuring the effectiveness of medical interventions: new expectations of health services research, *Health Serv Res* 25:691-696, 1990.
8. Pashos CL, McNeil BJ: Consequences of variation in treatment for acute myocardial infarction, *Health Serv Res* 25:717-722, 1990.
9. Johns L: Measuring quality in California, *Health Affairs* 266-270, 1992.

Chapter 14

ENDPOINTS FOR TRIALS OF REPERFUSION IN ACUTE MYOCARDIAL INFARCTION

Robert M. Califf
Lynn H. Woodlief

The goals of strategies to reperfuse the myocardium can be thought of as simple or complex, depending upon the level at which the effect of therapy needs to be understood. In simple terms, most clinicians and patients would agree that the goal of treatment of AMI is to allow the patient to live longer and feel better and, if at all possible, for the health care system to spend less money in the process. There are several problems with the simple approach, however. First, in order to demonstrate differences or lack of differences, such endpoints as death and cost require huge numbers of patients. Second, although the development of new therapies and the adoption of effective approaches would be enhanced if "surrogate" endpoints reflecting the intended biologic effect could be used to allow clinical trials to be done with smaller numbers of patients, in some cases a therapy will affect these endpoints in opposite directions, leaving an uncertain final interpretation of the value of the therapy. Third, for appropriate reasons we desire to understand why a therapy has improved outcome in order to provide insight into future therapeutic approaches and to ensure that the treatment effect is real and can be replicated. Accordingly this chapter will review the advantages and disadvantages of endpoints ranging from the simplest to the most complex clinical measurements.

Traditional clinical endpoints can be divided conceptually into five general categories: biochemical or hematologic, images, physiologic measurements, measures of

clinical complications, and survival. Each of these endpoints has its own profile of advantages and disadvantages. The critical endpoints of cost and quality of life are reviewed in Chapters 15 and 16.

BIOCHEMICAL AND HEMATOLOGIC MEASUREMENTS (TABLE 14-1)

Most therapeutic strategies for AMI and unstable angina include a component of antithrombotic effect. The impact of these therapies on the individual components of the coagulation system can be measured directly (see Chapter 38). Unfortunately, the relationship between any of these specific assays and the eventual clinical outcome is indirect at best.

Fibrinolytic agents produce variable degrees of breakdown of systemic fibrinogen and depletion of factors V and VIII. With the use of nonspecific fibrinolytic agents such as streptokinase, reperfusion is not successfully established unless a systemic fibrinolytic state is achieved.[1] Many developers of fibrin-specific agents have striven to achieve coronary thrombolysis without any disturbance of the systemic circulation. With fibrin-specific agents such as t-PA, the degree of fibrinogenolysis is highly variable and only modestly related to bleeding complications.[2-4]

Antithrombin therapy can be assayed using a variety of markers of thrombin activation (Fig. 14-1). After thrombolytic therapy administration a procoagulant state is produced, marked by increases in fibrinopeptide

149

Table 14-1. Coagulation measures

Measures	Normal values in acute phase of MI	Comments
Fibrinolysis		
Fibrinogen	200-300 ± 66 mg/dL	Depletion is a marker of lytic state; correlation with bleeding risk is only modest
Thrombin activity		
Fibrinopeptide A (FPA)	.5-1.3 ± .25 nM	Persistent elevation may be marker of failed reperfusion; recurrent elevation associated with reocclusion. Careful sampling critical; very sensitive to artifactual increase
Thrombin-antithrombin complex	0-3 μg/mL ± .17 μM	Same issues pertinent to FPA
Fragment 1.2 (F1.2)	.44-1.2 ± .20 nM	Same issues pertinent to TAT and FPA
D-Dimer		Provides evidence of fibrin breakdown
Plasminogen activator inhibitor (PAI)		Elevated baseline levels may correlate with persistent reocclusion
Platelet activity		
Platelet aggregation	Highly variable dependency on agonist	Desired value undefined
Bleeding time	2.5-10 min	Poor correlation with efficacy or bleeding
Factors V, VIII		Repletion is marker of lytic state

Markers of thrombin activity

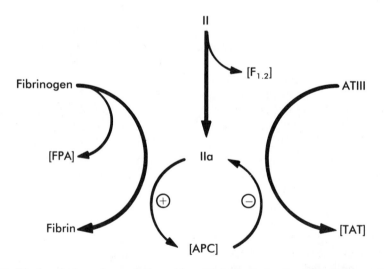

Fig. 14-1. Biochemical markers of thrombin activity include the following: prothrombin fragment 1.2 (F1.2), the cleavage peptide formed during activation of factor II; fibrinopeptide A (FPA), the cleavage peptide released by fibrinogen during fibrin formation; thrombin antithrombin complex (TAT), which forms as antithrombin III binds to and inactivates thrombin; and activated protein C, which both indirectly inhibits IIa and increases in response to increased thrombin activity.

A, thrombin-antithrombin complex, and F 1.2. This state has been attributed to the release of clot-bound thrombin, reexposure of the subendothelium to the circulating clotting factors, new thrombogenic surfaces produced by ischemic damage to the endothelium,[5] and activation of prothrombin by the lytic process itself.[6] Heparin does not suppress this state,[7] presumably because the large size of the heparin-antithrombin III complex prevents penetration of the clot. Other antithrombin agents such as hirudin and hirulog may suppress the procoagulant state, but the relationship of this suppression to clinical benefit is not defined.

Because of the beneficial effect of aspirin, more effective antiplatelet therapy is generally believed to be desirable. Antiplatelet therapy is commonly measured using ADP-induced platelet aggregation studies and bleeding times. The relationship of platelet aggregation studies to clinical outcomes in this setting has not been defined. In the setting of percutaneous revascularization procedures for acute ischemic syndromes, 80% inhibition of 20 micromolar ADP-induced platelet aggregation has been found to be associated with a 25% reduction in acute ischemic events,[8] but the value of even more extreme inhibition remains untested. Prolongation of bleeding time is associated with a modest increase in the risk of bleeding,[9] but increased bleeding time could also be associated with a higher initial perfusion rate and a reduction in the risk of reocclusion.

The major advantages of these coagulation marker endpoints are that they can be measured precisely and that differences between therapies can be demonstrated with small sample sizes. The management of blood samples is complex, however, because many of these assays either must be done on site or require extremely careful blood sampling, with meticulous handling after samples have been drawn. Most importantly, the "desired" level for each of these measures is not known, so whether the observed differences are good or bad can be discerned only by measuring the clinical endpoints. For this reason we advocate the measurement of coagulation markers in early pilot studies and in a subset of patients in larger trials, but these measures will not replace clinical endpoint measurement in the near future.

IMAGES
Measures of coronary perfusion

Angiographic endpoints. The goal of many therapies in AMI or unstable angina is to attain or maintain perfusion of the infarct-related coronary artery. From this perspective the direct measurement of perfusion should be considered the most direct measure of clinical efficacy, because a thrombolytic agent that did not result in high rates of coronary patency would be unlikely to result in improved survival or other positive clinical outcomes. Coronary perfusion as measured by angiog-

raphy currently has three dimensions: early patency, sustained patency, and myocardial perfusion at both time points.

Early patency has been the focus of most of the efforts in the thrombolytic arena. Initially enthusiasm was high that simply demonstrating a difference in patency would be adequate to prove that one agent was superior to another. These differences in early patency led to early termination of the TIMI-1 trial when t-PA was found to have a much higher early patency rate than streptokinase.[10] The GISSI-2[11] and ISIS-3[12] trials failed to demonstrate the mortality benefit of t-PA as compared with streptokinase despite clearcut differences from many trials, including TIMI, in early patency. The reasons for this discrepancy remain unclear, although it is likely that conventional t-PA dosing in the absence of intravenous heparin leads not only to a high early patency rate but also to a high reocclusion rate.

Reocclusion, or the absence of sustained patency, is an issue that has been somewhat neglected in the examination of efficacy of thrombolytic regimens. Early data from the TAMI trials indicate that when reocclusion occurs, the mortality rate is doubled.[13] However, the angiographic measurement of reocclusion is not as simple as it may seem. In order to make a valid assessment there must be documentation of a patent artery early in the hospital course and the patient must have another angiogram before hospital discharge. The likelihood of successfully obtaining both of these studies is only 70% to 90%, which means that the endpoint cannot be ascertained in a substantial number of patients entered into the study. The two most troublesome groups of dropouts are patients who have a reinfarction and either die or develop medical contraindications to follow-up angiography and patients who go on to have bypass surgery or angioplasty because of recurrent ischemia before the scheduled follow-up angiogram. Because of these problems we believe that a range of estimated reocclusion rates should be published that reflects the different possibilities engendered by the withdrawal bias that these complicating factors create. One analysis would report only patients with both studies (early and late patency); a second would report the "worst case" scenario, counting all patients lost to follow-up as having reocclusion; a third analysis would report the "best case" scenario of counting all patients lost to follow-up as not having reocclusion; and finally an imputed analysis would count all patients with fatal or nonfatal reinfarction as well as all patients who undergo early revascularization for recurrent ischemia as having reocclusion if they did not have angiographic follow-up.

One of the most important findings of the GUSTO-I trial[14] was the demonstration that mortality was directly related to early patency and, more specifically, to the TIMI grade perfusion at the 90-minute angiogram (Fig.

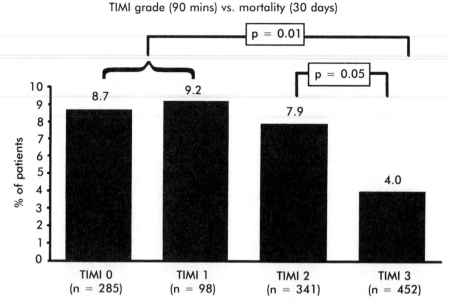

Fig. 14-2. Patients enrolled in the GUSTO-I trial who had TIMI grade 1 or 2 flow were at significantly greater risk of dying within 30 days of randomization than patients with TIMI 2 or 3 flow.

14-2). These results, combined with previous key studies,[15-17] demonstrate that TIMI grade 2 and 3 flow should no longer be lumped together, and that the primary goal of reperfusion therapy should be to establish TIMI grade 3 flow as rapidly as possible. The observed mortality result is also contingent upon reocclusion rates, however, and one of the surprising findings of the GUSTO-I trial was the absence of a difference in reocclusion rates across treatment groups. As long as the reocclusion rates are equivalent, the treatment with the highest TIMI-3 flow at 90 minutes should, and does, correspond to the treatment with the lowest mortality rate.

In future trials why not simply measure 60- or 90-minute perfusion, which was such a good surrogate for total mortality in the GUSTO-I trial? Unfortunately, most systemic therapies have the possibility of creating "unintended effects" through action on nontarget organs (e.g., bleeding in the brain), or through unanticipated physiologic effects on the target organ (e.g., higher risk of sudden ventricular fibrillation in patients treated with "antiarrhythmic" drugs). For this reason we believe that it will be essential to perform large-scale trials measuring clinically relevant endpoints before a new therapy should be recommended to the public in a disease as widespread as coronary artery disease. Carefully conducted angiographic trials focusing on early TIMI grade 3 flow may provide the best screen for therapies to consider in large-scale trials. It should be noted that although TIMI grade would appear to be a straightforward measurement, the few studies that have

evaluated interobserver and intraobserver reliability have shown that the differentiation of TIMI grades 2 and 3 can be subtle.[18] For this reason angiographic core laboratories are necessary, including quality control studies that demonstrate the variability of the measurements within the laboratory.

Contrast echocardiography. By creating microparticles with sonicated contrast material injected into the coronary arteries, tissue perfusion can be measured more directly. Using chest wall echocardiography, several preliminary studies have developed evidence to suggest that a substantial number of infarct-related arteries with TIMI grade 3 angiographic perfusion do not have tissue perfusion by contrast echocardiography.[19,20] These same patients do not have recovery of regional left ventricular function. Thus, contrast echocardiography may be the most sensitive measure of tissue level perfusion, but the technical difficulty of the measurement and the absence of substantial follow-up data to prove its clinical relevance make this technique a promising research method only.

Measures of left ventricular function (Table 14-2)

Left ventriculography. Contrast ventriculography remains the gold standard of left ventricular function measurement. Extensive previous research provides a natural interpretation for the clinical relevance of differences in global left ventricular function. Substantial information ties ejection fraction to risk of death and likelihood of other significant complications.[21]

Contrast left ventriculography also has important

Table 14-2. Imaging measures

Method of measurement	Usual values in acute phase of MI	Comments
Angiography		
Early TIMI grade 3	Placebo/heparin: 10%-20% SK: 30% APSAC, conventional t-PA: 40% Accelerated t-PA: 55%-60%	Key issue in reperfusion; studies with this endpoint will have incremental bleeding
Late TIMI grade 3 (beyond 12 hours)	80%-90%	Large dropout rate because of need for multiple angiograms
Contrast ventriculography		
Ejection fraction	50-58 ± 10%-14%	Large dropout rate
Regional wall motion	−2--2.8 ± 1.2--1.7 SD/chord	Relationship to outcome unclear
Radionuclide angiography	52-60 ± 10%-14%	
Thallium scintigraphy	10-20 ± 9%-11%	Cannot measure area at risk
Technetium sestamibi	10-20 ± 7%-20% of LV .55-.75 ± .35 salvage index	Area at risk measure requires pretreatment injection
Echocardiography	1.5-2.5 (wall motion score index)	Inadequate imaging in modest number of patients; difficult to quantitate

limitations. The procedure is expensive and carries some risk. The likelihood of completing a technically adequate pair of studies is generally on the order of 60% to 80%. Much of the shortfall is the result of patient refusal, but technical difficulties, patient death, and other clinical complications frequently prevent adequate follow-up studies. Patients at highest risk are most likely to drop out for clinical reasons or to have technically inadequate studies because patients with extensive anterior infarctions more often have difficulty with apical opacification, have complicating arrhythmias, and cannot tolerate repeat injections.

Compared with conservative therapy, thrombolytic administration has resulted in only a modest improvement in global left ventricular function (Fig. 14-3).[22] When trials measuring both mortality and left ventricular function were reviewed, the trials with mortality benefit seemed to show no left ventricular function difference and those showing left ventricular function improvement demonstrated no benefit in survival[23,24] (Fig. 14-4). This dissociation has been attributed for the most part to the fact that reperfusion allows patients with poor left ventricular function to survive and thus be available for follow-up left ventricular function measurement. In the control groups more patients with markedly impaired function caused by large infarction die before the follow-up examination.

Infarct zone regional left ventricular function has been touted as a more sensitive measure for detecting therapeutic effects. This endpoint can be quantified in several ways, but the most popular method, developed by Sheehan and Dodge,[25] divides the left ventricular contour into 100 radii, or chords. The inward excursion of each chord is compared with a database of normals, and the number of standard deviations away from the norm is calculated for each chord. The program then takes the general area of the infarction (anterior or inferior) and calculates the average number of standard deviations per chord away from normal for the worst 50% of chords in the infarct territory. The same measurements can then be made in the noninfarct territory. Although these measurements are scientifically appealing and provide insight into the mechanisms of therapeutic effect,[23] they are subject to all the limitations of left ventricular ejection fraction. Furthermore, they cannot be intuitively translated into clinical outcomes or clinical practice.

Long-term outcome studies have demonstrated that left ventricular volume is the most potent predictor of survival, with more prognostic information than left ventricular ejection fraction.[26] Unfortunately, measurement of end-systolic volume and end-diastolic volume requires compulsive calibration and filming of grids to ensure that comparable relationships are measured. For this reason volumes have not been used frequently as a major endpoint in therapeutic trials.

Radionuclide angiography. Radionuclide angiography can provide a measurement of systolic left ventricular function (ejection fraction) without the cost and risk of a contrast left ventriculogram. Extensive information

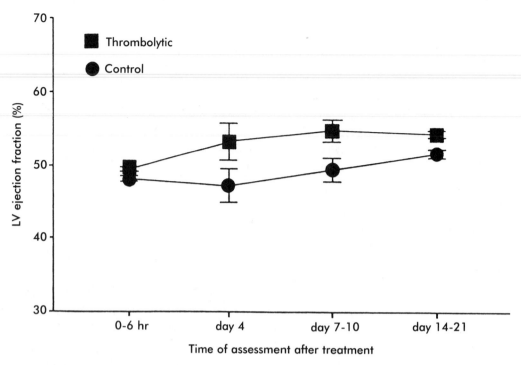

Fig. 14-3. Pooled analysis of left ventricular ejection fraction from randomized trials of thrombolytic therapy versus control: thrombolytic therapy results in significantly higher ejection fraction ($P \leq 0.001$ for each time point), and the difference between thrombolytic and control does not increase after day 4. Includes 3066 ventriculographic observations. (From Granger CB, Califf RM, Topol EJ: Thrombolytic therapy for acute myocardial infarction: a review, *Drugs* 44:293-325, 1992.)

exists to demonstrate the strong relationship of ejection fraction with subsequent survival.[27] This method generally yields ejection fraction measurements that are four or five points above the values calculated with contrast ventriculography.[28] Despite this difference, if left ventricular function were the only important clinical endpoint of a trial, radionuclide ventriculography would be superior to left ventriculography because of the higher rate of acquisition of follow-up studies. Unfortunately, in most cases the perfusion of the myocardium distal to the infarct-related artery is of paramount importance, so it remains essential to perform left ventriculography.

Thallium infarct size. Thallium-201 is a monovalent cation that follows the same course as potassium in terms of myocardial blood flow. In essence, thallium is distributed to myocardium in the same distribution as blood flow. The radionuclide is taken up by myocardium that is metabolically viable, so that areas of cellular necrosis do not take up thallium. Both animal and human studies have shown that thallium is taken up by stunned, noncontractile myocardium, providing evidence that thallium imaging can provide a reasonable estimate of myocardial infarction size that would not be susceptible to the problems of stunning that potentially could give a false impression with measures of systolic function. In animal models the relationship between quantitatively

assessed infarct size by thallium and other measures of infarct size has been excellent.[29,30] Thallium "washes out" rapidly from normal myocardium with a half-life that is dependent on hemodynamics.

In addition to the use of resting studies to assess infarct size, exercise thallium studies provide an excellent means of stratifying prognosis after myocardial infarction. Particularly when the intervention is designed to reduce postinfarction ischemia, exercise thallium provides a quantitative measure of efficacy. Paradoxically, many pharmacologic therapies designed to lead to earlier perfusion may actually *increase* the likelihood of late ischemia.

Echocardiography. Serial echocardiography is particularly attractive conceptually because it can be repeated many times to yield estimates of left ventricular shape and volume. Several small, single-center studies have found calculation of a wall motion score index to be useful in prediction of outcome with AMI.[31,32] Unfortunately no large studies have used serial echocardiography, except the GISSI study in which echocardiographic estimates of left ventricular function were used as a key component of a composite clinical endpoint.[33] A major concern with echocardiography is the high rate of technically inadequate studies, leaving the patient without key data after the point of randomization.

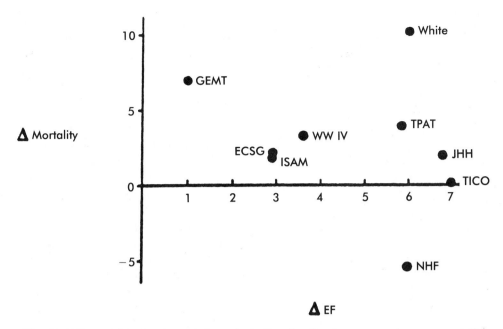

Fig. 14-4. Scatterplot showing relation of ejection fraction improvement versus mortality reduction in 10 placebo-controlled intravenous thrombolytic therapy reperfusion trials. The graph demonstrates lack of any clear relation and, if anything, a paradoxical inverse one. Trials that have shown the most benefit in terms of ejection fraction improvement over placebo (ΔEF) have tended to exhibit the least mortality reduction. It is important to point out these were trials of left ventricular ejection fraction and were not intended to detect differences of mortality. The trial abbreviations are as follows: ECSG, European Cooperative Study Group; TPAT, Tissue Plasminogen Activator—Toronto Trial; WWIV, Western Washington Intravenous Streptokinase Trial; GEMT, German Eminase Multicenter Trial; ISAM, Intravenous Streptokinase in Acute Myocardial Infarction; JHH, Johns Hopkins Hospital Trial; NHF, National Heart Foundation Trial; TICO, Thrombolysis in Coronary Occlusion Trial; White, White HD, Norris RM, Brown MA, et al: Effect of intravenous streptokinase on left ventricular function and early survival after acute myocardial infarction, *N Engl J Med* 317:850-855, 1987.

Technetium sestamibi. Hexakis (2-methoxy-isobutyl isonitrile) technetium (I), or Tc sestamibi, provides a unique ability to evaluate both final infarct size and area at risk during the period of infarct vessel occlusion. In contrast to thallium, Tc sestamibi has minimal redistribution after injection; imaging therefore can be delayed until after the acute phase of the infarction to obtain initial measurements. A predischarge measurement can then be used to determine the final infarct size. Extensive studies by Gibbons et al.[34] have documented the reasonable correlation of Tc sestamibi measures with other standard correlates of infarct size such as enzyme levels, end-systolic volume index, and left ventricular ejection fraction.

The extent of the defect can be calculated either acutely or predischarge by using tomography to acquire multiple images of the left ventricle. By assuming that the left ventricle is a hollow cylinder except at the apex, where it is believed to be a hollow cone, an estimate of the volume of nonperfused or nonviable myocardium can be made from representative imaging slices. The extent of collateral flow can be estimated by a series of measurements reflecting the degree of hypoperfusion of the infarct zone on the acute image.[35]

The major advantage of using Tc sestamibi in clinical trials is that it can markedly reduce the sample size required to demonstrate small effects on infarct size because the variance in the population is minimized by calculating the proportion of myocardium salvaged as a function of the amount of myocardium at risk. The major difficulty with the use of Tc sestamibi is that the first injection must be made before reperfusion therapy is initiated. Given current data on the importance of rapid treatment, no delay can be tolerated in initiating thrombolytic therapy in order for a technician to administer the Tc sestamibi. This practical constraint markedly reduces the number of patients who can be enrolled in clinical protocols using this method.

PHYSIOLOGIC MEASUREMENTS (TABLE 14-3)
Electrocardiographic monitoring

There is a fundamental physiologic difficulty with angiographic measurement of patency and perfusion. A number of studies have shown that a coronary angiogram

Table 14-3. Physiologic measurements

Method of measurement	Comments
Electrocardiographic monitoring	
Static 12-lead	Practice standard; good outcome studies
Continuous	
Holter	Only two leads; cannot analyze in real time; technology familiar to most staffs
12-lead (Mortara)	Complex attachment; frequent artifact; intuitively interpretable; real-time application
Vector (MIDA)	Not intuitively interpretable; real-time application
Myocardial enzymes	
Creatine kinase	Nonspecific
CK-MB	Standard diagnostic and enzyme-sizing tool
Troponin T	Very sensitive; not validated as measure of infarct size; detects unstable artery
HBDH	Of historical interest only

in the early phases of infarction is only a "snapshot" and that many episodes of opening and closing of the artery can occur. Because it is simply not feasible to perform serial coronary angiography multiple times during the early phase of MI, less expensive, less invasive, and less risky methods of following coronary perfusion are essential.

The ECG provides the opportunity to estimate coronary perfusion repeatedly during the clinical course. The simplest clinical approach, the routine static 12-lead ECG, has been demonstrated to be a marker of coronary perfusion when repeated within the first 60 to 90 minutes of reperfusion therapy.[36] Various studies have found different thresholds for best distinguishing levels of perfusion measured angiographically, so the exact ECG criteria for distinguishing the level at the bedside remains somewhat arbitrary. In general, however, failure to achieve a 50% reduction in the level of the ST segment in the first 90 minutes after initiation of therapy in the lead with the most elevation has been associated with a doubling of mortality as well as a substantial increase in heart failure[37] and a lower rate of angiographic reperfusion.[38]

Continuous electrocardiography is discussed in Chapter 37. The ability to measure time until reperfusion and to characterize multiple episodes of reperfusion and reocclusion makes this technique particularly attractive for pilot studies. Currently, continuous information can be garnered using standard Holter monitoring, continuous QRS vector monitoring, or continuous ST-segment monitoring. All three of these technologies have been validated in terms of a general relationship to reperfusion.[39-41] Comparative information is not available to allow a definitive assessment of which technology is superior.

The complexity of the information derived from continuous ECG monitoring points out the potential complexity of endpoint measurement. A pattern of intermittent reperfusion and reocclusion is often seen with as many as 5 to 10 cycles of reperfusion in the first 90 minutes after thrombolytic treatment is started. Although the simpler static ECG measure may be quite misleading compared with continuous ECG monitoring in the individual patient, in populations of patients the simple comparison at one point in time may be equally beneficial in terms of comparing one treatment with another. Ongoing research in this area should clarify the relative advantages and disadvantages of static and continuous ECG monitoring.

Myocardial enzymes

As the myocardium necroses, a variety of enzymes are released into the systemic circulation. The use of these enzymes to measure the perfusion of the myocardium is discussed in Chapter 37. Additionally, however, cardiac enzymes can estimate the amount of damage to the myocardium. Table 14-4 describes the properties of these enzymes.

In the United States total creatine kinase (CK) and CK-MB isoforms are routinely measured in patients with acute ischemic syndromes. CK-MB is specific to the myocardium and is released into the serum proportional to the amount of myocardial necrosis, although the presence and rate of reperfusion of the portion of the infarcted heart (greater proportional release with right ventricular infarction) have an impact on the peak CK-MB and the area under the curve of activity. A number of studies, both in the thrombolytic era[42] and before the thrombolytic era,[43,44] have demonstrated a significant relationship between various measures of CK-MB and clinical outcomes including mortality, left ventricular function, and clinical manifestations of congestive heart failure. Most recently, it was demonstrated that the accelerated t-PA arm of GUSTO-I was associated with decreases in area under the curve for both CK-MB and HBDH. Several isoforms of CK-MB are measurable; although these isoforms may be useful for assessing reperfusion, they are unlikely to be useful as a measure of infarct size.

Myoglobin is a nonspecific marker of muscle injury that has a low molecular weight and thus diffuses into the circulation quickly after myocardial damage.[45] Although it is perhaps the most effective early marker of myocardial damage and may have a role in assessing reperfusion, it has not been useful as a measure of infarct size.

HBDH, which is a measure of the action of lactate

Table 14-4. Plasma markers of myocardial necrosis

Constituent	Molecular weight (Da)	Cardiospecific	Commercial rapid assay*
Myoglobin	17,800	No	Yes
Total creatine kinase	85,000	No	No
Creatine kinase-MM subforms	85,000	No	No
Creatine kinase-MB	85,000	Yes	Yes
Creatine kinase-MB subforms	85,000	Yes	No
Troponin T	37,000	Yes	No
Myosin light chains	26,000	Yes	No

*Assay time < 20 minutes.

Table 14-5. Clinical endpoints

	Commonly observed rate	Sample size per group for 25% reduction	
		80% power	90% power
Death (30 days)	5%-10%	4341-2075	5758-2751
Re(infarction)	2%-6%	11,139-3586	14,778-4756
Stroke	0.1%-1.0%	153,600-22,470	203,400-29,813
Congestive heart failure	10%-20%	2075-942	2751-1248
Recurrent ischemia	10%-25%	2075-715	2751-947

dehydrogenase (LD) on α-ketobutyrate, has been used as a measure of myocardial infarct size. Now that LD can be measured accurately, its isoforms provide information about myocardial necrosis. The heart contains predominately LD1, although some LD2 is also contained. For diagnosis the ratio of LD1 to LD2 has been used, although this use is likely to be supplanted by Troponin T measurement. In general, the larger the infarction the more HBDH or LD1 will be released into the circulation.[46] This measure is mostly of historical interest now that CK-MB assays with much more specificity are available.

Troponin T is a component of the myocardial contractile apparatus that regulates the contractile process. Because cardiac Troponin T is relatively easily distinguishable from skeletal muscle isoforms, normal individuals have undetectable serum levels. Accordingly, Troponin T is an extremely sensitive marker for myocardial cell injury. Because of a relatively long half-life, it may be quite useful as a diagnostic test for patients reporting late with MI. However, fascinating data in patients with chest pain have demonstrated that Troponin T is a strong predictor of negative outcomes in patients with absent or low levels of CK-MB. Although the mechanism for this prognostic stratification remains unclear pending further research, it is likely that elevated Troponin T levels in patients with normal CK-MB represent unstable lesions creating "infarctlets" downstream as the result of platelet or platelet/fibrin emboli. It is critical in designing a clinical trial to

separate this type of prognostic marker from an enzyme marker of MI size. Low-level Troponin T may be an excellent surrogate marker to evaluate interventions designed to prevent acute events, whereas the area under the curve or peak enzyme level provides an estimate of MI size for interventions designed to provide or enhance reperfusion.

CLINICAL COMPLICATIONS (TABLE 14-5)

A variety of clinical endpoints can be measured with considerable frequency in patients with AMI. Both our group[23] and the TIMI group[47] have posited that combining clinical endpoints in a small trial into a composite measure can provide insight concerning the likely overall clinical benefit of a therapy. This concept is based on the belief that therapies with higher rates of early reperfusion and better left ventricular function will not only reduce mortality but also lower the risk of adverse nonfatal outcomes. In this sense clinical endpoints can be used as a "surrogate" for mortality. Extensive experience with surrogate endpoints in other aspects of cardiology has produced healthy skepticism about accepting anything short of mortality as definitive evidence that a therapy should be used in routine practice in a disease with the mortality rate of AMI.

Another consideration, however, is the use of nonfatal endpoints as simply another outcome measure, particularly for therapies unlikely to have a major impact on survival. Given two therapies with similar effects on survival, the preferred therapeutic approach would be

Table 14-6. Results of a survey of 407 cardiologists at the 1989 meetings of the American Heart Association

Outcome	Score*			Rank†		
	(25	50 (N = 407)	75)‡	(25	50 (N = 407)	75)‡
Death	10	10	10	1	1	1
Intracranial hemorrhage	9	9	10	1	2	2
Nonhemorrhagic stroke	7	8	9	2	4	7
Ejection fraction < 30%	7	8	9	3	4	7
Reinfarction	7	8	8	3	5	6
Heart failure	5	7	8	4	6	9
Pulmonary edema	5	7	8	4	6	9
Cardiac arrest	3	6	8	3	8	14
Emergency bypass surgery	5	6	8	4	7	11
Ischemia with electro-cardiographic changes (no reinfarction)	4	6	7	5	8	11
Reocclusion	4	6	7	7	9	12
Other						
Emergency PTCA	3	5	6	8	12	14
Ejection fraction < 45%	4	5	7	7	10	3
Ischemia without ST segment changes	3	5	6	9	11	14
Nonemergency CABG	3	5	6	7	11	13
Transfusion requirement	2	3	5	11	14	16

PTCA, percutaneous transluminal coronary artery angioplasty; CABG, coronary artery bypass graft surgery.
*Based on a score of 0-10, with 10 being the worst outcome.
†Based on assigning a rank of 1 to the outcome scored the highest (worst).
‡(25 50 75), 25% quartile, median, 75% quartile.
(From Califf RM, Harrelson-Woodlief L, Topol EJ: Left ventricular ejection fraction may not be useful as an end point of thrombolytic therapy comparative trials, *Circulation* 82:1847-1853, 1990.)

the one associated with less stroke, heart failure, or recurrent ischemia, especially if the cost was not different. This use of clinical events as an ancillary endpoint is a fundamentally different concept from the surrogate endpoint strategy. Table 14-6 demonstrates the approach we have taken to the development of a composite endpoint for AMI compared with the approach advocated by Braunwald (Table 14-7).

The interpretation of composite endpoints has been the subject of considerable discussion. Our view is that a prespecified composite can provide an excellent basis for interpretation of small or intermediate-size studies. The composite must always be judged as a whole first; then each component of the composite should be evaluated individually to determine whether the apparent treatment effect is uniform across different endpoints. A sense of how to evaluate a composite endpoint is given in Figure 14-5. First, the concordance of the point estimates and confidence limits can be assessed by visual inspection. If the point estimates are discordant and not much overlap exists between the confidence intervals (example A), the elements of the composite endpoint must be regarded with care in terms of a uniform interpretation. Secondly, a formal test for

heterogeneity can be done just as in metaanalysis, but these tests must be interpreted with caution because they are generally considered to be underpowered. When a study is sized to have power to detect a significant difference in a composite endpoint, enough power will not be present to evaluate each component statistically. However, by assessing an odds ratio plot a sense of the concordance of the composite can be gained.

An especially appealing composite endpoint is the occurrence of either death or (re)infarction. Both these endpoints can be measured objectively and carry consequences for the patient that cannot be disputed.

SURVIVAL

Survival is the most easily measured and universally agreed-upon endpoint in clinical trials evaluating therapy for AMI. In almost every circumstance individual patients, society, and physicians would see prolonged survival as advantageous. For this reason most investigators would agree that, if possible, new therapeutic advances should be evaluated in terms of their effect on survival. Several critical issues prevent this endpoint from being as simple as we would hope.

Table 14-7. Weighted unsatisfactory-outcome end points

Event	Score
Death	1.0
Intracranial hemorrhage with severe permanent neurologic deficit	1.0
Development of severe, sustained CHF or cardiogenic shock	0.8
Ejection fraction < 40% (or < 30% for second MI)	0.6
Reinfarction	0.5
Occlusion or reocclusion of the IRA 1-7 days after AMI	0.4
Major spontaneous hemorrhage; hematocrit drop > 15% or intracranial hemorrhage without severe or permanent neurologic deficit	0.3
Failure of early recanalization of IRA up to 2 hours after onset of therapy	0.2
None of the above	0

CHF, severe congestive heart failure; IRA, infarct-related artery.
(Reprinted with permission from Braunwald E, Cannon CP, McCabe CH: An approach to evaluating thrombolytic therapy in acute myocardial infarction: the "unsatisfactory-outcome" end point, *Circulation* 86:683-687, 1992.)

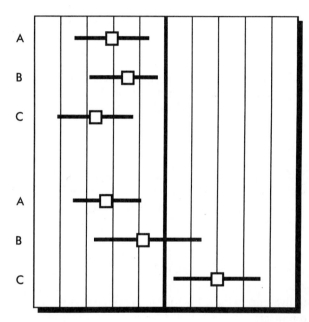

Fig. 14-5. This figure demonstrates a qualitative method for estimating whether a treatment effect is homogeneous. In example A although the point estimate of the treatment benefit is somewhat variable from subgroup to subgroup, the confidence intervals overlap, indicating that the best assumption is that the treatment effect is similar in all subgroups. In example B the confidence intervals do not overlap, indicating that a true qualitative treatment interaction may be present. A treatment interaction indicates that the effect of treatment is significantly different in one group versus another. This type of differential treatment effect is tested through formal statistical tests for interaction.

Clinicians inevitably seem drawn to the concept of measuring *disease-specific* mortality as the primary endpoint of a mortality trial. The general reasoning is that one should measure the outcome that the treatment is purported to ameliorate. One would not expect a

thrombolytic agent, for example, to reduce the risk of death from noncardiac causes. Unfortunately, several key issues provide a strong rationale for using *all-cause* mortality if the goal of the trial is to determine whether a therapy should be recommended in clinical practice. Therapies often have unintended effects on other organ systems that can lead to beneficial or detrimental effects on survival; the effect of thrombolytic agents on stroke, especially intracranial hemorrhage, is a classic example of this problem. In addition, separating cardiovascular from noncardiovascular causes of death can be difficult. In our current medical care system many deaths occur after prolonged hospitalization with multiple complications, leading to difficulty in isolating the proximate cause of death. Furthermore, unobserved deaths are very difficult to classify.

One additional issue that is often underappreciated in cardiovascular trials is the length of follow-up required to demonstrate the effect of revascularization procedures on survival. As shown in Figure 14-6, even in groups of patients with a documented benefit of bypass surgery the survival curves do not cross until 6 to 18 months after the procedure.[48] Therefore, a minimum of 1 year would be needed to demonstrate an effect of revascularization when it is associated with a significant procedural complication rate.

In the field of AMI trials studies may be sized for one of two objectives. Obviously in many situations the goal is to demonstrate a survival advantage. Our approach to this goal is to convene a group of practitioners to assess the magnitude of advantage that would be beneficial and worthwhile from the perspective of potential cost and difficulty in application of the therapy. In the GUSTO-I trial it was determined that a difference in absolute mortality of 1% or relative mortality of 15% would be worthwhile (Table 14-8). One can readily see the large number of patients required in mortality trials to

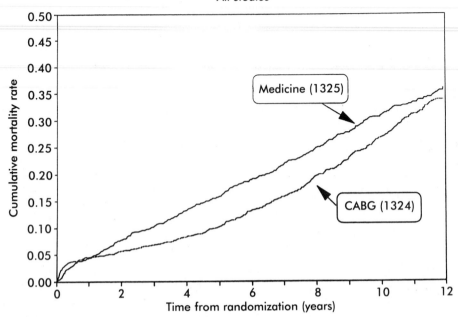

Fig. 14-6. Overall mortality up to 12 years from randomization from six trials that randomized patients with stable coronary artery disease to CABG or medical treatment. (From Yusuf S, Zucker D, Peduzzi P, et al. for the Coronary Artery Bypass Graft Surgery Trialists Collaboration: Overview of 10-year results from the randomized trials, 1993.)

Table 14-8. Sample sizes for mortality trial

Mortality rates		Sample size per group	
Control group	Treated group	80% power	90% power
10%	9%	13,687	18,225
	7%	1413	1869
	5%	464	608
7.5%	6.5%	10,406	13,863
	5%	1537	2031
5%	4%	6925	9203
	2.5%	962	1261

demonstrate expected benefits of particular interventions.

As therapies to improve quality of life or to provide a less expensive alternative are developed, more studies will be designed to demonstrate "equivalence," which is defined as proof that the new treatment is not inferior to the old treatment. In this type of endpoint one must avoid the trap of doing a small study, finding no significant difference, and concluding that the treatments are equivalent. Such a conclusion would be incorrect because of the Type II error. The proper design of such a trial would again involve reaching a consensus about the magnitude of difference that could be tolerated before calling a treatment equivalent. In the

Bypass Angioplasty Revascularization Investigation it was presumed that clinicians and patients would be satisfied if angioplasty was associated with a 5-year mortality rate within 2% of that for surgery on an absolute scale. In the field of thrombolytic therapy one can expect a 6% to 8% 30-day mortality in typical patients entered into clinical trials. Table 14-9 demonstrates sample size calculations needed to demonstrate equivalence within 1% to 2%; the large sample sizes are apparent.

(Re)infarction

One of the primary goals in a patient identified with an unstable ischemic syndrome is to prevent infarction in the case of unstable angina or to prevent reinfarction in the case of AMI. Reinfarction within the first 30 days after the index event is caused in general by recurrent occlusive thrombus at the site of the culprit lesion. Measurement of (re)infarction can be complex, especially in systems with a high rate of coronary intervention; the procedures themselves are frequently associated with small amounts of myocardial necrosis that do not have the same significance as *de novo* events. Increasingly sensitive enzyme tests have also contributed to difficulty in distinguishing artifact from a significant episode of myocardial necrosis with long-term consequences for the patient.

Table 14-9. Sample sizes for "equivalence"

Control mortality rate	Difference to be excluded	Total sample size	
		80% power	90% power
10%	1%	29,887	39,876
	2%	7868	10,466
7.5%	0.5%	90,560	120,960
	1%	23,484	31,304
	2%	6283	8345
5%	0.5%	63,233	84,381
	1%	16,684	22,200
	2%	4596	6085

For first infarction general agreement can be reached that elevation of the MB isoenzyme of creatine kinase above the upper limit of normal constitutes an event. Even this relatively simple construct can be complicated by the fact that different hospitals have different enzyme assays with different test operating characteristics. Using a core laboratory in a small study can obviate this problem, but the expense in a large study is generally prohibitive.

The detection of reinfarction is much more complex. If it is documented that the enzyme values have returned to normal, then reelevation as discussed for first infarction is an acceptable endpoint. However, if the enzymes become reelevated before returning to the normal range, there is no commonly accepted standard threshold for a binary cutoff for reinfarction. Based on expert consensus we have adopted the following standard: for a patient with MI at the time of enrollment and an initially elevated CK-MB, at least a doubling of the trough value is required to classify the event as a reinfarction.

A particularly thorny problem occurs in studies of unstable ischemic syndromes in which the patient is admitted and randomized into the study and then the enzymes turn positive 8 hours later. Was this an event after randomization or did the enzymes become positive as a manifestation of an event that occurred before randomization? Given the fact that in the absence of reperfusion appearance of CK-MB can be delayed for as long as 12 to 16 hours,[49] we have adopted the following convention: in order to determine whether the patient was indeed having an MI at the time of enrollment in an acute trial we have adopted the convention that an elevated CK-MB at baseline or 8 hours after enrollment will always be considered an entry MI. If the CK-MB first becomes elevated at 16 hours, it is classified as an entry MI if no signs or symptoms of reinfarction have occurred between hospital admission and the 16-hour sample.

There is unanimous agreement that the development of new .03- to .04-second Q waves heralds a new MI; this criterion should override all enzyme criteria.

There are many problems associated with data acquisition in assessing (re)infarction. Often enzyme samples are not drawn or fall prey to technical difficulties. Some patients with obvious clinical reinfarction die before enzymes can be drawn. No matter how carefully sampling times are constructed, clinical difficulties will lead to delays or other problems in timing.

Major complexities in classification are encountered when a patient undergoes myocardial revascularization. Some elevation of CK-MB occurs in 5% to 20% of patients undergoing percutaneous procedures, depending upon the procedure and the operator. Most of these cases have an enzyme rise of less than twice the upper limit of normal, which seems to have no measurable impact on left ventricular function or clinical course. In many of these situations the enzyme rise is secondary to transient coronary occlusion during the case, with eventual opening of the vessel and no significant residual stenosis. Because it is apparent that these events do not carry the same clinical significance as an enzyme elevation in a patient without coronary intervention, we have arbitrarily selected a threefold increase in CK-MB to designate a clinical event. Because enzyme elevation of any kind is clearly undesirable during a cardiac procedure, it remains important to record and report all enzyme elevations in clinical studies.

Coronary artery bypass grafting creates an elevation of CK-MB in almost every patient. In order to signify a significant clinical event the general convention is to require a new Q wave on the ECG, realizing that this measure will miss a modest number of MIs. Furthermore, the common occurrence of conduction disturbances in the perioperative period as the result of cardioplegia[50] makes new Q waves less specific than they are in the nonoperative setting.

In our opinion the decision about whether a patient has had a (re)infarction will inevitably require some clinical judgment. Therefore our policy is to establish a set of detailed guidelines for classification of potential nonfatal infarctions, and then to use a committee blinded to treatment to make the final determination. This process allows for an unbiased assessment that can be replicated by other studies evaluating the same or similar therapies.

Heart failure

Congestive heart failure is an excellent target for therapies of AMI. It occurs in 15% to 30% of patients and accounts for substantial morbidity, cost, and mortality. However, the accurate measurement of congestive heart failure is difficult. Patients are frequently recumbent and develop rales caused by atelectasis, making the chest examination an invalid measure. Blood pressure can drop for a variety of reasons in addition to heart failure. The chest x-ray can develop an interstitial pattern for a variety of reasons besides heart failure. Hemodynamic monitoring is not done often enough to make it an inclusive measure. In short, every clinician feels that he or she knows heart failure when it occurs, yet quantitative clinical measurements are difficult.

Our approach to this problem has been to require concordance of several measurements to justify the classification scheme, in particular the presence of alveolar or interstitial edema on the chest roentgenogram. In the GUSTO-II direct angioplasty substudy heart failure is defined as either of the following occurring after 72 hours: (1) pulmonary edema on chest x-ray in the absence of high suspicion for noncardiac origin or (2) at least two of the following: (a) rales greater than one third of the way up the lungfields believed to be caused by pulmonary edema; (b) pulmonary capillary wedge pressure > 18 mm Hg with cardiac index < 2.4 L/min/m^2; (c) dyspnea, with documented pO$_2$ < 80 mm Hg or O$_2$ saturation < 90%, without known preexisting lung disease; (d) use of furosemide to treat presumed pulmonary congestion in a patient not previously treated with furosemide.

Recurrent ischemia

Perhaps more than any other endpoint the measurement of recurrent ischemia is dependent upon the intensity of surveillance. Patients in the early postinfarction period have a variety of symptoms and electrocardiographic changes that could be diagnosed as recurrent ischemia. For clinically relevant endpoints we generally require both symptoms and electrocardiographic changes. As shown in Table 14-10, associated electrocardiographic and physical findings can provide powerful prognostic information. One must be careful, however, depending on the proposed mechanism of the therapy being evaluated. Therapies resulting in a higher early rate of reperfusion could easily increase the rate of symptomatic recurrent ischemia, because earlier, sustained opening would leave more vessels capable of reoccluding in a setting in which the downstream myocardium would be viable. If this occurred the increase in recurrent ischemia may be easier to detect with a small sample size than the decrease in mortality caused by the same therapy, because of a higher rate of perfused myocardium.

Stroke

Stroke is a more difficult clinical endpoint to define than most physicians appreciate, particularly in large simple trials. Experience in GUSTO-I demonstrated that 90% of 650 patients who were suspected of having a stroke were eventually proven to have had one but that the classification of type of stroke is difficult based on timing and clinical characteristics. For example, although strokes during the first day after thrombolysis are

Table 14-10. Recurrent ischemia

	Recurrent ischemia and MI	Recurrent ischemia only	Neither
Age (median)	61	60	57
Male gender	58%	74%	80%
Heart rate	80	75	76
Blood pressure	130	130	130
Anterior location	45%	48%	42%
Multivessel disease	50%	48%	46%
Ejection fraction	52%	51%	51%
Death*	23%	11%	4%
Heart failure†	48%	31%	17%
ICU stay (days)	6	4	3
Hospital stay (days)	14	10	9
Charges	$24,690	$23,609	$19,721

*$P < 0.0001$ (2 df)
†$P < 0.0001$ (2 df)

Table 14-11. Stroke disability

Clinical classification	N	Time trade-off
None	15/21	0.92 ± 0.17
Mild disability	60/80	0.89 ± 0.15
Moderate disability	32/67	0.81 ± 0.24
Severe disability	7/51	0.71 ± 0.31

generally believed to be hemorrhagic, in GUSTO-I 34% were nonhemorrhagic. For this reason we strongly recommend the mandatory use of brain imaging, either computed tomography or magnetic resonance imaging, and review by an independent committee when definitive clinical trials are done.

Although many healthy people would consider a stroke after MI to be worse than death, when interviewed directly patients with stroke estimated the value of their living as much closer to normal than to death. The critical issue is the degree of disability after recuperation from the stroke. Degrees of disability after hemorrhagic and nonhemorrhagic stroke are outlined in Table 14-11. We therefore recommend the use of disabling stroke as the critical endpoint in clinical trials, irrespective of the mechanism.

Bleeding

Everyone recognizes the importance of measuring bleeding complications in the assessment of acute reperfusion strategies, yet the actual measurement is fraught with subjectivity and variability (Table 14-12). When bleeding occurs, the quantification of the amount of bleeding by the appearance of the patient is notoriously unreliable. Human tissues can hide large amounts

Table 14-12. Bleeding measures

Measure	Comment
Nadir hematocrit/hemoglobin	Dependent on transfusion threshold
Drop in hematocrit/hemoglobin	Dependent on transfusion threshold
Units of red blood cells transfused	Dependent on transfusion threshold
Hematoma size	Subjective; no observer variability studies
Landefeld index (ΔHct/3 + units transfused)	Best overall measure of blood loss
TIMI criteria	
Major	Can be altered by different transfusion threshold
Minor	Includes wide spectrum of bleeding severity
TAMI criteria	
Mild	Very subjective
Moderate	Difficult to distinguish from mild
Severe	Objective; clearly demarcates serious bleeding
GUSTO-I criteria	
Mild	Includes spectrum of bleeding
Moderate	Subjective, dependent on transfusion threshold
Severe	Objective; clear

Table 14-13. Risk of viral transmission in blood products

	New infections per unit transfused	Percent infection per unit
HIV	1/225,000	.004
HTLV-I/II	1/60,000	.0016
Hepatitis B	1/200,000	.0005
Hepatitis C	1/3300	.03
Syphilis	Unknown	Unknown

of blood, making hematoma size estimation treacherous. Because of different thresholds for transfusion, driven by the clinical appearance of the patient and physician variability, using transfusion as an endpoint is dependent on subjective factors that do not directly reflect loss of blood. Nevertheless, blood transfusion has become a major concern of the patient. Table 14-13 depicts the estimated risk of transmission of viral infections in blood transfusions, so that ignoring this endpoint is not satisfactory for assessment of clinical value. Nadir hematocrit and change in hematocrit as endpoints are similarly unstable as true estimates of bleeding.

We have found the bleeding index as developed by Landefeld to be the best overall measure of bleeding because it reflects both the drop in hematocrit and the use of transfusions. This index includes the number of units of blood transfused plus the drop in hematocrit from admission to nadir divided by 3. The continuous number reflecting a clinical estimate of the number of units of blood lost has excellent properties for comparing therapies and covers the subjective determinations of when to transfuse.

Because of the complexity of bleeding measurements,

several study groups have developed criteria to categorize bleeding as mild, moderate, or severe. The TIMI study group[3] defined severe bleeding as intracranial or associated with a drop in the hemoglobin level of more than 5 grams. Moderate bleeding was defined as a 3-gram drop in hemoglobin requiring a transfusion; minor bleeding was classified as spontaneous blood loss observed as gross hematuria or hematemesis or a decrease in hemoglobin of more than 4 g/dL with no bleeding site identified. The TAMI study group[2] defined severe bleeding as intracranial or associated with sustained hemodynamic compromise. Moderate bleeding was defined as any other bleeding requiring transfusion, and mild bleeding was all other clinically identified bleeding. The GUSTO-I bleeding criteria defined severe bleeding as an intracranial bleed or bleeding causing hemodynamic compromise and requiring intervention, moderate bleeding as that requiring transfusion but not leading to hemodynamic compromise, and mild bleeding as bleeding not requiring transfusion and not leading to hemodynamic compromise.

Regardless of the primary measure for a clinical trial we have found that to develop a good understanding of the overall impact of a therapy on bleeding, multiple aspects of bleeding risk must be identified and evaluated. When consistency is observed across multiple measurements, great assurance can be expected that the result is durable. However, when an effect is seen with regard to one parameter of bleeding, such as "major bleed," but not in another such as "transfusion," one must be concerned that the result is caused by the subjective nature of the endpoint.

This review underscores the diversity of endpoints that could be designated in trials involving therapy for acute myocardial ischemia. The specific endpoints for a trial should be chosen only after considering the likely mechanism of action of the proposed treatment, the goal of the particular trial, and the resources available to ensure adequate data acquisition. In general we believe that early Phase II trials should focus on pathophysiologic mechanisms while observing clinical endpoints to guide future decisions. For a disease as epidemic as acute ischemic heart disease, any trial designed to determine whether a new therapy should be used in practice must include enough patients to allow clear measurement of the impact of the treatment on mortality, (re)infarction, and other relevant clinical endpoints.

REFERENCES

1. Hogg KJ, Gemmill JD, Burns JM, et al: Angiographic patency study of anistreplase versus streptokinase in acute myocardial infarction, *Lancet* 335:254-258, 1990.
2. Califf RM, Topol EJ, George BS, et al: Hemorrhagic complications associated with the use of intravenous tissue plasminogen activator in treatment of acute myocardial infarction, *Am J Med* 85:353-359, 1988.
3. Rao AK, Pratt C, Berke A, et al, for the TIMI Investigators: Thrombolysis in Myocardial Infarction (TIMI) trial -- Phase 1: Hemorrhagic manifestations and changes in plasma fibrinogen and the fibrinolytic system in patients treated with recombinant tissue plasminogen activator and streptokinase, *J Am Coll Cardiol* 11:1-11, 1988.
4. Sane DC, Califf RM, Sigmon KN, et al: Effect of heparin administration on fibrinogenolysis during thrombolytic therapy with tissue plasminogen activator for acute myocardial infarction, *Fibrinolysis* 7:103-107, 1993.
5. Eisenberg PR: Role of new anticoagulants as adjunctive therapy during thrombolysis, *Am J Cardiol* 67:19A-24A, 1991.
6. Eisenberg PR, Sobel BE, Jaffe AS: Activation of prothrombin accompanying thrombolysis with recombinant tissue-type plasminogen activator, *J Am Coll Cardiol* 19:1065-1069, 1992.
7. Heras M, Chesebro JH, Webster MW, et al: Hirudin, heparin, and placebo during deep arterial injury in the pig; the in vivo role of thrombin in platelet-mediated thrombosis, *Circulation* 82(4):1476-1484, 1990.
8. The EPIC Investigators: Use of a monoclonal antibody directed against the platelet glycoprotein IIb/IIIa receptor in high-risk coronary angioplasty, *New Engl J Med* 330:956-961, 1994.
9. Gimple LW, Gold HK, Leinbach RC, et al: Correlation between template bleeding times and spontaneous bleeding during treatment of acute myocardial infarction with recombinant tissue-type plasminogen activator, *Circulation* 80:581-588, 1989.
10. Chesebro JH, Knatterud G, Roberts R, et al: Thrombolysis in Myocardial Infarction (TIMI) Trial, Phase I: A comparison between intravenous tissue plasminogen activator and intravenous streptokinase, *Circulation* 76:142-154, 1987.
11. GISSI-2 (Gruppo Italiano per lo Studio della Sopravvivenza nell'Infarto Miocardico): GISSI-2: a factorial randomised trial of alteplase versus streptokinase and heparin versus no heparin among 12,490 patients with acute myocardial infarction, *Lancet* 336:65-71, 1990.
12. ISIS-3 Collaborative Group: ISIS-3: a randomised comparison of streptokinase vs tissue plasminogen activator vs anistreplase and of aspirin plus heparin vs aspirin alone among 41,299 cases of suspected acute myocardial infarction. ISIS-3 (Third International Study of Infarct Survival) Collaborative Group, *Lancet* 339:753-770, 1992.
13. Ohman EM, Califf RM, George BS, et al: The use of intraaortic balloon pumping as an adjunct to reperfusion therapy in acute myocardial infarction. The Thrombolysis and Angioplasty in Myocardial Infarction (TAMI) Study Group, *Am Heart J* 121:895-901, 1991.
14. The GUSTO Investigators: An international randomized trial comparing four thrombolytic strategies for acute myocardial infarction, *New Engl J Med* 329:673-682, 1993.
15. Karagounis L, Sorensen SG, Menlove RL, et al: Does thrombolysis in myocardial infarction (TIMI) perfusion grade 2 represent a mostly patent artery or a mostly occluded artery? Enzymatic and electrocardiographic evidence from the TEAM-2 study, *J Am Coll Cardiol* 19:1-10, 1992.
16. Anderson JL, Karagounis LA, Becker LC, et al for the TEAM-3 investigators: TIMI perfusion grade 3 but not grade 2 results in improved outcome after thrombolysis for myocardial infarction: ventriculographic, enzymatic, and electrocardiographic evidence from the TEAM-3 study, *Circulation* 87:1829-1839, 1994.
17. Lincoff M, Califf RM, Ellis SG, et al for the Thrombolysis and Angioplasty in Myocardial Infarction Study Group: Thrombolytic therapy for women with myocardial infarction: is there a gender gap? *J Am Coll Cardiol* 22:1780-1787, 1993.
18. Nissen SE, Gurley JC, Grimes C, et al: Observer variability in TIMI flow grading: comparison to a new computer method for measurement of reperfusion kinetics (abstract), *J Am Coll Cardiol* 13:91A, 1989.
19. Sabia PJ, Powers ER, Ragosta M, et al: An association between collateral blood flow and myocardial viability in patients with recent myocardial infarction, *New Engl J Med* 327:1825-1831, 1992.
20. Ito H, Tomooka T, Sakai N, et al: Lack of myocardial perfusion immediately after successful thrombolysis: a predictor of poor recovery of left ventricular function in anterior myocardial infarction, *Circulation* 85:1699-1705, 1992.
21. Multicenter Post-Infarction Research Group: Risk stratification and survival after myocardial infarction, *New Engl J Med* 309:321-336, 1983.
22. Granger CB, Califf RM, Topol EJ: Thrombolytic therapy for acute myocardial infarction: a review, *Drugs* 44:293-325, 1992.
23. Califf RM, Harrelson-Woodlief L, Topol EJ: Left ventricular ejection fraction may not be useful as an end point of thrombolytic therapy comparative trials, *Circulation* 82:1847-1853, 1990.
24. Van de Werf F: Discrepancies between the effects of coronary reperfusion on survival and left ventricular function, *Lancet* 1:1367-1369, 1989.
25. Sheehan FH, Bolson EL, Dodge HT, et al: Advantages and applications of the centerline method for characterizing regional ventricular function, *Circulation* 74:293-305, 1986.
26. White HD, Cross DB, Elliott JM, et al: Long-term prognostic importance of patency of the infarct-related coronary artery after thrombolytic therapy for acute myocardial infarction, *Circulation* 89:61-67, 1994.
27. Lee KL, Pryor DB, Pieper KS, et al: Prognostic value of radionuclide angiography in medically treated patients with coronary artery disease. A comparison with clinical and catheterization variables, *Circulation* 82:1705-1717, 1990.
28. Wackers FJ, Terrin ML, Kayden DS, et al: Quantitative radionuclide assessment of regional ventricular function after thrombolytic therapy for acute myocardial infarction: results of phase I Thrombolysis in Myocardial Infarction (TIMI) trial, *J Am Coll Cardiol* 13:998-1005, 1989.
29. Ohtani H, Callahan RJ, Khaw BA, et al: Comparison of technetium-99-m-glucarate and thallium-201 for the identification of acute myocardial infarction in rats, *J Nucl Med* 33:1988-1993, 1992.
30. Canby RC, Silber S, Pohost GM: Relations of the myocardial imaging agents 99mTc-MIBI and 201T1 to myocardial blood flow

in a canine model of myocardial ischemic insult, *Circulation* 81:289-296, 1990.

31. Gibson RS, Bishop HL, Stamm RB, et al: Value of early two-dimensional echocardiography in patients with acute myocardial infarction, *Am J Cardiol* 49:1110-1119, 1982.

32. Nishimura RA, Tajik AJ, Shub C, et al: Role of two-dimensional echocardiography in the prediction of in-hospital complications after acute myocardial infarction, *J Am Coll Cardiol* 4:1080-1087, 1984.

33. Maggioni AP, Franzosi MG, Santoro E, et al: The risk of stroke in patients with acute myocardial infarction after thrombolytic and antithrombotic treatment. Gruppo Italiano per lo Studio della Sopravvivenza nell'Infarto Miocardico II (GISSI-2), and The International Study Group, *New Engl J Med* 327:1-6, 1992.

34. Gibbons RJ: Technetium 99m sestamibi in the assessment of acute myocardial infarction, *Semin Nucl Med* 21:213-220, 1991.

35. Christian TF, Gibbons RJ: Detection of recanalization with the use of radioisotope techniques, *Cor Art Dis* 3:481-488, 1992.

36. Clemmensen P, Bates ER, Califf RM, et al: Complete atrioventricular block complicating inferior wall acute myocardial infarction treated with reperfusion therapy. TAMI Study Group, *Am J Cardiol* 67:225-230, 1991.

37. Barbash GI, Roth A, Hod H, et al: Rapid resolution of ST elevation and prediction of clinical outcome in patients undergoing thrombolysis with alteplase (recombinant tissue-type plasminogen activator): results of the Israeli Study of Early Intervention in Myocardial Infarction, *Br Heart J* 64:241-247, 1990.

38. Krucoff MW, Croll MA, Pope JE, et al: Continuously updated 12-lead ST-segment recovery analysis for myocardial infarct artery patency assessment and its correlation with multiple simultaneous early angiographic observations, *Am J Cardiol* 71:145-151, 1993.

39. Krucoff MW, Parente AR, Bottner RK, et al: Stability of multilead ST-segment "fingerprints" over time after percutaneous transluminal coronary angioplasty and its usefulness in detecting reocclusion, *Am J Cardiol* 61:1232-1237, 1988.

40. Krucoff MW, Croll MA, Pope JE, et al for the TAMI 7 Study Group: Continuous 12-lead ST segment recovery analysis in the TAMI 7 study: performance of a noninvasive method for real-time detection of failed myocardial reperfusion, *Circulation* 88:437-446, 1993.

41. Dellborg M, Riha M, Swedberg K: Dynamic QRS-complex and ST-segment monitoring in acute myocardial infarction during recombinant tissue-type plasminogen activator therapy. The TEA-HAT Study Group, *Am J Cardiol* 67:343-349, 1991.

42. Gore JM, Roberts R, Ball SP, et al: Peak creatine kinase as a measure of effectiveness of thrombolytic therapy in acute myocardial infarction, *Am J Cardiol* 59:1234-1238, 1987.

43. Sobel BE, Shell WE: Serum enzyme determinations in the diagnosis and assessment of myocardial infarction, *Circulation* 45:471, 1972.

44. Grande P, Hansen BF, Christiansen C, et al: Estimation of acute myocardial infarct size in man by serum CK-MB measurements, *Circulation* 65:756, 1982.

45. Ohman EM, Casey C, Bengtson JR, et al: Early detection of acute myocardial infarction: additional diagnostic information by serum myoglobin in patients without ST elevation, *Br Heart J* 63:335-338, 1990.

46. van der Laarse A, Hermens WT, Hollaar L: Assessment of myocardial damage in patients with acute myocardial infarction by serial measurement of serum a-hydroxybutyrate dehydrogenase levels, *Am Heart J* 107:248-260, 1984.

47. Braunwald E: Myocardial reperfusion, limitation of infarct size, reduction of left ventricular dysfunction, and improved survival: should the paradigm be expanded? *Circulation* 78:441-444, 1989.

48. Yusuf S, Personal communication, December 1, 1993.

49. Irvin RG, Cobb FR, Roe CR: Acute myocardial infarction and MB creatine phosphokinase. Relationship between onset of symptoms of infarction and appearance and disappearance of enzyme, *Arch Int Med* 140:329-334, 1980.

50. Chu A, Califf RM, Pryor DB, et al: Prognostic effect of bundle branch block related to coronary artery bypass grafting, *Am J Cardiol* 59:798-803, 1987.

Chapter 15

ECONOMIC ANALYSIS METHODS AND ENDPOINTS

Daniel B. Mark

Until very recently few physicians knew or thought they had a need to know the cost of the medical care they provided. Such is clearly no longer the case. The era of open-ended reimbursement in medicine is over. In its place we have fixed prospective payments, government-set fee schedules, and various forms of capitation. One of the major results of these ongoing reforms is to shift an increasing amount of the financial risks of health care from payors to providers (hospitals, physicians, managed care organizations). In addition, most of the current proposals for health care reform attempt to define limits for health care spending without providing any guidance about what types of care clinicians should no longer provide. A major assumption of the current health care reform movement is that much of the desired reduction in health care spending can be achieved by reducing all the waste in the medical care system. It is true that medical care is unlikely to be provided in a maximally efficient manner unless there are fairly strong incentives for this to occur; such incentives have been lacking until recently. However, in the discussion about medical "waste," distinctions are often not made between "no yield" medicine and "low yield" medicine. The former represents care that (almost) all practitioners would agree is unnecessary or wasteful; in the latter situation, the appropriateness of care is viewed differently by different practitioners (and patients). At present there are few guidelines to help a clinician negotiate the ever-changing minefield of balancing the medical care needs of their patients with the increased pressures for cost containment.[1]

Clinicians now clearly have a need to be informed about medical economics. If cost containment plans are created without appropriate clinical input the results may be deleterious both to patient care and to future medical progress. If physicians are to be full partners in the health policy debates to come, they must possess at least a basic understanding of the principles of medical economics and the goals of health policy. The purpose of this chapter is to provide a brief introduction to the former; more details can be found elsewhere.[2] Some health policy issues related to acute ischemic heart disease are discussed in Chapter 71, and translation of economic principles into cost containment strategies on the cardiac care unit is described in Chapter 69.

MAJOR COST CONCEPTS
General economic principles

To an economist a "cost" is the consumption of societal resources that have more than one possible use (as almost all resources do). Society consumes resources to satisfy its wants, including those for housing, food, clothing, and recreation, as well as for health care. In the conventional economic view, resources are finite, and because society cannot satisfy all its wants, it must make choices about how its resources will be used.[3,4] The classic example of this is the "guns-versus-butter" tradeoff used in freshman economics: resources applied to the production of weapons cannot also be used to produce food, and in a world of limited resources, more weapons may mean less food. Similarly, more resources devoted to health care may ultimately translate into less societal investment in education, housing, transportation, or other societal priorities. A major goal of health policy and medical economics is to define the proper level of societal investment in health care and the proper distribution of assigned resources among different aspects of health care.[4]

Resources are typically classified into large generic categories, such as labor, supplies, equipment, and land. Through the use of technology these resources can be combined to produce society's desired goods and services, including health care. Because resources come in many different forms, making tradeoffs among alternative uses requires a common means of valuation.[3] In the United States, Canada, and much of Europe resources are allocated using a market system. In this system the market price of a product or service reflects the economic value of the inputs used in producing it. According to the traditional economic model, in each sector of the economy the interplay of supply and demand determines the quantities of goods and services produced and their prices.

Theoretically at least, a perfectly competitive market produces an optimal pattern of resource allocation relative to society's wants. Unfortunately, the medical care marketplace deviates substantially from ideal conditions. For one, medical market prices (also known as *medical charges*) are a grossly distorted measure of medical resource consumption. The reason for the distortion in these prices is complex but derives in large part from the absence of true free-market competition. Until very recently there was little evidence that medical providers competed with each other on the basis of price.[5] (In the last few years health care providers have started competing on price for managed care contracts.[6]) Providers instead have competed by acquiring the latest high-technology items and by improving their facilities; they were able to do this because they were sure they could pass the costs of these enhancements along to consumers without fear that the buyers/consumers of health care would take their business elsewhere.

Economic theory also holds that informed consumers (patients) make rational choices among available alternatives and pay for their choices themselves.[3,7] This is also clearly not the case in the health care arena. Purchasing health care is a much more complicated proposition than purchasing in other sectors of the economy.[8] One does not need to be an auto mechanic or an engineer in order to be able to purchase an automobile intelligently. There is plenty of information available to the interested consumer that compares different automobiles on a variety of characteristics including quality and durability, and the consumer can test-drive the potential purchase before making any binding commitments. Health care is a much more arcane proposition for lay people to master. Compared with other segments of the economy, the field does not tend to lend itself (for a variety of reasons) to a

---

Major components of hospital charges for medical services
1. True costs to hospital of resources consumed (e.g., disposable supplies, personnel, equipment, allocated overhead)
2. Cost-shifting accounting maneuvers   Bad debts   Free services (e.g., indigent care, employees)   Disallowed costs by third-party payers
3. Replacement of existing equipment (depreciation)
4. Acquisition of new technologies (e.g., laser angioplasty, digital angiographic equipment)
5. Budgeting for expansion of services (e.g., more inpatient beds, more outpatient clinics)
Item 1: Cost for given hospital service.
Items 1 to 5: Charge or price for given hospital service.
Although the majority of U.S. hospitals are "nonprofit," items 3 to 5 are analogous to the functions that are served by profit in other sectors of the economy.

(From Mark DB, Jollis J: Economic aspects of therapy for acute myocardial infarction. In Bates ER, (ed): *Adjunctive therapy for acute myocardial infarction,* New York, 1991, Marcel Dekker.)

Consumer Reports type of evaluation nearly as well. And it is rarely possible to "test-drive" a particular health care service before making the final purchase decision. Finally, very few consumers of health care actually pay for the care themselves out of pocket. Most are insulated from at least the majority of the costs of their health care by some form of insurance.[9-11] If patients had to pay completely out of pocket for coronary angioplasty or coronary bypass surgery, for example, it is likely that either the prices (charges) for these services would be dramatically reduced or the consumption of these services would fall substantially below present levels. However, it is true that the demand for health care is unlike the demand for other goods and services in the economy in that failure to obtain appropriate health care may result in disability or even death. Thus, patients may be forced to seek certain kinds of care regardless of the price associated with that care.

In most parts of the economy the price of a product or service is equal to the true cost of producing that item plus some amount of profit. In the medical arena the discrepancy almost universally observed between hospital prices (or charges) and hospital costs (the true cost to the hospital of providing the medical service in question) is largely attributable to a set of accounting practices known as "cost-shifting."[2] These maneuvers are designed to shift costs from a variety of sources (see accompanying box) onto whichever group of payers is most willing and able to absorb them. The bottom-line goal of cost-shifting is to maintain the hospital's financial solvency and to help it meet whatever additional financial goals it has. The net effect of these cost-shifting practices is that the relationship between medical prices or charges and medical resource consumption or cost is distorted substantially. The practical import of all this is that clinicians must be extremely wary of medical charge data used either in analyses of potential cost savings associated with changes in clinical practice or in cost-effectiveness analyses designed to help health policy analysts set societal priorities for health care spending.

Medical cost terminology

To facilitate the analysis of the economic implications of different clinical strategies, medical costs can be subdivided in a number of different ways.[2,12-14] Perhaps the most useful classification is based on the behavior of cost as production of health services increases or decreases. *Variable costs* change with unit changes in service volume. For example, in a cardiac catheterization procedure the catheters, intravenous tubing, contrast dye, and any other disposable supplies used would be variable: the amount of those supplies needed would vary in direct proportion to the number of cases being done over any particular time period. *Fixed costs,* on the other hand, do not change with changes in service volume. For example, the cost of building a new cardiac care unit or interventional catheterization laboratory are fixed because they do not recur with each additional patient cared for.

Another set of terms separates costs into direct and indirect components according to the degree to which the costs can be traced to the production of specific health care services. A *direct cost* can be directly linked to the production of a given product or service. In the cardiac care unit the costs associated with the use of a unit bed ("hotel" costs) as well as the nursing care provided and the drugs administered would all be direct. *Indirect costs,* in contrast, cannot be directly associated with a specific service or product without resorting to some arbitrary assignment method. Depreciation or rent of the hospital building, electricity, laundry, maintenance, hospital administration, and medical records would all constitute indirect costs. The hospital knows the total costs for these items but not the costs for a specific patient. The direct-indirect cost distinction is primarily of importance to accountants and hospital administrators interested in making sure that expenditures and revenues match up in the hospital budget. The distinction can also be important in a cost-finding study that attempts to define in detail all the resources consumed (and their associated costs) in the production of a particular medical service. Related to this, the distinction has also recently become important to clinicians who are under increased pressure from hospital administrators (who are part of the indirect cost) to cut the direct costs associated with patient care. On the other hand, the distinction between variable and

fixed costs is critical to an understanding of the economic concepts of marginal and incremental costs.

Marginal cost analysis is a key concept used by economists to determine the variable costs (or cost savings) of doing one more (or one less) procedure or test.[13,15] For example, moving a patient from an aggressive reperfusion strategy with thrombolytic therapy routinely followed by catheterization at 18 to 48 hours (i.e., the TIMI II intermediate strategy) to a conservative strategy of thrombolytic therapy with catheterization reserved for patients demonstrating recurrent ischemia (i.e., the TIMI II conservative strategy) will save the variable costs of the extra catheterization procedure averted but not the fixed cost each hospital incurs by having a catheterization suite with its specially trained personnel. In many hospitals patient care personnel represent a fixed cost because they are paid to be at work whether there is a sufficient amount for them to do or not. Recently, in response to the increasing pressures for cost control, hospitals have begun to use more flexible staffing patterns and have converted many personnel over to a variable cost category, so that if patient volume is down, unit staffing is reduced proportionally for that particular time period.

The marginal cost of doing one additional procedure such as a coronary angiogram cannot be simply determined from medical bills (hospital and physician). Even if it were an absolutely accurate reflection of true hospital costs rather than the distorted charges as noted earlier, the hospital bill would still provide a measure of average cost rather than marginal cost. The distinction is important because average cost includes not only the marginal or variable components defined earlier, but also the patient's allocated share of fixed costs. These latter costs are not usually saved by changes in medical practice and therefore should not be included in a marginal cost analysis.[16] When large patient volume changes occur, however, even costs previously regarded as fixed may need to be included in the marginal cost analysis. For example, shifting enough CAD patients from CABG to PTCA at a particular medical center will eventually result in the closing of operating rooms and layoffs or reassignment of the associated personnel. Conversely, when the PTCA volume gets high enough, a new PTCA laboratory will need to be constructed and new personnel will need to be hired. In these situations marginal cost includes both fixed and variable components.

The concept of *one more or less* test or procedure is a useful construct in economic analysis, but in clinical practice the more practical question usually relates to the costs of shifting a *group* of patients from one diagnostic or therapeutic strategy to some alternative. In this setting the term *incremental* is often substituted for *marginal.*[15] *Incremental cost analysis* addresses the key question of the amount of savings available or costs added by adopting one clinical strategy over another. However, the methodology for doing such an analysis is relatively complex, and there are very few published examples of a true incremental cost analysis. Thus, despite the caveats just mentioned, most cost analyses in the medical literature use average costs (or average charges).

Medical cost estimation

The method of estimating medical costs we prefer for multicenter cost research uses a data collection system set up by the federal government. In the earlier (pre-prospective payment) era of Medicare, hospital reimbursements were based on the reasonable and necessary costs of providing care to patients in the program. Recognizing that these were not equivalent to hospital charges, Medicare developed an elaborate reporting system that required each hospital to file a cost report with the Health Care Financing Administration (HCFA) each year. This report details how hospital expenses for patient care, overhead, capital equipment, and so forth relate to billed charges. It also provides a set of ratios—the Medicare ratios of cost to charges (RCCs)—that can be used to convert charges to hospital costs. The HCFA also created a billing form, known as the *Uniform Billing Form of 1982 (UB 82)*, that attempted to standardize hospital billing practices. The UB 82 (now the *UB 92*) and the Medicare Cost Report can be used to make a reasonable estimate of hospital costs for any given hospital admission. The advantage of this methodology is that it can be applied to almost every hospital in the United States (excluding the Veterans Administration and military hospitals) and thus is particularly valuable for multicenter cost studies and for comparing costs measured in different hospitals. Some important limitations to this methodology should be kept in mind.[2] First, it provides a measure of average rather than marginal cost as noted previously and thus will typically overestimate potential cost savings to some degree. Second, Medicare cost reports resemble federal income tax forms in that, even within the regulations, there is a lot of room for individual hospitals to interpret the reporting instructions differently.

The degree of inaccuracy in cost estimates created by these deficiencies has not been studied adequately. To attempt to define more clearly the practical import of these distinctions, we recently compared charges for elective PTCA and CABG patients at Duke Hospital with costs calculated using the Medicare cost report and with true marginal cost estimated from pricing out individual resources.[17] In this sample, cost savings calculated using Medicare RCCs were intermediate between true marginal costs plus departmental overhead (true average cost) and charges. In a follow-up analysis

we have found close agreement of Medicare-estimated average costs with true hospital average costs measured using a detailed bottom-up hospital accounting system (Transition System 1).[18]

There are several other options for estimating cost besides the use of hospital billing data.[2] Perhaps the most common is the use of counts of "big-ticket" items (such as number of PTCAs, cardiac catheterizations, bypass surgery, and length of stay in the intensive care unit [ICU] and in the non-ICU hospital bed) and a standardized price list. Total cost is estimated by multiplying prices by quantities and summing. Although this is an attractive and seemingly simple way to get an estimate of cost and has the potential added advantage of eliminating some of the "noise" that exists in real-life billing data that may be extraneous to the inquiry at hand, there are also some important limitations that must be kept in mind. First, creation of the appropriate cost equation requires knowledge of the critical resource unit elements that must be in that equation. This presumes some prior economic evaluation of the clinical scenario under study, but in many cases no prior economic analysis is available and the investigator is left making an educated guess.

Second, in the United States there is no standard "price list" available to be applied in this sort of analysis. It is an oversimplification even to consider that one price will adequately summarize the resource inputs of a given "big-ticket" item. For example, in analyses of the Duke database experience we have found that the costs associated with coronary angioplasty are dependent on the extent of the underlying coronary disease as well as on the type of procedure attempted (simple angioplasty or angioplasty plus another interventional technique such as atherectomy or stent).[19] We have also found in the CAVEAT randomized trial that directional atherectomy was significantly more expensive than coronary angioplasty despite identical lengths of stay in hospital for patients randomized into the two arms of the trial.[20,21] The cost differences were derived from the cumulative effect of a number of smaller-ticket items. In the uncomplicated case, atherectomy was $400 to $500 more expensive than angioplasty because of the increased resource use required for that procedure. However, in higher-risk patients in whom there was an increased incidence of abrupt closure and emergency bypass surgery, there was a complex interplay between patient complications and resource use that accounted for the remaining cost difference seen in the trial. Costing out only big-ticket resources without accounting for the effects of these complications would not provide, at least in this case, an accurate assessment of the true cost difference between the two procedures. On the other hand, costing out resources and complications (e.g., adding extra cost if the patient had a reinfarction or abrupt closure) is problematic because of inability to account for overlap in these two types of cost drivers and therefore the possibility of double-counting of some costs. The "price × quantity" approach to cost estimation is often preferred because it requires less expense in data collection. However, we believe that for U.S. studies it is most appropriate when there have been previous detailed economic analyses that have identified all the important cost drivers and have created the appropriate weighted cost formula for use with price weights. Many economic investigators tend to derive price weights from whatever source is most convenient (such as their own hospital or an available claims database), but there is no guarantee that such price weights may be relevant to the study population at hand, much less be generalizable beyond that study population to the larger population of interest. In most non-U.S. countries there are no billing data available, and therefore this type of analysis is almost the only option for economic analysis. Some countries, such as Australia, have government-established price weights to be used in medical economic analyses.

A third option for cost estimation, at least for hospitalization episodes, is to assign hospitalizations to diagnosis related group (DRG) categories and then use DRG reimbursement rates as the summary price weight.[2] If DRGs did indeed describe homogenous hospitalization episodes this would be a reasonably good method of estimating cost. However, in our experience the DRG system is not nearly sensitive enough to discern important cost differences within DRG categories — that is, the categories are not economically homogenous. Therefore, using DRG cost weights in an economic analysis necessarily restricts the sensitivity of that analysis to the detection of patient shifts from one DRG category to another.

For estimation of physician fees there are two main options.[2] First, physician bills can be collected. However, there are two major problems with this: physician fees are often distorted now because of cost-shifting practices similar to that of hospitals, but there is no charge-to-cost conversion methodology for physician fees; and because many physicians still work in small independent groups, there is no centralized billing authority from which these data can be easily collected. Thus, collecting physician bills is many times more labor-intensive than collecting hospital billing information. The other major option for estimating physician cost is to use an enumeration of physician services along with resource-based relative value (RBRV) price weights.[22] This is essentially what the Medicare fee schedule is supposed to represent. Although there is controversy and continuing argument about the appropriate weights for some services and the conversion factor used to translate the work units of the schedule into dollars paid for individual services, this still probably represents the best available methodology for costing out physician services.

Types of cost analysis

The type of economic analysis most appropriate in a given situation depends on the questions being asked and on the underlying medical relationships. If a new technology or strategy is being compared with an older standard and the new technology is expected to provide additional benefits but at a clearly increased cost, then economic analysis has two parts: measurement of the cost difference as described previously, and cost-effectiveness analysis. If the two technologies compared are (or are believed to be) equivalent in effectiveness, then the principal economic question is which is less expensive — this is ascertained through a cost minimization analysis. In the unusual situation in which a new technology is both more effective and less expensive, economic analysis would consist of demonstrating the cost advantage through the techniques described earlier. It is important to keep in mind that economic analysis should always be done in relation to clinical evaluation of efficacy and effectiveness. A very inexpensive therapy may be judged not worthwhile if its effectiveness is inadequate, whereas a very expensive therapy may be judged as standard of care because it is highly effective.

One of the most commonly misunderstood issues in clinical economics is the role of cost-effectiveness analysis.[23] Many use the term *cost-effectiveness analysis* synonymously with the term *economic analysis,* but this is inaccurate. As noted previously, cost-effectiveness analysis is applicable in the specific situation in which the analyst wishes to determine whether additional medical benefits (improved effectiveness) are worth the additional cost that will be required to obtain them.[15] Cost-effectiveness analysis is a structured method of relating costs and medical effectiveness for the specific purpose of comparing alternative uses of scarce health care and other societal dollars.[13,15,24,25] The principal agenda of a cost-effectiveness analysis is to define the most efficient use of those health care dollars among the possible alternative spending options. Cost-effectiveness analysis therefore is a policy tool rather than a tool for clinical decision-making. Importantly, cost-effectiveness analysis does not indicate whether a particular medical practice is worthwhile; rather, it provides one of several pieces of data upon which such a judgment can be based.

Cost-effectiveness actually refers to a family of techniques for economic analysis.[26] As shown in Table 15-1 the principal result of a cost-effectiveness analysis is a cost-effectiveness ratio. This is simply the ratio of incremental cost, with the new technology being studied over standard therapy related to the corresponding incremental life expectancy. Life expectancy is the most common measure of effectiveness used in cost-effective-

Table 15-1. Cost-effectiveness, cost utility, and cost benefit: examples of calculations

Strategy	Treatment costs	Effectiveness (life expectancy)	Utility (QOL)	QOL-adjusted life expectancy	Benefits*
New technology	$20,000	4.5 years	0.80	3.6 QALYs	$4000
Standard therapy	$10,000	3.5 years	0.90	3.15 QALYs	$2000
Incremental cost-effectiveness ratio	$\dfrac{\$20,000 - \$10,000}{4.5 \text{ years} - 3.5 \text{ years}}$	$10,000 per life year saved			
Incremental cost utility ratio	$\dfrac{\$20,000 - \$10,000}{\$3.6 \text{ QALYs} - 3.15 \text{ QALYs}}$	$22,222 per QALY saved			
Incremental cost benefit ratio	$\dfrac{\$20,000 - \$10,000}{\$4000 - \$2000}$	5			

From Detsky AS, Naglie IG: A clinician's guide to cost-effectiveness analysis, *Ann Intern Med* 113:147-154, 1990.
*Shows health benefits valued in dollars.
Rx = treatment, QOL = quality of life, QALY = quality-adjusted life year.

Table 15-2. League table of cost-effectiveness ratios

New Rx	Comparison Rx	Patients	CE ratio ($)
CABG	Medicine	Left main disease	7000
Medical Rx	No Rx	Severe HBP	20,000
Dialysis	No dialysis	Chronic renal failure	35,000
Medical Rx	No Rx	Moderate HBP	40,000
Cholestyramine	No Rx	Cholesterol > 265 in men 45-60	180,000
Nonionic contrast	Ionic contrast	Low-risk patients	22,000

Data from Goldman L: Cost-effective strategies in cardiology. In Braunwald E, (ed): *Heart disease: a textbook of cardiovascular medicine*, ed 4, Philadelphia, 1992, WB Saunders; and Goel V, Deber RB, Detsky AS: Nonionic contrast media: a bargain for some, a burden for many, *Can Med Assoc J* 143:480-481, 1990.
CABG = coronary bypass surgery; HBP = hypertension; Rx = treatment; CE = cost effectiveness.

ness analysis, although theoretically any measure of effectiveness can be used to generate a ratio.[13] However, because the purpose of generating the cost-effectiveness ratio is to compare with other cost-effectiveness ratios (usually displayed in a so-called *league table* [Table 15-2]) to decide about spending priorities, it is usually necessary to create a ratio that has the same units as those with which it will be compared. In the vast majority of cases these units are dollars per additional life year saved.

In many cases, describing the incremental life expectancy attributable to some new strategy or technology provides an insufficient measure of the new technology's effect on medical outcomes. For this reason many analysts will use a modified form of cost-effectiveness analysis known as *cost utility analysis* (see Table 15-1), in which quality-of-life weights are combined with life expectancy to generate a compound measure of effectiveness, such as the quality-adjusted life year (QALY). The methods for estimating these quality-of-life or utility weights are discussed in the chapter on quality-of-life endpoints. The difference between cost-effectiveness and cost utility analysis is well illustrated in the example shown in Table 15-1. Taking into account only differ-

ences in life expectancy and costs yields a cost-effectiveness ratio of $10,000 per life year saved in the example shown. However, because the new technology results in a somewhat worse quality of life compared with the standard therapy (such as might occur from drug side effects), the benefits expressed in quality-adjusted life years are more modest than those expressed solely in life expectancy terms and the resulting cost utility ratio is $22,000 per quality-adjusted life year saved.

A third form of cost-effectiveness analysis that can be applied to medical problems is *cost benefit analysis*.[25] Many clinicians and others use the terms *cost benefit* and *cost-effectiveness* synonymously, but most economic analysts reserve the term *cost benefit* for the specific situation in which effectiveness or health benefits are valued in dollars. Thus, rather than estimating life expectancy or quality-adjusted life expectancy, cost benefit analysis would require the analyst to convert such measures to their equivalent dollar value. In other words, it requires the analyst to figure out how much a human life is worth in monetary terms. There are several techniques that have been applied for making this assessment.[2] For obvious reasons an analysis that

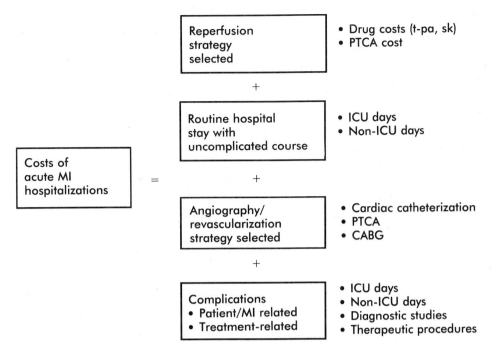

Fig. 15-1. Schematic diagram of the major cost components of a hospitalization for AMI.

requires valuation of human life in monetary terms is substantially more controversial than the other forms of cost-effectiveness analysis, and it is rarely applied in medical economics research. It does have one noteworthy advantage over the other forms of cost-effectiveness analysis described, however, and that is that it is suitable for informing spending decisions across the entire spectrum of societal decision-making rather than being restricted to health care. In other words, cost-effectiveness analysis, which produces a ratio of dollars per life years saved, can be used only to compare alternative expenditures that produce the same outcome. Cost benefit analysis, on the other hand, directly calculates society's gain or loss in terms of dollars invested vs. the monetary value of the return on investment. Thus, comparisons can theoretically be made between medical care expenditures and expenditures on defense, education, transportation, and so forth. There is also a theoretical argument that suggests that cost benefit analysis is a better tool than cost-effectiveness or cost utility analysis for achieving optimal efficiency in resource allocation, but this is primarily of interest to economists.[25]

COST STUDIES OF AMI THERAPIES
General issues

A major objective of an economic analysis for a new drug, device, or strategy is to discover the ways in which this innovation will alter costs relative to conventional or usual care. This in turn requires an in-depth understanding of effects on resource consumption patterns. Conceptually the cost of hospitalization for treatment of

AMI can be decomposed into four major resource/cost components (Fig. 15-1). The cost of the reperfusion strategy consists principally of the cost of the drug administered or the cost of an angioplasty procedure. Standard care in the United States for an AMI patient includes several days in the intensive care unit (the median length of stay in the American/GUSTO-I participants who did not undergo revascularization was 3 days) and some additional days in a non-ICU hospital setting, with a total length of stay typically ranging between 5 and 13 days. In the uncomplicated patient the cost of the revascularization strategy and the hospital stay would be the major components of the cost of the baseline hospitalization. However, there are two other important types of cost drivers that occur in these patients: complications and revascularization procedures. Complications can be of several different types and can have varying cost implications. There can be complications caused by the reperfusion strategy selected. In milder cases, such as minor bleeding, the complication may produce no discernible cost effects. However, major reperfusion-related complications are usually expensive. Thus, a major hemorrhagic event following thrombolytic therapy may necessitate emergency resuscitation with numerous blood products, emergency consultation with other specialists, and emergency diagnostic procedures (e.g., endoscopy, angiography, computed tomographic scanning). Direct PTCA may be complicated by abrupt reclosure necessitating further percutaneous procedures or even coronary bypass surgery. There are also complications resulting from the AMI itself that can have important cost implications. These include hemodynamically significant ventricular tachycardia or ventricular fibrillation, high-grade AV block, pulmonary edema, cardiogenic shock, acute mitral regurgitation, and acute ventricular septal rupture. Such complications may require advanced cardiac life support, intravenous drug therapy, temporary pacing, intubation and mechanical ventilation, placement of an intraaortic balloon pump, or even emergency surgery. Even when the complication does not generate a significant treatment expense, it can increase costs by delaying hospital discharge. Finally, there are complications that are primarily caused by a patient's noncoronary co-morbidity. Thus, severe chronic obstructive lung disease may predispose the AMI patient to a pulmonary infection or even respiratory failure. One of the biggest elements in the cost equation for AMI is the angiography/revascularization strategy selected. Two major alternatives are the aggressive strategy, in which most or all patients undergo angiography and revascularization (PTCA, CABG) and which is applied based on the technical findings at angiography; and the conservative strategy, in which angiography is reserved for complicated or high-risk patients.

As might be expected from these considerations, there is no one dollar figure that represents the cost of AMI. It is no more correct to assign a single figure to the cost of an AMI hospitalization than it is to assign a single mortality rate. It is possible to speak of a representative distribution of the cost for AMI that can be summarized with an average (i.e., mean) or typical (e.g., median) cost. The determinants of the cost of AMI have not been adequately investigated to date, hence it is still uncertain how true cost for this disorder should vary from one patient sample to the next. We have proposed that cost determinants should be analyzed in four major categories: patient-related, treatment-related, provider-related, and geographic–economic-related (see the accompanying box). Patient-related factors act on cost primarily by influencing the complication rates of the underlying disease process and the intensity of care required. For example, all other things being equal, an elderly patient with AMI is more likely to have a complicated course and a prolonged hospital stay than a younger patient. Treatment-related factors are substantial cost drivers because selection of an aggressive invasive strategy will increase costs substantially compared with selection of a conservative strategy. There is also a complex interaction between the treatment selected and patient characteristics that may increase or decrease the risk of treatment-related complications. Provider-related factors address the larger issues of quality of care (which may determine the rate of complications independent of patient- and treatment-related factors), efficiency of care, as well as the general type of care pattern selected. *Efficiency of care* in this context refers to the

---

Major categories of medical cost determinants

Patient-related

Age
Sex
Comorbidity
CAD severity
LV dysfunction

Treatment-related

Aggressive vs. conservative
Complications

Provider-related (MD, hospital)

Complications
Efficiency of care
Treatment strategies selected

Geographic/economic

Local costs of labor supplies

---

ability to provide the necessary care with a minimum of waste of medical resources. If one hospital is able to discharge uncomplicated AMI patients an average of 5 days after admission and a second hospital discharges the same type of patients an average of 8 days after admission, then the first hospital is more efficient from an economic point of view. Of course it is important to be sure that both hospitals are delivering the same quality of care and that the postdischarge complication rate in the first hospital is no higher than that of the second hospital.

That provider factors can be important independent determinants of medical resource use and consequently of cost has only recently been clearly demonstrated. In the TIMI II trial Feit et al. showed that among patients randomized to the conservative arm of the treatment protocol (i.e., catheterization only for recurrent ischemia or in high-risk situations), patients enrolled in community hospitals had a significantly lower rate of invasive procedures than patients enrolled in tertiary-care participating hospitals.[27] Furthermore, data from the Myocardial Infarction Triage Intervention (MITI) study and from New York state have independently shown that the availability of catheterization facilities at a hospital is a significant and independent determinant of whether or not an AMI patient undergoes coronary angiography.[28,29] Even after all these characteristics are accounted for, costs will still vary from one hospital to another because of true variations in the cost of labor in different geographic markets, and to a lesser extent because of variations in the purchase price of supplies (e.g., large consortia of health care buyers may get a better price from suppliers than small independent hospitals).

Thrombolytic therapy

Table 15-3 summarizes the available cost studies involving thrombolytic therapy compared with no reperfusion therapy as well as comparisons of different thrombolytic regimens. Of the fifteen studies listed, seven are cost-effectiveness models based on efficacy data from previously published literature and contain no empirical cost data. An additional seven were performed using efficacy data from randomized trials or from subsets of randomized trials: five of these were performed in Europe using a variety of different price weights and currencies. It is notable that there is no published study involving an empirical cost comparison of thrombolytic therapy vs. no thrombolytic therapy in U.S. patients. Furthermore, review of the published reports of the medical outcomes from the major randomized trials of thrombolysis often does not even provide any indication of differences between therapies in the use of big-ticket resource items.

Based on the current treatment trends with thrombolytic therapy, the most pressing cost and cost-effectiveness questions in this area deal with the use of intravenous streptokinase and intravenous t-PA. Although the cost of a streptokinase strategy relative to no reperfusion therapy has not been defined in the United States, we can get some insight into this area from an analysis like the one suggested Figure 15-1. The cost of the thrombolytic agent itself is quite modest, and although it has increased in recent years from less than $100 to its current average wholesale price of $320 per 1.5 million-unit dose,[30] it is still by far the cheapest thrombolytic regimen available. One major issue that has been debated in the literature over the years is whether or not thrombolytic therapy requires a greater use of angiography and revascularization than a no-reperfusion strategy. Metaanalysis of the available data by Naylor and Jaglal suggested that there was an 80% increase in the use of invasive procedures following thrombolysis.[31] The literature also suggests that, at least in the absence of early invasive procedures, complications related to the streptokinase therapy itself were relatively infrequent and usually successfully treatable. It is more difficult to get a handle on the effect of therapy on cost relating to changes in the natural history of AMI. The beneficial effects on left ventricular function were more modest than was initially anticipated. Some studies (but not all) have shown reduction in congestive heart failure and other major disease-related complications. Unfortunately, the published database is inadequate for the proper economic evaluation of this issue. For example, there is almost no information about the effect of streptokinase on length of stay in a hospital or intensive care unit. Thus, it is actually possible that streptokinase might be cost-saving relative to no therapy, but this is hard to prove because of the deficiencies of available data.

Assuming that streptokinase improves medical outcomes and at an increased cost relative to no reperfusion therapy, it is necessary to evaluate the cost-effectiveness of streptokinase relative to conservative care. Assuming a life expectancy of approximately 10 years for survivors, Naylor et al. estimated that substitution of intravenous streptokinase for no reperfusion therapy had a cost-effectiveness ratio ranging between $2000 and $4000 per additional life year saved.[32] Relative to other cost-effectiveness ratios this is an extraordinarily good value (see Table 15-2) and indicates that the decision to choose streptokinase over no therapy is likely to be one of the best buys that can be made in medicine.

Midgette et al. recently reported a cost-effectiveness analysis of intravenous streptokinase compared with no thrombolysis, looking specifically at the importance of infarct location on the resulting cost-effectiveness ratio.[33] Their base case analysis assumed, based on a literature metaanalysis, greater relative efficacy for streptokinase in anterior MIs than in inferior MIs (summary risk ratio 0.72 vs. 0.87, respectively). They also assumed that only 84% of treated patients in both groups would actually have a confirmed MI. In addition, their analyses only considered short-term (i.e., 30-day) survival differences. The marginal short-term cost-effectiveness ratios from this study were $9900 for anterior MI and $56,600 for inferior MI. Assuming a life expectancy for the added survivors of at least 5 years, these figures would be brought in the general range reported by Naylor et al.[32]

Krumholz et al. examined the cost-effectiveness of intravenous streptokinase versus no reperfusion therapy for elderly patients ($\geq$ age 75).[34] Based on GISSI and ISIS-2 data they assumed a 13% relative reduction in short-term mortality with streptokinase. They also assumed that only 83% of patients treated would subsequently prove to have an AMI. This analysis found a base case cost-effectiveness ratio of $21,200 for an 80-year-old (projected undiscounted life expectancy 2.7 years) and $21,600 for a 70-year-old (projected life expectancy 5.5 years).

Both the Midgette et al.[33] and the Krumholz et al.[34] analyses assumed a false-positive diagnosis rate of 16% to 17%. However, clinical trial data in the United States would suggest that this assumption is significantly higher than the rates seen in current clinical practice. Assuming greater clinical diagnostic accuracy would substantially reduce the cost-effectiveness ratios in both studies. In addition, these analyses point out that one limitation of cost-effectiveness analysis is the need to incorporate projected life expectancy into the cost-effectiveness ratio. Ratios expressed in terms of short-term survivors are particularly unfavorable for therapies that have a

Table 15-3. Cost studies of thrombolytic therapy

Study	Years of enrollment	Type of study	Sample size	Measure of costs	No reperfusion/placebo	t-PA	SK	UK	Combo	APSAC	IC SK
Laffel et al.[53]	NA	CE model	NA	Estimated costs (RCC method) using Brigham and Women's Hospital data (1986 U.S. $)	X	X	X				
Steinberg et al.[54]	NA	CE model	NA	DRG reimbursement rates for Baltimore (1988 U.S. $)	X	X	X				
Liu et al.[55]	NA	CE model	NA	Estimated costs (1987 Canadian $)	X	X	X				
Porath et al.[56]	NA	CE model	NA	N/A	X	X	X				
Vermeer et al.[57]; Simoons et al.[58]	1981-1985	RCT	533	Calculated from big-ticket items (1984 Dutch guilders)	X						X
Herve et al.[59]	1986-1987	Observational	162	Calculated from medical bills (British pounds)	X					X	
Goel and Naylor[37]	NA	CE model	NA	Estimated costs (1988 Canadian $)		X	X				
Levin and Jonsson[60]	1987-1988	RCT substudy of ASSET	313	Calculated from big-ticket items (1989 Swedish crowns)	X	X					
Machecourt et al.[61]	N/A	RCT	270	N/A	X	X	X				
Mark et al.[36]		RCT TAMI 5	575	Measured costs (RCC method)		X		X	X		
Fenn et al.[62]	N/A	RCT AIMS	NA	Prices from previous cost studies	X					X	
Castiel et al.[63]	N/A	RCT	167	N/A (U.S. $)							
Krumholz et al.[34]	N/A	CE model	N/A	Estimated costs using Beth Israel Hospital data (1990 U.S. $)	X		X			X	
Midgette et al.[33]	N/A	CE model	N/A	Average variable costs for Tufts Transition 1 System	X		X				
Mark et al.[40]	1990-1993	RCT GUSTO	2600	Average costs from Duke Transition System 1 (1994 U.S. $)		X	X				

(Modified from Mark DB: Medical economics and health policy issues for interventional cardiology. In Topol EJ (ed): *Textbook of interventional cardiology*, ed 2, Philadelphia, 1993, WB Saunders.)

NA = not applicable; N/A = not available.

high up-front cost (e.g., CABG, t-PA) but have a persisting benefit in a cohort that may have 10 to 20 more years to live. It is therefore crucial in interpretation of cost-effectiveness data to understand the time frame of the analysis.

Given that streptokinase is such a good buy, the next and more controversial question is whether substitution of accelerated t-PA for streptokinase is also a good societal investment. Note that at the *patient* decision level the GUSTO-I trial has clearly shown that for almost all subgroups the net benefit with accelerated t-PA (i.e., additional survivors minus additional disabling strokes) favors t-PA use (see Chapter 24). Although there are some who challenge the scientific interpretation of this study (as discussed in other sections of this book), for most clinicians the controversy surrounding t-PA is not whether it is more effective than streptokinase but whether it is sufficiently more effective to be "worthwhile." As noted earlier, cost-effectiveness analysis approaches this question from the point of view of society as a whole, not of an individual patient. The individual patient's interest is to spend whatever money is available to buy additional benefits, even if those benefits are relatively modest. Society, on the other hand, wishes to spend its money in the most efficient manner and theoretically wishes to buy the maximum amount of benefit available regardless of who individually profits and loses in the process.

Two studies have performed economic analyses that are relevant to the streptokinase–t-PA comparison. The TAMI 5 randomized trial enrolled 575 patients into three different thrombolytic regimens: standard t-PA, urokinase, and combination t-PA-UK.[35] This trial clinically showed a benefit in a composite outcomes event from combination thrombolytic therapy relative to monotherapy. Benefit was manifest primarily in a reduction of recurrent ischemic events. Economic analysis showed an equivalent overall hospital cost for the three thrombolytic regimens.[36] However, when the cost of the thrombolytic agents themselves was subtracted, there was a strong trend for the combination thrombolytic arm to have a less expensive hospital stay. This study reinforces the concepts presented in Figure 15-1 that costs for any thrombolytic regimen will represent a balance between the extra dollars required for the treatment regimen itself and for any complications produced vs. the complications and treatments averted.

Naylor et al. performed a cost-effectiveness analysis of t-PA vs. streptokinase before the release of the GUSTO-I results.[32,37] This analysis, which was based on the assumption that the primary hypothesis of the GUSTO-I trial would be confirmed (namely a 1% absolute reduction in mortality rate with the t-PA relative to streptokinase), reported a cost-effectiveness ratio of $28,000, assuming that the initial survival benefits of

t-PA would be sustained for 10 years. Recent results from the GUSTO-I trial have shown that the initial benefits of accelerated t-PA are maintained for at least 1 year following infarction; there are no data yet on the post–1-year differences in these two groups. Earlier data comparing thrombolytic therapy with placebo have suggested that the benefits of thrombolytic therapy, once established, are maintained for at least 5 years without attenuation; it seems reasonable to assume that benefits may persist significantly longer than this because there is no evidence of convergence of the survival curves on any study that has been published so far.[38,39]

Preliminary findings of the economic analysis of the GUSTO-I results in the United States show no significant differences in short-term or long-term resource use between the patients treated with streptokinase and those treated with t-PA.[40] Thus, the major difference in cost between the two arms remains the cost of initial therapy. Assuming that the initial medical benefit of accelerated t-PA is maintained indefinitely, and with an average life expectancy for the cohort exceeding 10 years, the incremental cost-effectiveness ratio for accelerated t-PA is approximately $29,000.[40] If a threshold cost-effectiveness ratio of $50,000 is used to define the category "best buy," then use of accelerated t-PA would fall into this category as long as the initial benefits reported in the GUSTO-I trial are maintained for approximately 5 years. One issue that has come up frequently in discussion about this analysis is whether there are subgroups of patients for whom t-PA is more or less cost-effective. The question is particularly directed toward the issue of whether treating the relatively low-risk inferior MI patients is cost effective or whether those patients should rather be treated with streptokinase. Although there was indeed less initial benefit with t-PA for inferior MIs (6 lives saved per 1000 vs. 19 lives saved per 1000 for anterior MI), because these patients are lower-risk, they also have a lower life expectancy than the higher-risk patients, so the cumulative count of life years added is more similar than might be expected from examination of the approximately threefold differences in initial benefit.

Direct coronary angioplasty

Direct coronary angioplasty has undergone a substantial revival in the last several years because of recent randomized trials that have all shown a consistent trend towards better outcomes relative to thrombolytic therapy. Five trials have included some form of economic analysis along with their assessments of medical outcomes (Table 15-4). The two most persuasive studies are the Mayo Clinic randomized trial and the PAMI randomized trial.[41-44] Although both these studies used charges rather than medical costs, and both had relatively small sample sizes, both were consistent in showing

Table 15-4. Cost studies of direct PTCA in AMI

Study	Years of enrollment	Type of study	Sample size	Measure of costs	Time frame of analysis	Hospital days		Costs	
						PTCA	Lytic Rx	PTCA	Lytic Rx
DeWood[64]	N/A	RCT (vs. t-PA)	54	Hospital charges	Initial hospitalization 1 year	N/A	N/A	H: $14,500 ± $5900 / 1 year: 18,200 ± 7900	19,000 ± 10,800 / 25,000 ± 12,400
O'Neill et al.[65]	1988-1990	RCT (vs. SK)	122	Hospital charges	Initial hospitalization	7.7 ± 4	9 ± 5	19,643 ± 7250	25,191 ± 15,368
Gibbons et al.[43]	1989-1991	RCT (vs. t-PA)	103	Hospital charges/ estimated costs	Initial hospitalization 6 months	7.7 ± 2.9	10.6 ± 8.1	H: 16,811 ± 8827 / F/U H: 480 ± 3609	21,400 ± 14,806 / 2738 ± 7666
Grines et al.[41] Browne et al.[42]	1990-1992	RCT (vs. t-PA)	358	Hospital charges, MD fees	Initial hospitalization	N/A	N/A	H: 24,569 MD: 4239 ± 3260 T: 28,808 ± 14,020	28,235 / 3263 ± 2708 / 31,498 ± 10,792
Mark et al.[45,46]	1990-1992	Prospective cohort	270	Hospital costs (RCC method) MD fees	Initial hospitalization; cumulative 6 months	9.1		H: 12,772 ± 8548 MD: 5522 ± 2570 F/U H: 3563 ± 6543 F/U MD: 1144 ± 2426	— — — —

(From Mark DB: Medical economics and health policy issues for interventional cardiology. In Topol EJ (ed): *Textbook of interventional cardiology,* ed 2, Philadelphia, 1993, WB Saunders.) *Abbreviations*: PTCA, percutaneous transluminal coronary angioplasty; AMI, acute myocardial infarction; Rx, treatment; RCT, randomized controlled trial; t-PA, tissue-type plasminogen activator; SK, streptokinase; MD, physician; N/A, not available; H, hospital; T, total; F/U, follow-up; RCC, cost/charge ratio; vs., versus.

Table 15-5. TIMI-2 cost substudy*

	Angiography-PTCA strategy		
	Immediate invasive (N = 66)	Delayed invasive (N = 160)	Conservative (N = 150)
Initial hospitalization			
Hospital days	10	9	9
PTCA performed (%)	67	58	21
CABG performed (%)	26	16	16
Hospital charges	14,552 ± 6890	14,471 ± 8377	13,372 ± 8354
Hospital costs	10,739 ± 5093	11,571 ± 6685	10,601 ± 6622
Professional fees	4548 ± 3068	3754 ± 2346	2698 ± 2649
Total costs	15,287	15,325	13,299
Follow-up (1 year) resource use			
Cardiac catheterization (%)	3	13.6	15.4
PTCA (%)	1.5	7.2	5.1
CABG (%)	6.6	6.4	6.8
Cardiac rehospitalization (%)			
1	19.7	20	22.2
>1	1.5	7.2	8.5
Cardiac-related hospital days (mean)	1.7 ± 4.9	2.2 ± 5.3	3.2 ± 8.1

(From Charles ED, Rogers WJ, Reeder GS, et al: Economic advantages of a conservative strategy for AMI management: rt-PA without obligatory PTCA [abstract], *J Am Coll Cardiol* 13:152A9; and Charles E, Mark DB: The economics of percutaneous intervention. In: Roubin G, Phillipa HR, III, O'Neill WW, et al, (eds): *Interventional cardiovascular medicine*, New York, 1993, Churchill Livingstone.)
Abbreviations: CABG, coronary artery bypass graft; PTCA, percutaneous transluminal coronary angioplasty; TIMI, Thrombolysis in Myocardial Infarction (Study); *X*, mean.
*Charges and costs reflect 1986 to 1988 dollars and are reported as medians. Note that figures do not include the cost of t-PA, which was provided without charge in this study. Hospital costs calculated from charges using RCC method. *Delayed invasive* and *Conservative* groups represent combination of TIMI-2A and TIMI-2 patients.

a trend towards $3000 to $6000 lower hospital charges in the direct angioplasty arm. We did a careful analysis of 270 patients in the primary angioplasty registry (PAR).[45,46] This study showed that the average hospital cost for a direct angioplasty strategy was approximately $12,800, with professional fees of $5500. Although this study did not include a comparison group treated with thrombolytic therapy alone, the cost figures are quite comparable with those reported by Charles et al. for the TIMI-II conservative care strategy.[47,48] Thus, at present it is not possible to say whether direct angioplasty is equivalent to or less expensive than thrombolytic therapy, but there are very suggestive data available that such may be the case. The ongoing GUSTO-II trial includes a substudy of 1500 patients randomized between thrombolytic therapy and direct coronary angioplasty, and we have planned a detailed economic analysis of this treatment strategy (including hospital cost data).

Adjunctive coronary angioplasty

The use of coronary angioplasty or other interventional procedures either to improve early coronary patency rates in patients treated with thrombolytic therapy (rescue angioplasty) or to ensure long-term patency after initial successful reperfusion has continued to be the subject of vigorous debate in recent years. As reviewed in Chapter 27, there is evidence for additional medical benefit associated with rescue PTCA in the setting of failed thrombolysis. The major economic limitation on this technology has been the need to perform coronary angiography on all patients in order to identify the subset requiring rescue angioplasty. The TAMI 5 randomized trial compared such a strategy involving acute angiography with a rescue PTCA performed only for occluded infarct arteries against a strategy of deferred angiography at 5 to 10 days.[35,36] The aggressive angiography strategy was approximately $3000 more expensive in hospital costs.[36] Importantly, this study tested the timing of angiography once the decision to do angiography in all patients had been made. Recent progress in our understanding of the evolution of reperfusion and its clinical correlates has allowed us to be significantly more selective in the patients we refer for emergency angiography and possible revascularization (see Chapter 37). Although economic analysis of this has not yet been done, it is possible that a selective angiography strategy with rescue PTCA might be substantially more cost-competitive with conservative care than was evident in the results of TAMI 5.

Charles et al. at the University of Alabama and the Mayo Clinic performed a cost study on 386 patients enrolled in the TIMI-II trial at their institutions[47,48]; the major economic results of this study are presented in Table 15-5. It is important to note that the cost figures do not include the cost of the t-PA, which was provided free to participants in this study. Overall the study shows a modest difference in hospital costs between the immediate invasive strategy and the conservative strategy, along with a twofold difference in professional fees. Thus, total costs were approximately $2000 lower for the conservative arm of the trial. In follow-up, catheterization and coronary angioplasty were more common in the delayed invasive and conservative arms and were associated with a somewhat higher rate of cardiac rehospitalization.

Adjunctive medical therapy

A number of medical interventions have become a standard part of the care of AMI, particularly after reperfusion therapy. These include antiplatelet therapy with aspirin and antithrombin therapy with heparin. Neither has been subjected to any form of economic analysis to date. Aspirin therapy in particular clearly falls in the "best buy" category because its cost is trivial and its benefits are substantial. Heparin therapy appears to be most important when used in conjunction with t-PA, and although its economic effects are unknown, it may be cost-saving if it prevents a significant number of infarct artery reocclusions as is currently believed. Newer, more effective, and more expensive antiplatelet and antithrombin agents are currently being tested. In particular, the GUSTO-II and the TIMI-9 studies evaluate hirudin vs. heparin in AMI patients. Both these studies also include economic and cost-effectiveness evaluations.

A number of other standard medical therapies are applied in the AMI patient, including nitrates, beta blockers, and calcium-channel blockers. The efficacy of these agents continues to be debated (as is discussed in other chapters), and none of these agents has been subjected to an economic evaluation. There has been one study on the cost-effectiveness of long-term oral beta blockers performed by Goldman et al.[49] They created a cost-effectiveness model of oral propranolol therapy started before discharge and continued for 6 to 15 years. With a dose of 240 mg per day of propranolol, the average cost in 10 retail pharmacies in the Boston area in 1987 was $208 per year. Assuming a 25% relative reduction in the annual mortality with treatment, these investigators reported cost-effectiveness ratios of $23,400 per life year saved in low-risk patients, $5900 in medium-risk patients, and $3600 in high-risk patients. Thus, judged against other medical interventions (see Table 15-2), long-term oral beta blockers appeared to be quite cost-effective in this analysis.

The delivery and funding of health care are in the midst of dramatic changes. Although it is clear that the status quo is viewed by policy makers and by the general public as untenable, there is little agreement about what a reformed health care delivery system should look like. Clinicians have been largely caught off guard by sudden demands that they prove that what they do adds "value" to the lives of their patients and to society. We feel that a basic understanding of economic analysis methods is as vital for the physician of the 1990s as a grounding in anatomy and physiology has been for previous generations. By understanding the language of the new debate on medical care, physicians can become part of the process shaping the new face of medicine. By questioning key assumptions made by nonmedical participants, physicians can ensure that health care reform does not discard the hard-won advances of medical technology in pursuit of economic efficiency and cost containment.

REFERENCES

1. Ginzberg E: High-tech medicine and rising health care costs, *JAMA* 263:1820-1822, 1990.
2. Mark DB: Medical economics and health policy issues for interventional cardiology. In Topol EJ, (ed): *Textbook of interventional cardiology,* ed 2, Philadelphia, 1993, WB Saunders.
3. Fuchs VR (ed): *The health economy,* Cambridge, Mass, 1986, Harvard University Press.
4. Feldstein PJ (ed): *Health care economics,* ed 4, Albany, New York, 1993, Delmar.
5. Robinson JC, Luft HS: Competition and the cost of hospital care, 1972 to 1982, *JAMA* 257:3241-3245, 1987.
6. Iglehart JK: Managed competition, *N Engl J Med* 328:1208-1212, 1993.
7. Feldstein PJ (ed): *Health care economics,* ed 3, New York, 1988, John Wiley & Sons.
8. Newhouse JP (ed): *Measuring medical prices and understanding their effects,* Santa Monica, Calif, 1988, Rand.
9. Iglehart JK: The American health care system: private insurance, *N Engl J Med* 326:1715-1720, 1992.
10. Iglehart JK: The American health care system: Medicare, *N Engl J Med* 327:1467-1472, 1992.
11. Iglehart JK: The American health care system: Medicaid, *N Engl J Med* 328:896-900, 1993.
12. Cleverley WO, (eds): *Essentials of health care finance,* ed 4, Gaithersburg, Md: 1992, Aspen.
13. Weinstein MC, Fineberg HV, Elstein AS, et al (eds): *Clinical decision analysis,* Philadelphia, 1980, WB Saunders.
14. Stewart RD, (eds): *Cost estimating,* ed 2, New York, 1991, John Wiley & Sons.
15. Eisenberg JM: Clinical economics. A guide to the economic analysis of clinical practices, *JAMA* 262:2879-2886, 1989.
16. Eisenberg JM: New drugs and clinical economics: analysis of cost-effectiveness in the assessment of pharmaceutical innovations, *Rev Infec Dis* 6:S905-S908, 1984.
17. Hlatky MA, Lipscomb J, Nelson C, et al: Resource use and cost of initial coronary revascularization. Coronary angioplasty versus coronary bypass surgery, *Circulation* 82 (suppl IV):IV208-IV213, 1990.
18. Lipscomb J, Cowper T, Mark DB: Comparison of hospital costs with Medicare cost to charge conversions versus a detailed hospital accounting system in patients being treated for ischemic heart

disease. Presentation at the Association for Health Services Research, San Diego, 1994.

19. Mark DB, Gardner LH, Nelson CL, et al: Long-term costs of therapy for CAD: a prospective comparison of coronary angioplasty, coronary bypass surgery and medical therapy in 2258 patients (abstract), Circulation 88 (Part 2):I480, 1993.

20. Topol EJ, Leya F, Pinkerton CA, et al: A comparison of directional atherectomy with coronary angioplasty in patients with coronary artery disease, *N Engl J Med* 329:221-227, 1993.

21. Mark DB, Talley JD, Lam LC, et al: Economic outcomes following coronary angioplasty versus coronary atherectomy: results from the CAVEAT randomized trial, *J Am Coll Cardiol* 23:284A, 1994.

22. Hsiao WC, Braun P, Dunn D, et al: Results and policy implications of the resource-based relative-value study, *N Engl J Med* 319:881-888, 1988.

23. Doubilet P, Weinstein MC, McNeil BJ: Use and misuse of the term "cost effective" in medicine, *N Engl J Med* 314:253-256, 1986.

24. Udvarhelyi IS, Colditz GA, Rai A, et al: Cost-effectiveness and cost-benefit analyses in the medical literature: are the methods being used correctly? *Ann Intern Med* 116:238-244, 1992.

25. Drummond MF, Stoddart GL, Torrance GW, (eds): *Methods for the economic evaluation of health care programmes,* Oxford, England, 1987, Oxford University Press.

26. Detsky AS, Naglie IG: A clinician's guide to cost-effectiveness analysis, *Ann Intern Med* 113:147-154, 1990.

27. Feit F, Mueller HS, Braunwald E, et al and the TIMI Research Group: Thrombolysis in myocardial infarction (TIMI) Phase II trial: outcome comparison of a "conservative strategy" in community versus tertiary hospitals, *J Am Coll Cardiol* 16:1529-1534, 1990.

28. Every NR, Larson EB, Litwin PE, et al for the Myocardial Infarction Triage and Intervention Project Investigators: The association between on-site cardiac catheterization facilities and the use of coronary angiography after acute myocardial infarction, *N Engl J Med* 329:546-551, 1993.

29. Blustein J: High-technology cardiac procedures. The impact of service availability on service use in New York State, *JAMA* 270(3):344-349, 1993.

30. *1993 Drug Topics Red Book,* Montvale, NJ, 1993, Medical Economics Data.

31. Naylor CD, Jaglal SB: Impact of intravenous thrombolysis on short-term coronary revascularization rates. A meta-analysis, *JAMA* 264:697-702, 1990.

32. Naylor CD, Bronskill S, Goel V: Cost-effectiveness of intravenous thrombolytic drugs for acute myocardial infarction, *Can J Cardiol* 9(6):553-558, 1993.

33. Midgette AS, Wong JB, Beshansky JR, et al: Cost-effectiveness of streptokinase for acute myocardial infarction: a combined meta-analysis and decision analysis of the effects of infarct location and of likelihood of infarction, *Med Decis Making* 14(2):108-117, 1994.

34. Krumholz HM, Pasternak RC, Weinstein MC, et al: Cost effectiveness of thrombolytic therapy with streptokinase in elderly patients with suspected acute myocardial infarction, *N Engl J Med* 327:7-13, 1992.

35. Califf RM, Topol EJ, Stack RS, et al: An evaluation of combination thrombolytic therapy and timing of cardiac catheterization in acute myocardial infarction: the TAMI 5 randomized trial, *Circulation* 85:1543-1556, 1991.

36. Mark DB, Lam LC, Hlatky MA, et al: Effects of three thrombolytic regimens and two interventional strategies on acute MI costs: results from a prospective randomized trial (abstract), *Circulation* 84:221, 1991.

37. Goel V, Naylor CD: Potential cost-effectiveness of intravenous tissue plasminogen activator versus streptokinase for acute myocardial infarction, *Can J Cardiol* 8:31-38, 1992.

38. Simoons ML, Vos J, Tijssen JGP, et al: Long-term benefit of early thrombolytic therapy in patients with acute myocardial infarction:

5-year follow-up of a trial conducted by the Interuniversity Cardiology Institute of the Netherlands, *J Am Coll Cardiol* 14:1609-1615, 1989.

39. Cerqueira MD, Maynard C, Ritchie JL, et al: Long-term survival in 618 patients from the Western Washington Streptokinase in Myocardial Infarction trials, *J Am Coll Cardiol* 20(7):1452-1459, 1992.

40. Mark DB, Naylor CD, Nelson CL, et al: Cost effectiveness of tissue plasminogen activator relative to streptokinase in acute myocardial infarction: results from the GUSTO Trial (abstract), *Circulation* 88:I144, 1993.

41. Grines CL, Browne KF, Marco J, et al: A comparison of immediate angioplasty with thrombolytic therapy for acute myocardial infarction, *N Engl J Med* 328:673-679, 1993.

42. Browne KF, Grines C, O'Neill W: Randomized trial of primary PTCA vs. thrombolytic therapy in acute myocardial infarction (PAMI)—six-month follow-up (abstract), *J Am Coll Cardiol* 21:176A, 1993.

43. Gibbons RJ, Holmes DR, Reeder GS, et al: Immediate angioplasty compared with the administration of a thrombolytic agent followed by conservative treatment for myocardial infarction, *N Engl J Med* 328:685-691, 1993.

44. Reeder GS, Bailey KR, Gersh BJ, et al for the Mayo Coronary Care Unit and Catheterization Laboratory Groups: Cost comparison of immediate angioplasty versus thrombolysis followed by conservative therapy for acute myocardial infarction: a randomized prospective trial, *Mayo Clin Proc* 69:5-12, 1994.

45. Mark DB, Brodie B, Ivanhoe R, et al: Effects of direct angioplasty on hospital costs in acute myocardial infarction; results from the multicenter PAR study (abstract), *Circulation* 2:257, 1991.

46. Mark DB, Brodie B, Ivanhoe R, et al: Follow-up cost and other economic outcomes in patients treated with direct angioplasty for acute myocardial infarction (abstract), *J Am Coll Cardiol* 21:176A, 1993.

47. Charles ED, Rogers WJ, Reeder GS, et al: Economic advantages of a conservative strategy for AMI management: rt-PA without obligatory PTCA (abstract), *J Am Coll Cardiol* 13:152A, 1989.

48. Charles E, Mark DB: The economics of percutaneous intervention. In Roubin G, Phillips HR III, O'Neill WW, et al (eds): *Interventional cardiovascular medicine,* New York, 1993, Churchill Livingstone.

49. Goldman L, Sia STB, Cook EF, et al: Costs and effectiveness of routine therapy with long-term beta-adrenergic antagonists after acute myocardial infarction, *N Engl J Med* 319:152-157, 1988.

50. Reference deleted in proofs.

51. Goldman L: Cost-effective strategies in cardiology. In Braunwald E, (ed): *Heart disease: a textbook of cardiovascular medicine,* ed 4, Philadelphia, 1992, WB Saunders.

52. Goel V, Deber RB, Detsky AS: Nonionic contrast media: a bargain for some, a burden for many, *Can Med Assoc J* 143:480-481, 1990.

53. Laffel GL, Fineberg HV, Braunwald E: A cost-effectiveness model for coronary thrombolysis/reperfusion therapy, *J Am Coll Cardiol* 10:79B-90B, 1987.

54. Steinberg EP, Topol EJ, Sakin JW, et al: Cost and procedure implications of thrombolytic therapy for acute myocardial infarction, *J Am Coll Cardiol* 12:58A-68A, 1988.

55. Liu P, Floras J, Haq A, et al: Cost-effective evaluation of thrombolytic therapy: comparison of current modalities and identification of critical cost factors—a Canadian perspective (abstract), *J Am Coll Cardiol* 11:186A, 1988.

56. Porath A, Wong JB, Selker HP, et al: Should patients with suspected acute myocardial infarction receive thrombolytic therapy? (abstract), *Med Decis Making* 9:318, 1989.

57. Vermeer F, Simoons ML, de Zwaan C, et al: Cost benefit analysis of early thrombolytic treatment with intracoronary streptokinase: twelve-month follow-up report of the randomised multicentre trial

conducted by the Interuniversity Cardiology Institute of the Netherlands, *Br Heart J* 59:527-534, 1988.

58. Simoons ML, Vos J, Martens LL: Cost-utility analysis of thrombolytic therapy, *Eur Heart J* 12:694-699, 1991.

59. Herve C, Castiel D, Gaillard M, et al: Cost-benefit analysis of thrombolytic therapy, *Eur Heart J* 11:1006-1010, 1990.

60. Levin LA, Jonsson B: Cost-effectiveness of thrombolysis—a randomized study of intravenous rt-PA in suspected myocardial infarction, *Eur Heart J* 13:2-8, 1992.

61. Machecourt J, Dumoulin J, Calop J, et al: Cost effectiveness of thrombolytic treatment for myocardial infarction: comparison of anistreplase, alteplase and streptokinase in 270 patients treated within 4 hours, *Eur Heart J* 14:75-83, 1993.

62. Fenn P, Gray AM, McGuire A: The cost-effectiveness of thrombolytic therapy following acute myocardial infarction, *BJCP* 45(3):181-184, 1991.

63. Castiel D, Herve C, Gaillard M, et al: Cost-utility analysis of early thrombolytic therapy, *PharmacoEconomics* 1(6):438-442, 1992.

64. DeWood MA: Direct PTCA vs. intravenous t-PA in acute myocardial infarction: results from a prospective randomized trial. Presented at the Sixth International Workshop on Thrombolysis and Interventional Therapy in Acute Myocardial Infarction, Dallas, Tex, 1990 (unpublished).

65. O'Neill WW, Weintraub R, Grines CL, et al: A prospective, placebo-controlled, randomized trial of intravenous streptokinase and angioplasty versus lone angioplasty therapy of acute myocardial infarction, *Circulation* 86:1710-1717, 1992.

Chapter 16

QUALITY OF LIFE ASSESSMENT

Daniel B. Mark

Life can be viewed conceptually as having two principal characteristics, quantity and quality.[1] Disorders of health can adversely affect both of these features. Over the last 200 years technologic medical advances have dramatically altered the prevailing view of what health is. Initially conceived as freedom from death (when mortality rates were high and life expectancy was short), and subsequently as freedom from disease, health is now often defined in terms of positive concepts such as functional excellence or happiness and well-being.[2,3] Advances in medical technology have provided cures for many acute illnesses, particularly infectious diseases, that were previously fatal. However, the prolonged life expectancy of the population has been accompanied by a rise in the prevalence of a host of previously uncommon chronic illnesses, particularly involving the cardiovascular, pulmonary, renal, skeletal and nervous systems. Medicine has made dramatic advances in control or palliation of these disorders over the last 50 years, but in many cases cure is still not possible. Thus, an increasing proportion of the adult population faces the prospect of spending a significant proportion of its life expectancy coexisting with one or more chronic illness. The notion of *quality of life* evolved in order to characterize the consequences of chronic disease on an individual or population.

The purpose of this chapter is to review the concepts and methods of assessment of quality of life and to describe some of the research on quality of life that has been done on patients with acute ischemic heart disease. The chapter is divided into four main sections. First, we briefly describe the historical background of quality of life assessment and consider what is meant by the term *quality of life*. Second, we examine the major reasons for measuring quality of life. Third, we outline the key issues relating to measurement of quality of life and describe the steps used in undertaking a new quality of life assessment. Finally, we review some of the literature on quality of life assessment in acute ischemic heart disease.

BACKGROUND AND DEFINITIONS
Historical background

In 1947 the World Health Organization set the stage for the modern debate on quality of life by defining health as ". . . not only the absence of infirmity and disease, but also a state of physical, mental, and social well being."[4] A year later Karnofsky published a performance status index that was designed to assess the usefulness of chemotherapy for cancer patients.[5] This index ranged from 0%, for death, to 100%, for an individual who has no complaints and no evidence of disease. The scale and its weighting scheme was devised based on clinical intuition and experience and was not subjected to any of the evaluative steps that would be required of a modern quality of life instrument; however, it has attained the status of a classic measure in the field and its use has extended widely beyond that for which it was initially designed. In 1964 the New York Heart Association proposed a refined version of its Functional

Supported in part by Research Grants HL36587, HL45702, and HL17670 from the National Heart, Lung and Blood Institute, Bethesda, Md.

Classification to assess the effects of cardiovascular symptoms on performance of physical activities.[6] The term *quality of life* was apparently coined in the early 1960s by a presidential commission set up by John Kennedy to define U.S. goals for the year 2000.[7]

During the mid- and late 1970s four separate groups of investigators developed the first generation of quality of life assessments that have influenced many of the subsequent efforts in the field. Bush and Kaplan created the Index of Well Being to provide a comprehensive measure of health that covered all possible levels of functioning and all possible symptoms; it also included "consumer ratings" of the desirability of each possible health state.[8] Bergner et al. developed the Sickness Impact Profile (SIP) to assess perceived health and sickness-related behavior in a "culturally unbiased" fashion.[9,10] The SIP has since become a standard that has been widely used in clinical trials and observational research. At the same time Ware et al. created a set of scales for the Rand Health Insurance Experiment that several generations later have evolved into the current Rand Short Forms that are now used very widely.[1,11] Finally, during this period Torrance began to adapt the axioms of utility theory to develop methods for measuring the health state preferences of individuals.[12]

One of the defining features of the field of quality of life is the number of different academic disciplines that have contributed to it: psychology, social psychology, sociology, anthropology, medicine, nursing, economics, and philosophy. Unfortunately, rather than working toward a common goal, investigators in different disciplines have tended to focus on their own preferred approaches to quality of life assessment. As a consequence the early quality of life instruments bore little resemblance to each other. More recently, investigators have attempted to find areas of common ground among these different academic cultures.[13] However, although there are now some instruments and approaches that are more popular than others, it still cannot be said that there is any broad consensus on the best approach to assessing quality of life.

Conceptual background

Quality of life is often equated with "health," but the term has actually been used to describe a much broader concept encompassing not only health but standards of living, quality of social relationships, financial status, and other aspects of life.[2,3] Although viewing quality of life in this broad fashion may be useful in some types of inquiries, for medical research and practice it makes sense to restrict the field of inquiry to aspects of quality of life that are most directly affected by health and that can be changed by medical intervention. To emphasize the distinction between the broader concept of quality of life and the latter narrower concept, the term *health-related quality of life (HRQL)* is often used. All references to quality of life in this chapter should be understood as referring to health-related quality of life.

However, even after having narrowed the field of concern in this fashion the notion of quality of life still lacks sharp definition or focus. The meaning of the term almost certainly differs from one individual to the next. In order to be useful in medical research and practice the concept must have an operational definition, which in turn drives the type of measurements used to represent the concept. These measurements can be divided into four major categories: (1) laboratory or diagnostic tests, (2) symptoms of illness, (3) adequacy of functioning, and (4) feelings of well-being.[3] The first category is now typically excluded from most formulations of health-related quality of life, and most investigators concentrate on one or more of the remaining areas of measurement relating to "subjective health."[3] Used in this sense the term *subjective health* refers to a measurement that has as its cardinal feature a judgment made by the patient or in some cases by another observer as contrasted with the type of measurement made by a technologic device in a laboratory test.[3] Thus it can include both phenomena that are observable (e.g., exercise performance) and phenomena that are not observable by anyone other than the affected individual (e.g., pain).

The heavy dependence of quality of life assessment on subjective judgments or measurements raises important questions about the validity and reliability of the whole field. The principal evidence that subjective judgments can provide a sound basis for assessing health-related quality of life has been provided by psychophysics.[3] By studying the relationships between physical stimuli and perception, psychophysics has generated a body of experimental data showing a predictable relationship between physical stimuli of varying intensities and the resulting sense perception.[3,14] Although the exact form of this relationship continues to be debated, the initial work in this field supports the contention that valid measurements can be made with the "human yardstick." Adaptation of the methods and concepts of psychophysics to the study of phenomena for which no physical scale exists has given rise to the field of psychometrics.[3]

WHY ASSESS QUALITY OF LIFE

There are three major reasons for measuring health-related quality of life (see the accompanying box). First, in order to define the medical care needs of an individual or population it is necessary to describe the health and health-related problems of that individual or group. To interpret such descriptions it is usually necessary to compare the patient or group under study with some reference standard (e.g., "normals," other patients with the disease in question or with other diseases or

Major issues in quality of life assessment

Purpose of assessment
Descriptive/discriminative
Evaluative
Predictive

Major methodology issues
Conceptual approach
Domains to be assessed
Profile vs. index vs. battery
Scoring/weighting of responses
Validity, reliability, responsiveness

Other methodology issues
Self-assessment vs. external observer
Time frame of assessment

disorders). This category of use has been referred to by Guyatt et al. as *discrimination*[15,16] and is typically performed both as part of the description of the natural history of the disorder under study and for the purpose of identifying areas of medical need. At the health policy level these data can be used to set regional or national priorities for health improvements of the population based on need. They can also be used to define current problems regarding access to adequate health care.

Second, repeated longitudinal measurements of quality of life can help further characterize the natural history of the health problem and can be used to monitor individuals or populations with a particular condition or disorder. This category of use has been termed *evaluation*[16] and includes randomized trials and observational studies that are designed to uncover quality of life (and other) differences between different treatment strategies. In addition the growth of the outcomes assessment and quality assurance movements over the last several years has placed increasing emphasis on assessing whether patients are "satisfied customers," largely by examining quality of life outcomes. At the health policy level these data can be used in conjunction with economic data to identify the most cost effective medical technologies and to help guide societal investment in health care.

The third major use of health-related quality of life measurements is to predict future health care outcomes and needs.[15] For example, the ability to predict future functional disability or premature departure from the work force could be used to target high-risk individuals or groups for more frequent follow-up or more aggressive therapy.[17] At the health policy level these data can help to define future spending priorities based on projected needs for access to different forms of health care.[14]

MEASUREMENT OF QUALITY OF LIFE

Measurement of health-related quality of life requires both a conceptual formulation of the problem to be studied and technical decisions about the measurement process itself. We referred earlier to three types of subjective measurements that, in varying combinations, make up health-related quality of life: symptoms of illness, adequacy of functioning, and feelings of well-being. In order to develop a quality of life assessment for a particular application it is necessary to decide how important each of these areas is to the problem at hand. Most quality of life assessments evaluate some aspect of patient symptoms, although such an evaluation is often limited to the general category of "pain." Most assessments also include measures relating to various aspects of functioning, particularly physical functioning and activities of daily living.[2] More recently, quality of life assessments have tended to include measures of positive health and well-being.[2]

Functioning and well-being represent two alternative conceptual approaches to quality of life.[14] Functioning is typically examined in terms of impaired performance of activities that should be performable for that individual or group (i.e., disability) and the resulting social and other consequences of that impaired performance.[2,3] Well-being or positive health goes beyond functional disability to the more nebulous concept of functional excellence and often includes concepts related to resilience and resistance to illness. It has also been interpreted by some to include the concept of satisfaction,[18] although still others consider well-being and satisfaction with life and health to be related but distinct concepts.[2,14,19] Although these latter measures are important because they emphasize that quality of life is more than the absence of disease, they are also problematic in that assessing positive health or well-being implicitly requires making subjective value judgments about the desirability of different health states, judgments that different individuals make differently. For example, for a new therapy to produce the side effect of major depression in a portion of patients treated would clearly be an adverse health outcome. Could the same be said of a difference in the percentage of patients who identified themselves as "happy" or "completely satisfied" with their current health? The notion of positive health is clearly complicated by the patient's own expectations. Two individuals with different expectations will have different judgments about what it means to be happy or satisfied. As a practical matter, however, many scales that purport to measure some aspect of well-being still primarily evaluate functional impairment. Thus it is useful to be aware of these distinctions but also of the problems involved in measuring and interpreting well-being. A third conceptual approach to quality of life assessment, utility, will be discussed later in this section.

Quality of life domains

Major domains

Physical functioning and mobility
Cognitive function
Emotional or psychologic status/well-being
Functioning in social and role activities
General perceptions of health/well-being
Disease specific symptoms/somatic discomfort

Domains less often included

Intimacy and sexual functioning
Economic status/personal productivity
Employment
Laboratory test values

Options for measurement

Regardless of the conceptual approach preferred in a health-related quality of life assessment, it is necessary to define further the aspects of functioning or well-being that are of concern to the investigation being performed. Traditionally quality of life measures have been segregated into discrete domains or dimensions.[1,20] There are both operational and conceptual motives for doing this. Although researchers still do not agree on how many distinct domains the concept of health-related quality of life entails, the accompanying box shows one of the more common classifications in use. A "comprehensive" quality of life assessment usually includes some measurement of each of the major domains mentioned in the accompanying box except for cognitive function (which is technically quite difficult to assess adequately).[1,21]

Besides being classified according to scope, quality of life assessments can be characterized in several other ways that are relevant to the design of a new investigation. As shown in Table 16-1 one important distinction is whether the assessment will adopt a generic or a disease-specific perspective.[7,16,22,23] A *generic* instrument applies equally to all diseases, conditions, and populations that might require a health-related quality of life assessment. In contrast, a disease-specific instrument is focused on a specific disease (e.g., AMI), condition (e.g., congestive heart failure), or population (e.g., subjects with heart disease). For example, a generic assessment of somatic symptoms might include the question: "How much bodily pain have you had in the last week?" Whereas a disease-specific instrument would include: "How frequently have you had chest pain (angina) in the last week?" or "How severe have your joint pains been in the last week?" The principal advantage of the generic approach is that it allows comparisons of individuals with different disorders (e.g., angina, arthritis) on the same scale. Also, generic assessment instruments tend to include most or all the major quality of life domains (aside from cognitive function). A frequent argument made in the literature is that use of such an instrument may uncover unanticipated (at least by the investigator) quality of life problems. This is most likely to be true in areas where little previous quality of life research has been done.

The major disadvantages of the generic instruments are their lower responsiveness to clinically relevant changes over time and their tendency to be perceived by patients and clinicians as less clinically relevant. The problem of responsiveness can be illustrated with a simple example: a patient with both angina pectoris and lower back pain (a not-uncommon combination) in a trial of antianginal therapy may report moderate bodily pain on both a baseline and a 6-month follow-up generic assessment. Yet that patient may have had class II angina at the time of the baseline assessment and no angina at 6 months. Concomitant variations in the severity of that patient's back pain could easily confound and obscure any evidence of therapeutic efficacy. In fact, the confounding effect of comorbidity on quality of life assessment has received far less attention than it deserves.

Disease-specific measures tend to be more acceptable to patients and clinicians because they appear more relevant; they also may be more responsive to change (see discussion of responsiveness that follows).[24] However, they also tend to be so narrowly focused (e.g., on physical functioning, chest pain, dyspnea) that they do not provide a comprehensive quality of life assessment. In addition, they cannot be compared across different diseases or conditions, which makes them less useful for public health and health policy purposes.

Another level of classification of quality of life instruments deals with their construction (Table 16-1). Questions in an instrument may be chosen using either empirical (pragmatic) or theoretic criteria.[3] Clinical researchers tend to favor the pragmatic approach whereas social scientists and psychologists often prefer instruments that have a clear relationship to a specific theory or model of health (Fig. 16-1). Unfortunately, there are almost as many models of health as there are quality of life instruments, which along with general unfamiliarity is perhaps why clinicians tend to avoid choosing quality of life instruments on theoretical grounds.

Quality of life instruments can be further classified according to the type of score they produce. A *single indicator,* such as bed days or disability days, may be useful in summarizing a particular concept or domain especially in population surveys, but will not be sufficient for the vast majority of clinical evaluations. A *health status index,* in contrast, summarizes all aspects of health or quality of life in one overall score. The appeal of such an index is that it reduces a complex multidimensional

Table 16-1. Taxonomy of health-related quality of life measures

Measure	Strengths	Weaknesses	Examples
Range of populations and concepts			
Generic: applies equally across diseases, conditions, and populations	Allows comparison across diseases Typically includes a comprehensive assessment of QOL domains Detection of unanticipated effects possible	Likely to be less responsive to changes over time May be less clinically relevant	Sickness Impact Profile Quality of Well-Being Index Nottingham Health Profile Short Form Health Survey (SF-36)
Specific: applies to a specific disease, condition, population, or domain	More acceptable to patients/clinicians May be more responsive to change	Cannot be compared across conditions or populations Narrowly focused, cannot detect unanticipated effects in other domains	New York Heart Association functional classification Specific Activity Scale (SAS) Rose chest pain questionnaire Duke Activity Status Index
Based on method of construction			
Empirical (pragmatic)	Most easily understood by clinicians/patients	Cannot be used to explain why outcomes are related to certain patterns of responses	Most QOL instruments
Theoretical (model)	Ties in with other psychosocial research and theory May allow explanation, rather than just description, of the patient's health state	Less easily understood by clinicians/patients	Quality of Well-Being Index Sickness Impact Profile
Based on method of scoring			
Single indicators (number summarizing one concept or domain)	Global evaluation Useful for population monitoring	Trends may be difficult to interpret May not be sensitive to changes over time	Mortality rate Disability days Disease prevalence
Health Status Index (single number summarizing multiple concepts or domains)	Represents net impact Useful for cost utility analysis	May not be able to identify contributions of individual domains to overall score May not be responsive to changes over time	Disability/Distress Index Quality of Well-Being Index Health Utilities Index EuroQOL
Health Profile (profile of interrelated scores)	Single instrument Contribution of domains to overall score can be determined	May not be responsive to changes over time May not have a summary score	Sickness Impact Profile Nottingham Health Profile Short-Form Health Survey (SF-36)
Battery of independent scores	Can be optimized for each application	No summary score No common interpretation of individual scores Multiple comparisons may be a problem May need to specify primary outcome	Quality of Life instruments used in: SOLVD CAST BARI GUSTO I
Weighting system			
Sum of item ratings or frequency of responses	Simpler scoring More familiar	May not reflect actual patient preferences for different health states	Almost all QOL measures
Utility or preference weights obtained from patients, providers, or community	Patient or consumer view incorporated	Most suitable source of weights not clear Measurement techniques complex	Standard gamble Time trade-off Health Utilities Index

Modified from Patrick DL, Erickson P: *Health status and health policy: quality of life in health care evaluation and resource allocation,* New York, 1993, Oxford University Press.

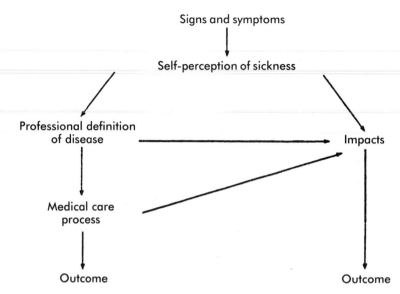

Fig. 16-1. Model for measuring sickness-related behavior upon which the development of the Sickness Impact Profile (SIP) was based. (From Bergner M et al: *Intl J Health Services* 6(3):393-415, 1976.)

problem to a single number. This is particularly useful in the form of economic analysis known as cost utility analysis. An important limitation of the health status index, however, is that it does not allow one to judge the contribution of individual domains (see the box on p. 186) to the overall score. In addition, all health status indexes are generic and therefore possess the general limitations of generic measures described previously.

A *health* or *quality of life profile* provides a set of scores that reflect a common development and scoring methodology and usually an underlying conceptual model that indicates how the component parts relate to "health." Like the health status indexes, all these measures are generic and have the associated limitations described earlier. Many of the health profiles have only domain-specific scores (Fig. 16-2) without an overall summary score, however, because they are not designed with any method that would allow fair determination of the relative importance of the component scales.

The most common quality of life assessment used for clinical trials and other forms of outcome studies is the *health* or *quality of life battery*. This instrument is an investigator-defined set of specific scales that ideally provides both a comprehensive generic assessment of the major quality of life domains along with sensitive disease-specific measures focused in areas of expected greatest importance or change. Most of the major cardiovascular randomized trials that have included a significant quality of life component have taken this approach.[25-31] The potential disadvantages of this approach are, first, that the investigator ends up with a sometimes large set of individual quality of life component scores that have no theoretic or constructional

relationship to each other. For example, a trial of therapy for angina pectoris might include both a measure of symptoms (including chest pain) and a measure of functioning. Which endpoint should be primary in the study analysis is not immediately clear. In addition, individual measures may change in different directions or amounts (e.g., improved chest pain, worse functional status) making interpretation problematic. Although such problems are particularly of concern to psychometricians, they tend to be less troubling for clinicians who are used to dealing with unrelated multidimensional outcomes data in daily practice.

The final classification of quality of life scales shown in Table 16-1 deals with the weighting system used in the scoring. The options for weighting quality of life scores depend first on what level of measurement the scores represent. Four levels are possible here.[3,32] *Nominal* or *categorical scales* use either numbers or words as labels for different response options but no ranking or mathematical relationship is present. Examples include: "yes-no"; "check all the symptoms you have experienced in the last week—chest pain, back pain, joint pains, headache, other"; "1 = male, 2 = female." The numerical values used here have no mathematical meaning and cannot be analyzed statistically as numbers. The second level of measurement possible is an *ordinal scale* in which response options reflect a hierarchical relationship. Examples include: "mild, moderate, or severe pain"; "at the present time my health is excellent, very good, good, fair, poor." Such responses, which are very commonly used in quality of life instruments, can be assigned numerical values (e.g., excellent = 5, very good = 4, and so forth). It is important to remember,

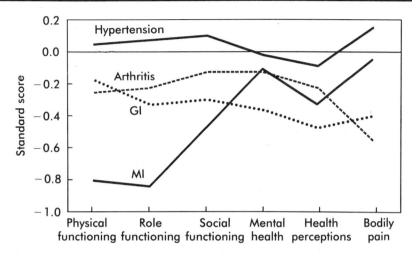

Fig. 16-2. Comparison of the health profiles of four chronic medical disorders using the Rand Medical Outcomes Study (MOS) Short Form General Health Survey. Dotted line indicates patients with no chronic medical conditions. MI = myocardial infarction in the past 12 months; GI = chronic gastrointestinal disorders (peptic ulcer, enteritis, or colitis). (From Stewart AL et al.: *JAMA* 262(7):907-913, 1989.)

however, that the distance between grades in ordinal data does not reflect any underlying measurement scale. That is, a change on an ordinal score from a value of 5 (e.g., excellent health) to 4 (e.g., very good health) may not represent the same magnitude of change as does a shift from 2 (e.g., fair health) to 1 (e.g., poor health). Thus it is technically incorrect to add or subtract item scores from ordinal questions or to calculate summary statistics such as means and standard deviations. Nonetheless, such mathematical manipulation of ordinal data is frequently done in quality of life research, with the justification offered that the resulting errors are small.[3] It is probably more correct to say that the level of error introduced is actually unknown in most cases and difficult to discern because of the absence of appropriate external gold standards.

Interval data have both rank ordering and a specification of the distance between items on a scale. It is, thus, appropriate to add and subtract values and to calculate summary statistics. What interval data lack is an absolute zero point. Therefore it is not possible to state, for example, that an interval level quality of life score of 24 is twice as good (or bad depending on the scale) as a score of 12. Few quality of life scales are actually constructed as interval measures (although many claim to be). The Sickness Impact Profile (SIP) scoring system was devised as an interval scale using a large number of judges who provided weights for each statement.[10] The Duke Activity Status Index (DASI) is scored using individual item weights derived by regres-

sion analysis against measured VO$_2$ max.[33] Some other scales have used factor analysis to derive weights.[7] Utility measures (see below) have also been suggested as examples of interval scale measures.

Ratio scale measures have the properties of an interval scale plus an absolute zero point. This allows judgments about the relative magnitude of changes or differences in a score (e.g., one value is twice as bad as a second value). In the physical realm time and dimensional measures (e.g., height, weight) meet these criteria. It is not clear that any subjective measures fulfill these criteria, although this is still a matter of controversy.

Most commonly, items in a quality of life score, index, or profile are ordinal measures that are treated like interval data and are all given the same weight. For example, in a 20-item scale with each item having response options from 1 (best) to 5 (worst), a total scale score is typically calculated as the simple algebraic sum of the individual item scores—in this case the scale would range from 20 (best possible outcome) to 100 (worst possible outcome). This type of scoring system assumes that the sum of item scores in a particular scale is linearly related to the concept or attribute being measured.[14] The vast majority of health-related quality of life measures are scored in this fashion. Some investigators transform the raw scores to a 0 to 100 scale, presumably because of the general familiarity of such a grading system.[34] The Rand Short Form 36 (SF-36) is a health profile that uses this transformation.[35] However, it is important not to be misled in interpreting scores presented in such an apparently familiar format; only by having reference data on normal or other relevant populations can such a score be interpreted correctly. In addition, a score of 50 on one part of the profile scored 0 to 100 (e.g., physical functioning) may have an entirely different connotation about the level of impairment than that same score on another scale from the same profile (e.g., emotional status). Each part of the profile must be interpreted separately with the relevant reference data.

A related problem in evaluating the typical ordinal or interval type of quality of life scale is determining the clinical relevance or importance of observed score differences or changes over time.[34] A 10-point improvement on a functional status scale ranging from 0 to 100 does not necessarily correspond to a 10% improvement in any standard clinical parameter. In addition, a 10-point change from 10 to 20 on the scale may not indicate the same amount of improvement as a change from 80 to 90.

The major alternative to the weighting schemes described previously is the use of utility weights. The term *utility* in this context is synonymous with preference weights or relative desirabilities of different health states.[36] The conceptual underpinnings of utility measurement are substantially different from the other types of quality of life measures thus far described and are derived from game theory, decision sciences, and economics.[14,16] Unlike other quality of life measures, utilities reflect both a multidimensional health state and the desirability of that health state relative to other possible health states. By convention, utilities are usually scored on an arbitrary 0 to 1 scale where 0 represents death and 1 represents excellent health. It is worth noting that health states with values worse than death are possible on a utility scale.[37] The primary application of utility scales is in economic analysis where they are used to provide a weighted summary of diverse health states on a common 0 to 100 scale that can be combined with survival data to yield an aggregate measure such as the quality adjusted life year (QALY). This is discussed further in the chapter on economic endpoints.

There are two major approaches to obtaining utility or preference weights for health states: direct assessment and use of a health utility index.[36,38] Direct assessment involves measuring utilities on a population of assessors. Most commonly, these assessors are patients in the given health state of interest who are asked to rate their own health state. However, it is also possible to use other raters who are asked to imagine being in the health state(s) of interest and to provide the required preference weights. To help these raters understand what they are rating, they are provided with descriptions that explicitly characterize the health state (e.g., class II angina pectoris) according to the level of health functioning or well being in some or all of the major quality of life domains (see box on p. 186). If the patient is assessing his or her own health state, it is often assumed that he or she is taking these dimensions into account in providing a rating without having them explicitly specified. It is not known whether personal experience of a given health state affects the rating assigned.[39,40]

The most common techniques of direct assessment of utilities are the standard gamble and the time trade-off. The standard gamble asks the rater to make a series of choices between a certain nonrisky outcome of intermediate desirability ("sure thing") and an uncertain or risky outcome (a gamble) where one specified outcome (e.g., immediate cure) is better than the sure thing and one is worse (e.g., immediate death).[14,41] As the assessment progresses the gamble is adjusted based on previous responses until the point of equivalence (indifference) is found between the gamble and the sure thing. This indifference point is the utility value of the "sure thing" option. As can be imagined, the standard gamble technique is complex and difficult for many raters to understand.[38] An alternative, somewhat simpler technique is the time trade-off.[42,43] This method asks in a series of questions how much time the rater would give up to live his or her remaining life expectancy in a healthier state (e.g., excellent health). For theoretical reasons many economists and decision analysts favor the standard gamble for obtaining utilities; it carries with it six axioms from game theory (sometimes referred to as *Von Neumann-Morgenstern axioms*) that collectively define a model of how decision makers *should* react in situations of uncertainty (i.e., specifically, they should select the option with the highest expected utility value). Recently the validity of the standard gamble has been challenged by observations that many decision makers do not behave according to the Von Neumann-Morgenstern axioms.[38] In particular, many individuals have been found to be inconsistent in their attitudes toward risk or gambling—the positive value of a gain of a certain magnitude is judged significantly lower than the negative value of a loss of equal magnitude. On the other hand, the time trade-off technique assumes that individuals value their future survival uniformly; in contrast, for most subjects the next year of survival will typically be much more important than a year of survival that occurs 9 years from now.

The major alternative to these direct utility assessment techniques is the use of a health utility index. Typically, a health utility index consists of a finite (and often limited) set of discrete health states based on combinations of possible health problems and utility weights for each state that were derived usually from the (nondiseased) general population. Thus new patients can be mapped into one of the prespecified multiattribute health states for which population preference weights already exist. There are four major health utility indexes: the Disability/Distress Index of Rachel Rosser and colleagues, the Quality of Well-Being (QWB) Index of Bush and Kaplan, the Health Utility Index of Torrance and coworkers, and the EUROQOL devised by a group of European investigators.[14,44-46] The major objection to these instruments for use in clinical studies is that they are a form of generic quality of life assessment and have the associated limitations described previously. In particular, the categories of health states contained in such indexes tend to have low resolution for clinically relevant differences—for example, all levels of functional impairment may be reduced to three or four categories, thereby substantially reducing the sensitivity of the instrument to change.

Recent investigations comparing health utility measures with more conventional quality of life measures have shown at best only modest levels of concordance.[47,48] Tsevat et al. found that time trade-off scores did not change in the face of clinically significant changes in functional status in post-MI patients.[49] Reduced responsiveness has been observed in other disease states as well.[50] The implications of this reduced sensitivity to change include a significant increase in the sample size required in a clinical trial to detect a specific clinical effect with a utility measure. In addition, aspects of health status (particularly depression) as well as demographics and education level have been shown to influence patient utilities measured with the standard gamble and the time trade-off.[47,50]

Assessing the quality of quality of life measures

Given the profusion of quality of life instruments and measurement approaches and the lack of consensus on the preferred approach for any particular problem or situation, it is reasonable to inquire whether there are standards for selecting among measures for one purpose or another. In fact, there is a large (and confusing) body of literature regarding the desirable performance characteristics of a quality of life measure. The most important characteristics are shown in the accompanying box.

According to the physical sciences, a measurement has three components: true value (which is only theoretically knowable), systematic measurement error or bias, and random measurement error or "noise." These concepts have been applied by psychometricians to subjective measurements of quality of life made with the "human yardstick." The *validity* of a scale or instrument is thus defined as the extent to which it measures what it is designed to measure (and nothing else) or its freedom from bias. To the confusion of nonpsychometricians, there are actually several forms of validity referred to in this area (see the accompanying box). Most exist because of the absence of a true gold standard against which new scales can be assessed. *Content validity* refers to the extent to which all relevant

---

Evaluation of the quality of health-related quality of life measures

Validity (freedom from systematic error or bias)
CONTENT VALIDITY
Reasonableness ("face validity")
CRITERION VALIDITY ("GOLD STANDARD")
Correlational evidence
Predictive evidence
CONSTRUCT VALIDITY
Correlational evidence
Convergence-divergence evidence

Reliability (freedom from random error)
Test-retest reproducibility
Inter-rater reproducibility
Inter-item consistency

Responsiveness (sensitivity to change)
Variability (distribution of responses)
Response bias

---

concepts are included in the measure.[3,34] The specification of what the relevant concepts are may be driven by a particular theory or model. Most often, however, a panel of experts is used to determine whether content validity has been achieved. Face validity is a type of content validity that refers to subjective assessment of whether the content is reasonable. There is no standard statistical method for assessing content validity.

Tests of *criterion validity* are applied when there is a gold standard available for the concept in question.[34] For example, if functional performance is conceptualized as maximal exercise capacity, there are several exercise test variables that could serve as a reasonable gold standard (e.g., exercise time, VO_2 max). If a new short form assessment of depression or anxiety is desired to replace a longer form, the latter can serve as the "gold standard" in the assessment of validity.

For most quality of life concepts, however, no suitable gold standard exists; therefore, *construct validity* assessment is substituted for criterion validity. Construct validity has been described as ". . . part science, but to a large extent an art form."[3] It is consequently seldom definitive and tends to be approached differently by different investigators. The basic issue addressed by construct validity is whether the quality of life measure in question relates to other measures in ways consistent with expectations.[51] For example, different measures of depression should be more strongly related to each other than to a measure of anxiety or a measure of physical functioning. Typically, construct validity is evaluated with the correlation coefficient. Measures hypothesized to reflect the same domain or concept should have a correlation coefficient ≥ 0.40, whereas measures reflecting different concepts should have a correlation that is as small as possible.[34]

Reliability reflects the other part of the measurement paradigm and refers to the freedom from random error (or noise). Synonyms commonly used in the quality of life literature include consistency, reproducibility, and repeatability.[34] Within this general notion of reliability, at least three different assessments are referred to (see box on p. 191). *Test-retest reproducibility* refers to the extent to which repeat administrations of the same quality of life measure yield the same result, assuming no underlying change has occurred. This type of reliability is typically assessed with a correlation coefficient or (better) an intraclass correlation coefficient or a κ statistic.[52] The major methodologic challenge here is to do the second test long enough after the first one so that the subject does not remember his or her original answers, but not so long that the subject's true condition under assessment has changed.[3] Typical reproducibility coefficients lie between 0.85 and 0.90. A second type of reliability is *inter-rater reproducibility*, which refers to the ability of different raters to obtain the same quality of life assessment.[48] Typical inter-rater reproducibility correlations range from 0.80 to 1.0.[34] The third type of reliability commonly referred to in the quality of life literature is *inter-item* or *internal consistency*, which refers to the extent to which all items in a given multiitem scale measure the same domain or concept. Heterogeneity among items will increase the measurement noise relative to a scale demonstrating high homogeneity.[34] Inter-item consistency can be tested by randomly forming two subscales from the scale in question and showing that the two have a high correlation (referred to as *split-half reliability*). More commonly, investigators use a statistic known as *Cronbach's coefficient alpha,* which gives the average correlation of all possible split-half samples.[32] Alpha coefficients of 0.50 or more are generally considered acceptable, whereas in most cases a value ≥ 0.70 is desirable.[34] Because this statistic indicates what the correlation would be between different versions of the same scale, it has been used by some as a "poor man's test-retest reliability measure."[3]

Besides validity and reliability, several other desirable properties have been identified for quality of life measures (see box on p. 191). One of the most important (and often least studied) for clinical purposes is *responsiveness* or sensitivity to clinically relevant changes over time.[2] The most common approach to assessing responsiveness is to make a set of measurements before and after application of a treatment of known efficacy.[52] Responsiveness may be quantitated by computation of the effect size (the change in mean score from baseline to follow-up divided by the standard deviation of the baseline score) or the Guyatt variant of effect size (substitutes the standard deviation of score changes from baseline to follow-up in stable subjects in the denominator).[52] If an external standard of clinical improvement is available the responsiveness of the quality of life measure can be assessed as a type of diagnostic test for change, with sensitivities and specificities defined according to the cutoff value used for indicating clinically significant improvement. With these data a receiver operating characteristic (ROC) curve can be constructed to provide a quantitative measure (the area under the ROC curve) of responsiveness.[52]

Two other qualities of health-related quality of life measures are discussed by some researchers (see box on p. 191). *Variability* or the distribution of responses refers to how well the full range of the score is reflected in the group under study and whether the scores have an approximately normal distribution.[34] Although some skewing is characteristically seen in many quality of life scales, a highly skewed distribution may result in what is known as "floor" or "ceiling" effects. These occur when baseline scores are concentrated around the bottom or top end of a scale, making it impossible for that measure to detect further deterioration or improvement.[14] The remedy for this problem is to add questions that expand the resolution of the scale at the low and high end, respectively.[34] *Response bias* refers to a form of systematic error that is common in self-report research.[2,34] For example, some individuals seek to present themselves in a favorable light or to give the "right" answer. This may be one situation in which self-administered questionnaires may be less susceptible to bias than direct interviews. Another form of response bias comes from individuals who agree with whatever they are asked. In both these situations careful construction of questions provides the best hope for minimizing the problem.

Selecting a quality of life assessment for clinical use

The details in the foregoing sections may make those not directly involved with the field feel as if quality of life assessment is a prohibitively confusing or complicated endeavor. The accompanying box outlines the major questions that an investigator needs to address when in the planning phase of a new quality of life assessment. After having identified the goals and, where appropriate, the hypotheses of the investigation, the researcher must decide whether a comprehensive or a limited assessment is most appropriate to achieve those goals. As noted previously, a comprehensive approach is preferred where the possibility exists of unexpected quality of life effects beyond those anticipated by the investigators. It is also necessary to select an instrument or battery for use. In general, we recommend "off the shelf" instruments because their validity, reliability, and (occasionally) responsiveness have been previously defined in the literature. Creation of new scales is a complex and time-consuming task that generally should be undertaken only

---

| Selection of a health-related quality of life instrument for clinical use |

Extent of assessment
Comprehensive
Limited

Which instrument(s) to use
Standard instrument(s)
Ad hoc battery

Method of administration
Direct observation
Face-to-face interview
Telephone interview
Self-administered questionnaire
Supervised self-administered questionnaire
Proxy respondent

Acceptability to target subjects
Respondent burden
Interviewer burden

Length and cost of administration
Completion rate
Quality of data

Modified from Patrick DL, Erickson P: *Health status and health policy: quality of life in health care evaluation and resource allocation.* New York, 1993, Oxford University Press.

by an experienced researcher. For clinical trials and most other clinical investigations, it has been our practice to create an ad hoc battery of validated instruments that includes a comprehensive generic assessment along with detailed disease-specific measures appropriate to the specific study question(s). A partial menu for such choices is presented in the box on p. 194. Where cost effectiveness analysis is one of the study goals, we also include either a direct utility assessment or a health utility index. In our view, however, utility instruments are complementary to but not substitutes for a battery of standard quality of life measures when detection of clinically relevant changes in health-related quality of life is desired.

Another important issue that needs to be addressed in planning is the method of administration (see the accompanying box). Having tried all the different methods, we now favor interviews (face-to-face or telephone) whenever the study budget permits. This gives us better control over the quality and completeness of responses and reduces the problem of assessing subjects who have poor reading skills. Self-administered questionnaires are cheaper to use but completeness rates are lower (both item completion and questionnaire completion). In addition, a follow-up assessment with a questionnaire

can take 3 months or more to reach acceptable completion rates (making the time point of assessment less precise). Proxies (e.g., household member, close relative) can be used when the subject is incapacitated or otherwise unable to participate but should be limited to the more objective parts of the assessment (e.g., employment status, activities of daily living).[53,54]

How many items to include in a quality of life assessment is another important issue in the planning phase. It is tempting to put together a large (and impractical) assessment, particularly when the investigation is not well-focused and is being used as a shotgun inquiry to flush out any unsuspected quality of life effects that may occur. This may particularly be a problem when assembling a battery of previously validated instruments for each domain of interest (see box on p. 194). If each domain is covered by a 20-item scale (and some domains may require multiple scales, such as a separate assessment of depression, anxiety, and emotional well-being), it is relatively easy to devise a very long battery that is burdensome both to the patients and to the research staff. It is crucial here to know something about the group being assessed. A sick in-patient group will have less tolerance for a long assessment than a relatively healthy outpatient group. However, if the quality of life assessment is tagged on at the end of a long medical evaluation, even relatively healthy patients may have reduced tolerance for a long instrument. The education level of the group being assessed will affect the decision about the best type of questions to use. For example, we have noted that patients with low education levels seem to have more trouble using a multi-level ordinal response (e.g., all of the time, most of the time, some of the time). Both the tolerability of the battery and the appropriateness for the target population should be assessed, whenever possible, in a pilot study. Finally, some clinical insight into expected quality of life outcomes is essential to guide selection of the most appropriate assessment instrument.

QUALITY OF LIFE IN ACUTE ISCHEMIC HEART DISEASE

Over the last two decades substantial and dramatic advances have been made in the therapeutics of acute ischemic heart disease. Hospital mortality in patients with acute myocardial infarction has fallen from 13% in conventionally treated patients in the GISSI I trial to 6.3% in patients in the GUSTO-I trial receiving accelerated t-PA. Current estimates of 30-day mortality for patients with unstable angina or non–Q wave myocardial infarction obtained from the recently completed TIMI 3 trial average around 2%. Although these figures are not yet low enough for clinicians to become complacent, they are low enough to make it very difficult to demonstrate further improvements in mortality across the spectrum

---

Sample quality of life assessment instruments by domain

Physical functioning/functional status

Duke Activity Status Index (DASI)[33]
Duke-UNC Health Profile Physical Function Scale[75]
Karnofsky Performance Scale[5]
Katz Index of Activities of Daily Living[76]
Older American's Resources and Services Schedule
  (OARS) Multidimensional Functional Assessment[77]
Rand Functional Limitations Battery
Rand Physical Capacities Battery
Rand Short Form-36 Physical Function Scale[11,96]
Sickness Impact Profile Physical Scale[10]
Six Minute Walk Test[78,79]
Specific Activity Scale (SAS)[80]

Cognitive function

Folstein Mini-Mental Status Examination

Emotional/psychologic status

Beck Depression Inventory[81]
Brief Carroll Depression Rating Scale[82]
Center for Epidemiologic Studies Depression Scale
  (CES-D)
General Health Questionnaire[83,84]
General Well-Being Schedule[85]
Hospital Anxiety and Depression Scale
Profile of Mood States (POMS)
Psychosocial Adjustment to Illness (PAIS)
Rand Mental Health Inventory (38 item, 5 item)[86,96]
Spielberger State Trait Anxiety Inventory (STAI)

Symptom Check List (SCL-90)
Zung Depression Scale

Social/role functioning

Rand Social Health Battery
Sickness Impact Profile Social Interaction Scale[10]
Sickness Impact Profile Recreation and Pastimes Scale[10]
Framingham Disability Study Social Interaction
  Scale[87,88]
Rand Short Form Role Functioning Scale[11,96]
Rand Short Form Social Functioning Scale[11,96]
Duke-UNC Health Profile Social Function Scale[75]

General health/well-being

Single item rating (excellent to poor)
General Well-Being Schedule[85]

Cardiac disease-specific scales

Rose Angina Questionnaire[89]
Rose Dyspnea Questionnaire[89]
New York Heart Association (NYHA) Functional Classifica-
  tion[6,90]
Canadian Cardiovascular Society (CCVS) Functional Classi-
  fication[91]
Specific Activity Scale (SAS)[80]
Minnesota Living with Heart Failure Questionnaire[92,93]
Duke Activity Status Index (DASI)[33]
Seattle Angina Questionnaire[94]
McMaster Quality of Life Post-MI[95]

This is not meant to be a comprehensive listing or a recommendation for use of any particular scale. Some scales appear in more than one list because of ambiguity about what they are measuring. It is possible to use domain-specific scales out of a health profile as part of a quality of life battery.

of acute ischemic heart disease. Because demonstrating further reductions in mortality now requires megatrials on the scale of GUSTO-I or ISIS-4, clinical investigators have recently become interested in the possibility of using quality of life as a potentially more sensitive indicator of therapeutic efficacy that might allow comparison of different therapies with smaller numbers of patients. However, although there are a number of observational studies on selected aspects of quality of life following AMI, surprisingly little empirical research has been reported on the effects of different therapeutic strategies on post-MI quality of life outcomes. Even less information is available on patients with unstable angina. Much of the existing quality of life literature in this area deals with very specific issues such as cardiac symptoms, psychologic status (and particularly depression), and return to work. The literature on angina following acute ischemic heart disease is voluminous and will not be reviewed here. Most of the available work was done as part of an assessment of "medical" outcomes rather than as a quality of life evaluation. Consequently, the most commonly used measures of anginal status have

been the NYHA or CCVS functional classifications (see the accompanying box).

A number of studies have evaluated the incidence and time course of depression and anxiety following acute MI.[55] Up to two thirds of MI patients have been found to have evidence of psychological distress, particularly in the early post-MI period. In one series of 283 consecutive AMI patients, 18% met criteria for major depression and an additional 27% had minor depression.[55] Interestingly, in this study depression did not correlate with the severity of MI but was associated with the extent of noncardiac comorbidity. At a repeat assessment 3 months post-MI, 15% of patients still had major depression and 18% had minor depression. Thus major depression tended to be persistent and it correlated with a significantly reduced likelihood of returning to work in previously employed patients. Recently Frasure-Smith et al. reported that post-MI major depression was associated with a significantly higher 6-month cardiac mortality rate (adjusted hazard ratio of 4.3).[56] Although it is tempting to postulate that the life disruption produced by an AMI caused the subsequent depression (and this may be true for minor depression and anxiety), observations in coronary disease patients without a recent MI show a similar incidence (18%) of major depression.[57] Thus the extent to which emotional status and well-being can be affected by medical interventions that improve clinical outcomes in acute ischemic heart disease remains to be defined.

One randomized trial has evaluated the effects of a brief cardiac rehabilitation program on quality of life in 201 post-MI patients with evidence of minor anxiety or depression.[58] By 8 weeks, patients randomized to the rehabilitation program had significantly improved emotional status. However, control patients also improved in this and other quality of life dimensions, and by 1 year there was no significant difference in any quality of life dimension between the two groups.

Return to work following acute MI has been studied fairly intensively. A complicated MI has been associated with a lower return-to-work rate, but among patients with an uncomplicated MI the extent of the left ventricular damage does not correlate with return rates.[59,60] In almost all analyses on the subject, education level comes out as one of the strongest predictor of return-to-work behavior. Older age at the time of infarction also predicts a decreased return rate. Job-related factors have been inconsistently related to work behavior. Some studies have found an effect of heavier physical demands on the job, blue collar vs white collar jobs, and job satisfaction. As noted above, psychological factors may also predict return-to-work behavior. In addition, one recent study has suggested that returning to work produces an improved emotional status.[61]

We have found return-to-work behavior to be an insensitive marker of therapeutic benefit following revascularization therapy of coronary disease.[62] Dennis et al. performed a randomized trial to determine if an occupational work evaluation (symptom-limited treadmill test and formal recommendation about suitability and timing of return-to-work) could shorten return to work times in patients with an uncomplicated AMI. They found that the intervention reduced the time to return to work by 25 days ($P < .002$) but did not significantly change the number of patients who went back to work.[63] However, when this occupational work evaluation was retested in four San Francisco Kaiser-Permanente medical centers the benefits were much lower (13 days) and were not statistically significant.[64] Oldridge et al. at McMaster found no evidence of benefit on return-to-work rates of an 8-week post-MI cardiac rehabilitation program.[58]

A group of Swedish investigators studied long-term quality of life post-MI using the Nottingham Health Profile. They found that compared to age- and sex-matched normals, at 5 years the MI survivors had the greatest impairments in the areas of energy, sleep, and mobility; these impairments had the greatest adverse effect on their sex life, hobbies, and recreational activities.[65] The presence of continued cardiac symptoms (dyspnea, angina) and anxiety were closely associated with lower quality of life scores. Similar outcomes were observed in a population of 397 patients with unstable angina.[66]

Olsson and colleagues created an ad hoc ordinal seven-level quality of life scale for use in a trial of metoprolol post-MI.[67] This scale combined death and nonfatal complications (reinfarction, stroke, CABG) with drug side effects and NYHA functional class. Survival time for each patient was apportioned as appropriate among the seven levels of this scale. Comparison of the two randomized groups using this scale suggested that the metoprolol group gained an average of 28 days of life for each 3 years of treatment and added 102 days of optimal functional capacity; however, they also added 30 days with class I functioning but suspected side effects of therapy.[67]

Elliott et al. compared quality of life outcomes following streptokinase or placebo in 145 AMI patients.[68] Streptokinase was associated with an increased ability to exercise on a treadmill and a reduced incidence of limiting dyspnea. Return to work and to sport and leisure activities occurred at the same rate in the two groups, but occurred earlier in the streptokinase-treated patients. In contrast, preliminary comparisons of quality of life following accelerated t-PA versus streptokinase in the Economics and Quality of Life substudy of the GUSTO-I trial (EQOL GUSTO) have shown no differences in a comprehensive assessment battery.[31] Specifically, the improved survival for the t-PA group did not appear to be produced at the expense of a lowered quality of life. In the smaller TAMI 5 trial we found no difference in quality of life up to 1 year associated with the three thrombolytic regimens (t-PA, urokinase, combination therapy) or the two catheterization strategies (immediate, deferred) tested. Finally, in the Primary Angioplasty Registry (PAR), using the same assessment instrument employed in TAMI 5, we found similar 6-month quality of life outcomes for primary angioplasty and thrombolytic therapy. Taken together these preliminary data suggest that whereas reperfusion may improve quality of life modestly relative to no reperfusion, different reperfusion strategies produce similar long-term health-related quality of life. In contrast, substantially different use of revascularization therapies post-MI as was seen in Canadian and U.S. patients in the GUSTO-I trial was associated with much larger differences in quality of life.[69]

Interesting data on the potential responsiveness of quality of life measures comes from a study by Neill et al. of 100 men with clinically stable CAD (one third with severe angina, one third with mild angina, and one third

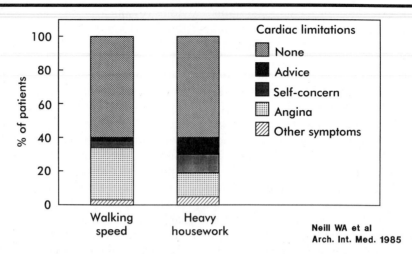

Reasons for cardiac limitations:
patient perceptions

Fig. 16-3. Coronary disease patients' perceptions of why they were limited in walking speed and heavy housework. (From Neill WA et al: *Arch Intern Med* 145:1642-1647, 1985.)

asymptomatic).[70] These investigators found that many aspects of daily functioning (such as household duties, social activities) had little or no relationship to objectively measured exercise capacity. In multivariable analysis the four predictors of lower exercise capacity assessed by treadmill testing in this population were severity of anginal symptoms, exercise-limiting angina, older age, and more severe angiographic CAD. In contrast, the predictors of lower patient functional status assessed by questionnaire were anginal severity, previous myocardial infarction, exercise-limiting angina, and lower education level. In this study patient perceptions of the reasons for functional limitations with cardiac disease were much more diverse and complex than many clinicians appreciate (Fig. 16-3). Patients usually keep their daily activity levels significantly below their true physical capacity, making it difficult for any self-report measure to assess functional capacity as thoroughly as an exercise test.[71,72]

Cardiovascular therapies can improve that part of functioning that is limited by cardiac symptoms. However, other perceived limitations (including both psychological and comorbidity effects) may be relatively resistant to such interventions. Thus the opportunity for new medical therapies to improve quality of life will vary according to the patient population treated, and the extent and type of pretreatment impairment present. For example, CABG or PTCA produce a clinically significant improvement in functional status in patients limited because of chronic coronary disease symptoms.[73] However, when applied to patients presenting with acute ischemic heart disease as the first clinical manifestation of CAD, these same procedures may be associated with

no change in functional status or even a modest net decrease. Simply put, if the patient was asymptomatic before his or her acute illness, the best that medical therapy can offer such a patient is restoration of premorbid quality of life. However, complications of the illness and of the procedures will keep some patients from being restored to this level. Similarly, treatment with enalapril has been reported to improve quality of life in patients with symptomatic left ventricular dysfunction (mostly NYHA class $\geq$ II) but not in patients with largely asymptomatic left ventricular dysfunction.[65] However, comparison of enalapril with hydralazine/isosorbide in the V-HeFT II trial (mostly NYHA Class II or III) showed no discernible differences in quality of life.[74]

CONCLUSIONS

The current emphasis on health care cost containment and on demonstrating value added for health care dollars spent has produced a dramatic change in attitudes about quality of life. Increasingly, payors are suggesting that they will only pay for those aspects of medical care that have demonstrated efficacy in improving either survival or quality of life. The Food and Drug Administration has made similar statements about the approval of new drugs and medical devices. As noted in the previous section, showing that a given therapy prolongs survival in therapeutic trials of acute ischemic heart disease has now become extremely difficult (and quite expensive). This has created a search for meaningful alternative endpoints. Clinicians still tend to favor composite clinical endpoints (see Chapter 14, Medical Endpoints), but there is also growing interest in using quality of life endpoints to assess therapeutic efficacy. Clearly, we still have much to learn about the measurement and interpretation of quality of life in cardiovascular disease. Until very recently physicians have generally regarded quality of life assessment as either too unscientific or too arcane to be useful. However, criticizing from the sidelines is unlikely to prove an effective strategy for changing policy. Physicians must either join the debate about what quality of life is and how it should be measured or cede this area to the nonclinicians who currently dominate it. This chapter attempts to demystify the notion of quality of life and offers a starting point for those wishing to improve their understanding of the field.

REFERENCES

1. Ware JE Jr: Standards for validating health measures definition and content, *J Chron Dis* 40:473-480, 1987.
2. Wilkin D, Hallam L, Doggett M (eds): *Measures of need and outcome for primary health care,* Oxford, 1992, Oxford University Press.
3. McDowell I, Newell C (eds): *Measuring health: a guide to rating scales and questionnaires,* New York, 1987, Oxford University Press.
4. Spitzer WO: State of science 1986: quality of life and functional status as target variables for research, *J Chron Dis* 40(6):465-471, 1987.
5. Schag CC, Heinrich RL, Ganz PA: Karnofsky Performance Status revisited: reliability, validity, and guidelines, *J Clin Oncol* 2(3):187-193, 1984.
6. Kossman CE, Chasis H, Connor CAR, et al (The Criteria Committee of the New York Heart Association) (eds): *Diseases of the heart and blood vessels. Nomenclature and criteria for diagnosis,* ed 6, Boston, 1964, Little, Brown.
7. Williams JI: Strategies for quality-of-life assessment—a methodologist's view, *Thor Surg* 6:152-157, 1991.
8. Kaplan RM, Bush JW, Berry CC: Health status: types of validity and the Index of Well-being, *Health Serv Res* 4:478-507, 1976.
9. Bergner M, Bobbitt RA, Kressel S, et al: The Sickness Impact Profile: conceptual formulation and methodology for the development of a health status measure, *Int J Health Serv* 6(3):393-415, 1976.
10. Bergner M, Bobbitt RA, Carter WB, et al: The Sickness Impact Profile: development and final revision of a health status measure, *Med Care* XIX:787-805, 1981.
11. Ware JE Jr, Snow KK, Kosinski M, et al (eds): *SF-36 Health Survey: Manual and interpretation guide,* Boston, 1993, Nimrod Press.
12. Torrance GW: Toward a utility theory foundation for health status index models, *Health Serv Res* Winter:349-369, 1976.
13. Bergner M, Kaplan RM, Ware JE Jr: Evaluating health measures. Commentary: Measuring overall health: an evaluation of three important approaches, *J Chron Dis* 40(suppl 1):23S-26S, 1987.
14. Patrick DL, Erickson P: *Health status and health policy: quality of life in health care evaluation and resource allocation,* New York, 1993, Oxford University Press.
15. Kirshner B, Guyatt G: A methodological framework for assessing health indices, *J Chron Dis* 38(1):27-36, 1985.
16. Guyatt GH, Feeny DH, Patrick DL: Measuring health-related quality of life, *Ann Intern Med* 118:622-629, 1993.
17. Mark DB, Lam LC, Lee KL, et al: Identification of patients with coronary disease at high risk for loss of employment: a prospective validation study, *Circulation* 86:1485-1494, 1992.
18. Gotay CC, Korn EL, McCabe MS, et al: Quality-of-life assessment in cancer treatment protocols: research issues in protocol development, *J Natl Cancer Inst* 84(8):575-579, 1992.
19. Shumaker SA, Anderson RT, Czajkowski SM: Psychological tests and scales. In Spilker B (ed): *Quality of life assessments in clinical trials,* New York, 1990, Raven Press.
20. Bergner M: Quality of life, health status, and clinical research, *Med Care* 27(3):S148-S156, 1989.
21. Robinson M, Blumenthal JA, Burker EJ, et al: Coronary artery bypass grafting and cognitive function: a review, *Cardiopul Rehabil* 10:180-189, 1990.
22. Patrick DL, Deyo RA: Generic and disease-specific measures in assessing health status and quality of life, *Med Care* 27(3):S217-S232, 1989.
23. Aaronson NK: Quality of life assessment in clinical trials: methodologic issues, *Controlled Clin Trials* 10:195S-208S, 1989.
24. Guyatt GH, Bombardier C, Tugwell PX: Measuring disease-specific quality of life in clinical trials, *Can Med Assoc J* 134:889-895, 1986.
25. Wiklund I, Gorkin L, Pawitan Y, et al for the CAST Investigators: Methods for assessing quality of life in the Cardiac Arrhythmia Suppression Trial (CAST), *Qual Life Res* 1:187-201, 1992.
26. Rogers WJ, Johnstone DE, Yusuf S, et al for the SOLVD Investigators: Quality of life among 5,025 patients with left ventricular dysfunction randomized between placebo and enalapril: the Studies of Left Ventricular Dysfunction, *J Am Coll Cardiol* 23(2):393-400, 1994.
27. Gorkin L, Norvell NK, Rosen RC, et al for the SOLVD Investigators: Assessment of quality of life as observed from the baseline data of the Studies of Left Ventricular Dysfunction (SOLVD), *Am J Cardiol* 71:1069-1073, 1993.
28. The BARI Investigators: Protocol for the Bypass Angioplasty Revascularization Investigation, *Circulation* 84 (suppl 6):1-27, 1991.
29. Cleary PD, Epstein AM, Oster G, et al: Health-related quality of life among patients undergoing percutaneous transluminal coronary angioplasty, *Med Care* 29(10):939-950, 1991.
30. Croog SH, Levine S, Testa MA, et al: The effects of antihypertensive therapy on the quality of life, *N Engl J Med* 314:1657-1664, 1986.
31. Mark DB, Clapp-Channing N, Hlatky MA, et al for the GUSTO Investigators: Quality of life outcomes with tissue plasminogen activator versus streptokinase in 3000 North American patients: the EQOL GUSTO substudy (abstract), *J Am Coll Cardiol* 1995 (in press).
32. Streiner DL, Norman GR (eds): *Health measurement scales. A practical guide to their development and use,* Oxford, 1989, Oxford University Press.
33. Hlatky MA, Boineau RE, Higginbotham MB, et al: A brief self-administered questionnaire to determine functional capacity (the Duke Activity Status Index), *Am J Cardiol* 64:651-654, 1989.
34. Stewart AL: Psychometric considerations in functional status instruments. In WONCA Classification Committee (ed): *Functional status measurement in primary care,* New York, 1990, Springer-Verlag.
35. Stewart AL, Ware JE Jr. (eds): *Measuring functioning and well-being. The Medical Outcomes Study approach,* Durham, NC, 1992, Duke University Press.
36. Froberg DG, Kane RL: Methodology for measuring health-state preferences-I: measurement strategies, *J Clin Epidemiol* 42:345-354, 1989.
37. Patrick DL, Starks HE, Cain KC, et al: Measuring preferences for health states worse than death, *Med Decis Making* 14:9-18, 1994.
38. Froberg DG, Kane RL: Methodology for measuring health-state preferences-II: scaling methods, *J Clin Epidemiol* 42:459-471, 1989.
39. Christensen-Szalanski JJJ: Discount functions and the measure-

ment of patients' values: women's decisions during childbirth, *Med Decis Making* 4:47, 1984.

40. Llewellyn-Thomas HA, Sutherland HJ, Thiel EC: Do patients' evaluations of a future health state change when they actually enter that state? *Med Care* 31:1002-1012, 1993.

41. Sox HC Jr, Blatt MA, Higgins MC, et al (eds): *Medical decision making*, Boston, 1988, Butterworths.

42. Torrance GW: Measurement of health state utilities for economic appraisal. A review, *J Health Econ* 5:1-30, 1986.

43. Torrance GW, Feeny D: Utilities and quality-adjusted life years, *Tech Assess Health Care* 5:559-575, 1989.

44. Kaplan RM, Anderson JP, Ganiats TG: The Quality of Well-being Scale: rationale for a single quality of life index. In Walker SR, Rosser RM (eds): *Quality of life assessment: key issues in the 1990s*, Dordrecht, 1993, Kluwer Academic Publishers.

45. Rosser R, Allison R, Butler C, et al: The Index of Health-related Quality of Life (IHQL): a new tool for audit and cost-per-QALY analysis. In Walker SR, Rosser RM (eds): *Quality of life assessment: key issues in the 1990s*, Dordrecht, 1993, Kluwer Academic Publishers.

46. Rosser R, Sintonen H: The EuroQol quality of life project. In Walker SR, Rosser RM (eds): *Quality of life assessment: key issues in the 1990s*, Dordrecht, 1993, Kluwer Academic Publishers.

47. Revicki DA: Relationship between health utility and psychometric health status measures, *Med Care* 30(5):MS274-MS282, 1992.

48. Tsevat J, Goldman L, Lamas GA, et al: Functional status versus utilities in survivors of myocardial infarction, *Med Care* 29(11):1153-1159, 1991.

49. Tsevat J, Goldman L, Soukup JR, et al: Stability of time-tradeoff utilities in survivors of myocardial infarction, *Med Decis Making* 13:161-165, 1993.

50. Katz JN, Phillips CB, Fossel AH, et al: Stability and responsiveness of utility measures, *Med Care* 32(2):183-188, 1994.

51. O'Brien BJ, Buxton MJ, Patterson DL: Relationship between functional status and health-related quality-of-life after myocardial infarction, *Med Care* 31(10):950-955, 1993.

52. Deyo RA, Diehr P, Patrick DL: Reproducibility and responsiveness of health status measures. Statistics and strategies for evaluation, *Controlled Clin Trials* 12:142S-158S, 1991.

53. Epstein AM, Hall JA, Tognetti J, et al: Using proxies to evaluate quality of life. Can they provide valid information about patients' health status and satisfaction with medical care? *Med Care* 27(3):S91-S98, 1989.

54. Rothman ML, Hedrick SC, Bulcroft KA, et al: The validity of proxy-generated scores as measures of patient health status, *Med Care* 29(2):115-124, 1991.

55. Schleifer SJ, Macari-Hinson MM, Coyle DA, et al: The nature and course of depression following myocardial infarction, *Arch Intern Med* 149:1785-1789, 1989.

56. Frasure-Smith N, Lesperance F, Talajic M: Depression following myocardial infarction. Impact on 6-month survival, *JAMA* 270(15):1819-1825, 1993.

57. Carney RM, Rich MW, teVelde A, et al: Major depressive disorder in coronary artery disease, *Am J Cardiol* 60:1273-1275, 1987.

58. Oldridge NB, Guyatt GH, Fischer ME, et al: Cardiac rehabilitation after myocardial infarction: combined experience of randomized clinical trials, *JAMA* 260:945-950, 1988.

59. Davidson DM: Return to work after cardiac events: a review, *J Cardiac Rehab* 3:60-69, 1983.

60. Smith GR, O'Rourke DF: Return to work after a first myocardial infarction. A test of multiple hypotheses, *JAMA* 259:1673-1677, 1988.

61. Rost K, Smith GR: Return to work after an initial myocardial infarction and subsequent emotional distress, *Arch Intern Med* 152:381-385, 1992.

62. Mark DB, Lam LC, Lee KL, et al: Comparison of coronary angioplasty, coronary bypass surgery and medical therapy on employment in patients with coronary artery disease: a prospective comparison study, *Ann Intern Med* 120:111-117, 1994.

63. Dennis C, Houston-Miller N, Schwartz RG, et al: Early return to work after uncomplicated myocardial infarction. Results of a randomized trial, *JAMA* 260:214-220, 1988.

64. Pilote L, Thomas RJ, Dennis C, et al: Return to work after uncomplicated myocardial infarction: a trial of practice guidelines in the community, *Ann Intern Med* 117:383-389, 1992.

65. Wiklund I, Herlitz J, Hjalmarson A: Quality of life five years after myocardial infarction, *Eur Heart J* 10:464-472, 1989.

66. Wiklund I, Herlitz J, Bengtson A, et al: Long-term follow-up of health-related quality of life in patients with suspected acute myocardial infarction when the diagnosis was not confirmed, *Scand J Prim Health Care* 9:47-52, 1991.

67. Olsson G, Lubsen J, van Es GA, et al: Quality of life after myocardial infarction: effect of long-term metoprolol on mortality and morbidity, *Br Med J* 292:1491-1493, 1986.

68. Elliott JM, Williams BF, White HD: Streptokinase and lifestyle outcome in survivors of myocardial infarction, *NZ Med J* May:163-164, 1992.

69. Mark DB, Naylor CD, Califf RM, et al: Less catheterization and revascularization following myocardial infarction in Canada is associated with more angina: initial results from the Canadian-US GUSTO substudy (abstract), *Circulation* 88:I-479, 1993.

70. Neill WA, Branch LG, De Jong G, et al: Cardiac disability. The impact of coronary heart disease on patients' daily activities, *Arch Intern Med* 145:1642-1647, 1985.

71. Oka RK, Stotts NA, Dae MW, et al: Daily physical activity levels in congestive heart failure, *Am J Cardiol* 71:921-925, 1993.

72. Smith RF, Johnson G, Ziesche S, et al for the V-HeFT VA Cooperative Studies Group: Functional capacity in heart failure. Comparison of methods for assessment and their relation to other indexes of heart failure, *Circulation* 1993; 87(suppl VI):88-93, 1993.

73. Mark DB, Nelson C, DeLong E, et al: Comparison of quality of life outcomes following coronary angioplasty, coronary bypass surgery and medicine (abstract), *J Am Coll Cardiol* 21(2):216A, 1993.

74. Rector TS, Johnson G, Dunkman B, et al for the V-HeFT VA Cooperative Studies Group: Evaluation by patients with heart failure of the effects of enalapril compared with hydralazine plus isosorbide dinitrate on quality of life, *Circulation* 87(suppl VI):71-77, 1993.

75. Parkerson GR Jr, Gehlbach SH, Wagner EH, et al: The Duke-UNC Health Profile: an adult health status instrument for primary care, *Med Care* 19(8):806-828, 1981.

76. Katz S, Downs TD, Cash HR, et al: Progress in development of the index of ADL, *Gerontologist* Spring:20-30, 1970.

77. Fillenbaum GG (ed): *Multidimensional functional assessment of older adults. The Duke Older Americans Resources and Services Procedures*, Hillsdale, NJ, 1988, Lawrence Erlbaum Associates, Inc.

78. Bittner V, Weiner DH, Yusuf S, et al for the SOLVD Investigators: Prediction of mortality and morbidity with a 6-minute walk test in patients with left ventricular dysfunction, *JAMA* 270(14):1702-1707, 1993.

79. Guyatt GH, Sullivan MJ, Thompson PJ, et al: The 6-minute walk: a new measure of exercise capacity in patients with chronic heart failure, *Can Med Assoc J* 132:919-923, 1985.

80. Goldman L, Hashimoto B, Cook EF, et al: Comparative reproducibility and validity of systems for assessing cardiovascular functional class: advantages of a new Specific Activity Scale, *Circulation* 64:1227-1134, 1981.

81. Beck AT, Kovacs M, Weissman A: Hopelessness and suicidal behavior: an overview, *JAMA* 234(11):1146-1149, 1975.

82. Koenig HG, Meador KG, Cohen HJ, et al: Self-rated depression scales and screening for major depression in the older hospitalized patient with medical illness, *J Am Geriatr Soc* 36:699-706, 1988.

83. Goldberg DP, Blackwell B: Psychiatric illness in general practice. A detailed study using a new method of case identification, *Br Med J* 2:439-443, 1970.
84. Goldberg DP, Hillier VF: A scaled version of the General Health Questionnaire, *Psychol Med* 9:139-145, 1979.
85. Fazio AF (ed): *A concurrent validation study of the NCHS general well-being schedule,* ed 2, Hyattsville, Md, 1977, US Department of HEW, National Center for Health Statistics.
86. Berwick DM, Murphy JM, Goldman PA, et al: Performance of a five-item mental health screening test, *Med Care* 29:169-176, 1991.
87. Pinsky JL, Jette AM, Branch LG, et al: The Framingham disability study: relationship of various coronary heart disease manifestations to disability in older persons living in the community, *Am J Public Health* 80:1363-1368, 1990.
88. Branch LG, Jette AM: The Framingham Disability Study: I. Social disability among the aging, *Am J Public Health* 71:1202-1210, 1981.
89. Rose GA, Blackburn H, Gillum RF, et al (eds): *Cardiovascular survey methods,* Geneva, 1982, World Health Organization.
90. Bruce RA: Evaluation of functional capacity and exercise tolerance of cardiac patients. I. Functional capacity, *Mod Concepts Cardiovasc Dis* 25(4):321-326, 1956.

91. Cox J, Naylor CD: The Canadian Cardiovascular Society grading scale for angina of effort: is it time for refinements? *Ann Intern Med* 117(8):677-683, 1992.
92. Rector TS, Kubo SH, Cohn JN: Patients' self-assessment of their congestive heart failure. Part 2: Content, reliability and validity of a new measure, The Minnesota Living with Heart Failure Questionnaire, *Heart Failure* Oct/Nov:198-209, 1987.
93. Rector TS, Kubo SH, Cohn JN: Validity of the Minnesota Living with Heart Failure Questionnaire as a measure of therapeutic response to enalapril or placebo, *Am J Cardiol* 71:1106-1107, 1993.
94. Spertus JA, Winder JA, Dewhurst TA, et al: Development and evaluation of the Seattle Angina Questionnaire: a new functional status measure for coronary artery disease, *Ann Intern Med* 1994 (in press).
95. L-Y Lim L, Valenti LA, Knapp JC, et al: A self-administered quality-of-life questionnaire after acute myocardial infarction, *J Clin Epidemiol* 46(11):1249-1256, 1993.
96. Stewart AL, Greenfield S, Hays RD: Functional status and well-being of patients with chronic conditions. Results from the Medical Outcomes Study, *JAMA* 262(7):907-913, 1989.

ACUTE CARDIAC ISCHEMIA TIME–INSENSITIVE PREDICTIVE INSTRUMENT (ACI-TIPI): A DECISION AID FOR EMERGENCY DEPARTMENT TRIAGE AND A MEASURE OF APPROPRIATENESS OF CORONARY CARE UNIT USE

Harry P. Selker
John L. Griffith
Joni R. Beshansky

In the United States, acute cardiac ischemia (ACI), here referring to both unstable angina pectoris and acute myocardial infarction (AMI), is a leading cause of morbidity and mortality and an enormous consumer of health care resources. The use of intensive care beds for patients suspected to have ACI is particularly expensive. Yet of the 1.5 million U.S. patients admitted to coronary care units (CCUs) for suspected ACI each year, more than half prove not to have true ACI,[1,2] and only about half of those with ACI have AMIs.[3-6] These unnecessary CCU admissions represent a substantial waste; in this country the direct costs alone may be as much as $3 billion annually.[7]

Although the high proportion of seemingly unnecessary admissions is not desired, it has been assumed that a more restrictive admission policy would increase the numbers of patients with AMI inappropriately sent home. Generally about 2% to 4% of those who do have AMIs are mistakenly sent home.[1,3,5,8] Beyond the cost and potential adverse effects of unnecessary false-positive CCU admissions and with the growing number of acute interventions for treating arrhythmias or preventing or reducing AMI size, there is also growing interest in changing the historically stable false-negative AMI discharge rate. Attempts to improve the accuracy of emergency department (ED) triage of patients with suspected ACI have included the use of identification of high-risk clinical indicators,[9,10] rapid determination of cardiac enzymes,[11,12] two-dimensional echocardiography,[13] and thallium-201 scintigraphy.[14] However, none of these has been shown prospectively to reduce the number of CCU admissions for patients without ACI.[1,15] In that context, in recent years there has been work to devise mathematically-based decision aids to try to improve ED triage.[1,2,4,15] (A review of the roles of clinical history, physical examination, the electrocardiogram [ECG], cardiac enzymes, and newer diagnostic decision aids for ED triage can be found in a recent review.[2])

GENERAL METHODOLOGIC ISSUES IN THE STUDY OF ED TRIAGE OF PATIENTS WITH SUSPECTED ACI

A number of methodologic issues are important to the study of triage of ED patients with suspected ACI. First, the prevalence of ACI among a population studied can dramatically alter the predictive value of a particular symptom, sign, or test.[16] For example, ST-segment depression may appear very predictive of infarction among *CCU patients* but would be much less predictive among *ED patients*. Similarly, even ED-based studies may not apply to EDs where the ACI prevalence is significantly different from the study sites. The setting and role of the study hospital (e.g., urban vs. rural or teaching vs. community hospital) may affect the generalizability of a study's findings, particularly by this mechanism. Optimally a range of hospitals with widely varying prevalence of ACI will be included.

Studies of ED triage can also be strongly affected by issues of inclusion criteria. For example, if only patients with chest pain are studied, the results may not apply to the 13% to 25% of patients with AMI who do not have chest pain.[1,17-19] Thus, entry criteria should be broad, including those patients whose ACI, and particularly AMI, manifests *without* chest pain, as well as those who have typical pain.

The definition of the diagnostic endpoint is also important in studies of ED triage. Many studies have focused on identifying or predicting only AMI.[4,16] However, diagnosing unstable or new-onset angina pectoris is also important, because it can lead to hospital monitoring and early therapy during a high-risk period and possibly prevent progression to AMI. Indeed, approximately 9% of patients admitted with new-onset or unstable angina progress to AMI.[20,21] Thus, the clinically relevant group for study of ED triage includes *all* ACI patients rather than only those who prove to have AMIs.

Completeness of follow-up in terms of both study subjects and key data is another critical ingredient of ED triage studies. For example, the occurrence of AMI may be seriously underestimated if patients are lost to follow-up (perhaps related to their having an AMI that includes sudden death) or if the follow-up evaluation does not include cardiac enzyme tests. Follow-up with repeat ECGs and cardiac enzyme analyses after the patient is admitted or sent home is therefore essential to such studies.

Finally, for ED decision aids, the validation of actual clinical impact is key. Although measuring the misclassification rate and performance characteristics in independent samples is important, even more critical is a *prospective trial of a decision aid's effects on patient care* in diverse settings.[22] To date, the only such tool to survive such a clinical trial is the ACI predictive instrument.[1,15]

MATHEMATICALLY-BASED DECISION AIDS FOR ACI

The goal of mathematically-based diagnostic aids for ACI and AMI is to improve physicians' use of clinical information. This may be done by directing attention to important variables, quantifying risk, and reassuring physicians in the face of uncertainty.[22] Early work suggests that of these potential functions, improving physicians' risk estimates may be the most important.[23]

The first diagnostic aid for suspected ACI was Sawe's "clinical diagnostic index," which predicted AMI based on nine clinical variables derived by discriminant analysis.[24] Important predictive variables in his model included ECG signs of AMI, extension of pain to the jaw or arms, a history of unstable angina, and a respiratory rate more than 16 breaths/min. Although when tested prospectively it was 100% sensitive for AMI, its poor specificity (16%) limited its practical value.

From multivariate analysis of 655 ED patients with chest pain, Tierney et al.[25] identified four variables with independent predictive values for infarction: ST-segment elevation, new Q waves, diaphoresis with chest pain, and history of AMI. Compared with physicians, this model was more specific (86% vs. 78%) but somewhat less sensitive (81% vs. 87%) and therefore was considered unlikely to significantly improve triage accuracy. A prospective trial of its clinical use has not been reported.

Using recursive partitioning analysis, Goldman et al.[4,16] developed computer-derived protocols to segregate ED patients with chest pain by their clinical manifestations and ECG findings into subgroups with different likelihoods of AMI. The protocols predicted AMI for those subgroups with a probability of 7% or greater. The earlier protocol's sensitivity (92%) and specificity (70%) did not differ from that of physicians.[4] More recently, this group[16] combined their earlier data to revise their protocol. In a hypothetical test on prospectively collected data from 4770 patients with chest pain admitted to six hospitals, the protocol's 88% sensitivity in predicting AMI was no different than physicians', but the protocol's specificity was better than physicians' (74% vs. 71%, respectively, $P < 0.001$). To date, results of a prospective clinical trial of the actual impact of either the original or revised tool have not been reported.

Using multivariable logistic regression, we[15] developed "predictive instruments" that provide ED physicians with a given patient's probability of ACI. These instruments incorporate clinical and ECG findings of ED patients with symptoms suggestive of ACI, including chest pain, abdominal pain or nausea, shortness of breath, and dizziness or lightheadedness. (These inclusion criteria were based on the Imminent Rotterdam MI[IMIR] Criteria, which have been shown to capture more than 90% of all patients in a community with ACI.[26]) In the controlled prospective trials of the instrument's use, first at Boston City Hospital[15] and then in six hospitals in diverse settings,[1] the use of the predictive instrument reduced false-positive CCU admissions by 30%, with no increase in false-negative discharges to home. This and related work are reviewed further later on.

DEVELOPMENT OF THE ACI TIME-INSENSITIVE PREDICTIVE INSTRUMENT (ACI-TIPI) AS AN ED TRIAGE DECISION AID
Original ACI predictive instrument and its prospective clinical trial

Given that more than half of admissions for presumed ACI prove to be false-positive, an ideal diagnostic aid for ACI would increase physicians' diagnostic specificity without decreasing their already high diagnostic sensitivity. Reasoning that a single numerical probability value might be easily incorporated into physicians' clinical decision-making processes, in the Boston City Hospital[15] and Multicenter Predictive Instrument Trials,[1] the aim was to develop and prospectively test a mathematical instrument that could provide ED physicians with a patient's calculated likelihood of having ACI. The Boston City Hospital study was the pilot for the larger study and had essentially the same results; only the multicenter trial is reviewed here. The Multicenter study had two 1-year phases: development of the predictive instrument and a prospective trial of its use in the participating hospitals' EDs.[1]

In phase 1, the predictive instrument was developed from data on the 2801 study subjects seen in the six participating hospitals' EDs from March 1979 through February 1980. Beginning with 59 clinical features available to ED physicians, including clinical manifestation, history, physical findings, ECG, sociodemographic characteristics, and coronary disease risk factors, we developed an equation that used only 7 variables that were applicable to all 6 hospitals. These variables

required that the clinician specify whether the patient had a chief complaint of chest discomfort, a history of heart attack or of nitroglycerine use, and features of the ECG ST segments and T waves. This mathematically-based instrument provided an estimate of a patient's likelihood of having true ACI expressed as a value between 0% and 100%. Once programmed into a hand-held calculator, into which the clinician enters yes or no responses regarding the presence of the variables, the actual use of the instrument required less than 20 seconds of computation time.

Phase 2 was an 11-month prospective trial of the predictive instrument's impact that included 2320 patients who were seen in the 6 hospitals' EDs: 1288 during experimental periods and 1032 during control periods. The instrument's use markedly improved physicians' *diagnostic performance*. Specificity was significantly superior during the experimental periods ($P = 0.002$), with no significant change in sensitivity. The false-positive diagnosis ("predictive") rate improved significantly ($P = 0.004$) without any deterioration in the false-negative diagnosis ("predictive") rate. In terms of actual *admission practices,* for patients who proved to have ACI, there was no difference between the experimental and control periods. However, for patients *without* ACI, CCU admission rates were significantly lower during the experimental periods ($P = 0.003$), dropping from 24% during the control periods to 17%, and their ED discharge rates to home increased from 44% during the control periods to 51%. This represents a *30% reduction in CCU admissions for patients without ACI.* Expressed using the CCU population as the denominator, the proportion of patients admitted to the CCU that did not have ACI fell from 44% to 33% ($P = 0.001$).

Further analysis was done to try to determine which patients benefitted most from the use of the predictive instrument. For patients whose likelihood of having ACI was *less than 50%,* there was a 22% reduction ($P = 0.0002$) in the false-positive diagnosis rate during the experimental periods, whereas for patients with likelihoods of having ACI exceeding 50%, the improvement did not reach statistical significance. Thus, the predictive instrument *was most helpful for correctly diagnosing patients with less definite signs and symptoms of ACI,* whereas physician judgment alone was sufficient to diagnose ACI correctly in patients with higher probabilities of ACI. This is consistent with more recent results suggesting that much of the predictive instrument's effect is due to reducing uncertainty for the patient for whom the "correct" clinical decision is not clear.[8,27]

Based on the more than 1.5 million patients with suspected ACI admitted to CCUs every year in this country, a nationwide reduction in admissions comparable with that seen in this study would reduce the number of CCU admissions by more than *250,000 each year*. Thus, if widely used, the predictive instrument for ACI would likely have important medical and financial benefit. However, despite considerable attention that was given the study on its release and continued interest, the instrument has not become widely used. It was the appreciation of the cumbersomeness of the programmable calculator version that led us to try to improve the attractiveness of its use, including the incorporation of a revised version of the original instrument, the acute cardiac ischemia time-insensitive predictive instrument (ACI-TIPI), into the electrocardiograph, as described later on.

Development and testing of the ACI-TIPI

Two general approaches have been tried to improve the appropriateness of CCU use: prospective real-time interventions, as described earlier, and retrospective assessment for feedback, as for utilization review. Although prospectively used clinical tools may seem more attractive than currently available feedback systems, feedback about triage performance based on retrospective analysis will remain important for physicians' and institutions' self-assessment, and this approach is now getting more attention as part of efforts to continuously improve quality of care. Moreover, the payors and organizations responsible for hospital and CCU use need a retrospective tool by which the appropriateness of CCU use can be accurately measured. Ideally a *single* tool should be able to serve *both* prospective (clinical) and retrospective purposes, but to date this has not been the case. Generally tools designed for real-time use, such as the original predictive instrument, have not been validated for retrospective medical record review. Conversely, tools developed for retrospective review of clinical practice have not been applicable to the real-time clinical setting, undermining clinicians' interest and confidence in such methods. Thus we sought to develop a new *time-insensitive* predictive instrument (TIPI), valid for *both* prospective real-time clinical use and retrospective medical record review, that would accurately predict a patient's likelihood of having ACI, as of the time of ED presentation.[28] Not only theoretically desirable as a tool usable by clinicians, hospital administrators, and payors, it might have the added benefit of promoting cooperation among these groups in optimizing CCU use. (This line of reasoning also was applied to the AMI mortality predictive instrument,[29] congestive heart failure predictive instrument,[30] and the thrombolytic predictive instrument,[31] which could prove to be of equal importance as tools for clinical use and for outcome assessment.)

Indeed, we initially investigated the use of the original predictive instrument for retrospective use, but, unfortunately, in preliminary investigations, two clinical history variables were found to be unreliable via medical

record review, thus precluding the instrument's retrospective use. Thus, we reformulated the instrument with a new set of clinical variables that were reliably available in the real-time clinical setting and by retrospective review. (In doing so, because of the potential ambiguity of the ECG reading of the "ST-segment straightening" variable in the original instrument, we also chose to eliminate this variable from a reformulated instrument.)

The 3453 patients seen during the original study's first year were the basis for the development of the new ACI-TIPI using multivariable logistic regression.[28] Starting with the most important variables from initial models, we tested candidate variables for their reliability of retrospective abstraction by two blinded independent reviewers who examined the ED records of 100 subjects. This allowed for the development of a final set of variables and a final logistic regression equation of the same format as the original instruments, requiring the input of the following seven clinical factors for a given patient: age; sex; the presence or absence of chest pain or pressure or left arm pain; whether or not chest pain or pressure was the patient's most important presenting symptom; the presence or absence of ECG Q waves; the presence and degree of ECG ST-segment elevation or depression; and the presence and degree of ECG T-wave elevation or inversion.

When the instrument was reformulated, an intentional change was made in the performance of the instrument. Although an instrument for CCU admission should properly identify all patients with *ACI* (and hopefully thereby help prevent progression to AMI in some), we designed the new instrument to give somewhat *higher probability predictions for patients with AMI* than those with unstable angina pectoris, to create bias against false-negative predictions for the more severe cases. This was accomplished by including more detail in the ACI-TIPI's specification of its ECG ST-segment and T-wave variables. For example, in the new instrument, ST-segment depression of 0.1 mV is given 1 point, depression of 0.2 mV is given 2 points, and so forth, whereas for the former instrument ST-segment depression was merely dichotomized as "yes" or "no" for depression of 0.1 mV or more.[28]

The diagnostic performance test phase included the application of the ACI-TIPI to the 2320 patients seen at the six study hospitals' EDs during the second year. The original predictive instrument had also been applied to these patients, allowing direct comparison, and ED physician diagnostic performance for ACI was also assessed for comparison to the instruments' predictions.

Calculation of the receiver-operating characteristic (ROC) curve area, which simultaneously evaluates sensitivity and specificity of a continuous scale test, yielded values of 0.88 to 0.89 for the ACI-TIPI and the original instrument, demonstrating excellent and very similar diagnostic performance by both. The fact that the instruments' ROC curve paths include the point depicting ED physicians' performance (sensitivity 95%, specificity 73%) suggests that the instruments perform comparably with physicians when one considers the probability scale as only "yes" or "no" diagnoses based on a single cut point (at probability 25%). Using such a single cut point classifies all scores higher than (and all scores lower than) the cut point as being equivalent; in other words, a 30% likelihood of ACI is considered diagnostically identical to 95% (and 20% is considered diagnostically identical to 5%) and ignores the large amount of clinical information contained in the instrument's full 0% to 100% probability scale. Thus, although direct comparison with physicians' performance is not possible, the ACI-TIPI clearly compares favorably. This is quite encouraging for a single equation based on a patient's age, gender, complaint of chest pain, ECG Q waves, ST segments, and T waves.

Although the full 0% to 100% probability range has more information, and for groups of patients will more accurately predict, than dichotomous or categorical diagnostic designations, in clinical and especially retrospective settings, specified probability cut-points that separate patients into different risk groups might be useful. In the ED, the terms "low," "medium," and "high" probability of ACI might be more intuitively helpful to some physicians than an actual probability value and might be more helpful as an aid to retrospectively review patient care. Such a risk stratification system was developed by dividing, in the Development Phase, the 3453 ED patients into four similar-sized groups based on the ACI-TIPI probability scale by cutting at 10%, 25%, and 55% to create higher and lower ACI probability groups. (When this was done, the actual midpoint of each probability range, 5%, 17.5%, 40%, and 77.5%, never differed by more than 1% from the actual observed proportion of patients with ACI, confirming the excellent calibration of ACI-TIPI's predictions.[28]) Given that such low, medium, and high probability categories might be used by themselves as a diagnostic tool, we believed that, like any other diagnostic test, such categories should be developed on one set of patients and then prospectively tested on an independent sample. When the accuracy of the four ACI probability groups was prospectively tested on year 2 patients, among the 552 patients in the low probability group, only 1.6% had ACI, of whom only 0.7% had AMIs, whereas among the 484 patients in the high probability group, 81.6% had ACI, including 53.3% with AMIs. Of note, because of the bias built into this instrument to give higher scores to patients with AMI, as desired, of those with ACI in each group, *the subproportions of those with AMI were disproportionately low in the lower probability groups and disproportionately high in the*

higher risk groups. The marked clinical difference between the high (ACI probability >55%) and low (ACI probability ≤10%) probability groups can be illustrated by comparing them with current ED triage practice. *If the entire high probability group were admitted to the CCU, this would reflect diagnostic performance superior to that of current CCU admitting practices. If all patients in the low probability group were sent home, fewer patients than at present would be sent home with ACI or AMI.*[28]

Given the very similar performance of the original and new instruments, the ACI-TIPI's use should result in the substantially improved CCU admitting practices demonstrated with the use of the original instrument. If any difference in the ACI-TIPI's impact in clinical use is to be expected, given its slightly higher scores for patients with AMI, there might actually be a tendency to improve rather than leave unchanged the sensitivity of CCU admission for AMI. Moreover, in settings where retrospective review of CCU admission practice is desired, clearly the ACI-TIPI would seem preferable. This is now being tested in a multicenter controlled clinical trial. Results of pilot trials at Harbor UCLA Medical Center and at the University of Geneva Hospital are outlined later on.

INCORPORATION OF THE ACI-TIPI INTO A COMPUTERIZED ELECTROCARDIOGRAPH: A USER-FRIENDLY DECISION AID TO ASSIST REAL-TIME ED TRIAGE DECISIONS

The original predictive instrument has been used in several ways. A physician can carry a calculator to allow quick access to the probability value. Alternatively, an ED triage nurse can compute the value and write it on the clinical record for the physician's use in a manner similar to vital signs recording. However, a more attractive method is the integration of the instrument into a computerized electrocardiograph: once the non-ECG clinical variables (age, sex, and chest pain) have been entered, the machine can automatically assess the ECG variables and compute a patient's probability of having ACI while generating the ECG. Convinced that the predictive instrument's probability would be more likely used if provided automatically, we incorporated the ACI-TIPI into a computerized electrocardiograph.[32] Comparing the electrocardiograph version of the ACI-TIPI to the generation of ACI probabilities based on the interpretations of an electrocardiographer showed exact agreement on 85% of 100 ECGs, and cases of disagreement were all on minor differences in ST-segment depression or T-wave flattening vs. inversion. For the ECGs on which the electrocardiographer and the computer disagreed, the average difference between probability values based on their respective interpretations was 2%. Samples of ACI-TIPI ECGs are shown in Fig. 17-1.

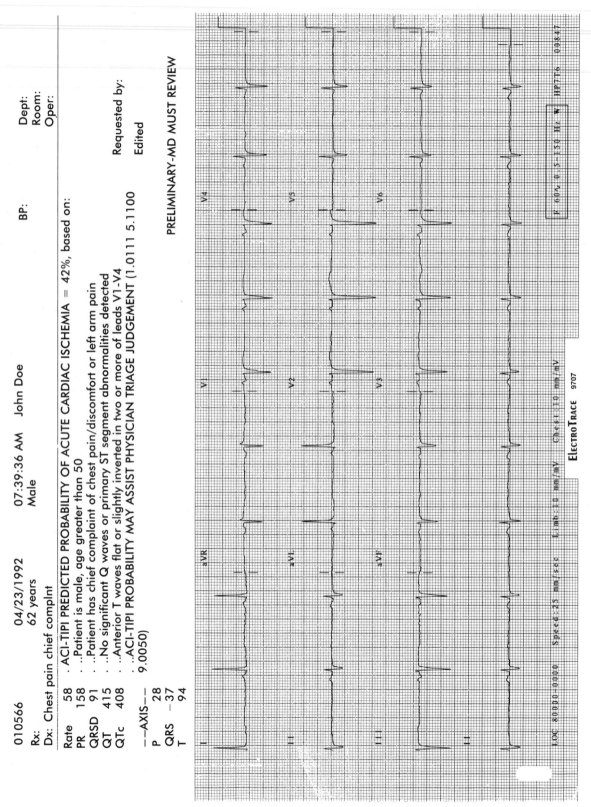

Fig. 17-1. Electrocardiogram from ACI-TIPI Electrocardiograph.

AMI and AMI–related complications as outcomes of importance in the use of the ACI-TIPI: pilot study at Harbor UCLA General Hospital

In a preliminary test of the ACI-TIPI electrocardiograph's performance, we performed a 3-month prospective study at the Harbor UCLA General Hospital. Included were all consenting ED patients 35 years old or older who had chest pain and no abnormalities on chest x-ray film or history of thoracic trauma.[33] For each study ED patient, an ECG with the ACI-TIPI's 0% to 100% probability was generated in real-time but was not provided to the ED physician. However, ED physicians recorded their own qualitative estimate of the probability of ACI (also expressed as a 0%-100% probability) to provide a comparison with the ACI-TIPI's performance. In this investigation, the primary interest was in AMI and complications of AMI rather than ACI per se, which had been the outcome used in our previous investigations. Thus, the diagnostic performance for the detection of AMI or acute complications of ACI were calculated for the ACI-TIPI prediction and physician triage. Characteristic creatine kinase MB (CK-MB) fraction elevations were used to define AMI, and acute complications of AMI were defined as the occurrence of life-threatening ventricular arrhythmias and congestive heart failure requiring continuous intravenous infusion and ICU care.

Of the 189 study patients, 101 were admitted, including 17 to ward beds (mean ACI-TIPI probability 21%; no AMIs, no complications), 38 to monitored telemetry beds (mean ACI-TIPI 41% ± 4; four AMIs, four complications), and 46 to CCU beds (ACI-TIPI 52%; 13 AMIs, 17 complications). There were 88 patients discharged home (mean ACI-TIPI 25%). As a "diagnostic test" for AMI or complications of ACI, the use of a "cut-off" ACI-TIPI probability of 38% had a sensitivity of 93%, specificity of 74%, a predictive value positive of 59%, and a predictive value negative of 96%. Physician triage for AMI and complications had a sensitivity of 83%, specificity of 69%, a predictive value positive of 52%, and a predictive value negative of 91%. The ROC area for predicting AMI and complications was 0.85 for ACI-TIPI and 0.64 for ED physicians.

Despite the limitations of this preliminary work, including having insufficient resources to follow-up nonadmitted patients, the ACI-TIPI did show utility as a diagnostic test in predicting which patients were at risk for AMI or ACI complications. For this reason, these outcomes will be studied further in subsequent ACI-TIPI trials.

This trial supported another potentially new area of improvement by the ACI-TIPI electrocardiograph: *the reduction of false-negative ED discharges of AMI patients to home.* We had hoped that the increased discrimination built into the ACI-TIPI formula for AMI,[28] as well as the increased sensitivity and reliability of ECG measurement of the computerized electrocardiograph, would avoid missing ECG abnormalities that are important for the predictive instrument,[34] thereby reducing false-negative discharges. During this preliminary trial we did find anecdotal support for this: in specific cases, unblinding the ACI-TIPI value after the physician triage decision had been made led to a changed decision to admit rather than send home.[33] This was particularly true with cases of "non-Q-wave" AMI, including one case where the ACI-TIPI electrocardiograph led to the detection of an otherwise unrecognized ominous ECG findings in a patient who developed ventricular fibrillation soon thereafter.[33]

Impact of the ACI-TIPI on the speed of ED triage: Geneva, Switzerland, ACI-TIPI trial

In collaboration with physicians at the University Hospital in Geneva, we recently completed another pilot study of the ACI-TIPI electrocardiograph.[35] This trial was designed and implemented in this hospital to address a different aspect of potential impact of the ACI-TIPI: its impact on the *speed of triage for patients with suspected ACI.* This hospital's practice is that patients are held in the ED until multiple CK tests are done to confirm the presence of an AMI before CCU admission. This has two results: there are fewer than half as many false-positive (non-ACI) CCU admissions as is typical of American hospitals, and patients spend much more time in the ED. Therefore, this trial was not directed at changing triage *disposition* but at changing *ED triage speed.* We wondered whether the additional information provided by the ACI-TIPI's probability value would prompt ED physicians and others involved in the care of a patient to triage more quickly. Specifically, this trial sought to determine the impact of the ACI-TIPI on the speed of ED triage and transfer from the ED for patients seen with symptoms suggesting ACI, particularly among physicians at earlier stages in their training.

The trial ran 7 months, with the ACI-TIPI electrocardiograph being set to provide its probability value every other month. Men and women more than 40 years of age with chest pain or other symptoms suggestive of ACI were included, totaling 605.

To test the hypothesis that the use of the ACI-TIPI changes physicians' ED triage speed, we used multivariate linear regression predicting patient time from ED manifestation to triage decision-making and to actual discharge from the ED (the results were consistent; only time to ED discharge is presented here). When the ACI-TIPI value was available, ED time to triage was decreased by 0.7 hour (18%) for patients with ACI seen by physicians in their first ED rotation ($P = 0.007$). Subanalyses by type of ACI revealed that the ACI-TIPI's use was associated with a 0.9-hour reduction (23%) for patients with unstable angina ($P = 0.01$), a 0.6-hour reduction (15%) for patients with AMI ($P = 0.1$), and a 1.1-hour reduction (24%) for AMI patients who received thrombolytic therapy ($P = 0.2$). (In addition to the ACI-TIPI use, important factors affecting ED time to triage were (1) patient's age greater than 65 years ($+0.9$ hour, $P = 0.0001$), (2) whether the CCU was full ($+0.5$ hour, $P = 0.05$), (3) night-time ED manifestation ($+0.8$ hour, $P = 0.0005$), and use of thrombolytic therapy (-1.7 hours, $P = 0.0001$).)

The 18% improvement in the speed of ED triage decision by use of the ACI-TIPI may have been the result of several mechanisms. It may be that in the ED triage clinical setting, where decisions are made under the stress of limited time and resources, a readily available "second opinion" based on explicit criteria may facilitate physician triage decision-making. Another hypothesis is that the impact of the ACI-TIPI might have resulted from directing physician attention to important clinical variables (age, sex, chest pain, and key ECG findings), by quantifying risk numerically, or by reassuring the physician in the face of uncertainty. In either case, it does not seem surprising that less experienced physicians benefitted more from the real-time availability of the ACI-TIPI than the more experienced residents or staff. These results suggest the need for more study of the ACI-TIPI's impact among physicians of diverse training backgrounds at different types of hospitals.

Given that the success of procedures to prevent or limit AMI (such as thrombolytic therapy) declines rapidly in the first few hours, any aid that speeds identification and treatment of patients with ACI should enhance the quality and success of acute cardiac care. Thus, the improvement in speed of triage provided by the ACI-TIPI may well have an impact on patient outcomes such as mortality and infarct size. This too deserves further study in a larger clinical trial.

This preliminary study in Geneva has important limitations. Among them is that there were relatively small numbers of patients in the study, especially in the different ACI subgroups, thus limiting the outcomes amenable to analysis. Another limitation is that it was conducted in only one hospital, and one not necessarily representative of any U.S. hospital. Clearly a trial at more hospitals representing a broader range of practice situations is needed.

USE OF THE ACI-TIPI TO RETROSPECTIVELY ASSESS APPROPRIATENESS OF CCU ADMISSION

In addition to its presentation of the ACI-TIPI's probability in real-time, the computerized electrocardiograph also has the capacity to support the creation of clinical feedback and operations reports. The computerized electrocardiographs that have the ACI-TIPI typi-

cally have standard personal computer "floppy disk" drives for data storage and transfer. Thus, the ACI-TIPI probability data, ECG data, and other information entered directly into the electrocardiograph in clinical use (e.g., presenting complaint, age, and sex) can be directly transferred to a personal computer, where they can be combined with other data and used for reports and analyses. Combining these tools allows the clinician and operations personnel of a hospital (and payors, HMOs, malpractice carriers, monitoring agencies, etc.) to use the same clinically valid risk-adjusted outcome prediction/measure, with no need for separate medical record–based data acquisition. This allows achievement of seven attributes that we sought to incorporate into the ACI-TIPI as a triage-appropriate assessment system to make it attractive to those who should be working together, namely, clinicians, administrators, consumers, and payors. These seven attributes are as follows:

To earn clinicians' trust and positive involvement, and unlike traditional quality assessment tools, a retrospective assessment system should be sufficiently accurate to also be also valid for clinical use. The ACI-TIPI's accuracy, its ease of use, and its growing evidence of clinical utility meet this criterion.[28]

A particular aspect of accuracy is "calibration," the property of having accurate predictions over the tool's full range of values. In the absence of good calibration, deviations from predicted outcome rates are more likely to reflect inadequacies of the tool than primary differences in quality of care. The Medicare Mortality Prediction System (MMPS), like many medical outcome predictive systems, having poor calibration for patients at both extremes of the mortality risk scale, illustrates the danger of this flaw.[36,37] Because it underpredicts the likelihoods of mortality for more severely ill patients and overpredicts the likelihoods of death for less ill patients, it creates two important biases: *hospitals taking care of more ill patients* will tend to have observed mortality rates above predicted, thus *will appear to be giving poor care;* and *hospitals taking care of less ill patients* will tend to have observed mortality rates lower than predicted and thus *will appear to be providing better than average care.* Unfortunately, in the context of quality assessment by such a system, this rewards hospitals who successfully avoid caring for more severely ill patients. The ACI-TIPI's excellent calibration guards against this problem.[28]

To avoid biases (intentional or unintentional) in the assignment of diagnoses related to individual and local practices, implications for triage opportunities in the real-time setting, and impact for reimbursement, a retrospective care review tool should not be dependent on medical record–based diagnoses.[38] Thus, it is important that the ACI-TIPI is applicable to any patient admitted to the ED with symptoms consistent with cardiac disease, regardless of the assigned or eventual coded ICD-9 diagnosis.

To accurately capture a patient's true presenting risk for ACI, a review tool should determine this risk as it was *at the very time of hospital admittance,* not based on a 24-hour or longer period as is used for the APACHE II, MMPS, and other such tools.[36,37,39-41] Including predictors of outcome severity over a period after hospital admittance may give predictive credit to what is actually already the outcome of poor quality care. This is especially so with cardiac disease, for which there is extensive evidence showing the importance of interventions in the first several hours and from which most deaths occur within the first 24 hours. The ACI-TIPI avoids this problem by using only data available within the first 10 or fewer minutes of care.

A clinical predictor to be used for review should not be affected by where in the hospital or even whether a patient is admitted as an inpatient. Because some patients admitted to hospitals do not generate inpatient hospital records because they are triaged to home or to another institution or because they do not survive sufficiently long, if a clinical outcome-reporting system requires full inpatient records, inclusion biases may contaminate hospital comparisons. Depending on the type of hospital, its aims, its role in the community, and the quality of its ED care, certain types of presenting patients may be more or less likely to be admitted following initial evaluation. Further, if the more detailed data generated in an intensive care unit (ICU) setting are likely to yield a higher severity score or different prediction than would have been generated for the same patient if admitted to a ward bed, there will be biases in retrospective review related to admission practice patterns. Thus, ideally systems should generate clinical predictions based on data generated independent of whether a patient is admitted to ICU, to a ward bed, or not admitted at all. This is the case for the data required for the ACI-TIPI: the chief complaint, age, sex, and the presenting ECG.

Related to the previous requirement, such tools should require only data that are universally collected for patients to whom they relate. Systems that give more weight to high technology or special tests (e.g., Medis-Groups' giving more severity credit to ascites detected by sonogram than to ascites determined by physical examination[42]) will reward hospitals for using more tests regardless of appropriateness. Unfortunately, this does not necessarily mean that using only the basic medical record itself avoids this bias. Clearly the quantity and quality of documentation vary among different hospitals, often in parallel with differences in patient populations because of referrals, physician practice types, the availability of special expertise and facilities, and with the use of physician trainees. Thus, ideally a clinical prediction

system should require minimal and universally collected, if any, information from the medical record. This is in fact the case with the ACI-TIPI.

Finally, to have any chance of widespread use, a clinical predictive reporting system must be easy to use and flexible. This is increasingly important given hospitals' increasing loads of reviews and reports mandated by payors and agencies. A retrospective review system that can be used quickly and reliably with commonly available equipment and (computerized) systems will be much more likely to have a positive impact. In this light, it is a distinct advantage that all of the ACI-TIPI's required data can easily be collected automatically via currently available computerized electrocardiographs without resorting to medical records. Given the time and expense of record handling that is saved, along with its automatic availability for real-time clinical use, we believe that such an implementation should provide an excellent opportunity for clinicians and reviewers of care to use the very same tool and to work together in assessing and, when necessary, improving care.

The ACI-TIPI electrocardiograph linked with a computerized reporting system could incorporate the previously cited desirable features of an "ideal" retrospective review system; however, such systems are only now being designed and built. Nonetheless, the needed components are available, and clinicians, investigators, hospitals, and other components of the health care system that participate in the creation of such systems should find their efforts well repaid.

FUTURE OF PREDICTIVE INSTRUMENTS AND ED DECISION AIDS

What is the current status of ED decision aids? The "ultimate measure of a prediction rule is its effect on patient care."[22] Before a decision aid is recommended for general use, clinical trials of any decision aid should demonstrate that it actually will safely improve ED triage and CCU admissions, especially given the risks inherent in reducing CCU admissions and the general lack of experience with such tools.[27]

To date, the ACI predictive instruments are the only such aids shown to be effective in such trials. A related AMI mortality TIPI that predicts cardiac mortality for presenting ED patients has been published[29] and presumably will also be incorporated into an electrocardiograph and then subjected to clinical trials. In addition, currently under development is the thrombolytic predictive instrument (TPI), which will provide ED clinicians with predictions printed on the ECG header of the likely benefit and adverse effects from the use of thrombolytic therapy for AMI for a given patient, again to assist real-time clinical decision-making.[31] Given the great importance of very rapid appropriate triage and treatment for patients with suspected ACI or AMI, these aids seem to hold considerable promise. Nonetheless, the results of clinical impact trials of these and other decision aids will provide a better picture of the proper role of such tools in the clinical setting. In conjunction with this, the use for feedback of those aids that are "time insensitive" will also need to be developed and tested further. Hopefully such feedback and reporting systems will also contribute to the improvement of direct clinical care, the overall management of care, and communication among those involved in the different facets of care. Only as all these development and evaluation efforts unfold will the full impact of TIPIs and other such tools be known.

REFERENCES

1. Pozen MW, D'Agostino, Selker HP, et al: A predictive instrument to improve coronary-care-unit admission practices in acute ischemic heart disease, *N Engl J Med* 310:1273-1278, 1984.
2. McCarthy BD, Wong JB, Selker HP: Detecting acute cardiac ischemia in the emergency department: a review of the literature, *J Gen Int Med* 5:365-373, 1990.
3. Schor S, Behar S, Modan B, et al: Disposition of presumed coronary patients from an emergency room. A follow-up study, *JAMA* 236:941-943, 1976.
4. Goldman L, Weinberg M, Weisberg M, et al: A computer-derived protocol to aid in the diagnosis of ER patients with acute chest pain, *N Engl J Med* 307:588-596, 1982.
5. Lee TH, Rouan GW, Weisberg MC, et al: Clinical characteristics and natural history of patients with acute myocardial infarction sent home from the emergency room, *Am J Cardiol* 60:219-224, 1987.
6. Selker HP, Griffith JL, Dorey FJ, et al: How do physicians adapt when the coronary care unit is full? A prospective multicenter study, *JAMA* 257:1181-1185, 1987.
7. Fineberg HV, Scadden D, Goldman L: Care of patients with a low probability of acute myocardial infarction: cost-effectiveness of alternatives to coronary-care-unit admission, *N Engl J Med* 310:1301-1307, 1984.
8. McCarthy BD, Beshansky JR, D'Agostino RB, et al: Missed diagnoses of acute myocardial infarction: results from a multicenter study, *Ann Emerg Med* 22:579-582, 1993.
9. Fuchs R, Scheidt S: Improved criteria for admission to cardiac care units, *JAMA* 246:2037-2041, 1981.
10. Nattel S, Warnica JW, Ogilvie RI: Indications for admission to a coronary care unit in patients with unstable angina, *Can Med Assoc J* 122:180-184, 1980.
11. Eisenberg JM, Horowitz LN, Busch R, et al: Diagnosis of acute myocardial infarction in the ER: a prospective assessment of clinical decision making and the usefulness of immediate cardiac enzyme determination, *J Community Health* 4:190-198, 1979.
12. Seager SB: Cardiac enzymes in the evaluation of chest pain, *Ann Emerg Med* 9:346-349, 1980.
13. Horowitz RS, Morganroth J: Immediate detection of early high-risk patients with an acute myocardial infarction using two-dimensional echocardiographic evaluation of left ventricular regional wall motion abnormalities, *Am Heart J* 103:814-822, 1982.
14. Wackers FJT, Lie KI, Liem KL et al: Potential value of thallium-201 scintigraphy as a means of selecting patients for the coronary care unit, *Br Heart J* 41:111-117, 1979.
15. Pozen MW, D'Agostino RB, Mitchell JB, et al: The usefulness of a predictive instrument to reduce inappropriate admissions to the coronary care unit, *Ann Intern Med* 92:238-242, 1980.
16. Goldman L, Cook EF, Brand DA, et al: A computer protocol to predict myocardial infarction in emergency department patients with chest pain, *N Engl J Med* 318:797-803, 1988.
17. Kinlen LJ: Incidence and presentation of myocardial infarction in an English community, *Br Heart J* 35:616-622, 1973.
18. Margolis JR, Kannel WB, Feinleib M, et al: Clinical features of unrecognized myocardial infarction-silent and symptomatic. Eighteen year follow-up: the Framingham Study, *Am J Cardiol* 32:1-6, 1973.
19. Uretsky BF, Farquhar DS, Berezin AF, Hood Jr WB: Symptomatic myocardial infarction without chest pain: prevalence and clinical course, *Am J Cardiol* 40:498-503, 1977.
20. Unstable angina pectoris: National Cooperative Study Group to compare medical and surgical therapy: IV. Results in patients with left descending coronary artery disease, *Am J Cardiol* 48:517-524, 1981.
21. Krause KR, Hutter Jr AM, DeSanctis RW: Acute coronary insufficiency. Course and follow-up, *Circulation* 45 and 46 (suppl I):166-171, 1972.
22. Wasson JH, Sox HC, Neff RK, et al: Clinical prediction rules: applications and methodological standards, *N Engl J Med* 313:793-799, 1985.
23. McNutt RA, Selker HP: How did the acute ischemic heart disease predictive instrument reduce unnecessary coronary care unit admissions? *Med Decision Making* 8:90-94, 1988.
24. Sawe U: Early diagnosis of acute myocardial infarction with special reference to the diagnosis of the intermediate coronary syndrome: a clinical study, *Acta Med Scand* 520(suppl):1-76, 1972.
25. Tierney WM, Roth BJ, Psaty B, et al: Predictors of myocardial infarction in emergency room patients, *Crit Care Med* 13:526-531, 1985.
26. Van der Does E, Lubsen J, Pool J, et al: Acute coronary events in a general practice: objectives and design of the Imminent Myocardial Infarction Rotterdam Study, *Heart Bull* 7:91-98, 1976.
27. Selker, HP: Coronary care unit triage decision aids: How do we know when they work?, *Am J Med* 87:491-493, 1989.
28. Selker HP, Griffith JL, D'Agostino RB: A tool for judging coronary care unit admission that is appropriate for both real-time and retrospective use: a time-insensitive predictive instrument (TIPI) for acute cardiac ischemia: a multicenter study, *Med Care* 29:610-627, 1991.
29. Selker HP, Griffith JL, D'Agostino RB: A time-insensitive predictive instrument for acute myocardial infarction mortality: a multicenter study, *Med Care* 29:1196-1211, 1991.
30. Selker HP, Griffith JL, D'Agostino RB: A time-insensitive predictive instrument for acute mortality due to congestive heart failure: development, testing, and use for comparing hospitals: a multicenter study, *Med Care* 32:(In Press), 1994.
31. Selker HP, Griffith JL, Beshansky JR, et al: The thrombolytic predictive instrument project: combining clinical study data bases to take medical effectiveness research to the streets. In *Medical effectiveness research data methods*, 1991, Rockville, Md, Agency for Health Care Policy and Research, DHHS.
32. Lobodzinski SM, Laks MM: Present and future concepts in computerized electrocardiography, *IM Intern Med Specialist* 8:152-192, 1987.
33. Cairns CB, Niemann JT, Selker HP, et al: A computerized version of the time-insensitive predictive instrument: use of the Q wave, ST segment, T wave and patient history in the diagnosis of acute myocardial infarction by the computerized ECG, *J Electrocardiol* 24(suppl):46-49, 1991.
34. Jayes RL, Larsen GC, Beshansky JR, et al: Physician electrocardiogram reading in the emergency department: accuracy and effect on triage decisions—findings from a multicenter study, *J Gen Int Med* 7:387-392, 1992.
35. Sarasin FP, Reymond JM, Griffith JL, et al: Impact of the acute cardiac ischemia time-insensitive predictive instrument (ACI-

TIPI) on the speed of triage decision making for emergency department patients presenting with chest pain: a controlled clinical trial, *J Gen Intern Med* 9:187-194, 1994.

36. Horn SD, Horn RA: The computerized severity index: a new tool for case-mix management, *J Med Sys* 10:73-78, 1986.

37. Daley J, Jencks SF, Draper D, et al: Predicting hospital-associated mortality for Medicare patients with stroke, pneumonia, acute myocardial infarction, and congestive heart failure, *JAMA* 260: 3617-3624, 1988.

38. Iezzoni LI, Burnside S, Sickles L, et al: Coding of acute myocardial infarction, *Ann Intern Med* 109:745-751, 1988.

39. Knaus WA, Draper EA, Wagner DP, et al: APACHE II: A severity of disease classification system, *Crit Care Med* 13:818, 1985.

40. Brewster AC, Karlin BG, Hyde LA, et al: MEDISGRPS: a clinically based approach to classifying hospital patients at admission, *Inquiry* 12:377-387, 1985.

41. Jencks SF, Daley J, Draper D, et al: Interpreting hospital mortality data: the role of clinical risk adjustment, *JAMA* 260:3611-3616, 1988.

42. Iezzoni LI, Moskowitz MA: A clinical assessment of MedisGroups, *JAMA* 260:3159-3163, 1988.

Part **II**

PREHOSPITAL AND ER PHASE

Chapter 18

SELECTION OF PATIENTS FOR REPERFUSION THERAPY

Cindy L. Grines

Several randomized, placebo-controlled trials have demonstrated unequivocally that patients with acute myocardial infarction (AMI) who are treated promptly with reperfusion therapy have a substantial reduction in mortality.[1-8] Furthermore, reperfusion therapy is associated with an improvement in both regional and global left ventricular function, as well as a reduction in in-hospital complications, such as the development of congestive heart failure, pulmonary emboli, and arrhythmias. It is also well recognized that thrombolytic agents have the potential for causing serious and even life-threatening complications. Thus appropriate patient selection is critical so that the maximal number of patients with AMI can benefit from this important therapeutic option with minimal side effects. It should be kept in mind, however, that thrombolytic ineligibility does not mean that the patient is ineligible for all forms of reperfusion therapy. Revascularization with coronary angioplasty, or even emergency bypass grafting, may be the preferential therapy for certain types of patients with AMI.

PROPORTION OF PATIENTS ELIGIBLE FOR THROMBOLYTIC THERAPY

The majority of patients who present with AMI are ineligible for thrombolytic therapy based on currently accepted criteria.[9] Recently the lay press has placed

The author gratefully acknowledges Phyliss McKinney for her expert manuscript preparation.

great emphasis on the lower percentage of patients treated in the United States as compared with Europe. As demonstrated in Table 18-1, however, the proportion of patients treated depends more upon how the infarct population is defined than on the country in which the patient is treated. Retrospective reviews, which use the discharge diagnosis of AMI, have shown that the minority of patients are treated with thrombolytic agents.[10-14] Series of patients discharged with a retrospective diagnosis of MI have included those with postoperative MIs, patients who presented with unstable angina or congestive heart failure and later were ruled in for MI based on enzymes, and a diverse array of other patients who did not meet the specific criteria for thrombolytic treatment. Conversely, prospective studies that have used coronary care unit (CCU) logs of patients acutely admitted with presumed or definite MI have shown a higher proportion of patients being treated (15% to 50%).[3-5,15-23] Although the majority of these prospective registries were conducted in Europe, two recent registries from the United States demonstrated that 30% to 39% of MI patients admitted to the CCU were treated with thrombolytics.

The difference between a CCU log and a retrospective review of patients discharged with the diagnosis of MI confirmed by CPK isoenzymes can be illustrated from our experience. Our CCU log includes approximately 250 patients per year compared with 600 patients per year who are discharged from our hospital with the diagnosis of MI. Approximately 125 patients

Table 18-1. Eligibility for thrombolysis

Retrospective studies	Location	Year	Eligible (%)
Worcester Heart Attack Study[10]	USA	1986	9.3
Doorey[11]	USA	1987	24.0
Worcester Heart Attack Study[10]	USA	1988	20.3
Althouse[12]	USA	1988	24.0
Cragg[13]	USA	1990	16.0
Worcester Heart Attack Study[10]	USA	1990	25.0
Morgan[14]	Canada	1992	21.5

Prospective studies			
Sainsous[15]	France	1985	15.0
GISSI-1[4]	Italy	1986	37.0
Murray[16]	UK	1987	14.0
Jagger[17]	UK	1987	51.0
ISAM[3]	Germany	1987	23.0
ASSET[5]	Europe	1988	38.0
GISSI-2[18]	Italy	1990	33.0
Behar[19]	Israel	1991	14.8
Karlson[20]	Sweden	1991	37.0
Greenbaum[21]	UK	1992	50.0
Paine[22]	USA	1992	30.0
Rogers[23]	USA	1992	39.0

Retrospective: Discharge diagnosis of MI (includes mixed population).
Prospective: CCU logs of patients acutely admitted with the diagnosis of MI.
ASSET: Anglo-Scandinavian Study of Early Thrombolysis.
GISSI-1: Gruppo Italiano per lo Studio della Streptochinasi nell'Infarto Miocardico.
ISAM: Intravenous Streptokinase in Acute Myocardial Infarction trial.
GISSI-2: Gruppo Italiano per lo Studio della Sopravvivenza nell'Infarto Miocardio.

receive reperfusion therapy each year, indicating that 50% of CCU infarcts are being treated, compared with only 21% of patients discharged with the diagnosis of MI. Thus differences in definitions make interpretation of treatment patterns quite difficult.

It does seem that with increasing awareness of the benefits of thrombolysis more patients are receiving treatment. The Worcester Heart Attack Study demonstrated that only 9.3% of patients with infarcts received thrombolytic therapy in 1986, compared with 20.3% and 25% in 1988 and 1990 respectively.[10] These data suggest that approximately 50% of patients who present with a clear diagnosis of MI and 25% of patients with a retrospective diagnosis of MI are currently receiving reperfusion therapy. Whether the remaining AMI patients have a favorable risk-benefit ratio for thrombolysis and thus should receive this therapy remains to be determined.

MORTALITY RATES OF ELIGIBLE VS. NONELIGIBLE PATIENTS

Many of the standard guidelines for the use of thrombolytic therapy were denied originally as entry

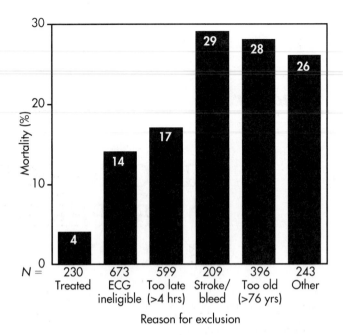

Fig. 18-1. Only the minority of patients who constituted a low-risk group were eligible and treated with thrombolytic therapy. Patients who were excluded from consideration for thrombolytic therapy had a high mortality rate, regardless of the reason for exclusion.

criteria for randomized clinical trials of these agents. To understand how thrombolytic therapy relates to the larger population of AMI patients, our group recently analyzed 1471 patients with AMI admitted during the recruitment period for the TIMI-2B study.[13] Among the 16% of patients who were eligible for the trial, the in-hospital mortality rate was 4% compared with 19% in ineligible patients. In-hospital mortality rates for excluded subgroups included 28% in the elderly, 29% in patients with stroke or increased bleeding risk, 17% in patients who presented more than 4 hours after the onset of chest pain, 14% in patients with an ineligible electrocardiogram, and 26% in patients with other reasons for exclusion (Fig. 18-1). When patients were deemed ineligible because of multiple exclusions, mortality increased as a function of the number of exclusions: 17% for patients with a single exclusion, 18% for patients with 2 exclusions, 24% for patients with 3 exclusions, and 27% for patients with 4 or more exclusions. Importantly, in light of the results of subsequent trials some of the exclusions for this early TIMI trial have been revised or eliminated, particularly the exclusion of the elderly and of patients beyond 4 hours from symptom onset.

To evaluate the use of thrombolytic therapy outside of investigational protocols, Pfeffer et al. collected data from 133 North American hospitals between 1987 and 1989.[24] They reported differences in the preinfarction characteristics of groups treated or not treated with thrombolytic drugs. Patients who were treated with thrombolytic therapy were significantly younger, less often female or diabetic, had a better functional status, used fewer cardiac medications, and were less likely to have a history of prior infarction or prior angina ($P < 0.005$) compared with patients who were not treated.

Therefore, in the United States both clinical and investigational use of thrombolytic therapy appears to be limited to a relatively low-risk group of patients. Even the Italian GISSI-I trial, which included high-risk subsets such as the elderly and those in cardiogenic shock, demonstrated a relatively high mortality rate (12.5%) in patients who were excluded primarily on the basis of low suspicion for MI or those who presented more than 4 hours from symptom onset.[4] Because the majority of patients with MI do not meet existing criteria for thrombolytic therapy and this group has a much higher mortality rate, it has been suggested that reperfusion therapy may have an even greater influence on mortality in such patients and should be pursued more aggressively.

TRADITIONAL INCLUSION AND EXCLUSION CRITERIA FOR THROMBOLYTIC THERAPY

The currently accepted inclusion and exclusion criteria for thrombolytic therapy have recently been compiled and published by the American College of Cardiology and the American Heart Association.[25] In addition, eligibility criteria from major clinical trials conducted in the United States, [e.g., Thrombolysis In Myocardial Infarction (TIMI) trials] are used by many practitioners to determine which patients to treat with thrombolytics.[26] Recommendations have included treatment of patients with prolonged chest pain in whom the prompt diagnosis of MI is established by ST-segment elevations in two contiguous leads. Because early studies demonstrated beneficial results only in patients treated in the early hours of onset of chest pain, patients who have presented later than 4 to 6 hours after symptom onset traditionally have been excluded. In addition, elderly patients have been considered ineligible for thrombolytic therapy by many experts because of the increased incidence of intracranial bleeding in this group. Additional contraindications have included a history of uncontrolled hypertension, recent surgery, noncompressible vascular punctures, cardiopulmonary resuscitation, and prior anticoagulation. It should be noted that many of these contraindications were based on historical recommendations with few scientific data to support them.

CONTROVERSIES REGARDING BENEFITS OF THROMBOLYSIS

If thrombolytic therapy were completely without risk it would be administered to every patient with suspected MI. However, because of the risks of therapy (catastrophic bleeding complications in particular) and the uncertainty of the risk-benefit "ratio" for individual patients, many physicians have limited its use.

Inferior MI

In the past considerable controversy existed with regard to whether patients with inferior infarction benefit from thrombolysis. Bates et al. reviewed the effect of thrombolytic therapy on left ventricular function in patients with inferior MI.[27] Seven placebo-controlled trials, four with streptokinase and three with tissue plasminogen activator, demonstrated either a trend or a significant difference in left ventricular function in favor of patients with inferior MI treated with thrombolytic therapy. The difference in ejection fraction between treated and placebo groups ranged from 2 to 8 percentage points. Furthermore, several additional trials demonstrated a significant improvement in infarction zone function after reperfusion therapy of inferior MI. Table 18-2 summarizes mortality results from nine placebo-controlled trials in patients with inferior MI.[2-8,28,29] The prognosis of typical patients with acute inferior MI, regardless of whether they were treated conservatively or with thrombolytic therapy, was substantially better than that of typical patients who presented with anterior MI. In addition, the reduction in mortality associated with thrombolysis after acute inferior MI was more modest. Given the low mortality rate in control groups after inferior MI, many studies have been too small to demonstrate a significant improvement in survival after thrombolysis. Pooled data involving more than 12,000 patients with inferior MI show a clinically relevant reduction in the mortality rate of the thrombolytic treatment group (6.8%) compared with the control group (8.7%, $P < 0.0001$).[9] Furthermore, no large mortality trial has found that patients with inferior MI have a worsened outcome as a result of the complications of thrombolysis. The most recent metaanalysis performed by the Fibrinolysis Trialists Collaboration continues to show a benefit in this group.

According to a substudy of the GISSI trial, the site of infarction is less important in determining early mortality (and consequently the benefits of therapy) than is the size of the infarction.[30] In this study infarction size was determined on the basis of the number of electrocardiographic (ECG) leads showing ST-segment elevation. Mortality correlated well with the size of infarction regardless of infarction site, increasing from 6.5% in patients with small MI (elevation in 2 to 3 leads), to 9.6% in patients with modest infarction (4 to 5 leads involved), to 14.3% in patients with large infarction (6 to 7 leads involved), to 21.7% in patients with extensive infarction (8 or 9 leads involved). Intravenous streptokinase therapy was associated with a statistically significant

Table 18-2. Mortality rates in inferior myocardial infarction in previous trials*

Study	Follow-up	Treated No.	(%)	Control No.	(%)	P Value
Kennedy et al.[2]	4 wks	0/71	0	3/63	4.8	0.06
Kennedy et al.[8]	2 wks	5/124	4.0	2/110	1.8	0.32
Vermeer et al.[28]	3 mos	6/129	4.7	14/138	10.1	0.09
European Coop[29]	6 mos	8/69	11.6	13/63	20.6	0.16
ISAM[3]	7 mos	46/448	10.3	61/429	14.2	0.07
GISSI-1[4]	1 yr	137/2009	6.8	145/2004	7.2	0.6
ISIS-II[7]	5 wks	150/2076	7.2	185/2112	8.8	0.06
ASSET[5]	1 mo	47/753	6.3	74/754	9.8	0.01
AIMS[6]	1 mo	11/329	3.3	26/333	7.8	0.01
Pooled		410/6008	6.8	523/6006	8.7	0.0001

AIMS: APSAC Interventional Mortality Study (APSAC = anisolyated plasminogen streptokinase activator complex)
ISIS-II: Second International Study of Infarct Survival.
European Coop: European Cooperative Study Group.
*Reprinted with permission from Grines CL, DeMaria AN: Optimal utilization of thrombolytic therapy for acute myocardial infarction: concepts and controversies, *J Am Coll Cardiol* 16:223-231, 1990.

reduction in mortality in patients with modest, large, and extensive infarction. In contrast, the mortality in patients with small infarctions was not reduced significantly regardless of infarction site. It must be emphasized, however, that these data do not prove that patients with small infarction failed to benefit. Rather, because of the low mortality at baseline, much greater numbers of patients were required to show a significant benefit of thrombolysis. These results do emphasize, however, that the size of infarction is a very important determinant of outcome and may be more relevant than infarction site in determining the risk-benefit ratio of thrombolytic therapy.

Absence of ST-segment elevation

Although it is well accepted that patients with ST-segment elevation generally benefit from thrombolysis, the absence of ST-segment elevation continues to be the focus of considerable interest[31] (Fig. 18-2).

Left bundle branch block. Because the presence of left bundle block may make the ST-segment changes difficult to interpret, patients with this finding have generally been excluded from thrombolytic trials. In contrast to the GISSI-I trial,[4] in which patients who presented with left bundle branch block appeared to have similar mortality rates in the treated and control groups, the ISIS-2 trial found these patients to be a very high-risk group, having a mortality rate of 28% in the absence of treatment.[5] In this trial patients who received streptokinase alone had a mortality rate of 19.8%, and the combination of streptokinase with aspirin further reduced the mortality to 14%. Pooled data on nearly 2000 patients with bundle branch block demonstrated a 17.1% mortality in thrombolytic-treated

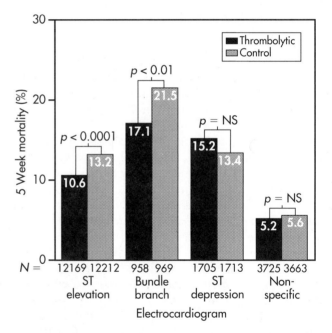

Fig. 18-2. Benefit of thrombolytic therapy based upon the admission ECG.

patients compared with a 21.5% mortality in the control group ($P < 0.01$)[32] (see Fig. 18-2). Thus, in the absence of contraindications, patients who present with a convincing clinical picture of MI and left bundle branch block on the 12-lead electrocardiogram should be treated with reperfusion.

Nonspecific ST- and T-wave changes. The Fibrinolysis Trialists recently performed a metaanalysis of all the major thrombolytic mortality trials; this analysis included 7288 patients with nonspecific ECG changes who received either thrombolytic therapy or placebo.[32] Compared with other patients in the analysis, this group appeared to be low-risk and had no mortality benefit from thrombolytic therapy (Fig. 18-2). Therefore patients who present with prolonged chest pain and nonspecific ST-segment changes generally should not be treated with thrombolytics. Importantly, however, the metaanalysis upon which these recommendations are based was limited by inadequate power to detect up to a 15% benefit of thrombolytic therapy.

ST-segment depression. Although patients with ST-segment depression generally are thought to represent a low-risk group composed primarily of patients with unstable angina, randomized MI trials have demonstrated a very high mortality rate in this subgroup (see Fig. 18-2). This finding may represent selection bias, whereby only the very sickest of patients with ST-segment depression were thought to be suffering from an acute myocardial infarction (AMI). Although it is generally believed that the sickest patients may have the most to gain from reperfusion therapy, AMI patients presenting with ST-segment depression appear to have a statistically insignificant increase in mortality with thrombolytic therapy (15.2%) compared with the control group (13.4%).

To determine why patients with AMI in the absence of ST-segment elevation may have a worse prognosis, we reviewed the records and angiograms of 76 patients who had confirmed diagnoses of infarction in the absence of ST-segment elevation.[33] Compared with a cohort of patients with AMI and ST-segment elevation, those patients who were ineligible on the basis of their ECGs were older (60 vs. 54 years, $P = .005$), included a higher proportion of females, had more prior myocardial infarctions and a higher prevalence of multivessel disease (68% vs. 50%, $P = .01$). Therefore it appears that patients with MI and ST-segment depression more often have multivessel disease and multiple previous infarctions resulting in the inability to develop ST-segment elevations. In light of their high-risk profile and poor outcomes, perhaps more aggressive and complete revascularization should be considered in patients who have ST-segment depression and convincing ongoing symptoms that are compatible with AMI.

Although patients who are diagnosed retrospectively as having infarction after presenting with ST-segment depression appear to have a poor outcome, it is unknown how many patients present with chest pain and ST-segment depression and do not go on to have an infarction. If one is to recommend aggressive treatment of this group, a method of precisely determining patients who are likely to develop infarction would be desirable.

Karlson et al. evaluated over 7000 patients who presented to the emergency room with chest pain.[34] Of these, 4690 patients were admitted to the hospital and 921 subsequently developed an AMI. The patients were prospectively classified in the emergency room on the basis of history, clinical examination, and ECG into one of four categories according to the initial degree of suspicion of MI. Of the 279 patients judged to have an "obvious" AMI, 88% were actually confirmed to have infarction. Of patients with a "strong suspicion" of AMI, 34% had enzymatic confirmation. "Strong suspicion" was defined as (1) a patient who presented with typical symptoms but whose ECG did not demonstrate ST-segment elevation, (2) a patient with atypical symptoms, with ST-segment changes consistent with acute ischemia, (3) the new onset of severe congestive heart failure without ST-segment elevation, or (4) unstable angina regardless of ECG changes. Of patients with a "vague" suspicion of AMI, 8% were confirmed; and of patients admitted with "no suspicion" of MI, 6% were later confirmed to have had myocardial necrosis. Therefore a low but significant percentage of patients with a normal initial ECG or a vague initial suspicion of MI developed a confirmed MI. The fact that the majority of patients who subsequently had AMI were judged appropriately by the admitting physician is encouraging. However, 66% of patients with a "strong suspicion" of MI did not develop evidence of myocardial necrosis. Using Karlson's criteria of treating all patients who have obvious or strong suspicion of AMI, 986 (21%) of the 4690 patients admitted would have been inappropriately treated with thrombolysis. Therefore a more specific method of detecting patients with ongoing infarction would be desirable.

Cannon evaluated 1247 patients enrolled in the TIMI-3B trial to determine whether the diagnosis of non–Q-wave myocardial infarction could be prospectively distinguished from unstable angina.[35] In this trial 32% of patients sustained an infarction on the basis of CK-MB enzymes. Logistic regression analysis demonstrated that the following three baseline variables were strongly predictive of the development of non–Q-wave MI: duration of pain greater than 120 minutes (odds ratio 3:2), ST-segment deviation (odds ratio 2:7), and male gender (odds ratio 1:6). In the absence of these three factors only 14% of patients had a non–Q-wave MI. Pain greater than 120 minutes in duration and associated with ST-segment deviation represented an infarction in 60% of women and 69% of men in whom these characteristics were present. Thus these clinical and electrocardiographic characteristics may be used to distinguish patients who are at high risk of having AMI in the absence of ST-segment elevation.

Additionally, some have recommended the use of echocardiograms obtained in the emergency room to determine regional wall motion abnormalities or the use of emergency catheterization to determine patency of the infarct vessel, left ventricular function, and the presence of multivessel disease (see Chapters 40 and 33). Although clinical, electrocardiographic, echocardiographic, or angiographic characteristics may prospectively define patients who are at risk of developing infarction, there is currently no evidence that reperfusion therapy is beneficial in the absence of occlusive coronary thrombosis. For these reasons we confine the use of thrombolytics to patients with ST-segment elevation of at least 1 mm in two contiguous leads, or left bundle branch block.

Delayed time to treatment

Many patients have been denied entry to thrombolytic trials because of presentation beyond the 4- to 6-hour time window. The rationale for exclusion includes the perceived lack of benefit of the treatment, and the belief that by surviving for several hours a patient has selected himself or herself to be in a low-risk category for death. However, it is now clear that patients who present late continue to have high mortality rates despite surviving the first several hours of infarction. In their review of 33 intravenous or intracoronary thrombolytic trials conducted in the early 1980s, Yusuf et al. reported improved survival in patients treated after 6 hours.[36] A survival advantage for patients treated late was also found in ISIS-2.[7] In contrast, the GISSI-1 trial showed no benefit from late treatment.[4]

With these conflicting results, the ISIS-3 "uncertain" arm as well as the EMERAS (Estudio Multicentrico Estreptoquinasa Republicas de America del Sur) and LATE (Late Assessment of Thrombolytic Efficacy) trials were undertaken. The EMERAS trial demonstrated a 17% reduction in mortality in patients treated with streptokinase after 6 to 12 hours of infarction; however, no reduction in mortality was seen after 12 hours.[37] The LATE trial was a double-blind placebo-controlled trial designed to determine the effects of tissue plasminogen activator (t-PA) therapy in patients who presented from 6 to 24 hours after the onset of AMI symptoms.[38] The overall mortality did not differ between the t-PA and the placebo groups. However, a significant mortality benefit (27% reduction) was observed for the subset of patients treated between 6 and 12 hours after symptom onset. This mortality reduction was maintained for the duration of the 1-year follow-up. A 2.25% incidence of overall stroke was noted in the t-PA group compared with a 1.1% incidence of stroke in the placebo group. Although an insignificant trend was observed for mortality reduction in the trial as a whole, a 27% reduction in mortality was observed in patients treated between 6 and 12 hours from symptom onset. This mortality benefit was maintained for 1 year. Although a significant excess of total strokes (2.25 vs. 1.1%) was observed with t-PA, the incidence of nonfatal disabling stroke was similar in the two groups.

In a metaanalysis of the available randomized data the ISIS study group concluded that treatment of the patient between 0 to 6 hours after AMI was definitely indicated, between 6 to 12 hours after AMI was probably indicated, and between 12 to 24 hours after AMI was possibly of benefit to patients.[32] They did, however, note a paradoxical increase in mortality in the first day after the administration of a thrombolytic agent. Patients treated late had a particular increase in this early hazard of death when compared with patients who were treated earlier. However, the later benefit from thrombolytic therapy was comparable regardless of when the patient was treated. Whether this early increase in mortality from thrombolysis is due to reperfusion injury, ischemia, or hemorrhagic infarction with rupture is not known. The mechanism responsible for the mortality benefit of late reperfusion is not entirely clear. It has been speculated that myocardial salvage occurs only when reperfusion occurs within the first few hours of coronary occlusion and the favorable outcome observed with late reperfusion may be because of improved healing of the damaged myocardium or preservation of the epicardial rim of myocardium following acute AMI.[39] Either mechanism may potentially inhibit left ventricular dilation, infarct expansion, and aneurysm formation, leading to a decrease in malignant arrhythmias and left ventricular thrombus formation and to an improvement in diastolic filling characteristics.

The current data strongly suggest that use of thrombolytic therapy between 6 to 12 hours after symptom onset will be of benefit on average. Patients likely to derive the greatest benefit are those with large infarction, stuttering onset of infarction in whom the infarct vessel may not have been completely occluded for the entire duration of pain, or those in whom collateral vessels may have resulted in persistent viable myocardium. The modest benefit derived from late reperfusion may be outweighed by the risks in patients who have one or more relative contraindications for thrombolysis. Patients with small areas of infarction who are severely hypertensive, elderly, or have debilitating illnesses may not be appropriate candidates for late treatment.

Prior coronary artery bypass grafting

Many thrombolytic trials have excluded patients with prior coronary artery bypass graft surgery (CABG), thus leaving unsettled the efficacy of reperfusion therapy in this population. Little et al. reviewed 40 patients with prior CABG who presented with AMI and had coronary angiography performed within 1 month (16 ± 14 days) after infarction.[40] They found that the MI was associated with graft occlusion in 66% of patients and occurred in an unbypassed native vessel in 34%. Crean et al. described angiographic findings 10 ± 3 days after MI in 52 patients with prior CABG.[41] They found that the culprit was an ungrafted coronary vessel in 23% of cases, a vein graft in 63% of cases, and disease in the native vessel distal to the graft insertion site in 15%. Crean reported a smaller infarct size in bypass patients compared with controls (as assessed by ST-segment elevation, development of Q-waves, peak creatine kinase, and ejection fraction). Importantly, patients with prior bypass grafting who are admitted to coronary care units with chest pain do not present as frequently with ST-segment elevation or have enzymatic confirmation of MI; however, their prognosis appears to be worse than MI patients who have not undergone prior bypass surgery because patients with previous CABG on average are older and have more multivessel disease and left ventricular dysfunction compared with patients with MI without prior CABG.[42,43] Therefore, defining the optimal treatment strategy for these patients is of great importance.

To ascertain the mechanisms responsible for AMI in patients with bypass grafting and to examine the potential for these patients to benefit from thrombolytic therapy we reviewed angiograms obtained between 1 hour and 7 days after AMI (median 1 day) in 43 patients.[44] Infarction was caused by recent occlusion of a vein graft in 63%, critical graft stenosis in 12% and recent occlusion of a native vessel in 19%. The infarct-related vessel could not be accurately determined in 7%. Angiographic evidence of huge thrombi with stagnant columns of blood was frequently observed in the vein grafts. Successful reperfusion occurred in only 2 of 8 (25%) grafts after intravenous thrombolytic therapy. Intragraft thrombolysis or angioplasty was successful in restoring flow in 8 of 10 (80%) grafts. It is possible that the absence of flow in the graft may result in an inadequate delivery of the thrombolytic agent when administered by the intravenous route. In addition, the large mass of thrombus and absent flow may require a higher thrombolytic dose, subselective drug infusion, or mechanical means of recanalization.

To date, limited information is available regarding this important subgroup of patients. We favor taking patients with prior CABG directly to the cardiac catheterization laboratory for intragraft thrombolytic therapy, extraction atherectomy, and/or angioplasty. If a cardiac catheterization laboratory is not readily available, there is no reason to withhold the thrombolytic therapy in this population because the infarction may be caused by a native vessel occlusion, which should respond well to IV thrombolysis. Furthermore, some case studies have reported successful reperfusion of vein grafts using intravenous thrombolytic therapy.[45]

Cardiogenic shock

Although it is generally believed that the sickest patients stand to benefit the most from thrombolytic therapy, patients with cardiogenic shock appear to have minimal benefit from thrombolytic therapy.[46] The Western Washington GISSI and ISIS trials have demonstrated that despite intracoronary streptokinase, intravenous streptokinase, or t-PA therapy, patients with cardiogenic shock continue to have a very high mortality.[2,4,7] It is possible that the low perfusion pressure results in an inadequate delivery of thrombolytic drug to the site of thrombus with resulting poor patency rates. However, the confidence limits for the treatment effect in patients with cardiogenic shock overlaps with the observed 25% to 30% mortality reduction seen in other patients with ST elevation. An alternative explanation is that the lack of a significant treatment effect with thrombolytic therapy is because of chance and that with more patients involved in trials, a benefit would be observed. Conversely, coronary angioplasty of the infarct vessel has been reported to reduce the mortality rate to approximately 50%, compared with an expected mortality of 80% to 90%.[47] Based on these data patients who present in cardiogenic shock should have fluid resuscitation as well as vasopressor drugs and intraaortic balloon counterpulsation initiated. Because thrombolytic drugs appear to offer little advantage in this clinical situation, mechanical reperfusion strategies including PTCA or emergency bypass grafting in the event of severe multivessel disease should be aggressively pursued, even if this requires interhospital transfer.

If a patient cannot be transported expeditiously to an interventional facility, we use streptokinase preferentially because both the GISSI-2 international trial and the GUSTO trial demonstrated a nonsignificant trend towards a greater benefit with this drug than with t-PA. Before a decision is made to pursue the aggressive route of reperfusion therapy in a patient with profound cardiogenic shock, the physician should carefully review the overall quality of life and medical condition of the patient, including significant comorbid conditions. The patient's previously expressed preferences for aggressive care should also be assessed because the course will frequently be complicated and will require a prolonged stay in the intensive care unit.

CONTROVERSIES REGARDING RISKS OF THROMBOLYSIS

Of all the complications of thrombolytic therapy, bleeding (particularly central nervous system hemorrhage) is the most feared. Because of concern about bleeding complications, traditional thrombolytic guidelines have established multiple contraindications including age > 70 years, severe hypertension, recent cardiopulmonary resuscitation or surgery, a history of previous cerebral ischemia or infarction, as well as conditions that are clearly associated with an unacceptable risk of hemorrhage, such as active internal bleeding, and known intracranial abnormalities such as an aneurysm or neoplasm. Several studies have attempted to identify conditions that predispose patients to an increased risk of bleeding. Increased doses[26] and a prolonged infusion of t-PA[48] have been associated with bleeding, as have the use of adjunctive heparin,[31] invasive procedures, and patient factors such as hypertension, older age, female gender, and low body weight.[49,50] Clearly, life-threatening bleeding such as intracranial or gross gastrointestinal bleeding is far more serious than bleeding that occurs at the site of an invasive procedure. Therefore reperfusion therapy should be selected to avoid these life-threatening bleeding complications.

Historically the contraindications for thrombolytic therapy were based on studies that identified risk factors for spontaneous hemorrhage. One of the largest series is that of Brott et al. who reviewed 154 cases of spontaneous intracranial hemorrhage.[51] They found that 46% of patients were elderly, 45% had a history of hypertension, and 54% were hypertensive at the time of presentation. A prior cerebral event or neoplasm was present in 27% of cases. Despite an extensive evaluation for potential risk factors, 41% of patients had no predisposing conditions.

The most common risk factors for spontaneous intracranial hemorrhage are age and hypertension. Longstanding hypertension can produce distinct changes in small intracerebral arteries. The incidence of these lesions increases with elevating blood pressure and age, and they may be the site of bleeding when intracerebral hemorrhage occurs.

The risk of intracranial bleeding also depends on the thrombolytic drug used and its dosage. Intravenous streptokinase therapy is associated with a low rate of intracranial bleeding.[47] t-PA was associated with a higher incidence of stroke compared with streptokinase in GISSI-2 (1.3% vs. 1%) and ISIS-3 trials (1.5% vs. 1.1%, $P = 0.00001$).[18,31,52] When higher doses of t-PA are used (such as the 150-mg dose used early in the TIMI-2B study), an even greater incidence of intracranial bleeding was observed (1.9%).[26] In addition, intravenous heparin therapy further increases the rate of stroke, presumably because of intracranial bleeding.[53] For these reasons, when considering a patient who may be at high risk of developing bleeding complications (i.e., an elderly patient with longstanding hypertension), it would be prudent to choose therapies known to have a lower risk of serious bleeding (e.g., coronary angioplasty[54] or intravenous streptokinase therapy).[18,31,52]

Elderly patients

Elderly patients traditionally have been excluded from thrombolytic therapy because of the perceived increased risk of intracranial hemorrhage. Indeed, Montague et al. found that only 4% of patients over the age of 70 with AMI received thrombolytics[55] compared with 20% of patients younger than 70 years, ($P < .001$). In addition, elderly patients were significantly less likely to receive aspirin, nitrates, and β-blockers and to undergo stress testing or cardiac catheterization. Similarly, Weaver et al. found that 29% of younger patients were treated with thrombolytic drugs compared with only 5% of patients over age 70.[56]

The explanation for physicians not using diagnostic tests or treatment modalities in elderly patients may relate to their attitudes. A high proportion of physicians appear to believe that life-style interventions may not be beneficial in elderly patients. However, it should be noted that in 1987, 57% of all patients hospitalized with an AMI in the United States were 65 years of age or older.[57] In addition, the average life expectancy of a 65-year-old member of the general U.S. population is an additional 16.9 years, and that of a 75-year-old is an additional 10.7 years.[58] Many of these patients are active and pursue vigorous and productive lives. Furthermore, of elderly patients who were discharged following MI, 65% of late deaths were sudden or caused by new myocardial infarction.[59] Their findings suggest that diagnostic studies are needed to identify high-risk patients suitable for revascularization procedures that may prevent the late mortality.

It is clear that the in-hospital mortality rate in older age groups is much greater than the overall group of patients with MI.[3-7] If the difference in mortality rates between placebo and treatment groups is calculated to determine the lives saved per 100 patients treated, it becomes apparent that the greatest absolute benefit of thrombolytic therapy is in the elderly. As demonstrated in Table 18-3, the life-saving potential for the elderly appears to be two to three times that of younger age groups. In addition, pooled data from five trials demonstrate a significant reduction in mortality after thrombolytic therapy in the elderly (17.9% compared with 22.1% in control patients, $P < .0001$). The ISIS study group recently analyzed pooled mortality data considering only patients who presented with ST-segment elevation or bundle branch block[32] (Fig. 18-3). It is clear from these data that both the elderly (age 65 to 74) and the ultraelderly (age >75 years) have improved survival with thrombolytic therapy. Finally, in a recent decision analysis thrombolytic therapy using streptokinase was found to be a beneficial and cost-effective treatment for suspected MI in the elderly.[60] Therefore age in and of itself should not be considered a contraindication to thrombolytic therapy.

Despite wanting to treat more elderly patients with thrombolytics, we have found substantial obstacles to this policy. Although we do not exclude patients on the basis of age alone, in a recent review we found that only 7% of the elderly (≥76 years) were eligible for

Table 18-3. Mortality: effect of age in previous trials*

Study	Age (yr)	No. of deaths (%)		Lives saved†	P Value
		Treatment	Control		
ISAM[3]	<70	37/728(5.1)	48/726(6.6)	1.5	0.21
	70-75	17/131(13.0)	15/156(9.6)	−3.4	0.37
GISSI[4]	<75	457/5268(8.7)	552/5226(10.6)	1.9	0.001
	>75	171/592(28.9)	206/623(33.1)	4.2	0.11
ISIS-II[7]	<70	482/6897(7.0)	659/6879(9.6)	2.6	0.0001
	>70	309/1695(18.2)	370/1716(21.6)	3.4	0.01
ASSET[5]	<66	92/1711(5.4)	104/1641(6.3)	0.9	0.24
	66-75	90/827(10.8)	140/852(16.4)	5.6	0.001
AIMS[6]	<65	21/405(5.2)	35/411(8.5)	3.3	0.06
	65-70	11/90(12.2)	26/86(30.2)	18.0	0.003
Pooled	Not elderly	1089/15009(7.3)	1398/14883(9.4)	2.1	0.0001
	Elderly	598/3335(17.9)	757/3433(22.1)	4.1	0.0001

*Reprinted with permission from Grines CL, DeMaria AN: Optimal utilization of thrombolytic therapy for acute myocardial infarction: concepts and controversies, *J Am Coll Cardiol* 16:223-231, 1990.
†Number of lives saved per 100 patients treated (control group mortality-treatment group mortality).

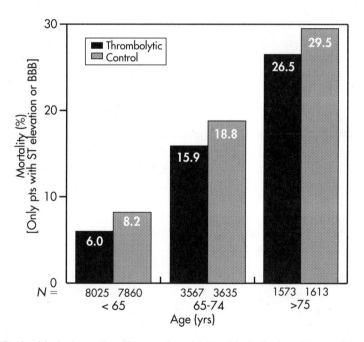

Fig. 18-3. Both elderly (age 65 to 74 years) and ultraelderly (age > 75 years) benefit from thrombolytic therapy.[32]

thrombolytic therapy compared with 22% of the younger population.[61] Bleeding risks resulted in a higher rate of exclusion in the elderly (32 vs. 17%, P < 0.0001), while the ECG was not diagnostic in 43% of elderly patients compared with 33% of the younger cohort (P = 0.003). In addition, elderly patients are less likely to have classical cardiac pain on presentation and often have atypical or no chest pain or congestive heart failure as the primary symptom.[55,56,62] Many elderly patients have longstanding hypertension, previous strokes, and other debilitating illnesses that make them ineligible for

thrombolysis. An aspect of assessment of the elderly that is difficult to portray in the literature is the frequent presence of multiple relative contraindications in the same patient. Therefore the intention to treat more elderly patients is hampered by the higher incidence of complicating illness and the frequent atypical presentations in this group.

When considering treatment of the elderly patient, we make a quick assessment of comorbidities that may place the patient at high risk of bleeding complications. In addition, we attempt to understand the patient's lifestyle and preferences. For example, if the patient is bedridden in a nursing home, we are less likely to choose an aggressive approach to treatment. In elderly patients with significant comorbidities that may predispose them to bleeding, thrombolytics are avoided and the patient is taken directly to the cardiac catheterization laboratory for mechanical reperfusion. For the low-risk elderly patient, thrombolytic therapy is acceptable; we prefer to use streptokinase therapy because of its lower incidence of intracranial bleeding. An alternative approach is to perform angioplasty to achieve reperfusion even if the patient is eligible for thrombolysis, since angioplasty appears to be associated with a lower risk of intracranial bleeding.[54]

Hypertension

Patients have traditionally been excluded from thrombolytic therapy if they have evidence of uncontrolled hypertension (usually thought to be a blood pressure > 200 mm Hg systolic or 110 mm Hg diastolic). The rationale for excluding these patients is that both spontaneous and thrombolytic intracranial bleeding occur more frequently in patients who have a longstanding history of hypertension or uncontrolled hypertension at the time of presentation. Althouse, Weaver, and Kennedy reported a relationship between intracranial hemorrhage after thrombolytic therapy and transient diastolic blood pressure elevation (≥ 120 mm Hg).[63] However, their conclusion was based on observations in only two patients. Furthermore, they found that up to 10% of patients with symptoms of MI had transiently elevated diastolic blood pressures in this range. Anderson et al. reported that age greater than 70 years and elevated blood pressure ($\geq 150/95$ mm Hg) are important risk factors for intracerebral hemorrhage.[64] Many have questioned the validity of these reports because they involve so few patients. Recently, data were reported on 20,768 patients enrolled in the GISSI-2 and International study group. In this study a total of 236 (1.14%) patients had strokes in the hospital (0.36% confirmed hemorrhage strokes, 0.48% ischemic strokes, and 0.30% strokes of undefined cause). Patients treated with t-PA had an excess of strokes (odds ratio 1:42); in addition, older age, higher Killip Class, and occurrence of anterior MI significantly increased the risk of stroke. Interestingly, a history of hypertension had no relationship to occurrence of stroke in these patients, all of whom received either intravenous streptokinase or t-PA. Similarly, the ISIS-2 trial reported the outcome of patients based on their blood pressure at the time of presentation.[7] Although "severe, persistent hypertension" was a relative contraindication in that trial, among the 1141 patients who presented with a systolic blood pressure greater than 175 mm Hg, streptokinase therapy resulted in an improved mortality rate compared with

placebo control (5.7% vs. 8.7%, respectively). Therefore the data regarding an increased risk of stroke in patients with "moderate" hypertension remains controversial. Furthermore, the mortality rate remains lower after treatment of the moderately hypertensive patient compared with that in patients in whom thrombolytic therapy is withheld.

Further data on the relationship between hypertension and intracranial bleeding are needed before firm conclusions can be drawn. Our approach is to treat the patient aggressively with medications to reduce pain and anxiety and to lower blood pressure. These medications include morphine, intravenous nitroglycerin, and intravenous beta blockade (which may also be associated with a reduced rate of stroke).[26] If the systolic blood pressure drops below 180 mm Hg and the diastolic drops below 105 mm Hg, thrombolytic therapy is considered. An alternative approach is to take the patient to the catheterization laboratory for primary angioplasty.

Cardiopulmonary resuscitation

Cardiopulmonary resuscitation (CPR) is often considered a contraindication for thrombolytic therapy because of the fear of producing hemorrhagic pericardial tamponade. Tenaglia et al. reported 59 patients who required less than 10 minutes (median duration of 1 minute) of CPR before receiving thrombolytic therapy.[65] They compared their outcome to 649 patients who had no CPR with an average of two cardioversions performed. Patients who required more than 10 minutes of CPR were excluded. There were no bleeding complications directly attributed to CPR. In particular, the decrease in hematocrit and need for transfusion were the same in both groups, and there were no cases of pericardial tamponade, pneumothorax, or hemothorax.

Scholz et al.[66] reported 43 patients who underwent prolonged CPR either following or during administration of thrombolytic therapy. As opposed to the study by Tenaglia et al.[65] the mean duration of CPR in this series was 36 minutes. Despite an often traumatic CPR with rib fractures verified in 17 patients, no bleeding complications were directly related to performance of CPR. Furthermore, there was no difference in the rate of bleeding complications for patients with ($N = 43$) and without ($N = 57$) resuscitation.

These data suggest that in patients with AMI cardiac arrest preceding or during the thrombolytic infusion requiring CPR and cardioversion should not be considered a contraindication for thrombolytic therapy. Furthermore, CPR following thrombolytic therapy appears to be quite safe. Our approach is not to exclude patients who have undergone brief periods of CPR. However, if the patient has had prolonged periods of CPR with a significant decrease in the mental status, we tend to avoid thrombolytic therapy. These patients are generally taken to the catheterization laboratory and triaged to the appropriate reperfusion strategy.

Prior stroke

Patients with a previous stroke have frequently been excluded from thrombolytic therapy; therefore data regarding their risk of having a second stroke is difficult to ascertain. In addition, among the more liberal European trials that did not exclude patients with a history of prior stroke,[7,52] baseline demographic information is often lacking. In a study reported by O'Connor et al.[67] 18 patients with a history of prior (>6 mos) stroke or TIA received t-PA with or without adjunctive urokinase, as well as aspirin and full-dose heparin. None of them developed intracranial hemorrhage or stroke on follow-up. Similarly, the ISIS-3 uncertain arm found that patients with a prior history of stroke had no excess in bleeding, and the authors concluded that they should not be excluded from receiving thrombolytic therapy.[32]

It appears that patients with a remote (>2 to 6 mos) history of an ischemic stroke probably have no increased risk of intracranial bleeding with thrombolytic therapy. Therefore, these patients should not be excluded from treatment. Any patient who has had a prior intracranial bleed (at any time) should not receive thrombolytic therapy.

Prior surgery, trauma, or GI bleed

Obviously, thrombolytic therapy is absolutely contraindicated in patients with active internal bleeding. However, patients with a past history of peptic ulcer disease often have been excluded from thrombolytic therapy. The ISIS-3 uncertain arm found that there was no excess in bleeding in patients with a previous history of ulcer, and they suggested that these patients should not be excluded from thrombolytic therapy.[32] However, in the ISIS-3 trial it was left up to the enrolling physician to determine whether he or she was "uncertain" regarding the risk-to-benefit ratio of thrombolytic therapy. It is entirely possible that in a patient who had a recent GI bleed, the physician felt "certain" that thrombolytics should not be administered. Therefore it is difficult to determine precisely which of these patients should receive treatment. In general, patients with active peptic ulcer disease who were treated should heal well within 1 month. For that reason we will treat patients who have had no signs of active bleeding in the past month.

Many thrombolytic trials have excluded patients who have recent trauma or surgery. However, the time frame has been quite variable, ranging from 1 week to 3 months. In a recent study published by Verstraete et al.[68] 34 patients were treated with t-PA for a massive pulmonary embolism, some of whom had undergone a surgical procedure within the previous 15 days. Of the 34 patients 4 (12%) had major bleeding. All 4 of these

patients had had a major operation an average of 7.5 days (range 2 to 13 days) before treatment with heparin and t-PA. In 7 other patients who had undergone recent surgery (range 3 to 15 days), either minor or no bleeding was observed. These data suggest that in patients who present with AMI within 10 days of a recent surgery or trauma, thrombolytic therapy should probably be deferred. Alternative interventions such as primary PTCA would be an appropriate reperfusion strategy.

Other relative contraindications

Numerous other relative contraindications to thrombolytic therapy have been proposed. These include puncture of a noncompressible vessel, patients who may be at risk of having left heart thrombus, prior anticoagulation with warfarin, and menstruating women. Very little data exist regarding bleeding risks in any of these subsets. We do not exclude patients who have had a puncture of a subclavian or internal jugular vein unless it is known to be a traumatic procedure. In our opinion patients who have been on prior warfarin therapy are not considered ineligible for thrombolytic therapy. Conversely, we believe that if they have not bled despite systemic anticoagulation with warfarin, they may be less likely to bleed with thrombolytic therapy. However, a recent report from the Netherlands found warfarin therapy to be associated with an increased risk of intracranial bleeding, but this study only had a small number of patients, making the estimate of excess bleeding unreliable. Patients who have a high likelihood of a left heart thrombus (mitral stenosis with atrial fibrillation) have also been considered poor candidates for thrombolytic therapy because there might be partial lysis of the thrombus and embolization resulting in stroke. Once again, data on this entity are limited.

Whether menstruating women who sustain an AMI should be considered candidates for thrombolytic therapy has also been debated. We have not routinely excluded patients who are menstruating and have in fact treated a few such patients. Although an increase in menstrual flow was noted, we did not observe any serious bleeding in these women. A report from the GUSTO trial found no evidence of excess bleeding in 12 women treated with thrombolytic therapy.[69]

CONCLUSION

Given the data from recently completed trials,[31,32,37,38] indications for reperfusion therapy should be reassessed (Table 18-4). Patients who present with chest pain of greater than 30 minutes' duration with ST segment elevation (regardless of location) will generally benefit from reperfusion therapy. Special consideration should be given to patients with good clinical evidence for infarction and whose ECGs manifest left bundle branch block. Recent metaanalyses and randomized

Table 18-4. Patient selection for thrombolytic therapy

Indications

1. Chest pain > 20 min
2. ECG:
   ST ↑ ≥1 mm in two contiguous leads
   Left bundle branch block
   Questionable: anterior ST ↓ consistent with true posterior MI
3. Time window:
   <12 hours → all eligible patients
   12-24 hours → high-risk patients, continued CP
4. Special subsets (treat in absence of other contraindications):
   Remote (>6 mos) history of nonhemorrhagic stroke
   Past history (>2 mos) of gastrointestinal bleed
   Elderly
   Hypotension or moderate hypertension
   Cardiopulmonary resuscitation (nontraumatic, <10 minutes)

Contraindications

1. Absolute:
   Active internal bleeding
   Prior intracranial bleed, cerebral neoplasm, or other major intracranial pathology
   Stroke or head trauma (within 6 mos)
   Known allergy to a drug considered for use
2. Relative:
   Recent (<2 mos) surgery, gastrointestinal bleed
   Pregnancy, or within 1 month postpartum
   Severe, persistent hypertension (diastolic BP >110 mm Hg)
   Recent (<2 wks) trauma including CPR with rib fractures

trials suggest that the time window for treatment should be extended to 12 hours from symptom onset. Because there is some evidence to suggest that patients may continue to benefit beyond 12 hours, reperfusion therapy should be considered in this group if the patient is high risk, has stuttering onset of chest pain, or has evidence of continued ischemia. Furthermore, there are special subsets traditionally excluded from reperfusion therapy in whom the benefit may outweigh the risk. These subsets include the elderly, patients who present with hypertension, and those who have undergone CPR.

Although the indications for thrombolytic therapy should be expanded, given the lack of controlled scientific data determination of risk-to-benefit ratio for a patient with one or more relative contraindications remains difficult. It is important to point out that patients who are perceived as being at high risk for bleeding complications should not be denied reperfusion therapy. In these high-risk subsets strong consideration should be given to performance of emergency catheterization and percutaneous or surgical revascularization when appropriate.

REFERENCES

1. Simoons ML, Serruys PW, van den Brand M, et al: Early thrombolysis in acute myocardial infarction: limitation of infarct size and improved survival, *J Am Coll Cardiol* 7:717-728, 1986.
2. Kennedy JW, Ritchie JL, Davis KB, et al: Western Washington randomized trial of intracoronary streptokinase in acute myocardial infarction, *N Engl J Med* 309:1477-1482, 1983.
3. Schroder R, Neuhaus K-L, Leizorovicz A, et al for the ISAM Study Group: A prospective placebo-controlled double-blind multicenter trial of intravenous streptokinase in acute myocardial infarction (ISAM): long-term mortality and morbidity, *J Am Coll Cardiol* 9:197-203, 1987.
4. Gruppo Italiana per lo Studio della Streptochinasi nell'Infarto Miocardico (GISSI): Effectiveness of intravenous thrombolytic treatment in acute myocardial infarction, *Lancet* 1:349-360, 1986.
5. Wilcox RG, Olsson CG, Skene AM, et al for the ASSET Study Group: Trial of tissue plasminogen activator for mortality reduction in acute myocardial infarction, *Lancet* 1:525-530, 1988.
6. AIMS Trial Study Group: Effect of intravenous APSAC on mortality after acute myocardial infarction: preliminary report of a placebo-controlled clinical trial, *Lancet* 1:545-549, 1988.
7. ISIS-2 (Second International Study of Infarct Survival) Collaborative Group: Randomised trial of intravenous streptokinase, oral aspirin, both, or neither among 17,187 cases of suspected acute myocardial infarction: ISIS-2, *Lancet* 2:349-360, 1988.
8. Kennedy JW, Martin GV, Davis KB, et al: The Western Washington intravenous streptokinase in acute myocardial infarction randomized trial, *Circulation* 77:345-352, 1988.
9. Grines CL, DeMaria AN: Optimal utilization of thrombolytic therapy for acute myocardial infarction: concepts and controversies, *J Am Coll Cardiol* 16:223-231, 1990.
10. Goldberg RJ, Alpert JS: Worcester Heart Attack Study (unpublished data), 1992.
11. Doorey AJ, Michelson EL, Weber FJ, et al: Thrombolytic therapy of acute myocardial infarction: emerging challenges of implementation, *J Am Coll Cardiol* 10:1357-1360, 1987.
12. Althouse R, Maynard C, Olsufka M, et al: Incidence of contraindications to thrombolysis in patients with myocardial infarction, *Circulation* 78:(suppl II)II-211, 1988.
13. Cragg DR, Friedman HZ, Bonema JD, et al: Outcome of patients with acute myocardial infarction who are ineligible for thrombolytic therapy, *Ann Intern Med* 115:173-177, 1991.
14. Morgan C, Dombrower H, Choi E, et al: Thrombolytic therapy for acute myocardial infarction: is it under used? (abstract), *J Am Coll Cardiol* 19:A-20, 1992.
15. Sainsous J, Serradimigni A, Richard JL, et al: How many patients with acute myocardial infarction could be treated in France by intravenous streptokinase? Results of a prospective trial (abstract), *Eur Heart J* 6:I-67, 1985.
16. Murray N, Lyons J, Layton C, et al: What proportion of patients with myocardial infarction are suitable for thrombolysis? *Br Heart J* 57:144-147, 1987.
17. Jagger JD, Murray RG, Davies MK, et al: Eligibility for thrombolytic therapy in acute myocardial infarction, *Lancet* 1:34-35, 1987.
18. Gruppo Italiano per lo Studio della Sopravvivenza nell'Infarto Miocardico (GISSI-2): A factorial randomized trial of alteplase versus streptokinase and heparin versus no heparin among 12,490 patients with acute myocardial infarction, *Lancet* 336:65, 1990.
19. Behar S, Hod H, Barbash G, et al: Incidence of and reasons for excluding patients with acute myocardial infarction from thrombolytic therapy, *Isr J Med Sci* 27:121-123, 1991.
20. Karlson BW, Herlitz J, Edvardsson N, et al: Eligibility for intravenous thrombolysis in suspected acute myocardial infarction, *Circulation* 82:1140-1146, 1990.
21. Greenbaum R, Sritara P, Shanit D, et al: Acute myocardial

infarction in greater London, 1980-1989, reduced mortality with general adoption of thrombolytic therapy: scope for increased use in the elderly (abstract), *J Am Coll Cardiol* 29:21A, 1992.

22. Paine TD, Maske LE, Bradley EL Jr, et al: Community practice patterns in the management of prolonged ischemic chest pain with or without ST elevation (abstract), *J Am Coll Cardiol* 29:21A, 1992.
23. Rogers WJ, Chandra NC, Tiefenbrunn AJ, et al: Practice patterns in the management of patients with acute myocardial infarction: report of a registry of 74,237 patients (abstract), *J Am Coll Cardiol* 16:223, 1990.
24. Pfeffer MA, Braunwald E, Cuddy TE, et al: Selection bias in the use of thrombolytic therapy in acute myocardial infarction (abstract), *Circulation* 80:II-522, 1989.
25. Gunnar RM, Bourdillon PDV, Dixon DW, et al: A report of the American College of Cardiology/American Heart Association Task Force on Assessment of Diagnostic and Therapeutic Cardiovascular Procedures (Subcommittee to Develop Guidelines for the Early Management of Patients with Acute Myocardial Infarction). Guidelines for the early management of patients with acute myocardial infarction, *J Am Coll Cardiol* 16:249-292, 1990.
26. The TIMI Study Group: Comparison of invasive and conservative strategies after treatment with intravenous tissue plasminogen activator in acute myocardial infarction. Results of the Thrombolysis in Myocardial Infarction (TIMI) Phase II trial, *N Engl J Med* 320:618-627, 1989.
27. Bates ER: Reperfusion therapy in inferior myocardial infarction, *J Am Coll Cardiol* 12:44A-51A, 1988.
28. Vermeer F, Simoons ML, Bar FW, et al: Which patients benefit most from early thrombolytic therapy with intracoronary streptokinase? *Circulation* 74:1379-1389, 1986.
29. European Cooperative Study Group for Streptokinase Treatment in Acute Myocardial Infarction: Streptokinase in acute myocardial infarction, *N Engl J Med* 301:797-802, 1979.
30. Mauri F, Gasparini M, Barbonaglia L, et al: Prognostic significance of the extent of myocardial injury in acute myocardial infarction treated by streptokinase (the GISSI trial), *Am J Cardiol* 63:1291-1295, 1989.
31. Third International Study of Infarct Survival Collaborative Group: ISIS-3: a randomised comparison of streptokinase vs tissue plasminogen activator vs anistreplase and of aspirin plus heparin vs aspirin alone among 41,299 cases of suspected acute myocardial infarction, *Lancet* 339:753-770, 1992.
32. Fibrinolytic Therapy Trialists' (FTT) Collaborative Group: Indications for fibrinolytic therapy in suspected acute myocardial infarction: collaborative overview of early mortality and major morbidity results from all randomised trials of more than 1000 patients, *Lancet* 343:311-322, 1994.
33. MacDonnel AH, Grines CL: Absence of ST elevation during myocardial infarction identifies a patient population with advanced age and increased need for revascularization, *J Am Coll Cardiol* 17:45A, 1991.
34. Karlson BW, Herlitz J, Wiklund O, et al: Early prediction of acute myocardial infarction from clinical history, examination, and electrocardiogram in the emergency room, *Am J Cardiol* 68:171-175, 1991.
35. Cannon CP, McCabe CH, Chaitman B, et al for the TIMI-3B investigators. Clinical variables that distinguish non–Q-wave MI from unstable angina in patients with acute coronary ischemia: an analysis from the TIMI-3B trial, *Circulation* 86:I-388, 1992.
36. Yusuf S, Collins R, Peto R, et al: Intravenous and intracoronary fibrinolytic therapy in acute myocardial infarction: overview of results on mortality, reinfarction, and side effects from 33 randomized controlled trials, *Eur Heart J* 6:556-585, 1985.
37. EMERAS (Estudio Multicentrico Estreptoquinasa Republicas de America del Sur) Collaborative Group: Randomised trial of late

thrombolysis in patients with suspected acute myocardial infarction, *Lancet* 342:767-772, 1993.
38. LATE (Late Assessment of Thrombolytic Efficacy) Study Group: Late assessment of thrombolytic efficacy (LATE) study with alteplase 6-24 hours after onset of acute myocardial infarction, *Lancet* 342:759-766, 1993.
39. Braunwald E: Myocardial reperfusion, limitation of infarct size, reduction of left ventricular dysfunction, and improved survival. Should the paradigm be expanded? *Circulation* 79:441-444, 1989.
40. Little WC, Gwinn NS, Burrows MT, et al: Cause of acute myocardial infarction late after successful coronary artery bypass grafting, *Am J Cardiol* 65:808-810, 1990.
41. Crean PA, Waters DD, Bosch X, et al: Angiographic findings after myocardial infarction in patients with previous bypass surgery: explanations for smaller infarcts in this group compared with control patients, *Circulation* 71:693-698, 1985.
42. Maynard C, Weaver WD, Litwin P, et al for the MITI Investigators: Prior coronary artery surgery and acute myocardial infarction: patient characteristics, treatment, and outcome, *J Am Coll Cardiol* 17:65A, 1991.
43. Cox DA, Davis WR, Williams JA, et al: How do patients with prior coronary artery bypass grafting and severe chest pain differ in presentation, management, and outcome? *Circulation* 86:I-196, 1992.
44. Grines CL, Booth DC, Nissen SE, et al: Mechanism of acute myocardial infarction in patients with prior coronary artery bypass grafting and therapeutic implications, *Am J Cardiol* 65:1292-1296, 1990.
45. Kleiman NS, Berman DA, Gaston WR, et al: Early intravenous thrombolytic therapy for acute myocardial infarction in patients with prior coronary artery bypass grafts. *Am J Cardiol* 63:102-104, 1989.
46. Bates ER, Topol EJ: Limitations of thrombolytic therapy for acute myocardial infarction complicated by congestive heart failure and cardiogenic shock, *J Am Coll Cardiol* 18:1077-1084, 1991.
47. O'Neill WW: Angioplasty therapy of cardiogenic shock: are randomized trials necessary? *J Am Coll Cardiol* 19:915-917, 1992.
48. Schumacher RR, Smalling RW, Morris DC, et al: A multicenter, randomized comparison of two doses of recombinant tissue plasminogen activator in treatment of myocardial infarction (abstract), *Circulation* 78:II-275, 1988.
49. Califf RM, Topol EJ, George BS, et al and the Thrombolysis and Angioplasty in Myocardial Infarction Study Group: Hemorrhagic complications associated with the use of intravenous tissue plasminogen activator in treatment of acute myocardial infarction, *Am J Med* 85:353-359, 1988.
50. Bovill EG, Terrin ML, Stump DC, et al for the TIMI Investigators: Hemorrhagic events during therapy with recombinant tissue-type plasminogen activator, heparin, and aspirin for acute myocardial infarction, *Ann Int Med* 115:256-265, 1991.
51. Brott T, Thalinger K, Hertzberg V: Hypertension as a risk factor for spontaneous intracerebral hemorrhage, *Stroke* 17:1078-1083, 1986.
52. Maggioni AP, Granzosi MG, Santoro E, et al for the GISSI-2 and the International Study Group: The risk of stroke in patients with acute myocardial infarction after thrombolytic and antithrombotic treatment, *N Engl J Med* 327:1-6, 1992.
53. Granger CB, O'Connor CM, Bleich SD, et al: An overview of the effect of intravenous heparin on clinical endpoints following thrombolytic therapy for acute myocardial infarction (abstract), *Circulation* 86:I-259, 1992.
54. Grines CL, Browne KF, Marco J, et al for the Primary Angioplasty in Myocardial Infarction (PAMI) Study Group: A comparison of immediate angioplasty with thrombolytic therapy for acute myocardial infarction, *N Engl J Med* 328:673-679, 1993.
55. Montague TJ, Ikuta RM, Wong RY, et al: Comparison of risk and

patterns of practice in patients older and younger than 70 years with acute myocardial infarction in a two-year period (1987-1989), *Am J Cardiol* 68:843-847, 1991.

56. Weaver WD, Litwin PE, Martin JS, et al for the MITI Project Group: Effect of age on use of thrombolytic therapy and mortality in acute myocardial infarction, *J Am Coll Cardiol* 18:657-662, 1991.

57. National Center for Health Statistics 1987 Summary: National Hospital Discharge Survey. Advance Data from Vital and Health Statistics, DHHS Publication 88-1250; 159:1-16.

58. Black JS, Sefcik T, Kapoor W: Health promotion and disease prevention in the elderly. Comparison of house staff and attending physician attitudes and practices, *Arch Intern Med* 150:389-393, 1990.

59. Smith SC, Jr, Gilpin E, Ahnve S, et al: Outlook after acute myocardial infarction in the very elderly compared with that in patients aged 65 to 75 years, *J Am Coll Cardiol* 16:784-792, 1990.

60. Krumholz HM, Pasternak RC, Weinstein MC, et al: Cost effectiveness of thrombolytic therapy with streptokinase in elderly patients with suspected acute myocardial infarction, *N Engl J Med* 327:7-13, 1992.

61. Devlin W, Cragg DR, Jacks MJ, et al: Outcome of aged with myocardial infarction in the lytic era (abstract), *J Am Coll Cardiol* 21:482A, 1993.

62. Yang XS, Willems JL, Pardaens J, et al: Acute myocardial infarction in the very elderly. A comparison with younger age groups. *Acta Cardiol* XLII(42):59-68, 1987.

63. Althouse R, Weaver WD, Kennedy JW: Transient elevation of diastolic blood pressure in acute myocardial infarction—a contraindication to thrombolytic therapy? *Circulation* 76:IV-306, 1987.

64. Anderson JL, Karagounis L, Allen A, et al: Older age and elevated blood pressure are risk factors for intracerebral hemorrhage after thrombolysis, *Am J Cardiol* 68:166-170, 1991.

65. Tenaglia AN, Califf RM, Candela RJ, et al: Thrombolytic therapy in patients requiring cardiopulmonary resuscitation, *Am J Cardiol* 68:1015-1019, 1991.

66. Scholz KH, Tebbe U, Herrmann C, et al: Frequency of complications of cardiopulmonary resuscitation after thrombolysis during acute myocardial infarction, *Am J Cardiol* 69:724-728, 1992.

67. O'Connor CM, Califf RM, Massey EW, et al: Stroke and acute myocardial infarction in the thrombolytic era: clinical correlates and long-term prognosis, *J Am Coll Cardiol* 16:533-540, 1990.

68. Verstraete M, Miller GA, Bounameaux H, et al: Intravenous and intrapulmonary recombinant tissue-type plasminogen activator in the treatment of acute massive pulmonary embolism, *Circulation* 77:353-360, 1988.

69. Karnash SL, Granger C, Kline-Rogers E, et al: Menstruating women may be safely and effectively treated with thrombolytic therapy: experience from the GUSTO trial, *J Am Coll Cardiol* 23:315A, 1994.

Chapter 19

TWELVE-LEAD ECG AND EXTENT OF MYOCARDIUM AT RISK OF ACUTE INFARCTION

Galen S. Wagner
Ronald H. Selvester
Richard D. White
Nancy B. Wagner

In a patient with symptoms of acute myocardial ischemia-infarction (AMI-I), the 12-lead electrocardiogram (ECG) is the most important commonly available clinical test. When the patient is first seen, it is most appropriate to use the term AMI-I, because the diagnosis of infarction cannot be made with certainty, and the progression from ischemia to infarction may not have occurred. A significant relationship has been established between the initial changes in ST-segment deviation and the final extent of infarcted myocardium in patients who do not receive reperfusion therapy.[1-3] Consideration of this relationship might (1) provide a rationale for deciding which patients with AMI-I might and which might not benefit from acute interventions to achieve myocardial reperfusion[4] and (2) facilitate the assessment of both the benefit and cost of such interventions.[5,6]

The ventricular myocardium receives its electrical current from the endocardial Purkinje network. Although this network is minimally vulnerable to AMI-I,[7] the subendocardium into which the Purkinje fibers insert is extremely vulnerable because it is composed of working myocardial cells at the distal aspect of the coronary arterial perfusion bed. AMI-I may slow con-

duction in this subendocardial layer and delay the electrical activation of the deeper myocardial layers.[8] The effect of diminished blood flow on intra-Purkinje, Purkinje-to-myocardium, and transmyocardial activation and recovery determines the behavior of the "cardiac electrical generator" during the processes of ischemia and infarction. The geometric and conductive properties of the torso determine the final waveforms recorded via the ECG leads on the body surface.[9]

The purpose of this chapter is to provide insight into the relationships between the timing and extent of AMI-I and the changes that appear on the patient's presenting ECG.

REGIONAL MYOCARDIAL SUBDIVISIONS

Considerable inconsistency and ambiguity currently exist in the literature regarding the nomenclature of the myocardial regions. For effective communication about the interpretation of diagnostic tests, it is essential to have a set of clearly defined terms for the various regions that are generally agreed on and used by consensus.

The report of the Committee on Nomenclature of Myocardial Wall Segments of the International Society of Computerized Electrocardiography addressed this

Segment subdivision

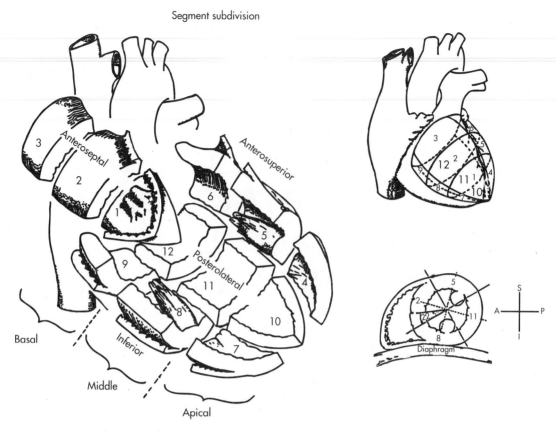

Fig. 19-1. The 12-segment subdivision of the left ventricle of Ideker et al. is presented in three diagrams. The center of the septum is the reference point for constructing eight circumferential (octant) subdivisions in serial bread-loaf cross sections of the left ventricle (LV) (*lower right*). Each two adjacent octants are combined to provide quadrant subdivisions (*solid lines*): anteroseptal (*A*), anterosuperior (*S*), posterolateral (*P*), and inferior (*I*). The LV is further divided from apex to base into three approximately equal parts by passing planes at right angles to its internal long axis (*upper right*). (From Ideker RE, Wagner GS, Ruth WK, et al: *Am J Cardiol* 49:1604, 1982. Used by permission.)

specific problem.[10] This committee recommended the adoption of a 12-segment subdivision of the left ventricle (LV) based on the method of Ideker et al.,[11] which is a modification of the method of Horan et al.[12] The Ideker et al.[11] method uses eight circumferential (octant) subdivisions starting with a line 22.5 degrees posterior to the middle of the septum in serial bread-loaf cross sections of the heart. This is shown in the lower right diagram in Fig. 19-1. This line was chosen because it is located approximately at the junction between the perfusion beds of the septal-perforating branches of the left anterior descending (LAD) and posterior descending (PD) arteries. Continuing in a clockwise direction around these cross sections (as viewed from below), each two adjacent octants are combined to provide four quadrants: anteroseptal, anterosuperior, posterolateral, and inferior. The LV is further subdivided into three regions from apex to base (apical, middle, and basal) by construction of planes at right angles to its internal long

axis, as shown in the upper right diagram in Fig. 19-1. This produces the final 12 segments of approximately equal volume shown at the left of the figure. An analogous recommendation for subdivisions also appeared at about the same time from the Committee on Nomenclature and Standards of the American Society of Echocardiography.[13] The nomenclature and definitions of the four quadrants and 12 subdivisions shown in Fig. 19-1 are used throughout this chapter.

CORONARY ARTERIAL ANATOMY

A Mercator projection of the epicardial surface of the LV based on the Ideker et al.[11] subdivisions is depicted in Fig. 19-2, showing the typical distributions of the three major coronary arteries. The anteroseptal and antero-superior quadrants are perfused by the LAD, which also typically supplies the apical segments of both the posterolateral and inferior quadrants (about 60% of the LV). The base of the anterosuperior wall has a dual

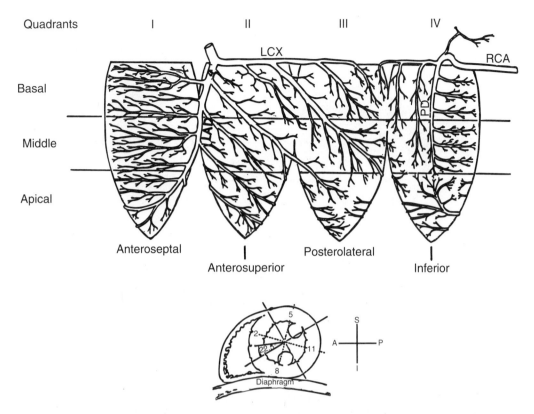

Fig. 19-2. Mercator projection of the epicardial surfaces of the Ideker et al. quadrants of the left ventricle (LV) is shown, with the typical distributions of the three major coronary arteries. The inferior portion of the septum, which is perfused by the posterior descending (*PD*) branch of the right coronary artery (*RCA*), is included in the inferior quadrant (IV). The left anterior descending (*LAD*) artery typically supplies the anteroseptal (I) and anterosuperior (II) quadrants and most of the apical segments of the posterolateral (III) and inferior (IV) quadrants (> 50% of the LV). The base of the anterosuperior quadrant has a dual blood supply from both the LAD and left circumflex (*LCX*) branches. Except for their apical segments, the posterolateral quadrant is supplied by the LCX and the inferior quadrant by the RCA. Each of these arteries typically supplies about 20% of the LV.

blood supply from both the LAD and left circumflex (LCX). The LCX supplies the basal and middle segments of the posterolateral quadrant (about 20% of the LV). The basal and middle segments of the inferior quadrant are perfused by the PD (about 20% of the LV).

There is variability throughout the population in the coronary artery distributions to the various myocardial areas. This is particularly true in the apical segments of the posterolateral and inferior quadrants, which may be supplied by the distal LAD, the PD branch of the RCA, or the obtuse marginal branch of the LCX. In a small percentage of patients, the RCA is unusually dominant, supplying much of the middle and basal segments of the posterolateral quadrant. In the 10% to 15% of the patients with a left dominant coronary circulation, the PD is a branch of the LCX.

MI-I ANATOMY

The regional distributions of wall motion abnormalities caused by MI-I in the three primary coronary arterial areas, as seen in biplane ventriculograms in the Rancho Los Amigos (USC) population,[14] are presented in Fig. 19-3. When a coronary artery is acutely occluded, the entire area of its supply is potentially at risk of infarction. The more proximal the occlusion, the larger the risk area. The typical sizes of the risk areas (expressed as percentage of the LV) in the distributions of the major coronary arteries are LAD 50%, RCA 20%, and LCX 20%. These sizes are similar to the risk areas documented by Gibbons et al.[15] using technetium-99m–labeled sestamibi imaging of patients with acute coronary occlusions.

In the absence of reperfusion via the acutely occluded artery, myocardial salvage within the risk area depends on collateral flow from other arterial beds. This reperfusion via collateral arteries typically produces salvage of approximately 50% of the risk area. This would result in anterior infarcts in the distribution of the LAD with a median extent of 25% of the LV, and inferior or posterolateral infarcts in the distributions of the RCA or

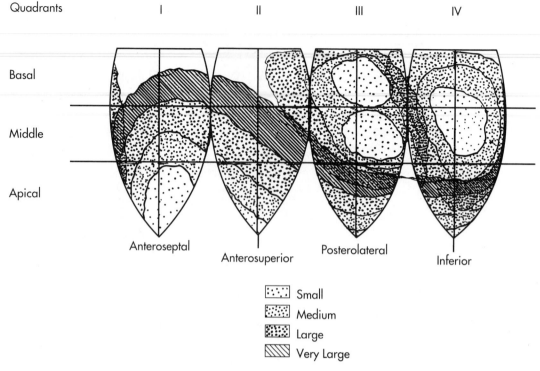

Fig. 19-3. Mercator projection of the epicardial surface of the left ventricle (LV) (as in Fig. 2-2), with the regional distribution of single infarcts as seen on biplane ventriculograms in the Rancho/USC series. The majority of infarcts involved less than half of the potential risk area and were localized to the distal distribution of their particular vascular beds. Large to very large infarcts involving more than 30% of the LV occurred in less than one fifth of this patient population. (From Wagner GS, Cowan MJ, Flowers NC, et al: Nomenclature of myocardial wall segments: committee report. In Selvester RH [ed]: *Proceeding of the 1983 Engineering Foundation Conference, computerized interpretation of the ECG VIII,* New York, 1983, Engineering Foundation Press, p 222. Used by permission.)

LCX of 10% of the LV. These sizes are similar to those documented anatomically by Sevilla et al.[16] and ventriculographically by Selvester et al.[14] Table 19-1 presents the distributions of the sizes of wall motion abnormalities produced by healed infarcts in the various myocardial locations. The Rancho Los Amigos (USC) population presented in Table 19-1 and Fig. 19-3 was studied before the introduction of therapeutic reperfusion therapies.[14]

There is great variability of the extent of reperfusion of the risk area via either collateral arteries or the acutely occluded artery. The collaterals could be so effective that the entire risk area is salvaged and no infarct occurs. If reperfusion via the occluded artery is achieved within minutes, complete salvage could also occur.

Acute occlusion of the proximal LAD coronary artery not accompanied by reperfusion via either collaterals or the acutely occluded vessel typically results in large to very large areas of infarction (Fig. 19-3). When reperfusion accomplishes extensive salvage, the resulting

infarcts are small to medium and are confined mainly to the endocardial half of the myocardium in the distal distribution of a particular vascular bed. The two areas of small infarcts in the LCX distribution relate to occlusions of the obtuse marginal and distal divisions, respectively; both areas would be involved with occlusions of the proximal LCX.

Very large infarcts—involving more than 30% of the LV with severe dysfunction and ejection fraction less than 35%—occurred in less than one fifth of patients, most of whom had anterior locations. Acute occlusion of an "unusually dominant RCA" or a dominant LCX also produced very large "inferoposterior" infarcts.

PURKINJE SYSTEM ANATOMY

The projection of the left ventricle shown in Fig. 19-4 provides a view of its endocardial surface. The 12 subdivisions are the same as those presented in Fig. 19-1. The multifascicular left bundle and its regional insertions into the endocardium are shown. These insertions tend to cluster on the anteroseptal quadrant

Table 19-1. Percentage of left ventricle infarcted

Infarct location	All sizes (%)	%			
		Small (<12%)	Moderate (13%-21%)	Large (22%-32%)	Very large (>33%)
Anterior	40	11	16	8	5
Inferior	39	22	14	3	0
Posterolateral	21	14	6	1	0

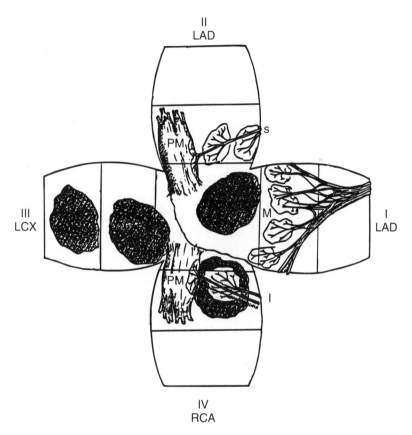

Fig. 19-4. In this subendocardial view of the left ventricle, the four quadrants and their apical, middle, and basal segments are the same as those in previous figures. The shaded areas represent the typical sites of small infarcts in each of the three major coronary artery distributions. The two areas shown in the left circumflex (*LCX*) area represent the distal perfusion beds of its main marginal and distal branches. The sites of endocardial insertion of the superior (*S*), middle (*M*), and inferior (*I*) fascicles of the left bundle are shown. The left anterior descending (*LAD*) artery supplies all of quadrants I and II and most of the apical segments of quadrants III and IV. *PM,* Papillary muscles of the mitral valve.

near the junction of its apical and middle segments, and adjacent to the papillary muscles on the middle segments of both the inferior and anterosuperior quadrants. There are multiple individual fascicles clustered within each of the three main subdivisions of the left bundle. The cluster on the anteroseptal quadrant would be most appropriately termed the "middle fascicles," the cluster on the anterosuperior quadrant the "anterosuperior fascicles," and the cluster on the inferior quadrant the "posteroinferior fascicles." The right bundle branch inserts into the apical segment near the base of the papillary muscle on the right septal surface. All of these Purkinje fascicles insert into myocardium supplied by the LAD except for the posteroinferior fascicles of the left bundle, which insert into the center of the endocardial region supplied by the PD. A peripheral network of Purkinje fibers extends beyond the insertions of these fascicles to supply rapid electrical activation to the remainder of the endocardial surfaces of both ventricles.

ANATOMIC CONSIDERATIONS AND THE PRESENTING ECG DURING AMI-I

AMI-I can be associated with intraventricular conduction delays because of blocks within the proximal bundle branches and their fascicles caused by occlusion of the blood supply to the basal segment of the anteroseptal quadrant.[17] New-onset right bundle branch block, left bundle branch block, or left anterosuperior fascicular block are therefore indicative of a very large area of AMI-I. Isolated left posteroinferior fascicular block almost never results from direct interference with the Purkinje system blood supply.[17] However, when these conduction abnormalities appear on the presenting ECG, it is possible to determine whether they are old or new only if a recent previous ECG is available for comparison. Various combinations of bundle branch and fascicular blocks appear early during AMI-I and then persist or recur during evolution of the infarction.[17,18] When both right and left bundle branches are involved, the patient is at risk for sudden occurrence of complete atrioventricular block. These conduction abnormalities typically occur with large anterior infarcts resulting from main left or proximal LAD occlusion but may rarely occur with large inferior infarcts that extend into the base of the anteroseptal quadrant.

AMI-I can also produce intraventricular conduction delays when subendocardial ischemia impedes the spread of electrical activation from the insertions of the various Purkinje fascicles into the myocardium. This phenomenon was initially described during acute infarction and termed "periinfarction block" by First et al.[19] in 1950. The schematic view of the endocardial surface of the LV as viewed from above in Fig. 19-4 provides

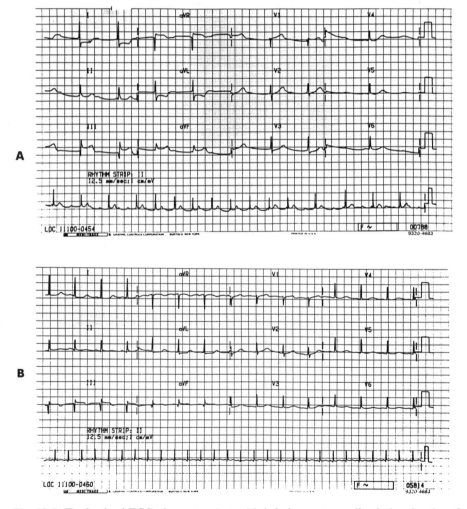

Fig. 19-5. Twelve-lead ECGs from a patient with inferior acute cardiac ischemia when first seen (**A**) and on the second day of treatment (**B**). Note the vertical QRS axis in **A** and the shift leftward in **B**. This shift is accompanied by resolution of the intraventricular conduction disturbance, as indicated by decrease in QRS duration from 0.10 to 0.08 second.

visualization of the relationships between the fascicular insertions and the most common sites of AMI-I in the various arterial distributions. An understanding of these relationships elucidates the meaning of the changes that may appear on the ECG almost immediately after sudden complete occlusion of the various arteries.

AMI-I IN THE INFERIOR QUADRANT

The endocardial area at greatest risk for inferior quadrant AMI-I is located at the site of the insertion of the inferoposterior fascicles of the left bundle. Thus, even minimal inferior AMI-I may be associated with disruption of the normal electrical activation of this region, producing a conduction disturbance that mimics block in the inferoposterior fascicles themselves (Fig. 19-5). The classic changes on the ECG of inferoposterior fascicular block are (1) wide separation of the initial and terminal 30 msec of the QRS complex in the frontal plane with Q waves and late R waves in leads II, III, and aV_F, (2) slight increase in QRS duration to 100 to 110 msec, and (3) a rightward and inferior axis shift to greater than plus 60 degrees.[20]

The changes in QRS morphology resulting from AMI-I in this region are variations on the classic changes of inferoposterior fascicular block. During the earliest phase of AMI-I there is transmural ischemia, which is most profound in the interior subendocardial regions. The Purkinje fibers insert into this ischemic myocardium, which then conducts very slowly into the deeper layers. Terminal inferior and rightward forces are produced by the delayed activation of the deeper layers

of myocardium in the inferior quadrant, closely mimicking the changes typical of inferoposterior fascicular block (see Figs. 19-2 to 19-5, A). Previous terms such as "inferior periinfarction block"[19] and "left posterior hemiblock"[20] have been applied, but a more appropriate term is "inferior ischemic block."

During the later phases of AMI-I, as infarction evolves and extends transmurally and basally, it significantly eliminates any activation of these regions (see Figs. 19-2 to 19-5, B). The mean QRS axis then shifts back leftward and occasionally even moves superiorly. A small inferior and rightward terminal activation front produces a slight QRS prolongation and usually persists throughout the evolutionary process because the infarct rarely becomes completely transmural at the base.

AMI-I IN THE ANTEROSUPERIOR QUADRANT

Only a large area of AMI-I could interrupt endocardial conduction from the anterosuperior fascicles into the underlying myocardium, producing a change in activation similar to that of left anterosuperior fascicular block. The classic changes seen on the ECG are (1) wide separation of the initial and terminal 30 msec of the QRS with Q waves and late R waves in leads I and aV_L, (2) modest increase in QRS duration to 100 to 110 msec, and (3) leftward and superior axis deviation greater than -30 degrees. The changes in QRS resulting from AMI-I in this region are variations of the classic changes of anterosuperior fascicular block, depending on the extent of the subendocardial involvement. Previous terms such as "lateral periinfarction block,"[19] "left anterior hemi-

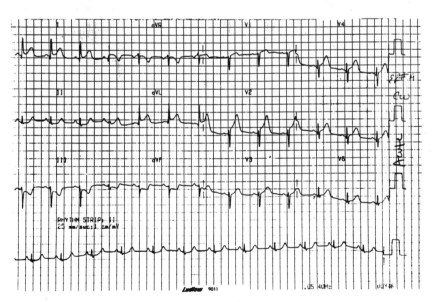

Fig. 19-6. Presenting 12-lead ECG from a patient with extensive anterosuperior AMI-I. Note the intraventricular conduction disturbance (QRS 0.10 second), with late forces directed toward the area of involvement, producing a leftward axis deviation. This change could represent true left superior fascicular block or its mimic caused by AMI-I of the anterosuperior endocardium into which the fascicle inserts.

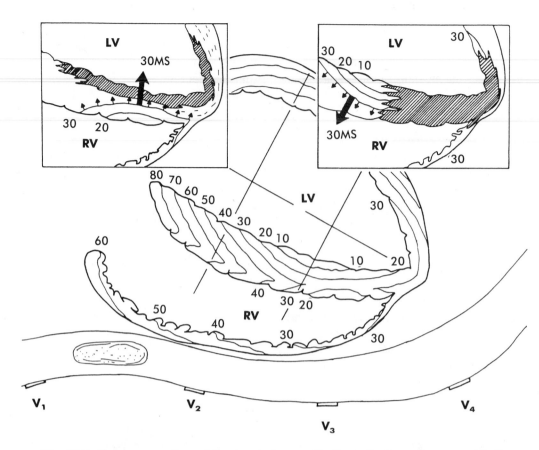

Fig. 19-7. Transverse section of the heart shown with the activation sequences of both ventricles. Activation by way of the middle fascicles of the left bundle begins on the left septal surface at the junction of the middle and apical segments. The right bundle activates its more distal site of insertion on the right septal surface about 10 ms later. Subendocardial AMI-I that disrupts the left septal activation (*left insert*) can lead to posteriorly directed 30-ms vectors from the unopposed right septal activation. Conversely, transmural AMI-I that preserves the left septal activation (*right insert*) but disrupts the right septal activation can lead to an anteriorly directed 30-ms vector. V_1-V_4, Leads on body surface; *LV,* left ventricle; *RV,* right ventricle.

block,"[20] and "parietal block"[21] have been applied, but a more appropriate term is "anterosuperior ischemic block." Because the base of the anterosuperior quadrant usually survives even a very large anterior infarct, an abnormal leftward and superior axis typically persists throughout the evolution of the infarct (Fig. 19-6).

AMI-I IN THE ANTEROSEPTAL QUADRANT

A moderate-sized area of AMI-I involving the mid-septum and extending into the region of the insertion of the middle fascicles of the left bundle may disrupt the normal activation of the endocardium (see Fig. 19-4) and simulate "middle fascicular block." This can lead to augmentation of the normal posteriorly directed activation fronts from the right septal activation, as shown for the 30-msec front in the left insert of Fig. 19-7. There may be diminished R waves or even Q waves in the right precordial leads. A study by Hassett et al.[22] has documented such changes transiently during AMI-I that did not progress to infarction.

In comparison with the left bundle, the right bundle inserts more distally on its septal surface and provides myocardial activation about 10 msec later (Fig. 19-7). Because of this bilateral septal activation, there is normally cancellation of QRS forces. As shown in the right insert, a moderately large transmural area of anterior AMI-I that disrupts the right but not the left septal activation can augment the anteriorly directed activation fronts throughout the early to mid-QRS, producing increased R and decreased S waves in leads V_1 and V_2. These changes may suggest incomplete RBBB. However, the typical late R' wave of RBBB is not prominent because the normal activation of the right ventricular free wall has not been disturbed (Fig. 19-8).

These conduction disturbances are commonly observed transiently during the hyperacute and acute phases of AMI-I. They typically disappear when the acute ischemia is either reversed or evolves into infarction.

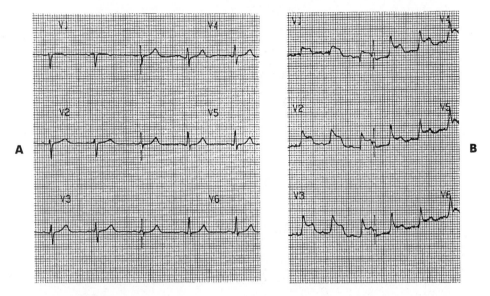

Fig. 19-8. The baseline appearance of the horizontal plane **(A)** is presented as reference for the changes that evolve after four minutes of angioplasty balloon occlusion of the proximal LAD **(B)**. Note the loss of S waves and terminal R′ waves in leads V1 and V2 during the transmural ischemia. This represents the shift in QRS forces toward the involved myocardial area caused by the "current of injury" and also a disturbance in intraventricular conduction, most likely at the site of insertion of the right bundle into the septum (see right insert in Fig. 19-7).

AMI-I IN THE POSTEROLATERAL QUADRANT

The posterolateral quadrant is located in the left ventricular free wall between the papillary muscles. This region is activated relatively late because it does not receive a cluster of fascicles from the left bundle branch. Therefore, AMI-I in the posterolateral quadrant is less likely to be accompanied by ischemia-induced conduction delays that mimic fascicular blocks. However, this area is supplied by the peripheral Purkinje network, and acute ischemia in this region may cause as much as 50 msec of late activation to be added to the QRS duration.

CARDIAC ANATOMY AND ECG LEAD LOCATIONS

Orthogonal transaxial (transverse plane) and coronal (frontal plane) magnetic resonance imaging (MRI) of the heart[23] offers a new perspective for understanding the orientation of the heart relative to the surface of the body. Visualization of the relationships of the frontal and precordial leads of the standard ECG to the cardiac anatomy may elucidate the characteristic ECG changes resulting from infarcts in the distribution of the three major coronary arteries. However, because the positioning of the heart in the body varies with individual patients, these relationships can be discussed only in general.

An evaluation of the relationships of the precordial ECG leads and the LV by transaxial MRI indicates that leads V_1 through V_6 roughly follow the course of the LAD coronary artery along the interventricular groove. Leads V_1 and V_2 are placed directly over the basal third of the interventricular septum (proximal LAD distribution) and opposite the posterolateral wall of the LV located between the papillary muscles (Fig. 19-9, A). This perspective elucidates the importance of observing ECG changes that are exactly opposite those of anteroseptal involvement when the myocardium is evaluated in the left circumflex (LCX) distribution. Leads V_3 and V_4 override the middle third of the interventricular septum in the mid-LAD distribution (Fig. 19-9, B and C). Leads V_5 and V_6 overlie the anterior superior and posterolateral aspects of the LV apex, respectively, in the distal LAD distribution (Fig. 19-9, C). Because the precordial leads are perpendicular to the inferior region of the LV, they would not be expected to effectively record ischemic events in this quadrant.

The inferior portion of the interventricular septum and the immediately adjacent free wall are best visualized on coronal MR images (frontal plane, Fig. 19-10, A and B). Leads II, III, and aV_F are directed at these regions, which are usually supplied by the distal distribution of a dominant RCA. The basal and middle aspects of these regions are best viewed in the frontal plane because of their inferior position in the in situ heart. Leads I and aV_L are oriented superoleftward and

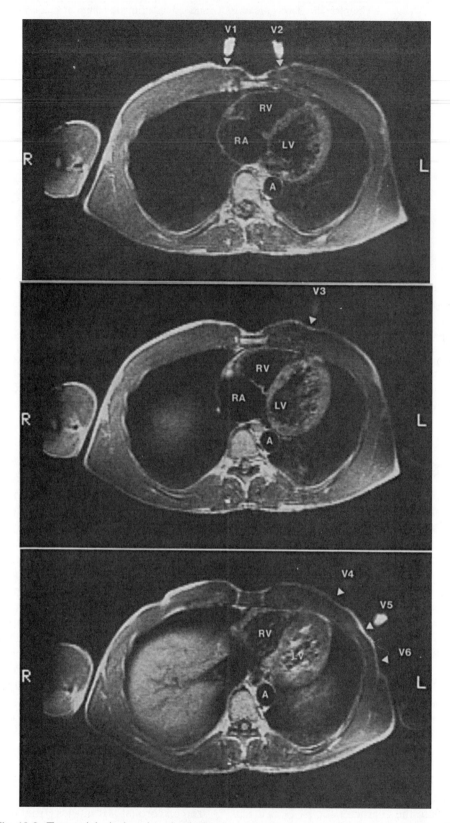

Fig. 19-9. Transaxial, single spin-echo (echo time 30 ms), electrocardiogram-gated magnetic resonance images (1 cm thick) from a normal volunteer. The orientations of the precordial leads (V_1-V_6) are indicated. The left and right ventricles (*LV* and *RV*), right atrium (*RA*), and thoracic aorta (*A*) are labeled. In these three sequential images, the normal positions of the precordial leads are demonstrated by markers on the chest wall. Leads V_1 and V_2 are found directly over the basal interventricular septum (proximal–left anterior descending [LAD] distribution) and opposite the posterolateral wall (left circumflex distribution). Leads V_3 and V_4 (*top* and *bottom*) override the middle portion of the septum (mid-LAD distribution), and leads V_5 and V_6 (*bottom*) overlie the apex (distal-LAD distribution).

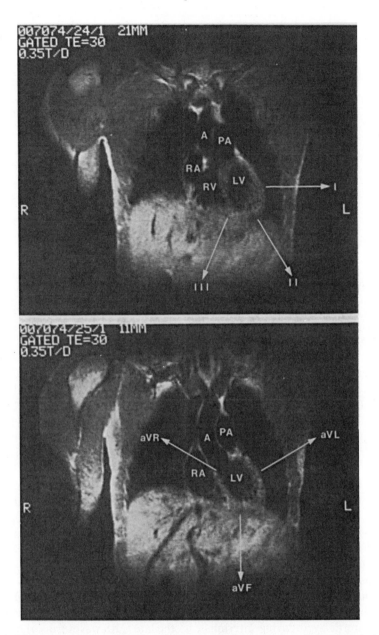

Fig. 19-10. These two consecutive coronal images demonstrate the relationships between the frontal leads (*arrows* indicate direction of positive polarity) and regions of the left ventricle (LV). Leads II, III, and aV_F would reflect ischemic changes in the inferior region lying adjacent to the diaphragm and in the interoseptal region of the LV (distal distribution of a dominant right coronary artery [RCA]). Changes in leads I and aV_L would be most indicative of damage in the anterosuperior region in the basal and middle thirds of the LV (proximal diagonal branches of left anterior descending and/or proximal obtuse marginal branches of the left circumflex). Thoracic aorta (*A*), left and right ventricles (*LV* and *RV*), right atrium (*RA*), and main pulmonary artery (*PA*) are labeled.

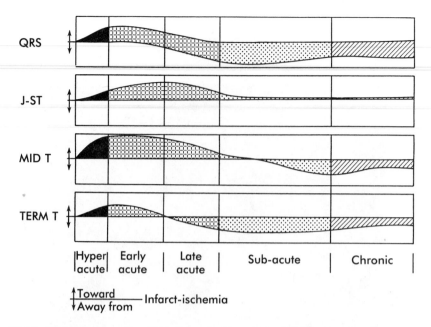

Fig. 19-11. Diagram shows the four electrocardiographic (ECG) phases of acute coronary occlusion. Panels showing the evolution of the acute infarct to its chronic, stable phase are indicated at the bottom. Each panel illustrates the typical change in direction and amplitude of the QRS complex, J point and ST segment, and middle and terminal T wave. A shift toward the ischemic/infarcted area is indicated by an upward-pointing arrow; a shift away from this area is indicated by a downward-pointing arrow.

are directed at the anterosuperior quadrant in the basal and middle thirds of the LV. This region is supplied by either the optional diagonal branch of the LAD or marginal branch of the LCX.

PHASES OF SERIAL ECG CHANGES DURING AMI-I

There are ECG changes associated with the ischemia, necrosis, and healing process that can be generally classified into four phases: hyperacute, acute, subacute, and chronic (Fig. 19-11). In general, the ischemic process is potentially reversible in the hyperacute phase, with progressive infarction occurring throughout the acute phase. The healing process begins during the subacute phase and continues through the chronic phase. The time courses of these phases vary with individuals. Further, the time courses are delayed during intermittent coronary occlusion and accelerated by prompt reperfusion.

Hyperacute phase

Within seconds after occlusion there typically is a significant increase in T-wave amplitude directed toward the epicardial surface in the center of the ischemic area (Fig. 19-12). This change—generally termed "hyperacute T"—resembles the hyperkalemic T wave and may represent local shifts of potassium in the extracellular space. These changes are seen in anterior precordial leads (especially V_2-V_4) in acute occlusion of the LAD;

in leads II, III, and aV_F in occlusion of the RCA or PD; and as mirror image, inverted T waves in leads V_1 and V_2 in LCX occlusion. Ischemic conduction delays may also be evident at this time. These delays can be quite location-specific, giving early clues to the site of the advancing necrosis. This initial phase usually lasts only minutes but may persist if the occlusion develops intermittently.

With the appearance of the hyperacute T waves, the entire ST segment also begins to shift ("current of injury") toward the area of myocardium at risk. The ST segment may become curved upward, merging with the T wave to produce one continuous waveform. When this current of injury is large, indicating severe regional ischemia, it "carries" the QRS waveforms toward the area at risk. This injury current has its maximal effect on the late QRS waveforms, requiring that their amplitudes be measured from the ST rather than the PR baseline. However, this current may also effect early QRS waveforms, masking the development of abnormal Q waves. Using continuous recordings of orthogonal leads, Sederholm[24] has shown that the peak spatial magnitude of the ST-segment shift may be quite transient, often lasting less than 2 hours.

Acute phase

The terminal portion of the T wave begins to decrease in amplitude first, leaving the J point, ST segment, and mid–T wave elevated (Fig. 19-13). In the early part of

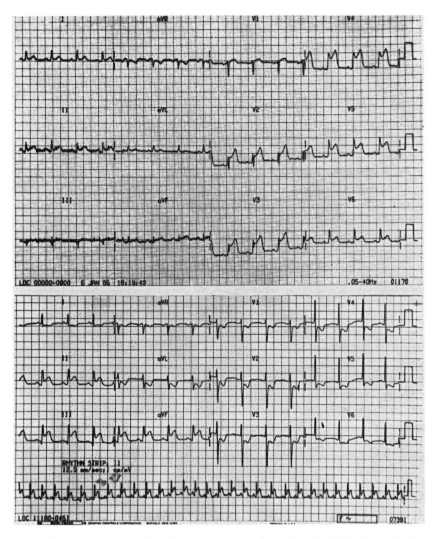

Fig. 19-12. Hyperacute phase. *Top,* Anterior acute cardiac ischemia (ACI). Note the dramatic elevation in ST segment in leads V_2 to V_5, which "carry" the contiguous aspects of the QRS complex waveforms along. *Bottom,* Inferior ACI. ST-segment elevation is present in leads II, III, and aV_F, with reciprocal depression and/or posterior involvement indicated by ST depression in the precordial leads. In both examples there are no QRS changes of myocardial infarction.

this phase the ischemic process may still be reversible. The specific QRS changes of local infarction begin to appear and progress, reaching their full extent by the end of the acute phase. As the current of injury subsides, the QRS complex shifts away from the area at risk, revealing or "unmasking" abnormal Q waves, decreased or notched R waves, and altered terminal forces. The precise changes depend on the location and size of the AMI-I process. Typically there are prominent Q waves or loss of R waves in anterior and leftward leads with LAD occlusion and abnormal Q waves in the inferior leads with RCA occlusion. However, with LCX occlusion there is loss of the middle to late activation fronts from the middle and basal segments of the posterolateral quadrant. This results in (1) increased middle to late R or R′ waves and decreased S waves in the anterior

precordial leads V_1 and V_2 and (2) decreased R and R/S ratios in leftward leads (I, V_5, and V_6).

Subacute phase

Early in the subacute phase the terminal portion of the T wave becomes negative, and the J point, ST segment, and mid–T wave return toward normal (Fig. 19-14). The typical regional QRS changes are usually well-established and remain stable unless the patient develops recurrence of the AMI-I process. The ischemic myocardium has become, in general, irreversibly infarcted, and early healing has begun. The J-point and ST-segment abnormalities have usually stabilized and may be either normal or remain directed slightly toward the infarct. The T wave is directed maximally away from the infarct by the end of this phase.

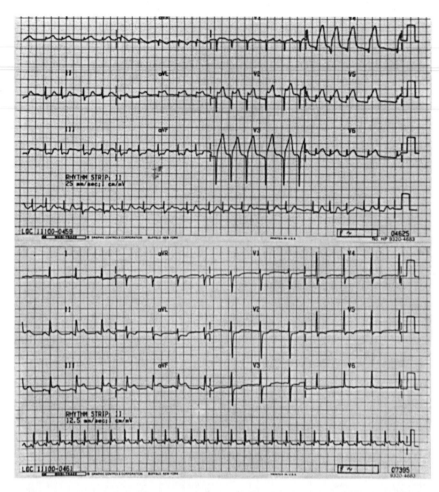

Fig. 19-13. Acute phase. **Top,** Anterior acute cardiac ischemia (ACI). **Bottom,** Inferior ACI. Significant ST-segment elevation persists throughout this phase as the typical QRS changes of the evolving myocardial infarction begin to appear.

Chronic phase

During the chronic phase, the changes on the ECG caused by the infarct have stabilized (Fig. 19-15). If there is no recurrence of ischemia, these changes will gradually evolve toward resolution. The T wave will remain directed away from the area of infarction unless influenced by local ischemia elsewhere, left ventricular hypertrophy, or bundle branch block. It remains to be determined if the timing of this normalization process is related to the extent of the infarcted myocardium.[25,26]

IMPLICATIONS OF THESE OBSERVATIONS FOR MANAGEMENT OF PATIENTS

Currently most investigators use the "time from onset of chest pain" as the primary criterion for decisions regarding acute intervention. However, chest pain onset is not always a reliable marker, because many patients experience nonspecific or intermittent symptoms or episodes of "silent ischemia." Further, the time course of occlusion may either occur abruptly or intermittently over several hours. There are also other important factors on the presenting ECG that should be considered in the decision to administer reperfusion therapy, such as the extent of ST-segment deviation, the number of leads involved, and anterior vs. inferior vs. posterolateral location. The optimal clinical decision requires consideration of the ECG phase in the ischemia/infarction/healing process. Although variable amounts of jeopardized myocardium are potentially salvageable in the earliest phases of acute MI, no significant salvage can occur during the subsequent phases. Possible benefits of reperfusion occurring during a later phase would be prevention of MI extension and enhancement of the healing process.[25,26]

Immediate reperfusion therapy would be recommended during the hyperacute phase when there are no QRS changes caused by infarction, although significant transient QRS changes may be produced by the acute ischemia. One can postulate that the quantity of these transient changes in the QRS complex may be related to

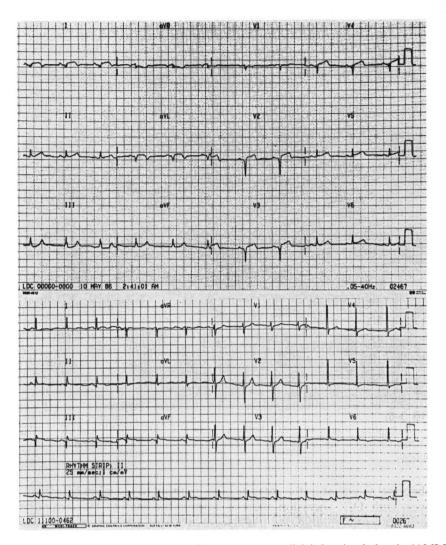

Fig. 19-14. Subacute phase. **Top,** Anterior acute myocardial infarction-ischemia (AMI-I). **Bottom,** Inferior AMI-I. QRS changes of MI are well established in this phase with minimal persistent ST elevation. The T wave begins to shift away from the infarct/ischemia zone.

the amount of myocardium at risk. In the acute phase, the decision whether to intervene is most complex and requires careful examination of a variety of parameters. Early in this phase, intervention would be indicated, because patients typically have extensive ST-segment deviation but minimal QRS changes of infarction. During the later acute phase, as significant QRS changes appear, reperfusion therapy would be less likely to limit the size of the MI.

ECG INDICES OF THE AMI-I PROCESS

1. Admission prediction of the final infarct size in the absence of reperfusion via the acutely occluded coronary artery[2]:
   a. Anterior location:
      Initial predicted % LV infarcted = 3(1.5 [number of leads with ST elevation

   ≥ 0.1 mV] $- 0.4$)
   b. Inferior location:
      Initial predicted % LV infarcted = 3(0.6 [Σ ST elevation in II, III, aV$_F$] + 2.0)
2. Prehospital discharge estimation of final infarct size[28]:
      Final % LV infarcted = 3(Selvester QRS score)
3. Prehospital discharge estimation of myocardial salvage attained via acute reperfusion therapies[5]:
      % salvage = 100 (initial ST predicted % infarcted $-$ final QRS estimated % infarcted)

SUMMARY

For an individual patient, the ECG is influenced by variations in lead placement, phase of respiration, abdominal distention, degree of recumbency, and the technical quality of the recording. Optimal quantifica-

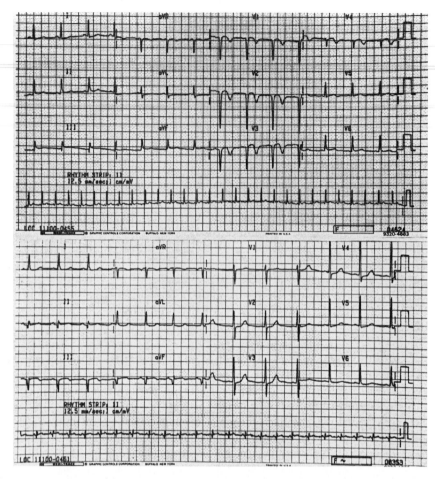

Fig. 19-15. Chronic phase. **Top,** Anterior acute myocardial infarction-ischemia (AMI-I). **Bottom,** Inferior AMI-I. Typical stable electrocardiogram changes of the completed MI are seen. There is little or no residual ST-segment elevation, the T waves are directed away from the zone of infraction, and the QRS changes indicative of MI are fully developed.

tion of the information on the ECG requires standardization of these factors. Improved understanding of the relationships between the positions of the surface ECG leads and the cardiac anatomy is also necessary. One should consider that the amount of myocardium in jeopardy may be related to both the extent of ST-T changes[27] and the location of the AMI-I, with the anterior area at risk typically twice as large as either the inferior or posterolateral areas. Studies now in progress may provide methods for quantifying the extents of both the infarcted and ischemic myocardium during the hyperacute and acute phases, which may be useful in determining the extent to which an individual patient is likely to benefit from reperfusion therapy.

REFERENCES

1. Sederholm M, Erhardt L, Sjögran A: Continuous vectorcardiography in acute myocardial infarction. Natural course of ST and QRS vectors, *Int J Cardiol* 4:53-63, 1983.
2. Aldrich HR, Wagner NB, Boswick J, et al: Use of initial ST segment for prediction of final electrocardiographic size of acute myocardial infarcts, *Am J Cardiol* 61:749-763, 1988.
3. Hackworthy RA, Vogel MB, Harris, PJ: Relationship between changes in ST segment elevation and patency of the infarct-related coronary artery in acute myocardial infarction, *Am Heart J* 112:279, 1986.
4. Bar FW, Vermeer F, De Zwaan C, et al: Value of admission electrocardiogram in predicting outcome of thrombolytic therapy in acute myocardial infarction: a randomized trial conducted by The Netherlands Interuniversity Cardiology Institute, *Am J Cardiol* 59:6-13, 1987.
5. Clemmensen P, Grande P, Saunamaki K, et al: Effect of intravenous streptokinase on the relationship between initial ST predicted and final QRS estimated size of acute myocardial infarcts, *J Am Coll Cardiol* 16:1252-1257, 1990.
6. Sevilla DC, Wagner NB, Pieper KS, et al: Use of the 12-lead electrocardiogram to detect myocardial reperfusion and salvage during acute myocardial infarction, *J Electrocardiol* 25:281-286, 1992.
7. Hackel DB, Wagner GS, Ratliff NB, et al: Anatomic studies of the cardiac conducting system in acute myocardial infarction, *Am Heart J* 83:77-81, 1972.
8. Selvester RH, Wagner NB, Wagner GS: Ventricular excitation during percutaneous transluminal angioplasty of the left anterior descending coronary artery, *Am J Cardiol* 62:1116-1121, 1988.
9. Selvester RH, Kalaba R, Collier CR, et al: A digital computer

model of the vectorcardiogram with distance and boundary effects: simulated myocardial infarction, *Am Heart J* 74:792-808, 1967.

10. Wagner GS, Cowan MJ, Flowers NC, et al: Nomenclature of myocardial wall segments: committee report. In Selvester RH (ed): *Proceeding of the 1983 Engineering Foundation Conference, computerized interpretation of the ECG VIII*, New York, 1983, Engineering Foundation Press, p 222.

11. Ideker RE, Wagner GS, Ruth WK, et al: Evaluation of a QRS scoring system for estimating myocardial infarct size: II. Correlation with quantitative anatomic findings for anterior infarcts, *Am J Cardiol* 49:1604-1614, 1982.

12. Horan LG, Flowers NC, Johnson JC: Significance of the diagnostic Q wave of myocardial infarction, *Circulation* 43:448, 1971.

13. Henry WL, DeMaria A, Feigenbaum H, et al: Identification of myocardial wall segments: report of the ASE Committee on Nomenclature and Standards, Raleigh, NC, 1982, American Society of Ecocardiography.

14. Selvester RH, Sanmarco ME, Solomon JC, et al: The ECG: QRS change. In Wagner GS (ed): *Myocardial infarction: measurement and intervention*, The Hague, 1982, Martinus Nijhoff, pp 23-50.

15. Christian TF, Clements IP, Gibbons RJ: Noninvasive identification of myocardium at risk in patients with acute myocardial infarction and nondiagnostic electrocardiograms with technetium-99m-sestamibi, *Circulation* 83:1616-1620, 1991.

16. Sevilla DC, Wagner NB, White RD, et al: Anatomic validation of electrocardiographic estimation of the size of acute or healed myocardial infarcts, *Am J Cardiol* 65:1301-1307, 1990.

17. Hindman MC, Wagner GS, JaRo M, et al: The clinical significance of bundle branch block complicating acute myocardial infarction: I. Clinical characteristics, hospital mortality, and one year follow-up, *Circulation* 58:679-688, 1978.

18. Hindman MC, Wagner GS, JaRo M, et al: The clinical significance of bundle branch block complicating acute myocardial infarction: II. Indication for temporary and permanent pacemaker insertion, *Circulation* 58:689-699, 1978.

19. First SR, Bayley RH, Bedford DR: Peri-infarction block: electrocardiographic abnormality occasionally resembling bundle branch and local ventricular block of other types, *Circulation* 2:31-36, 1950.

20. Rosebaum MB: The hemiblocks: diagnostic criteria and clinical significance, *Mod Concepts Cardiovasc Dis* 12:141-146, 1970.

21. Grant RP: *Clinical electrocardiography*, New York, 1957, McGraw-Hill, pp 129-136.

22. Hassett MA, Williams RR, Wagner GS: Transient QRS changes simulating acute myocardial infarction, *Circulation* 62:975-979, 1980.

23. White RD, Lipton MJ, Higgins CB: Magnetic resonance imaging for evaluation of myocardial ischemia and infarction. In Califf RM, Wagner GS (eds): *Acute Coronary Care 1986*, Boston, 1985, Martinus Nijhoff, pp 145-162.

24. Sederholm M: Evolution of ischemia and necrosis in acute myocardial infarction as assessed by continuous vectorcardiography, thesis. Stockholm, 1984, Karolinska University.

25. Reimer KA, Jennings RB: Myocardial ischemia, hypoxia, and infarction. In Fozzard HA, et al (eds): *The heart and cardiovascular system*, New York, 1986, Raven Press, pp 1133-1201.

26. Jeremy RW, Hackworthy RA, Bautovich G, et al: Infarct artery perfusion and changes in left ventricular volume in the month after acute myocardial infarction, *J Am Coll Cardiol* 9:989-995, 1987.

27. Bar FW, Vermeer F, De Zwaan C, et al: Value of admission electrocardiogram in predicting outcome of thrombolytic therapy in acute myocardial infarction: a randomized trial conducted by the Netherlands Interuniversity Cardiology Institute, *Am J Cardiol* 59:6-13, 1987.

28. Hindman NB, Schocken DD, Widmann M, et al: Evaluation of a QRS method scoring system for estimating myocardial infarct size: V. Specificity and method of application of the complete system, *Am J Cardiol* 55:1485-1490, 1985.

Chapter 20

PREHOSPITAL EVALUATION AND TREATMENT OF PATIENTS WITH SUSPECTED ACUTE MYOCARDIAL INFARCTION

W. Douglas Weaver

The goals of managing patients with suspected acute myocardial infarction have changed from the management of arrhythmia, limitation of myocardial oxygen consumption by using beta-blockers and nitrates, and pain management to identification of those patients most likely to benefit from administration of thrombolytic therapy and use of direct angioplasty to reestablish coronary perfusion. Lysis of an occlusive thrombus has been shown to reduce mortality, limit infarct size, and preserve left ventricular function.[1-13] In an overview of the relationship between time to treatment and outcome, it is clear that the greatest opportunity for maximizing the result of thrombolytic therapy is in the first hour of symptoms (Fig. 20-1). Unfortunately, few patients arrive at the hospital or are managed expeditiously enough to permit treatment of any significant proportion within this period. In the GUSTO-I trial, which probably reflects typical delays in the United States, the average delay from symptom onset until treatment was 2.8 hours, and only 3% of patients were treated within the first hour of symptoms.[14]

This chapter outlines the components of delay until treatment and the current state of knowledge of the means to modify them. They include the patient component, the role of prehospital diagnosis and treatment by paramedics, and the current shortcomings of most hospitals in providing timely treatment.

PATIENT-RELATED DELAYS AND MEANS TO SHORTEN THEM

Of the three components of delay from symptom onset to initiation of treatment, patient delay is the single largest, encompassing almost two thirds of the total delay from symptom onset to initiation of treatment. Past attempts at reducing the delay from symptom onset until admission, by using the media or other targeted interventions to the lay public, have either been small studies too short to make a meaningful impact or uncontrolled/poorly controlled studies whose effects cannot be adequately assessed. They have demonstrated variable success. Most of the existing large studies aimed at assessing techniques for reducing this component of delay have been done in other countries and in health care systems that differ considerably from that of the United States. Therefore the results of these media educational efforts may not be indicative of what might be expected in our population. For example, in the United States the current role of the general practitioner is a relatively small one compared with most other Western countries, whereas professional paramedic-based emergency med-

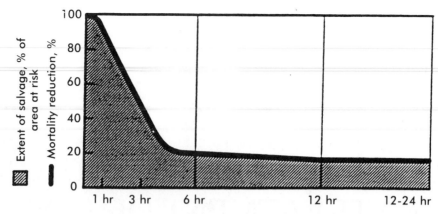

Fig. 20-1. Curve of hypothetical relationship between duration of symptoms and mortality reduction and myocardial salvage after treatment with thrombolytic therapy. Very early benefits appear most related to myocardial salvage, whereas the relationship between time and effect at 6 hours or longer is more constant.[9]

ical systems are widespread throughout both urban and suburban settings, and efficient volunteer emergency services are present in most rural communities. Lastly, hospital emergency department care is widely available and encouraged for patients for both medical and surgical emergencies.

Any successful program that reduces the time from symptom onset to hospital arrival or access to the emergency medical system is likely not only to increase the number of candidates eligible for reperfusion treatments but also to decrease the number of patients with out-of-hospital sudden death associated with acute infarction. In the recently completed GUSTO-I trial there was a 1% higher mortality per hour of delay until treatment, independent of treatment regimen and equal, in fact, to the amount of added benefit associated with t-PA versus streptokinase.[15] Therefore, reducing time to treatment by influencing the patient's decision to seek emergency medical care is possibly as significant as further refinements of the treatment regimen used.

Earlier studies evaluating patient delay times have shown marked variability (from 4.6 to 21 hours), probably because of the heterogeneous populations studied.[16,17] More recent studies have demonstrated that the distribution of delay times is not a normal one, and median delays (a better measure) are reported to be from 2.2 to 6.4 hours.[17-20]

Two contemporary registries of less-selected patients with AMI provide some additional insight into the problem of delay in the United States. The National Registry of Myocardial Infarction, which is sponsored by Genentech but carried out by ClinTrials, contains a small amount of identifying and treatment data about patients with AMI. Although the Registry under-represents very small hospitals (100 or fewer beds) and may overrepresent patients who receive thrombolytic therapy, it is widely used in all states. In slightly over 2

years the Registry contained data from over 178,000 patients admitted to 1081 hospitals. One quarter of all patients identified as having AMI received treatment with thrombolytic therapy. As might be expected, there were substantial differences between delays reported in the thrombolysis-treated patients versus those who were not eligible and were not treated. The mean and median delays for treated patients were 2 hours, 50 minutes and 1 hour, 34 minutes respectively, compared with times of 6 hours, 9 minutes and 2 hours, 41 minutes for those patients not treated. The 25th to 75th percentiles of delay for all patients ranged from 1.1 hours to 5.9 hours. Although 20% of patients arrived at a hospital within 1 hour of symptom onset, 25% had not arrived by 6 hours, and 13% were not present until after 12 hours, by which time reperfusion may no longer be useful. The average delay for women was also significantly longer than for men (5.7 vs. 4.9 hours). Only 50% of patients with findings of AMI called 911 or emergency services, despite the fact that the likelihood of mortality is highest in the first hour.[21]

The MITI Registry was also a contemporary community-based study of patients with AMI in the greater Seattle metropolitan area carried out from 1988 through 1993. Although a shortcoming is that it represented a single "high-tech" community, the data are complete and include consecutive patients. The patient delays in Seattle were remarkably similar to those from the National Registry; 22% of patients with a discharge diagnosis of AMI received thrombolytic therapy; only 48% with AMI called 911 despite the fact that Seattle has one of the original paramedic programs in the country. The median delay for all patients was 2.5 hours and was substantially longer for patients who "walked in" (3.5 hours) than for those who called 911 (1.5 hours). As was shown in earlier studies, delay increased with age, female sex, African-American race, and in patients with lower social economic status.[20,22] Thus, the recently collected data from unselected patients with AMI clearly demonstrate an opportunity to reduce the time to treatment if appropriate patients can be motivated to act sooner.

Previous community-based attempts at reducing delay

In general, most attempts at using the media to reduce the time delay have been made outside the United States, in countries with more homogeneous populations and considerably different communication methods and medical systems from those in this country. The largest study, Heart Pain 90,000 (Göteborg, Sweden), was carried out for 1 year, using a before-and-after design to measure its effectiveness. The study employed mass media, including radio, print, and billboard advertising. Several of its findings are relevant: during an intense radio campaign there was a marked increase in the number of patients arriving at the emergency room with symptoms of chest pain, but the majority of this increase were patients without coronary disease. Although this number declined weekly after the radio campaign was discontinued, it points out the potential for an imperfect intervention to significantly increase the number of inappropriate hospital evaluations for non-cardiac chest pain and to overburden the hospitals. This could outweigh any benefit to patients with AMI in terms of costs, loss of productivity, and inconvenience to society. The campaign also failed to increase the proportion of patients arriving by ambulance. On the other hand, delay to hospital admission for patients with AMI declined from 3 hours to 2 hours 20 minutes.[23,24]

An 8-week campaign was carried out in Nova Scotia, Canada, using television and radio public service announcements (PSAs).[25] The study was small and included 471 patients, of whom 101 were assessed prior to the test campaign. As in Göteborg, the number of patients who presented to the emergency department more than doubled during the campaign compared with the pretest period. Similar proportions of patients (22.8%) were admitted as before the campaign, suggesting again that the greatest effect of the media campaign was on patients without AMI. However, an encouraging finding was that significantly more persons (both those with cardiac disease and those without) presented to the emergency department within 2 hours (31% compared with a baseline 15.8%). A reduction in the time to patient action was directly related to the campaign, as determined by information obtained from patient interviews.[25]

In the United States even fewer attempts have been made to influence patient delays. Moses reported on a study of a small community (Jacksonville, Illinois) using a before-and-after design.[26] The media included brochures, posters, and PSAs aired on radio and television.

There was little change in utilization of hospitals or in patient delay. The study, however, was too small to be conclusive.

In Seattle a 6-week radio and print media campaign was carried out in cooperation with the state American Heart Association affiliate.[27] It was aimed at increasing the number of calls to 911 and reducing the time to admission of patients with suspected infarction. A random telephone survey was done to determine penetration of the message. There was a marked increase in the proportion of people who had heard information about the treatment of heart attacks during the media blitz (from 52% to 73%); however, there was no change in the proportion of patients who called 911, nor in the time to admission of patients with AMI.

A more recent study was carried out by Eisenberg in the Seattle metropolitan area (Call Fast/Call 911). This study may be the largest attempt in the United States to change lay awareness of the symptoms of heart attack. Two strategies were tested and included a media intervention and individual interventions in a higher-risk subset of patients recently discharged from hospital. For the media intervention, three different strategies were tested in serial mass mailings to households with people over the age of 50 years. One of the interventions was strictly informational or cognitive in content, a second was emotion-based and aimed at reducing delay by addressing fear or denial about the illness, and the third was primarily aimed at bystanders and was based on the concept that the sooner a person having chest pains tells someone else, the shorter the delay.[28] The first phase of the campaign used a 6-week multimedia awareness campaign consisting of television or radio advertisements. Both sets of PSAs were scheduled to air during programs most likely to reach the targeted audience of individuals 50 years of age and older. During the intense media campaign the number of 911 calls increased significantly; however, this was primarily for patients without evidence of AMI. Following the campaign the number dropped precipitously, pointing out the need for any media campaign to be either continuous or repetitive. The study is currently in the last part of follow-up and results should be reported soon. The results of these earlier studies have prompted the NHLBI to sponsor a multicenter community-based trial to further define means as well as the effectiveness of mass educational strategies to reduce the time from symptom onset to hospital admission. Clearly this is an extremely important area of research, which if successful could have major public health importance in reducing mortality and morbidity from MI.

PREHOSPITAL TREATMENT TRIALS

One means to reduce the time to treatment of patients, and particularly to increase the proportion treated within the first hour, would be to administer thrombolytic therapy in the prehospital setting. Several small studies carried out a few years ago demonstrate the feasibility of this approach; they also suggest that prehospital-initiated treatment may result in significant reduction in infarct size, preservation of left ventricular function, and reduction of mortality.[29-32] Complications were uncommon in these studies and a significant time savings (about 1 hour) occurred.

More recently, three randomized trials of prehospital vs. hospital-initiated thrombolytic therapy have been reported.[12,33,34] Two were done in Europe: one involved the initiation of treatment by general practitioners and the second by a physician in the ambulance in countries offering mobile coronary care. The third trial was carried out in the United States, where paramedics both selected and treated patients under the direction of a remote emergency physician who directed care using the telephone.

GREAT

The Grampian Region Early Anistreplase Trial (GREAT) was a randomized double-blind trial in which 311 patients with suspected AMI were treated initially either by general practitioners at home or after hospital arrival in a rural part of Scotland.[33] The primary endpoint of the trial was the incidence of Q-wave MI. Although an ECG was routinely obtained, diagnostic ST elevation was not required; it was present in about half of patients treated. Treatment at home routinely resulted in time savings of over 2 hours in the delivery of thrombolytic therapy (median 103 vs. 240 minutes). Fewer patients treated at home developed Q-wave infarction than those who were treated after arriving in hospital (53% vs. 68%, $P < 0.02$). Left ventricular function, assessed by Doppler cardiac output, was not significantly higher in the early treatment group. There was a reduction in mortality in those patients treated at home, particularly in those patients treated within 2 hours of symptom onset. Outcome at 1 year also favored prehospital-initiated treatment.[36] This finding, like the summary of findings by Gersh and Anderson,[36] points out the magnitude of benefit attainable with treatment in the first 1 to 2 hours.

EMIP

The largest trial of prehospital-initiated thrombolytic therapy is the European Myocardial Infarction Project (EMIP).[34] This study, which initially intended to enroll 11,000 patients, was terminated prematurely after randomizing 5429 patients in a double-blind, double-dummy placebo-controlled trial of prehospital- vs. hospital-initiated anistreplase. Prehospital screening, diagnosis, and designation of patients for treatment were accomplished jointly by nurses, ambulance attendants,

and physicians. Aspirin was given to all patients and heparin use was not specified. Eighty-seven percent of the patients had ST-segment elevation and a similar proportion showed evidence of AMI before discharge or death.

The prehospital screening process consumed 25 minutes and prehospital treatment resulted in a mean savings of 55 minutes relative to treatment initiated in-hospital. Despite this approach, few patients were treated within the first hour of symptom onset. Although hypotension and minor bleeding were more common in those treated early, there were no differences in major adverse events. At 30 days total mortality (the primary endpoint) was reduced by 13% (9.7% vs. 11.1%; $P = 0.08$). The greatest benefit of prehospital-initiated treatment occurred when time to hospital vs. prehospital treatment was 90 minutes or longer (a 45% lower mortality associated with prehospital treatment).

MITI

In the United States prehospital care is most commonly provided by paramedics and sometimes nurses. Except for management of cardiac arrest, all medical care delivered is under the direction of a physician, in most cases an emergency physician in a base hospital. Because of this, initiating thrombolytic therapy in the prehospital setting is more complex. A system that ensures careful and consistent patient screening must be in place; the ECG must be either interpreted automatically by a computer algorithm on site or transmitted to the physician for interpretation. The Myocardial Infarction, Triage, and Intervention (MITI) Prehospital Trial was a prospective evaluation of both the feasibility and effectiveness of prehospital-initiated treatment.[12] The rapid and accurate interpretation of the ECG was mandatory in selecting appropriate patients for treatment in the MITI Trial.[37] The best method for doing this is controversial. Both paramedics and emergency physicians are likely to be less skilled in interpreting ECGs with more subtle findings of acute injury than is an electrocardiographer.[38] Serious errors in interpretation have resulted in up to 23% of patients with chest pain being managed inappropriately.[39] On the other hand, it is the unusual setting in which expert consultation by an electrocardiographer is immediately available. Computerized ECG interpretation provides a means to solve this problem and was used in the MITI trial to minimize the number of patients treated who did not have infarction (2%). The current diagnostic accuracy of available algorithms is still less than perfect but nonetheless useful in this setting — one in which the objective is to identify the subset of patients with uncontroversial evidence of acute infarction. In a preliminary validation of the algorithm, 71% of all consecutive patients with AMI who had been screened by paramedics had 1 mm or more of ST-

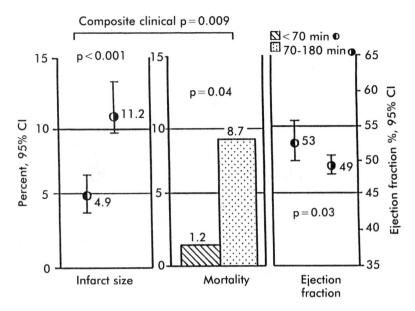

Fig. 20-2. Secondary analysis of time to treatment and infarct size, mortality, and ejection fraction in the MITI Prehospital Trial. Time to treatment averaged 90 minutes, 96% of patients were treated within 3 hours. There was a marked change in outcome at 60 to 80 minutes (not a gradual one). Patients treated very early (<70 minutes) had over a 50% reduction in infarct size as well as lower mortality and more preserved left ventricular function.

segment elevation. The electrocardiographer identified 61% of the individuals correctly, with a 4% false-positive rate.[37] The computer algorithm, by contrast, was accurate in identifying 52%, but at a lower false-positive rate (2%). These findings lead us to believe that accurate computer-interpreted electrocardiography can be an important tool for the initial rapid identification of patients who are eligible to receive thrombolytic therapy and to prevent errors in interpretation and treatment.

The MITI Prehospital Trial enrolled 360 patients in an open single-blind randomized controlled trial. A composite endpoint, which included death, stroke, serious bleeding, and infarct size, was used to measure possible differences in outcome between treatment groups. Infarct size has been shown in other studies to correlate with long-term survival and may be a far more sensitive indicator of therapeutic effect in this setting than ejection fraction.[40] In addition, the study was sized to show a five percent or greater difference in infarct size (SPECT thallium imaging) and a four-point difference in ejection fraction (MUGA), which were performed and interpreted in a core laboratory that was blinded to treatment assignment. The baseline characteristics of the patients were well matched. Of note, the median time from symptom onset to treatment was barely over 1 hour (77 minutes). There was no difference in the composite endpoint (death, stroke, major bleeding, and infarct size) or in ejection fraction between the two randomized groups. Prehospital identification of patients in the trial markedly shortened hospital treatment

times from a median of 60 minutes (time to treatment for patients not in the trial) to 20 minutes. There was a 33-minute time savings with prehospital-initiated treatment instead of the expected 1 hour.[12,22]

The data from both randomized groups were combined to evaluate the effect of time to treatment on infarct size, ejection fraction, and mortality. Half the patients were treated within 90 minutes of symptom onset and almost all (96%) were treated within 3 hours. The relationship between time and measures of infarct size limitation and outcome changed markedly, not gradually, at, before, and after 60 to 80 minutes. At the best cutpoint (70 minutes), infarct size was 50% smaller, ejection fraction was 5 points higher, and even mortality was lower in those patients treated *very* early (Fig. 20-2).

The randomized trials of prehospital-initiated thrombolysis treatment have shown us that prehospital treatment is feasible and may be effective in further limiting infarct size and lowering mortality, particularly when a substantial number of patients can be treated within the first hour. A metaanalysis of the effects of prehospital treatment, which is understandably weighted with the EMIP experience, suggests overall that prehospital treatment may further reduce mortality by 18%.[34] It is also clear that all of the available trials were all underpowered to measure an effect of treatment on mortality. The very means of having these patients in a protocol that emphasizes time to treatment serves to minimize the time savings. A definitive study would require 10,000 patients or more. Such a study is not likely to be done,

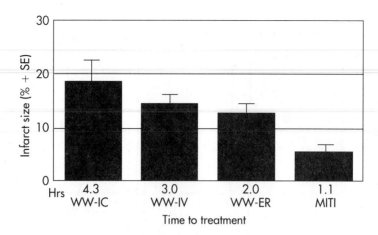

Fig. 20-3. Infarct size vs. time to treatment in Western Washington trials. In the MITI trial, in which time to treatment was just over an hour, over 40% of patients had no infarct discernible by SPECT thallium tomographic imaging.

however. Given the current interest in direct angioplasty as a means to improve mortality over the results of thrombolytic therapy, it might be more insightful to conduct a trial of prehospital-initiated thrombolytic therapy (the best that can be achieved in terms of minimizing time to treatment) and direct PTCA (the best that can be currently expected in terms of reperfusion).

IS PREHOSPITAL THERAPY NECESSARY?

Very early treatment with thrombolytic therapy results in the greatest reduction in infarct size and mortality (Fig. 20-3).[8,11,13,36] No prehospital trial in and of itself has shown unequivocal reductions in mortality (Table 20-1). Instead, research suggests that, except where because of logistics the delay until hospital arrival would be 1 hour or more, providing an "early warning" to hospitals by prehospital diagnosis of eligible patients is sufficient to minimize the time to treatment in order to obtain maximal results from therapy.[12,41] However, unless a time-conscious protocol is in place, routine hospital delays may be too excessive to match the results of prehospital approaches. Given early reports describing hospital delays in many U.S. cities, time from hospital arrival to treatment remains inexplicably long.[42,43] Without a designated team approach, conscious effort, and continued monitoring, hospital delays seem unlikely to change.[44] There are two impediments to routine prehospital-initiated treatment. First, with few exceptions, cardiologists are not involved in the prehospital medical care delivery systems. To be successful a prehospital program requires input from knowledgeable cardiologists and emergency physicians in setting goals and monitoring the quality of care in the protocols for patients with acute coronary syndromes. This duty, except in unusual settings, should not be relegated to a less-than-expert physician—it requires an expert in the care of patients with MI and one who is well-read

Potential benefits of prehospital electrocardiography in patients with suspected AMI:
- more rapid treatment with thrombolytic drugs after hospital arrival
- improved recognition of AMI patients with evolving but borderline ECG changes
- ECG documentation of ischemia prior to any treatment
- triage of patients with MI at high risk (anterior ST elevation, hemodynamic instability, systolic BP < 100 mmHg, heart rate > 100 bpm) to tertiary cardiac facilities, so that angiography, coronary angioplasty, and surgery can be accomplished rapidly if needed.

in the continuous refinement of treatment of MI. Second, the ongoing debate on the best thrombolytic regimen or means of reperfusion also impedes the widespread use of a prehospital protocol. If a paramedic system serves many different hospitals and practitioners, all of whom have different treatment protocols and regimens, the situation is too complex to lend itself to prehospital implementation. If further studies in the coming years demonstrate one superior approach applicable for most patients, then a common prehospital protocol can be developed and implemented.

IMPROVEMENTS IN PREHOSPITAL IDENTIFICATION OF AMI

The widespread use of prehospital electrocardiography to identify and hasten both prehospital and hospital management of patients with suspected AMI is recommended (see accompanying box). Several studies have shown that prehospital electrocardiography speeds the care of patients who are eligible for reperfusion treatments after arriving in the hospital.[12,38,41,45-47] Although not currently used for

Table 20-1. Results of clinical trials comparing prehospital and in-hospital thrombolytic therapy*

Study	Treatment	Interval (min)[†]	Total short-term mortality[‡]		Odds ratio (95% CI)	P value
			Prehospital group	Hospital group		
			no. of deaths/no. randomized			
Castaigne et al.[51]	Anistreplase (30 IU, IV bolus)	60	3/50	2/50	1.53 (0.25-9.56)	0.60
Schofer et al.[29]	Urokinase ($2 \times [10^6]^6$ IU, IV bolus)	43	1/40	2/38	0.46 (0.04-5.11)	0.50
GREAT[33]	Anistreplase (30 IU, IV bolus)	130	11/163	17/148	0.56 (0.25-1.23)	0.10
MITI[22]	Aspirin (325 mg) plus alteplase (100 mg/3 hr)	33	10/175	15/185	0.69 (0.30-1.57)	0.40
EMIP[34]	Anistreplase (30 IU, IV bolus)	55	266/2750	303/2719	0.85 (0.72-1.01)	0.08

Total adjusted proportional reduction in risk. 17% (95% CI, 2%-29%; $P = 0.03$)

*CI denotes confidence interval; IV, intravenous; GREAT, Grampian Region Early Anistreplase Trial; and MITI, Myocardial Infarction Triage and Intervention trial.[23] The study by Castaigne et al. and the MITI study were not double-blinded. Patients were randomly assigned to receive treatment either before or after hospital admission. In all studies with the exception of GREAT, prehospital treatment was administered by the staff of the mobile emergency unit in the presence of a physician (except MITI, in which paramedical staff were present); in GREAT, therapy was administered by general practitioners.
†The median interval between the prehospital and in-hospital interventions.
‡Short-term mortality was defined as 30-day or hospital mortality.

this purpose, prehospital diagnostic capability also permits triage of patients at high risk of mortality (e.g., those with anterior ST-segment elevation and hemodynamic compromise) to hospitals with tertiary cardiac services in communities having hospitals of varied capability. Although not of proven benefit, it is probably better to manage such patients initially when angiography is readily available, instead of transferring a patient later, which is difficult, more cumbersome, and potentially risky to the patient. Such an approach has been used by the American College of Surgeons for the past decade to appropriately triage traumatized patients. Cardiovascular medicine has lagged, and yet there are patients with MI in whom angiography and mechanical means of reperfusion are preferred. Other noninvasive markers of infarction that are in development, such as serial ST-segment monitoring and enzyme and protein markers of necrosis, also lend themselves to improving prehospital triage as these markers are made more simple for bedside testing.[48-50]

In summary, the role of prehospital identification of patients with suspected MI is now certain. In the coming years this capability needs to become routine in all settings and the tools improved to maximize their utility.

REFERENCES

1. AIMS Study Group: Effect of intravenous APSAC on mortality after acute myocardial infarction: preliminary report of a placebo-controlled clinical trial, *Lancet* 317:545-549, 1988.
2. Guerci AD, Gerstenblith G, Brinker JA, et al: A randomized trial of intravenous tissue plasminogen activator for acute myocardial infarction with subsequent randomization to elective coronary angioplasty, *N Engl J Med* 317:1613-1618, 1987.
3. O'Rourke M, Baron D, Keogh A, et al: Limitation of myocardial infarction by early infusion of recombinant tissue-type plasminogen activator, *Circulation* 77:1311-1315, 1988.
4. Rentrop KP, Blanke H, Karsch KR: Effects of nonsurgical coronary reperfusion on the left ventricle in human subjects compared with conventional treatment, *Am J Cardiol* 49:1-8, 1982.
5. Smalling RW, Fuentes F, Matthews MW, et al: Sustained improvement in left ventricular function and mortality by intracoronary streptokinase administration during evolving myocardial infarction, *Circulation* 68:131-138, 1983.
6. Sheehan FH, Mathey DG, Schofer J, et al: Effect of interventions in salvaging left ventricular function in acute myocardial infarction: a study of intracoronary streptokinase, *Am J Cardiol* 52:431-438, 1983.
7. Spann JF, Sherry S, Carabello BA, et al: Coronary thrombolysis by intravenous streptokinase in acute myocardial infarction: acute and follow-up studies, *Am J Cardiol* 43:655-661, 1984.
8. Gruppo Italiano per lo Studio della Streptochinasi nell'Infarto Miocardico (GISSI): Effectiveness of intravenous thrombolytic treatment in acute myocardial infarction, *Lancet* 2:349-360, 1986.
9. Kennedy JW, Ritchie JL, David KB, et al: Western Washington randomized trial of intracoronary streptokinase in acute myocardial infarction, *N Engl J Med* 309:1477-1482, 1983.
10. Mathey DG, Schofer J, Sheehan FH, et al: Improved survival up to four years after early coronary thrombolysis, *Am J Cardiol* 61:524-529, 1988.
11. Second International Study of Infarct Survival Collaborative Group (ISIS-2): Randomized trial of intravenous streptokinase, oral aspirin, both, or neither among 17,187 cases of suspected acute myocardial infarction, *Lancet* 2:349-360, 1988.

12. Weaver WD, Cerqueria M, Hallstrom AP, et al. for the MITI Project Group: Early treatment with thrombolytic therapy: results from the Myocardial Infarction, Triage, and Intervention Prehospital Trial, *JAMA* 270:1211-1216, 1993.

13. Hermens WT, Willems GM, Nijssen KM, et al: Effect of thrombolytic treatment delay on myocardial infarct size, *Lancet* 340;1297, 1992.

14. The GUSTO investigators: An international randomized trial comparing four thrombolytic strategies for acute myocardial infarction, *N Engl J Med* 329:673-682, 1993.

15. Rutsch W, Pfisterer M, Weaver WD, et al. for the GUSTO Trial Investigators: Earlier time to treatment is associated with lower mortality and greater benefit of accelerated t-PA (abstract). *Circulation* 88:I-17, 1993.

16. Moss AJ, Goldstein RE: The pre-hospital phase of acute myocardial infarction, *Circulation* 41:737-742, 1970.

17. Cooper CW, Hays RB: Emergencies in general practice, *Med J Aust* 156:541, 544-548, 1992.

18. Rawles JM, Haites NE: Patient and general practitioner delays in acute myocardial infarction, *BMJ* 296:882-884, 1988.

19. Turi ZG, Stone PH, Muller JE, et al and the MILIS Study Group: Implications for acute intervention related to time of hospital arrival in acute myocardial infarction, *Am J Cardiol* 57:203-209, 1986.

20. Maynard C, Althouse R, Olsufka M, et al: Early versus late hospital arrival for acute myocardial infarction in the Western Washington thrombolytic therapy trials, *Am J Cardiol* 63:1296-1300, 1989.

21. Weaver WD, for the National Registry of Myocardial Infarction Investigators: Factors influencing the time to hospital administration of thrombolytic therapy: results from a large national registry (abstract), *Circulation* 86(suppl I):60, 1992.

22. Weaver WD, Eisenberg MS, Martin JS, et al: Myocardial Infarction Triage and Intervention Project—Phase I: patient characteristics and feasibility of prehospital initiation of thrombolytic therapy, *J Am Coll Cardiol* 15:925-931, 1990.

23. Herlitz J, Karlson BW, Liljeqvist J-A, et al: Early identification of acute myocardial infarction and prognosis in relation to mode of transport to hospital, *Am J Emerg Med* 10:406-412, 1992.

24. Blohm M, Herlitz J, Hartford M, et al: Consequences of a media campaign focusing on delay in acute myocardial infarction, *Am J Cardiol* 69:411-413, 1992.

25. Mitic WR, Perkins J: The effect of a medical campaign on heart attack delay and decision times, *Can J Pub Hlth* 75:414-418, 1984.

26. Moses HW, Engelking N, Taylor GJ, et al: Effect of a two-year public education campaign on reducing response time of patients with symptoms of acute myocardial infarction, *Am J Cardiol* 68:249-251, 1991.

27. Ho MT, Eisenberg MS, Litwin PE, et al: Delay between onset of chest pain and seeking medical care: the effect of public education, *Ann Emerg Med* 18:727-730, 1989.

28. Meischke H, Eisenberg M, Larsen MP: Prehospital delay interval for patients who use emergency medical services: the effect of heart-related medical conditions and demographic variables, *Ann Emerg Med* 22:109-113, 1993.

29. Schofer J, Buttner J, Geng G, et al: Prehospital thrombolysis in acute myocardial infarction, *Am J Cardiol* 66:1429-1433, 1990.

30. Koren G, Weiss AT, Hasin Y, et al: Prevention of myocardial damage in acute myocardial ischemia by early treatment with intravenous streptokinase, *N Engl J Med* 313:1384-1389, 1985.

31. Barbash GI, Roth A, Hod H, et al: Improved survival but not left ventricular function with early prehospital treatment with tissue plasminogen activator in acute myocardial infarction, *Am J Cardiol* 66:261-266, 1990.

32. McNeill AJ, Cunningham SR, Flannery DJ, et al: A blind placebo-controlled study of early and late admission of recombinant tissue plasminogen activator in acute myocardial infarction, *Br Heart J* 61:316-321, 1980.

33. The GREAT Group: Feasibility, safety, and efficacy of domiciliary thrombolysis by general practitioners: Grampian Region Early Anistreplase trial, *BMJ* 305:548-553, 1992.

34. The European Myocardial Infarction Project Group (EMIP Group): Early prehospital intervention in patients with suspected acute myocardial infarction: results from a randomized controlled trial, *N Engl J Med* 329(6):383-389, 1993.

35. Rawles J: Halving of mortality at 1 year by domiciliary thrombolysis in the Grampian Region Early Anistreplase Trial (GREAT), *J Am Coll Cardiol* 23(1):1-5, 1994.

36. Gersh BJ, Anderson JL: Thrombolysis and myocardial salvage: results of clinical trials and the animal paradigm—paradoxic or predictable? *Circulation* 88:296-306, 1993.

37. Kudenchuk PJ, Ho MT, Weaver WD, et al: Accuracy of computer-interpreted electrocardiography on time to in-hospital thrombolytic therapy in acute myocardial infarction, *J Am Coll Cardiol* 17:1486-1491, 1991.

38. Aufderheide TP, Hendley GE, Thakur RK, et al: The diagnostic impact of prehospital 12-lead electrocardiography, *Ann Emerg Med* 19:1280-1287, 1990.

39. Jayes RL, Larson GC, Beshansky RJ, et al: Physician electrocardiogram reading in the emergency department—accuracy and effect on triage decision, *J Gen Intern Med* 7:387-393, 1992.

40. Cerquiera MD, Maynard C, Ritchie JL, et al: Long-term survival in 618 patients from the Western Washington streptokinase in myocardial infarction trials, *J Am Coll Cardiol* 20:1452-1459, 1992.

41. Karagounis L, Ipsen SK, Jessop MR, et al: Impact of field-transmitted electrocardiography on time to in-hospital thrombolytic therapy in acute myocardial infarction, *Am J Cardiol* 66:786-791, 1990.

42. Kereiakes DJ, Weaver WD, Anderson JL, et al: Time delays in the diagnosis and treatment of acute myocardial infarction: a tale of eight cities, *Am Heart J* 120:773-780, 1990.

43. Sharkey SW, Brunette DD, Ruiz R, et al: An analysis of time delays preceding thrombolysis for acute myocardial infarction, *JAMA* 262:3171-3174, 1989.

44. Pell ACH, Miller HC, Robertson CE, et al: Effect of "fast track" admission for acute myocardial infarction on delay to thrombolysis, *BMJ* 304:83-87, 1992.

45. Gibler WB, Kereiakes DJ, Dean EN, et al and the investigators of the Cincinnati Heart Project and the Nashville Prehospital TPA Trial: Prehospital diagnosis and treatment of acute myocardial infarction: a North-South perspective, *Am Heart J* 12:1-11, 1991.

46. Arntz H-R, Stern R, Linderer T, et al: Efficiency of a physician-operated mobile intensive care unit for prehospital thrombolysis in acute myocardial infarction, *Am J Cardiol* 70:417-420, 1992.

47. Bouten MJM, Simoons ML, Hartman JAM, et al: Prehospital thrombolysis with alteplase (rt-PA) in acute myocardial infarction, *Euro Heart J* 13:925-931, 1992.

48. Krukoff MW, Croll M, O'Connor CM, et al: Prediction of infarct vessel patency early after thrombolysis with continuous 12-lead ST-segment monitoring: results of the TAMI 7 trial (abstract). *Eur Heart J* 12(suppl):442, 1992.

49. Katus HA, Remppis A, Neumann FJ, et al: Diagnostic efficiency of Troponin-T measurements in acute myocardial infarction, *Circulation* 83:902-912, 1991.

50. Hamm CW, Ravkilde J, Gerhardt W, et al: The prognostic value of serum Troponin-T in unstable angina, *N Engl J Med* 327:146-150, 1992.

51. Castaigne AD, Herve C, Douval-Moulin AM, et al: Prehospital use of APSAC: results of a placebo-controlled study, *Am J Cardiol* 64:30A-33A, 1993.

Chapter 21

EMERGENCY ROOM EVALUATION AND TRIAGE STRATEGIES FOR PATIENTS WITH ACUTE CHEST PAIN: LESSONS FROM THE PRE-THROMBOLYTIC ERA

Jean-Michel Gaspoz
Thomas H. Lee
Lee Goldman

Before the thrombolytic era, physicians were faced with essentially a straightforward issue when a patient was admitted to the emergency department with symptoms suggestive of acute myocardial infarction (AMI): first and foremost, a prompt decision had to be made about whether or not to admit the patient to the hospital. Although diagnostic acumen was important, the precise diagnosis was less important than appropriate triage decisions. Treatment in the emergency department was reactive, was in response to manifest problems, and, except in the sickest patients, carried less strategic consequences than the inappropriate decision of sending home a patient with AMI who might suffer an arrhythmic death shortly thereafter.

Thrombolysis, with its known benefits but also its risks, has changed the situation in three ways. First, treatment is now a major focus of attention. Second, thrombolysis decisions depend on the accuracy with which the diagnosis of AMI can be established in the emergency room. Because the diagnosis may not be certain, both risks and benefits must be weighed, with due consideration to the recommended indications and established contraindications for thrombolysis. Third, because the benefits of thrombolysis decline if treatment is delayed, substantial time pressure may influence the medical decision-making of emergency department physicians.

In this chapter, we first review the relative value of clinical information, the initial electrocardiogram (ECG), and laboratory data in assessing the probability of AMI in the emergency department and in assisting triage decisions for patients with suspected AMI. We then put this information in the perspective of thrombolysis.

CLINICAL INFORMATION
Prior history

In patients with a history of known angina pectoris or prior AMI, comparison with prior symptoms of ischemia allows identification of a group with about a 15%

Table 21-1. Clinical characteristics predictive of acute myocardial infarction in emergency department patients with chest pain

	Probability of acute myocardial infarction (%)
Description of the pain	
Pressure, tightness, crushing	24
Burning, indigestion	23
Ache	13
Sharp, stabbing	5
Partially pleuritic or positional	7
Fully pleuritic or positional	1
Radiation of the pain to the jaw, neck, left arm, or left shoulder	19
Reproducibility	
Pain partially reproducible by chest wall palpation	6
Pain fully reproducible by chest wall palpation	5
Combination of variables	
Sharp or stabbing pain; no prior angina or myocardial infarction; pain pleuritic, positional, or reproducible by palpation	0

probability of AMI if the current pain is similar to pain of a prior MI or is similar to but worse than the patient's chronic angina in terms of severity, duration, frequency, or failure to respond to usual treatment.[1] Epidemiologic risk factors such as smoking status, hypertension, hyperlipidemia, and family history, although important in predicting the long-term likelihood of coronary artery disease, are not particularly helpful in the emergency department setting because other historical and ECG characteristics are more predictive of AMI.

Presenting symptoms

Nature of the pain. Typical symptoms of AMI have been described as crushing pain, pressure, and tightness. However, only 24% of emergency room patients who use such descriptions are having an AMI (Table 21-1).[2] Discomfort described as "burning," "indigestion," or "numbness" or that the patient cannot describe with any usual adjective is equally as predictive, because MI was also diagnosed in 23% of the patients using such terms. The probability of acute MI is lower, 13%, in patients with a complaint of "chest ache" and the lowest, 5%, in patients who describe a sharp or stabbing pain. If the chest discomfort is partially reproduced by respiration (pleuritic) or is exacerbated by changes in position (positional), the probability of AMI is about 7%. It is the lowest, 1%, if the pain is fully pleuritic or positional. The location of the patient's discomfort is critically important, as are its reproducibility by palpation and the

radiation of the pain.[2-4] Most MIs manifest with substernal or left precordial chest pain. If such a symptom is not reproducible on local palpation and radiates to the neck, the left shoulder or the left arm, the likelihood of MI increases threefold to fourfold. On the contrary, MI is significantly less frequent if chest wall palpation fully or partially reproduces the pain (see Table 21-1).

When the decision under consideration is related not to thrombolytic treatment but to whether to admit or discharge, combinations of clinical variables are more valuable than any single variable for identifying patients with a low probability of AMI. The combination of three variables—sharp or stabbing pain, no history of angina or MI, and pain that is reproduced by chest wall palpation or that is partially or fully pleuritic or positional—identifies the lowest-risk group (see Table 21-1). In a report from the Multicenter Chest Pain Study,[2] none of 48 emergency room patients with such characteristics had MI, unstable angina, or stable angina. Only this combination of clinical variables yielded a probability of AMI as low as a normal ECG (probability of AMI <1%).

Responses to empiric therapy such as antacids, nitroglycerin, or analgesics are rarely helpful and sometimes misleading. Pain may not respond to nitroglycerin because it results from AMI rather than angina or because it is not ischemic in origin. A response to antacids is often interpreted as being pathognomonic of a gastrointestinal cause. However, a substantial fraction of patients with AMI have chest discomfort that seems to respond to antacids, sometimes because of a placebo effect, because some relief is provided by subsequent belching or because the pain coincidentally subsides.

Physical examination

Because there are no pathognomonic clinical signs of AMI, the physical examination will rarely help in making that diagnosis. The physical examination may, however, be helpful in revealing a nonischemic cause of the chest discomfort or in finding areas of localized tenderness that may fully or partially reproduce the chest discomfort.

INITIAL ECG

Using various criteria, both univariate[3] and multivariate analyses[4-9] consistently show that the initial ECG is helpful in the diagnosis and in the prognostic stratification of emergency department patients with suspected acute AMI (see also Chapter 2). Recent investigations have also shown that the availability of a prior ECG during the emergency department evaluation improves diagnostic accuracy, particularly among patients whose current tracings are abnormal. In the Multicenter Chest Pain Study, patients who did not have AMI but whose emergency department ECGs

Table 21-2. Relation between ECG interpretations and diagnosis of MIs[4]

ECG finding	% of patients who had MIs (positive predictive value)	% of MI patients (sensitivity)
1. ≥1 mm ST elevation or Q waves in ≥2 leads (not known to be old)	76	45
2. New ischemia or strain ≥1 mm ST depression in ≥2 leads (not known to be old)	38	20
3. Other ST or T wave changes of ischemia or strain not known to be old	21	14
4. Old infarction, ischemia or strain	8	5
5. Other new or old abnormality	5	5
6. Nonspecific ST-T changes only	5	7
7. Normal	2	3.4

From Rouan GW, Lee TH, Cook EF, et al: *Am J Cardiol* 64:1087-1092, 1989.
*ECG, Electrocardiographic; MI, myocardial infarction.

showed changes consistent with ischemia or infarction were more than twice as likely to be discharged (26% vs. 12%) and 1.5 times as likely to avoid admission to the coronary care unit (39% vs. 27%) if a prior tracing were available for comparison.[10]

In the Multicenter Chest Pain Study,[1,2,8] an initial ECG showing ST-segment elevations of more than 1 mm or Q waves in two or more leads that were not known to be old was the single best predictive variable for AMI; 73% to 78% of the patients with these findings had AMIs. Other ECG findings were less helpful (Table 21-2). Signs of new ischemia or strain are important predictors of both AMI or unstable angina except in a patient at an exceptionally low risk according to a combination of clinical variables and for whom the ECG may be misleading. However, almost no combination of clinical factors is sufficiently reassuring to warrant discharge of a patient who has chest pain and ischemic ST-T-wave changes that are not known to be old.

On the other end of the ECG spectrum, abnormalities known to be old, nonspecific ECG abnormalities, and a normal ECG should not be used to exclude MI. Up to 7% of patients with signs of ischemia, strain, or infarction known to be old have MI; this proportion rises to 15% if their current pain is the same as a prior MI or similar to but worse than their usual angina.[10,11] The probability of acute MI in patients with chest pain and an initially normal ECG is about 3% but varies from 1% to 17%, depending on such clinical characteristics as age, sex, and the type and radiation of the pain.[12] In these patients, historical features are more helpful in the prediction of MI than in patients with highly suggestive ECGs. Of all the patients with AMI in the Multicenter Chest Pain Study,[1,2,8,10-12] about 60% had significant new ST-segment elevations or new Q waves on their initial ECG, and 25% had new ECG signs of ischemia or strain, whereas 15% had initial ECGs without any new changes of ischemia, strain, or infarction. Thus, reliance on the ECG alone would have missed about 15% of AMIs.

EFFECTS OF AGE, GENDER, AND RACE

Although older age is associated with an increased probability of AMI among emergency department patients,[2] the same clinical and ECG features are associated with increased relative risks for MI in patients older than 65 years of age and younger patients.[13] The relative risks for classic clinical features[2] are, however, closer to 1.0 among older patients, so that the diagnosis of acute chest pain is especially difficult in the elderly who, as a result, are more likely to be admitted to the hospital and to the coronary care unit in the absence of AMI or even unstable angina.[13]

Clinical factors that predict MI in men predict MI in women to a similar degree.[14] However, because of the lower prior probability of coronary artery disease in women, in the absence of classic changes in the emergency room ECG, women have about a 40% lower risk of AMI than men even after adjusting for other clinical factors.

Interest in the manifestation and natural history of coronary artery disease in patients of different races has been stimulated in recent years by data demonstrating that black patients admitted to the hospital for ischemic heart disease are less likely to have cardiac procedures than white patients.[15] Whether this pattern reflects bias in the use of procedures is unclear, because other data indicate that black emergency department patients with acute chest pain have about half the risk (17% vs. 33%) of having AMI or unstable angina as white patients.[16] This difference may reflect differences in access to care among patients with varying socioeconomic status. Multivariate analyses of emergency department data show that after differences in presenting symptoms and signs are adjusted for, blacks and whites have similar rates of AMI.[16]

CARDIAC ENZYMES

In most hospitals today, rapid automated assays of total serum creatine kinase (CK) and quantitative

Table 21-3. Sensitivity and specificity of CK and CK-MB in the emergency room*

Threshold for admission	Sensitivity† (%)	Specificity‡ (%)
Total CK >normal limit	38	80
Total CK >2 times normal limit	24	95
Total CK >normal limit and		
CK-MB >5% of total CK	34	88
CK-MB >7% of total CK	30	96
CK-MB >9% of total CK	21	98

From Lee TH, Goldman L: *Pract Cardiol* 14:47-56, 1988, used by permission.
*CK, Creatine kinase; CK-MB, creatine kinase subunits M and B; AMI, acute myocardial infarction.
†Sensitivity is defined as the number of patients with AMI and an abnormal test result divided by the number of patients with AMI.
‡Specificity is defined as the number of patients without AMI and with a normal test result divided by the number of patients without AMI.

CK-MB levels are available during the emergency department evaluation. Assays of lactate dehydrogenase (LDH) and aspartate aminotransferase (AST) can also be obtained. Data from the Multicenter Chest Pain Study and elsewhere[2,17,18] show that regardless of the cutoff value chosen, single determinations of total CK, LDH, and AST cannot detect MI with a high sensitivity and a low false-positive rate. The initial CK level is elevated in only 39% of patients with MI, but it is also elevated in 22% of patients without MI.[2] In patients seen more than 12 hours after the onset of symptoms, the AST level is significantly more accurate than in patients seen before 12 hours have elapsed, but total CK levels are still unreliable. In one series of 80 patients, the availability of cardiac enzyme levels in the emergency department might have prevented the discharge of 1 patient with AMI but could have led to the inappropriate discharge of 5 other patients with MIs and to the inappropriate admission of 11 patients without MIs.[18]

Among all patients with AMI, only 34% have an elevated total CK level and a CK-MB level greater than 5% in the emergency department, whereas similar enzymatic patterns are also found in 12% of patients without AMI.[19] A strategy using abnormal CK levels only is slightly more sensitive for detecting MI than the one requiring both elevated total CK and CK-MB levels of 5% or more but has substantially more false-positive results. Analysis of receiver operating characteristic (ROC) curves shows that both strategies are better than chance in diagnosing AMI but that a strategy using both an elevated total CK level and a CK-MB level of 5% or more performs significantly better than the strategy using an elevated total CK level only.[19] Table 21-3 shows the respective sensitivity and specificity of these two strategies, as well as the decrease in sensitivity but increase in specificity of higher CK-MB thresholds. The sensitivity of both strategies improves for patients seen more than 12 hours after the onset of symptoms. However, the prevalence of MI among emergency department patients declines in parallel with the time elapsed since the onset of symptoms, which results in a progressively lower pretest probability of MI. A Bayesian analysis therefore shows that the overall predictive value of such enzyme level determinations does not change based on time, because the increased sensitivity of the test is offset by the declining prevalence of AMIs.[19]

Radioimmunoassays of CK-MB and newer solid-phase immunoradiometric assays have increased the sensitivity and specificity of this test for detecting AMI.[20,21] Their impact in the emergency department remains limited, however, by the fact that less than half of AMI patients have abnormal total CK levels when admitted.

Although most hospitals do not assay CK-MB levels in the absence of elevated total CK levels, increased CK-MB levels in the absence of abnormal total CK levels can reflect AMI, especially in elderly patients.[21,22] Although such patients seem to have a worse prognosis than patients with suspected MI and normal CK-MB levels,[21-23] it is still unclear whether determining this apparently small amount of myocardial damage would modify management after all other clinical data are taken into account.

Determination of the CK-MM isoform profile in a single blood sample taken when the patient is seen initially has been shown to have greater sensitivity for diagnosing AMI in the early hours after symptoms onset than CK-MB levels, but it also has a lower specificity.[24] CK-MB isoform profiles have a better specificity.[25] The usefulness of routine determination of both CK-MM and CK-MB isoforms, as well as of other markers of ischemic injury such as myoglobin or troponin-T,[26,27] is yet to be determined.

Measurements of serum total CK and CK-MB levels continue to be the most widely available tests. Although serial measurements of serum levels of these cardiac enzymes are important for the diagnosis of AMI, single determinations of their serum levels are of limited value in the emergency department setting, not only because of high false-negative rates but also because of high false-positive rates in a population with a high prevalence of noncardiac conditions that may be associated with skeletal muscle injury.[2,17,19] Enzyme level determinations in the emergency department should not be relied on as a guide in choosing treatment options or in deciding not to admit a patient. They might, however, have a role in determining which patients should not be sent home, because a very positive CK-MB level in an otherwise low-risk patient raises the probability of AMI sufficiently to warrant admission.

TRIAGE AND MANAGEMENT STRATEGIES

In the Multicenter Chest Pain Study, 4% of the patients admitted to an emergency department with an AMI were sent home.[28] Despite less typical and lower-risk manifestations, their mortality rate within 72 hours of the initial emergency department visit (23%) was significantly higher, after adjustment for possible confounders, than for AMI patients admitted to the hospital (mortality rate at 72 hours 12%). Emergency department physicians are therefore likely to admit a patient, often to the coronary care unit, if there is any reasonable suspicion of AMI. Today the proportion of coronary care unit patients who "rule in" for AMI is only about 30%[29]; patients who "rule out" in such a unit have few life-threatening complications and a good short-term prognosis, but they account for a large proportion of the coronary care unit charges.[30]

Decision aids

To assist physicians in the diagnosis of emergency department patients with suspected AMI and to achieve more appropriate triage, a number of decision aids have been developed* to incorporate both clinical and ECG data from the initial evaluation. For example, Pozen et al.[5,31] derived a mathematical instrument based on nine clinical historical and ECG variables to generate probabilities of acute ischemic heart disease. When emergency department physicians of six teaching and nonteaching hospitals were provided with these probabilities, which were generated by a hand-held programmable calculator, rates of false-positive diagnosis decreased with no increase in the rates of false-negative diagnosis. Coronary care unit admissions of patients without acute ischemic heart disease decreased by 11%. Using recursive partitioning analysis, Goldman et al.[1,8] constructed a decision protocol in the format of a single flowchart on the basis of nine clinical factors to predict the probability of AMI in emergency room patients with chest pain (Fig. 21-1). When prospectively tested on 4770 patients at 2 university and 4 community hospitals, the computer-derived protocol had sensitivity similar to emergency room physicians for detecting AMI (88.0 vs.

87.8) but significantly higher specificity (74.0 vs. 71.0), which would have resulted in a 11.5% reduction in coronary care unit admissions of patients without AMI. More recently, neural networks, which are designed to consider a wide range of interactions among factors, have been used to derive decision aids,[32] but the weighting of the clinical factors and the applicability of this "black box" approach to other settings is unclear.

Alternatives to coronary care unit admissions

Not only can these aids help in making a decision about admitting a patient to the hospital, they can also determine a group of patients for whom the probability of AMI and of complications is too low for coronary care unit admission to be cost-effective yet too high for discharge to be safe. Such patients may benefit from admission to intermediate care units with monitoring and resuscitation capabilities but without the other expensive services provided in coronary care units. A cost-effectiveness analysis showed that at probabilities of infarction up to about 20%, admission to an intermediate care unit rather than to the coronary care unit was a cost-effective strategy.[33] A later study confirmed the safety of admission to intermediate care units of such initially uncomplicated patients.[34] Triage of low-risk patients to monitored short-stay units instead of coronary care or intermediate care units may be preferable, because these short-stay units provide equal safety but at lower costs than intermediate or coronary care units.[35,36]

Duration of observation period

One of the major goals of admitting patients with suspected AMI is to detect arrhythmias and prevent sudden death as a result of myocardial damage. The duration for which patients were observed before the diagnosis of MI was considered excluded (or ruled out) was formerly highly variable, but multicenter data have demonstrated that a 24-hour observation period has a high sensitivity for detecting MI.[37] More recently, the safety and effectiveness of a 12-hour observation period for admitted patients with a low ($\leq 7\%$) initial risk of AMI was evaluated using prospective data from the Multicenter Chest Pain Study.[38] This analysis indicated that a 12-hour observation period was appropriate for low-risk patients, whereas patients with a higher initial risk of AMI should be observed for 24 hours. These data do not imply that patients should be discharged at the end of these observation periods but that patients can be considered for transfer out of a monitored setting while further evaluation (e.g., exercise testing) is pursued.

THROMBOLYTIC ERA

Since the widespread use of thrombolysis, the focus of attention in the emergency room has become prompt administration of intravenous thrombolytic agents to

---

*References 1, 3, 5, 7, 8, 31, 32.

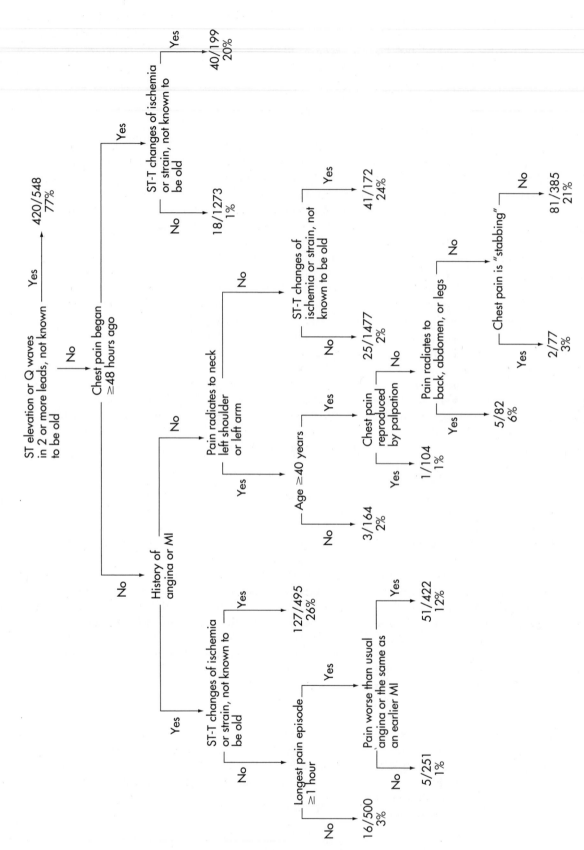

Fig. 21-1. Prospectively validated multivariate algorithm for the prediction of a patient's risk of acute myocardial infarction (*AMI*) on the basis of emergency room data. On the basis of the algorithm, patients can be assigned to 1 of 14 subgroups, each of which has been classified as having a low (≤7%) or a high (>7%) risk of AMI. The values shown for each subgroup are the number of patients with AMI, divided by the total number of patients in a subgroup of 6149 patients enrolled in the Chest Pain Study, with the corresponding percentages. "Pain worse than usual angina" denotes worse in frequency, severity, or duration, or failure to respond to usual measures. (From Lee TH, Juarez G, Cook EF, et al: *N Engl J Med* 324:1239-1246, 1991. Used by permission.)

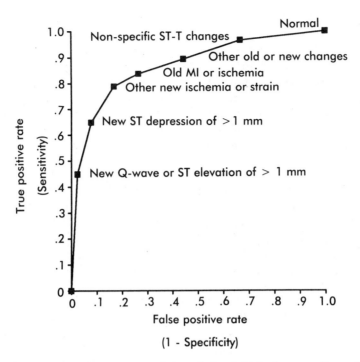

Fig. 21-2. Receiver operating characteristics of the initial electrocardiographic (ECG) interpretation. The cumulative sensitivity (number of myocardial infarction [*MI*] patients with the finding divided by all patients with MI) of ECG interpretations is on the y axis and is plotted against the cumulative false positive rate (number of noninfarction patients with the finding divided by all patients without MI) on the x axis. The ECG interpretations that were considered highly suggestive of MI (new ST elevation, new ST depression, or other new ischemia or strain) had a cumulative sensitivity of 79% (i.e., they correctly identified 79% of MIs) and had an associated false-positive rate of 17% (i.e., incorrectly classified 17% of noninfarction patients). (From Rouan GW, Lee TH, Cook EF, et al: *Am J Cardiol* 64:1087-1092, 1989. Used by permission.)

suitable candidates with symptoms and signs suggestive of AMI. In this perspective, thrombolysis does not alter but instead highlights the relevance of the lessons learned in the prethrombolytic era about the predictive value of clinical, ECG, and enzymatic data available in the acute setting. This information can be used to determine the probability of AMI for an individual patient, as well as to assess the sensitivity and specificity of current and future eligibility criteria for thrombolysis.

Shortly after the Gruppo Italiano per lo Studio della Streptochinasi nell'Infarto Miocardico (GISSI) trial,[39] the accepted eligibility criteria for intravenous thrombolysis became age 75 or younger, time since onset of symptoms 4 hours or less, and an emergency room ECG showing ST-segment elevation of 1 mm or more in two or more leads not known to be old. Of 1118 acute MI patients in the Multicenter Chest Pain Study from December 1983 to August 1985, 261 (23%) patients were 75 years of age or younger, were seen within 4 hours of the onset of symptoms, and had ECGs that were interpreted as showing AMI (ST-segment elevation ≥ 1 mm or pathologic Q waves in two or more leads not

known to be old).[40] Sixty (0.9%) of the 6616 patients without AMI also met these criteria, resulting in a positive predictive value of 81% (confidence interval 77%-86%). It was therefore estimated that for every eight true-positive patients, two false-positive patients also would have been eligible according to these criteria. If patients suspected of having AMI on the basis of new pathologic Q waves in the absence of ST-segment elevation were excluded, 250 (22%) patients with infarction and 46 (0.7%) patients without infarction would have been candidates for thrombolysis (positive predictive value 84%; confidence interval 80%-89%). Because about one third of patients who meet the eligibility criteria just listed have other contraindications to thrombolysis, only about 15% of AMI patients were estimated to represent suitable candidates for thrombolysis.[40]

Recent evidence of the benefits of thrombolysis for patients older than 75 years of age and for patients seen later after the onset of symptoms[41] has led to the broadening of the eligibility criteria. The lengthening of the time interval since the onset of symptoms during which AMI patients are considered candidates for thrombolysis will result in the treatment of not only more patients with MI but also of more patients without it, because the prevalence of MI decreases with the time since the onset of symptoms,[19] and the probability of an helpful ECG does not correlate with the time since the onset of symptoms.[12] For example, moving the time limit since the onset of symptoms from 4 to 6 hours and keeping the criteria for age and ECG findings unchanged would have led to the treatment of 23 (6%) additional patients with AMI in the study cited before[40] but also of 6 (5%) other patients without it, a ratio of true positive/false positive similar to during the first 4 hours. Because the current trend is to consider treating patients up to 12 hours and sometimes 24 hours after the onset of symptoms, a risk/benefit analysis of various time limits is warranted, taking into account the declining benefits and the increasing risk of cardiac rupture related to thrombolysis for patients with AMI, as well as the risks for patients inappropriately treated.

Because the clinical and ECG features predictive of the presence or the absence of acute MI in younger patients are applicable in the elderly,[13] disappearance of an age limit for thrombolysis is not likely to modify significantly the positive predictive value of current eligibility criteria. A decision analysis model assessing the role of thrombolytic therapy in patients greater than 75 years of age with suspected AMI suggests that such a strategy provides a significant survival advantage to elderly patients and may be cost effective.[42]

Thrombolysis does not seem to offer any benefit to patients with unstable angina[43,44] or to AMI patients without new ST-segment elevation or new Q waves.[39] If further studies were to contradict these findings, a broadening of the ECG eligibility criteria would considerably increase the proportion of false-positive rates, depending on which ECG changes would enter into consideration, given the receiver operating characteristics curve of the initial ECG interpretation (Fig. 21-2). For example, if ST-segment elevation or depression or T-wave abnormalities consistent with ischemia or strain not known to be old were accepted as ECG eligibility criteria for thrombolysis, 73% of AMI patients would be eligible for thrombolysis, as well as 15% of the patients without AMI (positive predictive value of these ECG criteria 44%).[40] Patients with a bundle branch block on the initial ECG and a clinical manifestation highly suggestive of AMI seem to benefit from thrombolysis; the consequences in terms of true-positive and false-positive rates of this new indication for thrombolysis require further study.

In light of the current eligibility criteria for thrombolysis, decision aids developed to achieve more appropriate triage in the emergency departments[1,5,8,31] can also be used to identify patients with a high probability of MI who are candidates for immediate thrombolysis.

These approaches also can identify patients for whom close observation is required to monitor for signs of recurrent ischemia and the subsequent development of MI, which may require the later use of thrombolytic agents. These decision aids can also help identify low-risk patients, who not only are not candidates for thrombolysis but who are suitable either for discharge or for short-stay admission to cost-effective alternatives to coronary care units.

REFERENCES

1. Goldman L, et al: A computer-derived protocol to aid in the diagnosis of emergency room patients with acute chest pain, *N Engl J Med* 307:588-596, 1982.
2. Lee TH, et al: Acute chest pain in the emergency room. Identification and examination of low-risk patients, *Arch Intern Med* 45:65-69, 1985.
3. Behar S, et al: Evaluation of electrocardiogram in emergency room as a decision-making tool, *Chest* 71:486-491, 1977.
4. Pipberger HV, Klingeman JD, Cosma J: Computer evaluation of statistical properties of clinical information in the differential diagnosis of acute chest pain, *Methods Inf Med* 7:79-92, 1968.
5. Pozen MW, et al: The usefulness of a predictive instrument to reduce inappropriate admissions to the coronary care unit, *Ann Intern Med* 92:238-242, 1980.
6. Lubsen J, Pool J, Van der Does E: A practical device for the application of a diagnostic or prognostic function, *Methods Inf Med* 17:127-129, 1978.
7. Patrick EA, et al: Pattern recognition applied to early diagnosis of heart attacks. In *Proceedings of the International Medical Information Processing Conference,* Toronto, 1977, vol 2, pp 203-207.
8. Goldman L, et al: A computer protocol to predict myocardial infarction in emergency department patients with chest pain, *N Engl J Med* 318:797-803, 1988.
9. Yusuf S, et al: The entry electrocardiogram in the early diagnostic and prognostic stratification of patients with acute myocardial infarction, *Eur Heart J* 5:690-696, 1984.
10. Lee TH, et al: Impact of the availability of a prior electrocardiogram on the triage of the patient with acute chest pain, *J Gen Intern Med* 5:381-388, 1990.
11. Goldman L: Acute chest pain: emergency room evaluation, *Hosp Prac* 7:94A-94T, 1986.
12. Rouan GW, et al: Clinical characteristics and outcome of acute myocardial infarction in patients with initially normal or non-specific electrocardiograms (a report from the Multicenter Chest Pain Study), *Am J Cardiol* 64:1087-1092, 1989.
13. Solomon CG, et al: Comparison of clinical presentations of acute myocardial infarction in patients older than 65 years of age to younger patients: the Multicenter Chest Pain Study experience, *Am J Cardiol* 63:772-776, 1989.
14. Cunningham MA, et al: The effect of gender on the probability of myocardial infarction among emergency department patients with acute chest pain. A report from the Multicenter Chest Pain Study, *J Gen Intern Med* 4:392-398, 1989.
15. Wenneker MB, Epstein AM: Racial inequalities in the use of procedures for patients with ischemic heart disease in Massachusetts, *JAMA* 261:253-257, 1989.
16. Johnson PA, et al: Impact of race on the clinical presentation, natural history and access to medical care and procedures in emergency department patients with acute chest pain. (Submitted.)
17. Lee TH, Goldman L: Serum enzyme assays in the diagnosis of acute myocardial infarction. Recommendations based on quantitative analysis, *Ann Intern Med* 105:221-233, 1986.

18. Eisenberg JM, et al: Diagnosis of acute myocardial infarction in the emergency room, *J Community Health* 4:190-198, 1979.

19. Lee TH, et al: Evaluation of creatine kinase and creatine kinase–MB for diagnosing myocardial infarction. Clinical impact in the emergency room, *Arch Intern Med* 147:115-121, 1987.

20. Al-Sheikh W, et al: Evaluation of an immunoradiometric assay specific for the CK-MB isoenzyme for the detection of acute myocardial infarction, *Am J Cardiol* 54:269-273, 1984.

21. Clyne CA, Medeiros LJ, Marton K: The prognostic significance of immunoradiometric CK-MB assay (IRMA) diagnosis of myocardial infarction in patients with low total CK and elevated MB isoenzymes, *Am Heart J* 118:901-906, 1989.

22. White RD, et al: Diagnostic and prognostic significance of minimally elevated creatine kinase-MB in suspected acute myocardial infarction, *Am J Cardiol* 55:1478-1484, 1985.

23. Yusuf S, et al: Significance of elevated MB isoenzyme with normal creatine kinase in acute myocardial infarction, *Am J Cardiol* 59:245-250, 1987.

24. Jaffe AS, et al: Diagnostic changes in plasma creatine kinase isoforms early after the onset of acute myocardial infarction, *Circulation* 74:105-109, 1986.

25. Puleo PR, et al: Early diagnosis of acute myocardial infarction based on assay for subforms of creatine kinase-MB, *Circulation* 82:759-764, 1990.

26. Katus HA, et al: Diagnostic efficiency of troponin T measurements in acute myocardial infarction, *Circulation* 83:902-912, 1991.

27. Ellis AK: Serum protein measurements and the diagnosis of acute myocardial infarction, *Circulation* 83:1107-1109, 1991.

28. Lee TH, et al: Clinical characteristics and natural history of patients with acute myocardial infarction sent home from the emergency room, *Am J Cardiol* 60:219-224, 1987.

29. Lee TH, Goldman L: The Coronary Care Unit turns 25. Historical trends and future directions, *Ann Intern Med* 108:887-894, 1988.

30. Detsky AL, et al: Prognosis, survival, and the expenditure of hospital resources for patients in an intensive-care unit, *N Engl J Med* 305:667-672, 1989.

31. Pozen MW, et al: A predictive instrument to improve coronary-care-unit admission practices in acute ischemic heart disease. A prospective multicenter clinical trial, *N Engl J Med* 310:1273-1278, 1984.

32. Baxt WG: Use of an artificial neural network for the diagnosis of myocardial infarction, *Ann Intern Med* 115:843-848, 1991.

33. Fineberg HV, Scadden D, Goldman L: Care of patients with a low probability of acute myocardial infarction. Cost effectiveness of alternatives to coronary-care-unit admission, *N Engl J Med* 310:1301-1307, 1984.

34. Fiebach NH, et al: Outcomes in patients with myocardial infarction who are initially admitted to stepdown units: data from the Multicenter Chest Pain Study, *Am J Med* 89:15-20, 1990.

35. Gaspoz JM, et al: Outcome of patients who were admitted to a new short-stay unit to "rule-out" myocardial infarction, *Am J Cardiol* 68:145-149, 1991.

36. Gaspoz JM, et al: Cost-effectiveness of a new short-stay unit to rule-out acute myocardial infarction, *Clin Res* 39:222A, 1991.

37. Lee TH, et al: Sensitivity of routine clinical criteria for diagnosing myocardial infarction within 24 hours of hospitalization, *Ann Intern Med* 106:181-186, 1987.

38. Lee TH, et al: Ruling-out acute myocardial infarction. A prospective validation of a 12-hour strategy for low-risk patients, *N Engl J Med* 324:1239-1246, 1991.

39. Gruppo Italiano per lo Studio della Streptochinasi nell'Infarto Miocardico (GISSI): Long term effects of intravenous thrombolysis in acute myocardial infarction: final report of the GISSI study, *Lancet* 2:871-874, 1987.

40. Lee TH, et al: Candidates for thrombolysis among emergency room patients with acute chest pain. Potential true- and false positive rates, *Ann Intern Med* 110:957-962, 1989.

41. ISIS-2 (Second International Study of Infarct Survival) Collaborative Group: Randomized trial of intravenous streptokinase, oral aspirin, both or neither among 17,187 cases of suspected acute myocardial infarction: ISIS-2, *Lancet* 2:349-360, 1988.

42. Krumholz HM, Pasternak RC, Weinstein MC, et al: Cost effectiveness of thrombolytic therapy with streptokinase in elderly patients with suspected acute myocardial infarction, *N Engl J Med* 327:7-13, 1992.

43. Freeman MR, et al: Thrombolysis in unstable angina. Randomized double-blind trial of t-PA and placebo, *Circulation* 85:150-157, 1992.

44. Leinbach RC: Thrombolysis in unstable angina, *Circulation* 85:376-377, 1992.

Chapter 22

STRATEGIES TO DECREASE TREATMENT DELAYS IN PATIENTS RECEIVING THROMBOLYTIC THERAPY FOR ACUTE MYOCARDIAL INFARCTION

Eva Kline
Deborah Smith
Jenny Martin
Kathleen Dracup

Thrombolytic therapy significantly reduces morbidity and mortality associated with acute myocardial infarction (AMI). However, the benefits of this therapy are time-dependent[1-5]: early treatment results in preservation of more myocardium and improved clinical outcomes. Sources delaying initiation of thrombolytic therapy need to be identified and reduced. These delays can be divided into three areas: patient delays in seeking treatment, prehospital delays, and in-hospital delays.

The longest delays occur in the area of the patient seeking treatment. Although not as significant, prehospital delays contribute to the overall delay time and could be reduced by increasing the public's use of emergency medical systems (EMSs), thereby facilitating rapid identification and treatment. Delays within the hospital system may be the ones most easily targeted for strategies aimed at delay reduction. The emergency department (ED) is the most common point of hospital entry for the majority of patients. Several groups have

reported reduced time delays by implementing a team approach using standard protocols for acute MI patients. The purpose of this chapter is to describe the components of delays in treating patients with thrombolytic therapy and to recommend potential strategies to reduce these delays.

MORTALITY REDUCTION

The DeWood et al.[6] pivotal study in 1980 was the catalyst that led to the vigorous investigation of thrombolytic agents for mortality reduction in AMI. In this study, total thrombotic coronary occlusion was demonstrated in 87% of 126 patients who underwent coronary angiography within 4 hours of symptom onset of AMI. This was the first conclusive clinical evidence to link the cause of MI to coronary thrombosis, thus suggesting that thrombolytic agents could play a role in treatment of AMI. Multiple large-scale, randomized trials of thrombolytic therapy have demonstrated effectiveness in reducing deaths in patients with AMI. The results of three recent international megatrials of thrombolytic therapy, with combined recruitment of greater than 100,000 patients,[2,3,5] further validate the benefits of thrombolytic therapy for mortality reduction in AMI, particularly in patients treated within the first hour of symptoms. In the Gruppo Italiano per lo Studio della Streptochinasi nell'Infarto Miocardico (GISSI-1) Study, patients who were treated within 1 hour of the onset of symptoms demonstrated a 47% reduction in in-hospital mortality.[1] In comparison, patients treated within 3 to 6 hours had a 17% reduction.

Several contemporary trials have also demonstrated significant mortality reduction in patients treated soon after symptom onset.[5,7,8] Honan et al.[4] examined the relation between the risk of cardiac rupture and the timing of thrombolytic therapy of AMI. They found that thrombolytic therapy early after AMI improves survival and decreases the risk of cardiac rupture. This clinical experience confirms the fundamental findings of Reimer and Jennings,[9] who demonstrated in the canine model that myocardial necrosis after coronary artery occlusion is a dynamic process occurring gradually from endocardium to epicardium and is near completion at 4 to 6 hours. Therefore, it is apparent that to reduce morbidity and mortality, rapid diagnosis and initiation of therapy will facilitate early reperfusion of ischemic myocardium.

PATIENT DELAYS IN SEEKING TREATMENT

Patient delay in recognition of symptoms and seeking care is the largest component of delays to treatment of AMI. The median time between the onset of symptoms indicative of acute MI and admittance to a medical care facility is 4 hours.[10] Several investigators have attempted to delineate the factors that contribute to this delay.

Although studies have been completed identifying variables that affect delay times, methodologic differences and study limitations make comparisons across studies difficult and confusing. Dracup and Mosher[11] reviewed all related literature and drew some conclusions regarding the effect of selected variables on prehospital delay time. The variables listed in Table 22-1 have been identified as contributing to prehospital delays. Table 22-2 lists those variables that decrease delay times according to Dracup and Moshers'[11] analyses.

The following four recommendations have been made by Dracup and Mosher[11] based on the previous findings:
1. Target individuals at high risk for delays. These are patients with a history of heart disease, who are 65 years of age and older, are black, or have a history of angina, diabetes, or hypertension. Specific instructions regarding how to access the EMS and how to differentiate between chronic and acute symptoms should be given to these high-risk groups. In addition,

Table 22-1. Variables that contribute to prehospital delays

Older age
Black race
Patients who have documented hypertension, diabetes, or angina
Consultation with physician or family member about decision to seek treatment
Patients experiencing acute myocardial infarction symptoms during daylight hours
Patients' decision to try self-treatment for symptoms

Adapted from Dracup K, Moser DK: *Heart Lung* 20:570, 1991.

Table 22-2. Variables that decrease prehospital delays

Hemodynamically unstable patients
Patients with large infarcts
Patients who recognize their symptoms as being cardiac in origin
Severity of chest pain when accompanied by hemodynamic instability
Asking unrelated individuals for advice

Adapted from Dracup K, Moser DK: *Heart Lung* 20:570, 1991.

the issue of self-treatment should be discussed to reduce prolonged delays while patients wait for their regular medications to relieve symptoms.
2. Emphasize emergency medical systems. Several researchers found that consultation with a primary care physician resulted in prolonged delay times. Educational programs should emphasize the need to seek immediate emergency care in the face of cardiac symptoms. These messages need to include specific signs and symptoms of AMI to avoid overloading the EMSs with patients who have noncardiac symptoms.
3. Implement educational campaigns. Public educational campaigns are often used to increase public knowledge about a particular disease state with recommendations for an appropriate course of action. Several such campaigns have studied the effect of disseminating knowledge regarding the signs and symptoms of AMI with an emphasis on the importance of a rapid decision to seek medical care. One study conducted in Göteborg, Sweden, analyzed the effect of a media campaign on delay times and ambulance use in suspected AMI. The intention of the study was to shorten delay times and increase ambulance use in patients with suspected AMI. The results of the study demonstrated a significant reduction in delay time after the onset of the campaign. This reduction was most marked in patients who had confirmed AMI (the median delay time was reduced from 3 hours to 2 hours). However, the absolute number of patients with AMI remained stable, and

"Call fast, Call 9-1-1" trial

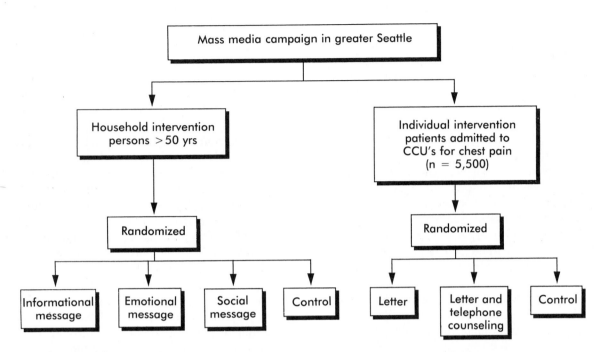

Fig. 22-1. Two strategies employed in the Seattle campaign include (1) a general mailing to all households to alert them to symptoms of acute myocardial infarction, randomizing into a control and three "treatment" approaches and (2) a targeted approach to high-risk patients who are also randomized into a control and two "treatment" groups.

there was a temporary increase in the number of patients with noncardiac chest pain in the emergency department.[12] In addition, no data regarding the long-term outcomes were reported. The results from the Swedish study were similar to those of a Canadian study that reported that a radio and television campaign resulted in reduced delay times but also increased the number of patients with chest pain arriving at the ED.[13] These studies suggest that delay times in AMI can be reduced by an intense public information campaign, although at the cost of an increase in the number of patients with noncardiac chest pain in the ED.

Another educational campaign in the Seattle area was effective in increasing the public's awareness and knowledge of symptoms; however, delays in seeking care and EMS use were not affected. Greater than 40% of patients delayed more than 4 hours and more than 50% of patients did not use the EMS after the campaign.[14] Evidence gathered thus far demonstrates that educational campaigns have the potential for increasing knowledge without changing behavior. Future campaigns may need to focus on the emotional reasons that people resist calling the EMS (e.g., embarrassment or fear) rather than on didactic information.[11]

4. Focus on family members as potential witnesses. It is particularly important that educational campaigns target potential witnesses because most people experience symptoms of an acute MI in the company of others. Alonzo[15] found an increased delay when patients asked family members to help them evaluate their symptoms; the delay was decreased when the decision to call was given to the family member. Witnesses need to be instructed to take charge when an individual experiences a cardiac event.

Currently a large prospective randomized, controlled trial is underway in the Seattle area aimed at increasing the use of EMS for people with symptoms of AMI and to decrease the duration from symptom onset before seeking medical care. The "Call Fast, Call 9-1-1" study will employ two strategies: household interventions using a mass mailing approach and an individual intervention for patients considered at risk for AMI using personal telephone calls and correspondence (Fig. 22-1).

The household interventions are targeted at households where one resident is at least 50 years old. The intervention consists of three different messages randomly assigned to households in the Seattle area. This approach explores a relatively inexpensive mode of educating the community and uses three different messages: informational, emotional, and social messages. The individual intervention consists of personal letters or letters plus personal telephone contact that will be randomly assigned to patients discharged from area hospital coronary care units (CCUs). This intervention, targeted at patients with known disease, is more intensive and thus more expensive. The contact will contain the same three messages as already described: informational, emotional, and social. Results from this portion of the study will define whether this method of mass mailings is effective and which message or messages are most effective in stimulating the public to seek care earlier after symptoms begin.

Each intervention group also has a control group, allowing the potential interaction between the two educational methods to be examined. The study was preceded by a community-wide mass media campaign using television, radio, and newsprint. This campaign was meant to increase awareness and sensitize individuals for the subsequent randomized trial. A surveillance system (registry) involving all hospitals located in Seattle/King County, Washington, allows the investigators to measure outcomes before, during, and after the interventions to understand which intervention best accomplishes the aims of the study.

ROLE OF EMERGENCY MEDICAL SERVICES

Several trials have shown the benefit of early thrombolytic therapy.[1-5] The GISSI-1 Trial demonstrated a mortality reduction of nearly 50% when patients were treated within 1 hour of symptom onset. A more contemporary trial, the 41,000-patient international Global Utilization of Streptokinase and t-PA for Occluded Coronary Arteries (GUSTO-I) Trial has also shown a significant reduction in mortality in those patients treated soon after symptom onset.[5] The GUSTO-I Trial also validated, using angiography, the concept that achieving coronary perfusion is the mechanism for the greatest survival benefit.

Several groups interested in treating patients very early after symptom onset have designed trials to evaluate the role of prehospital health care personnel in the diagnosis and treatment of acute MI. One study in the United States, the Myocardial Infarction Triage and Intervention (MITI) project, based in Seattle, Washington, developed a checklist for paramedics to screen patients for thrombolytic eligibility as well as to obtain and transmit an electrocardiogram (ECG) to an emergency physician before hospital arrival. Three hundred and sixty patients were randomized to receive either thrombolytic therapy and aspirin before hospital arrival by paramedics under remote prescription of a physician or after hospital arrival. Overall findings demonstrated that prehospital administration of thrombolytic therapy was safe, although no difference in outcome was observed between the two groups. However, in a second analysis of time to treatment, those patients treated early had smaller infarcts when measured by single photon emission computed tomography (SPECT). And although the trial was not designed to show a mortality difference, a 1% mortality rate was seen in patients treated early—within 60 to 90 minutes of symptom onset—compared with 8.7% in patients treated later.[7]

The largest prehospital trial to date, the European Myocardial Infarction Project (EMIP), enrolled nearly 6000 patients. In this trial, general practitioners (physicians) responding to ambulance calls randomized suspected AMI patients into a double-blind study of anistreplase given either before or after hospital arrival. Cardiac mortality was marginally lower in prehospital-treated patients ($P = 0.049$).[8] Both trials also demonstrated rapid treatment times after hospital arrival. In the EMIP Trial patients treated in-hospital received treatment within 15 minutes of arrival, and in the MITI Trial patients were treated within 30 minutes. The MITI investigators also noted treatment times of greater than 60 minutes in patients treated outside of the study in the same hospitals. These results indicate that prehospital screening of patients and protocol-driven care can help to decrease in-hospital treatment times dramatically.

LIMITATIONS OF PREHOSPITAL TREATMENT

Despite the potential beneficial effects of prehospital diagnosis and treatment, these strategies can be used in only the portion of acute MI patients who use the EMS. Several studies throughout the world have shown that the rate of EMS use for patients with chest pain as the primary symptom is less than 50% in metropolitan areas,[12,13,16,17] even in communities such as Seattle where active public awareness campaigns have been performed. In addition, the structure of EMSs varies from one geographic area to the next. Not all communities can afford sophisticated EMSs.

Another limitation of prehospital administration of thrombolytic therapy may be that it could be carried out only in large urban or suburban areas where skilled personnel are available. In addition, the expense of educating paramedics or nurses and acquiring portable ECG equipment with telephone transmission capabilities may be prohibitive for many systems. Other considerations relating to prehospital thrombolysis include the cost of maintaining a stock of drug, overhead expenses, misdiagnosis, potential litigation expenses if an unfavorable outcome results from inappropriate patient selection, and administration of thrombolytic therapy in the field.[18]

IN-HOSPITAL DELAYS

In contrast to prehospital drug administration, the ED is the common hospital entry point for all patients. In most studies the delay from ED arrival until initiation of thrombolytic therapy is approximately 50 to 100 minutes.[18] If this time delay can be significantly reduced, the ED is the most practical site in which to alter the chain of events to reduce time delays. It may also be the most cost-effective strategy, because identification and analysis of time delays with implementation of strategies to reduce the delays may only require more efficient use of existing staff and equipment.

Several groups have attempted to quantify the variability in time from patient arrival in the ED to treatment with thrombolytic therapy. The median time to treatment in the Thrombolysis and Angioplasty in Myocardial Infarction (TAMI) Trials was 80 minutes. Time to treatment was longer (92 minutes) in those patients who were seen within 2 hours of symptom onset vs. those seen more than 3 hours of symptom onset (57 minutes). In addition, time to treatment was longer in community hospitals (83 minutes) compared with large referral hospitals (69 minutes).[19]

The Minnesota TIMI (Thrombolysis in Myocardial Infarction) II Clinical Unit compiled a detailed analysis of data regarding the source and magnitude of the delays in initiation of thrombolytic therapy in their institutions. Data obtained from the two academic and two private hospitals revealed that in-hospital delays accounted for more than half of the total time from the onset of symptoms to initiation of thrombolytic therapy. Patients waited an average of 19.9 ± 17.9 minutes for the initial ECG after arrival in the ED. Once diagnosed with an AMI, patients waited an additional 70 ± 40 minutes before thrombolytic therapy was begun. The time delay between the initial ECG and initiation of therapy was less for patients treated in the ED (46.8 minutes) compared with those patients treated in the CCU (82.1 minutes).[20]

To demonstrate that treatment delays are a universal problem, Kereiakes et al.[21] analyzed both retrospective and prospective data from several hospitals around the United States to assess the time delays in the diagnosis and treatment of AMI. Of 3715 patients from eight cities, the average time from EMS activation to patient arrival at the hospital was 46.1 ± 6.2 minutes; the time from admission to the hospital to initiation of thrombolytic therapy was 83.8 ± 55 minutes in a subgroup of 730 patients from the 6 different cities. In addition, both the prehospital and hospital time delays were much longer than those perceived by both the paramedics and the ED directors.[21]

One group of investigators further quantified in-hospital delays by examining the time from ED arrival to initial ECG (mean time 11 ± 15 minutes), time from initial ECG to the decision to treat with thrombolytics (31 ± 35 minutes), time from decision to treat to administration of thrombolytics (23 ± 16 minutes), and time from ED arrival to administration of thrombolytics

Table 22-3. Factors that contribute to in-hospital time delays

Registration time
Nurse and physician evaluation
Obtaining and interpreting an electrocardiogram
Informed consent
Intravenous access
Obtaining blood samples for admission laboratory data
Obtaining a chest x-ray film
Administering other drugs (e.g., morphine and lidocaine)
Waiting for a cardiologist to assess patient and/or approve administration of the drug
Drug preparation and administration time
Waiting for the drug to arrive from pharmacy

Adapted from Ornato JP: *Clin Cardiol* 13:V48-V52, 1990; Sharkey SW, Brunette DD, Ruiz E: *JAMA* 120:773, 1990, Martin JS, Novotny-Dinsdals V, Jensen SK, et al: *J Emerg Nurs* 16:195, 1990.

(64 ± 42 minutes). According to this study of 210 patients, variables that significantly correlated with a reduction in in-hospital delays were using a hospital in an urban location, using a hospital with a teaching hospital status, using a hospital with a high AMI case volume, stocking the drug in the ED instead of the pharmacy, initiating the drug in the ED, and having the ED physician make the decision to treat without involving other physicians.[22]

In the recently completed international GUSTO-I Trial, the median time from patient arrival in the ED to initiation of thrombolytic therapy was 65 minutes in more than 41,000 AMI patients enrolled worldwide.[5] In addition, the median time from symptom onset to initiation of thrombolytic therapy was 165 minutes, supporting the fact that the greatest delays occur outside of the hospital. Half (51%) of all patients in the GUSTO trial were treated within 2 to 4 hours of symptom onset, whereas 27% were treated within 2 hours or less and 19% within 4 to 6 hours of symptom onset.[5]

Several factors have been identified as contributing to the in-hospital time delays and are listed in Table 22-3. In addition to these factors, necessary equipment and personnel are not always immediately available because the ED staff are responsible for treating many patients simultaneously. Current fiscal hospital constraints and diminishing governmental financial support are indirectly contributing to delays by creating an environment in which rapid triage and treatment are difficult. ED overcrowding and an insufficient number of trained personnel capable of rapidly intervening with AMI patients are an increasing problem. Only 4% to 5% of all patients who are seen in the ED complaining of chest pain will actually be eligible for thrombolytic therapy. A negative reinforcement for the triage nursing staff exists because the system will be activated 20 times for every case. Also, the overcrowded, busy environment creates greater litigation potential for the physician and nurse,[23] thereby leading to an overly cautious attitude resulting in unnecessary consultation and testing.

GENERALIZED APPROACH TO DECREASING DELAYS IN THE ED

Several guidelines for minimizing in-hospital treatment delays have been formulated by evaluating the factors that contribute to delays. One suggestion is the development of a "trauma team" type of response for suspected AMI patients, thereby allowing a more rapid triage. This approach includes the use of standard protocols that have been developed and approved jointly by nurses, emergency physicians, and cardiologists.[24] Standard protocols can delineate specific activities to be delegated to appropriate team members to facilitate the treatment process. An effective standard treatment protocol should (1) establish a mechanism for proper patient identification and selection; (2) delineate specific tasks for staff members; and (3) translate tasks into time and personnel needs, assuring efficiency in manpower use.[25]

One example of the trauma team approach is the heart team currently being used in Seattle.[24] The heart team consists of an intravenous (IV) therapy nurse, an ECG technician, an x-ray technician, a pharmacist with a "clot box" (contains all necessary drugs and equipment for initiation of therapy), a nursing supervisor, and a critical care unit nurse. The prehospital team calls ahead to notify the ED of the patient with AMI. The physician notifies the triage nurse, who then informs the heart team, which assembles in the ED 5 minutes before arrival of the patient. Once the patient arrives, the team acts quickly to diagnose and initiate treatment. Unlike trauma victims who require multiple team members for long durations, AMI patients can be quickly diagnosed when proper equipment and personnel are present and treated by as few as two to three nurses or team members working together for less than 30 minutes. Once therapy is initiated, a single staff member can manage the care of the AMI patient.[25]

Establishment of protocols, procedures, and educational training for ED personnel can significantly shorten the time to treatment. One group decreased the time between ED arrival and initiation of thrombolytic therapy from 91 to 52 minutes after a conscious effort was made to reduce the time to treatment by including a training program for ED and coronary care staff.[26]

Implementation of a chest pain emergency department is another effective strategy being used is the United States. Hospitals that have implemented this approach have a dedicated area within or adjacent to the ED that is used specifically to triage patients with chest pain.[27] Hospital personnel are trained to triage and treat this specialized patient population rapidly and efficiently.

Another approach aimed at reducing in-hospital delays is the development of a quality improvement program. Because timing is crucial in treatment with thrombolytic therapy, emergency personnel need to evaluate their care delivery systems to ensure that the standard of care provides maximal patient benefits, that is, that AMI patients are rapidly triaged and treated. One way to achieve this goal is to develop a quality improvement program focused on the AMI patient. The primary purpose of any quality improvement program is to continuously evaluate and improve the quality of care delivered through consistent standardized monitoring.[28] This results in practice changes, with the outcome being the highest achievable standard of care.

SPECIFIC STRATEGIES FOR DECREASING DELAYS IN THE ED

The first prospective randomized trial designed to decrease time to treatment in patients receiving thrombolytic therapy for AMI was recently completed. The purpose of the GUSTO-I Time to Treatment Study was to determine the duration of treatment delays within the medical system, to identify factors associated with delays, and to evaluate the effectiveness of interventions targeted to decrease these delays (Fig. 22-2). The Time to Treatment Study included two phases. During phase 1, the preintervention phase, the source of time delays was assessed in participating hospitals. In the second phase, the intervention phase, hospitals were randomized to one of two strategies: intervention (time delays were evaluated for each hospital, and corresponding interventions were implemented to decrease these delays) and control (no feedback or communication with sites, although sites continued to collect data on time delays).

The preliminary results of phase 1 are displayed in Table 22-4. The median time to treatment for 1423 patients was 70 minutes. Also, less than 5% of all patients were treated within 35 minutes.[29]

Seventy-eight hospitals in North America participated in the Time to Treatment Study. Of these hospitals, 35 were randomly assigned to the intervention strategy and 34 to control. Hospitals that were randomized to the intervention strategy were given a detailed description of their time delays for variables listed on the Time to Treatment data form (Fig. 22-3). The times for all patients enrolled were averaged for each hospital, and the median delay time was displayed for each variable next to the "ideal" times. The ideal times were derived from the top 25th percentile of patients enrolled from all sites with the shortest time delays. In addition, the overall perceived time to treatment for each site was provided for comparison with actual delay times. Sites

Gusto time to treatment study

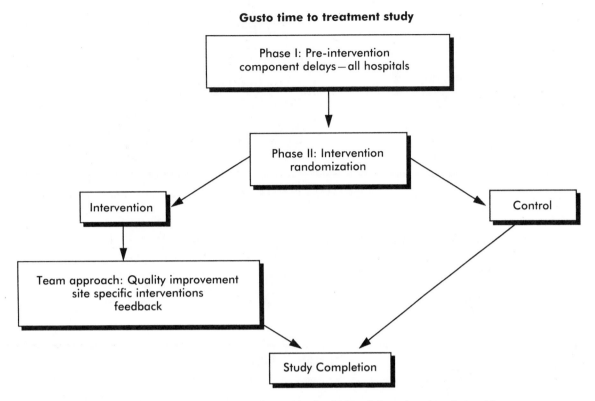

Fig. 22-2. Patients in the GUSTO Study seen in the 78 North American hospitals taking part in the Time to Treatment Substudy received similar treatment. After the determinants of treatment delays in the hospitals were assessed in phase 1, 35 hospitals implemented interventions designed to decrease the delays, whereas 34 served as controls from the start of phase 2 until completion of the substudy.

Table 22-4. GUSTO Time to Treatment Study: preliminary results of phase 1

	Percentile*				
	5th	10th	25th	50th	75th
ED physician examination†	0	0	3	10	16
ECG obtained†	1	2	5	11	19
Laboratory values drawn	3	5	12	21	35
Decision to treat	6	10	18	33	59
Consent signed	13	17	25	40	70
Cardiologist consulted	10	15	27	48	85
Treatment					
Mixed	17	21	33	50	77
Initiated	35	41	52	70	96

*Time delay in minutes, *n* equal 1423.
†*ED*, Emergency department; *ECG*, electrocardiogram.

generally perceived that their time to treatment was better than the data revealed. The investigators then discussed with the site study coordinators each delay as it compared with ideal times. Both the study coordinator and the Time to Treatment investigator mutually decided which delays would be targeted for interventional strategies.

An assessment strategy was developed by the Time to

Treatment investigators to examine each participating hospital's current system to determine appropriate interventions because each system is highly variable and resources used according to internal hospital structures, policies, and politics. This assessment allowed personalization of the intervention strategies, which helped to avoid unreasonable expectations. As an example, cellular transmission of prehospital-acquired ECGs has been

Time to Treatment Site Data

GUSTO
Global Utilization of Streptokinase and t-PA
For Occluded Coronary Arteries

Site #: _____
Study Coordinator: _____
Date: _____
Co-Investigator: _____
Number of Patients Tallied: _____

TREATMENT DELAYS

A. Perceived Time to Treatment (SIS) _____

B. Average Time to Treatment* _____

C. Ideal Time to Treatment** _____ 54 mins. _____

DELAY TIMES

Delays	Average Time* (minutes)	Ideal Time** (minutes)
3. Seen by Triage/First Health Care Professional	_____	_____
4. RN: History and Physical Performed	_____	_____
5. ED MD: History and Physical Performed	_____	_____
6. Cardiologist: History and Physical Performed	_____	_____
7. ECG Obtained	_____	_____
8. Decision to Treat with Lytics	_____	_____
9. Chest X-ray Obtained	_____	_____
10. Consent Signed	_____	_____
11. Admission/Pretreatment Labs	_____	_____
12. Lytic Therapy Ordered/Mixed	_____	_____

*Time from patient presentation in the Emergency Department until task completed. Times for all patients have been averaged; this number represents the median.

** Based on the top 25th percentile for all Time to Treatment sites (n = 436).

Fig. 22-3. Time to Treatment Site Data Form, showing a detailed description of each site's delays and a comparison to the "ideal" times.

shown to decrease delay time in the ED. However, this intervention may not be either feasible, available, or cost-effective for all hospitals.

The assessment strategy consisted of a series of standardized questions for each delay. For a delay in obtaining an ECG, the investigator asked the following questions: "Who obtains the ECG? Is an ECG machine available in the ED or is one shared between units? Who is trained and authorized to read the ECG? Who makes the diagnosis?" After assessing the system for each delay, the investigator gave the site suggestions for interventions based on a standardized list developed for each delay variable. The study coordinator and investigator then defined goals and a projected time line for implementation of intervention strategies. As part of the intervention process, study coordinators, in the unique position of interacting with all team members during the patient's treatment, were then encouraged to present the delay times to the ED staff, management, administration, and key team members responsible for caring for the patient.

The intervention strategy was based on a quality improvement approach similar to Edward Deming's Theory of Continuing Quality Improvement,[30] which proceeds through three phases. First, analyze the steps; the investigator assisted the study coordinator to closely examine the process of admitting and treating AMI patients with thrombolytic therapy. Second, collate data; the investigator provided each site with time delay data that reflected the effectiveness of the system for treating patients rapidly. Finally, change the process; the investigator provided the sites with specific interventions to improve time delays.

Strong administrative support is an important element when implementing a team approach to improving patient care, such as that suggested for the AMI patient. In a recently published report, one group of investigators discovered an average delay time of 86 minutes from arrival in the ED to treatment with lytic therapy in 816 patients and subsequently implemented special measures to increase the speed of therapy. Although these efforts included standard protocols, giving the ED physician decision-making authority, storing drugs in the ED, and implementing other interventions, no improvement was noted in time to treatment during the first year. At that time, hospital administration became actively involved in coordinating the efforts of the staff by forming an efficiency committee (composed of representatives from all disciplines involved in the patients' care) to implement the protocol, conduct inservice training for ED staff and review results on a bimonthly basis. These measures led to a significant reduction in time to treatment (34 ± 5 minutes).[31]

The Time to Treatment study combined the team approach with quality improvement feedback to facili-

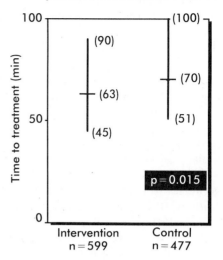

Gusto time to treatment study phase II, randomized results

Fig. 22-4. Average time delay in minutes from patient preparation in the ED to diagnostic and treatment strategies. Patients seen in the hospitals involved in the intervention arm of the substudy received treatment significantly sooner than patients in control hospitals: 63 vs. 70 minutes ($P = 0.015$).

tate each hospital's efforts in reducing time delays. Despite the fact that 85% of the hospitals in the Time to Treatment Substudy had a standard thrombolytic protocol in place, the average time to treatment before the intervention phase was 68 minutes.

The 35 hospitals randomized to the intervention strategy enrolled 599 patients during the Intervention Phase; the control hospitals enrolled 477 patients during the same time period. Despite the fact that only 50% of the hospitals randomized to the intervention strategy actually implemented one or more of the site-specific interventions, there was a significant time difference between the two groups (Fig. 22-4). In addition, several important factors associated with prolonged delays were identified. If thrombolytic therapy was started in the CCU, the treatment time was 90 minutes vs. 65 minutes if it was started in the ED. If a cardiologist made the decision to treat, the median treatment time was 69 vs. 60 minutes if the ED physician decided. Patients who arrived as "walk-ins" to the ED were treated in 73 vs. 66 minutes for patients transported via EMSs. If an ECG was acquired before arrival, the average time to treatment for these patients was 60 vs. 70 minutes if no prehospital ECG was done.[32]

TIME TO TREATMENT: ASSESSMENT AND INTERVENTION STRATEGIES

Site-specific interventions were devised and implemented after a thorough assessment of the treatment process at each site. The following paragraphs describe the areas most frequently assessed and targeted for interventions.

TRIAGE AND DIAGNOSIS

The registration process for a walk-in patient with chest pain may be prolonged by an admission clerk who is unable to recognize a patient's AMI symptoms and the urgency for treatment. Acute MI patients are often overlooked or triaged inappropriately because they lack visible signs of bleeding or fractured limbs. Assessment of the triage system needs to include an examination of the training and knowledge level of the personnel initially in contact with the patient. Are chest pain patients given high priority for treatment? Is there a system in place for rapid treatment? Basic educational programs should be designed for registration personnel and triage nurses to improve their ability to recognize patients with AMI and the need for rapid treatment.

In a published study regarding treatment delays and thrombolytic therapy, one hospital implemented a thrombolytic program designed to address the nursing staff's concerns about administering thrombolytic agents. Three educational sessions focused on pathophysiology and diagnosis of AMI, recognition of eligible thrombolytic candidates, the sequence of thrombolytic therapy treatment, and the management of potential complications. Each nurse was given a certification examination after completing the course. Education of the nursing staff resulted in increased awareness of treatment of AMI patients; the nurses also felt more comfortable recognizing and treating AMI patients.[33]

Assessment by the ED nurse and physician is another area that needs streamlining. Of primary importance should be the confirmation of the diagnosis and identification of risk factors that may exclude the patient from receiving thrombolytic therapy. Assessment tools and checklists can facilitate this process by listing the signs and symptoms of AMI, as well as the inclusion and exclusion criteria for thrombolytic therapy (Fig. 22-5).

DECISION TO TREAT

A common perception of some cardiologists is that ED physicians do not appreciate the subtle aspects of ECG interpretation necessary for diagnosing an AMI.[34] Such perceptions have led to the policy of consulting a cardiologist to assess the patient before thrombolytic therapy can be initiated, which results in a prolonged delay before the decision to treat is made. The median time from ED presentation to consultation by the cardiologist was 48 minutes in phase 1 of the GUSTO Time to Treatment Study. Interestingly, 89% of these patients had average blood pressure and were Killip class I and II on admission.[32]

Although it has been shown that ED physicians missed 5% of the AMIs diagnosed by official ECG overreaders and were correct in only 29% as opposed to 71% of the official overreaders in discordant ECG readings in one study, the official readers may have been biased, as they knew the patient's subsequent outcome and diagnosis.[35] The study did indicate the need for ED physicians to consult cardiologists for uncertain ECGs and for increased knowledge of ECG interpretation by the ED physicians.

Ornato,[36] in a unique position as both a cardiologist and an ED physician, has closely examined the decision-making process and asserts that there are only four reasons why an ED physician should consider consulting a cardiologist or internist before initiating thrombolytic therapy. These reasons are listed in Table 22-5. If a cardiology consult is indicated, it should be requested immediately, and if the cardiologist is not readily available, the ED physician should be given the authority to make the decision to treat. Many hospitals on the Time to Treatment Study set a time limit, usually 5 minutes, after which the ED physician made the decision if the cardiologist had not responded.

Cardiologists can play a vital role in developing educational programs for the ED physicians through ECG courses, as well as case discussions in which ED physicians can benefit from the cardiologists' expertise and can ask questions in a nonacute setting. This is particularly important if the cardiologists are concerned about the skill level of the ED physicians. The staff at one hospital significantly improved the time to treatment by reviewing cases during CCU rounds and examining undue delays. After each delay was investigated, suggestions and instructions were given as appropriate.[37] Open communication between cardiologists and ED physicians is critical to improve treatment times. In the Time to Treatment Study, communication between cardiology departments and EDs in many hospitals was not ideal: both were quick to blame the other for treatment delays. Protocols and streamlined systems should be mutually developed to ensure success.

LABORATORY RESULTS AND INTRAVENOUS THERAPY

Another delay in the decision to treat can occur when treatment is withheld until results of diagnostic tests are available. Generally the decision to treat should not be delayed for unknown laboratory results. In addition, admission laboratory values should be drawn immediately when the patient arrives using a "double team" approach in which more than one nurse starts IV lines and draws blood from the same line. Having nurses assume accountability for blood drawing can decrease the delay time frequently seen when waiting for ancillary personnel. If laboratory personnel must draw blood, a priority system should be established through team meetings to facilitate a rapid response to acute MI patients. A box with all the equipment for rapid blood drawing should be readily accessible. This could include specific packets with laboratory slips for each test

Emergency Department
Thrombolytic Worksheet

Treatment Criteria

BP _____

Weight _____

☐ Ongoing chest pain > 30 min and < 6 hrs

☐ ST elevation > 2 mm in two anterior leads
  or > 1 mm in two inferior leads

Contraindications

☐ SBP < 90 (unresponsive to fluid or
  vasopressors) or > 180 mmHg

☐ DBP > 110 mmHg

Within the previous two weeks:

☐ GI bleed

☐ Surgery, biopsies

☐ Non-compressible central lines

☐ Trauma

☐ Recent internal bleeding

Medical history of:

☐ CVA, TIA, Hx of head injury/surgery

☐ Recent CPR > 10 minutes

☐ Hemorrhagic retinopathy

☐ Recent pericarditis

☐ Terminal illness

☐ Left heart thrombus

Time to Treatment Evaluation

Note Time	Initials	
___:___	_____	Arrival in ER
___:___	_____	Triage nurse evaluation
___:___	_____	Nursing H/P
___:___	_____	ASA given
___:___	_____	ECG obtained
___:___	_____	ED physician H/P
___:___	_____	MD consult, if ordered
___:___	_____	Drug ordered from Pharmacy
___:___	_____	Standing orders signed
___:___	_____	IV access
___:___	_____	Baseline labs drawn: CBC, PTT, FDP, Fibrinogen, CK, CK-MB, Chem Panel
___:___	_____	Heparin _____ u bolus and infusion begun
___:___	_____	Thrombolytic infusion begun
___:___	_____	CCU bed arranged
___:___	_____	Transferred to CCU

Decision to Treat

With lytic: _____ (type)   ☐ Yes ☐ No

WARNINGS The risks of thrombolytic therapy may be increased and should be weighed against the anticipated benefits in any condition in which bleeding constitutes a significant hazard or would be particularly difficult to manage because of its location.

Fig. 22-5. Checklist of inclusion and exclusion criteria for thrombolysis.

Table 22-5. Reasons why ED physicians should consult a cardiologist before initiating thrombolytic therapy*

To call the patient's personal physician to verify past medical history or prior ECG findings

To request a cardiologist's consult in interpreting a complex or subtle ECG

To ask assistance from an internist or cardiologist in estimating the time of onset of infarction in a stagger-start manifestation

To seek consult from the patient's personal physician, an internist, or cardiologist in difficult cases where the diagnosis is unclear, when there is a relative contraindication to thrombolytic therapy, or when other therapy may be a wise option

From Ornato J: *Am J Emerg Med* 9:86, 1991. Used by permission.
*ED, Emergency department; ECG, electrocardiogram.

required for the acute MI patient. To assist nurses in determining the number of IV lines needed and to consolidate medications, IV compatibility charts specific to thrombolytic therapy and commonly used drugs for acute MI patients should be easily accessible.

OBTAINING AN ECG

The 12-lead ECG is the most critical diagnostic tool for patients with suspected acute MI. Although obtaining a prehospital ECG has been shown to reduce delays, it is not always feasible or cost-effective. Therefore, rapidly obtaining and interpreting an ECG should be two of the highest priorities for every suspected AMI patient in the ED. Many hospital EDs do not have a dedicated ECG machine and are dependent on an ECG technician to come to the ED with a machine. This becomes a severe problem at night or on weekends when machines and technicians may be limited. As an alternative, nursing staff can be trained to obtain 12-lead ECGs and to recognize significant ST-segment elevation. The intent is not to shift the responsibility of the ECG interpretation to the nursing staff but to increase the nurses' awareness of acute changes so that rapid treatment can be anticipated.

Interpretation of the ECG in difficult cases may cause further delays. A cardiologist needs to be available in the hospital by beeper. A facsimile machine can be used to send an ECG to a remote cardiologist for an immediate decision. Cardiologists, nurses, and ED physicians should meet regularly to discuss difficult cases to enhance rapid decision-making in future cases. Quick reference posters that show ECG changes consistent with AMI should be made available as reminders to staff.

INFORMED CONSENT

Obtaining informed consent can be one of the most time-consuming parts in the assessment and treatment

process of AMI patients. Written informed consent should be avoided when standard lytic therapy is used. Of course, patients and families should be informed verbally of the benefits and risks of thrombolytic therapy. If written informed consent is necessary in a study protocol, staff should be able to present a concise synopsis of the procedure or study as opposed to reading the consent word for word. A brief one-page summary containing all of the key points should be developed and used by the staff to shorten the time required to obtain consent. This method worked well to reduce consent delays in the hospitals that participated in the Time to Treatment Study. In addition, the consent should be presented to the patient or family by whomever can do it most effectively and rapidly in layman's terms that the patient can easily understand.

TREATMENT PROCESS

Standard orders and thrombolytic protocols (Fig. 22-6) have been shown to decrease delay times, particularly in ordering and mixing the thrombolytic therapy for AMI patients. Staff should be thoroughly oriented to familiarize them with all aspects of the standard protocol. A thrombolytic resource manual that contains the thrombolytic protocol, standing orders, ED triage checklist, drug compatibility information, dosage and mixing guide for thrombolytics, laboratory forms, and helpful hints for patient care can provide the staff with a resource. The manual should be shared with all new staff during orientations to the ED and should be kept in an accessible area. Printed pocket cards with the protocol or directions for reconstituting and administering the drug can also assist staff.

Thrombolytic supplies need to be standardized and organized in one location so that equipment is ready for rapid initiation of therapy. One successful method of doing this is by using a clot box or thrombolytic cart. Contents could include the thrombolytic drug, heparin, syringes, IV tubing, flush bags, pump, blood drawing supplies, copies of protocol and checklists, weight-dose charts, and a list of contraindications to thrombolytic therapy. If the pharmacy must mix the drug, ED staff representatives should meet with them to discuss ways of decreasing delay times and implementing a system to get the drug to the ED quickly and to assure coverage on off shifts when the pharmacy is understaffed. When delays do occur, feedback to the pharmacy and problem-solving with the staff are recommended.

NATIONAL HEART ATTACK ALERT PROGRAM

Because significant delays in treatment adversely affect morbidity and mortality of AMI patients and most of these delays are preventable, the National Heart, Lung, and Blood Institute (NHLBI) has recently launched an initiative entitled the National Heart Attack

Sample Standing Orders for the Acute MI Patient

☐ Patient screened, 12-lead ECG obtained

☐ Aspirin: 160 mg chewed STAT; then ASA 325 mg po qd

☐ Patient has no known contraindications to thrombolytic therapy

☐ Start 2 – 3 IV lines

☐ Prior to beginning infusion, draw CCU MI admission labs including aPTT

☐ Heparin: a. 80 u/kg bolus (rounded to nearest 50 units) = _____ units
                 b. 15 u/kg/hr starting infusion (rounded to nearest 50 units) = _____ units/hr
                 c. draw aPTT at 2 hrs and q6h x 24 hrs; then qd while heparinized
                 d. follow heparin protocol for aPTT< 60 only, for first 24 hours
                   → DO NOT ADJUST FOR aPTT > 100 DURING FIRST 24 HOURS
                 e. follow heparin protocol for aPTT < 60 or > 100 after first 24 hours

Notify pharmacy to mix, deliver drug and administer when applicable:

Thrombolytic Agent (check one)

☐ "front loaded" rt-PA   15 mg bolus over 1–2 minutes
(100 mg/100 ml IV PB)   0.75 mg/kg over 30 minutes (NTE 50 mg)
                       0.50 mg/kg over 60 minutes (NTE 35 mg)

☐ rt-PA reconstitute 1 mg/ml	pts > 65 kgs (143 lbs) 100 mg total dose	pts < 65 kgs (143 lbs) 1.25 mg/kg total dose
	6 mg bolus over 1–2 minutes 54 mg IVPB over 1 hour 40 mg IVPB over 2 hours	6 mg bolus over 1–2 minutes 54% IVPB over 1 hour 40% IVPB over 2 hours

☐ streptokinase (SK)   1.5 million units diluted in 50 ml D5W IVPB over 60 minutes

☐ Administer thrombolytic infusion via controlled infusion pump. At end of infusion (bag empty), add 30 cc NS to the bag and continue infusing to flush tubing

☐ Repeat 12-lead ECG at 3, 6, 12 and 24 hours after admission or if any chest pain reoccurs

☐ Vital signs with neuro checks every 15 mins x 4; then every 30 mins x 2; then every 2 hours x 18; then routine, CCU vital signs

☐ Gulac all stools and emesis x 2 days

☐ Heme-test urine x 24 hours

☐ No radial artery or femoral artery punctures

☐ No subclavian or I.J. lines

☐ Notify MD STAT if evidence of significant internal bleeding occurs or there is a change in neurologic status. Stop heparin and thrombolytic agents

☐ Notify MD STAT if chest pain reoccurs

MD signature: _____   Date: _____

Fig. 22-6. Sample standard orders and thrombolytic protocol for patients with acute MI.

Table 22-6. Objectives of the national heart attack alert program*

Increase awareness and knowledge of the symptoms and signs of AMI among those at increased risk and those around them.

Promote immediate action by patients and those around them at the first symptoms and signs of AMI.

Promote immediate identification and treatment of patients with suspected AMI or sudden death by health care professionals in prehospital and hospital emergency systems.

Collaborate with other state and federal agencies to promote the appropriate use of enhanced EMSs.

Consider, when the time is appropriate, a public education campaign to complement the objectives.

From Somelofski CA, Osguthorpe S: *Heart Lung* 20:535, 1991. Used by permission.

*AMI, Acute myocardial infarction; EMSs, emergency medical systems.

Alert Program (NHAAP) aimed at identifying and reducing treatment delays. Several task forces have been assembled, with the focus being (1) improved patient recognition of life-threatening symptoms, (2) access to EMSs, (3) early defibrillation, (4) improved EMS response to patients, and (5) expeditious and dignified treatment of patients in EDs. Table 22-6 summarizes the objectives of the NHAAP.[38] The NHAAP members have formulated initiatives to target four groups: health professionals, high-risk patients, EMS managers, and the public. The intended outcomes of targeting these individuals and groups are to decrease delays in all areas, thereby significantly impacting the outcome of AMI patients.[39]

SUMMARY AND CONCLUSIONS

Benefits of thrombolytic therapy in AMI patients are time-dependent. Recently much attention has been focused on identifying time delays associated with the initiation of thrombolytic therapy and finding pragmatic solutions for reducing these delays. Despite increased awareness in the average clinical setting, little improvement has been seen in decreasing treatment delays. Three areas have been identified as potential sources for delays: patient delays in seeking treatment, transport delays, and delays within the hospital system in delivering thrombolytic therapy.

Patient delays may be reduced by (1) targeting individuals at high risk for delays (age ≥ 65 years, black race, individuals with a history of angina, diabetes, or hypertension), (2) emphasizing the use of EMSs, (3) creating educational campaigns that support behavior change, and (4) focusing on family members as potential witnesses.

Recommendations to reduce prehospital delays include training prehospital staff to evaluate suspected

acute MI patients rapidly through the use of screening checklists, obtaining a prehospital ECG that can be transmitted to a remote physician, and initiating thrombolytic therapy in the prehospital setting. Of primary importance is continuing to emphasize the use of EMSs.

Several strategies may be implemented to reduce hospital delays. Generalized strategies include plans to:
1. Develop a team approach to treating suspected AMI patients.
2. Devise standard protocols and procedures to establish a mechanism for patient identification and selection and to delineate specific tasks for staff members.
3. Provide educational training for emergency medical personnel.
4. Develop a quality improvement program to provide timely feedback.

In addition, more specific strategies may be employed to target problem areas that have been identified during recent attempts to qualify hospital time delays. These recommendations include efforts to:
1. Ensure rapid triage and diagnosis of suspected AMI patients by emphasizing quick action by admitting personnel.
2. Allow ED physicians to make the decision to treat; a cardiologist need be consulted by telephone only in difficult cases or after treatment has started.
3. Initiate thrombolytic therapy without waiting for laboratory results unless absolutely necessary.
4. Obtain an ECG within 5 minutes of patient's arrival to the ED by procuring a dedicated ECG machine and training nursing staff to obtain and interpret ECG results.
5. Streamline the process of obtaining informed consent by training appropriate staff to present a brief synopsis of the procedure or study.
6. Store the thrombolytic therapy in the ED.
7. Initiate therapy in the ED as opposed to the CCU.

Perhaps the strongest message from the Time to Treatment Study is that only 5% of hospitals are treating patients within 30 minutes of hospital arrival. Inefficient hospital systems and lack of commitment to reduce treatment delays are costing patients' lives. Much time and effort have been spent investigating which thrombolytic regimen is optimal for patient outcome. However, the beneficial effects of the best thrombolytic regimen are negated or minimized by prolonged treatment delays. Each hospital must take the time to focus on the issue of treatment delays. Success is possible only through a concentrated team effort to first identify and then target specific interventions to decrease treatment delays.

A critical emerging issue in the 1990s with regard to treatment with thrombolytic therapy in AMI is identifying and reducing treatment delays. Health care providers can and must implement changes to facilitate rapid identification and treatment of these patients.

REFERENCES

1. Gruppo Italiano per lo Studio della Streptochinasi nell'Infarto Miocardico (GISSI): Effectiveness of intravenous thrombolytic treatment in acute myocardial infarction, *Lancet* I:397-401, 1986.
2. Gruppo Italiano per lo Studio della Sopravvivenza nell'Infarto Miocardico: GISSI-2. A factorial randomized trial of alteplase versus streptokinase and heparin versus no heparin among 12,490 patients with acute myocardial infarction, *Lancet* 336:65-71, 1990.
3. Third International Study of Infarct Survival (ISIS-3): a randomised comparison of streptokinase vs tissue plasminogen activator vs anistreplase and of aspirin plus heparin vs aspirin alone among 41,299 cases of suspected acute myocardial infarction, ISIS-3, *Lancet* 339:753-770, 1992.
4. Honan MB, Harrell FE, Reimer KA, et al: Cardiac rupture, mortality and the timing of thrombolytic therapy: a meta-analysis, *J Am Coll Cardiol* 16:359-367, 1990.
5. The GUSTO Investigators: An international randomized trial comparing four thrombolytic strategies for acute myocardial infarction, *N Engl J Med* 329:673-382, 1993.
6. DeWood MA, Spores J, Motske R, et al: Prevalence of total coronary occlusion during the early hours of transmural myocardial infarction, *N Engl J Med* 303:897-902, 1980.
7. Weaver WD, Cerqueira M, Hallstrom AP, et al: Prehospital-initiated vs hospital-initiated thrombolytic therapy, The Myocardial Infarction and Triage (MITI) Trial, *JAMA* 270:1211-1216, 1993.
8. The European Myocardial Infarction Project Group: Pre-hospital thrombolytic therapy in patients with suspected acute myocardial infarction, *N Engl J Med* 329:383-389, 1993.
9. Reimer KA, Jennings RB: The "wavefront phenomenon" of myocardial ischemic cell death, *Lab Invest* 40:633, 1979.
10. Ho MT: Delays in the treatment of acute myocardial infarction: an overview, *Heart Lung* 20:566-570, 1991.
11. Dracup K, Moser DK: Treatment-seeking behavior among those with signs and symptoms of acute myocardial infarction, *Heart Lung* 20:570-575, 1991.
12. Herlitz J, Hartford M, Blohm B, et al: Effect of a media campaign on delay times and ambulance use in suspected acute myocardial infarction, *Am J Cardiol* 64:90-93, 1989.
13. Mitic WR, Perkins RRT: The effect of a media campaign on heart attack delay and decision times, *Can J Public Health* 75:414-418, 1984.
14. Ho MT, Eisenberg MS, Litwin PE, et al: Delay between onset of chest pain and seeking medical care: the effect of public education, *Ann Emerg Med* 18:727-731, 1989.
15. Alonzo AA: The impact of the family and lay others on care-seeking during life-threatening episodes of suspected coronary artery disease, *Soc Sci Med* 22:1297-1311, 1986.
16. Weaver WD, Mickey SE, Martin JS, et al: Myocardial infarction triage and intervention project—phase I: patient characteristics and feasibility of prehospital initiation of thrombolytic therapy, *J Am Coll Cardiol* 15:925-931, 1990.
17. Leitch JW, Birbara J, Freedman B, et al: Factors influencing the time from onset of chest pain to arrival at hospital, *Med J Aust* 150:6-10, 1989.
18. Ornato JP: Role of emergency department in decreasing the time to thrombolytic therapy in acute myocardial infarction, *Clin Cardiol* 13:V48-V52, 1990.
19. Mantell SJ, Flanagan CH, Berrios ED, et al: Delay in treatment with thrombolytic therapy: the time cushion effect, *Circulation* 80:II391, 1989.
20. Sharkey SW, Brunette DD, Ruiz E: An analysis of time delays preceding thrombolysis for acute myocardial infarction, *JAMA* 262:3171-3174, 1989.
21. Kereiakes DJ, Weaver WD, Anderson JL, et al: Time delays in the diagnosis and treatment of acute myocardial infarction: a tale of eight cities. Report from the Prehospital Study Group and the Cincinnati Heart Project, *Am Heart J* 120:773-780, 1990.
22. Gonzalez ER, Ornato JP, Jones LA, et al: Prospective multicenter assessment of critical factors delaying hospital thrombolytic therapy, *J Am Coll Cardiol* 17:247A, 1991.
23. Ornato JP: Problems faced by the urban emergency department in providing rapid triage and intervention for the patient with suspected acute myocardial infarction, *Heart Lung* 20:584-588, 1991.
24. Martin JS, Novotny-Dinsdale V, Jensen SK, et al: Early triage and treatment of the acute myocardial infarction patient: How fast is fast? *J Emerg Nurs* 16:195-202, 1990.
25. Martin LH: Implementation of a thrombolytic protocol in the emergency department, *J Emerg Nurs* 15:182-187, 1989.
26. Althouse R, Maynard C, Olsufka M, et al: The Western Washington tissue plasminogen activator emergency room study, *J Am Coll Cardiol* 13:94A, 1989.
27. Bahr RD: Early cardiac care centers, *Circulation* 79:463, 1989.
28. Schell C, Uibel I: The patient with acute myocardial infarction: assessing quality of care in one emergency department, *J Emerg Nurs* 16:208-211, 1990.
29. Kline E, Smith D, Martin J, et al: In-hospital treatment delays in patients treated with thrombolytic therapy: a report of the GUSTO time to treatment substudy (abstract), *Circulation* 86(suppl I):I-702, 1992.
30. Deming WE: *Quality, productivity, and competitive position,* Cambridge, Mass, 1986, Massachusetts Institute of Technology, Center for Advanced Engineering Study.
31. Moses H, Bartolozzi J, et al: Reducing delay in the emergency room in administration of thrombolytic therapy for myocardial infarction associated with ST elevation: brief reports, *Am J Cardiol* 68:251-253, 1991.
32. Kline E: GUSTO time to treatment substudy: randomized results. Paper presented at the American Federation for Clinical Researchers Annual Meeting, Washington DC, April 30, 1993.
33. Pierleoni L, Pace M: Implementation of a thrombolytic program: one hospital's experience, *J Emerg Nurs* 15:188-195, 1989.
34. Eisenberg M, Smith M: The farmer and the cowman should be friends: emergency physicians and cardiologists must work together to ensure rapid initiation of thrombolytic therapy, *Ann Emerg Med* 17:155-156, 1988.
35. Lee TH, Weisberg MC, Brand DA, et al: Candidates for thrombolysis among emergency room patients with acute chest pain, potential true- and false-positive rates, *Ann Intern Med* 110:957-962, 1989.
36. Ornato J: The role of emergency department in thrombolytic therapy in acute myocardial infarction, *Am J Emerg Med* 9:86-87, 1991.
37. MacCullum AG, Stafford PJ, et al: Reduction in hospital time to thrombolytic therapy by audit of policy guidelines, *Eur Heart J* 11(F):48-52, 1990.
38. Somelofski CA, Osguthorpe S: Symposium proceedings: early hospital arrival and treatment of patients with acute myocardial infarction: practice management and your role in thrombolytic therapy, *Heart Lung* 20:535-537, 1991.
39. Lenfant C, LaRosa JH, Horan MJ, et al: Considerations for a national heart attack alert program, *Clin Cardiol* 13:VIII9-11, 1990.

Chapter 23

CODE R: RESPONDING TO THE EMERGENCY IN THE HOSPITAL

Seth Joseph Worley
Donald A. Berkow
Wendy S. Fitts

Patients presenting to the emergency department with chest pain have the potential to benefit from the administration of thrombolytic therapy, which can enhance survival and reduce both heart failure and arrhythmias.[1,2] However, these benefits accrue to only those patients who have ST-segment elevation on the electrocardiogram[3] and do not have a major contraindication to thrombolysis. Furthermore, although there is debate as to which thrombolytic agent is best, there is no question that the sooner thrombolytic therapy is administered, the greater the effect on outcome.[4,5] Figures 23-1 and 23-2 demonstrate the importance of time to treatment from two perspectives. Figure 23-1 shows the relationship between time to randomization and the mortality reduction from randomized trials of thrombolytic therapy vs. placebo. This information is derived from the Fibrinolytic Therapy Trialists Collaboration, a combined analysis of all available controlled studies on the topic; the power of this comparison is somewhat diminished by "dilution bias" because the only available data represent time to *randomization,* not time to treatment. Figure 23-2 shows the relationship between risk of 30-day mortality and time to treatment from GUSTO-I. Although the relationship is not linear, the risk of death increases incrementally with longer time to treatment, even after adjusting for other differences in baseline characteristics. Therefore it is critical to minimize the time from presentation of a patient to the delivery of thrombolytic therapy.[6-9] This process involves ensuring that adequate personnel are available to minimize the time to appropriate diagnosis, to maximize the accuracy of the diagnosis, and to reduce the time to administration of therapy as much as possible once the decision to treat is made.

TEAM APPROACH

In the emergency department the patient with chest pain is approached in a fashion similar to patients presenting with major trauma or cardiac arrest. A team of medical professionals is assembled to provide the care necessary to initiate thrombolytic therapy in the most efficient way possible. This team approach, which is called *Code R* (*R* symbolizing reperfusion), was initiated at Lancaster General Hospital in May of 1989. Since then over 400 patients have been treated using this trauma-team approach.

This approach does not alter the fact that the emergency department staff must sort out thrombolytic candidates from the much larger number of patients with chest pain. It is important to emphasize that the Code R process does not obligate the patient to thrombolytic therapy. In many cases the emergency physician must evaluate a patient with chest pain while handling a crowded emergency department. Once the presumptive diagnosis of AMI is established, activation of the Code R team allows the emergency physician time to deal with

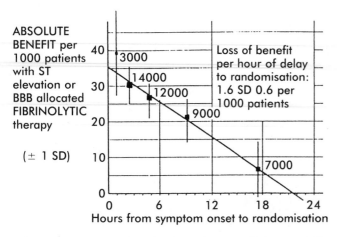

Fig. 23-1. Absolute reduction in 35-day mortality versus delay from symptom onset to randomization among 45,000 patients with ST elevation or BBB. Area of black square and extent to which it influences line drawn through five points is approximately proportional to number of patients it is based on. (Formally, area is inversely proportional to variance of absolute benefit it describes, and slope is inverse-variance-weighted least squares regression line.) (From Fibrinolytic Therapy Trialists' (FTT) Collaborative Group: Indications for fibrinolytic therapy in suspected acute myocardial infarction: collaborative overview of early mortality and major mobidity results from all randomised trials of more than 1000 patients, *Lancet* 343:311-322, 1994.)

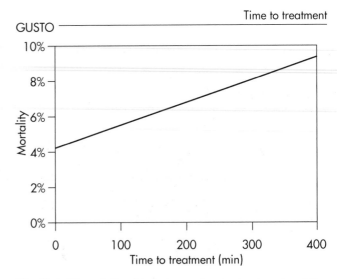

Fig. 23-2. The relationship between time to treatment and the risk of mortality within 30 days in the 41,000-patient GUSTO trial.

the other patients or to proceed with further evaluation of the MI patient without delaying treatment. Even if the patient ultimately is not a suitable candidate for thrombolytic therapy, the Code R team efficiency still offers the maximal medical therapy in the shortest period of time. The importance of such an approach has been highlighted by the recent finding from the GUSTO-I trial that patients with the most to benefit from rapid administration of therapy are often treated the latest.[10] As shown in Table 23-1, patients in shock, the elderly, and women are treated later than hemodynamically stable patients, younger patients, and men. Convening a larger group of caregivers for the brief but crucial time of thrombolytic administration ensures that the treatment is given in a timely fashion without distracting the emergency department personnel, who may have to deal with other medical issues to stabilize the patient.

In addition to the emergency department physician and nurse, the Code R response team consists of the following five people: the IV therapy nurse, the phlebotomist, the pharmacy representative, the critical care nurse designated to receive the patient upon admission to the hospital, and the patient's attending cardiologist. Each member of the team has assigned tasks and therefore does not need to worry about the broader overview of the patient.

The following sequence of events in a Code R proceeds in an orderly fashion. A patient presenting to

the emergency department with chest pain is immediately regarded as a potential candidate for thrombolytic therapy. An electrocardiogram is quickly obtained and reviewed by the emergency physician. On the basis of the history and ECG the emergency physician makes the diagnosis of AMI, then quickly assesses for contraindications to thrombolytic therapy and calls the Code R. The hospital operator is notified and announces "Code R — emergency department" by hospital intercom and pages each of the individual members of the response team. The IV therapist arrives and starts the additional IVs necessary to initiate thrombolytic therapy. The phlebotomist is available as the IVs are started so that blood can be withdrawn into syringes from the intravenous cannulas and placed in the appropriate tubes so that admission laboratory studies can be performed without additional venipuncture. The critical care nurse presents to the emergency department and helps the staff with the initiation of medications such as the intravenous nitroglycerin and the thrombolytic agent. Before the final decision to give thrombolytic therapy is made, the pharmacy representative mixes thrombolytic agents, knowing that if thrombolytic therapy is not ultimately decided upon, the cost of the drug will be reimbursed by the pharmaceutical firm. While the IVs are being started and the heparin is being initiated, the attending cardiologist examines the patient and reviews the patient's potential contraindications to thrombolytic therapy. The attending cardiologist and emergency physician review the data and, if appropriate, thrombolytic therapy is initiated. In the event the attending cardiologist is not immediately available, lytic therapy is typically initiated before his or her arrival, unless there is a question about the ECG or the clinical situation.

Table 23-1. Time to treatment in GUSTO-I

Baseline	N		Time to treatment (min. hospital arrival to initiation of lytic)			
Characteristics		Mortality*	Median	25th	75th	P value
Men	2446	5.5%	66	49	92	P < .001
Women	879	11.3%	73	55	103	
Age ≤ 75	2947	5.1%	67	50	75	
Age ≥ 75	378	20.6%	95	57	101	
Anterior MI	2048	9.9%	66	49	91	P = .001
Inferior MI	1188	5.0%	70	51	100	
Killip I	2928	5.1%	68	50	95	P = .01
Killip II	329	13.8%	67	50	91	
Killip III	38	31.6%	100	52	120	
Killip IV	24	57.6%	86	72	114	

From Smith DD, Martin JS, Kline-Rogers E, for the GUSTO Trial Investigators/Study Coordinators: Excess delays in treatment in high-risk patients in the GUSTO time to treatment substudy, *J Am Coll Cardiol* 23:313A, 1994 (abstract).
*Mortality of group in overall GUSTO trial (*N* = 41,021).

Once the thrombolytic agent is started, the patient is admitted to the critical care unit. At Lancaster General Hospital the time to assemble the Code R members, including the cardiologist, at the patient's bedside is 5 minutes.

RESPONSE TEAM MEMBERS

The rationale for each of the Code R response team members is as follows:

Critical care nurse: The critical care nurse assists with medication administration. In addition, the Code R patient is given priority admission status to the critical care unit. As a member of the Code R team, the critical care nurse has firsthand knowledge of the patient's clinical situation; thus report and transfer of responsibilities are facilitated. For each shift in the critical care unit, the nurse assigned to receive the next admission is designated as the Code R nurse for that shift.

Pharmacy representative: Mixing the thrombolytic agent is a time-consuming process and occupies one person full-time. If the thrombolytic agent is mixed while the intravenous cannulas are being inserted and the drip is being started, the lytic agent will be ready when the final decision to give therapy is made. If the thrombolytic agent is not mixed until the final decision is made, mixing will add 5 to 10 minutes to delivery time. If t-PA is chosen as the thrombolytic agent, the cost is reimbursed by Genentech Corporation should the mixed drug not be used. The cost of streptokinase is not prohibitive. The likelihood of using the lytic agent is greater than 90%, thus the current practice is to mix the drug at the initiation of the Code R. In patients enrolled in studies of AMI, such as GUSTO-I, the final decision on the thrombolytic agent to be delivered is not made until the patient is enrolled in the study, which alters the process somewhat.

IV therapy nurse: Several IVs (three to five) are necessary to initiate thrombolytic therapy. Delays may occur in delivering the thrombolytic therapy because of difficult IV access. The IV therapist is the most experienced in starting IVs. The IV therapist, working with emergency department nurses, reduces the time to have adequate IV access available to start thrombolytic therapy.

Phlebotomy team: As the IVs are started the phlebotomist is available to receive blood withdrawn via syringe from the inserted intravenous cannula. In this way, subsequent venipuncture is avoided.

Attending cardiologist: The patient's attending cardiologist is paged to the emergency room as part of the Code R team. Recognition that the call is for an AMI allows the attending cardiologist to prioritize the call and minimize the time to respond to the emergency room. In hospitals in which a cardiologist is not immediately available, the emergency department physician should fulfill this role.

PROTOCOL

The use of Code R standing orders ensures that no vital treatment is delayed or forgotten (Fig. 23-3).

The 48 patients enrolled in the GUSTO-I study using the Code R protocol had an average time from presentation to the receipt of thrombolytic therapy of 41 minutes. This figure compared with an average of over 60 minutes in the trial as a whole and placed Lancaster General Hospital in the 10th percentile for time to treatment. In this environment, adhering to the GUSTO-I protocol delayed the time to delivery of thrombolytic therapy because once the final decision to give thrombolytic therapy was made, a call to the randomization center was required to assign a kit number before the kit could be retrieved and thrombolytic agent(s) mixed. In nonstudy patients, thrombolytic therapy is usually being mixed while the final decision is made. A time savings of

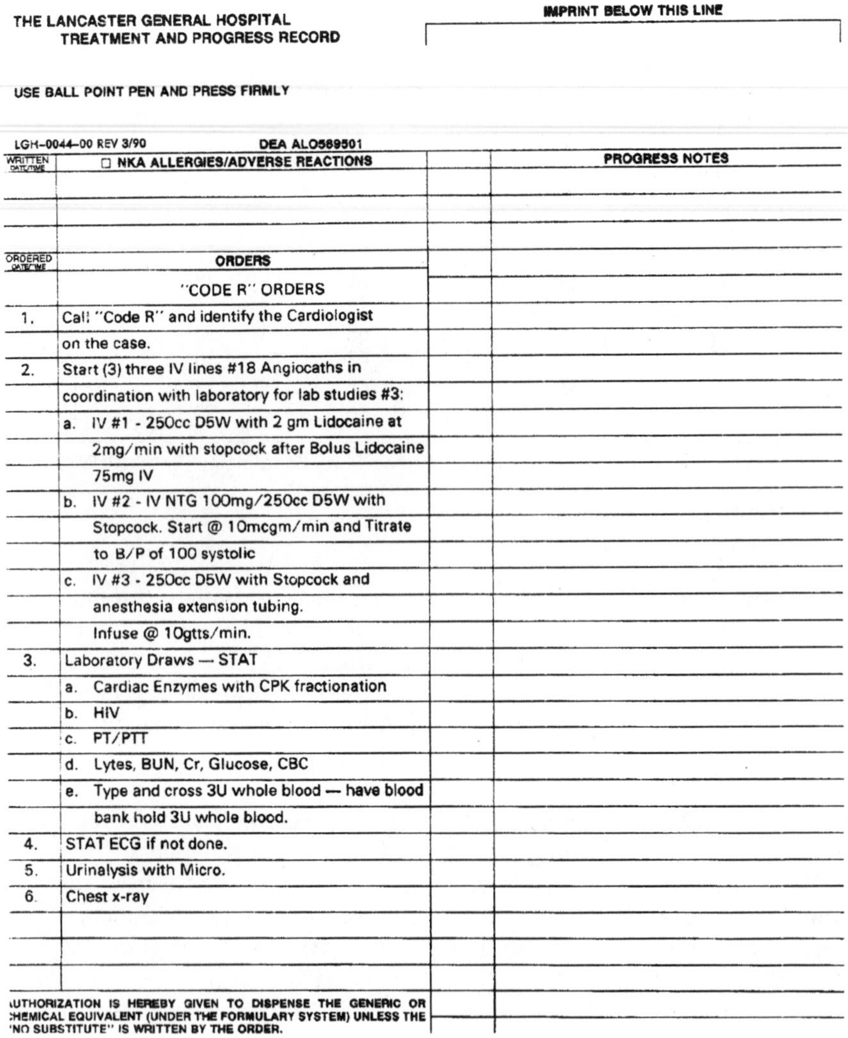

THE LANCASTER GENERAL HOSPITAL
TREATMENT AND PROGRESS RECORD

IMPRINT BELOW THIS LINE

USE BALL POINT PEN AND PRESS FIRMLY

LGH-0044-00 REV 3/90   DEA AL0589501

WRITTEN DATE/TIME	☐ NKA ALLERGIES/ADVERSE REACTIONS		PROGRESS NOTES
ORDERED DATE/TIME	**ORDERS**		
	"CODE R" ORDERS		
1.	Call "Code R" and identify the Cardiologist		
	on the case.		
2.	Start (3) three IV lines #18 Angiocaths in		
	coordination with laboratory for lab studies #3:		
	a. IV #1 - 250cc D5W with 2 gm Lidocaine at		
	2mg/min with stopcock after Bolus Lidocaine		
	75mg IV		
	b. IV #2 - IV NTG 100mg/250cc D5W with		
	Stopcock. Start @ 10mcgm/min and Titrate		
	to B/P of 100 systolic		
	c. IV #3 - 250cc D5W with Stopcock and		
	anesthesia extension tubing.		
	Infuse @ 10gtts/min.		
3.	Laboratory Draws — STAT		
	a. Cardiac Enzymes with CPK fractionation		
	b. HIV		
	c. PT/PTT		
	d. Lytes, BUN, Cr, Glucose, CBC		
	e. Type and cross 3U whole blood — have blood		
	bank hold 3U whole blood.		
4.	STAT ECG if not done.		
5.	Urinalysis with Micro.		
6.	Chest x-ray		

AUTHORIZATION IS HEREBY GIVEN TO DISPENSE THE GENERIC OR
CHEMICAL EQUIVALENT (UNDER THE FORMULARY SYSTEM) UNLESS THE
"NO SUBSTITUTE" IS WRITTEN BY THE ORDER.

Fig. 23-3. Code R standing orders as used at Lancaster General Hospital ensure that patients are treated appropriately and quickly upon their presentation in the emergency room.

approximately 5 to 8 minutes on average is estimated for patients not involved in a clinical trial that requires randomization.

Code R reduces the time between presentation to the emergency room and the delivery of thrombolytic therapy in patients with AMI. Code R is cost-effective; all the health care professionals involved in the Code R are already on staff, and they are used in a more efficient fashion with Code R. Code R also enhances the transfer of patients from the emergency department to the critical care unit/cath lab by facilitating patient report and providing early notification of a need for a critical care bed and/or cath lab slot.

REFERENCES

1. Gruppo Italiano per lo Studio della Streptochinasi nell'Infarto Miocardico (GISSI): Effectiveness of intravenous thrombolytic treatment in acute myocardial infarction, *Lancet* 1:397-402, 1986.
2. ISIS-2 (Second International Study of Infarct Survival) Collabo-rative Group: Randomized trial of intravenous streptokinase, oral aspirin, both, or neither among 17,187 cases of suspected acute myocardial infarction: ISIS-2, *Lancet* 2:349-360, 1988.
3. Fibrinolytic Therapy Trialists' (FTT) Collaborative Group: Indi-cations for fibrinolytic therapy in suspected acute myocardial infarction: collaborative overview of early mortality and major morbidity results from all randomised trials of more than 1000 patients, *Lancet* 343:311-322, 1994.
4. Rutsch W, Pfisterer M, Weaver WD, et al. for the GUSTO Trial Investigators: Earlier time to treatment is associated with lower mortality and greater benefit of accelerated t-PA, *Circulation* 88(suppl I):I-17, 1993.
5. Linderer T, Schroder R, Arntz R, et al: Pre-hospital thrombolysis: beneficial effects of very early treatment on infarct size and left ventricular function, *J Am Coll Cardiol* 22:1304-1310, 1993.
6. Braunwald E: Myocardial reperfusion, limitation of infarct size, production of left ventricular dysfunction, and improved survival: should the paradigm be expanded? *Circulation* 79:441-444, 1989.
7. Lincoff AM, Topol EJ: Illusion of reperfusion: does anyone achieve optimal reperfusion during acute myocardial infarction? *Circulation* 88:1361-1374, 1993.
8. Califf RM, Topol EJ, Gersh BJ: From myocardial salvage to

patient salvage in acute myocardial infarction: the role of reperfusion therapy, *J Am Coll Cardiol* 14:1382-1388, 1989.

9. Sharky SW, Brunette DD, Ruiz E: An analysis of time delays preceding thrombolysis for acute myocardial infarction, *JAMA* 262:3171-3174, 1989.

10. Smith DD, Martin JS, Kline-Rogers E, for the GUSTO Trial Investigators/Study Coordinators: Excess delays in treatment in high-risk patients in the GUSTO time to treatment substudy, *J Am Coll Cardiol* 23:313A, 1994 (abstract).

HOSPITAL PHASE

Chapter 24

CURRENT THROMBOLYTIC AGENTS: FIBRIN-SPECIFIC

Frans Van de Werf
Marc Verstraete

The difference between fibrin-selective and non-fibrin-selective plasminogen activators is explained on the basis of an independent binding to fibrin by the former, whereas fibrin acts as a cofactor for the formation of plasmin, preferentially on the fibrin surface. However, fibrin selectivity is only relative and all of the thrombolytic agents at doses currently used for *rapid* thrombus dissolution activate plasminogen, although with a different intensity. Thus, the infusion of these agents at the high doses presently recommended results in two types of activity: local thrombolytic activity (fibrinolysis) and systemic plasma proteolytic activity as usually measured by the extent of fibrinogen decrease and the appearance of fibrinogen degradation products. In practice the fibrinogenolytic effect of prourokinase and tissue-type plasminogen activator (t-PA) is about one third when compared with streptokinase or urokinase.

SINGLE-CHAIN UROKINASE-TYPE PLASMINOGEN ACTIVATOR

Single-chain urokinase-type plasminogen activator (scu-PA, prourokinase) is a naturally occurring human protein first isolated from natural sources[1] and then produced through recombinant technology.[2] The human gene responsible for its synthesis is located on chromosome 10, is about 6.4 kb long, is organized in 11 exons, and gives rise to a 2.5-kb long messenger RNA, which transcribes a single-chain glycosylated polypeptide.[3-5] Evidence for the signal transduction pathways involved in regulation of the u-PA gene has to date demonstrated three mechanisms that are dependent, respectively, on activation of cyclic adenosine monophosphate (cAMP) protein kinase, protein kinase C, and an as yet uncharacterized protein kinase.[6]

The single-chain protein is synthesized principally by renal and vascular endothelial cells but also from a variety of cultured normal, transformed, and malignant cell types.[7,8] The level of production of scu-PA is about ten times higher in tumor cell lines compared with normal tissues and further stimulated by prolactin and pituitary gland extracts,[9] interleukin-1,[10] a number of cytokines, including phorbol esters, transforming growth factor-β (TGF-β), lipopolysaccharides (LPS), and tumor necrosis factor-α (TNF-α).[11]

scu-PA has also been expressed by gene cloning techniques in *Escherichia coli* bacteria.[12]

Physicochemical properties

The glycosylated natural scu-PA is a single-chain glycoprotein with a molecular weight of 54 kD containing 411 amino acid residues.[13] The N-terminal domain has a homology with the growth factor domain of other proteins, followed by a kringle domain, homologous to plasminogen, t-PA, and other proteins involved in coagulation.[14]

However, the single trisulfide-bonded kringle domain of scu-PA does not contain a lysine-binding site, and it does not confer fibrin-binding properties to the enzyme.[15]

The single glycosylation site of the glycoprotein is located at asparagine 302. The molecule expressed by *E.*

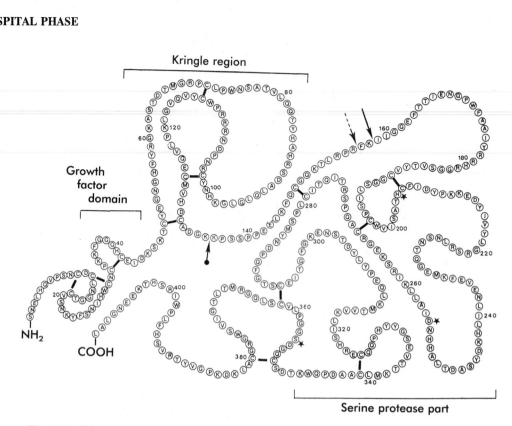

Fig. 24-1. Schematic representation of the primary structure of single-chain urokinase-type plasminogen activator (scu-PA). The amino acids are represented by their single-letter symbols and black bars indicate disulfide bonds. The active site residues His^{204}, Asp^{255}, and Ser^{356} are indicated with asterisks. The arrows indicate the plasmin cleavage sites for conversion of relative molecular mass (M_r) 54 kD scu-PA to M_r 54 kD tcu-PA and of M_r 54 kD tcu-PA to M_r 33 kD tcu-PA (↓), for conversion to inactive M_r 54 kD tcu-PA by thrombin (↓), and for conversion to M_r 32 kD scu-PA by an unidentified protease (↓).

coli lacks the glycosyl group, which reduces the molecular weight to 47 kD (specific activity 175,000 units/mg).

scu-PA is the native zymogenic precursor of urokinase. Limited hydrolysis by plasmin or kallikrein of the Lys^{158}-Ile^{159} peptide bond converts the molecule to two-chain urokinase-type plasminogen activator (tcu-PA), which is held together by one disulfide bond that is essential for the thrombolytic activity (Fig. 24-1). A fully active tcu-PA derivative is obtained after additional proteolysis at position Lys^{135}-Lys^{130}.

The kinetics of activation of scu-PA by full-length plasmin have been reported not to follow Michaelis kinetics, whereas addition of ε-amino caproic acid changes the kinetic pattern to the Michaelis form.[16] Plasmin that is lacking the kringle domains 1 to 4 (miniplasmin) activates scu-PA according to Michaelis kinetics, leading to the hypothesis of an interaction between scu-PA and the kringles of plasmin.[16]

Specific hydrolysis of the Glu^{143}-Leu^{144} peptide bond in scu-PA by an unidentified protease yields a low-molecular-weight scu-PA of 32 kD (scu-PA-32k).[17] Thrombin, on the other hand, cleaves the Arg^{156}-Phe^{157} peptide bond in scu-PA, resulting in an inactive double-chain molecule.[18]

Mechanism of plasminogen activation

Studies on the intrinsic functional activity of scu-PA have been hampered because the single-chain form is too readily activated by plasmin to the two-chain form of urokinase. Therefore, aprotinin has been used to block plasmin and dansyl-glutamyl-glycyl-arginine-chloromethylketone to inhibit tcu-PA, or site-directed mutant forms of scu-PA were used, rendering these molecules incapable of conversion by plasmin to tcu-PA. scu-PA does not have a specific affinity for fibrin.[16] In purified systems, scu-PA has some intrinsic plasminogen-activating potential, which is, however, 1% or less of that of tcu-PA.[19] Conversion of scu-PA to tcu-PA in the vicinity of a fibrin clot apparently constitutes a significant positive feedback mechanism for clot lysis in human plasma in vitro.[13,19] This conversion may, however, play a less important role in in vivo thrombolysis because of preferential fibrin-associated activation of plasminogen by scu-PA.

Several cell types express specific high-affinity binding sites on their surface for scu-PA and tcu-PA, such as human peripheral monocytes, fibroblasts, and Bowes melanoma cells. The interaction between these plasminogen activators and the receptor were recently summarized[20]: (1) receptor binding does not require the active site of the enzymes, (2) scu-PA binds with the same affinity as tcu-PA, (3) receptor-bound scu-PA can be activated on the site of the receptor, (4) the region of scu-PA that binds to the receptor is located in the cysteine-rich amino-terminal fragment peptide (residues 12-32), (5) this region shows sequence homology to that part of the epidermal growth factor (EGF) that is responsible for the binding of EGF to the EGF receptor (but EGF does not bind to the scu-PA receptor), (6) bound scu-PA dissociates very slowly from the cell surface and is not appeciably degraded, and (7) receptor binding does not shield scu-PA from the action of plasminogen activator inhibitor-1 (PAI-1) and PAI-2. Enzyme inhibitor complexes are bound with about ten times lower affinity compared with the enzyme itself. Cell-bound scu-PA and tcu-PA are thought to be involved in the generation of pericellular proteolysis during cell migration and tissue remodeling.[21,22]

Studies with scu-PA in thrombotic animal models

Low relative molecular mass scu-PA (scu-PA-32k), purified from the conditioned medium of a human lung adenocarcinoma cell line[18] or prepared by recombinant DNA technology[23] had a fibrinolytic capacity in a rabbit jugular vein thrombosis model comparable with that of wild-type recombinant scu-PA.[46] The relative fibrin specificity of scu-PA compared with tcu-PA was maintained at thrombolytic doses. Provided this relative fibrin specificity also holds for patients with thromboembolic disease, scu-PA-32k might be a practical alternative molecule for the large-scale production of a fibrin-specific thrombolytic agent by recombinant DNA technology.

Pharmacokinetics

scu-PA is rapidly cleared from the blood after disappearance kinetics, which can be described by two exponential terms with half-lives of 7.9 ± 1.2 and 48 ± 8 minutes, respectively. NH$_2$-terminal recognition sites and carbohydrate moieties appear not to be critical for clearance, because the pharmacokinetics of natural glycosylated scu-PA,[24] of recombinant nonglycosylated scu-PA, and of the truncated low-molecular-weight variant scu-PA-32k are identical.[17] These findings suggest the need for continuous intravenous infusion to achieve and maintain steady-state plasma levels required for thrombolytic efficacy. Postinfusion clearance of scu-PA occurs with similar rapidity, suggesting nonsaturability of the clearance mechanism.

Dose of saruplase

There is still limited clinical experience with recombinant scu-PA. The generic name for full-length unglycosylated human recombinant scu-PA obtained from *E.* *coli* is saruplase. With a preparation containing 160,000 units/mg, the dose used successfully in patients with acute myocardial infarction (AMI) was 20 mg given as a bolus and 60 mg in the next 60 minutes, immediately followed by an intravenous heparin infusion (20 IU/kg/hr) for 72 hours.[25-27] This dosage regimen was found to cause a clear systemic activation of the fibrinolytic system and fibrinogen degradation. This may result, at least in part, from conversion of scu-PA to tcu-PA in the circulation.

Adverse effects of saruplase

In a direct double-blind comparison between intravenous saruplase (80 mg over 60 minutes) and streptokinase (1.5 million IU over 60 minutes) in 401 patients with AMI, a somewhat smaller reduction in circulating fibrinogen levels was observed in patients treated with saruplase. There were significantly less bleeding episodes in the saruplase group vs. the streptokinase group (14% vs. 25%), and less transfusion requirement (4% vs. 11%).[25]

t-PA

The plasminogen activator, which is synthesized by endothelial cells and secreted into the blood, has been identified as t-PA. Antigen levels of t-PA in normal plasma are about 5 ng/ml. t-PA has been purified from the tissue culture fluid of stable human melanoma cell lines in sufficient amounts to study its biochemical and biologic properties[28]; it is presently produced for clinical use by recombinant DNA technology.[29] The human t-PA gene, located on chromosome 8 (bands 8.p.12 $\rightarrow$ 9.11.2), is divided into 14 exons that code for specific domains of the protein.[30]

Physicochemical properties

t-PA is a serine proteinase with a molecular weight of about 70 kD, composed of a single polypeptide chain of 527 amino acids with Ser as the NH$_2$-terminal amino acid. The complete 2530-base pair complementary DNA sequence has been elucidated.[30] It was subsequently shown that native t-PA contains an NH$_2$-terminal extension of three amino acids (Gly-Ala-Arg-).[31]

The mature, secreted molecule contains five domains (Fig. 24-2): (1) a 43-residue long NH$_2$-terminal region (F domain) that is homologous with the finger domain responsible for the fibrin affinity of fibronectin[32]; (2) residues 44 to 91 (E domain) that are homologous with human EGF, which is also present in many other serine proteases and cell membrane receptors; (3) two disulfide-rich regions of 82 amino acids each (residues 92-173 and 180-261) (K$_1$ and K$_2$ domains) that share a high degree of homology with the kringles of urokinase, plasminogen, prothrombin, Hageman factor, and apolipoprotein a; and (4) a serine proteinase domain (amino

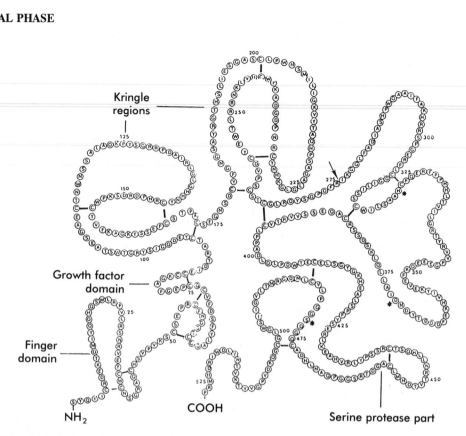

Fig. 24-2. Schematic representation of the primary structure of tissue-type plasminogen activator (t-PA). The amino acids are represented by their single letter symbols, and black bars indicate disulfide bonds. Active site residues His^{322}, Asp^{371}, and Ser^{478} are indicated with asterisks. The arrow indicates the plasmin cleavage site for conversion of single-chain t-PA to two-chain t-PA.

acids 276-527) with the active site residues His^{322}, Asp^{371}, and Ser^{478}, which is homologous with other serine proteinases.

The t-PA gene is assembled according to the "exon shuffling" principle. The different structural domains of the heavy chains (F, E, K$_1$, and K$_2$) are indeed encoded by a single exon or by two adjacent exons. Because of the striking correlation between the intron-exon distribution of the gene and the putative domain structure of the protein, it was suggested that these domains would harbor autonomous functional entities ("modules"). This concept implies that these structural domains of t-PA are involved in most of its functions and interactions, including its enzymatic activity, binding to fibrin, stimulation of plasminogen activation by fibrin, inhibition by PAI-1, binding to endothelial cells, and in vivo clearance of t-PA. The validity of the "exon-shuffling" concept for t-PA has been investigated by the construction of mutants with precise domain deletions, insertions, or substitutions and the evaluation of the fibrin affinity, the fibrin specificity, and the pharmacokinetic and thrombolytic properties of such mutants. The two-chain form of t-PA arises from cleavage of the Arg^{275}-Ile^{276} peptide bond by endogenous proteinases, most efficiently by plasmin.

The t-PA of saliva from the vampire bat *Desmodus rotundus* (bat-PA) is highly homologous with human t-PA but lacks K$_2$ and the plasmin cleavage site for conversion to a two-chain form.[33,34] It was found to be stimulated 45,000-fold by fibrin and to constitute a potent and fibrin-specific thrombolytic agent in rabbits and dogs with femoral arterial thrombosis.

Fibrin affinity of t-PA

The structures involved in the fibrin binding of t-PA are fully comprised within the NH$_2$-terminal (heavy) chain, as evidenced by the intact fibrin affinity of the heavy chain isolated after mild reduction of tcu-PA. Evidence obtained with domain deletion mutants of t-PA indicated that its affinity for fibrin is mediated via the finger domain and mainly via the second kringle domain.[35]

It has been suggested that in the process of fibrinolysis, binding of t-PA to intact fibrin would initially be mediated by the F domain. Subsequently, on partial fibrin digestion by plasmin, increased binding of t-PA to newly exposed COOH-terminal lysine residues would occur via the lysine-binding site in the K$_2$ domain. During degradation of fibrin(ogen) by plasmin, new t-PA-binding sites with markedly lower dissociation constants (2-4 orders of magnitude) are formed, but the increased binding of t-PA does not involve a lysine-binding site.[36]

Some authors have not found a difference between the fibrin-binding properties of single-chain and two-chain t-PAs, whereas another study reported a significant difference. Binding of t-PA to fibrin appears to be a dynamic interaction, which may be modulated during fibrinolysis by partial degradation of fibrin and by conversion of single-chain to two-chain t-PA.

Mechanism of plasminogen activation

In the absence of fibrin, t-PA is a poor plasminogen activator, mainly because of a low affinity for its substrate.[37] Single-chain t-PA is less active toward low-molecular-weight substrates and inhibitors, but its activity toward plasminogen was shown to be comparable with that of the two-chain form. The intrinsic enzymatic activity of single t-PA was confirmed by the construction of recombinant t-PA (rt-PA) mutants in which the plasmin cleavage site for conversion to two-chain t-PA was destroyed by site-specific mutagenesis of Arg^{275} to Glu. Such mutants were demonstrated to have lower activity than two-chain t-PA in the absence of fibrin but full plasminogen-activating activity in the presence of fibrin.[38] Inhibition by PAI-1 was also comparable for the wild-type and mutant t-PA. In contrast to other zymogen precursors of serine proteinases, the single-chain form of t-PA thus appears to be an active enzyme.

In the presence of fibrin, t-PA is a potent plasminogen activator, mainly because of a strongly enhanced affinity for its substrate.[37] The isolated proteinase part of two-chain t-PA, which is fully active, is not stimulated by fibrin, indicating that the structures involved in the fibrin stimulation are localized in the NH_2-terminal region. The kinetic data suggest that the fibrin stimulation of plasminogen activation by t-PA occurs by sequential-ordered addition of t-PA and plasminogen to fibrin, producing a thermodynamically more stable cyclic ternary complex.[37]

Pharmacokinetics

Single-chain t-PA (alteplase) has a significantly shorter half-life in humans (4.3 minutes, α-phase; 36.5 minutes, β-phase) compared with two-chain t-PA, the earlier product made available for clinical use (5.2 minutes, α-phase; 46.2 minutes, β-phase).[38,39] Whether this difference is related to the chain composition or to other factors such as glycosylation remains unclear. When the latter material was studied in healthy human volunteers, the mean clearance (of antigen) was 620 ± 70 ml/min, the volume of distribution at steady state was 8.1 ± 0.8 L, and the initial volume of distribution was 4.4 ± 0.6 L.[40]

Animal experiments have indicated that rapid clearance of t-PA occurs via the heavy chain and primarily via hepatocytes.[41,42] Although a receptor for t-PA has not yet been definitively identified, the rapid uptake probably involves receptor-mediated endocytosis and lysosomal degradation. Large doses of unlabeled t-PA administered concomitantly with radiolabeled t-PA in mice do not affect clearance, suggesting that hepatic binding and catabolism are not saturated by usual therapeutic doses. Two different mechanisms for removal of t-PA have been characterized, a protein-mediated pathway via hepatocytes and a carbohydrate-mediated pathway via endothelial cells in the liver.[43] Recently, studies with rt-PA deletion mutants suggested that interaction of t-PA with hepatocytes would involve primarily kringle 1 (where residue Asn^{117} anchors a high-mannose carbohydrate side chain) but in addition occur via the F and E domains, whereas binding to endothelial cells would occur mainly via the F and E domains.

PAI-1 neutralizes single-chain t-PA, two-chain t-PA, and urokinase very rapidly.[44] To design mutants of t-PA that are resistant to inhibition by PAI-1, Madison et al.[45] have modeled the interactions between the active site of t-PA and PAI-1 based on the known three-dimensional structure of the trypsin-trypsin inhibitor complex. They have identified specific amino acids (residues Lys^{296}-His-Arg-Arg-Ser-Pro-Gly^{302} and Arg^{304}) in t-PA, which interact with PAI-1 but not with the substrate plasminogen. Mutants of rt-PA obtained by site-specific mutagenesis in this region were shown to be fully active toward substrates but to display significant resistance to inhibition by PAI-1.[45,46] In view of the large excess of t-PA over PAI-1 achieved during thrombolytic therapy, resistance of t-PA mutants to PAI-1 may not directly constitute a significant advantage over wild-type t-PA. High PAI-1 levels may contribute to the occurrence of reocclusion, however, and PAI-1-resistant mutants of rt-PA may be useful for maintenance infusion after initial thrombolysis.

Resistance to PAI-1 has been combined with prolonged half-life in a molecule in which Thr^{103} is substituted by Asn (prolonged half-life), and the sequence Lys^{296}-His-Arg-Arg is mutagenized to Ala-Ala-Ala-Ala (resistance to PAI-1). This mutant was indeed shown to have a reduced plasma clearance and an increased potency on platelet-rich plasma clots (rich in PAI-1) in animal models.[47]

Dosage

The recommended dose of alteplase (Activase, Actilyse) for the treatment of AMI is 100 mg administered as 60 mg in the first hour (of which 6-10 mg is administered as a bolus over the first 1-2 minutes), 20 mg over the second hour, and 20 mg over the third hour. More recently it was proposed to give the same total dose of 100 mg but "front-loaded," starting with a bolus of 15 mg, followed by 50 mg in the next 30 minutes and the remaining 35 mg in the following 60 minutes.[48] A 15-mg intravenous bolus of alteplase, followed by 0.75 mg/kg over 30 minutes (not to exceed 50 mg) and then 0.50 mg/kg over 60 minutes (not to exceed 35 mg), has been successfully tested in the large-scale Global Utilization of Streptokinase and Tissue-Type Plasminogen Activator for Occluded Coronary Arteries (GUSTO) trial. Whatever the dose regimen used, it is important to coadminister intravenous heparin during and after alteplase treatment. For catheter-directed local thrombolysis with alteplase in patients with recent peripheral arterial occlusion, the dose of 0.05 to 0.10 mg/kg/hr over 8 hours is usually recommended.

Duteplase is the generic name for rt-PA, produced in its two-chain form by the Burroughs-Wellcome Company. It also differs from recombinant human alteplase because of a substitution of methionine for valine in position 245 in the amino acid sequence and is therefore a variant of the naturally occurring human t-PA. The specific activity of duteplase is approximately 300,000 units/mg of protein, but different production lots may have specific activities that vary as much as ± 100,000 units.[49] For this reason the dosage of duteplase is given in megaunits per kilogram of body weight (0.6-1.0 megaunit/kg over 4 hours).[50] In ISIS-3 the lower dose of duteplase (0.6 megaunit/kg over 4 hours) was used, which corresponds to about 83% of the thrombolytic activity of 100 mg of alteplase but to a dose of 2 mg/kg (160 mg in the average 80-kg patient).

Adverse effects

Bleeding complications are the most common and feared side effects with any thrombolytic agent, including alteplase. The reported rates of bleeding during treatment with thrombolytic agents depend on the methods of data collection, which can be very elaborate in trials on a limited number of patients, or limited in megatrials including thousands of patients. Valid conclusions can therefore be drawn only from direct comparisons between drugs in a given trial. In a recent large trial directly comparing alteplase and streptokinase, the reported incidence of cerebral bleeding (confirmed by computed tomographic scan and necropsy) was similar for the two thrombolytic agents, but, overall, significantly more strokes were reported in the alteplase group.[51] For both agents there was an excess of strokes in patients greater than 70 years of age (> 70 years: 2.7% alteplase; 1.6% streptokinase; ≤ 70 years: 0.9% alteplase; 0.8% streptokinase). Significantly more major bleeds occurred in patients allocated to streptokinase. However, the total number of bleeds (minor plus major) was significantly higher with alteplase (4.2% vs. 3.3%). More allergic reactions (0.2% vs. 1.7%) and hypotension

(1.7% vs. 3.8%) were seen with streptokinase in this large international trial. In the ISIS-3 trial the incidence of cerebral bleeding was 0.3%, 0.5%, and 0.6% in patients treated with streptokinase, anistreplase, and duteplase, respectively.[52] Bleeding and other complications can be avoided by carefully observing the relative and absolute contraindications to thrombolysis.

REFERENCES

1. Bernik MB, Oller EP: Plasminogen activator and proactivator (urokinase precursor) in lung cultures, *J Am Med Wom Assoc* 31:465-472, 1976.
2. Nolli ML, Sarubbi E, Corti A, et al: Production and characterization of human recombinant single chain urokinase-type plasminogen activator from mouse cells, *Fibrinolysis* 3:101-106, 1989.
3. Günzler WA, Steffens GJ, Ötting F, et al: Structural relationship between human high and low molecular mass urokinase, *Hoppe-Seylers Z Physiol Chem* 363:1155-1165, 1982.
4. Tripputi P, Blasi F, Verde P, et al: Human urokinase gene is located on the long arm of chromosome 10, *Proc Natl Acad Sci USA* 82:4448-4452, 1985.
5. Verde P, Stoppelli MP, Galeffi P, et al: Identification of primary sequence of an unspliced human urokinase poly(A)$^+$ RNA, *Proc Natl Acad Sci USA* 81:4727-4731, 1988.
6. Scully MF: Plasminogen activator–dependent pericellular proteolysis, *Br J Haemotol* 79:537-543, 1991.
7. Eaton DL, Scott RW, Baker JB: Purification of human fibroblast urokinase proenzyme and analysis of its regulation by proteases and protease nexin, *J Biol Chem* 259:6241-6247, 1984.
8. Nielsen LS, Hansen JG, Skriver L, et al: Purification of zymogen to plasminogen activator from human glioblastoma cells by affinity chromatography with monoclonal antibody, *Biochemistry* 24:6410-6415, 1982.
9. Mira-y-Lopez R, Reich E, Ossowski L: Modulation of plasminogen activators in rodent mammary tumors by hormones and other effectors, *Cancer Res* 43:5467-5477, 1983.
10. Michel JB, Quertermous T: Modulation of mRNA levels for urinary- and tissue-type plasminogen activator and plasminogen activator inhibitors 1 and 2 in human fibroblasts by interleukin 1, *J Immunol* 143:890-895, 1989.
11. Sawdy M, Podor TJ, Loskutoff DJ: Regulation of type I plasminogen activator inhibitor gene expression in cultured bovine aortic endothelial cells, *J Biol Chem* 264:10396-10401, 1989.
12. Holmes WE, Pennica D, Blaber M, et al: Cloning and expression of the gene for pro-urokinase in *Escherichia coli*, *Biotechnology* 3:923-929, 1985.
13. Declerck PJ, Lijnen HR, Verstreken M, et al: A monoclonal antibody specific for two-chain urokinase-type plasminogen activator. Application to the study of the mechanism of clot lysis with single-chain urokinase-type plasminogen activator in plasma, *Blood* 75:1794-1800, 1990.
14. Patthy L, Traxler M, Vali Z, et al: Kringles: modules specialized for protein binding. Homology of the gelatin-binding region of fibronectin with the kringle structures of proteins, *FEBS Lett* 171:131-136, 1984.
15. Lijnen HR, Zamarron C, Blaber M, et al: Activation of plasminogen by pro-urokinase: I. Mechanism, *J Biol Chem* 261:1253-1258, 1986.
16. Scully MF, Ellis V, Watahiki Y, et al: Activation of pro-urokinase by plasmin: non-Michaelian kinetics indicates a mechanism of negative cooperation, *Arch Biochem Biophys* 268:438-446, 1989.
17. Stump DC, Lijnen HR, Collen D: Purification and characterization of single-chain urokinase-type plasminogen activator from human cell cultures, *J Biol Chem* 261:1274-1278, 1986.

18. Ichinose A, Fujikawa K, Suyama T: The activation of pro-urokinase by plasma kallikrein and its inactivation by thrombin, *J Biol Chem* 261:3486-3489, 1986.

19. Lijnen HR, Van Hoef B, De Cock F, et al: The mechanism of plasminogen activation and fibrin dissolution by single chain urokinase-type plasminogen activator in a plasma milieu in vitro, *Blood* 73:1864-1872, 1989.

20. Kirchheimer JC, Binder BR: Function of receptor-bound urokinase, *Semin Thromb Hemost* 17:246-250, 1991.

21. Danø K, Andreasen PA, Grøondahl-Hansen J, et al: Plasminogen activators, tissue degradation and cancer, *Adv Cancer Res* 44:139-266, 1985.

22. Saksela O, RIfkin DB: Cell-associated plasminogen activation: regulation and physiological functions, *Annu Rev Cell Biol* 4:93-126, 1988.

23. Lijnen HR, Nelles L, Holmes WE, et al: Biochemical and thrombolytic properties of a low molecular weight form (comprising Leu[144] through Leu[411]) of recombinant single-chain urokinase-type plasminogen activator, *J Biol Chem* 263:5594-5598, 1988.

24. Collen D, De Cock F, Lijnen HR: Biological and thrombolytic properties of proenzyme and active forms of human urokinase: II. Turnover of natural and recombinant urokinase in rabbits and squirrel monkeys, *Thromb Haemost* 52:24-26, 1984.

25. PRIMI Trial Study Group: Randomised double-blind trial of recombinant pro-urokinase against streptokinase in acute myocardial infarction, *Lancet* 1:863-868, 1989.

26. Kasper W, Meinertz T, Hohnloser S, et al: Coronary thrombolysis in man with pro-urokinase: improved efficacy with low dose urokinase, *Klin Wochenschr* 66(suppl XII):109-114, 1988.

27. Diefenbach C, Erbel R, Pop T, et al: Recombinant single-chain urokinase-type plasminogen activator during acute myocardial infarction, *Am J Cardiol* 61:966-970, 1988.

28. Collen D, Rijken DC, Van Damme J, et al: Purification of human tissue-type plasminogen activator in centigram quantities from human melanoma cell culture fluid and its conditioning for use in vivo, *Thromb Haemost* 48:294-296, 1982.

29. Ny T, Elgh F, Lund B: The structure of the human tissue-type plasminogen activator gene: correlation of intron and exon structures to functional and structural domains, *Proc Natl Acad Sci USA* 81:5355-5359, 1984.

30. Pennica D, Holmes WE, Kohr WJ, et al: Cloning and expression of human tissue-type plasminogen activator cDNA in *E. coli*, *Nature* 301:214-221, 1983.

31. Joernvall H, Pohl G, Bergsdorf N, et al: Differential proteolysis and evidence for a residue exchange in tissue plasminogen activator suggest possible association between two types of protein microheterogeneity, *FEBS Lett* 156:47-50, 1983.

32. Patthy L: Evolution of the proteases of blood coagulation and fibrinolysis by assembly from modules, *Cell* 41:657-663, 1985.

33. Gardell SJ, Duong LT, Diehl RE, et al: Isolation, characterization, and cDNA cloning of a vampire bat salivary plasminogen activator, *J Biol Chem* 264:17947-17952, 1989.

34. Krätzschmar J, Haendler B, Langer G, et al: The plasminogen activator family from the salivary gland of the vampire bat *Desmodus rotundus*: cloning and expression, *Gene* 105:229-237, 1991.

35. van Zonneveld AJ, Veerman H, Pannekoek H: On the interaction of the finger and the kringle-2 domain of tissue-type plasminogen activator with fibrin. Inhibition of kringle-2 binding to fibrin by E-amino caproic acid, *J Biol Chem* 261:14214-14218, 1986.

36. Higgins DL, Vehar GA: Interaction of one-chain and two-chain tissue plasminogen activator with intact and plasmin-degraded fibrin, *Biochemistry* 26:7786-7791, 1987.

37. Hoylaerts M, Rijken DC, Lijnen HR, et al: Kinetics of the activation of plasminogen by human tissue plasminogen activator. Role of fibrin, *J Biol Chem* 257:2912-2919, 1982.

38. Verstraete M, Bounameaux H, De Cock F, et al: Pharmacokinetics and systemic fibrinolytic effects of recombinant human tissue-type plasminogen activator (rt-PA) in humans, *J Pharmacol Exp Ther* 235:506, 1985.

39. Garabedian HD, Gold HK, Leinbach RC, et al: Comparative properties of two clinical preparations of recombinant human tissue-type plasminogen activator in patients with acute myocardial infarction, *J Am Coll Cardiol* 9:599-607, 1987.

40. Tanswell P, Seifried E, Su PCAF, et al: Pharmacokinetics and systemic effects of tissue-type plasminogen activator in normal subjects, *Clin Pharmacol Ther* 46:155-162, 1989.

41. Korninger C, Stassen JM, Collen D: Turnover of human extrinsic (tissue-type) plasminogen activator in rabbits, *Thromb Haemost* 46:658-661, 1981.

42. Rijken DC, Emeis JJ: Clearance of the heavy and light polypeptide chains of human tissue-type plasminogen activator in rats, *Biochem J* 238:643-646, 1986.

43. Kuiper J, Otter M, Rijken DC, et al: Characterization of the interaction in vivo of tissue-type plasminogen activator with liver cells, *J Biol Chem* 263:18220-18224, 1988.

44. Kruithof EKO, Tran-Thang C, Ransijn A, et al: Demonstration of a fast-acting inhibitor of plasminogen activators in human plasma, *Blood* 64:907-913, 1984.

45. Madison EL, Goldsmith EJ, Gerard RD, et al: Amino acid residues that affect interaction of tissue-type plasminogen activator with plasminogen activator inhibitor 1, *Proc Natl Acad Sci USA* 87:3530-3533, 1990.

46. Bennett WF, Paoni NF, Keyt BA, et al: High resolution analysis of functional determinants on human tissue-type plasminogen activator, *J Biol Chem* 266:5191-5201, 1991.

47. Refino CJ, Paoni NF, Keyt BA, et al: A mutant of human tissue plasminogen activator with decreased plasma clearance and greater fibrin specificity has increased potency and limited systemic activation in vivo when administered as a bolus [abstract 65]. *Fibrinolysis* 6(suppl 2):26, 1992.

48. Neuhaus KL, Feuerer W, Jeep-Tebbe S, et al: Improved thrombolysis with a modified regimen of recombinant tissue-type plasminogen activator, *J Am Coll Cardiol* 14:1566-1569, 1989.

49. Christodoulides M, Boucher DW: The potency of tissue-type plasminogen activator (TPA) determined with chromogen and clot lysis assay, *Biologicals* 18:103-111, 1990.

50. Grines CL, for the Burroughs Wellcome Study Group: Efficacy and safety of weight adjusted dosing of a new tissue plasminogen activator preparation in acute myocardial infarction [abstract]. *Circulation* 78(suppl II):127, 1988.

51. International Study Group: In-hospital mortality and clinical cause of 20,891 patients with suspected acute myocardial infarction randomised between alteplase and streptokinase with or without heparin, *Lancet* 336:71-75, 1990.

52. Third International Study of Infarct Survival Collaborative Group: ISIS-3: a randomized comparison of streptokinase versus tissue plasminogen activator versus anistreplase and of aspirin plus heparin versus aspirin alone among 41,299 cases of suspected acute myocardial infarction, *Lancet* 339:753-770, 1992.

Chapter 25

STREPTOKINASE AND ANISTREPLASE

Harvey D. White
Victor J. Marder

Although the various thrombolytic agents differ in their cell of origin and pharmacologic profiles, the aspects that influence the occurrence of adverse effects, the blood changes, and the details of actual use such as optimal infusion time and clinical benefits and complications induced by the agents are more similar than different. Based solely on their relative tendency to activate plasma plasminogen and to degrade fibrinogen to degradation products, the plasminogen activators are termed *fibrin-specific* or *non–fibrin-specific*. These terms imply that fibrin but not fibrinogen is degraded, but in reality this is a relative rather than an absolute distinction and could perhaps better be termed *fibrinogen-sparing* or *non–fibrinogen-sparing*. This terminology does not imply or indicate any specificity of one or another agent for thrombus dissolution (thrombolysis) over disintegration of a hemostatic plug (bleeding complication) (Table 25-1). The agents streptokinase and anistreplase have striking effects on plasma fibrinogen, more than those induced by tissue plasminogen activator (rt-PA), and therefore fall into the category of nonfibrin-specific agents.

This work was supported in part by grant HL-30616 from the National Heart, Lung and Blood Institute, National Institutes of Health, Bethesda, MD.
Editors' Note: Interpretation of the results of thrombolytic clinical trials has been a source of controversy. While we disagree with some of the views expressed in this chapter, we consider it important that they be presented.

PHARMACOLOGY

Streptokinase is derived from Lancefield group C β-hemolytic streptococci and activates the fibrinolytic system indirectly by combining with plasminogen to form an activator complex (Fig. 25-1). This complex has plasminogen activator activity and converts both plasma- and thrombus-bound plasminogen to the active enzyme plasmin. Plasmin degrades plasma coagulation proteins (especially fibrinogen), inducing the so-called *plasma proteolytic state*,[1] as well as fibrin within a thrombus or a hemostatic plug. Antiplasmin tends to neutralize plasmin, but as the plasma concentration of this inhibitor is only half that of plasminogen, the effect of systemic infusion of a massive amount of streptokinase (or any other therapeutic activator) is to exceed the neutralizing capacity of α_2 antiplasmin and produce the lytic state.

Anistreplase is a chemically inert plasminogen-streptokinase activator complex whose catalytic site is rendered inactive by acylation with an anisoyl group. The compound is inactive until deacylation occurs upon solution of the lyophilized material and continues in the blood after intravenous injection. The half-life of anistreplase is longer than that of streptokinase (90 vs. 23 minutes) and it can therefore be injected by a simple bolus intravenous push rather than by continuous infusion over 30 to 60 minutes or 90 to 180 minutes for the short-acting agents such as rt-PA.

The lytic state is more profound with streptokinase and anistreplase than with rt-PA, but there is no relationship between the degree of this lytic state and the incidence or severity of bleeding complications. This

Table 25-1. Pharmacologic features of thrombolytic agents

	Streptokinase	Anistreplase	rt-PA
Half-life (minutes)	23	90-150	5
Antigenicity	Yes	Yes	No
Specificity: clot vs. hemostatic plug	None	None	None
Fibrinogenolysis	+ + + +	+ + + +	+ +
Platelet activation	+ + +	+ + +	+ + +

disparity is explained by the fact that bleeding results from hemostatic plug disintegration at sites of vascular injury independent of changes in the blood, actions that reflect proteolysis of distinctly different anatomic entities. In fact the hypocoagulable lytic state may be advantageous[2,3] in protecting against reocclusion of reperfused infarct-related arteries. Once the infusion of plasminogen activator is complete, and following an interval of nadir plasminogen concentration that reflects the half-life of the activator, fibrinogen concentrations are gradually replenished by hepatic synthesis, a process that is completed in 36 to 48 hours.

REPERFUSION

The 90-minute patency or reperfusion rate has been used in many thrombolytic trials to evaluate the efficacy

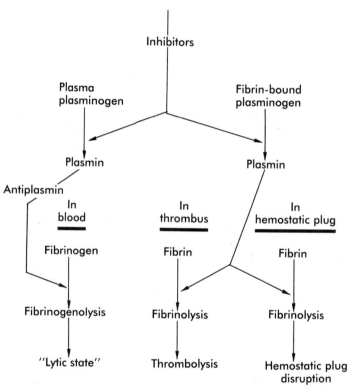

Fig. 25-1. Plasminogen activator action in blood, thrombus, and hemostatic plug. The tendency of a given plasminogen activator to induce the "lytic state," relative to its capacity to induce thrombolysis, defines the concept of a "fibrin-specific" or "fibrinogen-sparing" agent. When used at dosages chosen to induce effective thrombus dissolution, all the plasminogen activators cause the lytic state to some degree, but this effect is more marked with SK (streptokinase), UK (urokinase), and APSAC (anistreplase) than with t-PA (tissue plasminogen activator) or pro-UK (pro-urokinase). The "inhibitors" that may impair or block the action of a plasminogen activator include antibodies against exogenous agents such as SK and its derivative form anistreplase, and PAI-1 (plasminogen activator inhibitor type 1), which is a natural inhibitor of rt-PA. Antiplasmin (α_2-plasmin inhibitor) blocks the action of plasmin when in solution (in blood) much more efficiently than when plasmin is bound to fibrin (in thrombus or in hemostatic plug), an effect that tends to promote fibrin rather than fibrinogen degradation. All the plasminogen activators used for therapeutic purposes produce approximately equivalent therapeutic benefit (vascular reperfusion) via thrombolysis and complications (bleeding) via hemostatic plug disruption.

of thrombolytic agents. The data show that the administration of the standard regimen of rt-PA over 3 hours or streptokinase over 1 hour results in equivalent efficacy as judged by this endpoint when treatment is delayed for less than 2 hours after the onset of symptoms.[4] When therapy is begun more than 2 hours after symptom onset, rt-PA lyses thrombi more rapidly than streptokinase (Fig. 25-2). However, because the amount of salvageable myocardium decreases rapidly with time[5,6] this lytic advantage may be small in respect to patient benefit. Figure 25-2 shows that maximal patency is achieved at 90 minutes with rt-PA and that a constant patency rate is maintained thereafter as further thrombolysis is balanced by reocclusion. Slower progressive reperfusion is achieved with streptokinase, but there is a progressive increase in patency with streptokinase[7-10] so that 3 hours have elapsed after treatment, patency rates are the same for rt-PA- and streptokinase-treated patients, even when rt-PA is given in an accelerated regimen.[11] Perhaps the lower reocclusion rate with streptokinase[12] explains this "catch-up" of the patency rate using streptokinase.[4,13,14] The difference noted for rt-PA and streptokinase at 90 minutes may actually be less in respect to sustained patency because rt-PA-reperfused infarct-related arteries may have intermittent perfusion more often than streptokinase-reperfused arteries.[15]

Early (90-minute) patency rates with anistreplase tend to be higher than[9] or equivalent[8] to those with streptokinase and equivalent to those achieved 24 hours after using rt-PA.[16] One unblinded study using a rapid-administration rt-PA regimen showed a higher patency rate with rt-PA than with anistreplase.[17]

LEFT VENTRICULAR FUNCTION

A major effect of thrombolytic therapy on mortality after MI has been the decrease in the numbers of patients dying from cardiac failure.[18,19] In the thrombolytic era left ventricular function has remained the most important long-term prognostic factor[20-26] and in four large trials both left ventricular function and survival have been improved.[11,18,27,28]

Left ventricular function trials are the most powerful statistically, as ejection fraction and end-systolic volume (which may be the most important prognostic factor)[29] are measured as continuous variables. An improvement in ejection fraction from 50% to 53% requires only 300 randomized patients with a power of 80% and $P < 0.05$; however, to have the same power would require 1784 patients to show an improvement in patency from 70%

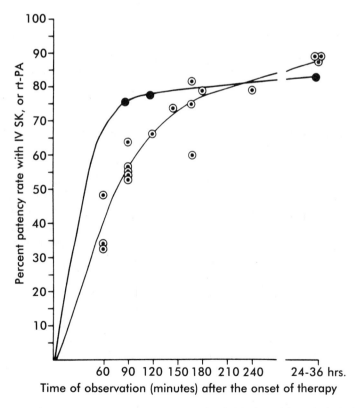

Fig. 25-2. Change in coronary artery patency rates after initiation of thrombolytic therapy with intravenous SK (⊙) or with standard rt-PA (•) per the elapsed time after the initiation of therapy. (Reproduced with permission from Sherry S, Marder VJ: Streptokinase and recombinant tissue plasminogen activator (rt-PA) are equally effective in treating acute myocardial infarction, *Ann Intern Med* 114:417-423, 1991.)

to 76% and 10,000 to 20,000 patients to show a 15% reduction in the mortality rate (21,490 if mortality is 5% and 10,726 if mortality is 10.5%).

Thrombolytic therapy has been shown to preserve left ventricular function following streptokinase,[18,30,31] rt-PA,[32-36] and anistreplase.[37] Interestingly, streptokinase has been shown to reduce infarct size in animals with nonreperfused infarct-related arteries[24] as well as in animals with patent infarct-related arteries. This may relate to a reduction in plasma and blood viscosity,[39-41] which may improve the microcirculation in the marginal infarct zone and decrease total peripheral resistance.

Comparative trials have shown that, given the standard regimens, the various agents have similar effects on preservation of left ventricular function.[42-44] These trials have been consistent with the mortality data from over 60,000 randomized patients in large mortality trials showing the agents to have equal efficacy using rt-PA in a standard regimen over 3 hours,[43,45,46] and are supported by the GUSTO-I trial, in which the combination limb received a regimen similar to the standard rt-PA regimen plus a million units of streptokinase, with no significant mortality advantage.[11a]

MORTALITY

There is no evidence of any difference between the thrombolytic agents in reducing mortality when standard regimens are used.[43,45,46] In GISSI-2 20,749 patients admitted within 6 hours of symptom onset were randomized to receive either streptokinase (1.5 million units over 30 to 60 minutes) or rt-PA (100 mg over 3 hours). The mortality rates were 8.9% for rt-PA and 8.5% for streptokinase.[45] Mortality was similar in patients treated with or without heparin administered subcutaneously (12,500 U twice daily) beginning 12 hours after onset of thrombolytic treatment. The lowest mortality occurred in patients treated with streptokinase plus heparin (7.9%) compared with patients treated with rt-PA plus heparin (9.2%).[45]

In ISIS-3 over 40,000 patients were randomized to receive no heparin or subcutaneous heparin begun 4 hours after starting a thrombolytic agent. Streptokinase was compared with duteplase (double-stranded rt-PA) infused over 4 hours and with anistreplase (30 U by bolus injection over 5 minutes). Thirty-five-day mortality was equivalent for the three groups: 10.5% for streptokinase, 10.3% for duteplase and 10.6% for anistreplase.[46] Table 25-2 compares the clinical features of the nonfibrin-specific agents streptokinase and anistreplase with standard-dose rt-PA.

ADVERSE EFFECTS
Bleeding complications

The most important adverse effect of thrombolytic therapy is bleeding, particularly hemorrhagic stroke. Bleeding is usually related to lysis of a hemostatic plug

Table 25-2. Comparison of clinical features of thrombolytic agents

	Streptokinase	Anistreplase	rt-PA*
Patency† (%)			
90 minutes	65	70	75
3 hours	85	85	85
Left ventricular function preservation	+ + +	+ + +	+ + +
Survival benefit	+ + +	+ + +	+ + +
Ease of administration	+ + +	+ + + +	+
Cost	+	+ + +	+ + + +

*Using standard dosage regimens.
†TIMI 2 and 3 flow.[11] In GUSTO-I, 90-minute patency with accelerated rt-PA was 81% vs. 54% with streptokinase plus subcutaneous heparin; the rates at 3 hours were 76% vs. 73%, respectively. Thirty-day mortality rates with these regimens were 6.3% with rt-PA and 7.4% with streptokinase.[11a]

at a site of previous trauma or injury[47] and occurs at about the same rate with all the agents, as shown in the large comparative trials.[43,45,46] However, the incidence of cerebrovascular accident with rt-PA or anistreplase has been higher than with streptokinase: 1.3% alteplase vs. 1% streptokinase in GISSI-2,[45] 1.4% duteplase and 1.3% anistreplase vs. 1.1% streptokinase in ISIS-3.[46] In ISIS-3 there were more cases of intracranial hemorrhage with rt-PA and anistreplase (0.7% and 0.6% respectively) compared with streptokinase (0.3%, $P < 0.0001$) although the underlying lesion predisposing to intracranial bleeding is not known. Of those patients affected by intracranial hemorrhage, about one half die of the lesion, one quarter suffer permanent disability, and one quarter recover without sequelae.[48] In the GUSTO-I trial there was an excess of total stroke with the accelerated rt-PA regimen vs. the ISIS-3 regimen of streptokinase plus delayed subcutaneous heparin (1.55% vs. 1.22%, $P = 0.09$) and also of hemorrhagic stroke (0.72% vs. 0.49%, $P = 0.03$).[11a] This excess bleeding must be balanced against the potential survival benefit of the accelerated rt-PA regimen in an individual patient.

Allergic reactions

Streptokinase and anistreplase can cause an allergic reaction with fever, nausea, or skin rash, but anaphylactic reactions are rare. There were no confirmed episodes of anaphylactic shock in 8592 treated patients in ISIS-2,[48] only 7 in 5860 patients in GISSI-1,[49] and only 0.3% using streptokinase and 0.5% with anistreplase in ISIS-3.[46] None of these reactions caused the death of the patient.

ADJUNCTIVE HEPARIN THERAPY

Intravenous heparin regimens may improve the time to patency and result in greater myocardial salvage.[50,51]

Table 25-3. Incidence of adverse effects and recommended treatment

Complication	Incidence*	
Hemorrhagic stroke	Streptokinase 0.3% Anistreplase 0.6%	1. Stop thrombolytic agent, aspirin, and heparin. 2. Reverse heparin with protamine sulphate. 3. Administer fresh frozen or freeze-dried plasma to replete clotting factors and fibrinogen.
Noncerebral bleeding (requiring transfusion)	Streptokinase 0.9% Anistreplase 1.0%	4. Consider aminocaproic acid. 5. Consider fresh platelet transfusion.
Hypotension (requiring treatment)	Streptokinase 6.7% Anistreplase 7.0%	Usually stopping the infusion and elevation of the patient's legs is all that is required. Volume loading may be necessary.
Major allergy	Streptokinase 0.3% Anistreplase 0.5%	Intravenous antihistamines and hydrocortisone may help. If severe, adrenaline 0.5-1 ml of 1:10,000 should be given intravenously and repeated every 3 minutes as necessary.

*Data from ISIS-3.[46]

ISIS-3,[46] GISSI-2,[43] and the international study[45] showed that subcutaneous heparin administered either 4 or 12 hours after beginning thrombolytic therapy was moderately beneficial, with a reduction in mortality (4 to 5 patients saved per 1000 patients treated) and reinfarction (1 to 3 fewer reinfarcts per 1000 patients) and no overall increase in total stroke. There was, however, an increased requirement for blood transfusions (3 to 5 patients per 1000 treated). In the GUSTO-I trial there was no evidence that the addition of intravenous heparin to streptokinase, compared with subcutaneous heparin, was advantageous for mortality or reinfarction.[11a] However, 36% of the patients randomized to receive subcutaneous heparin also received intravenous heparin, confounding assessment of the efficacy and safety of a more aggressive heparin regimen. This comparison was therefore not to the ISIS-3 regimen, but to a subcutaneous regimen with aggressive use of intravenous heparin if judged appropriate. Despite this, patency at 5 to 7 days (TIMI 2 and TIMI 3) was 12% higher in patients treated with intravenous heparin (72% subcutaneous vs. 84% intravenous heparin, $P = 0.032$).[11]

Although the different half-lives of the drugs and different effects on platelets and plasma clotting factors could require individualization for heparin therapy, there are no data showing that this is indeed the case, and current information indicates that heparin therapy has similar clinical results with streptokinase, rt-PA, and anistreplase. Heparin is clearly not an ideal agent, and the new thrombin inhibitors hirulog and hirudin may have major advantages by more effectively inhibiting clot-bound thrombin and thrombin-induced platelet aggregation. It is possible that these agents could dramatically improve early patency with streptokinase without increasing bleeding.

DOSAGE AND ADMINISTRATION

The recommended dosage of intravenous streptokinase is 1.5 million units infused over 30 to 60 minutes.

The faster the infusion, the higher the incidence of hypotension (up to 5% to 10%), but faster infusion may result in better reperfusion rates and clinical benefit.[18] Aspirin (150 to 300 mg) should be coadministered. Prophylactic hydrocortisone is unnecessary. Hypotension occurred in 4.3% of patients treated with rt-PA compared with 6.7% for streptokinase and 7.0% with the use of anistreplase in ISIS-3 (Table 25-3).

Following the administration of streptokinase or anistreplase, antibodies are induced within 3 to 4 days with titers sufficient to neutralize a standard dose of streptokinase or anistreplase. These antibodies persist for at least 4 years.[52,53] Although it has not been demonstrated that such antibodies cause allergic reactions, the risk that treatment of a patient previously exposed to streptokinase or anistreplase would be ineffective because of a high titer of neutralizing antibody warrants the use of a nonstreptokinase kind of agent such as rt-PA or urokinase for retreatment.

PLACE OF STREPTOKINASE AND ANISTREPLASE IN CLINICAL PRACTICE

Streptokinase is the most widely used thrombolytic agent worldwide and is also the cheapest. The use of rt-PA is associated with an excess of total stroke of 4 per 1000 patients treated.[54] Streptokinase is therefore the agent of choice in patients whose mortality risk is low, such as those with small to moderate infarcts or those aged less than 55 years, because an iatrogenically-induced stroke in a patient with a good outcome is unacceptable. Streptokinase is also the agent of choice in patients with an increased risk of stroke, such as those who have had a previous stroke or hypertension on admission that is subsequently controlled.

Thrombolytic therapy reduces mortality in patients treated (with streptokinase or rt-PA) within 12 hours of the onset of chest pain.[55] There are, however, no comparative trials of these agents for patients treated between 6 and 12 hours. It is interesting that for patients treated after 6 hours in the GUSTO-I trial, mortality was similar among the rt-PA-treated patients and the streptokinase-treated patients (10.4% rt-PA vs. 8.3% streptokinase).[11a] The aim of late therapy is to open the occluded infarct-related artery so as to reduce mortality through the mechanisms of decreased re-modeling and left ventricular dilatation, decreased arrhythmogenesis, and the provision of collaterals to another coronary artery territory if further infarction occurs.[55] As time to patency is not crucial to achieve these benefits, and because streptokinase and rt-PA achieve the same patency rates at 3 hours,[11] the agent with the lowest risk of adverse effects (particularly of stroke) should be used. In the LATE trial the incidence of stroke at 35 days was 2.29% with standard rt-PA vs. 1.18% with placebo, an excess over placebo of 9 strokes per 1000 patients treated,[56] whereas in the EMERAS trial[57] the incidence of stroke was 1.5% with streptokinase vs. 1.1% with placebo, an excess of 4 strokes per 1000 over placebo. Exceptions to routine use of streptokinase for patients presenting after 6 hours would be for patients who require retreatment that would necessitate the use of rt-PA or urokinase. Anistreplase is indicated where rapid completion of thrombolytic therapy may be desirable, such as in community administration.

REFERENCES

1. Sherry S, Fletcher AP, Alkjaersig N: Fibrinolysis and fibrinolytic activity in man, *Physiol Rev* 39:343-382, 1959.
2. Marder VJ, Sherry S: Thrombolytic therapy: current status, *N Engl J Med* 318:1512-1520, 1585-1595, 1988.
3. Rapaport E: Thrombolysis, anticoagulation, and reocclusion, *Am J Cardiol* 68:17E-22E, 1991.
4. Sherry S, Marder VJ: Streptokinase and recombinant tissue plasminogen activator (rt-PA) are equally effective in treating acute myocardial infarction, *Ann Intern Med* 114:417-423, 1991.
5. Reimer KA, Lowe JE, Rasmussen MM, et al: The wavefront phenomenon of myocardial ischemic cell death: myocardial infarct size vs. duration of coronary occlusion in dogs, *Circulation* 56:786-794, 1977.
6. Reimer KA, Jennings RB: The "wavefront phenomenon" of myocardial ischemic cell death: transmural progression of necrosis within the framework of ischemic bed size (myocardium at risk) and collateral flow, *Lab Invest* 40:633-644, 1979.
7. Six AJ, Louwerenburg HW, Braams R, et al: A double-blind randomized multicenter dose-ranging trial of intravenous streptokinase in acute myocardial infarction, *Am J Cardiol* 65:119-123, 1990.
8. Hogg KJ, Gemmill JD, Burns JMA, et al: Angiographic patency study of anistreplase versus streptokinase in acute myocardial infarction, *Lancet* 335:254-258, 1990.
9. Pacouret G, Charbonnier B, for the IRS II study: Multicentre European randomized trial of anistreplase versus streptokinase in acute myocardial infarction (abstract), *Circulation* 80 (suppl II):II-40, 1989.
10. Anderson JL, Sorensen SG, Moreno F, et al and the TEAM-2 investigators: Quantitative assessment of coronary stenosis after thrombolysis in acute myocardial infarction: results of a randomized study of anistreplase and streptokinase (abstract), *J Am Coll Cardiol* 15 (suppl A):218A, 1990.
11. The GUSTO Angiographic investigators: The effects of tissue plasminogen activator, streptokinase, or both on coronary-artery patency, ventricular function, and survival after acute myocardial infarction, *N Engl J Med* 329:1615-1622, 1993.
11a. The GUSTO investigators: An international randomized trial comparing four thrombolytic strategies for acute myocardial infarction, *N Engl J Med* 329:673-682, 1993.
12. Chesebro JH, Knatterud G, Roberts R, et al: Thrombolysis in myocardial infarction (TIMI) trial, phase I: a comparison between intravenous tissue plasminogen activator and intravenous streptokinase: clinical findings through hospital discharge, *Circulation* 76:142-154, 1987.
13. White H: GISSI-2 and the heparin controversy, *Lancet* 336:297-298, 1990.
14. PRIMI trial study group: Randomised double-blind trial of recombinant pro-urokinase against streptokinase in acute myocardial infarction, *Lancet* 1:863-868, 1989.
15. Kwon K-I, Freedman B, Wilcox I, et al: The unstable ST segment early after thrombolysis for acute infarction and its usefulness as a marker of recurrent coronary occlusion, *Am J Cardiol* 67:109-115, 1991.
16. Anderson JL, Becker LC, Sorensen SG, et al for the TEAM-3 investigators: Anistreplase versus alteplase in acute myocardial infarction: comparative effects on left ventricular function, morbidity and 1-day coronary artery patency, *J Am Coll Cardiol* 20:753-766, 1992.
17. Neuhaus KL, von Essen R, Tebbe U, et al: Improved thrombolysis in acute myocardial infarction with front-loaded administration of alteplase: results of the rt-PA-APSAC patency study (TAPS), *J Am Coll Cardiol* 19:885-891, 1992.
18. White HD, Norris RM, Brown MA, et al: Effect of intravenous streptokinase on left ventricular function and early survival after acute myocardial infarction, *N Engl J Med* 317:850-855, 1987.
19. Simoons ML, Serruys PW, van den Brand M, et al: Improved survival after early thrombolysis in acute myocardial infarction, *Lancet* 2:578-581, 1985.
20. White HD: Relation of thrombolysis during acute myocardial infarction to left ventricular function and mortality, *Am J Cardiol* 66:92-95, 1990.
21. Sheehan FH, Doerr R, Schmidt WG: Early recovery of left ventricular function after thrombolytic therapy for acute myocardial infarction: an important determinant of survival, *J Am Coll Cardiol* 12:289-300, 1988.
22. Simoons ML, Vos J, Tijssen JGP, et al: Long-term benefit of early thrombolytic therapy in patients with acute myocardial infarction: 5-year follow-up of a trial conducted by the Interuniversity Cardiology Institute of the Netherlands, *J Am Coll Cardiol* 14:1609-1615, 1989.
23. Topol EJ, Califf RM, George BS, et al: Insights derived from the thrombolysis and angioplasty in myocardial infarction (TAMI) trials, *J Am Coll Cardiol* 12:24A-31A, 1988.
24. Flygenring BP, Althouse RG, Sheehan FH, et al: Does vessel patency at the time of hospital discharge following thrombolytic therapy predict survival? (abstract), *J Am Coll Cardiol* 15:202A, 1990.
25. Zaret BL, Wackers FJ, Terrin M, et al and the TIMI investigators: Does left ventricular ejection fraction following thrombolytic therapy have the same prognostic impact described in the prethrombolytic era? Results of the TIMI II trial (abstract), *J Am Coll Cardiol* 17:214A, 1991.
26. Muller OW, Topol EJ, George BS, et al and the Thrombolysis and Angioplasty in Myocardial Infarction study group: Long-term follow-up in the thrombolysis and angioplasty in myocardial infarction (TAMI) trials: comparison with trials of thrombolysis alone (abstract), *Circulation* 80 (suppl II): 2068, 1980.
27. Serruys PW, Simoons ML, Suryapranata H, et al: Preservation of

global and regional left ventricular function after early thrombolysis in acute myocardial infarction, *J Am Coll Cardiol* 7:729-742, 1986.

28. Van de Werf F, Arnold AER, for the European cooperative study group for recombinant tissue type plasminogen activator (rt-PA): Intravenous tissue plasminogen activator and size of infarct, left ventricular function, and survival in acute myocardial infarction, *Br Med J* 297:1374-1379, 1988.

29. White HD, Norris RM, Brown MA, et al: Left ventricular end-systolic volume as the major determinant of survival after recovery from myocardial infarction, *Circulation* 76:44-51, 1987.

30. ISAM study group: A prospective trial of intravenous streptokinase in acute myocardial infarction (ISAM): mortality, morbidity and infarct size at 21 days, *N Engl J Med* 314:1465-1471, 1986.

31. Kennedy JW, Martin GV, Davis KB, et al: The western Washington intravenous streptokinase in acute myocardial infarction randomized trial, *Circulation* 77:345-352, 1988.

32. Bassand J-P, Faivre R, Becque O, et al: Effects of early high-dose streptokinase intravenously on left ventricular function in acute myocardial infarction, *Am J Cardiol* 60:435-439, 1987.

33. Guerci AD, Gerstenblith G, Brinker JA, et al: A randomized trial of intravenous tissue plasminogen activator for acute myocardial infarction with subsequent randomization to elective coronary angioplasty, *N Engl J Med* 317:1613-1618, 1987.

34. O'Rourke M, Baron D, Keogh A, et al: Limitation of myocardial infarction by early infusion of recombinant tissue-type plasminogen activator, *Circulation* 77:1311-1315, 1988.

35. National Heart Foundation of Australia Coronary Thrombolysis Group: Coronary thrombolysis and myocardial salvage by tissue plasminogen activator given up to 4 hours after onset of myocardial infarction, *Lancet* 1:203-208, 1988.

36. Armstrong PW, Baigrie RS, Daly PA, et al: Tissue plasminogen activator: Toronto (TPAT) placebo-controlled randomized trial in acute myocardial infarction, *J Am Coll Cardiol* 13:1469-1476, 1989.

37. Bassand JP, Machecourt J, Cassagnes J, et al: Multicenter trial of intravenous anisoylated plasminogen streptokinase activator complex (APSAC) in acute myocardial infarction: effects on infarct size and left ventricular function, *J Am Coll Cardiol* 13:988-997, 1989.

38. Kopia GA, Kopaciewicz LJ, Ruffolo RR Jr: Coronary thrombolysis with intravenous streptokinase in the anesthetized dog: a dose-response study, *J Pharmacol Exp Ther* 244:956-962, 1988.

39. Brogden RN, Speight TM, Avery GS: Streptokinase: a review of its clinical pharmacology, mechanism of action and therapeutic uses, *Drugs* 5:357-445, 1973.

40. Arntz R, Heitz J, Schäfer H, et al: Hemorrheology in acute myocardial infarction: effects of high-dose intravenous streptokinase, *Circulation* 72:III-417, 1985.

41. Moriarty AJ, Hughes R, Nelson SD, et al: Streptokinase and reduced plasma viscosity: a second benefit, *Eur J Haemol* 41:25-36, 1988.

42. White HD, Rivers JT, Maslowski AH, et al: Effect of intravenous streptokinase as compared with that of tissue plasminogen activator on left ventricular function after first myocardial infarction, *N Engl J Med* 320:817-821, 1989.

43. Gruppo Italiano per lo Studio della Sopravvivenza nell'Infarto Miocardico: GISSI-2: a factorial randomised trial of alteplase versus streptokinase and heparin versus no heparin among 12,490 patients with acute myocardial infarction, *Lancet* 336:65-71, 1990.

44. Machecourt J, Cassagnes J, Bassand JP, et al: Results of a randomized trial comparing APSAC and rtPA for the preservation of left ventricular function after acute myocardial infarction (abstract), *J Am Coll Cardiol* 15:214A, 1990.

45. International study group: In-hospital mortality and clinical course of 20,891 patients with suspected acute myocardial infarction randomised between alteplase and streptokinase with or without heparin, *Lancet* 336:71-75, 1990.

46. ISIS-3 (Third International Study of Infarct Survival) collaborative group: a randomised comparison of streptokinase vs. tissue plasminogen activator vs. anistreplase and of aspirin plus heparin vs. aspirin alone among 41,299 cases of suspected acute myocardial infarction, *Lancet* 339:1-18, 1992.

47. Marder VJ: The use of thrombolytic agents: choice of patient, drug administration, laboratory monitoring, *Ann Int Med* 90:802-808, 1979.

48. ISIS-2 (Second International Study of Infarct Survival) collaborative group: Randomised trial of intravenous streptokinase, oral aspirin, both, or neither among 17,187 cases of suspected acute myocardial infarction, *Lancet* 2:349-360, 1988.

49. Gruppo Italiano per lo Studio della Streptochinasi nell'Infarto Miocardico (GISSI): Effectiveness of intravenous thrombolytic treatment in acute myocardial infarction, *Lancet* 1:397-402, 1986.

50. Melandri G, Branzi A, Semprini F, et al: Enhanced thrombolytic efficacy and reduction of infarct size by simultaneous infusion of streptokinase and heparin, *Br Heart J* 64:118-120, 1990.

51. Col J, Decoster O, Hanique G, et al: Infusion of heparin conjunct to streptokinase accelerates reperfusion of acute myocardial infarction: results of a double blind randomized study (OSIRIS) (abstract), *Circulation* 86:I-259, 1992.

52. Lynch M, Littler WA, Pentecost BL, et al: Immunoglobulin response to intravenous streptokinase in acute myocardial infarction, *Br Heart J* 66:139-142, 1991.

53. Elliott JM, Cross DB, Cederholm-Williams SA, et al: Neutralizing antibodies to streptokinase four years after intravenous thrombolytic therapy, *Am J Cardiol* 71:640-645, 1993.

54. Fibrinolytic therapy trialists' (FTT) collaborative group: Indications for fibrinolytic therapy in suspected acute myocardial infarction: collaborative overview of results on mortality and major morbidity from the randomised trials of more than 1000 patients, *Lancet* 343:311-322, 1994.

55. White HD: Thrombolytic therapy for patients with myocardial infarction presenting after six hours, *Lancet* 340:221-222, 1992.

56. The LATE steering committee: Late assessment of thrombolytic efficacy (LATE) study with alteplase 6-24 hours after onset of acute myocardial infarction, *Lancet* 342:759-766, 1993.

57. EMERAS (Estudio Multicentrico Estreptoquinasa Republicas de America del Sur) collaborative group: Randomised trial of late thrombolysis in patients with suspected acute myocardial infarction, *Lancet* 342:767-772, 1993.

Chapter 26

PRIMARY ANGIOPLASTY FOR ACUTE MYOCARDIAL INFARCTION

Robert A. Harrington
Robert M. Califf
Harry R. Phillips
Daniel B. Mark

The landmark observation by DeWood et al. that acute myocardial infarction (AMI) was caused by acute coronary thrombosis[1] led to trials of intracoronary thrombolysis for the treatment of acute infarction.[2] Although intracoronary thrombolytic therapy was effective in achieving coronary patency, the necessity for acute cardiac catheterization made its widespread use appear to be impractical. International megatrials subsequently showed that intravenous thrombolytic therapy was effective in reducing mortality in AMI.[3,4] More recently the GUSTO-I (Global Utilization of Streptokinase and t-PA for Occluded Coronary Arteries) trial has shown that the combination of accelerated t-PA, intravenous heparin, and aspirin is associated with a low mortality rate (6.3% at 30 days) and acceptable stroke rate (1.55%).[5] Perhaps most impressively, the GUSTO-I trial clarified the importance of achieving rapid and complete perfusion, demonstrating that TIMI grade 3 flow in the infarct-related artery was the critical determinant of survival.[6]

Immediate infarct vessel angioplasty for patients with AMI has been reported in multiple observational studies over the past decade. With a better understanding of the importance of achieving optimal reperfusion, the potential to use primary percutaneous transluminal coronary angioplasty (PTCA) to treat patients with AMI has become more appealing. Recently several randomized but small clinical trials have suggested benefit from an immediate PTCA strategy compared with thrombolytic therapy in patients with AMI. This chapter will critically review the practical implications of the use of primary coronary angioplasty to achieve early and sustained reperfusion for AMI.

THROMBOLYTIC LIMITATIONS

Although use of intravenous thrombolytic therapy has revolutionized the treatment of AMI, significant limitations remain. Despite increasing data that document the safety of thrombolytic therapy, significant numbers of AMI patients do not receive treatment either because of true contraindications to therapy or due to physician preference. Often the patient has an array of relative contraindications, none of which alone would dissuade the clinician from using thrombolytic therapy, but which when taken together constitute an excessive risk of bleeding. Additionally, although more aggressive thrombolytic strategies result in very high patency rates, a significant minority of patients, perhaps 10% to 20%, fail to achieve acute reperfusion and have worse clinical outcomes.[7] After successful reperfusion occurs, and despite treatment with heparin and aspirin, patients remain at risk for recurrent ischemia and reinfarction.[8]

Califf et al. have recently reported that recurrent ischemia even without infarction is associated with worse clinical outcomes and a more expensive hospital course.[9] In a separate analysis of the Thrombolysis and Angioplasty in Myocardial Infarction (TAMI) population Ohman et al. have shown that reocclusion commonly follows thrombolysis and is associated with a substantial increase in morbidity and mortality.[10] Finally, the main limitation of thrombolytic therapy is bleeding; the most feared complication, intracranial hemorrhage, occurs in 0.20% to 0.94% of patients.[11,12]

OVERVIEW OF PTCA IN AMI

Primary coronary angioplasty should not be confused with angioplasty in conjunction with thrombolytic therapy. As reviewed in Chapter 34, early angioplasty after successful reperfusion is not beneficial and may be detrimental. Deferred angioplasty before hospital discharge has been examined in multiple clinical trials[13-15] without evidence of substantial benefit. It should be noted, however, that these were trials of automatic PTCA in patients with reperfusion but without regard to other clinical parameters, such as the number of diseased vessels, evidence of recurrent ischemia, or status of functional testing. When thrombolytic reperfusion fails, "rescue" angioplasty to establish perfusion appears to be beneficial, especially when the size of the infarction is large (see Chapter 27). The results with direct angioplasty appear to be much more promising than these other applications. The milieu of the infarct vessel following treatment with thrombolytic therapy may explain some of the discrepancy between the results of salvage PTCA versus primary PTCA. Thrombolytic therapy probably disrupts the ruptured plaque with superimposed thrombus, and may cause hemorrhage under the plaque, making PTCA a less beneficial endeavor. The ongoing lytic state may also contribute to other adverse procedural outcomes, like bleeding.

PRIMARY PTCA FOR AMI

The early perceived potential advantages of primary PTCA over thrombolytic therapy for the treatment of AMI included treatment of patients with thrombolytic contraindications, early confirmation of the diagnosis, ability to achieve high initial patency rates, and a decreased risk of bleeding complications, including intracranial hemorrhage. Whether these perceived advantages would translate into an improvement in left ventricular function and more important, in mortality, was uncertain. A number of single-center observational studies have been reported and are summarized in Table 26-1.[16-28] Taken together, these trials suggested that primary PTCA for AMI results in a high initial success rate, a low reocclusion rate, and a dramatic improvement in left ventricular function. The mortality rates were

Table 26-1. PTCA success and in-hospital deaths in studies of primary PTCA

Study	Patients	Deaths (%)	PTCA success (%)
O'Neill et al.[16]	29	7	83
Hartzler et al.[17]	442	8	93
Kimura et al.[18]	58	—	88
Flaker et al.[19]	93	14	—
Marco et al.[20]	43	14	95
Ellis et al.[21]	271	13	—
Rothbaum et al.[22]	151	9	87
Brodie et al.[23]	383	9	>90
Bittl[24]	20	9	>90
Kahn et al.[25]	614	8	>90
Beauchamp, Vacek, and Robuck[26]	214	8	>90
Williams et al.[27]	226	5	>90
Topol et al.[28]	47	6	86

acceptable, although their interpretation was clouded by the reported inclusion of a disproportionate number of patients with marked hemodynamic compromise compared with contemporaneous thrombolytic trials.

These single-center studies did not address whether the majority of AMI patients would be eligible for this treatment; only patients with an attempted angioplasty were reported, and patients in whom angioplasty was judged not to be feasible after the performance of an emergency angiogram were not included in these studies. The likelihood of achieving the same results in a multicenter study was uncertain because the centers reporting excellent results were technically expert. Whether the high initial angiographic success would translate into a mortality benefit could only be addressed by a carefully controlled trial. None of these studies addressed the restenosis rate or the relative economic costs of direct PTCA.

PRIMARY PTCA FOR AMI: RECENT RANDOMIZED CLINICAL TRIALS

Four recently published randomized trials compared primary PTCA with thrombolytic therapy for the treatment of AMI. The strategies and endpoints are summarized in Table 26-2. Grines et al., in the Primary Angioplasty in Myocardial Infarction (PAMI) trial, randomized 395 patients who were within 12 hours of their infarct onset to treatment with single-chain t-PA (alteplase, 100 mg/3 hours) or to acute cardiac catheterization and primary angioplasty.[29] A composite of death, reinfarction, and recurrent ischemia was the primary endpoint. Compared with a group that received thrombolytic therapy, the PAMI group reported a higher procedural success rate (97%), a lower combined incidence of reinfarction and death (5.1% vs. 12.0%, $P = 0.02$), and a significant decrease in intracranial

Table 26-2. Strategies in recent randomized trials of primary PTCA vs. thrombolysis

Trial	Patients	Thrombolytic agent	Primary endpoint
PAMI	395	t-PA	Death + Reinfarction + Recurrent Ischemia
Mayo	97	t-PA	Tc-sestamibi Infarct Size
Dutch	142	SK	MUGA LV Ejection Fraction

bleeding (0% vs. 2.0%, $P = 0.05$) in the PTCA arm. The Dutch group randomized 142 patients within 6 hours of infarction (24 hours if active ischemia) to streptokinase (1.5 million units/1 hour) or primary PTCA.[30] The study's primary endpoints (recurrent ischemia, radionuclide left ventricular ejection fraction, and infarct-vessel patency) all strongly favored PTCA over thrombolytic therapy. The Mayo group randomized 108 patients within 12 hours of infarction to double-chain t-PA (duteplase, 0.6 million units/kg/4 hours) or primary PTCA.[31] There was no difference between treatment groups in the change in sestamibi-determined myocardial perfusion defect, the study's primary endpoint. The major clinical endpoints of the trials are outlined in Table 26-3, along with the pooled odds ratios of these outcomes in patients treated with direct angioplasty vs. thrombolytic therapy. A recent trial reported from Brazil did not demonstrate such promising results.[32]

Although the aggregated results of these randomized prospective trials are dramatically positive for direct PTCA, the results should be interpreted with caution for several reasons. First, the studies, and in particular the PAMI and Dutch trials, were performed at sites with a strong interest in primary PTCA and a high degree of experience and expertise. Although a cursory analysis found no relationship between volume and outcome within PAMI, the sample sizes of these studies were inadequate for this purpose and none of the centers was low-volume by national standards; therefore, the generalizability of the results remains in question. Secondly, the markedly positive results favoring PTCA are driven largely by the dramatic differences observed in the PAMI trial. The very low mortality and absence of stroke in the PTCA group and the high intracranial hemorrhage rate in the t-PA–treated group are much different from those of previous clinical trials, including the larger trials of thrombolytic therapy. Additionally, none of the PTCA trials compared the PTCA strategy with accelerated t-PA given with intravenous heparin, the thrombolytic regimen associated with the lowest mortality in GUSTO-I.

Finally, two large registries comparing PTCA with thrombolytic therapy for AMI have found a nonsignificant trend towards better outcomes with thrombolysis over a 1-year follow-up period.[33,34] In the state of Alabama, an ongoing registry (ARMI) provided a chance to evaluate community use of primary angioplasty in a contemporary population. The Myocardial Intervention and Triage Investigation (MITI) also provided complete baseline characteristics and follow-up of a cohort treated at experienced centers with primary angioplasty. The Alabama registry used multivariable analysis to adjust for baseline risk; the MITI investigators used a case-control design.

PRIMARY ANGIOPLASTY REGISTRY (PAR) TRIAL

Simultaneous with the performance of the four randomized primary PTCA trials, the Primary Angioplasty Registry (PAR) collected information on patients undergoing primary PTCA for AMI in a nonrandomized study involving six experienced, high-volume angioplasty sites.[35] All the data were prospectively collected and then audited, reviewed, and analyzed by an independent coordinating center. The PAR study is distinguished from most other primary PTCA studies in that it evaluated the *strategy* of primary PTCA rather than the results of actual attempted PTCA. Because the physician cannot know whether the patient will be suitable for PTCA when the decision to forego treatment with thrombolytic therapy has to be made, it is critical to understand the implications of a policy to go to cardiac catheterization with an intent to perform primary PTCA. Knowing the outcomes of only patients who were actually treated with primary PTCA would be misleading if patients taken to the catheterization laboratory and then excluded from the procedure had particularly bad outcomes.

Over a period of 19 months a total of 271 patients were enrolled in the PAR trial. Of these 271 patients, 245 (90%) actually underwent primary PTCA as treatment for MI. The reasons for not performing primary angioplasty are outlined in Figure 26-1, which demonstrates that the vast majority of patients presenting with symptoms compatible with AMI and ST-segment elevation will be candidates for primary angioplasty. Some patients will have severe multivessel disease that would be most suitable for coronary bypass grafting; early identification of such patients could be a major advantage of the primary PTCA strategy. Additionally, a small percentage of patients will not have an MI despite suggestive histories; electrocardiograms and the primary PTCA strategy can spare these patients the risk of thrombolytic therapy.

The median time from onset of chest pain to emergency room arrival was just under 2.5 hours. Median time from presentation in the emergency room

Table 26-3. Outcomes in recent randomized trials of direct PTCA vs. thrombolytic therapy (TT)

	PAMI		Mayo		Dutch		Total		Odds ratio*
	PTCA (n = 195)	TT (n = 200)	PTCA (n = 47)	TT (n = 50)	PTCA (n = 72)	TT (n = 70)	PTCA (n = 314)	TT (n = 320)	(95% CI)
Death	5	13	2	2	0	4	7	19	2.7 (1.2-6.4)
Reinfarction	5	8	0	2	0	9	5	19	5.0 (2.1-12)
Recurrent ischemia	20	56	—	—	6	27	26	83	4.1 (2.6-6.5)
Stroke	0	4	0	0	0	2	0	6	7.0 (0.8-57.6)
Transfusion	24	16	—	—	2	6	26	22	0.8 (0.5-1.5)

*Odds of outcome for thrombolytic therapy relative to direct PTCA.

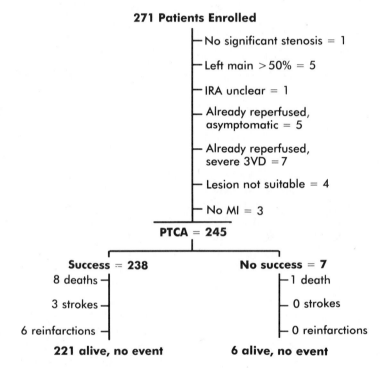

Fig. 26-1. Reasons for not performing primary PTCA in the Primary Angioplasty Registry (PAR) trial.

to the first angiogram was 1.3 hours, yielding a time from presentation to reperfusion similar to that of thrombolytic therapy—median time to treatment after emergency room arrival of more than 1 hour[36] plus average time from thrombolytic administration to reperfusion of 45 minutes.

Angiographic success (residual stenosis ≤ 50%), as determined by a core lab, was accomplished in 216 patients (88%) with 97% of all patients who underwent primary PTCA achieving TIMI grade 3 flow. This finding is particularly important in light of the recent report that TIMI grade 3 flow is associated with better clinical outcomes and greater left ventricular function preservation than TIMI grade 2 flow.[6] Rates of death, reinfarction, and recurrent ischemia were low, especially

when compared with previous trials of thrombolytic therapy (Table 26-4). The need for repeat invasive procedures was low, with only 5% of the patients with an initial successful procedure requiring repeat PTCA. The rate of bypass surgery was only 9%, comparing favorably with rates of 10% to 15% in most thrombolytic trials.[28,37-42] The risk of bleeding with primary PTCA was higher than anticipated, with transfusions being required in 18% of patients overall and in 14% of patients treated without bypass surgery.

Of the 271 patients enrolled in the trial, 6-month follow-up data were available on 267 (99%). Although recurrent angina and repeat PTCA were relatively common (22% and 16% in the overall population, 23% and 18% in the PTCA group), the rates of death, MI,

Table 26-4. In-hospital clinical outcomes from the primary angioplasty registry (PAR)

	No PTCA	Any PTCA	Total
Number of patients	26	245	271
Death	1(4%)	9(4%)	10(4%)
Reinfarction	1(4%)	6(2%)	7(3%)
Stroke			
Hemorrhagic	0	1(0.4%)	1(0.4%)
Nonhemorrhagic	0	2(0.8%)	2(0.7%)
Heart failure	9(35%)	46(19%)	55(20%)
Recurrent ischemia	2(8%)	24(10%)	26(10%)
Arrhythmias			
Ventricular fibrillation	3(12%)	17(7%)	20(7%)
Sustained VT	1(4%)	18(7%)	19(7%)
Supraventricular tachycardia*	5(19%)	35(14%)	40(15%)
Pericarditis	1(4%)	9(4%)	10(4%)
Respiratory failure	2(8%)	12(5%)	14(5%)
Dialysis	0	2(1%)	2(1%)

*PAT or A Fib/A Flutter

Table 26-5. Major hospital resource consumption and hospital costs in PAR and TAMI 5

	PAR	TAMI 5
	$N = 270$	$N = 575$
Total LOS (mean ± SD)	9.3 ± 7.4 days	12.3 ± 8.7 days
ICU/CCU LOS (mean ± SD)	5.5 ± 4.0 days	3.9 ± 4.5 days
Diagnostic catheterizations		
0	0%	1%
1	91%	64%
≥2	9%	35%
Revascularization pattern		
No PTCA/ CABG	5%	30%
PTCA only	85%	49%
CABG only	4%	17%
Both PTCA and CABG	6%	4%
Hospital costs		
Mean	$13,113	$18,357
Median	$10,548	$16,091
MD fees		
Mean	$5694	—
Median	$4907	—

Figures inflated to 1991 dollars. *LOS,* Length of stay.

bypass surgery, and heart failure were low. Restenosis rates ranged from 40% to 52%, depending on the definition used. Overall, the 6-month follow-up data show excellent clinical outcomes, which despite a substantial restenosis rate, suggest that relative to thrombolytic therapy the results of primary PTCA are likely to be sustained.

Because an important consideration in choosing primary PTCA over thrombolytic therapy for AMI therapy is cost, a detailed economics and quality-of-life (EQOL) substudy was carried out in the PAR trial. Of the patients enrolled in the overall study, 270 participated in the PAR EQOL substudy. In order to make a comparison with thrombolytic therapy, results from the 270 PAR EQOL patients were compared with those from the 575 patients participating in the TAMI 5 trial, a randomized trial involving a comparison of three thrombolytic regimens and two catheterization strategies in a 3 × 2 factorial design.[40] Baseline demographic and clinical outcomes were comparable in the two studies. Repeat angioplasty was more common in TAMI 5 (12% vs. 5%). Major hospital resource consumption and baseline medical costs are detailed in Table 26-5. The 6-month quality-of-life outcomes as measured by work status, general health status, functional status, and psychological status were similar between the two populations. Thus, these data suggest that primary PTCA in experienced centers can yield at least an equivalent

medical outcome to thrombolytic therapy and at a competitive cost.

PTCA IN CARDIOGENIC SHOCK

Despite the introduction of thrombolytic therapy for the treatment of AMI, the incidence of cardiogenic shock complicating AMI remains very high.[43] Although the mortality from cardiogenic shock remains unacceptably high, no clinical trial of thrombolytic therapy has had sufficient statistical power to detect a significant benefit of thrombolytic therapy in patients suffering from this complication. A number of small, single-center observational studies have reported marked improvement in survival in cardiogenic shock patients who have successful reperfusion of the infarct-related artery (IRA) with primary PTCA[21,23,44-51] (Table 26-6). These reports suffer from problems of retrospective review, varying definitions of cardiogenic shock, and selection bias in determining which patients were offered a more aggressive treatment strategy.[52] No randomized trial has been performed evaluating the strategy of early catheterization with immediate revascularization via either angioplasty or bypass surgery in these patients. Bengtson et al.[53] recently reported that in-hospital mortality from cardiogenic shock is strongly associated with patency of the IRA, with a mortality rate of 33% in patients with an open IRA compared to 75% when the vessel remains occluded. Despite the lack of definitive randomized

Table 26-6. Impact of coronary angioplasty on survival in cardiogenic shock

Reference	N	Overall survival (%)	Reperfusion (%)	Survival with reperfusion (%)	Survival without reperfusion (%)
O'Neill	27	70	88	75	33
Lee	24	50	54	83	25
Shani	9	66	66	83	0
Heuser	10	70	60	100	25
Brown	28	43	61	58	18
Brodie	22	50	68	NR	NR
Ellis	60	68	NR	NR	NR
O'Keefe	40	59	NR	NR	NR
Lee	69	55	71	69	20
Moosvi	38	NR	78	56	8
Total	327	59	64	73	22

NR = not reported.
(Reprinted from O'Neill WW: Angioplasty therapy of cardiogenic shock: are randomized trials necessary? *J Am Coll Cardiol* 19:915-917, 1992. With permission of the author and publisher.)

clinical trial evidence, the observational experience supports a strategy of early, aggressive intervention and revascularization in patients suffering from cardiogenic shock.

LIMITATIONS OF PRIMARY PTCA

Only a limited number of hospitals in the United States have the facilities and staff to perform coronary angioplasty. An even smaller percentage have the ability to perform primary PTCA on a 24-hour basis.[54] With the accumulating evidence that procedural outcome is strongly associated with procedural volume,[55] it is difficult to support universal application of a primary PTCA strategy when many centers will not be able to maintain the requisite experience to perform the procedure safely. In large centers with experienced operators and staff, primary PTCA, when feasible, seems to be a reasonable choice for the treatment of AMI; however, when the catheterization lab is not immediately available or a less experienced operator is on call, the value of primary PTCA is much less certain, whereas the benefits of thrombolytic therapy in even less sophisticated environments have been documented. This issue will become even more complex when prehospital diagnosis and therapy are possible. Finally, although the cost of primary PTCA may be comparable with that of thrombolysis on a per-patient basis, the cost of building more angioplasty facilities is substantial. This fixed cost cannot be ignored from a health-policy perspective and results of the studies to date do not justify such expansion of facilities for invasive cardiac care.

PATIENT SELECTION AND TECHNICAL CONSIDERATIONS IN PRIMARY ANGIOPLASTY

There are few absolute contraindications to primary angioplasty. Primary angioplasty should not be performed without surgical backup, especially if the patient is a good candidate for thrombolytic therapy. In selected circumstances when two hospitals are in close proximity, a carefully orchestrated plan for surgical backup at a second hospital has been shown to be effective.[56] Active bleeding that prohibits the use of high-dose heparin (i.e., to yield an ACT > 350 seconds) is a contraindication to either primary angioplasty or thrombolytic therapy. Patients with known severe peripheral vascular disease that is likely to limit vascular access options should be considered for thrombolytic therapy instead of primary PTCA. Patients with contraindications to thrombolytic therapy should be considered for primary PTCA, as should patients in whom the diagnosis is uncertain.

Because the goal of AMI treatment is the rapid restoration of infarct vessel blood flow, any delays in the ability to proceed immediately to the catheterization laboratory argues in favor of administering thrombolytic therapy. During working hours, when the catheterization laboratory and experienced angiographers are readily available, primary PTCA may be the preferred treatment of the AMI patient. At other times the decision to proceed to the laboratory and forgo thrombolytic therapy is more difficult. If the delay in moving to the laboratory will be more than 60 minutes, we believe that thrombolytic therapy is the preferred treatment option. In the absence of experienced and dedicated personnel, thrombolytic therapy is always preferred unless a contraindication to its use exists.

In preparation for the interventional procedure, the patient should be treated with oxygen, weight-adjusted heparin (we typically use a 65 units/kg IV bolus followed by a 17 units/kg/hr infusion), aspirin, intravenous nitrates, and intravenous beta blockade, if not contraindicated. Hypotension (systolic blood pressure ≤ 90 mm Hg) should be treated with volume repletion and vasopressor agents such as dopamine to help maintain coronary perfusion pressure. Diphenhydramine is given to minimize the risk of contrast dye reactions. Speed in moving to the interventional laboratory is critical, since outcome is probably a reflection of time to reperfusion, as with thrombolytic therapy. In general the emergency department staff should be preparing the patient for the procedure while the cardiologist and angiographic support team are in transit to the laboratory. Inordinate amounts of time spent attempting to achieve hemodynamic stability are inappropriate because the best treatment for hypotension in this setting is restoration of myocardial blood flow.

In the interventional laboratory, an intraaortic balloon pump should be placed in those patients who are hemodynamically unstable. Femoral access is obtained in both the artery and the vein. Venous access allows central delivery of medications, volume replacement, and emergency pacemaker placement. We do not routinely place prophylactic pacemakers before performing primary PTCA except in shock patients. Coronary arteriography is performed in the standard fashion. We first image the non-infarct vessel so as to have the anatomic information available if emergency bypass surgery becomes necessary during angioplasty of the infarct vessel, using 6- or 7-French diagnostic catheters, and then proceed to the suspected infarct-related artery using 7- or 8-French guiding catheters to minimize the time to attempt PTCA. Once diagnostic images have been obtained and the infarct vessel is proven to be occluded and suitable for PTCA, we cross and dilate the lesion using an appropriate over-the-wire balloon catheter system. In the acute setting we prefer 1- to 3-minute balloon inflations in an attempt to restore perfusion rapidly. Prolonged dilations (15 to 60 minutes) can be useful in the treatment of dissections and abrupt closure.[57] The decision as to the timing of the ventriculogram must be individualized to the clinical situation. We typically perform this after the angioplasty as the final stage of the procedure, but a ventriculogram can and should be performed before attempted PTCA if there is any question of a mechanical complication, such as acute mitral regurgitation or ventricular septal rupture, that may influence treatment strategies. Post-procedure sheaths should remain in place overnight, and anticoagulation with heparin should be continued to maintain an activated partial thromboplastin time (aPTT) of 60 to 85 seconds.

Much controversy exists regarding the routine use of nonionic contrast agents during routine coronary arteriography and elective PTCA. Although the high-osmolality ionic agents are associated with more electrophysiological (bradycardia) and hemodynamic (peripheral vasodilatation and myocardial depression) abnormalities than the low-osmolality nonionic agents, studies to date have failed to demonstrate any difference among agents with regard to clinical outcomes.[58,59] One small study[60] has suggested that there is a higher rate of thrombus formation using nonionic contrast media during PTCA, but no study has shown any significant difference in clinical outcomes regardless of the agents used.[61] Because these patients are typically unstable we prefer to use low-osmolality nonionic contrast agents during acute catheterization and PTCA to minimize the hemodynamic effects of the ionic dyes. The cost-effectiveness of this approach needs to be studied more.[62]

The use of adjunctive medications in these patients centers on drugs to reduce ischemia, drugs to improve PTCA outcomes, and agents that have been associated with a mortality reduction in AMI. All patients should be treated with nitrates and β-blockers, if not contraindicated by heart failure, heart block, or coexisting reactive pulmonary disease. Aspirin is standard therapy in these patients, improving the outcome of PTCA and the mortality in AMI.[63] The aspirin-allergic patient can be treated with ticlopidine, although the full antiplatelet effects will not occur for several days.[64] During the procedure the activated clotting time (ACT) should be maintained at ≥ 350 seconds with heparin in an effort to reduce ischemic complications of PTCA.[65]

Upon completion of the procedure, consideration should be given to prophylactic intraaortic balloon pump (IABP) placement to reduce the incidence of reocclusion. Balloon counterpulsation is useful following salvage angioplasty, and current data support its routine use following primary PTCA.[66] We favor balloon pump use with any evidence of hemodynamic instability, a suboptimal angiographic result, or a large area of myocardium at risk of reocclusion (i.e., proximal left anterior descending artery infarct). The ongoing PAMI-2 trial is testing the strategy of routine IABP placement following direct PTCA in high-risk patients to improve ischemic outcomes.

RECOMMENDATIONS

To use acute catheterization and primary angioplasty routinely requires a strong commitment on the part of the entire interventional laboratory staff, from technicians to physicians. These patients often arrive with little warning and each patient with AMI can become critically ill and hemodynamically unstable. The entire staff must be trained to react quickly and appropriately so that the procedure can be performed effectively in a minimal amount of time. Patient outcome is related to the experience of the operator and the volume of the center. Minimal guidelines should be established to accredit hospitals and operators who desire to treat AMI patients with a primary PTCA strategy.

Recent data from the GUSTO-I trial demonstrate the importance of achieving early and rapid infarct vessel patency, and so it is difficult to justify a major health policy shift away from rapid treatment with thrombolytic therapy at the majority of acute-care hospitals. Particularly if a strategy of primary PTCA would require the patient to be transferred to a tertiary-care facility, the simplicity of thrombolytic therapy is attractive. In hospitals with technical capabilities and experienced operators, however, primary PTCA may well be the preferred treatment strategy for patients with AMI.

The ongoing GUSTO-II trial will address many of these practical issues by randomizing 1200 patients with a compatible history and ST-segment elevation to direct angioplasty or thrombolytic therapy. The 50 centers participating in the trial represent a spectrum of large and small hospitals in the United States, Canada, and Europe. The minimal requirements for the performance of PTCA are those outlined by the American College of Cardiology/American Heart Association guidelines. If the results of this trial are as positive as the smaller trials described above, serious consideration will need to be given to increasing accessibility to institutions with these capabilities.

A strategy of acute catheterization, with its ability to define coronary anatomy, provide hemodynamic support, and delineate revascularization options, is especially appealing for patients with hemodynamic instability. Although we favor a primary PTCA strategy for patients with cardiogenic shock, more investigation needs to be done to define better what groups of patients may particularly benefit from such an aggressive approach.

REFERENCES

1. DeWood MA, Spores J, Notske R, et al: Prevalence of total coronary occlusion during the early hours of transmural myocardial infarction, *N Engl J Med* 303:897-902, 1980.
2. Rentrop KP, Feit F, Blanke H, et al: Effects of intracoronary streptokinase and intracoronary nitroglycerin infusion on coronary angiographic patterns and mortality in patients with acute myocardial infarction, *N Engl J Med* 311:1457-1463, 1984.
3. Gruppo Italiano per lo Studio della Streptochinasi nell'Infarto Miocardico (GISSI): Effectiveness of intravenous thrombolytic treatment in acute myocardial infarction, *Lancet* 1:397-402, 1986.
4. ISIS-2: Randomised trial of intravenous streptokinase, oral aspirin, both, or neither among 17,187 cases of suspected acute myocardial infarction: ISIS-2, *Lancet* 2:349-360, 1988.
5. The GUSTO Investigators: An international randomized trial comparing four thrombolytic strategies for acute myocardial infarction, *N Engl J Med* 329:673-682, 1993.
6. The GUSTO Angiographic Investigators: The effects of tissue plasminogen activator, streptokinase, or both on coronary-artery patency, ventricular function, and survival after acute myocardial infarction, *N Engl J Med* 329:1615-1622, 1993.
7. Granger CB, Califf RM, Topol EJ: Thrombolytic therapy for acute myocardial infarction: a review, *Drugs* 44:293-325, 1992.
8. Muller DW, Topol EJ, Ellis SG, et al: Determinants of the need for early acute intervention in patients treated conservatively after thrombolytic therapy for acute myocardial infarction—TAMI-5 Study Group, *J Am Coll Cardiol* 18:1594-1601, 1991.
9. Califf RM, Topol EJ, Ohman EM, et al: Isolated recurrent ischemia after thrombolytic therapy is a frequent, important and expensive adverse clinical outcome (abstract), *J Am Coll Cardiol* 19:301A, 1992.
10. Ohman EM, Califf RM, Topol EJ, et al: Consequences of reocclusion after successful reperfusion therapy in acute myocardial infarction—TAMI Study Group, *Circulation* 82:781-791, 1990.
11. Califf RM, Fortin DF, Tenaglia AN, et al: Clinical risks of thrombolytic therapy, *Am J Cardiol* 69:12A-20A, 1992.
12. Sane DC, Califf RM, Topol EJ, et al: Bleeding during thrombolytic therapy for acute myocardial infarction: mechanisms and management, *Ann Intern Med* 111:1010-1022, 1989.
13. TIMI Study Group: Comparison of invasive and conservative strategies after treatment with intravenous tissue plasminogen activator in acute myocardial infarction. Results of the thrombolysis in myocardial infarction (TIMI) phase II trial, *N Engl J Med* 320:618-627, 1989.
14. SWIFT Group: SWIFT trial of delayed elective intervention versus conservative treatment after thrombolysis with anistreplase in acute myocardial infarction, *Br Med J* 302:555-560, 1991.
15. Barbash GI, Roth A, Hod H, et al: Randomized controlled trial of late in-hospital angiography and angioplasty versus conservative management after treatment with recombinant tissue-type plasminogen activator in acute myocardial infarction, *Am J Cardiol* 66:538-545, 1990.
16. O'Neill W, Timmis GC, Bourdillon PD, et al: A prospective randomized clinical trial of intracoronary streptokinase versus coronary angioplasty for acute myocardial infarction, *N Engl J Med* 314:812-818, 1986.
17. Hartzler GO, Rutherford BD, McConahay DR, et al: Percutaneous transluminal coronary angioplasty with and without thrombolytic therapy for treatment of acute myocardial infarction, *Am Heart J* 106:965-973, 1983.
18. Kimura T, Nosaka H, Ueno K, et al: Role of coronary angioplasty in acute myocardial infarction (abstract), *Circulation* 74(suppl I):II-22, 1986.
19. Flaker GC, Webel RR, Meinhardt S, et al: Emergency angioplasty in acute anterior myocardial infarction, *Am Heart J* 118:1154-1160, 1989.
20. Marco J, Caster L, Szatmary LJ, et al: Emergency percutaneous transluminal coronary angioplasty without thrombolysis as initial therapy in acute myocardial infarction, *Int J Cardiol* 15:55-63, 1987.
21. Ellis SG, O'Neill WW, Bates ER, et al: Coronary angioplasty as primary therapy for acute myocardial infarction 6 to 48 hours after symptom onset: report of an initial experience, *J Am Coll Cardiol* 13;1122-1126, 1989.
22. Rothbaum DA, Hodes ZI, Linnemeier TJ, et al: Percutaneous transluminal coronary angioplasty for acute myocardial infarction, *Cardiol Clin* 7:837-851, 1989.
23. Brodie BR, Weintraub RA, Stuckey TD, et al: Outcomes of direct coronary angioplasty for acute myocardial infarction in candidates and noncandidates for thrombolytic therapy, *Am J Cardiol* 67:7-12, 1991.
24. Bittl JA: Indications, timing, and optimal technique for diagnostic angiography and angioplasty in acute myocardial infarction, *Chest* 99:150S-156S, 1991.
25. Kahn JK, Rutherford BD, McConahay DR, et al: Results of primary angioplasty for acute myocardial infarction in patients with multivessel coronary artery disease, *J Am Coll Cardiol* 16:1089-1096, 1990.
26. Beauchamp GD, Vacek JL, Robuck W: Management comparison for acute myocardial infarction: direct angioplasty versus sequential thrombolysis-angioplasty, *Am Heart J* 120:237-242, 1990.
27. Williams DO, Holubkov AL, Detre KM, et al: Impact of pretreatment by thrombolytic therapy upon outcome of emergent direct coronary angioplasty for patients with acute myocardial infarction (abstract), *J Am Coll Cardiol* 17:337A, 1991.

28. Topol EJ, Califf RM, George BS, et al: A randomized trial of immediate versus delayed elective angioplasty after intravenous tissue plasminogen activator in acute myocardial infarction, *N Engl J Med* 317:581-588, 1987.

29. Grines CL, Browne KF, Marco J, et al: A comparison of immediate angioplasty with thrombolytic therapy for acute myocardial infarction—the Primary Angioplasty in Myocardial Infarction Study Group, *N Engl J Med* 328:673-679, 1993.

30. Zijlstra F, de Boer MJ, Hoorntje JC, et al: A comparison of immediate coronary angioplasty with intravenous streptokinase in acute myocardial infarction, *N Engl J Med* 328:680-684, 1993.

31. Gibbons RJ, Holmes DR, Reeder GS, et al: Immediate angioplasty compared with the administration of a thrombolytic agent followed by conservative treatment for myocardial infarction—the Mayo Coronary Care Unit and Catheterization Laboratory Groups, *N Engl J Med* 328:685-691, 1993.

32. Ribeiro EE, Silva LA, Carneiro R, et al: Randomized trial of direct coronary angioplasty versus intravenous streptokinase in acute myocardial infarction, *J Am Coll Cardiol* 22:376-380, 1993.

33. Taylor HA, Wool KJ, Burgard SL, et al: Race and treatment strategy in acute myocardial ischemia (abstract), *Circulation* 86(suppl I):I-196, 1992.

34. Maynard C, Litwin PE, Martin JS, et al: Treatment and outcome of acute myocardial infarction in women 75 years and older: results from the MITI Registry (abstract), *Circulation* 86(suppl I):I-196, 1992.

35. O'Neill WW, Brodie BR, Ivanhoe R, et al: Primary coronary angioplasty for acute myocardial infarction (The Primary Angioplasty Registry), *Am J Cardiol* 73:627-634, 1994.

36. Kline EM, Smith DD, Martin JS, et al: In-hospital treatment delays in patients treated with thrombolytic therapy: a report of the GUSTO time to treatment substudy (abstract), *Circulation* 86(suppl I):I-702, 1992.

37. Topol EJ, Califf RM, George BS, et al: Coronary arterial thrombolysis with combined infusion of recombinant tissue-type plasminogen activator and urokinase in patients with acute myocardial infarction, *Circulation* 77:1100-1107, 1988.

38. Topol EJ, George BS, Kereiakes DJ, et al: A randomized controlled trial of intravenous tissue plasminogen activator and early intravenous heparin in acute myocardial infarction, *Circulation* 79:281-286, 1989.

39. Topol EJ, Ellis SG, Califf RM, et al: Combined tissue-type plasminogen activator and prostacyclin therapy for acute myocardial infarction. Thrombolysis and Angioplasty in Myocardial Infarction (TAMI) 4 Study Group, *J Am Coll Cardiol* 14:877-884, 1989.

40. Califf RM, Topol EJ, Stack RS, et al: Evaluation of combination thrombolytic therapy and timing of cardiac catheterization in acute myocardial infarction. Results of thrombolysis and angioplasty in myocardial infarction—phase 5 randomized trial. TAMI Study Group, *Circulation* 83:1543-1556, 1991.

41. Topol EJ, Califf RM, Vandormael M, et al: A randomized trial of late reperfusion therapy for acute myocardial infarction. Thrombolysis and Angioplasty in Myocardial Infarction-6 Study Group, *Circulation* 85:2090-2099, 1992.

42. Williams DO, Topol EJ, Califf RM, et al: Intravenous recombinant tissue-type plasminigen activator in patients with unstable angina pectoris: results of a placebo-controlled randomized trial, *Am J Cardiol* 65:124-131, 1990.

43. Goldberg RJ, Gore JM, Alpert JS, et al: Cardiogenic shock after acute myocardial infarction: incidence and mortality from a community-wide perspective, 1975 to 1988, *N Engl J Med* 325:1117-1122, 1991.

44. O'Neill W, Topol E, George B, et al: Improvement in left ventricular function after thrombolytic therapy and angioplasty: results of the TAMI study (abstract), *Circulation* 76(suppl IV):IV-259, 1987.

45. Lee L, Bates E, Pitt B, et al: Percutaneous transluminal coronary angioplasty improves survival in acute myocardial infarction complicated by cardiogenic shock, *Circulation* 78:1345-1351, 1988.

46. Shani J, Rivera M, Greengart A, et al: Percutaneous transluminal coronary angioplasty in cardiogenic shock, *J Am Coll Cardiol* 7:149A, 1986. (abstract)

47. Heuser R, Maddoux G, Gross J, et al: Coronary angioplasty in the treatment of cardiogenic shock: the therapy of choice (abstract), *J Am Coll Cardiol* 7:219A, 1986.

48. Brown T, Gordon D, Wheeler W, et al: Percutaneous myocardial reperfusion (PMR) reduces mortality in acute myocardial infarction (MI) complicated by cardiogenic shock (abstract), *Circulation* 72(suppl III):III-309, 1985.

49. O'Keefe JH, Rutherford BD, McConahay DR, et al: Early and late results of coronary angioplasty without antecedent thrombolytic therapy for acute myocardial infarction, *Am J Cardiol* 64:1221-1230, 1989.

50. Lee L, Erbel R, Brown TM, et al: Multicenter registry of angioplasty therapy of cardiogenic shock: initial and long-term survival, *J Am Coll Cardiol* 17:599-603, 1991.

51. Moosvi AR, Khaja F, Villanueva L, et al: Early revascularization improves survival in cardiogenic shock complicating acute myocardial infarction, *J Am Coll Cardiol* 19:907-914, 1992.

52. O'Neill WW: Angioplasty therapy of cardiogenic shock: are randomized trials necessary? *J Am Coll Cardiol* 19:915-917, 1992.

53. Bengtson JR, Kaplan AJ, Pieper KS, et al: Prognosis in cardiogenic shock after acute myocardial infarction in the interventional era, *J Am Coll Cardiol* 20:1482-1489, 1992.

54. Lange RA, Hillis LD: Immediate angioplasty for acute myocardial infarction, *N Engl J Med* 328:726-728, 1993.

55. Jollis JG, DeLong ER, Collins SR, et al: The relationship between angioplasty volume and outcome in the elderly in the Medicare database (abstract), *Circulation* 88:I-480, 1993.

56. Weaver WD, Litwin PE, Maynard C: Primary angioplasty for AMI performed in hospitals with and without on-site surgical backup (abstract), *Circulation* 84(suppl II):II-526, 1991.

57. Jackman JD, Jr, Zidar JP, Tcheng JE, et al: Outcome after prolonged balloon inflations of greater than 20 minutes for initially unsuccessful percutaneous transluminal coronary angioplasty, *Am J Cardiol* 69:1417-1421, 1992.

58. Davidson CJ, Mark DB, Pieper KS, et al: Thrombotic and cardiovascular complications related to nonionic contrast media during cardiac catheterization: analysis of 8,517 patients, *Am J Cardiol* 65:1481-1484, 1990.

59. Brogan WC, Hillis LD, Lange RA: Contrast agents for cardiac catheterization: conceptions and misconceptions, *Am Heart J* 122:1129-1135, 1991.

60. Gasperetti CM, Feldman MD, Burwell LR, et al: Influence of contrast media on thrombus formation during coronary angioplasty, *J Am Coll Cardiol* 18:443-450, 1991.

61. Lembo NJ, King SB, Roubin GS, et al: Effects of nonionic versus ionic contrast media on complications of percutaneous transluminal coronary angioplasty, *Am J Cardiol* 67:1046-1050, 1991.

62. Hlatky MA: Economic evaluation of low osmolality contrast media, *J Am Coll Cardiol* 21:1710-1711, 1993.

63. Fuster V, Dyken ML, Vokonas PS, et al: Aspirin as a therapeutic agent in cardiovascular disease, *Circulation* 87:659-675, 1993.

64. Defreyn G, Bernat A, Delebassee D, et al: Pharmacology of ticlopidine: a review, *Semin Thromb Hemost* 15:159-166, 1989.

65. Narins CR, Hillegass WB Jr, Nelson CL, et al: Activated clotting time predicts abrupt closure risk during angioplasty, *J Am Coll Cardiol* (suppl)23:470A, 1994.

66. Ohman EM, George BS, White CJ, et al: The use of aortic counterpulsation to improve sustained coronary artery patency during myocardial infarction: results of a randomized trial (abstract), *J Am Coll Cardiol* 21:397A, 1993.

Chapter 27

RESCUE CORONARY ANGIOPLASTY: THE PRESENT STATUS

Stephen G. Ellis

There is now no dispute that treatment of patients with AMI with appropriately applied intravenous thrombolytic therapy decreases both short- and intermediate-term mortality by approximately 25%.[1-3] There is further evidence that restoration of brisk antegrade flow is the primary means by which this form of therapy is effective.[4,5] Yet the importance of achieving infarct artery patency at 90 minutes after treatment onset, which is the primary endpoint of many clinical trials, remains debatable for many patients who present relatively late (>4 hr) after infarction. This forms the basis for conjecture and disagreement about the cost-effective need for the strategy of rescue coronary angioplasty after failed thrombolytic therapy.

The means by which an infarct artery is opened, thrombolytic therapy or balloon angioplasty, appears to matter little when it comes to short- and long-term prognosis.[6] Therefore, when one is considering which patients might benefit most from a strategy of rescue angioplasty, it is worthwhile to consider which patients benefit most from thrombolytic therapy: those with anterior MI (6% absolute reduction in in-hospital mortality), those with extensive inferior MI with "reciprocal" ST-segment depression in the anterior precordial ECG leads (5% absolute reduction in mortality), those presenting with left bundle branch block (4.4% absolute reduction in mortality), patients treated over the age of 64 (3% absolute reduction in mortality), and patients presenting within 6 hours of the onset of chest pain onset (2.7% absolute reduction in mortality).[7] Although treat-

ment benefit is also seen for patients with smaller inferior-wall MI, for those presenting 7 to 12 hours after chest pain onset, and for those under the age of 65, absolute benefit is more modest.[7]

POTENTIAL NEED FOR RESCUE ANGIOPLASTY

Based upon usage patterns of thrombolytic agents in 1990 it has been estimated that as many as 65,000 patients treated for conventional indications annually in the United States might require rescue PTCA because of a closed vessel 90 minutes following institution of therapy.[8] Further, many assert that thrombolytic therapy is underutilized in this country. The worldwide need is more difficult to ascertain. If, however, infarct artery patency achieved by 3 hours after treatment imparts the same benefit as patency achieved by 90 minutes, then the number of patients requiring rescue angioplasty would decrease appreciably.

RATIONALE FOR RESCUE ANGIOPLASTY

It is well established that the restitution of thrombolysis in myocardial infarction (TIMI) Grade 3 coronary flow in the infarct artery is associated with improved patient survival.[4] For example, the Thrombolysis in Angioplasty in Myocardial Infarction (TAMI) Study Group analyzed predictors of in-hospital mortality in the first three TAMI trials and found that patient age, left ventricular ejection fraction, the number of diseased vessels, and TIMI 3 flow correlated independently (*P* < 0.05) with in-hospital survival.[4] Importantly, infarct artery patency defined as TIMI 2 or 3 flow was not a significant predictor of outcome. These findings with regard to in-hospital mortality have been substantiated by the recent work of Vogt[9] and Simes et al.[10] Furthermore, even when TIMI 3 flow is established too late to affect improvement in left ventricular ejection fraction, complete reperfusion has been associated with improved 1-year survival compared with partial or no reperfusion ($P = 0.008$).[5] Second, even delayed reperfusion appears to improve infarct healing and to decrease infarct expansion. This has been demonstrated in several animal models, which concluded that left ventricular dimensions are improved by reperfusion established too late to decrease infarct size.[11,12] Third, reperfusion decreases the susceptibility of postinfarct patients to the occurrence of abnormal signal-averaged electrocardiograms[13] and electrophysiologic study-induced ventricular tachycardia or fibrillation,[14,15] thereby implying a reduced susceptibility to malignant ventricular arrhythmias causing sudden death. For example, in a relatively small study Kersschot found that patients randomized to streptokinase with reperfusion had only a 24% likelihood of developing ventricular tachycardia with two extra stimuli by a standard protocol compared with 79% of patients who were nonreperfused ($P < 0.001$).[15] Similarly, Sager et al. demonstrated that despite equal post-infarction left ventricular function, patients treated with thrombolytic therapy had an 8% incidence of inducible ventricular tachycardia compared with an 88% incidence in patients not treated with thrombolytic therapy ($P = 0.0008$).[14] In this study all patients had left ventricular aneurysms, the average ejection fraction in the thrombolytic therapy group was $28\% \pm 9\%$, and the average ejection fraction in the group that received no thrombolytic therapy was $30\% \pm 8\%$ ($P = $ ns).[14] Finally, an artery opened by rescue angioplasty, even if delayed to the extent that left ventricular systolic or diastolic function cannot be improved, might provide important collateral blood flow in the event of progression of other stenoses.

RATIONALE AGAINST RESCUE ANGIOPLASTY

Those who suggest that rescue angioplasty might not be beneficial point to several lines of reasoning. First, it is apparent that rapid infusion or other new methods of administering thrombolytic therapy or new adjunctive therapy might improve reperfusion and patency rates to the point that rescue angioplasty might need to be considered very infrequently and therefore would be cost-ineffective. For instance, Neuhaus et al. recently reported a 91% patency rate with a front-loaded regimen of recombinant tissue-type plasminogen activator (rt-PA).[16] Other groups have reported patency rates >80% with front-loaded t-PA regimens.[10,17,18] Second, it is quite possible that delayed thrombolytic-induced reper-

fusion might be sufficient to achieve a nearly optimal rate of in-hospital patient survival. The PRIMI trial investigators were the first to report a "catch up" phenomenon wherein the 24-hour infarct artery patency increased from 64% at 90 minutes to 85% after intravenous streptokinase,[19] suggesting that high rates of infarct artery patency may be achieved by agents that produce only modest patency rates at the standard 90-minute evaluation time. Clarification of the time course of this phenomenon occurred in the GUSTO-I trial, wherein the 3-hour patency rate with streptokinase approximated that seen with front-loaded t-PA.[10] For patients unlikely to regain systolic function by virtue of their late presentation, this delayed recanalization with streptokinase appeared sufficient in GUSTO-I (there was no difference between patients treated with streptokinase and those treated with t-PA presenting >4 hours after onset of chest pain).[20] Third, it may be argued that it is difficult to establish the need for rescue angioplasty by currently available techniques. This results in a possibly cost-ineffective triage of most patients to the catheterization laboratory for an early look at the infarct artery. However, despite the fact that routine bedside ECG monitoring as well as chest pain assessment is not accurate in the prediction of infarct artery patency,[21] it is likely that improved bedside techniques, including rapid assay of creatinine kinase isoenzymes or myoglobin enzymes as well as signal-averaged ECG,[22] may soon allow reliable detection of patients requiring urgent intervention.[23,24] Fourth, the potential harm from attempted but unsuccessful angioplasty might possibly outweigh the benefit from successful rescue angioplasty in aggregate. Although the exact cause is uncertain, failed rescue angioplasty has been associated with in-hospital mortality rates as high as 39%. This is particularly worrisome because these rates appear to be much higher than those expected from patients presenting with the same clinical characteristics. For example, of the 23 patients from the TAMI study group with failed rescue angioplasty (mean ejection fraction = 48%) there was a 39% mortality,[6] an incidence much higher than the expected 4% to 6% based upon their presenting ejection fraction.[25] Failed rescue angioplasty may be particularly detrimental in patients with a proximal right coronary artery occlusion.[26] However, it is important to note that the success rates for rescue angioplasty seem to be increasing. Our own data suggest that success rates have increased from 81% to 87% when outcomes from 1981 to 1986 vs. 1987 to 1991 are compared. A concordant reduction in mortality from 12% to 6% has also been observed. Finally, rescue angioplasty may not be worth the costs associated with its application in this era in which necessary limitations of resources have begun to impose constraints on the application of "high-tech" medicine.

Table 27-1. Metaanalysis of reported results of rescue coronary angioplasty

References	Number of patients	Thrombolytic regimen	Success (%)	Reocclusion (%)	ΔEF	Mortality (%)
Ellis[8]	109	rt-PA	79	20	+1	10.1
	5	rt-PA + UK	80	20	+2	20
	59	SK	76	18	+4	10.2
Belenkie[28]	16	SK	81	NR	+2	· 6.7
Topol[40]	86	rt-PA	73	29	−1	10.4
Califf[41]	15	rt-PA	87	15	+1	NR
	25	UK	84	12	+1	NR
	12	rt-PA + UK	92	0	+2	NR
Fung[42]	13	SK	92	0	+2	6.7
Topol[43]	22	rt-PA + UK	86	3	+5	0
Grines[44]	12	rt-PA + SK	90	12	−5	10
Holmes[45]	34	SK	71	NR	−11	11
Grines[46]	10	rt-PA + SK	90	12	+5	10
O'Connor[47]	90	SK	89	14	−1	17
Baim[48]	37	rt-PA	92	26	NR	5.4
Whitlow[49]	26	rt-PA	81	29	−2	NR
	18	UK	89	25	+1	NR
Pooled SK, UK, or combination	308*		260/308 (84%)†	31/223 (14%)†	−1	11.2
Pooled rt-PA only	252‡		191/252 (76%)†	38/157 (24%)†	−1	9.5
Total	560*†		451/560 (80%)	69/380 (18%)	−1	10.6

*Five patients included in both the series of Topol et al.[43] and this series are counted separately; †*P* = 0.01; ‡21 patients included in both the series of Califf et al.[41] and this series are counted separately; ΔEF = the change in left ventricular ejection fraction from baseline to the measurement before hospital discharge; NR = not reported; rt-PA = recombinant tissue-type plasminogen activator; SK = streptokinase; UK = urokinase.

NONRANDOMIZED STUDIES OF RESCUE PTCA

Very limited data have been published to allow one to judge appropriately whether or not, and to whom, rescue angioplasty should be applied. In aggregate, only slightly more than 500 patients have been reported (Table 27-1). In early studies, procedural success rates seem to be higher, and reocclusion rates lower, with systemically applied thrombolytic agents as opposed to fibrin-specific agents. In aggregate, left ventricular function does not seem to be improved, at least as rescue angioplasty was applied in these studies. The overall in-hospital mortality rate of 10.7% is somewhat difficult to put into perspective, in that this is generally a high-risk patient population. Comparison of in-hospital mortality of patients undergoing successful versus failed angioplasty suggests that the greatest difference is seen for patients with anterior wall MI or large inferior wall MI, and that little or no difference can be demonstrated for patients with inferior wall MI and no "reciprocal" anterior ST-segment depression.[27] These nonrandomized data suggest a relative benefit of successful vs. failed rescue angioplasty for patients treated even in the 6- to 24-hour time frame.[27]

RANDOMIZED STUDIES OF RESCUE ANGIOPLASTY

To date, the results of only a single small randomized trial of rescue angioplasty have been presented. Belenkie

randomized 28 patients presenting 3 to 6 hours after symptom onset. Angioplasty was successful in 13 of 16 attempts and was associated with a somewhat lower in-hospital mortality than was no coronary angioplasty (7% vs. 33%, *P* = 0.13), but there was no difference between patients with and without angioplasty with regard to late left ventricular systolic function.[28] The rationale and overall study design of the ongoing RESCUE trial has been described.[8]

THE PRACTICE OF RESCUE ANGIOPLASTY

With full recognition of the foregoing limitations regarding our understanding of the benefit of rescue angioplasty, we generally advocate early angiography for all patients presenting with cardiogenic shock after AMI and those presenting within the first 8 to 12 hours of symptom onset with anterior wall MI, apparently large inferior wall MI, or hemodynamic instability. Patients with multiple-lead ST-segment elevation inferior wall MI whose angina and/or ST-segment elevation persists are often also taken to the laboratory for emergency angiography.

Direct angioplasty is then undertaken as soon as possible after the administration of systemically active thrombolytic agents, except when bypass surgery is thought to be a superior alternative (significant left main obstruction or in the presence of a mechanical defect such as a ventricular septal defect), the anatomy is extremely disadvantageous for successful angioplasty (very large clot burden, occlusion beyond areas of extreme tortuosity or in small vessels),[29] or if the occlusion site proves to be more distal than one would have thought on the basis of the patient's clinical presentation. After the assurance that the patient has received aspirin and that the occlusion is not responsive to the intracoronary administration of nitrates, a temporary pacemaker is placed for proximal right coronary occlusions and dilatation is begun. Hemodynamic support in the form of intraaortic balloon counterpulsation is often applied if there is any evidence of hemodynamic instability. This form of therapy may also decrease the likelihood of coronary reocclusion after rescue angioplasty.[30,31] Consideration for the use of other support devices, such as percutaneous coronary bypass or coronary sinus retroperfusion, is usually limited to patients with cardiogenic shock and multivessel disease or inaccessible left anterior descending occlusions, respectively. In our hands, success rates exceeding 90% can be achieved using current over-the-wire systems and standard technique. One may prudently elect to accept a result that might not be considered optimal in the elective circumstance as long as TIMI 3 flow has been restored, because the production of angiographically evident dissection is associated with a much higher likelihood of later reclosure.[32] In the event of a large residual thrombus burden, equivocal result, or failed angioplasty caused by persistent thrombotic occlusion, some consideration should probably be given to prolonged intracoronary administration of thrombolytic agents. This has been quite successful in a limited number of procedures in our experience. Finally, following successful dilatation it is important to administer intravenous heparin guided by activated partial thromboplastin time or activated clotting time for at least 2 days.

Preliminary data suggests that the adjunct delivery of Fluosol[33] or perhaps other agents such as adenosine[34] as the initial reperfusate may improve myocardial salvage with rescue angioplasty, but this is not current practice at our institution.

Patients who have initially successful rescue PTCA and develop clinical signs or symptoms of recurrent ischemia appear to benefit from rapid triage back to the catheterization laboratory for repeat dilatation. One modest series suggests that successful treatment initiated within 90 minutes of recurrent ischemia leads to a less than 5% mortality, whereas delayed successful or unsuccessful recanalization or "retrieval" angioplasty may be associated with in-hospital mortality rates as high as 20%.[35] Repeat administration of thrombolytics is often effective for recurrent ischemia after primary thrombolysis,[36,37] albeit with high likelihood of the need for further revascularization, but data are insufficient to recommend its use after rescue angioplasty.

Finally, the issues related to the need for predischarge cardiac catheterization remain highly controversial. Such aggressive management can certainly be justified for patients with a prior MI,[38] large amounts of ischemic but salvaged myocardium,[39] and those with abnormal functional testing before hospital discharge.

CONCLUSIONS

The understanding and potential benefit of rescue angioplasty continues to evolve. At least until the results of ongoing randomized trials are made available, most interventionalists will continue to attempt to achieve infarct artery patency by this technique in patients presenting relatively early after symptom onset who have moderate or severe impairment of left ventricular function on the basis of ischemia. Whether this approach can be shown to improve patient outcome and whether it will be supported by third-party reimbursement agents in the future are important questions to be resolved jointly by the interventional cardiology community and the public health sector.

REFERENCES

1. GISSI: Effectiveness of intravenous thrombolytic treatment in acute myocardial infarction, *Lancet* 1:397-402, 1986.
2. ISIS-2: Randomized trial of intravenous streptokinase, oral aspirin, both, or neither among 17,187 cases of suspected acute myocardial infarction: ISIS-2, *Lancet* 2:349-360, 1988.
3. Wilcox RG, Olsson CG, Skene AM, et al: Trial of tissue plasminogen activator for mortality reduction in acute myocardial infarction. Anglo-Scandinavian study of early thrombolysis (ASSET), *Lancet* 2:525-530, 1988.
4. Topol EJ, Califf RM, George BS, et al for the TAMI Study Group: Insights from the Thrombolysis and Angioplasty in Myocardial Infarction (TAMI) Trials, *J Am Coll Cardiol* 12:24A-31A, 1988.
5. Kennedy JW, Ritchie JL, Davis KB, et al: The Western Washington randomized trial of intracoronary streptokinase in acute myocardial infarction: a 12-month follow-up report, *N Engl J Med* 312:1073-1078, 1985.
6. Abbottsmith CW, Topol EJ, George BS, et al: Fate of patients with acute myocardial infarction with patency of the infarct-related vessel achieved with successful thrombolysis versus rescue angioplasty, *J Am Coll Cardiol* 16:770-778, 1990.
7. Peto R: Unpublished observations.
8. Ellis SG, Van de Werf F, Ribeiro da Silva E, et al: Present status of rescue coronary angioplasty: current polarization of opinion and randomized trials, *J Am Coll Cardiol* 19:681-686, 1992.
9. Vogt A, von Essen R, Tebbe U, et al: Impact of early perfusion status of the infarct-related artery on short-term mortality after thrombolysis for acute myocardial infarction: retrospective analysis of four German multicenter studies, *J Am Coll Cardiol* 21:1391-1395, 1993.
10. Simes J, Ross AM, Simoons M et al for the GUSTO Investigators: Mortality reduction with accelerated tissue plasminogen activator is explained by early coronary patency (abstract), *Circulation* 88:I-291, 1993.
11. Hochman JS, Choo H: Limitation of myocardial infarct expansion by reperfusion independent of myocardial salvage, *Circulation* 75:299-306, 1987.
12. Brown EJ, Swinford RD, Gadde P, et al: Acute effects of delayed

reperfusion on myocardial infarct shape and left ventricular volume: a potential mechanism of additional benefits from thrombolytic therapy, *J Am Coll Cardiol* 17:1641-1650, 1991.

13. Eldar M, Leor J, Hod H, et al: Effect of thrombolysis on the evolution of late potentials within 10 days of infarction, *Br Heart J* 63:273-276, 1990.

14. Sager PT, Perlmutter RA, Rosenfeld LE, et al: Electrophysiologic effects of thrombolytic therapy in patients with a transmural anterior myocardial infarction complicated by left ventricular aneurysm formation, *J Am Coll Cardiol* 12:19-24, 1988.

15. Kersschot IE, Brugada P, Ramentol M, et al: Effects of early reperfusion in acute myocardial infarction on arrhythmias induced by programmed stimulation: a prospective, randomized study, *J Am Coll Cardiol* 7:1234-1242, 1986.

16. Neuhaus K-L, Tebbe U, Gottwik M, et al: Intravenous recombinant tissue plasminogen activator (rt-PA) and urokinase in acute myocardial infarction: results of the German Activator Urokinase Study (GAUS), *J Am Coll Cardiol* 12:581-587, 1988.

17. Carney R, Brandt T, Daley P, et al: Increased efficacy of rt-PA by more rapid administration: the RAAMI trial (abstract), *Circulation* 82:III-538, 1990.

18. Wall TC, Califf RM, George BS, et al: Accelerated plasminogen activator dose regimens for coronary thrombolysis, *J Am Coll Cardiol* 19:482-489, 1992.

19. PRIMI Trial Study Group: Randomized double-blind trial of recombinant pro-urokinase against streptokinase in acute myocardial infarction, *Lancet* 1:863-867, 1989.

20. The GUSTO Investigators: An international randomized trial comparing four thrombolytic strategies for acute myocardial infarction, *N Engl J Med* 329:673-682, 1993.

21. Califf RM, O'Neill W, Stack RS, et al: Failure of simple clinical measurements to predict perfusion status after intravenous thrombolysis, *Ann Intern Med* 108:658-662, 1988.

22. Krucoff MW, Croll MA, Pope JE, et al: Continuously updated 12-lead ST-segment recovery analysis for myocardial infarct artery patency assessment and its correlation with multiple simultaneous early angiographic observations, *Am J Cardiol* 71:145-151, 1993.

23. Ellis AK, Little T, Masud ARZ, et al: Early noninvasive detection of successful reperfusion in patients with acute myocardial infarction, *Circulation* 78:1352-1357, 1988.

24. Krucoff MW, Jackson YR, Burdette DL, et al: Digital real-time 12-lead ST segment trends: a bedside noninvasive monitor of infarct vessel patency (abstract), *Circulation* 80 (suppl II):II-354, 1989.

25. Kelly MJ, Thompson PL, Quinlan MF: Prognostic significance of left ventricular ejection fraction after acute myocardial infarction—a bedside radionuclide study, *Br Heart J* 53:16-24, 1985.

26. Gacioch GM, Topol EJ: Sudden paradoxic clinical deterioration during angioplasty of the occluded right coronary artery in acute myocardial infarction, *J Am Coll Cardiol* 14:1202-1209, 1989.

27. Ellis SG, O'Neill WW, Bates ER, et al: Implications for patient triage from survival and left ventricular functional recovery analyses in 500 patients treated with coronary angioplasty for acute myocardial infarction, *J Am Coll Cardiol* 13:1251-1259, 1989.

28. Belenkie I, Knudtson ML, Hall CA, et al: Vessel patency, rescue PTCA and mortality in acute myocardial infarction: results from a prospective randomized reperfusion trial (abstract), *Clin Invest Med* 13:157, 1990.

29. Ellis SG, Topol EJ, Gallison L, et al: Predictors of success for coronary angioplasty performed for acute myocardial infarction, *J Am Coll Cardiol* 12:1407-1415, 1988.

30. Ishihara M, Sato H, Tateishi H, et al: Intraaortic balloon pumping as the post-angioplasty strategy in acute myocardial infarction (abstract), *J Am Coll Cardiol* 17:115A, 1991.

31. Ohman EM, George BS, White CJ, et al for the Randomized IABP Study Group: Reocclusion of the infarct-related artery after primary or rescue angioplasty: effect of aortic counterpulsation (abstract), *Circulation* 88:I-107, 1993.

32. Ellis SG, Gallison L, Grines CL, et al: Incidence and predictors of early recurrent ischemia after successful coronary angioplasty for acute myocardial infarction, *Am J Cardiol* 63(5):263-268, 1989.

33. Forman MB, Perry JM, Wilson BH, et al: Demonstration of myocardial reperfusion injury in humans: results of a pilot study utilizing acute coronary angioplasty with perfluorochemical in anterior myocardial infarction, *J Am Coll Cardiol* 18:911-918, 1991.

34. Ely SW, Berne RM: Protective effects of adenosine in myocardial ischemia, *Circulation* 85:893-904, 1992.

35. Ellis SG, Debowey BS, Bates ER, et al: Treatment of recurrent ischemia after thrombolysis and successful reperfusion for acute myocardial infarction—effect on in-hospital mortality and left ventricular function, *J Am Coll Cardiol* 17:752-757, 1991.

36. White HD, Norris R, Brown MA, et al: Left ventricular end-systolic volume as the major determinant of survival after recovery from myocardial infarction, *Circulation* 76:44-51, 1987.

37. Barbash GI for the Israeli Investigators: Rescue thrombolysis in reinfarction (abstract), *Circulation* 88:I-491, 1993.

38. Mueller H, Cohen L, Williams D, et al: Subgroup analysis of the TIMI II study, *J Am Coll Cardiol* 17:167, 1991.

39. GISSI: Long-term effects of intravenous thrombolysis in acute myocardial infarction: final report of the GISSI study, *Lancet* 2:871-874, 1987.

40. Topol EJ, Califf RM, George BS, et al: A randomized trial of immediate versus delayed elective angioplasty after intravenous tissue plasminogen activator in acute myocardial infarction, *N Engl J Med* 317:581-588, 1987.

41. Califf RM, Topol EJ, Stack RS, et al: An evaluation of combination thrombolytic therapy and timing of cardiac catheterization in acute myocardial infarction: the TAMI 5 randomized trial, *Circulation* 83:1543-1556, 1991.

42. Fung AY, Lai P, Topol EJ, et al: Value of percutaneous transluminal coronary angioplasty after unsuccessful intravenous streptokinase therapy in acute myocardial infarction, *Am J Cardiol* 58:686-691, 1986.

43. Topol EJ, Califf RM, George BS, et al and the TAMI Study Group: Coronary arterial thrombolysis with combined infusion of recombinant tissue-type plasminogen activator and urokinase in patients with acute myocardial infarction, *Circulation* 77:1100-1107, 1988.

44. Grines CL, Nissen SE, Booth DC, et al and the KAMIT Study Group: A prospective randomized trial comparing combination half-dose tPA with streptokinase to full-dose tPA in acute myocardial infarction: preliminary report (abstract), *J Am Coll Cardiol* 15:4A, 1990.

45. Holmes DR Jr, Gersh BJ, Bailey KR, et al: "Rescue" percutaneous transluminal coronary angioplasty after failed thrombolytic therapy: 4-year follow-up (abstract), *J Am Coll Cardiol* 13:193A, 1989.

46. Grines CL, Nissen SE, Booth DC, et al and the KAMIT Study Group: A new thrombolytic regimen for acute myocardial infarction using combination half-dose tissue-type plasminogen activator with full-dose streptokinase: a pilot study, *J Am Coll Cardiol* 14:573-580, 1989.

47. O'Connor C, Mark DB, Hinohara T, et al: Rescue coronary angioplasty after failure of intravenous streptokinase in acute myocardial infarction: in-hospital and long-term outcomes, *J Invasive Cardiol* 1:85-95, 1989.

48. Baim DS, Diver DJ, Knatterud GL, and the TIMI II-A Investigators: PTCA "salvage" for thrombolytic failure: implications from TIMI II-A (abstract), *Circulation* 78 (suppl II):II-112, 1988.

49. Whitlow PL: Catheterization/Rescue Angioplasty Following Thrombolysis (CRAFT) study: results of rescue angioplasty (abstract), *Circulation* 82 (suppl III):III-308, 1990.

Chapter 28

ANTITHROMBOTIC THERAPY AS AN ADJUNCT TO THROMBOLYTIC THERAPY IN ACUTE MYOCARDIAL INFARCTION

Jack Hirsh
Allan Ross

The rationale for using antithrombotic therapy as an adjunct to thrombolytic therapy in patients with acute myocardial infarction (AMI) is based on the premise that rapid coronary thrombolysis is important and that the beneficial effects of rapid coronary thrombolysis are reversed by early reocclusion. There is evidence that thrombosis occurs while thrombolytic agents are being administered, since episodes of transient reperfusion followed by reocclusion often precede sustained reperfusion.[1] In the Thrombolysis and Angioplasty in Myocardial Infarction (TAMI) Phase 1-4 trials of 733 patients receiving intravenous thrombolytics, 12% developed reocclusion despite the concomitant use of aspirin, 325 mg/day, and intravenous heparin, 1000 U/hr.[2] Other studies have reported recurrent ischemic events within 7 days of successful reperfusion[3-5] in 11% to 21% of patients despite the concurrent use of aspirin and heparin. These patients have a higher in-hospital mortality rate than those who have sustained reperfusion,[2] a finding that supports the contention that maintaining the patency of a successfully reperfused artery is an important goal of coronary thrombolysis.

Patients who have had successful coronary thrombolysis are especially vulnerable to reocclusion because the process of coronary thrombolysis produces conditions in the newly opened coronary artery that can favor rethrombosis. Thus during coronary thrombolysis blood perfusing the reopened artery is exposed to thrombin, which is absorbed onto fibrin on the surface of the lysing coronary thrombus and on the surface of soluble fibrin fragments. These fragments are generated during thrombolysis and are present in high concentrations in the vicinity of the lysing coronary thrombus. The thrombin bound to exposed fibrin and to fibrin degradation products is enzymatically active and can interact with plasma fibrinogen and platelets and so lead to rethrombosis.[6-11] More importantly, the fibrin-bound thrombin in the vicinity of the lysing thrombus amplifies its own production many thousandfold by activating factors V and VIII and so produces an explosive burst of thrombin activity through an autocatalytic process.[12-14] In addition, plasmin released from the lysing clot has the potential to activate blood coagulation and so lead to more thrombin generation[6,15] (Fig. 28-1). There is biochemical evidence that the induction of coronary thrombolysis is accompanied by new fibrin formation[6,7,9,15-17] and platelet activation,[18] events that could contribute to recurrent thrombosis and reocclusion.[18-23]

Coagulation

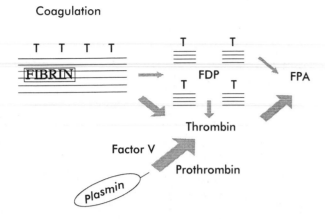

Fig. 28-1. Mechanism of thrombin formation and generation during thrombolysis: roles of clot-bound thrombin and plasma. *T,* thrombin; *FDP,* fibrin degradation products.

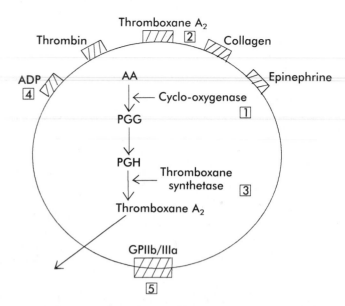

Fig. 28-2. Sites of inhibition of platelet function. Numbers in □ correspond to numbers designating inhibitors in Table 28-2.

Thrombin is fundamental to the process of reocclusion and contributes to this complication by converting fibrinogen into fibrin, activating factors V and VIII; this in turn amplifies thrombin generation, activating factor XIII, a process that renders the fibrin more resistant to lysis, and activating platelets to produce platelet aggregation. Thrombin binds to receptors on the platelet surface,[24] where it activates platelets and stimulates the release of adenosine diphosphate (ADP) and the synthesis and release of thromboxane A_2 (TXA$_2$).[25] These three platelet agonists, (thrombin, ADP, and TXA$_2$), bind to their specific receptors on the platelet surface and trigger a series of intracellular biochemical events that culminate in the exposure of a fibrinogen glycoprotein receptor Glycoprotein IIb/IIIa (GPIIb/IIIa) on the platelet surface.[25,26] Plasma fibrinogen, a bivalent ligand, binds to its receptors on the surface of adjacent platelets and links them together to form platelet aggregates.[26] Evidence from recent studies indicates that thrombin also exposes a thrombospondin receptor that is not blocked by ligands and that binds GPIIb/IIIa. These potential mechanisms for reocclusion are shown in Figure 28-2.

Many different approaches have the potential to accelerate thrombolysis and to reduce reocclusion.[20,22,27-35] Some of these have been studied clinically but most investigations have been in experimental animal models. Three approaches have been tested. The first is to increase the intensity of thrombolysis (to accelerate lysis) or to prolong the period of thrombolysis (to reduce the incidence of reocclusion); this approach can produce excessive bleeding.[29,31] The second is to inhibit thrombin formation or thrombin activity by using adjunctive treatment with heparin, low-molecular-weight heparins (LMWHs), direct thrombin inhibitors, and direct factor Xa inhibitors and other inhibitors of thrombin generation, including activated protein C

(APC) and tissue-factor pathway inhibitor (TPI). In general the heparins have been shown to be less effective than the other anticoagulants, possibly because both clot-bound thrombin and factor Xa are protected from inactivation by heparin/antithrombin III complex. The third approach is to inhibit platelet function with aspirin, specific thromboxane inhibitors, or agents that inhibit fibrinogen binding to its platelet glycoprotein receptor. In general the direct thrombin inhibitors have been more effective than antiplatelet agents, although there is evidence that the two approaches might be synergistic.[33,36]

Clinical experience with adjunctive antithrombotic therapy is limited to heparin and aspirin. Both are used routinely as adjuncts to thrombolytic therapy in patients with MI. Both have been shown to be effective clinically, but both have limitations that could, in theory, be overcome by a number of newer classes of antithrombotic agents.

Heparin suppresses the burst of thrombin activity that accompanies coronary thrombolysis,[16,17] improves patency after rt-PA–induced coronary thrombolysis, and reduces recurrent myocardial ischemia.[37-42] Even in subtherapeutic doses it has a small effect on reducing reinfarction and mortality after coronary thrombolysis, which is matched by a small increase in the rate of major bleeding including cerebral hemorrhage.[43,44] Subgroup analysis of a prospective study suggests that the effectiveness of heparin in improving coronary patency and reducing recurrent ischemia is critically dependent on obtaining an adequate anticoagulant effect, reflected in the activated thromboplastin time (aPTT).[41] Therapeutic (high) doses of heparin are required to improve early

Table 28-1. Inhibitors of coagulation

Inhibitor	Anticoagulant effect
Heparin	Nonbound thrombin
	Nonbound factor Xa
	(Factors IXa + XIa)
LMW heparins	Nonbound factor Xa
	Nonbound thrombin
	(Factor IXa + XIa)
Hirudin	
Hirudin fragments	Fibrin-bound thrombin
PPACKlike molecules	Free thrombin
Tick anticoagulant protein (TAP)	Factor Xa bound in pro-thrombinase complex
Antistasin	Free factor Xa
Tissue pathway inhibitor (TPI)	Tissue factor/factor VIIa complex
Activated protein C (APC)	Factors Va + VIIIa

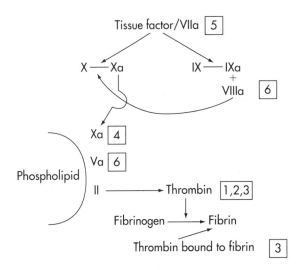

Fig. 28-3. Sites of inhibition of coagulation. Numbers in □ correspond to numbers designating inhibitors in Table 28-1.

patency.[41] Whether the potential benefits of achieving a "therapeutic" anticoagulant effect will be offset by an increase in "major bleeding" is an unanswered question that is being addressed by the Global Utilization of Streptokinase and t-PA for occluded coronary arteries (GUSTO-I) study.

Although heparin is an effective inhibitor of free thrombin, it does not inhibit fibrin-bound thrombin when used in pharmacologic concentrations.[10,11,45,46] In contrast the direct thrombin inhibitors, including hirudin and its derivatives, the chlormethylketones, and related small peptides, are able to inhibit fibrin-bound thrombin and soluble thrombin equally well.[10,45,47] Activated protein C (APC), a natural anticoagulant that has now been produced by recombinant DNA technology, inactivates activated factors V and VIII and is an effective inhibitor of thrombin-induced autocatalysis.[48] Novel direct factor Xa inhibitors derived from ticks and leeches[49-53] and tissue-factor pathway inhibitor have also been produced by recombinant DNA technology.[47] These new anticoagulants have been shown to be more effective than heparin in accelerating lysis and/or preventing rethrombosis in experimental models of thrombolysis.[11,33,54,55] The sites of action of these inhibitors are shown in Table 28-1 and Figure 28-3.

Aspirin inhibits TXA$_2$ synthesis but does not interfere with the other two pathways of thrombin-induced platelet aggregation.[25] There is very good evidence that aspirin is very effective clinically in reducing mortality and reinfarction after thrombolytic therapy.[56] The new antiplatelet agents, such as ticlopidine, and the platelet GPIIa/IIIb-receptor inhibitors have the potential to be more effective than aspirin because they block all three mechanisms of platelet aggregation.[25,54,57-60] In some but not all experimental models of arterial thrombolysis, the GPIIa/IIIb-receptor inhibitors have been shown to be more effective than either aspirin or heparin in

preventing reocclusion. Ridogrel, a combined thromboxane A$_2$ synthetase inhibitor and receptor antagonist, also shows promise.[61] The site of action of these inhibitors is shown in Table 28-2 and Figure 28-2.

In this chapter we will review (1) the mechanism of action and relevant pharmacokinetics for heparin and aspirin, (2) the results of clinical studies evaluating heparin and aspirin as adjuncts to thrombolytic therapy in MI, (3) the mechanism of action of the new anticoagulants and antiplatelet agents, and (4) the results of experimental studies evaluating these new agents in animal models of thrombolysis.

HEPARIN

Heparin has the potential to prevent reocclusion by inactivating free thrombin formed in the vicinity of the lysing thrombus, but it is ineffective as an inhibitor of fibrin-bound thrombin[10,45,47] and so has limitations as an adjunctive agent. These limitations are evident in studies in which heparin was shown to be less effective than the direct thrombin inhibitors and new platelet aggregation inhibitors in accelerating lysis and preventing reocclusion of experimental arterial thrombi in animals.[33,54,55]

Structure and mechanism of action of heparin

Heparin is a glycosaminoglycan (GAG) composed of chains of alternating residues of D-glucosamine and a uronic acid.[62] Its major anticoagulant effect is accounted for by a unique pentasaccharide with a high-affinity binding sequence for antithrombin III (ATIII).[63-72] The unique sequence is present in only one third of heparin molecules.[63,70,73-77] The anticoagulant effect of heparin is mediated largely through its interaction with ATIII;[20,75-78] this produces a conformational change in ATIII[79-81] and so markedly accelerates its ability to inactivate the coagulation enzymes thrombin (factor

Table 28-2. Inhibitors of platelet function

Inhibitor	Effect
Aspirin	Thromboxane A_2 synthesis
	Prostaglandin G_2 + H_2 synthesis
	Prostaglandin I_2 synthesis
Thromboxane A_2 receptor antagonists	Thromboxane A_2-mediated platelet activation
Thromboxane A_2 synthetase inhibitors	Thromboxane A_2 synthesis
Ticlopidine	Inhibition of platelet aggregation by ADP and
Clopidogrel	other agonists (mechanism unknown)
Glycoprotein IIb/IIIa inhibitors	Inhibit platelet aggregation induced by ADP, thrombin, thromboxane A_2, and collagen

IIa), factor Xa, and factor IXa.[71] Of these three enzymes, thrombin is the most sensitive to inhibition by heparin/ATIII.[13,14,71,82-84]

Heparin catalyzes the inactivation of thrombin by ATIII by acting as a template to which both the enzyme and inhibitor bind to form a ternary complex* (Fig. 28-4A). In contrast, the inactivation of factor Xa by ATIII/heparin complex is achieved by binding of the enzyme to ATIII only and does not require ternary complex formation† (Fig. 28-4B). Heparin also catalyzes the inactivation of thrombin by a second plasma cofactor, heparin cofactor II (HCII).[89] This second anticoagulant effect of heparin is specific for thrombin, it does not require the unique ATIII-binding pentasaccharide, and is achieved only at very high doses of heparin.[90-93]

Heparin is heterogeneous with respect to molecular size, anticoagulant activity, and pharmacokinetic properties. The molecular weight of heparin ranges from 5000 to 30,000 with an mean molecular weight of 15,000 (approximately 50 monosaccharide chains).[94-96] The anticoagulant activity of heparin is heterogeneous because: (1) only one third of the heparin molecules administered to patients have anticoagulant activity; (2) the anticoagulant profile of heparin is influenced by the chain length of the molecules; and (3) the clearance of heparin depends on molecular size, with higher-molecular-weight species cleared first. This differential clearance phenomenon results in an accumulation in vivo of the lower-molecular-weight species, which have a reduced ratio of antithrombin to antifactor Xa activity. This effect is responsible for the differences observed when the relationship between the heparin level and the activated partial thromboplastin time (aPTT) is as-

*References 14, 71, 76, 78, 85, 86.
†References 62, 64, 66, 67, 87, 88.

sessed in vivo and in vitro, since the lower-molecular-weight species that are retained in vivo are measured in the antifactor Xa heparin assay but have minimal effects on the aPTT.

Administration, pharmacokinetics, and pharmacodynamics

The two preferred routes of administration of heparin are by continuous intravenous infusion and subcutaneous injection. The efficacy and safety of heparin administered either by the continuous intravenous method or by the subcutaneous route are comparable provided that the dosage is adequate.[97,98] However, if the subcutaneous route is selected the initial dose must be sufficiently high to counteract the reduced bioavailability that occurs when heparin is administered by the subcutaneous route.[99] If an immediate anticoagulant effect is required and heparin is administered by subcutaneous injection the initial dose should be accompanied by an intravenous bolus injection because an anticoagulant effect from subcutaneous heparin is delayed for 1 to 2 hours.

Following its injection and passage into the blood stream, heparin binds to a number of plasma proteins including histidine-rich glycoprotein (HRGP),[100-102] platelet factor 4 (PF4),[100,103] vitronectin,[104] fibronectin,[105] and von Willebrand factor (VWF).[106] The binding of heparin to these proteins contributes to its reduced plasma recovery (bioavailability) at low concentrations, to the variability of the anticoagulant response to fixed doses of heparin in patients with thromboembolic disorders,[107] and to the laboratory phenomenon of heparin resistance.[108] Binding of heparin to VWF results in the inhibition of VWF-dependent platelet function.[106]

Heparin also binds to endothelial cells and macrophages,[109] a property that contributes to its complicated pharmacokinetics. Heparin is cleared through a combination of a rapid saturable and a much slower first-order mechanism of clearance.[110-115] The saturable phase of heparin clearance is thought to be the result of heparin binding to receptors on endothelial cells[116,117] and macrophages,[118] where it is internalized, depolymerized, and metabolized into smaller and less sulfated forms.[119,120] Clearance through the slower nonsaturable mechanism is largely renal. At therapeutic doses a considerable proportion of the administered heparin is cleared through the rapid saturable dose-dependent mechanism of clearance. Because of these kinetics, the anticoagulant response to heparin at therapeutic doses is not linear but increases disproportionally both in intensity and duration with dose increases. Thus the apparent biologic half-life of heparin increases from approximately 30 minutes with an intravenous bolus of 25 U/kg, to 60 minutes with an intravenous bolus of 100 U/kg and to 150 minutes with a bolus of 400 U/kg.[110,114,115]

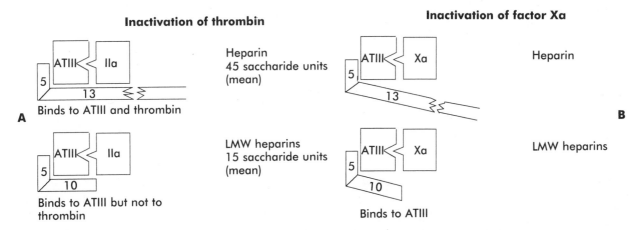

Fig. 28-4. A, To inactivate thrombin, heparins must bind to ATIII through the high-affinity pentasaccharide and to thrombin through an additional 13 saccharide units. LMWHs that contain fewer than 18 saccharide units cannot bind to thrombin and therefore are unable to inactivate thrombin. **B,** To inactivate factor Xa, heparins must bind to ATIII through the high-affinity pentasaccharide but do not need to bind to factor Xa. Therefore both heparin and LMWHs are able to inactivate factor Xa.

The plasma recovery of heparin is reduced when the drug is administered by subcutaneous injection in low doses (e.g., 5000 U/12 hr) or moderate doses of 12,500 U/12 hr[121] or 15,000 U/12 hr.[99] However, at high therapeutic doses of heparin (>35,000 U/24 hr) the plasma recovery is almost complete.[98] The poor bioavailability of heparin when administered by subcutaneous injection occurs because as heparin enters the intravascular space slowly from subcutaneous depots, it binds to saturable sites on endothelial cells and macrophages where it is internalized and metabolized. Circulating plasma levels are achieved only after these cell surface receptors are saturated, either by a large loading dose, or by the cumulative effects of a number of moderately high doses. The difference between the bioavailability of heparin when administered by subcutaneous or intravenous injection was demonstrated strikingly in a study of patients with venous thrombosis.[99] The patients were randomized to receive either 15,000 U/12 hr of heparin by subcutaneous injection or 30,000 U of heparin by continuous intravenous infusion; both regimens were preceded by a intravenous bolus dose of 5000 U. Therapeutic heparin levels and aPTT ratios were achieved at 24 hours in only 37% of patients who were randomized to receive subcutaneous heparin, whereas therapeutic heparin levels and aPTT ratios were achieved at 24 hours in 71% of patients given an identical dose of heparin by continuous intravenous infusion.

Laboratory monitoring and dose response relationships of heparin

The anticoagulant effects of heparin are usually monitored by the aPTT, a test that is sensitive to the inhibitory effects of heparin on thrombin, Factor Xa, and Factor IXa. When heparin is administered in fixed doses the anticoagulant response to heparin varies among sick patients, including those with acute venous thromboembolism[122] and with myocardial ischemia.[38,39,41,42] This variability is caused by differences between patients in the plasma concentrations of heparin-neutralizing plasma proteins and in the rates of heparin clearance. There is evidence from subgroup analysis of cohort studies that a relationship exists between the clinical effectiveness of heparin and its effect ex vivo on the aPTT for the following conditions: prevention of recurrent thrombosis in patients with proximal vein thrombosis,[99,123] prevention of mural thrombosis in patients with AMI,[121] prevention of recurrent ischemia in patients following streptokinase therapy for AMI,[38,42] and in the prevention of coronary artery reocclusion after thrombolytic therapy with tissue plasminogen activator[39,41] (Table 28-3). For this reason the dose of heparin administered to patients should be monitored by laboratory testing and adjusted to achieve a therapeutic level; this anticoagulant effect is referred to as the *therapeutic range*. The recommended therapeutic range for the aPTT for the treatment of venous thrombosis is based on a study performed in rabbits[124] that demonstrated that thrombus extension was prevented by a heparin dose that prolonged the aPTT ratio to 1.5 to 2.5, corresponding to a heparin level by protamine titration of thrombin time of 0.2 to 0.4 U/mL.

Unfortunately the different commercial aPTT reagents vary in their responsiveness to heparin.[125] For many aPTT reagents a therapeutic effect is achieved with an aPTT ratio of 1.5 to 2.5 (measured by dividing the observed aPTT by the mean of the laboratory control aPTT). With very sensitive aPTT reagents the

Table 28-3. Relationship between failure to reach lower limit of therapeutic range and thromboembolic events from subgroup analyses of prospective studies

Study	Type of patients	Outcome	N	Relative risk
Hull et al.[99]	DVT	Recurrent VTE	115	15.0
Basu et al.[123]	DVT	Recurrent VTE	157	10.7
Turpie et al.[121]	AMI	LVMT	112	22.2*
Kaplan et al.[42]	AMI	Recurrent MI/AP	75	6.0†
Camilleri et al.[38]	AMI	Recurrent MI/AP	70	13.3
De Bono et al.[39]	AMI	Coronary artery patency, PAI, t-PA	109	2.5
Hsia et al.[40]	AMI	Coronary artery patency, post–t-PA	94	9

DVT, deep vein thrombosis; AMI, acute myocardial infarction; VTE, venous thromboembolism; LVMT, left ventricular mural thrombosis; AP, angina pectoris.
*Estimated by assuming a normal distribution of the reported heparin levels.
†Kaplan used a PTT measurement and reported the relative risk associated with PTT values less than 50 seconds compared with PTT values of more than 100 seconds.

therapeutic range is higher than a ratio of 1.5 to 2.5, whereas for insensitive reagents the therapeutic range is lower. The difference in responsiveness of various aPTT test systems to the anticoagulant effects heparin is shown in Figure 28-5. Technical variables that affect the aPTT response to heparin are the type of clot-detection system and the composition of the aPTT reagent.[126]

Standardization of aPTT reagent can be achieved by calibrating it against the heparin level (therapeutic range 0.2 to 0.4 U/mL by protamine titration or 0.3 to 0.7 U/mL by antifactor Xa chromogenic assay) in a plasma system by addition of a range of clinically relevant concentrations of heparin.

Although there is good evidence that aPTT ratios above the lower limit of the therapeutic range are associated with protection against thrombosis,* maintaining the aPTT in the therapeutic range does not guarantee protection from bleeding complications. The risk of bleeding complications is increased with increasing heparin dose[127,128] (which in turn is related to the anticoagulant response), the concomitant use of thrombolytic therapy, recent surgery, trauma, invasive procedures, or a generalized hemostatic abnormality.[129]

A rapid therapeutic heparin effect is achieved by commencing with a loading dose of 5000 U as an intravenous bolus followed by 32,000 U/24 hr by continuous infusion.[122] A lower dose of 24,000 U/24 hr should be used immediately after thrombolytic therapy. The aPTT should be performed approximately 6 hours after the bolus and the heparin dose adjusted according to the result obtained. A heparin dose adjustment nomogram has been developed for aPTT reagents for which the therapeutic range is 1.9 to 2.7 times control [based on a heparin level of 0.2 to 0.4 U/mL (Table 28-4)]. This nomogram is not applicable to all aPTT reagents and should be adapted to the responsiveness

*References 38-42, 99, 121, 123.

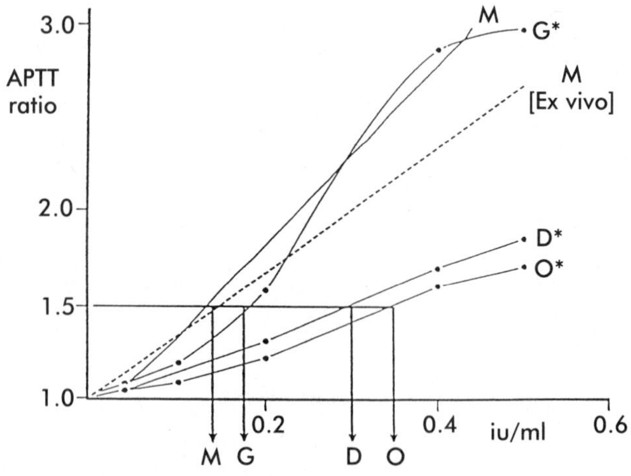

Fig. 28-5. aPTT ratios from surveys from the College of American Pathologists (CAP) and UK external quality assessment showing responses to in vitro heparinized samples. The dotted line indicates the Manchester aPTT response on fresh plasma from heparinized patients. The concentration of heparin giving a 1.5 aPTT ratio with the individual reagents is indicated by vertical arrows: M, Manchester; G, GD Automated; O, Ortho.

of the local thromboplastin to heparin. In patients with AMI who receive thrombolytic therapy, the lytic state often induces a transient coagulation defect that can prolong the aPTT for up to 24 hours.[130] Therefore the dose of heparin should only be adjusted upwards in the first 24 hours if the aPTT is below the therapeutic range.

It is also possible to achieve therapeutic heparin levels with subcutaneous injection. The anticoagulant effects of subcutaneous heparin are delayed for approximately 1 hour and peak levels occur at approximately 3 hours. A high initial dose should be used (35,000 U/24 hr in two divided doses) to overcome the poor bioavailability of moderate doses.[98] Monitoring is performed 6 hours after

Table 28-4. Heparin dose adjustment protocol

| Patient's aPTT* | Dosing instructions | | | |
	Repeat bolus dose	Stop infusion (minutes)	Change rate (dose) of infusion mL/hr† (U/24 hr)	Timing of next aPTT
<50	5000U	0	+3 (+2880)	6 hr
50-59	0	0	+3 (+2880)	6 hr
60-85‡	0	0	0	Next morning
86-95	0	0	−2 (−1920)	Next morning
96-120	0	30	−2 (−1920)	6 hr
>120	0	60	−4 (−3840)	6 hr

Starting dose of 5000 U IV bolus followed by 31,000 U/24 hr as a continuous infusion. First aPTT performed 6 hours after the bolus injection, dosage adjustments made according to protocol, and the aPTT repeated as indicated.
*Normal range for aPTT with Dade Actin FS reagent is 27-35 seconds.
†40 U/mL.
‡Therapeutic range of 60-85 seconds equivalent to a heparin level of 0.2-0.4 U/mL by protamine titration or 0.35-0.7 U/mL as an antifactor Xa level. Therapeutic range will vary with the responsiveness of the aPTT reagent to heparin.

injection with the aim of maintaining the aPTT in the therapeutic range at this time.[99,122]

ASPIRIN
Mechanism of action and dose-response relationships

Aspirin inhibits platelet aggregation by irreversibly inhibiting the enzyme cyclooxygenase.[131,132] Cyclooxygenase is responsible for the conversion of arachidonic acid to TXA_2 in the platelet; in vascular wall cells it is responsible for the conversion of arachidonic acid to PGI_2.[131,133-141] TXA_2 induces platelet aggregation and vasoconstriction; PGI_2 inhibits platelet aggregation and induces vasodilation.[138,142] Thus, aspirin has the potential to be both antithrombotic and thrombogenic.

Aspirin is rapidly absorbed in the stomach and upper intestine. Peak plasma levels occur 15 to 20 minutes after aspirin ingestion; inhibition of platelet function is evident by 1 hour. The plasma concentration of aspirin decays with a half-life of 15 to 20 minutes. Despite the rapid clearance of aspirin from the circulation, the platelet-inhibitory effect lasts for the life span of the platelet because it irreversibly inactivates platelet cyclooxygenase.[132,136] Aspirin also acetylates cyclooxygenase in megakaryocytes before new platelets are released into the circulation.[132,143] The mean lifespan of the human platelet is approximately 10 days, therefore approximately 10% of circulating platelets are replaced every 24 hours. However, virtually complete inhibition of platelet TXA_2 synthesis persists for approximately 48 hours after a single dose of 300 mg of aspirin, because the newly released platelets have had their prostaglandin synthetic mechanism inactivated before they are released from megakaryocytes.[143-146] A comparison has been performed of the effects of a range of very low doses of aspirin (20 mg twice daily, 40 mg daily, 80 mg every second day, and 324 mg daily) on thromboxane and prostacylin metabolism, on collagen-induced platelet aggregation, and on the bleeding time.[147] All doses of aspirin suppressed thromboxane excretion by more than 80%. Suppression of prostacyclin excretion was more pronounced with the 324-mg dose of aspirin than with the other doses that had similar effects. Aspirin in a dose of 20 mg inhibited platelet aggregation to a moderate degree but did not prolong the bleeding time. All the other dosages tested inhibited platelet aggregation and prolonged the bleeding time in a dose-related manner, with the dose of 324 mg being marginally more effective than the lower doses.[145]

Clarke et al.[145] performed a study to determine whether thromboxane A_2 formation could be inhibited without affecting prostacyclin production. Aspirin is subject to extensive first-pass metabolism in the liver to salicylate.[148] Therefore, by limiting the rate of drug delivery by using a controlled-release aspirin preparation the researchers reasoned that it might be possible to inhibit platelet prostaglandin G/H synthase in the prehepatic circulation while reducing the exposure of the systemic vascular endothelium to aspirin in the posthepatic circulation.[149] Accordingly, a controlled-release formulation containing 75 mg of aspirin was compared with a conventional immediate-release 75-mg dose of aspirin in normal volunteers. Steady-state inhibition of serum thromboxane A_2 was delayed with both 75-mg preparations and was slower with controlled-release aspirin than with the same amount of immediate-release aspirin. Maximal inhibition (greater than 95%) was achieved rapidly by adding a single loading dose of 162.5 mg of immediate-release aspirin to the regimen. Basal prostacyclin biosynthesis stimulated by bradykinin was preserved with the controlled-release aspirin but was inhibited with 75 mg of immediate-release aspirin.

Thus, rapid inhibition of platelet thromboxane A_2 production requires a dose that is greater than 75 mg and is acquired with a dose of 162.5 mg.

Aspirin is an effective antithrombotic agent when used in doses of 100 mg/day,[150] 75 mg/day,[151] 70 mg/day,[152] and possibly in doses as low as 30 mg/day.[153] Thus aspirin in a dose of 100 mg/day markedly augmented the effectiveness of warfarin in preventing systemic embolism and vascular death in patients with prosthetic heart valves[150]; aspirin in a dose of 75 mg/day was shown to be effective in reducing the risk of AMI and death in patients with unstable angina[151]; aspirin in a dose of 70 mg/day was shown to be effective in preventing recurrent cerebral ischemia in patients with minor stroke.[152] In a study of 3131 patients with transient cerebral ischemia or minor stroke, aspirin in a dose of 30 mg/day was compared with a dose of 300 mg/day and no difference was found in the incidence of the combined outcome of vascular death, stroke, or MI.[153]

Clinical trials of coronary thrombolysis evaluating adjunctive treatment with aspirin and heparin

Both heparin and aspirin have been evaluated as adjunctive antithrombotic agents in clinical trials of thrombolytic therapy in patients with AMI. Two types of outcome measures have been used: the angiographic endpoint of coronary artery patency[39-41] and the clinical endpoints of reinfarction and death.[43,44] Heparin has been shown to improve patency,[37,39-41] but its overall benefit in reducing mortality and major morbidity is controversial. Aspirin has been shown to reduce reinfarction and death,[56] but appears to be less effective than heparin in maintaining patency.[39-41]

In the recently completed GUSTO-I study[154] all four groups received heparin. No advantage was observed with immediate continuous intravenous heparin over subcutaneous heparin commencing 4 hours after thrombolytic therapy in the patients randomized to receive streptokinase (SK). Although there was a lower mortality in patients receiving t-PA than in either streptokinase arm, it is uncertain whether the greater efficacy is because of the accelerated t-PA regimen or the concomitant intravenous heparin regimen. Thus the role of adjuvant heparin in thrombolytic therapy for AMI is unresolved.

A role for aspirin as adjunctive therapy for coronary thrombolysis is accepted but the role of heparin is controversial and is currently being evaluated from the GUSTO-I data. Interest in this topic has intensified following the publication of the GISSI-2[43,155] and ISIS-3 studies.[44] In the GISSI-2 study[43,155] there was no apparent benefit from heparin in patients treated with rt-PA but there was evidence that heparin reduced mortality in patients treated with SK. The ISIS-3 study[44] showed that patients treated with thrombolytic therapy who were randomized to receive subcutaneous heparin had a modest reduction in reinfarction and a modest improvement in survival, which was offset in part by a small increase in major bleeding (including hemorrhagic stroke).

The question of need or lack of need for heparin cannot be separated from the fundamental questions of dosage of heparin, intensity of anticoagulant effect, and timing and route of heparin administration. It has been argued that the timing, dosage, and route of heparin administration in both the GISSI-2 study and the ISIS-3 study were suboptimal.[156] Furthermore, it has been argued that the failure to use an optimal heparin regimen may have compromised patients randomized to receive rt-PA more than those randomized to receive SK because rt-PA has less of a systemic anticoagulant effect than SK. On the other hand, because even subtherapeutic doses of heparin resulted in a small increase in the incidence of major bleeding in the ISIS-3 study, it is possible that some of the potential benefits of a more intensive intravenous heparin regimen (as was used in the GUSTO-I study) will be offset by an increased incidence of bleeding. Thus, the future of heparin as an adjuvant agent following coronary thrombolysis will depend on whether or not the anticipated reduction in mortality will offset the anticipated increase in the rate of major bleeding.

Patency

Five studies have investigated the effect of heparin on coronary artery patency after thrombolytic therapy with t-PA. In the first study, a single intravenous bolus of 10,000 U did not appear to influence coronary artery patency at 90 minutes.[35] In the other four studies heparin was administered either during or at the end of the t-PA infusion as a bolus of 5000 U IV followed by 1000 U/hr as a continuous infusion. The dose of heparin was adjusted to maintain the aPTT at 1.5 to 2 times control. In the Heparin-Aspirin Reperfusion trial[40] of 205 patients, the comparative group received 80 mg of ASA/day. Coronary artery patency at 18 hours was 82% in the heparin group and 52% in the aspirin group ($P < 0.0002$). In the trial reported by Bleich et al.[37] of 83 patients, the comparative group received no treatment. Patency at 2 days was 71% in the heparin group and 44% in the control group ($P < 0.023$). In the European Coronary Study Group-6 (ECSG-6) trial all 687 patients received aspirin and were randomized to heparin or no heparin.[39] Patency at a mean of 81 hours was 80% in the heparin group and 75% in the comparative group ($P < 0.01$). In the Australian National Heart Study trial all 202 patients received heparin for 24 hours.[157] They were then randomized to either continuous IV heparin or a combination of aspirin (300 mg) and dipyridamole (300 mg) daily. Patency at 1 week was 80% in both

Table 28-5. Subgroup analysis: angiography at 18 hrs in the HART Study[40]

	aPTT < 45 sec	aPTT > 45 sec	aPTT > 60 sec
Patency	45%	88%	95%

The relationship between the aPTT and coronary artery patency from subgroup analysis of a cohort who received rt-PA and heparin 5000 U bolus IV and 1000 U/hr by continuous infusion.

groups. The results of these studies suggest that heparin in a dose of 5000 U by IV bolus and 1000 U/hr by continuous infusion increases patency during the first few days after coronary thrombolysis with t-PA, probably by preventing rethrombosis.

Subgroup analysis of the ECSG-6 and the HART study[39,40] revealed some interesting and provocative findings. In both studies heparin was given intravenously in a fixed dose. The aPTT was performed but was not used to adjust the dose of heparin in a systematic manner. The subgroup of patients whose aPTT ratio was considered optimal had a significantly higher patency rate than those whose aPTT ratio was suboptimal[41] (Table 28-5). These findings suggest that the effectiveness of heparin in maintaining patency is critically dependent on maintaining an aPTT in the therapeutic range.

Mortality

The effectiveness of aspirin as adjunctive treatment to SK was clearly shown in the ISIS-2 study.[56] There were 17,187 patients randomized to SK, aspirin 160 mg/day, neither, or both. The vascular mortality was reduced from 12% to 9.2%, a 23% risk reduction ($P < 0.00001$) by SK compared with no SK, and from 13.2% to 8%, a 39% risk reduction ($P < 0.00001$) by the combination of SK and aspirin compared with no SK or ASA. This impressive result is supported by the proven efficacy of aspirin in reducing mortality in patients with coronary artery disease.

The efficacy of heparin on reinfarction or death after thrombolytic therapy for AMI has been evaluated in a number of randomized studies. In the ISIS-2 study[56] half of the patients were allocated to IV heparin over 48 hours in a 3 × 2 factorial design that included SK and aspirin; heparin treatment was associated with a nonsignificant decrease in infarction. In the Studio Sulla Calciparina Nell'Angina e Nella Trombosi Ventricolare Nell'Infarto (SCATI) study,[158] in which the control group received no treatment, the mortality was reduced significantly in patients randomized to receive heparin (2000 U IV bolus followed by 12,500 SC/12 hr) after thrombolytic therapy for AMI. The same trend was seen with SK but not with t-PA on the subgroup analysis

of the Gruppo Italiano per lo Studio della Sopravvivenza nell'Infarto Miocardico (GISSI-2)/International Study.[43,155] Among the patients who received SK and heparin (90% of whom also received aspirin), the mortality rate was 7.9% (408/5191) whereas it was 9.2% (479/5205) in the group that received SK alone ($P < 0.02$). When patients who died before heparin was started were excluded from the analysis, the same trend was still apparent: 5% (254/5037) vs. 6.2% (311/5037) ($P < 0.02$). The mortality rate in the GISSI-2/International Study among the patients who received rt-PA and heparin was 9.2% (476/5170); in those who received rt-PA not followed by heparin it was 8.7% (453/5202) ($P = 0.393$). After excluding the patients who died before heparin was started, the mortality rates were 5.9% (294/4988) among those who received heparin and 5.9% (298/5047) among those who did not ($P = 0.984$).

The recently completed ISIS-3 study[44] provides additional important information on the relative safety and efficacy of adjuvant heparin and on the relative safety of SK and t-PA. The addition of heparin (12,500 U SC/12 hr starting 4 hours after commencing thrombolytic therapy) to aspirin and thrombolytic therapy produced a small excess of major noncerebral bleeds (1% compared to 0.8%; $P < 0.01$) and of cerebral bleeds (0.56% to 0.40%; $P < 0.05$). Thus, the addition of heparin resulted in an excess of 3.6 per 1000 serious bleeding events. On the other hand, the addition of heparin resulted in a reduction of reinfarction of 3.1 events per 1000 treated ($P < 0.09$) and a reduction in 35-day mortality of 3 events per 1000 treated (ns). The incidence of stroke and stroke from presumed cerebral hemorrhage was significantly less in patients receiving SK over t-PA or APSAC. Thus, compared with SK, t-PA was associated with an excess of 3.5 strokes per 1000 and 4.2 episodes of presumed hemorrhagic strokes per 1000 (stroke 1.04% for SK and 1.39% for t-PA; cerebral hemorrhage 0.24% for SK and 0.66% for t-PA; $P < 0.05$ for both).

Based on these findings it is possible that any additional benefit from higher-dose and monitored IV heparin will be associated with an increase in hemorrhagic stroke. It is possible, however, that the benefits of heparin (in terms of mortality and reinfarction) when the aPTT is maintained in the therapeutic range will more than offset any increase in the incidence of cerebral hemorrhage.

Bleeding

The results of the GISSI-2 study and the ISIS-3 study show that the addition of heparin therapy to thrombolytic treatment increases the risk of bleeding[43,155] (Table 28-6): the reported incidence of minor bleeds was 594/6195 (9.6%) among patients who received heparin and 328/6206 (5.3%) among those who did not (RR 1.88, $P < 0.001$, GISSI centers only) and that of major bleeds

Table 28-6. Influence of heparin on incidence of bleeding

Study	Regimen	Major bleeding-noncerebral (%)			Intracranial bleeding (%)		
		Heparin	Control	Diff	Heparin	No heparin	Diff
GISSI-2[43]	12,500 U SC/12 hr, starting 12 hrs after TT	0.99	0.55 P < 0.001	0.44	0.35	0.37 NS	(0.02)
ISIS-3[44]	12,500 U SC/12 hr, starting 4 hrs after TT	1.02	0.75 P < 0.01	0.27	0.56	0.40 P < 0.05	0.16

The patients in the GISSI-2 trial were randomly allocated to receive either streptokinase or rt-PA treatment and those in the ISIS-3 trial to receive streptokinase, rt-PA, or APSAC treatment, independent of the allocation to heparin treatment (factorial design). *TT,* Thrombolytic therapy.

was 103/10361 (1%) in the heparin group and 57/10407 (0.5%) in the nonheparin group (RR 1.79, $P < 0.01$). The results of the ISIS-3 study[44] show that heparin produced a small but significant excess of episodes of major bleeding and of cerebral hemorrhage.

NEW ANTITHROMBOTIC AGENTS AND THEIR POTENTIAL AS ADJUVANT ANTITHROMBOTIC AGENTS

The benefits and limitations of heparin and aspirin as adjunctive agents to thrombolysis have stimulated the development of new antithrombotic compounds. The most promising of these are the ATIII-independent thrombin inhibitors, LMWHs, activated protein C, ATIII-independent factor Xa inhibitors, tissue-factor pathway inhibitor, platelet fibrinogen receptor inhibitors, and inhibitors of thromboxane A_2 (see Tables 28-1 and 28-2; Figs. 28-2 and 28-3).

New anticoagulants

The limitations of heparin are its highly variable anticoagulant response in sick patients, its poor bioavailability at low doses, its complicated dose-dependent clearance, its narrow benefit- (antithrombotic) to-risk (bleeding) ratio, and the interference of its anticoagulant effect by platelets, fibrin, and vascular surfaces. Some of these limitations can be overcome by three new classes of anticoagulants: the LMWHs, the ATIII-independent thrombin inhibitors, and the ATIII-independent factor Xa inhibitors. LMWHs have a more predictable anticoagulant response to fixed doses, a better bioavailability at low doses, a mechanism of clearance that is dose-independent, and a broader benefit-to-risk ratio.[159] The ATIII-independent thrombin inhibitors are equally effective against free and fibrin-bound thrombin and are not inhibited by platelets. The ATIII-independent factor Xa inhibitors are able to inhibit factor Xa in the prothrombinase complex and therefore have potential advantages over heparin and LMWHs. These properties might explain why heparin is less effective than direct thrombin inhibitors and direct factor Xa inhibitors at preventing arterial and venous thrombosis in experimental animals, and why the ATIII-independent inhibitors are more effective than heparin in preventing reocclusion after experimental coronary thrombolysis.[33,53-55]

Low-molecular-weight heparin

LMWHs are fragments of standard heparin produced by either chemical or enzymatic depolymerization.[159,160] They are approximately one third the size of heparin and have a mean molecular weight of 4000 to 5000. Depolymerization of heparin results in a change in its anticoagulant profile, its bioavailability and pharmacokinetics, and its effects on platelet function and experimental bleeding.

Like heparin, LMWHs produce their major anticoagulant effect by binding to antithrombin ATIII through a unique pentasaccharide sequence[75-78] that is present on less than one third of LMWH molecules. A minimum chain length of 18 saccharides is required for the inactivation of thrombin. In contrast, inactivation of factor Xa by ATIII does not require binding of the heparin molecules to the clotting enzyme,[71,76,78,85,86] and is therefore achieved by small-molecular-weight heparin fragments, provided that they contain the high-affinity pentasaccharide. Compared with heparin, LMWHs have a reduced antifactor Xa to anti-IIa ratio (see Fig. 28-3).

LMWHs have superior bioavailability at low doses and a more predictable anticoagulant response than heparin[161] because they do not bind to heparin-binding proteins.[105] LMWHs also do not bind to endothelial cells in culture,[109,162,163] a property that could account for their longer plasma half-life than heparin.[62,112,164-171] LMWHs produce less bleeding than heparin with equivalent antithrombotic effects in experimental animals,[88,172-179] a property that has been attributed to their different effects on platelet function,[106,172,180,181] their reduced binding to von Willebrand factor,[106] and reduced vascular permeability.[182] LMWHs have been investigated in man and have been shown to be very effective in the prevention and treatment of venous thrombosis.[159] Their potential role in the treatment of arterial thrombosis and as an adjunct to thrombolytic therapy is unknown.

ATIII-INDEPENDENT INHIBITORS

Several ATIII-independent inhibitors are now available. These include hirudin, hirudin fragments, argatroban, and the peptide chloromethyl ketone inhibitor D-phe-pro-argCH$_2$Cl (PPACK) and its derivatives. Although all these inhibitors bind directly to thrombin they have different mechanisms of action as described next. The potential advantage of the ATIII-independent inhibitors is that unlike heparin these agents can access and inactivate thrombin that is bound to fibrin.[10] As a result these inhibitors have proved to be more effective than heparin in experimental animal models of venous and arterial thrombosis[45,183,184] and as adjuncts to tissue plasminogen activator-induced thrombolysis using a variety of model systems.[55,60] These observations illustrate the importance of inhibiting fibrin-bound thrombin to achieve optimal antithrombotic effects.

Hirudin and its derivatives. Hirudin is a 65-amino acid residue protein isolated from the salivary glands of the medicinal leech. It is a potent and specific thrombin inhibitor that is now available through recombinant DNA technology. It forms an essentially irreversible, stoichiometric complex with thrombin. Analysis of the crystal structure of the thrombin-hirudin complex illustrates the extensive contact that hirudin makes with thrombin, as it binds both to the active center and to the substrate recognition site of the enzyme.[185] It inhibits thrombin by forming a stoichiometric complex with a dissociation constant that has been reported to be as low as 20 fmol.[186] The action of hirudin on thrombin is bivalent: it binds both to the anionic exosite (which is the substrate recognition site) and to the catalytic center.

Synthetic C-terminal peptide fragments of hirudin have been developed to study the interactions of hirudin with the anion-binding exosite of thrombin[187-189] and to design a novel class of bivalent thrombin inhibitors.[190,191] The first of these fragments is hirugen, a synthetic dodecapeptide comprising residues 53 to 64 of the carboxy-terminal region of hirudin.[191] Unlike hirudin, this peptide does not interact with the catalytic center of thrombin. Instead, hirugen binds to the nearby substrate recognition site, thereby blocking thrombin interaction with its substrates. By adding D-phe-pro-arg-pro-(gly)$_4$ to the amino-terminal region, hirugen has been converted from a weak competitive inhibitor to a potent bivalent inhibitor known as *hirulog*.[190] Like hirudin, this inhibitor blocks both the active center and the substrate recognition site. However, active site inhibition is transient because once complexed, thrombin can slowly cleave the pro-arg bond on the amino-terminal extension, thereby converting hirulog to a hirugenlike species.

Argatroban. This synthetic arginine derivative is a relatively weak competitive inhibitor of thrombin.[192] Argatroban interacts with the active site of thrombin and has a half-life of only a few minutes.

PPACK and its derivatives. The tripeptide chloromethyl ketone, PPACK, irreversibly inhibits thrombin by alkylating the active center histidine.[193] Because thrombin binds to fibrin through a site distinct from its catalytic center, PPACK readily inhibits clot-bound thrombin.[10] Recently a PPACK derivative, D-phe-pro-arg-borate, has been developed that is a more specific inhibitor of thrombin than the parent molecule.[194] Bagdy et al. have demonstrated that two synthetic peptides, D-Phe-Pro-Arg-H and D-MePhe-Pro-Arg-H, have anticoagulant and antiplatelet effects when administered both intravenously and orally in a number of animal species.[195]

A number of studies have been performed in animal models comparing the relative efficacy of the direct thrombin inhibitors with heparin, aspirin or platelet GPIIb/IIIa receptor antagonists in accelerating t-PA–induced thrombolysis or preventing reocclusion. In all of these studies the direct thrombin inhibitors proved to be more effective than the other antithrombotic agents. In a coronary thrombosis model in dogs Haskel et al.[36] showed that hirudin was more effective than heparin, aspirin, and SC 47643 (a peptide mimetic analogue of RGD that is a platelet GPIIb/IIIa fibrinogen receptor antagonist) in accelerating t-PA–induced thrombolysis. Fitzgerald et al. have reported that heparin in doses that produce a sixfold prolongation of the aPTT failed to prevent reocclusion after thrombolysis.[28] Similarly, studies from Fuster's group showed that hirudin was much more effective than high-dose heparin[45] and aspirin[196] in reducing platelet deposition and thrombosis after angioplasty in pigs. In contrast to the effectiveness of hirudin, argatroban in doses that prolonged the aPTT twofold to fourfold did not appear to be effective in preventing coronary reocclusion in dogs. Recently Klement et al.,[55] using a rat aortic thrombosis model, compared the effects of heparin, hirudin, the synthetic hirudin-derived peptide hirulog, and PPACK in accelerating thrombolysis and preventing reocclusion following t-PA–induced thrombolysis. Compared with saline control, heparin had no significant effect on time to reperfusion or reocclusion. All three of the direct thrombin inhibitors tested decreased the number of reocclusions; hirulog and PPACK accelerated thrombolysis. The superiority of hirudin over heparin in preventing thrombosis during and after thrombolysis and in permanently inactivating clot-bound thrombin has also been demonstrated in a study using a rabbit jugular vein model.[184]

ACTIVATED PROTEIN C

Natural and recombinant forms of activated protein C (APC) have been developed and studied in experimental models of thrombosis and hemostasis. APC inhibits coagulation and prolongs the aPTT by inactivating activated factors V and VIII (factor Va and factor VIIIa) on endothelial and platelet surfaces. By so doing APC inhibits thrombin generation induced by thrombin and factor Xa. APC has been shown to inhibit platelet deposition in a baboon model of acute arterial thrombosis,[197,198] to prevent experimental venous thrombosis, and to prevent rethrombosis after experimental thrombolysis.[199] The relative antithrombotic efficacy of combining APC and urokinase has been evaluated in an experimental model using a Dacron vascular graft incorporated into a chronic exteriorized femoral arteriovenous access shunt in baboons. APC and urokinase had additive effects in preventing the accumulation of fibrin and platelets onto the graft. These findings suggest that APC might be effective as an adjuvant antithrombotic agent during and following thrombolytic therapy.[199]

DIRECT FACTOR XA INHIBITORS

Two ATIII-independent factor Xa inhibitors have been developed: the tick anticoagulant peptide (TAP) and the leech anticoagulant peptide (antistasin). TAP is a 60-amino acid polypeptide that was originally isolated from the soft tick *Ornithodoros moubata*[200] and subsequently made recombinantly in yeast (rTAP).[201] It is a potent and selective inhibitor of factor Xa, which unlike heparin can access and inhibit factor Xa in the prothrombinase complex. rTAP has been shown to prevent venous thrombus formation effectively in rabbits,[53] to suppress systemic elevations in FPA induced by intravenous administration of thromboplastin in conscious Rhesus monkeys,[201] and to inhibit thrombosis in a silastic femoral arteriovenous (AV) shunt in baboons; the latter model has been used extensively[202,203] to stimulate arterial thrombosis produced under conditions of high shear.

The relative effects of TAP, rHirudin, and heparin have also been compared in a model of rt-PA–mediated thrombolysis and subsequent acute reocclusion in a canine model of platelet-dependent coronary artery thrombosis.[33,36] Both rTAP and rHIR, but not heparin, significantly accelerated rt-PA–mediated thrombolysis and prevented acute reocclusion. Heparin had a modest effect on enhancing thrombolytic reperfusion but surprisingly failed to prevent or significantly delay reocclusion even in doses that elevated the aPTT to approximately eightfold over baseline values.

Like TAP, recombinant antistasin (rATS) is a potent and selective inhibitor of factor Xa. Antistasin was originally isolated from the Mexican leech *Haementeria*

officinalis.[49-52] rATS has a molecular weight of 13,341 and produces potent anticoagulant properties for a period of greater than 30 hours following a single subcutaneous administration. This long duration of action reflects a prolonged period of absorption coupled with a rather long plasma half-life.[204] rATS exhibits no detectable inhibition of thrombin at molar ratios as high as 500 to 1.[49] The in vivo antithrombotic effects of rATS following continuous intravenous infusion have been demonstrated in a rabbit model of venous thrombosis[53] and a rhesus monkey model of mild disseminated intravascular coagulation (DIC).[51]

The failure of heparin (relative to rTAP and rHIR) to prevent experimental arterial thrombosis and reocclusion in these models may be a reflection of the inability of the heparin-antithrombin III complex to directly access factor Xa assembled in the prothrombinase complexes[82,84,205,206] and thrombin bound to fibrin within the residual thrombus.[10] In addition, release of platelet factor 4 by platelets in the thrombi could result in high levels of this heparin-neutralizing protein locally and so interfere with the anticoagulant effect of heparin.[207,208]

Tissue factor pathway inhibitor

One of the potential mechanisms of reocclusion following successful thrombolysis is through exposure of tissue factor in the subendothelium and in the depths of the lipid-rich atherosclerotic plaque.[47,209-211] Tissue pathway inhibitor (TPI) (formerly known as *lipoprotein-associated coagulation inhibitor* or *LACI*)[212,213] forms a complex with activated factor X that binds to and inhibits tissue factor/activated factor VII complex and so inhibits thrombin generation at one of the early steps in the activation of blood coagulation. TPI has been cloned, and limited studies with recombinant TPI have been performed in a canine femoral artery model. Thrombosis was induced by two methods and recanalization was produced by t-PA infusion. TPI infusion prevented reocclusion following t-PA in the arteries subjected to intimal injury.[47] These findings support a potential role in reocclusion for tissue factor exposure after successful thrombolysis.

New antiplatelet agents

There is evidence that platelets are activated during thrombolysis[25,28] and that the formation of new platelet aggregates at the site of the lysing thrombus both delays thrombolysis and leads to reocclusion; therefore, agents that inhibit platelet function have the potential to both accelerate thrombolysis and prevent reocclusion.

Platelets adhere to the ligands, collagen, and von Willebrand factor that are exposed on subendothelial surfaces of atherosclerotic coronary arteries. At low shear rates the adhesion of platelets to these proteins is mediated by platelet glycoprotein (GP) receptors (GPIa/IIa and GPIV for collagen; GPIb for von Willebrand factor).[25] Synthetic glycoprotein Ib receptor antagonists, engineered with sequence homology to von Willebrand factor, have been developed and are in an early stage of evaluation. Platelet aggregation is mediated through the platelet glycoprotein receptor GPIIb/IIIa, a member of the integrin family of receptors. At high sheer rates platelet adhesion is also mediated by binding to GPIIb/IIIa.[214-216] In contrast to GPIb receptor, which is functional on the resting platelet, the GPIIb/IIIa receptor becomes functional only after the platelet surface has been activated by exposure to platelet agonists, such as adenosine diphosphate (ADP), epinephrine, collagen, or thrombin.[25] Thromboxane A_2 can also activate platelets and expose the GPIIb/IIIa complex.[25] Each of these platelet agonists binds to its specific receptor on the platelet surface and stimulates intracellular events that lead to the exposure of GPIIb/IIIa. The exposed GPIIb/IIIa receptors bind the large adhesive glycoproteins, fibrinogen, von Willebrand factor, fibronectin, and vitronectin, which promote platelet aggregation. Of these, fibrinogen is present in the blood in by far the highest concentration and is the most important mediator of platelet aggregation.[25]

Aspirin is a very selective inhibitor of platelet function because it inhibits only platelet aggregation mediated through activation of the arachadonic acid/thromboxane A_2 pathway. This selective activity may explain the limited effectiveness of aspirin in inhibiting reocclusion clinically[39-41] and in experimental models of thrombolysis.[21,22] Nevertheless, because aspirin is effective in preventing death and reinfarction after coronary thrombolysis[56] there is considerable current interest in developing new and more potent inhibitors of platelet aggregation. The most promising group of platelet aggregation inhibitors are those that compete with fibrinogen and the other adhesive proteins for binding to the platelet glycoprotein receptor GPIIb/IIIa. Selective platelet GPIIb/IIIa fibrinogen receptor antagonists* have been shown to prevent experimental arterial thrombosis in several experimental studies.

Three broad classes of fibrinogen-receptor blocking agents, all of which share the recognition sequence arginine-glycine-aspartate (RDG sequence) for the GPIIb/IIIa binding site, have been developed. These are Fab fragments of monoclonal antibodies to the platelet fibrinogen GP,[54,59,217,218,219] nonenzymatic snake venom proteins that have high affinity for the platelet fibrinogen GP receptor[220-222] by virtue of containing the fibrinogen RGD binding sequence, and synthetic peptides that compete with fibrinogen for binding to the platelet fibrinogen GP receptor.[36,223,224]

_____
*References 33, 36, 54, 59, 203, 217, 218.

These antagonists of platelet GPIIb/IIIa receptor binding are very potent inhibitors of platelet aggregation because binding of these adhesive proteins to the platelet membrane receptor is a common pathway through which thrombin, adenosine diphosphate, thromboxane A_2, and collagen induce platelet aggregation. On the other hand, these GPIIb/IIIa receptor antagonists do not inhibit platelet release reaction or platelet thromboxane synthesis.

Inhibition of the platelet GPIIb/IIIa receptor by murine monoclonal antibodies (7E3-F[ab$'$]$_2$ [7E3] and 10E5-F[ab$'$]$_2$) has been shown in experimental models to prevent platelet thrombus formation after vascular injury[54,58,225] and to significantly shorten the time to reperfusion after thrombotic coronary occlusion.[54] In studies in dogs with experimental coronary thrombosis, 7E3 F(ab$'$)2 accelerated initial thrombolysis and prevented rethrombosis.[54,58] In other studies[218] the 7E3 F(ab$'$)2 shortened the time to reperfusion and prevented reocclusion in a canine model of coronary occlusion induced by electrical injury. The efficacy of 7E3 in combination with t-PA is currently being tested in patients with AMI.

Limited experience has been obtained with the synthetic peptides that mimic the RGD-containing sequence on fibrinogen and other adhesive proteins.[33,36,223-224] In vitro they have similar activity to the 7E3 F(ab$'$)2 product and inhibit platelet aggregation in man in a dose-related manner. These peptide mimetics are also active in experimental animals.[33,36,223] The receptor antagonist arginine-glycine-aspartate-0-methyltyrosine amide (SC 47643) is a tetrapeptide analogue of the adhesive protein recognition sequence RGD. This platelet antagonist has been shown to prevent reocclusion caused by platelet-rich thrombi after successful t-PA–induced thrombolysis in the femoral arteries of dogs,[223] but to be no more effective than aspirin and less effective than hirudin in preventing reocclusion after thrombolysis of coronary artery thrombi in dogs.[36] The peptide mimetic bistatin[33] has been shown to augment the effect of heparin in accelerating thrombolysis and preventing reocclusion following t-PA–induced thrombolysis in a canine model of coronary thrombolysis. Studies performed with the cyclic heptapeptide MK-852, which is another antagonist of GPIIb/IIIa binding, indicate that this is a potent antithrombotic compound in experimental models of arterial thrombosis.[226]

A number of snake venoms competitively inhibit the binding of fibrinogen to its platelet receptor. These naturally occurring inhibitors of the GPIIb/IIIa receptor include the snake venom peptides trigramin,[221] bititstatin,[33,222] echistatin,[220] and applaggin,[227] all of which inhibit platelet aggregation; some also accelerate experimental t-PA–induced thrombolysis and prevent reocclusion. Most experience has been obtained with Trigramin, an inhibitor from *Trimeresurus gramnes* snake venom.[228,229]

THROMBOXANE A₂ SYNTHETASE INHIBITORS

Studies performed in experimental animals using models of thrombolysis and in man using activation markers suggest that reocclusion after thrombolytic therapy may be the result not only of thrombin-induced fibrin formation and platelet activation but also of thromboxane A_2 production and release at the site of the lysing coronary thrombus.[25,230] Thrombin and thromboxane A_2 are important mediators of platelet activation.[231-233] Thromboxane A_2 causes platelet activation and coronary vasoconstriction. Both the activity of thrombin and thromboxane A_2 increase after administration of thrombolytic agents,[18,23] and there is experimental evidence that inhibition of both thromboxane A_2 and thrombin activity may be more effective than inhibition of either one alone in shortening the time to reperfusion and preventing reocclusion.[20-22,36,234,235] Recent studies showed that ridogrel, a combined thromboxane A_2 synthetase inhibitor and receptor antagonist,[124,236] when added to hirulog reduced the frequency of reocclusion after t-PA–induced lysis of coronary arteries of experimental thrombi in dogs more effectively than hirulog and t-PA. In the model, inhibition of thrombin alone or thromboxane A_2 alone did not prevent reocclusion. These findings suggest that both thromboxane A_2 and thrombin contribute to the process of reocclusion. Ridogrel[237,238] was more effective than either a thromboxane receptor antagonist[61] or a thromboxane synthetase inhibitor[239] when either of these classes of thromboxane inhibitors was used alone.

CONCLUSION

The aim of using adjunctive antithrombotic therapy in patients with AMI who are treated with thrombolytic agents is to accelerate lysis and prevent reocclusion. The concomitant use of aspirin improves survival and reduces the rate of reinfarction. Intravenous heparin is more effective than aspirin in maintaining early patency, but when used in moderate doses by subcutaneous injection produces only marginal improvement in survival at the cost of a small increase in major bleeding. High-dose intravenous heparin is usually more effective than moderate-dose subcutaneous heparin but is likely to produce more bleeding.

Studies in experimental animal models of arterial thrombolysis indicate that newly developed antithrombotic agents including ATIII-independent thrombin inhibitors, antithrombin III-independent factor Xa inhibitors, and agents that interfere with platelet aggregation by blocking fibrinogen binding to the platelet glycoprotein receptor GPIIa/IIIb are more effective than heparin and aspirin. Studies are under way to determine whether these compounds are effective as adjuvant antithrombotic agents in man.

REFERENCES

1. Gold HK, et al: Acute coronary reocclusion after thrombolysis with recombinant human tissue-type plasminogen activator: prevention by a maintenance infusion, *Circulation* 73:347-352, 1986.
2. Ohman EM, et al: Consequences of reocclusion following successful perfusion therapy in acute myocardial infarction, *Circulation* 82:781-791, 1990.
3. Ellis SG, et al: Recurrent ischemia without warning: analysis of risk factors for in-hospital ischemic events following successful thrombolysis with intravenous tissue plasminogen activator, *Circulation* 80:1159-1165, 1989.
4. The TIMI Study Group: The thrombolysis in myocardial infarction (TIMI) trial. Phase I findings, *N Engl J Med* 312:932-936, 1985.
5. Topol EJ, et al: A randomized trial of immediate versus delayed elective angioplasty after intravenous tissue plasminogen activator in acute myocardial infarction, *N Engl J Med* 317:581-588, 1987.
6. Eisenberg PR, Sherman LA, Jaffe AS: Paradoxic elevation of fibrinopeptide A: evidence for continued thrombosis despite intensive fibrinolysis, *J Am Coll Cardiol* 10:527-529, 1987.
7. Eisenberg PR, et al: Importance of continued activation of thrombin reflected by fibrinopeptide A to the efficacy of thrombolysis, *J Am Coll Cardiol* 7:1255-1262, 1986.
8. Francis CW, et al: Thrombin activity of fibrin thrombi and soluble plasmic derivatives, *J Lab Clin Med* 102:220-230, 1983.
9. Gulba DC, et al: Increased thrombin levels during thrombolytic therapy in acute myocardial infarction, *Circulation* 83:937-944, 1991.
10. Weitz JI, et al: Clot-bound thrombin is protected from inhibition by heparin-antithrombin III but is susceptible to inactivation by antithrombin III-independent inhibitors, *J Clin Invest* 86:385-391, 1990.
11. Weitz JI, Leslie B, Hudoba M: Thrombin remains bound to soluble fibrin degradation products and is partially protected from inhibition by heparin-antithrombin III (abstract), *Thromb Haemost* 65:931, 1991.
12. Buchanan MR, et al: The relative importance of thrombin inhibition and factor Xa inhibition to the antithrombotic effects of heparin, *Blood* 198-201, 1985.
13. Ofosu FA, et al: Unfractionated heparin inhibits thrombin-catalyzed amplification reactions of coagulation more efficiently than those catalyzed by factor Xa, *Biochem J* 257:143-150, 1989.
14. Ofosu FA, et al: The inhibition of thrombin-dependent feedback reactions is critical to the expression of anticoagulant effects of heparin, *Biochem J* 243:579-588, 1987.
15. Eisenberg PR, Miletich JP: Induction of marked thrombin activity by pharmacologic concentrations of plasminogen activators in non-anticoagulated whole blood, *Thromb Res* 55:635-643, 1989.
16. Rapold HJ: Promotion of thrombin activity by thrombolytic therapy without simultaneous anticoagulation, *Lancet* 1:481-482, 1990.
17. Rapold HJ, et al: Monitoring of fibrin generation during thrombolytic therapy of acute myocardial infarction with recombinant tissue-type plasminogen activator, *Circulation* 79:980-989, 1989.
18. Fitzgerald DJ, et al: Marked platelet activation in vivo after intravenous streptokinase in patients with acute myocardial infarction, *Circulation* 77:142-50, 1988.
19. Badimon L, et al: Residual thrombus is more thrombogenic than

severely damaged vessel wall (abstract), *Circulation* 78(suppl II):II-119, 1988.

20. Fitzgerald DJ, FitzGerald GA: Role of thrombin and thromboxane A₂ in reocclusion following coronary thrombolysis with tissue-type plasminogen activator, *Proc Natl Acad Sci USA* 86:7585-7589, 1989.

21. Golino P, et al: Mediation of reocclusion by thromboxane A₂ and serotonin after thrombolysis with tissue-type plasminogen activator in a canine preparation of coronary thrombosis, *Circulation* 77:678-684, 1988.

22. Golino P, et al: Simultaneous administration of thromboxane A₂- and serotonin S₂-receptor antagonists markedly enhances thrombolysis and prevents or delays reocclusion after tissue-type plasminogen activator in a canine model of coronary thrombosis, *Circulation* 79:911-919, 1989.

23. Owen J, et al: Thrombolytic therapy with tissue plasminogen activator or streptokinase induces transient thrombin activity, *Blood* 72:616-20, 1988.

24. Hung DT, et al: "Mirror image" antagonists of thrombin-induced platelet activation based on thrombin receptor structure, *J Clin Invest* 89:444-450, 1992.

25. Coller BS: Platelets and thrombolytic therapy, *N Engl J Med* 322:33-42, 1990.

26. Coller BS, et al: Abolition of in vivo platelet thrombus formation in primates with monoclonal antibodies to the platelet GPIIb/IIIa receptor: correlation with bleeding time, platelet aggregation, and blockade of GPIIb/IIIa receptors, *Circulation* 80:1766-1774, 1989.

27. Bang NU, Wilhelm OG, Clayman MD: After coronary thrombolysis and reperfusion, what next? *J Am Coll Cardiol* 14:837-849, 1989.

28. Fitzgerald DJ, Wright F, FitzGerald GA: Increased thromboxane biosynthesis during coronary thrombolysis: evidence that platelet activation and thromboxane A₂ modulate the response to tissue-type plasminogen activator in vivo, *Circ Res* 65:83-94, 1989.

29. Fox KAA, et al: Prevention of coronary thrombosis with subthrombolytic doses of tissue-type plasminogen activator, *Circulation* 72:1346-1354, 1985.

30. Fuster V, et al: Antithrombotic therapy after myocardial reperfusion in acute myocardial infarction, *J Am Coll Cardiol* 12:78A-84A, 1988.

31. Johns JA, et al: Prevention of coronary artery reocclusion and reduction in late coronary artery stenosis after thrombolytic therapy in patients with acute myocardial infarction, *Circulation* 78:546-556, 1988.

32. Shebuski RJ, et al: Influence of selective endoperoxide/ thromboxane A₂ receptor antagonism with sulotroban on lysis time and reocclusion rate after tissue plasminogen activator-induced coronary thrombolysis in the dog, *J Pharmacol Exp Ther* 246:790-796, 1988.

33. Shebuski RJ, et al: Acceleration of recombinant tissue-type plasminogen activator-induced thrombolysis and prevention of reocclusion by the combination of heparin and the Arg-Gly-Asp-containing peptide bitistatin in a canine model of coronary thrombosis, *Circulation* 82:169-177, 1990.

34. Topol EJ, et al: Combined tissue-type plasminogen activator and prostacyclin therapy for acute myocardial infarction, *J Am Coll Cardiol* 14:877-884, 1989.

35. Topol EJ, et al and the TAMI Study Group: A randomized controlled trial of intravenous tissue plasminogen activator and early intravenous heparin in acute myocardial infarction, *Circulation* 79:281-286, 1989.

36. Haskel EJ, et al: Relative efficacy of antithrombin compared with antiplatelet agents in accelerating coronary thrombolysis and preventing early reocclusion, *Circulation* 83:1048-1056, 1991.

37. Bleich SD, et al: Effect of heparin on coronary arterial patency after thrombolysis with tissue plasminogen activator in acute myocardial infarction, *Am J Cardiol* 66:1412-1417, 1990.

38. Camilleri JF, et al: Thrombolyse intraveineuse dans l'infarctus du myocarde. Influence de la qualite de l'antiocoagulation sur le taux de recidives precoces d'angor ou d'infarctus, *Arch Mal Coeur* 81:1037-1041, 1988.

39. de Bono DP, et al: Effect of early intravenous heparin on coronary patency, infarct size, and bleeding complications after alteplase thrombolysis: results of a randomised double-blind European Cooperative Study Group Trial, *Br Heart J* 67:122-128, 1992.

40. Hsia J, et al for the Heparin-Aspirin Reperfusion Trial (HART) Investigators: A comparison between heparin and low-dose aspirin as adjunctive therapy with tissue plasminogen activator for acute myocardial infarction, *N Engl J Med* 323:1433-1437, 1990.

41. Hsia J, et al: Heparin-induced partial thromboplastin time after thrombolysis: prolongation magnitude determines coronary patency (abstract), *Circulation* 84(suppl II):II-116, 1991.

42. Kaplan K, et al: Role of heparin after intravenous thrombolytic therapy for acute myocardial infarction, *Am J Cardiol* 59:241-244, 1987.

43. Gruppo Italiano per lo Studio della Sopravvivenza nell'Infarto Miocardico. GISSI-2: a factorial randomized trial of alteplase versus streptokinase and heparin versus no heparin among 12,490 patients with acute myocardial infarction, *Lancet* 336:65-71, 1990.

44. ISIS-3 Study Group: A randomised comparison of streptokinase vs. tissue plasminogen activator vs anistreplase and of aspirin plus heparin vs aspirin alone among 41,299 cases of suspected acute myocardial infarction, *Lancet* 339:753-770, 1992.

45. Heras M, et al: Effects of thrombin inhibition on the development of acute platelet-thrombus deposition during angioplasty in pigs. Heparin versus recombinant hirudin, a specific thrombin inhibitor, *Circulation* 79:657-665, 1989.

46. Hogg PJ, Jackson CM: Fibrin monomer protects thrombin from inactivation by heparin-antithrombin III: implications for heparin efficacy, *Proc Natl Acad Sic USA* 86:3619-3623, 1989.

47. Haskel EJ, et al: Prevention of arterial reocclusion after thrombolysis with recombinant lipoprotein-associated coagulation inhibitor, *Circulation* 84:821-827, 1991.

48. Esmon NL, Owen WG, Esmon CT: Isolation of a membrane-bound co-factor for thrombin-catalyzed activation of protein C, *J Biol Chem* 257:859-864, 1982.

49. Dunwiddie CT, et al: Antistasin, a leech-derived inhibitor of factor Xa: kinetic analysis of enzyme inhibition and identification of the reactive site, *J Biol Chem* 264:16694-16699, 1989.

50. Nutt EM, et al: The amino acid sequence of antistasin, *J Biol Chem* 263:10162-10167, 1988.

51. Nutt EM, et al: Purification and characterization of recombinant antistasin: a leech-derived inhibitor of coagulation factor Xa, *Arch Biochem Biophys* 285:37-44, 1991.

52. Tuszynski G, Gasic T, Gasic G: Isolation and characterization of antistasin, *J Biol Chem* 262:9718-9723, 1987.

53. Vlasuk GP, et al: Comparison of the in vivo anticoagulant properties of standard heparin and the highly selective factor Xa inhibitors antistasin and tick anticoagulant peptide (TAP) in a rabbit model of venous thrombosis, *Thromb Haemost* 65:257-262, 1991.

54. Gold HK, et al: Rapid and sustained coronary artery recanalization with combined bolus injection of recombinant tissue-type plasminogen activator and monoclonal antiplatelet GPIIb/IIIa antibody in a canine preparation, *Circulation* 77:670-677, 1988.

55. Klement P, et al: The effect of thrombin inhibitors on tissue plasminogen activator-induced thrombolysis in a rat model, *Thromb Haemost* 68(1):64-68, 1992.

56. ISIS-2 (Second International Study of Infarct Survival) Collaborative Group: Randomised trial of intravenous streptokinase, oral

aspirin, both, or neither among 17,187 cases of suspected myocardial infarction: ISIS-2, *Lancet* 2:349-360, 1988.

57. Ellis SG, et al: Antiplatelet GP IIb/IIIa (7E3) antibody in elective PTCA: safety and inhibition of platelet function (abstract), *Circulation* 82:III-755, 1990.

58. Yasuda T, et al: Monoclonal antibody against the platelet glycoprotein after reperfusion with recombinant tissue-type plasminogen activator in dogs, *J Clin Invest* 81:1284-1291, 1988.

59. Yasuda T, et al: Kistrin, a polypeptide platelet GPIIb/IIIa receptor antagonist, enhances and sustains coronary arterial thrombolysis with recombinant tissue-type plasminogen activator in a canine preparation, *Circulation* 83:1038-1047, 1991.

60. Yasuda T, et al: Comparative effects of aspirin, a synthetic thrombin inhibitor and a monoclonal antiplatelet glycoprotein IIb/IIIa antibody on coronary artery reperfusion, reocclusion and bleeding with recombinant tissue-type plasminogen activator in a canine preparation, *J Am Coll Cardiol* 16:714-22, 1990.

61. Yao SK, et al: Combined thromboxane A₂ synthetase inhibition and receptor blockade are effective in preventing spontaneous epinephrine-induced canine coronary cyclic flow variations, *J Am Coll Cardiol* 16:705-713, 1990.

62. Choay J, Petitou M: The chemistry of heparin: a way to understand its mode of action, *Med J Aus* 144(HS):7-10, 1986.

63. Atha DH, et al: Contribution of 3-0-and 6-0-sulfated glycosamine residues in the heparin-induced conformational change in antithrombin III, *Biochemistry* 26:6454-6461, 1987.

64. Casu B, et al: The structure of heparin oligosaccharide fragments with high anti-factor Xa activity containing the minimal anti-thrombin III-binding sequence, *Biochem J* 197:599-609, 1981.

65. Choay J, et al: Structural studies on a biologically active hexasaccharide obtained from heparin, *Ann NY Acad Sci* 370:644-649, 1981.

66. Choay J, et al: Structure-activity relationship in heparin: a synthetic pentasaccharide with high affinity for antithrombin III and eliciting high anti-factor Xa activity, *Biochem Biophys Res Comm* 116:492-499, 1983.

67. Ellis V, Scully MF, Kakkar VV: The relative molecular mass dependence of the anti-factor Xa properties of heparin, *Biochem J* 238:329-333, 1986.

68. Hook M, et al: Anticoagulant activity of heparin: separation of high-activity and low-activity heparin species by affinity chromatography on immobilized antithrombin, *FEBS Lett* 66:90-93, 1976.

69. Lindahl U, et al: Structure of the antithrombin-binding site of heparin, *Proc Natl Acad Sci USA* 76:3198-3202, 1979.

70. Lindahl U, et al: Extension and structural variability of the antithrombin-binding sequence in heparin, *J Biol Chem* 259:12368-12376, 1984.

71. Rosenberg RD: The heparin-antithrombin system: a natural anticoagulant mechanism. In Colman RW, Hirsh J, Marder VJ, et al (eds): *Hemostasis and thrombosis: basic principles and clinical practice,* ed 2, Philadelphia, 1987, JB Lippincott.

72. Rosenberg RD, Lam L: Correlation between structure and function of heparin, *Proc Natl Acad Sci USA* 76:1218-1222, 1979.

73. Oosta GM, et al: Multiple functional domains of the heparin molecule, *Proc Natl Acad Sci USA* 78:829-833, 1981.

74. Petitou M: Synthetic heparin fragments: new and efficient tools for the study of heparin and its interactions, *Nouv Rev Fr Hematol* 26:221-226, 1984.

75. Rosenberg RD, Damus PS: The purification and mechanism of action of human antithrombin-heparin cofactor, *J Biol Chem* 248:6490-6506, 1973.

76. Rosenberg RD, et al: High active heparin species with multiple binding sites for antithrombin, *Biochem Biophys Res Commun* 86:1319-1324, 1979.

77. Thunberg L, Backstrom G, Lindahl U: Further characterization of antithrombin-binding sequence in heparin, *Carbohydr Res* 100:393-410, 1982.

78. Bjork I, Lindahl U: Mechanism of the anticoagulant action of heparin, *Mol Cell Biochem* 48:161-162, 1982.

79. Nordenman B, Bjork I: Binding of low-affinity and high-affinity heparin to antithrombin. Ultraviolet difference spectroscopy and circular dichroism studies, *Biochemistry* 17:3339-3344, 1978.

80. Olson ST, et al: Binding of high-affinity heparin to antithrombin III: stopped flow kinetic studies of the binding interaction, *J Biol Chem* 256:11073-11079, 1981.

81. Villanueva GB, Danishefsky I: Evidence for a heparin-induced conformational change on antithrombin III, *Biochem Biophys Res Commun* 74:803-809, 1977.

82. Beguin S, Lindhout T, Hemker HC: The mode of action of heparin in plasma, *Thromb Haemost* 60:457-462, 1988.

83. Beguin S, et al: The mode of action of low molecular weight heparin preparation (PK 10169) and two of its major components on thrombin generation in plasma, *Thromb Haemost* 61:30-34, 1989.

84. Hemker HC: The mode of action of heparin in plasma. In Verstraete M, Vermylen J, Lijnen HR, et al (eds): *XIth Congress on Thrombosis and Haemostasis,* Brussels, 1987, Leuven University Press.

85. Danielsson A, et al: Role of ternary complexes in which heparin binds both antithrombin and proteinase, in the acceleration of the reactions between antithrombin and thrombin or factor Xa, *J Biol Chem* 261:15467-15473, 1986.

86. Olson ST, Shore JD: Demonstration of a two-step reaction mechanism for inhibition of α-thrombin by antithrombin III and identification of the step affected by heparin, *J Biol Chem* 257:14891-14895, 1982.

87. Holmer E, et al: Anticoagulant activities and effects on platelets of a heparin fragment with high affinity for antithrombin, *Thromb Res* 18:861-869, 1980.

88. Holmer E, Matsson C, Nilsson S: Anticoagulant and antithrombotic effects of low molecular weight heparin fragments in rabbits, *Thromb Res* 25:475-485, 1982.

89. Tollefsen DM, Majerus DW, Blank MK: Heparin cofactor II. Purification and properties of thrombin in human plasma, *J Biol Chem* 257:2162-2169, 1982.

90. Hurst RE, Poon MC, Griffith MJ: Structure-activity relationships of heparin. Independence of heparin charge density and antithrombin binding domains in thrombin inhibition by antithrombin and heparin cofactor II, *J Clin Invest* 72:1042-1045, 1983.

91. Maimone MM, Tollefsen DM: Activation of heparin cofactor II by heparin oligosaccharides, *Biochem Biophys Res Commun* 152:1056-1061, 1988.

92. Petitou M, et al: Is there a unique sequence in heparin for interaction with heparin cofactor II? Structural and biological studies of heparin-derived oligosaccharides, *J Biol Chem* 263:8685-8690, 1988.

93. Sie P, et al: Studies on the structural requirements of heparin for the catalysis of thrombin inhibition by heparin cofactor II, *Biochem Biophys Acta* 966:188-195, 1988.

94. Andersson L-O, et al: Molecular weight dependency of the heparin potentiated inhibition of thrombin and activated factor X. Effect of heparin neutralization in plasma, *Thromb Res* 115:531-541, 1979.

95. Harenberg J: Pharmacology of low molecular weight heparins, *Sem Thromb Hemost* 16:12-18, 1990.

96. Johnson EA, Mulloy B: The molecular weight range of commercial heparin preparations, *Carbohydr Res* 51:119-27, 1976.

97. Hirsh J: Heparin, *N Engl J Med* 324:1565-1574, 1991.

98. Pini M, et al: Subcutaneous vs intravenous heparin in the

treatment of deep venous thrombosis—a randomized clinical trial, *Thromb Haemost* 64:222-226, 1990.

99. Hull RD, et al: Continuous intravenous heparin compared with intermittent subcutaneous heparin in the initial treatment of proximal-vein thrombosis, *N Engl J Med* 315:1109-1114, 1986.

100. Lane DA, et al: Neutralization of heparin-related saccharides by histidine-rich glycoprotein and platelet factor 4, *J Biol Chem* 261:3980-3986, 1986.

101. Lijnen HR, Hoylaerts M, Collen D: Heparin-binding properties of human histidine-rich glycoprotein. Mechanism and role in the neutralization of heparin in plasma, *J Biol Chem* 258:3803-3808, 1983.

102. Peterson CB, Morgan WT, Blackburn MN: Histidine-rich glycoprotein modulation of the anticoagulant activity of heparin, *J Biol Chem* 262:7567-7574, 1987.

103. Holt JC, Niewiarowski S: Biochemistry of alpha granule proteins, *Semin Hematol* 22:151-163, 1985.

104. Preissner KT, Muller-Berghaus G: Neutralization and binding of heparin by S-protein/vitronectin in the inhibition of factor Xa by antithrombin III, *J Biol Chem* 262:12247-12253, 1987.

105. Dawes J, Pavuk N: Sequestration of therapeutic glycosaminoglycans by plasma fibronectin (abstract), *Thromb Haemost* 65:829, 1991.

106. Haskel EJ, et al: Prevention of arterial reocclusion after thrombolysis with recombinant lipoprotein-associated coagulation inhibitor, *Circulation* 84:821-827, 1991.

107. Hirsh J, et al: Heparin kinetics in venous thrombosis and pulmonary embolism, *Circulation* 53:691-695, 1976.

108. Young E, Petrowski P, Hirsh J: Heparin binding to plasma proteins an important mechanism for heparin resistance, *Thromb Haemost* 67(6):639-643, 1992.

109. Barzu T, et al: Binding and endocytosis of heparin by human endothelial cells in culture, *Biochem Biophys Acta* 845:196-203, 1985.

110. Bjornsson TO, Wolfram BS, Kitchell BB: Heparin kinetics determined by three assay methods, *Clin Pharmacol Ther* 31:104-113, 1982.

111. Boneu B, et al: Effects of heparin, its low molecular weight fractions and other glycosaminoglycans on thrombus growth in vivo, *Thromb Res* 40:81-89, 1985.

112. Boneu B, et al: Pharmacokinetic studies of standard unfractionated heparin, and low molecular weight heparins in the rabbit, *Sem Thromb Hemost* 14:18-27, 1988.

113. Boneu B, Caranobe C, Sie P: Pharmacokinetics of heparin and low molecular weight heparin. In Hirsh J (ed): *Bailliere's Clinical haematology: antithrombotic therapy.* London, 1990, Bailliere Tindall.

114. de Swart CAM, et al: Kinetics of intravenously administered heparin in normal humans, *Blood* 60:1251-1258, 1982.

115. Olsson P, Lagergren H, Ek S: The elimination from plasma of intravenous heparin. An experimental study on dogs and humans, *Acta Med Scand* 173:619-630, 1963.

116. Glimelius B, Busch C, Hook M: Binding of heparin on the surface of cultured human endothelial cells, *Thromb Res* 12:773-782, 1978.

117. Mahadoo J, Hiebert L, Jaques LB: Vascular sequestration of heparin, *Thromb Res* 12:79-90, 1977.

118. Friedman Y, Arsenis C: Studies on the heparin sulphamidase activity from rat spleen. Intracellular distribution and characterization of the enzyme, *Biochem J* 139:699-708, 1974.

119. Dawes J, Pepper DS: Catabolism of low-dose heparin in man, *Thromb Res* 14:845-860, 1979.

120. McAllister BM, Demis DJ: Heparin metabolism: isolation and characterization of uroheparin, *Nature* 212:293-294, 1966.

121. Turpie AGG, et al: Comparison of high-dose with low-dose subcutaneous heparin to prevent left ventricular mural thrombosis in patients with acute transmural anterior myocardial infarction, *N Engl J Med* 320:352-394, 1989.

122. Cruickshank MK, et al: A standard heparin nomogram for the management of heparin therapy, *Arch Intern Med* 151:333-337, 1991.

123. Basu D, et al: A prospective study of the value of monitoring heparin treatment with the activated partial thromboplastin time, *N Engl J Med* 287:324-327, 1972.

124. De Clerck F, et al: R68070: thromboxane A_2 synthetase inhibition and thromboxane A_2/prostaglandin in endoperoxide receptor blockage combined in one molecule. II: Pharmacological effects in vivo and ex vivo, *Thromb Haemost* 61:43-49, 1989.

125. Shojania AM, Tetreault J, Turnbull G: The variations between heparin sensitivity of different lots of activated partial thromboplastin time reagent produced by the same manufacturer, *Am J Clin Pathol* 89:19-23, 1988.

126. Hirsh J, et al: Heparin: mechanism of action, pharmacokinetics, dosing considerations, monitoring, efficacy and safety, *Chest* 102(4):3375-3515, 1992.

127. Levine MN, Hirsh J, Kelton JG: Heparin-induced bleeding. In Lane DA, Lindahl U, editors: *Heparin: chemical and biological properties, clinical applications,* London, England, 1989, Edward Arnold.

128. Morabia A: Heparin doses and major bleedings, *Lancet* 1:1278-1279, 1986.

129. Landefeld S, et al: Identification and preliminary validation of predictors of major bleeding in hospitalized patients starting anticoagulant therapy, *Am J Med* 82:703-723, 1987.

130. Magnani B, for the PAIMS Investigators: Plasminogen Activator Italian Multicenter Study (PAIMS): Comparison of intravenous recombinant single-chain human tissue type plasminogen activator (rt-PA) with intravenous streptokinase in acute myocardial infarction, *J Am Coll Cardiol* 13:19-26, 1989.

131. Burch JW, Majerus PW: The role of prostaglandins in platelet function, *Semin Hematol* 16:196-207, 1979.

132. Burch JW, Stanford PW: Inhibition of platelet prostaglandin synthetase by oral aspirin, *J Clin Invest* 61:314-319, 1979.

133. Burch JW, et al: Sensitivity of fatty acid cyclooxygenase from human aorta to acetylation by aspirin, *Proc Natl Acad Sci USA* 75:5181-5184, 1978.

134. FitzGerald GA, et al: Endogenous biosynthesis of prostacyclin and thromboxane and platelet function during chronic administration of aspirin in man, *J Clin Invest* 71:678-688, 1983.

135. Kyrle PA, et al: Inhibition of prostaglandin and thromboxane A_2 generation by low-dose aspirin at the site of plug formation in man in vivo, *Circulation* 75: 1025-1029, 1987.

136. Majerus PW: Arachidonate metabolism in vascular disorders, *J Clin Invest* 72:1521-1525, 1983.

137. Moncada S, Vane JR: The role of prostacyclin in vascular tissue, *Fed Proc* 38:66-71, 1979.

138. Moncada S, Vane JR: Pharmacology and endogenous roles of prostaglandin endoperoxides, thromboxane-A_2 and prostacyclin, *Pharmacol Rev* 30:293-331, 1978.

139. Patignani P, Filabozzi P, Patrono C: Selective cumulative inhibition of platelet thromboxane production by low-dose aspirin in healthy subjects, *J Clin Invest* 69:1366-1372, 1982.

140. Preston FE, et al: Inhibition of prostacyclin and platelet thromboxane A_2 after low-dose aspirin, *N Engl J Med* 304:76-79, 1981.

141. Weksler BB, et al: Differential inhibition by aspirin of vascular and platelet prostaglandin synthesis in atherosclerotic patients, *N Engl J Med* 308:800-805, 1983.

142. Moncada S, Vane JR: Mode of action of aspirin-like drugs. In

Stollerman GH (ed): *Cardiovascular drugs,* vol 24, New York 1982, Adis Press.

143. Demers LM, Budin R, Shaikh B: The effects of aspirin on megakaryocyte prostaglandin production, *Blood* 50(suppl 1):239, 1977.

144. Cerskus AL, et al: Possible significance of small numbers of functional platelets in a population of aspirin-treated platelets in vitro and in vivo, *Thromb Res* 18:389-397, 1980.

145. Clarke RJ, et al: Suppression of thromboxane A_2 but not of systemic prostacyclin by controlled-release aspirin, *N Engl J Med* 325:1137-1141, 1991.

146. O'Brien JR: Effects of salicylates on human platelets, *Lancet* 1:779-783, 1986.

147. Lorenz RL, et al: Superior antiplatelet action of alternative day pulsed dosing versus split dose administration of aspirin, *Am J Cardiol* 64:1185-1188, 1989.

148. Rowland M, et al: Absorption kinetics of aspirin in man following oral administration of an aqueous solution, *J Pharm Sci* 61:379-385, 1972.

149. Pedersen AK, FitzGerald GA: Dose-related kinetics of aspirin: presystemic acetylation of platelet cyclooxygenase, *N Engl J Med* 311:1206-1211, 1984.

150. Turpie AGG, et al: Reduction in mortality by adding acetylsalicylic acid (100 mg) to oral anticoagulants in patients with heart valve replacement (abstract), *Can J Cardiol* 7(suppl A):95A, 1991.

151. The RISC Group: Risk of myocardial infarction and death during treatment with low-dose aspirin and intravenous heparin in men with unstable coronary artery disease, *Lancet* 336:827-830, 1990.

152. The SALT Collaborative Group: Swedish Aspirin Low-Dose Trial (SALT) of 75 mg aspirin as secondary prophylaxis after cerebrovascular ischaemic events, *Lancet* 338:1345-1349, 1991.

153. The Dutch TIA Trial Study Group: The effects of 30 mg versus 300 mg acetylsalicylic acid, and of 50 mg atenolol versus placebo on mortality, stroke and myocardial infarction after TIA or minor ischemic stroke, *N Engl J Med* 325:1261-1266, 1991.

154. The GUSTO investigators: An international randomized trial comparing four thrombolytic strategies for acute myocardial infarction, *N Engl J Med* 329:673-682, 1993.

155. The International Study Group: In-hospital mortality and clinical course of 20,891 patients with suspected acute myocardial infarction randomised between alteplase and streptokinase with or without heparin, *Lancet* 336:71-75, 1990.

156. Prins MH, Hirsh J: Heparin as an adjunctive treatment after thrombolytic therapy for acute myocardial infarction, *Am J Cardiol* 67:3A-11A, 1991.

157. The Australian National Heart Study Trial: A randomized comparison of oral aspirin/dipyridamole versus intravenous heparin after rt-PA for acute myocardial infarction (abstract), *Circulation* 80(suppl II):II-114, 1989.

158. The SCATI (Studio sulla Calciparina nell'Angina e nella Thrombosi Ventriculare nell'Infarto) Group: Randomised controlled trial of subcutaneous calcium-heparin in acute myocardial infarction, *Lancet* 2:182-186, 1989.

159. Hirsh J, Levine MN: Low molecular weight heparin, *Blood* 79(1):1-17, 1992.

160. Ofosu FA, Barrowcliffe TW: Mechanisms of action of low molecular weight heparins and heparinoids. In Hirsh J (ed): *Antithrombotic therapy, Bailliere's Clinical haematology,* vol 3, London, 1990, Bailliere Tindall.

161. Handeland GF, et al: Dose-adjusted heparin treatment of deep venous thrombosis: a comparison of unfractionated and low molecular weight heparin, *Eur J Clin Pharmacol* 39:107-112, 1990.

162. Barzu T, et al: Binding of heparin and low molecular weight heparin fragments to human vascular endothelial cells in culture, *Nouv Rev Fr Haematol* 26:243-247, 1984.

163. Barzu T, et al: Heparin degradation in the endothelial cells, *Thromb Res* 47:601-609, 1987.

164. Bara L, et al: Comparative pharmacokinetics of low molecular weight heparin (PK 10169) and unfractionated heparin after intravenous and subcutaneous administration, *Thromb Res* 39:631-636, 1985.

165. Bara L, Samama MM: Pharmacokinetics of low molecular weight heparins, *Acta Chir Scand* 543:65-72, 1988.

166. Bradbrook ID, et al: ORG 10172: a low molecular weight heparinoid anticoagulant with a long half-life in man, *Br J Clin Pharmacol* 23:667-675, 1987.

167. Bratt G, et al: Low molecular weight heparin (KABI 2165, FRAGMIN): pharmacokinetics after intravenous and subcutaneous administration in human volunteers, *Thromb Res* 42:613-620, 1986.

168. Briant L, et al: Unfractionated heparin and CY216. Pharmacokinetics and bioavailabilities of the anti-Factor Xa and IIa. Effects of intravenous and subcutaneous injection in rabbits, *Thromb Haemost* 61:348-353, 1989.

169. Frydman A, et al: The antithrombotic activity and pharmacokinetics of enoxaparin, a low molecular weight heparin, in man given single subcutaneous doses of 20 up to 80 mg, *J Clin Pharmacol* 28:608-618, 1988.

170. Matzsch T, et al: Effect of an enzymatically depolymerized heparin as compared with conventional heparin in healthy volunteers, *Thromb Haemost* 57:97-101, 1987.

171. Stiekema JC, et al: Safety and pharmacokinetics of the low molecular weight heparinoid ORG 10172 administered to healthy elderly volunteers, *Br J Clin Pharmacol* 27:39-48, 1989.

172. Andriuoli G, et al: Comparison of the antithrombotic and hemorrhagic effects of heparin and a new low molecular weight heparin in the rat, *Haemostasis* 15:324-330, 1985.

173. Bergqvist D, et al: The effects of heparin fragments of different molecular weight in experimental thrombosis and haemostasis, *Thromb Res* 38:589-601, 1985.

174. Cade JF, et al: A comparison of the antithrombotic and haemorrhagic effects of low molecular weight heparin fractions: the influence of the method of preparation, *Thromb Res* 35:613-625, 1984.

175. Carter CJ, et al: The relationship between the hemorrhagic and antithrombotic properties of low molecular weight heparins and heparin, *Blood* 59:1239-1245, 1982.

176. Esquivel CO, et al: Comparison between commercial heparin, low-molecular weight heparin and pentosan polysulphate on haemostasis and platelets in vivo, *Thromb Res* 28:389-399, 1982.

177. Henny CP, et al: A randomized blind study comparing standard heparin and a new low molecular weight heparinoid in cardiopulmonary bypass surgery in dogs, *J Lab Clin Med* 106:187-196, 1985.

178. Hobbelen PM, Vogel GM, Mueleman DG: Time courses of the antithrombotic effects, bleeding enhancing effects and interactions with factors Xa and thrombin after administration of low molecular weight heparinoid ORG 10172 or heparin to rats, *Thromb Res* 48:549-558, 1987.

179. Ockelford PA, et al: Discordance between the anti-Xa activity and antithrombotic activity of an ultra-low molecular weight heparin fraction, *Thromb Res* 28:401-409, 1982.

180. Fabris F, et al: Normal and low molecular weight heparins: interaction with human platelets, *Eur J Clin Invest* 13:135-139, 1983.

181. Fernandez F, et al: Hemorrhagic doses of heparin and other glycosaminoglycans induce a platelet defect, *Thromb Res* 43:491-495, 1986.

182. Blajchman MA, Young E, Ofosu FA: Effects of unfractionated

heparin, dermatan sulfate and low molecular weight on vessel wall permeability in rabbits, *Ann NY Acad Sci* 556:245-254, 1989.

183. Agnelli G, et al: The comparative effects of recombinant hirudin (CGP 39393) and standard heparin on thrombus growth in rabbits, *Thromb Haemost* 63:204-207, 1990.

184. Agnelli G, et al: Sustained antithrombotic activity of hirudin after its plasma clearance:comparison with heparin, *Blood*, 1992.

185. Rydel TJ, et al: The structure of a complex of recombinant hirudin and human α-thrombin, *Science* 249:277-280, 1990.

186. Stone SR, Hofsteenge J: Kinetics of the inhibition of thrombin by hirudin, *Biochemistry* 25:4622-4628, 1986.

187. Bourdon P, Fenton JW II, Maraganore JM: Affinity labelling of lysine-149 in the anion-binding exosite of human α-thrombin with an N^a-(dinitrofluorobenzyl) hirudin C- terminal peptide, *Biochemistry* 29:6379-6384, 1990.

188. Chang J-Y, et al: The structural elements of hirudin which bind to the fibrinogen recognition site of thrombin are exclusively located within its acidic C-terminal tail, *FEBS Lett* 261:287-290, 1990.

189. Krstenansky JL, Mao SJT: Antithrombin properties of C-terminus of hirudin using synthetic unsulfated N^a-acetyl-hirudin 45-65, *FEBS Lett* 211:10-16, 1987.

190. Maraganore JM, et al: Design and characterization of hirulogs: a novel class of bivalent peptide inhibitors of thrombin, *Biochemistry* 29:7095-7101, 1990.

191. Maraganore JM, et al: Anticoagulant activity of synthetic hirudin fragments, *J Biol Chem* 264:8692-8698, 1989.

192. Kikumoto R, et al: Selective inhibition of thrombin by (2R,4R)-4-methyl-1[N^2-[(3-methyl-1,2,3,4-tetrahydro-8-quinolinyl) sulfonyl]-L-arginyl)]-2-piperidinecarboxylic acid, *Biochemistry* 23:85-90, 1984.

193. Kettner C, Shaw E: D-Phe-Pro-ArgCh₂Cl. A selective affinity label for thrombin, *Thromb Res* 14:969-73, 1979.

194. Kettner C, Mersinger L, Knabb R: The selective inhibition of thrombin by peptides of boroarginine, *J Biol Chem* 265:18289-18297, 1990.

195. Bagdy D, et al: In vivo anticoagulant and antiplatelet effect of D-Phe-Pro-Arg-H and D-MePhe-Pro-Arg-H, *Thromb Haemost* 67(3):357-365, 1992.

196. Lam JYT, et al: Is vasospasm related to platelet deposition? Relationship in a porcine preparation of arterial injury in vivo, *Circulation* 75:243-248, 1987.

197. Gruber A, et al: Inhibition of platelet dependent thrombus formation by human activated protein C in a primate model, *Blood* 73:639-642, 1989.

198. Gruber A, et al: Inhibition of thrombus formation by activated recombinant protein C in a primate model of arterial thrombosis, *Circulation* 82:578-585, 1990.

199. Gruber A, et al: Antithrombotic effects of combining activated protein C and urokinase in nonhuman primates, *Circulation* 84:2454-2464, 1991.

200. Waxman L, et al: Tick anticoagulant peptide (TAP) is a novel inhibitor of blood coagulation factor Xa, *Science* 248:593-596, 1990.

201. Neeper MP, et al: Characterization of recombinant tick antico-agulant peptide, *J Biol Chem* 265:17746-17752, 1990.

202. Hanson SR, Harker LA: Interruption of acute platelet-dependent thrombosis by the synthetic antithrombin D-phenylalanyl-L-propyl-arginyl chloromethyl ketone, *Proc Natl Acad Sci USA* 85:3184-3188, 1988.

203. Hanson SR, et al: Effects of monoclonal antibodies against the platelet glycoprotein IIb/IIIa complex on thrombosis and hemo-stasis in the baboon, *J Clin Invest* 82:149-158, 1988.

204. Dunwiddie CT, et al: Anticoagulant efficacy and immunogenicity of the selective factor Xa inhibitor antistasin following subcuta-

205. Marciniak E: Factor X_a inactivation by antithrombin III: evidence for biological stabilization of factor X_a by factor V-phospholipid complex, *Br J Hematol* 24:391-400, 1973.

206. Teitel JM, Rosenberg RD: Protection of factor Xa from neutralization by the heparin-antithrombin complex, *J Clin Invest* 71:1383-1389, 1983.

207. Lane DA: Heparin binding and neutralizing protein. In Lane DA, Lindahl U (ed): *Heparin: chemical and biological properties, clinical applications,* London, 1989, Edward Arnold.

208. Lane DA, et al: Anticoagulant activities of heparin oligosaccha-rides and their neutralization by platelet factor 4, *Biochem J* 218:725-732, 1984.

209. Weiss HJ, et al: Evidence for the presence of tissue factor activity on subendothelium, *Blood* 73:968-975, 1989.

210. Wilcox JN, et al: Localization of tissue factor in the normal vessel wall and in the atherosclerotic plaque, *Proc Natl Acad Sci USA* 86:2839-2843, 1989.

211. Zeldis SM, et al: Tissue factor (thromboplastin): localization to plasma membranes by peroxidase-conjugated antibodies, *Science* 175:766-768, 1972.

212. Broze GJ, et al: The lipoprotein-associated coagulation inhibitor that inhibits the factor VII-tissue factor complex also inhibits factor Xa: insight into its possible mechanism of action, *Blood* 71:335-343, 1988.

213. Rapaport SI: Inhibiton of factor VIIa/tissue factor-induced blood coagulation: with particular emphasis upon a factor Xa-dependent inhibitory mechanism, *Blood* 73:359-365, 1989.

214. Lawrence JB, Gralnick HR: Monoclonal antibodies to the glycoprotein IIb-IIIa epitopes involved in adhesive protein binding: effects on platelet spreading and ultrastructure on human arterial subendothelium, *J Lab Clin Med* 109:495-503, 1987.

215. Sakariassen KS, et al: The role of platelet membrane glycopro-teins Ib and IIb-IIIa in platelet adherence to human artery subendothelium, *Br J Haematol* 63:681-691, 1986.

216. Weiss HJ, et al: Fibrinogen-independent platelet adhesion and thrombus formation on subendothelium mediated by glycopro-tein IIb-IIIa complex at high shear rate, *J Clin Invest* 83:288-297, 1989.

217. Coller BS, et al: Antithrombotic effect of a monoclonal antibody to the platelet glycoprotein IIb/IIIa receptor in an experimental animal model, *Blood* 69:783-786, 1986.

218. Mickelson JK, et al: Antiplatelet antibody [7E3 F(ab')2] pre-vents rethrombosis after recombinant tissue-type plasminogen activator-induced coronary artery thrombolysis in a canine model, *Circulation* 81:617-627, 1990.

219. Ruoslahti E, Pierschbacher MD: New perspectives in cell adhesion: RGD and integrins, *Science* 238:491-497, 1987.

220. Bush LR, et al: Antithrombotic profile of echistatin, a snake venom peptide and platelet fibrinogen receptor antagonist in the dog (abstract), *Circulation* 80(suppl II):II-23, 1989.

221. Cook JJ, et al: Inhibition of platelet hemostatic plug formation by trigramin, a novel RGD-peptide, *Am J Physiol* 256:H1038-1043, 1989.

222. Mellott MJ, et al: Effects of bitistatin, a snake venom peptide and platelet fibrinogen receptor antagonist in a canine model of thrombolysis and reocclusion (abstract), *Circulation* 80(suppl II):II-216, 1989.

223. Haskel EJ, et al: Prevention of reoccluding platelet-rich thrombi in canine femoral arteries with a novel peptide antagonist of platelet glycoprotein IIb/IIIa receptors, *Circulation* 80:1775-1782, 1989.

224. Shebuski RJ, et al: Demonstration of Ac-Arg-Gly-Asp-Ser-NH₂

as an antiaggregatory agent in the dog by intracoronary administration, *Thromb Haemost* 61:183-188, 1989.

225. Gold HK, et al: Phase I human trial of the potent anti-platelet agents, 7E3-F(ab')2, a monoclonal antibody to the GP IIb/IIIa receptor (abstract), *Circulation* 80(suppl II):II-267, 1989.

226. Davidson JT, et al: Inhibition of arterial thrombus formation with a novel GP-IIb/IIIa fibrinogen receptor antagonist in a baboon model of platelet-dependent arterial thrombosis (abstract), *Circulation* 84:II-122, 1991.

227. Chao BH, et al: *Agkistrodon piscivorus piscivorus* platelet aggregation inhibitor: a potent inhibitor of platelet activation, *Proc Natl Acad Sci USA* 86:8050-8054, 1989.

228. Huang TF, et al: Trigramin. A low molecular weight peptide inhibiting fibrinogen interaction with platelet receptors expressed on glycoprotein IIb-IIIa complex, *J Biol Chem* 262:16157-16163, 1987.

229. Ouyang C, Huang T: Potent platelet aggregation inhibitor from *Trimeresurus gramnes* snake venom, *Biochem Biophys Acta* 757:332-341, 1983.

230. Willerson JT, et al: Role of new antiplatelet agents as adjunctive therapies in thrombolysis, *Am J Cardiol* 67:12A-18A, 1991.

231. Ganguly P: Binding of thrombin to human platelets, *Nature* 247:306-307, 1974.

232. Hamberg M, Svensson J, Sameulsson B: Thromboxanes: a new group of biologically active compounds derived from prostaglandin endoperoxides, *Proc Natl Acad Sci USA* 72:2994-2998, 1975.

233. Moncada S, Vane JR: Arachidonic acid metabolites and the interactions between platelets and blood vessel walls, *N Engl J Med* 300:1142-1147, 1979.

234. Yao SK, et al: Thrombin inhibition enhances recombinant tissue-type plasminogen activator-induced thrombolysis and delays reocclusion, *Am J Physiol* 262:374-379, 1992.

235. Yao SK, et al: Combination of inhibition of thrombin and blockade of thromboxane A_2 synthetase and receptors enhances thrombolysis and delays reocclusion in canine coronary arteries, *Circulation* 86:1993-1999, 1992.

236. De Clerck F, et al: R68070: thromboxane A_2 synthetase inhibition and thromboxane A_2/prostaglandin endoperoxide receptor blockade combined in one molecule. I:Biochemical profile in vitro, *Thromb Haemost* 61:35-42, 1989.

237. Ashton JH, et al: Inhibition of cyclic flow A_2/prostaglandin H_2 receptor antagonists, *Circ Res* 59:568-578, 1986.

238. Bush LR, et al: Effects of the selective thromboxane synthetase inhibitor dazoxiben on variations in cyclic blood flow in stenosed canine coronary arteries, *Circulation* 69:1161-1170, 1984.

239. Golino P, et al: Endogenous prostaglandin endoperoxides and prostacyclin modulate the thrombolytic activity of tissue plasminogen activator: effects of simultaneous inhibition of thromboxane A_2 synthetase and blockade of thromboxane A_2/prostaglandin H_2 receptors in a canine model of coronary thrombosis, *J Clin Invest* 86:1095-1102, 1990.

Chapter 29

ANTIPLATELET THERAPY IN THE SETTING OF ACUTE MYOCARDIAL INFARCTION

Neal S. Kleiman

As our understanding of the pathophysiology of acute myocardial infarction (AMI) has evolved, the need to find new agents to advance treatment of this syndrome has broadened. In particular, since the advent of reperfusion therapy and the recognition that persistent arterial patency is associated with improved survival after MI,[1-4] increased awareness of the central role of platelets in the occurrence and recurrence of arterial thrombosis has led to a need to explore new potent inhibitors of platelet aggregation, as well as to define the clinical role of existing agents. Although the role of platelet-inhibiting agents in classical secondary prevention after AMI has been appreciated for more than 10 years, such therapy has in recent years been extended to treatment of the acute phase of MI.

PATHOPHYSIOLOGY

Although the role of thrombus in the pathogenesis of AMI had been debated until the late 1970s, the importance of the atherosclerotic plaque was well recognized, and pathologists in the mid-1960s were aware that atherosclerotic plaques of patients undergoing autopsy soon after AMI were covered with a layer of adherent platelets.[5,6] Friedman and Van den Bovenkamp, early proponents of thrombus as a central factor in the occurrence of MI, reported the universal presence of plaque rupture into the arterial lumen from what they described as "atheromatous abscesses." The site of rupture was characterized by mixtures of lipid, cholesterol, and cellular debris, which were covered with a layer of adherent platelets. This area, termed the "body" of the thrombus, was found to be largely platelet-rich, whereas the areas both proximal and distal consisted mainly of fibrin and erythrocytes.[6] More recent autopsy studies of patients who have died after AMI have consistently revealed plaque rupture and deep fissuring, with exposure of plaque contents, subendothelial material, and overlying thrombus in the coronary artery responsible for the infarction.[7-9] Other techniques including biochemical assays of thromboxane A_2 metabolites and postmortem autoradiography have provided confirmatory evidence of platelet activation in patients with MI.

Platelet activity after arterial injury

Platelet activity has received even more attention since thrombolytic therapy (both with and without angioplasty) has become a mainstay in the treatment of AMI. It is now clear that platelet aggregation plays a central role in the initiation of arterial thrombosis. After endothelial injury and exposure of the subendothelium, platelets adhere to the damaged surface. Under conditions of laminar flow, this process occurs through the interaction of specific platelet receptors with the subendothelial extracellular matrix. Under conditions of turbulent flow (high shear) as is seen at the site of a high-grade arterial narrowing, the interaction of the platelet glycoprotein Ib receptor with high-molecular-weight von Willebrand factor appears to predominate.[10] High-molecular-weight von Willebrand factor is produced by the endothelium and secreted into the subendothelium; interaction between this molecule and glycoprotein Ib leads to platelet deposition, which is increased several-fold over that which occurs in settings of laminar flow.[11,12] After the rupture of a plaque and the subsequent protrusion of its contents into the arterial lumen, it is likely that both mechanisms are involved.

In a process known as activation, platelets subsequently undergo cytoskeletal alterations responsible for platelet spreading along the damaged surface, for the expression of surface receptor proteins, and for release of the contents of α-granules and dense granules.[13] The granules contain vasoconstrictor and proaggregatory substances that effectively provide feedback amplification for the activation process already in progress and help recruit additional platelets. Activation of circulating platelets occurs in response to a variety of biologic stimuli, including thrombin, plasmin, the catecholamines, collagen, adenosine diphosphate (ADP), serotonin (5-hydroxytryptamine), thromboxane A_2, platelet-activating factor, and von Willebrand factor. Specific receptors that mediate the platelet response to some of these agonists have been identified. These receptors include glycoprotein Ia, whose interaction with collagen mediates platelet adhesion,[14] and the recently isolated and cloned glycoprotein receptor for thrombin.[15] In addition, the glycoprotein complex IIb/IIIa has been shown to interact with von Willebrand factor and may play a role in platelet adhesion.[16] Regardless of the pathway of activation, the final result of this process is the release of calcium from the sarcoplasmic reticulum into the cytoplasm and a series of reactions that culminates in activation of the intracellular contractile apparatus.

Specific receptors that signal inhibition of platelet activation have also been identified (e.g., the receptor for prostaglandin [PGI_2, or prostacyclin]) and share the common mechanism of increasing intracellular concentrations of cyclic adenosine monophosphate (cAMP), which inhibits calcium-mediated responses, as well as intracellular cyclic guanine monophosphate (cGMP), which limits platelet response to several agonists.[17]

The receptors that are ultimately expressed on the platelet surface as a result of activation consist of the complexed glycoproteins IIb and IIIa. The IIb/IIIa complex (also known as integrin $\alpha_{IIb}\beta_3$) is a member of a larger family of intercellular adhesion molecules known as integrins and is believed to be almost solely responsible for platelet aggregation. Expression of the IIb/IIIa complex and binding of fibrinogen is the final common pathway through which platelet aggregation and the formation of a platelet-rich thrombus occur. This complex binds arginine-glycine-asparagine (RGD)

amino acid sequences, which are located on the alpha- and gamma-chains of circulating fibrinogen.[10,18] However, it is known to bind von Willebrand factor, fibronectin, vitronectin, and collagen as well,[19] probably through recognition of the same RGD sequence on these molecules. The fibrinogen molecule thus acts as a meshwork that stabilizes the platelet plug.

At the same time that activation occurs, platelets secrete coagulation factor V, which, when activated to factor Va along with calcium (also secreted from platelet granules during activation) and factor Xa, form the prothrombinase complex.[20] When assembled on the platelet surface, the prothrombinase complex is a potent catalyst for the formation of thrombin from prothrombin. Thrombin, in turn, catalyzes the formation of fibrin and, in addition, is itself an extremely potent stimulus for platelet activation. Thus, platelet activation and aggregation are intimately tied to activation of the soluble coagulation system and the formation of the occlusive thrombus. In addition to exerting a direct prothrombotic effect, platelet activation has several indirect effects that promote thrombus formation. The contents of platelet granules include ADP, serotonin, thromboxane A_2, and other potent vasoconstrictors, which may lead to further stasis and coagulation of intraarterial blood after their secretion. Two other secretagogues, platelet factor 4 and thrombospondin, may exert antiheparin effects. Finally, transforming growth factor-β, a constituent released from platelet α-granules, has been shown to stimulate secretion of plasminogen activator inhibitor-1 (PAI-1) by hepatocytes and endothelial cells.[21,22]

Platelet activation may also establish conditions conducive to thrombus formation by modulating vascular tone. In a canine model of high-grade arterial stenosis with underlying endothelial damage, Folts et al.[23] demonstrated cyclic reductions in antegrade flow in the portion of the artery distal to an artificially created obstruction. These reductions are the direct consequence of shear-induced platelet adhesion to the site of the stenosis and of distal embolization of platelet plugs. Treatment with aspirin and a variety of other platelet antiaggregants, including antagonists of thromboxane A_2 and serotonin, eliminate these flow variations.[24,25] A mild degree of vasoconstriction occurs in such a model; the addition of local thrombosis and arterial injury produce considerably greater vasoconstriction than is associated with a narrowing alone.[25] After even brief periods of ischemia and reperfusion, the vascular endothelium is damaged and endothelium-dependent relaxation is impaired. Consequently, arterial segments become hyperreactive in response to thrombin and other substances that would normally serve as vasodilators.[26,27] Activated platelets enhance these increases in vasomotion,[28] which may, in turn, impede the restoration and maintenance of antegrade coronary arterial flow.

Platelet activation after thrombolysis

Several lines of evidence implicate enhanced platelet activity as a factor in both failure to achieve recanalization after thrombolytic therapy and reocclusion after thrombolysis. During pharmacologic lysis of a thrombus, the process of arterial recanalization is dynamic; periods of reperfusion are frequently followed by reocclusion and subsequent reperfusion until a steady state of either persistent patency or occlusion is reached.[29] Thrombolytic drugs have been reported to both enhance and inhibit platelet aggregation during the acute phase of thrombolysis,[30-37] and different degrees of enhanced or inhibited aggregation have been reported with different agents.[38,39] During the early phases of thrombolysis, platelet thromboxane A_2 activity is increased, suggesting that platelet activation is occurring.[32,33] It is also likely that thrombin (which is generated in increased quanti-

Table 29-1. Platelet-inhibiting agents shown experimentally to decrease time to lysis with plasminogen activators and to decrease the frequency of reocclusion*

TXA_2 inhibition
  TXA_2 receptor blockers
  Combined thromboxane synthase and thromboxane receptor inhibitors
  Iloprost
  Prostaglandin E_1
Serotonin receptor blockade
Combined serotonin and TXA_2 receptor blockade
Adhesion receptor blockade
  Aurin tricarboxylic acid
  Monoclonal anti-Ib receptor antibody
Aggregation receptor blockade
  Snake venom–derived RGD peptides
  Synthetic RGD peptides
  Anti-IIb/IIIa monoclonal antibody (7E3)

TXA_2, Thromboxane A_2; RGD, arginine-glycine-asparagine.

ties during thrombolysis) contributes significantly to enhanced platelet aggregation.[40-42]

In numerous animal and in vitro models of thrombotic occlusion followed by pharmacologic reperfusion, the addition of a platelet-inhibiting drug has been shown to shorten the time within which reperfusion occurs, to increase the number of subjects in which reperfusion occurs, and to limit the number of subjects in which reperfusion is followed by reocclusion (Tables 29-1 and 29-2).[36,43-56] Morphologic findings in both animals and humans also support the role of platelet involvement in resistance to thrombolysis. In a rabbit arterial model, erythrocyte-rich thrombi are more susceptible to thrombolysis than are platelet-rich thrombi.[57] Autopsy data obtained from patients who have died despite receiving thrombolytic therapy also indicate that intravascular thrombi in these patients are approximately three times more likely to be platelet-rich than thrombi in autopsy specimens from patients who were not treated with thrombolytic therapy.[58,59] It would thus seem logical that interference with platelet activity would be helpful in preventing reocclusion and in increasing the rapidity of lysis.

PRIMARY TREATMENT
Prostacyclin analogues and thromboxane A_2 antagonists

Several studies to date have examined the mechanisms by which platelet antagonists may interact with plasminogen activators in patients with AMI. *Prostaglandin E_1 (PGE$_1$)* is a vasodilator[60] and in vitro is a mild antagonist of platelet adhesion and aggregation. Its action is believed to occur through stimulation of platelet adenyl cyclase activity,[61] which ultimately antagonizes the calcium-induced release of thromboxane A_2. Its actions in vitro are potentiated by the phosphodiesterase inhibitors dipyridamole and theophylline.[62,63]

Table 29-2. Platelet inhibitors studied in acute myocardial infarction

Agent	Clinical setting studied			
	1° treatment	2° treatment	With lysis	Without lysis
Prostacyclin analogues				
Prostacyclin	+		+	+
Prostaglandin E_1	+		+	
Cyclooxygenase inhibitors				
Sulfinpyrazone		+		
Aspirin	+	+	+	+
Thromboxane antagonists				
Ridogrel	+		+	
Phosphodiesterase inhibitors				
Dipyridamole		+		+
Integrin-specific blockers	+			
Monoclonal 7E3			+	

Approximately two thirds of a venous dose of PGE_1 is metabolized on first pass through the pulmonary circulation.[64] High concentrations of PGE_1 have been shown both in vitro[56] and in vivo[48] to accelerate thrombolysis with tissue-type plasminogen activator (t-PA). Sharma et al.[65] administered 20 ng of intracoronary PGE_1/kg to patients receiving intracoronary streptokinase for acute MI. The study included 24 sequentially-assigned control patients who received intracoronary streptokinase alone. The time to reperfusion was shortened and the rate of reocclusion was lower in patients receiving PGE_1.[65] Studies with intravenously administered PGE_1 have been performed, and results are currently being analyzed and should be forthcoming in the near future.

Prostacyclin, an endogenous metabolite of arachidonic acid, is produced by the vascular endothelium and media and is a potent vasodilator. Its antiaggregatory effect occurs through a mechanism similar to that of PGE_1 and is potentiated by aspirin[62]; however, in vitro its effects are up to 100 times more pronounced.[66] In patients with acute MI, infusion of 4 ng of prostacyclin/kg/min produces marked vasodilation and antagonism of ADP-induced platelet aggregation but is also associated with frequent hypotension and nausea.[67] Intracoronary PGI_2 given to patients with acute MI did not lead to reperfusion in vessels with occlusion refractory to streptokinase, although it was a powerful coronary vasodilator.[68] In a small placebo-controlled study of patients with acute MI, intravenous infusion of 4 ng of prostacyclin/kg/min for 24 hours did not limit infarct size, postinfarction arrhythmias, or clinical events.[69] The Thrombolysis and Angioplasty in Acute Myocardial Infarction (TAMI) investigators administered iloprost, a stable synthetic PGI_2 analogue titrated to an infusion rate of 2 ng/kg/min in a randomized double-blind fashion to patients receiving t-PA for acute MI. The study was terminated prematurely because of an unacceptable incidence of side effects (primarily fever, nausea, and diarrhea) in patients receiving iloprost. Arterial patency rates were lower in patients receiving prostacyclin, and no improvement in left ventricular ejection fraction could be shown.[70] At high doses, prostacyclin has been shown to increase catabolism of t-PA in experimental models,[71] but this effect has not been demonstrated in humans.[72] In a more recent study of 80 patients, conjunctive use of the PGI_2 analogue *taprostene* in patients treated with single-chain urokinase plasminogen activator (scu-PA) appeared to be well tolerated and produced high early reperfusion rates that correlated with inhibition of ADP-induced platelet aggregation and eliminated reocclusion.[73] In a larger study, the combination of streptokinase with the thromboxane synthase inhibitor *ridogrel* did not enhance reperfusion when compared with streptokinase combined with aspirin.[74]

Aspirin

In contrast to the prostacyclin analogues, the clinical benefits of the prostaglandin pathway antagonist aspirin have been appreciated for nearly 10 years in patients with unstable angina.[75,76] Aspirin eliminates in vitro aggregation in response to the agonist arachidonic acid, although its effect is more modest after stimulation with other agonists. In the Folts model,[23] it eliminates cyclic flow variations at the site of severe arterial narrowing, but catecholamine stimulation can restore these responses.[24] Aspirin acts by irreversibly acetylating both the tissue and platelet forms of the enzyme prostaglandin G/H synthase (cyclooxygenase), which catalyzes the formation of cyclic endoperoxides from arachidonic acid.[77] These compounds are intermediates in the formation of both thromboxane A_2 and prostacyclin. Aspirin in vitro inhibits reformation of pharmacologically-lysed clots formed in platelet-rich plasma but does not accelerate thrombolysis.[56] In most in vivo models of thrombolysis of a thrombus superimposed on a severe narrowing, it limits reocclusion less well than some of the novel platelet inhibitors tested.[78]

Pharmacokinetics

After ingestion of aspirin, platelet production of thromboxane B_2, the principal metabolite of thromboxane A_2, is inhibited before aspirin can be detected in the circulation. This action is believed to occur in the portal circulation[79,80] and is termed presystemic acetylation. The dose-response curve for aspirin-induced inhibition of platelet production of thromboxane A_2 is linear from doses of 6 to approximately 100 mg,[81,82] and numerous investigations have attested to comparable degrees of platelet aggregation inhibition and of thromboxane A_2 antagonism after chronic administration of doses between 20 and 1000 mg.[81-85] Alternate-day regimens of 80 mg[86] and every-third-day regimens of 325 mg[87] have also been shown to inhibit thromboxane A_2 production and to prolong the bleeding time.[88] In some studies, steady-state inhibition has occurred more slowly at doses less than 100 mg.[88,89]

Although the antiaggregatory efficacy of both water-soluble and enteric-coated preparations of aspirin (at relatively high doses of each) are comparable, earlier peaks in plasma salicylate levels (20-30 minutes vs. 4-6 hours)[90-92] and earlier peak inhibition of aggregation (1 hour vs. 24 hours)[90,91] and thromboxane B_2 production[62] occur with the water-soluble forms. However, when enteric-coated preparations are chewed[92] or an oral loading dose of water-soluble aspirin is used,[88] inhibition of aggregation occurs considerably earlier. Aggregation and thromboxane A_2 production return to baseline values approximately 1 week after treatment is stopped.[88,92] The bioavailability of aspirin has been

Table 29-3. Gastrointestinal complications in trials of high- and low-dose aspirin*

Trial	Dose	Follow-up interval	% GI complaints		% GI bleeding		% requiring transfusion
Dutch TIA (1991)†	30 mg qd	2.6 yr	ASA 30 mg	10.5	ASA 30 mg	1.9	(1.3)
			ASA 283 mg	11.4	ASA 283 mg	1.9	(1.5)
SALT (1990)†	75 mg qd	32 mo	ASA	12.5	ASA	1.6	(1.3)
			PL	10.7	PL	0.6	(0.6)
RISC (1991)	75 mg qd	1.0 yr	ASA	3.8	ASA	0.7	
			PL	2.8			
UK-TIA (1988)†	75 mg qd	4 yr	ASA 75 mg	29	ASA 75 mg	2.6	(1.5)
	1200 mg qd		ASA 1200 mg	39	ASA 1200 mg	4.7	(2.3)
			PL	24	PL	1.6	(0.9)
PARIS-I (1980)	324 mg tid	41.0 mo	A-D	20.7	A-D	5.9	
	(+Dip 75 mg)		ASA	18.1	ASA	6.4	
			PL	13.4	PL	2.5	
PARIS-II (1986)	324 mg tid	23.4 mo	A-D	15.2	A-D	3.4	
	(+Dip 75 mg)		PL	9.8	PL	3.2	
AMIS (1980)	500 mg bid	3.0 yr	ASA	23.7	ASA	7.6	(1.0)
			PL	14.9	PL	4.6	(0.4)

*GI, Gastrointestinal; *TIA*, transient ischemic attack; *ASA*, aspirin; *SALT*, Swedish Aspirin Low-dose Trial; *PL*, placebo; *RISC*, Research Group on Instability in Coronary Artery Disease; *PARIS*, Persantine Aspirin Reinfarction Study; *A-D*, aspirin and dipyridamole; *Dip*, dipyridamole; *AMIS*, Aspirin Myocardial Infarction Study.
†Trials in patients with cerebrovascular disease.

reported to be similar in both volunteers and patients with stable coronary artery disease.[93]

Debate has continued for nearly 15 years about the optimal dose of aspirin. Inhibition of cyclooxygenase metabolism limits production of prostacyclin by the arterial wall, as well as of platelet thromboxane A_2.[82] Although the vascular store of cyclooxygenase is renewable, kinetic studies have shown that platelet thromboxane A_2 production is inhibited for the life of the platelet.[94] Thus, it might be expected that lower doses of aspirin would have antiaggregatory effects with minimal vasoconstrictive effects. Doses of aspirin between 10 and 30 mg inhibit thromboxane A_2 selectively while producing minimal inhibition of tissue prostacyclin production.[82,83,94,95] To date, no clinically detrimental effect of prostacyclin inhibition has been demonstrated.

Clinical efficacy

Clinically important reductions in death and nonfatal infarction among patients with unstable angina have been shown to result from aspirin doses as high as 1300 mg/day[76] and as low as 75 mg/day.[96] In patients with cerebrovascular disease, 30 mg/day of aspirin was as effective as 283 mg/day in preventing mortality from vascular causes.[97] The reported frequency of side effects, predominantly gastrointestinal, is dose-dependent. Gastrointestinal upset occurs in as many as 39% of patients treated chronically with 1200 mg/day[98] and has been reported in 10.5% of patients treated receiving 30 mg/day.[97] However, a significant proportion of placebo-treated patients also complain of similar symptoms,

leading to only a slight excess of complaints attributable to aspirin (Table 29-3). In at least one study, these symptoms were considerably less common than those attributed to antiischemic drugs.[96] The incidence of gastrointestinal bleeding requiring transfusion or hospitalization is increased by aspirin and, although uncommon (<2%), also appears to be dose-related.[98] In shorter-term studies, gastric complaints occurred in 5% to 7% of patients receiving aspirin.[96,99]

It would therefore seem logical that treatment should be undertaken at the lowest effective dose. However, in patients with AMI, rapid onset of action is essential, which may be dose-dependent. Unfortunately, the dose-related efficacy of aspirin in the early period after administration has not been completely studied. Even after intravenous aspirin infusion, inhibition of platelet aggregation and thromboxane production has been reported to be time-dependent.[100] Complete inhibition of arachidonate-induced aggregation has been shown 4 hours after 325 mg of aspirin,[101] and when the aspirin preparation is chewed, inhibition of aggregation in response to modest concentrations of ADP occurs as quickly as within 15 minutes.[92,102] Although inhibition of thromboxane A_2 production has been detected within 5 minutes of administration of 20 mg of aspirin,[79,94] the extent to which platelet function is inhibited early after *low-dose* aspirin (i.e., ≥160 mg) is not established. In one study, a single 20-mg oral dose of aspirin inhibited serum thromboxane B_2 by 18% at 5 minutes and by 48% at 30 minutes, with 73% inhibition occurring after a second dose and 89% after a third dose.[94] In another

Table 29-4. Effect of 162 mg of aspirin on hospital event rate in acute myocardial infarction: ISIS-2*

Event	No. of events (%)			
	ASA	PL	SK-ASA	PL-PL
Vascular death†	804 (9.4%)	1016 (11.8%)	343 (8.0%)	568 (13.2%)
Nonfatal reinfarction	83 (1%)	170 (2%)	46 (1.1%)	61 (1.4%)
Stroke	47 (0.6%)	81 (1%)	25 (0.6%)	45 (1.1%)
Hemorrhagic stroke	5 (0.05%)	2 (0.02%)	5 (0.12%)	0 (0%)
Major bleeding	31 (0.37%)	33 (0.37%)	24 (0.57%)	11 (0.26%)

*ISIS, International Study of Infarct Survival; ASA, aspirin; PL, placebo aspirin tablet; SK-ASA, streptokinase-aspirin.
†Vascular mortality is within 5 weeks; all other events are by the time of hospital discharge.

study 25 mg of aspirin/day produced 97% inhibition of thromboxane A_2 but only after 4 days of treatment.[103] It is not certain whether this degree of inhibition is sufficient to inhibit platelet activity in humans; it is likely that although some aspirin-induced inhibition of platelet aggregation occurs when thromboxane A_2 production is inhibited by two thirds, at least 95% inhibition appears necessary to achieve maximal inhibition.[104,105] In one study in which ex vivo aggregation studies were performed on human blood within the early hours after low-dose aspirin administration, 40 mg of aspirin produced a modest decrease in ADP and epinephrine-induced aggregation that lasted less than 24 hours, whereas 325 mg of aspirin produced more marked inhibition lasting 7 days.[106] In a more recent study, oral doses of 81, 162, and 324 mg of aspirin produced comparable inhibition of arachidonate and ADP-induced platelet aggregation in volunteer subjects within 15 minutes after ingestion.[102]

The extension of these findings to patients with MI were made obvious in the Second International Study of Infarct Survival (ISIS-2) (Table 29-4).[107] In this study, 17,187 patients with suspected AMI underwent a factorial 2-by-2 randomization to aspirin 162 mg chewed immediately, 1.5 million units intravenous of streptokinase, neither, or both. Treatment with streptokinase led to a mortality reduction of 25%. Mortality in patients receiving aspirin was reduced by 23% compared with the placebo group, and unlike the effect seen after streptokinase administration, this reduction was independent of time from the onset of symptoms. The group of patients receiving both streptokinase and aspirin had a 42% reduction in mortality. This effect was accompanied by a 0.3% excess of major bleeding events and a 0.1% excess of hemorrhagic strokes. The differences between groups were sustained over 2 years. Interpretation of the mechanism of the ISIS-2 results may be partially clouded by the fact that confirmation of infarction was not mandatory in this study and that some of the benefit from aspirin may have occurred in patients with less specific electrocardiographic (ECG) signs of infarction who had unstable angina.

The use of aspirin during the acute phase of MI has not been addressed directly among patients receiving t-PA. In a report from the Thrombolysis and Myocardial Infarction Phase II Trial (TIMI II), however, arterial patency rates determined at 18 to 48 hours after receiving t-PA were equal regardless of whether oral aspirin had been taken before treatment,[108] and in a report from the first four phases of the TAMI studies, early reocclusion was not less common in patients who had used aspirin before the onset of their infarction.[109] In both studies, all patients were treated with intravenous heparin begun concommittantly with t-PA. A recent angiographic study demonstrated that beginning 48 hours after thrombolysis, 300 mg of aspirin daily was superior to both placebo and coumadin in maintaining arterial patency and preventing recurrent clinical events at 3 months.[110] In another angiographic study, 80 mg of aspirin daily begun concommittantly with t-PA was associated with more reocclusions than heparin alone within the first 18 hours after thrombolysis but with fewer reocclusions from that period to hospital discharge.[111] A recent metaanalysis in which trials of t-PA with and without aspirin were compared indicated that both reocclusions and recurrent ischemic events were reduced by approximately 50% when aspirin was used.[112]

In view of these findings, aspirin should be administered as rapidly as possible to all patients undergoing evaluation for suspected AMI. Chewing of the tablets is recommended to hasten absorption. Although the dose is probably not critical, a *minimal* dose of 160 mg should be used to assure adequate absorption by all individuals, whereas after the third hospital day, 80 mg daily is likely to be adequate. Aspirin is also likely to be useful in patients undergoing primary angioplasty for AMI and in the 10% to 15% of patients who require coronary angioplasty after thrombolysis.[113,114] Platelet deposition at the site of angioplasty occurs extremely rapidly[85,115]; one of the most frequent complications of this procedure in patients with AMI is the rapid reaccumulation of intraarterial thrombus after dilation. Data from studies of elective angioplasty indicate that aspirin reduces the frequency of abrupt closure associated with the procedure.[116,117] Although this issue has not been addressed directly in primary angioplasty, extrapolation of these data, as well as data from ISIS-2, would dictate that patients in whom direct angioplasty is planned receive a dose of aspirin as soon as possible. Because inhibition of platelet aggregation is probably necessary before the angioplasty procedure is begun (i.e., usually within the first hour after manifestation), a minimum dose of 325 mg chewed would seem indicated based on the small amount of platelet aggregation data available during this period.

Direct inhibitors of adhesion and aggregation

Most investigation to date has been directed toward agents that inhibit platelet aggregation through modulation of the cyclooxygenase pathway. Although such agents can abolish arachidonic acid–induced platelet aggregation in vitro, aggregation still occurs in response to such other agonists as thrombin, epinephrine, collagen, and ADP. Thus, their antiplatelet efficacy is somewhat limited. Attention has recently been focused on agents whose actions are directed toward the platelet surface receptors responsible for interactions between platelets and between platelets and the vessel wall. A variety of antibodies and peptides are currently being developed that are designed to act as competitive antagonists of these receptors. For example, a number of peptides derived from the venom of vipers are potent antagonists of glycoprotein IIb/IIIa, and analogues of these peptides that share the RGD sequence can be produced synthetically. In addition, aurin tricarboxylic acid, an antagonist of von Willebrand factor that binds to the glycoprotein Ib receptor responsible for platelet adhesion to the vascular wall under conditions of high shear, has been shown to prevent cyclic flow reductions in the Folts model of arterial stenosis and thrombosis.[118-120]

One clinical study has been performed in which a direct antagonist of the final common pathway for aggregation (the glycoprotein IIb/IIIa receptor) was used. In this study, the Fab fragment of a murine-derived monoclonal antibody (7E3) was administered to patients with acute MI who received treatment with t-PA. The antibody was administered in a dose-escalation fashion until nearly 90% median inhibition of baseline aggregation could be achieved and was then administered at progressively shorter time intervals after t-PA administration. The frequencies of major and minor bleeding events and of transfusion were similar among control patients receiving heparin, aspirin, and t-PA alone and those receiving 7E3 as well. Prolongation of the bleeding time was not associated with an increased risk of bleeding. Neither angiographic mechanisms nor clinical efficacy were the primary outcome variables of this study, but angiographic patency was present in 91% of

patients treated with 7E3. The incidence of recurrent ischemic events was also found to be lower than the expected 20% to 30%[84] in patients receiving the dose of the drug that consistently abolished in vitro platelet aggregation.[121] Other RGD sequence–containing peptides that antagonize the IIb/IIIa receptor are likely to undergo similar study in the near future.

SECONDARY PREVENTION

The role of antiplatelet therapy after hospital discharge after AMI has been a topic of investigation since the role of thrombosis in AMI was first appreciated. When aspirin was found to have platelet-inhibiting properties, it became apparent that administration of this agent to patients at risk for recurrent infarction might have a beneficial effect. At the same time, awareness of the role of platelet aggregates in stroke and transient ischemic attacks led to a number of randomized trials of aspirin in patients with ischemic cerebrovascular disease. The results are by and large concordant in suggesting limitation of death and nonfatal reinfarction by aspirin therapy. Although nearly all trials of secondary prevention by platelet inhibition after MI demonstrated trends toward event reduction, statistical significance was present in only one, probably as a consequence of the size of the studies.[122] Outcomes of the seven largest trials are shown in Table 29-5.[122-128] Several additional points are also evident. The most dramatic reductions in event rates are found in the studies in which enrollment occurred soon after the index infarction, presumably because most events during this period are secondary to rethrombosis. Interestingly, important subanalyses of the last trial, the Persantine Aspirin Reinfarction Study (PARIS) II, indicated that patients at low risk (i.e., those with New York Heart Association class I symptoms, those not requiring digitalis, and those with non-Q-wave infarction) had the most pronounced benefit.[122] Although it may at first seem surprising that the most benefit occurred in the lowest-risk patients, these findings may be explained by the greater susceptibility of patients in these groups to recurrent ischemia and infarction and proportionally lower susceptibility to death from such aspirin-insensitive causes as pump failure or arrhythmias, as might occur in patients with larger infarctions or more severe heart failure. In addition, in those studies from which analyses of results in different age groups are available, it is apparent that mortality reduction is more pronounced with increasing age.[124,125]

In 1988, the Antiplatelet Trialists' collaborators performed a metaanalysis of 25 placebo-controlled trials in which a total of 29,000 patients were enrolled after either stroke or infarction. In the majority of these trials, aspirin (in doses of at least 300 mg/day) was used as antiplatelet treatment, whereas in a few studies sulfinpyrazone or dipyridamole either alone or in combination

Table 29-5. Trials of aspirin as secondary prophylaxis after myocardial infarction*

Trial (yr)	No.	Dose	Enrollment interval	Follow-up interval	Nonfatal (%)	Mortality (%)
Ellwood (1974)	1239	300 mg qd	Open	12 mo	—	ASA 8.3 PL 10.9
Ellwood (1979)	1682	300 mg tid	<7 days	12 mo	ASA 10.9 PL 7.1	ASA 12.3 PL 14.8
CDP (1976)	1629	324 mg tid	>60 mo	10-28 mo	ASA 3.7 PL 4.2	ASA 5.8 PL 8.3
AMIS (1980)	4524	500 mg bid	8 wk-5.5 yr	3 yr	ASA 9.5 PL 11.6	ASA 10.8 PL 9.7
GAAT (1980)	946	500 mg tid	30-42 days	2 yr	ASA 7.5 PL 7.1 WAR 10.0	ASA 8.6 PL 10.3 WAR 12.2
PARIS-I (1980)	2026	324 mg tid (and Dip 75 mg tid)	8 wk-60 mo	41 mo	ASA 6.9 PL 9.9 A-D 7.9	ASA 10.5 PL 12.8 A-D 10.7
PARIS-II (1986)	3128	330 mg tid (and Dip 75 mg tid)	4 wk-4 mo	23.4 mo	A-D 5.2 PL 8.2	A-D 7.1 PL 7.3

*MI, Myocardial infarction; ASA, aspirin; PL, placebo; CDP, Coronary Drug Project; AMIS, Aspirin Myocardial Infarction Study; GAAT, German-Austrian Aspirin Trial; WAR, warfarin; PARIS, Persantine Aspirin Reinfarction Study; Dip, dipyridamole; A-D, aspirin and dipyridamole.

with aspirin were chosen. Antiplatelet therapy reduced the likelihood of vascular death by 15% and of nonfatal stroke or MI by 30%. For patients receiving aspirin after MI, the risk of vascular death was reduced by 14%, with reductions of 31% in the risk of nonfatal MI and 40% in the risk of nonfatal stroke. Given estimated 2-year rates of 12% mortality and 9% nonfatal MI, effective antiplatelet therapy would prevent one lethal MI and two nonfatal vascular events per 2 years per 100 patients treated.[129] Although the doses of aspirin used in these studies were relatively high by modern standards, it would seem reasonable to extrapolate to this setting both platelet aggregation data and the findings of recent studies of unstable angina[96] and transient ischemic attack[110,130] to use low-dose aspirin (80-160 mg) on a chronic basis. At a cost of $1.00 per 100 tablets, this intervention can be performed for $730 per 100 patients.

A minority of patients, unfortunately, are unable to take aspirin. True aspirin intolerance (either asthma or angioneurotic edema) occurs in 0.5% of the population[131] and has been estimated to occur in 5% to 20% of known adult asthmatics.[132] Other nonsteroidal antiinflammatory agents are also able to inhibit platelet aggregation (through inhibition of prostaglandin G/H synthase)[133-135]; however, these drugs also produce angioneurotic edema and exacerbations of asthma in aspirin-sensitive patients.[131,132] Because aspirin ingestion in these patients can provoke severe episodes of bronchospasm or angioneurotic edema, aspirin should obviously be avoided in this setting. Unfortunately, there are at the present time few other approved rapidly-acting inhibitors of platelet aggregation. Nitroglycerin is a mild

inhibitor of platelet aggregation and limits platelet deposition at the site of deep arterial injury.[136] This action occurs in vitro at suprapharmacologic concentrations.[137] Whether this effect is clinically significant is controversial, although in two clinical studies, thrombin and ADP-induced aggregation were inhibited at commonly-used clinical doses.[138,139] The mechanism appears to be related to nitrate-induced increases in platelet cGMP,[140,141] possibly induced by endothelial and smooth muscle cell production of nitric oxide.[140,142] This action may be synergistic with prostacyclin agonists.[143] Parenteral nitroglycerin may have beneficial effects on myocardial infarct size and favorable effects on remodeling[144] and mortality after infarction,[145] although some of these effects may be consequent to its ability to reduce ventricular preload and to dilate epicardial coronary arteries. In a small uncontrolled study, intracoronary isosorbide dinitrate led to persistent patency of vessels that had undergone cyclic occlusion and reocclusion during intracoronary streptokinase administration.[29] In many patients with infarction, intravenous nitroglycerin may be indicated for hemodynamic management or for relief of angina; in patients intolerant of aspirin, nitroglycerin, at doses titrated to reduce the systolic blood pressure by 10%, should be considered for use as a platelet inhibitor. In those patients also undergoing anticoagulation with heparin, activated partial thromboplastin times should be monitored closely in the event that nitroglycerin-induced heparin resistance occurs.[146]

Secondary prevention in aspirin-intolerant patients may be possible with the thienopyridine derivative ticlopidine. This agent is a powerful inhibitor of ADP-induced platelet aggregation. Its mechanism of action is not entirely understood, although it is believed to inhibit fibrinogen binding to glycoprotein IIb/IIIa on the platelet surface[147] and has been shown to inhibit the reduction in cAMP levels induced by ADP stimulation.[148] In addition, the drug has been shown to reduce levels of circulating fibrinogen.[149] Ticlopidine (250 mg twice daily) has been shown to be effective in reducing combined stroke, MI, and vascular death rates compared with placebo in patients with a recent stroke[150] and to be slightly more effective than aspirin in preventing stroke or death in patients with cerebral or retinal transient ischemic attacks.[151] Ticlopidine therapy was also associated with a 46.3% reduction in combined rates of death and nonfatal MI after 6 months in a study of 652 patients with unstable angina[152] and a 43% reduction in cardiac mortality in a study of 627 patients with intermittent claudication.[153] Approximately one third of the patients in the former study had prior MI and experienced a reduction in recurrent events similar to that in the overall cohort of patients. The antiplatelet effect of ticlopidine is relatively slow in onset (peak effect in 3 to 5 days[154]; thus, its usefulness as a primary adjunctive therapy in acute MI is limited. The principal side effects of treatment with ticlopidine are severe neutropenia (1%); rash (14%); and gastrointestinal upset, predominantly diarrhea (20%)[151]; although in the study of unstable angina, withdrawal for adverse drug effects was required in only 5% of patients.[152] At the current time, ticlopidine is approved for secondary prophylaxis for cerebral ischemia in patients unable to take aspirin.

REFERENCES

1. Kennedy JW, Ritchie JL, Davis KB, et al: The western Washington randomized trial of intracoronary streptokinase in acute myocardial infarction. A 12-month follow-up report, *N Engl J Med* 312:1073-1078, 1985.
2. Simoons ML, Serruys PW, Van Den Brand M, et al: Early thrombolysis in acute myocardial infarction: limitation of infarct size and improved survival, *J Am Coll Cardiol* 7:717-728, 1986.
3. Dalen JE, Gore JM, Braunwald E, et al: Six-and twelve-month follow-up of the phase I Thrombolysis in Myocardial Infarction (TIMI) trial, *Am J Cardiol* 62:179-185, 1988.
4. Simoons ML, Vos J, Tussen JGP, et al: Long-term benefit of early thrombolytic therapy in patients with acute myocardial infarction: 5 year follow-up of a trial conducted by the interuniversity cardiology institute of the Netherlands, *J Am Coll Cardiol* 14:1609-1615, 1989.
5. Chapman I: Morphogenesis of occluding coronary artery thrombosis, *Arch Pathol Lab Med* 80:256-261, 1965.
6. Friedman M, Van den Bovenkamp GJ: The pathogenesis of a coronary thrombus, *Am J Pathol* 48:19-44, 1966.
7. Davies MJ, Thomas A: Thrombosis and acute coronary-artery lesions in sudden cardiac ischemic death, *N Engl J Med* 310:1137-1140, 1984.
8. Davies MJ, Thomas AC: Plaque fissuring-the cause of acute myocardial infarction, sudden ischaemic death, and crescendo angina, *Br Heart J* 53:363-373, 1985.
9. Onodera T, Fujiwara H, Tanaka M, et al: Cineangiographic and pathological features of the infarct related vessel in successful and unsuccessful thrombolysis, *Br Heart J* 61:385-389, 1989.
10. Hawiger J: Adhesive interactions of platelets and their blockade, *Ann NY Acad Sci* 614:270-278, 1991.
11. Meyer D, Pietu G, Fressinaud E, et al: Von Willebrand Factor: structure and function, *Mayo Clin Proc* 66:516-523, 1991.
12. Badimon L, Fuster BV: Thrombogenesis and inhibition of platelet aggregation. Experimental aspects and future approaches, *Z Kardiol* 79:133-145, 1990.
13. Hawiger J: Formation and regulation for platelet and fibrin hemostatic plug, *Hum Pathol* 18:111-122, 1987.
14. Fuster V, Badimon L, Cohen M, et al: Insights into the pathogenesis of acute ischemic syndromes, *Circulation* 77:1213-1220, 1988.
15. Hung DT, Vu TKH, Wheaton VI, et al: Cloned platelet thrombin receptor is necessary for thrombin-induced platelet activation, *J Clin Invest* 89:1350-1353, 1992.
16. Fressinaud E, Baruch D, Girma J-P, et al: Von Willebrand factor mediated platelet adhesion to collagen involves platelet membrane glycoprotein IIb/IIIa as well as glycoprotein Ib, *J Lab Clin Med* 112:58-67, 1988.
17. Kroll MH, Schafer AI: Biochemical mechanisms of platelet activation, *Blood* 74:1181-1195, 1989.
18. Phillips DR, Charo IF, Scarborough RM: GPIIb-IIIa: the responsive integrin, *Cell* 65:359-362, 1991.
19. Ginsberg MH, Loftus JC, Plow EF: Cytoadhesins, integrins, and platelets, *Thromb Haemost* 59:1-6, 1988.
20. Monkovic DD, Tracy PB: Functional characterization of human platelet-released factor V and its activation by factor Xa and thrombin, *J Biol Chem* 265:17132-17140, 1990.
21. Fujii S, Lucore CL, Hopkins WE, et al: Potential attenuation of fibrinolysis by growth factors released from platelets and their pharmacologic implications, *Am J Cardiol* 63:1505-1511, 1989.
22. Fujii S, Hopkins WE, Sobel BE: Mechanisms contributing to increased synthesis of plasminogen activator inhibitor type 1 in endothelial cells by constituents of platelets and their implications of thrombosis, *Circulation* 83:645-651, 1991.
23. Folts JD, Crowell EB, Rowe GG: Platelet aggregation in partially obstructed vessels and its elimination with aspirin, *Circulation* 54:365-370, 1976.
24. Folts J: An in vivo model of experimental arterial stenosis, intimal damage, and periodic thrombosis, *Circulation* 83(suppl IV):IV3-IV14, 1991.
25. Golino P, Ashton JH, Glas-Greenwalt P, et al: Mediation of reocclusion by thromboxane A$_2$ and serotonin after thrombolysis with tissue-type plasminogen activator in a canine preparation of coronary thrombosis, *Circulation* 77:678-684, 1988.
26. Ku DD: Coronary vascular reactivity after acute myocardial ischemia, *Science* 218:576-578, 1982.
27. VanBenthuysen KM, McMurtry IF, Horwitz LD: Reperfusion after acute coronary occlusion in dogs impairs endothelium-dependent relaxation to acetylcholine and augments contractile reactivity in vitro, *J Clin Invest* 79:265-274, 1987.
28. Pearson PJ, Schaff HV, Vanhoutte PM: Acute impairment of endothelium-dependent relaxations to aggregating platelets following reperfusion injury in canine coronary arteries, *Circ Res* 67:385–393, 1990.
29. Hackett D, Davies G, Chierchia S, et al: Intermittent coronary occlusion in acute myocardial infarction, *N Engl J Med* 317:1055-1059, 1987.
30. Fitzgerald DJ, Catella F, Roy L, et al: Marked platelet activation in vivo after intravenous streptokinase in patients with acute myocardial infarction, *Circulation* 77:142-150, 1988.
31. Ohlstein EH, Storer B, Fujita T, et al: Tissue-type plasminogen activator and streptokinase induce platelet hyperaggregability in the rabbit, *Thromb Res* 46:575-585, 1987.

32. Kerins DM, Roy L, Fitzgerald GA, et al: Platelet and vascular function during coronary thrombolysis with tissue-type plasminogen activator, *Circulation* 80:1718-1725, 1989.

33. Fitzgerald DJ, Wright F, Fitzgerald GA: Increased thromboxane biosynthesis during coronary thrombolysis. Evidence that platelet activation and thromboxane A_2 modulate the response to tissue-type plasminogen activator in vivo, *Circ Res* 65:83-94, 1989.

34. Fitzgerald DJ, Fitzgerald GA: Role of thrombin and thromboxane A_2 in reocclusion following coronary thrombolysis with tissue-type plasminogen activator, *Proc Natl Acad Sci USA* 86:7585-7589, 1989.

35. Niewiarowski S, Senyi AF, Gillies P: Plasmin-induced platelet aggregation and platelet release reaction: effects on hemostasis, *J Clin Invest* 52:1647-1659, 1973.

36. Shebuski RJ, Storer BL, Fujita T: Effect of thromboxane synthase inhibition on thrombolytic action of tissue-type plasminogen activator in a rabbit model of peripheral arterial thrombosis, *Throm Res* 52:381-392, 1988.

37. Rudd MA, George D, Amarante P, et al: Temporal effects of thrombolytic agents on platelet function in vivo and their modulation by prostaglandins, *Circ Res* 67:1175-1181, 1990.

38. Terres W, Umnus S, Mathey DG, et al: Effects of streptokinase, urokinase, and recombinant tissue plasminogen activator on platelet aggregability and stability of platelet aggregates, *Cardiovasc Res* 24:471-477, 1990.

39. Vaughan DE, Van Houtte E, Declerck PJ, et al: Streptokinase-induced platelet aggregation prevalence and mechanism, *Circulation* 84:84-91, 1991.

40. Eisenberg PR, Sherman LA, Jaffe AS: Paradoxic elevation of fibrinopeptide A after streptokinase: evidence for continued thrombosis despite intense fibrinolysis, *J Am Coll Cardiol* 10:527-529, 1987.

41. Winters KJ, Santoro SA, Miletich JP, et al: Relative importance of thrombin compared with plasmin-mediated platelet activation in response to plasminogen activation with streptokinase, *Circulation* 84:1522-1560, 1991.

42. Aronson DL, Chang P, Kessler CM: Platelet-dependent thrombin generation after in vitro fibrinolytic treatment, *Circulation* 85:1706-1712, 1992.

43. Schumacher WA, Lee EC, Lucchesi BR: Augmentation of streptokinase-induced thrombolysis by heparin and prostacyclin, *J Cardiovasc Pharmacol* 7:739-746, 1985.

44. Gold HK, Coller BS, Yasuda T, et al: Rapid and sustained coronary artery recanalization with combined bolus injection of recombinant tissue-type plasminogen activator and monoclonal antiplatelet GPIIb/IIIa antibody in a canine preparation, *Circulation* 77:670-677, 1988.

45. Shebuski RJ, Smith Jr JM, Storer BL, et al: Influence of selective endoperoxide/thromboxane A_2 receptor antagonism with sulotroban on lysis time and reocclusion rate after tissue plasminogen activator-induced coronary thrombolysis in the dog, *J Pharmacol Exp Ther* 246:790-796, 1988.

46. Schumacher WA, Heran CL: Effect of thromboxane antagonism on recanalization during streptokinase-induced thrombolysis in anesthetized monkeys, *J Cardiovasc Pharmacol* 13:853-861, 1989.

47. Golino P, Ashton JH, McNatt J, et al: Simultaneous administration of thromboxane A_2- and serotonin S_2-receptor antagonists markedly enhances thrombolysis and prevents or delays reocclusion after tissue-type plasminogen activator in a canine model of coronary thrombosis, *Circulation* 79:911-919, 1989.

48. Vaughan DE, Plavin SR, Schafer AI, et al: PGE_1 accelerates thrombolysis by tissue plasminogen activator, *Blood* 73:1213-1217, 1989.

49. Fujita T, Hasan S, Storer BL, et al: Effect of selective endoperoxide/thromboxane A_2 receptor antagonism with sulotroban on tPA-induced thrombolysis in a rabbit model of

femoral arterial thrombosis, *Fund Clin Pharmacol* 3:643-653, 1989.

50. Shebuski RJ, Stabilito IJ, Sitko GR, et al: Acceleration of recombinant tissue-type plasminogen activator-induced thrombolysis and prevention of reocclusion by the combination of heparin and the arg-gly-asp-containing peptide bitistatin in a canine model of coronary thrombosis, *Circulation* 82:169-177, 1990.

51. Yasuda T, Gold HK, Yaoita H, et al: Comparative effects of aspirin, a synthetic thrombin inhibitor and a monoclonal antiplatelet glycoprotein IIb/IIIa antibody on coronary artery reperfusion, reocclusion and bleeding with recombinant tissue-type plasminogen activator in a canine preparation, *J Am Coll Cardiol* 16:714-722, 1990.

52. Golino P, Rosolowsky M, Yoa SK, et al: Endogenous prostaglandin endoperoxides and prostacyclin modulate the thrombolytic activity of tissue plasminogen activator: effects of simultaneous inhibition of thromboxane A_2 synthase and blockade of thromboxane A_2/prostaglandin H_2 receptors in a canine model of coronary thrombosis, *J Clin Invest* 86:1095-1102, 1990.

53. Holahan MA, Mellott MJ, Garsky VM, et al: Prevention of reocclusion following tissue type plasminogen activator-induced thrombolysis by the RGD-containing peptide, echistatin, in a canine model of coronary thrombosis, *Pharmacology* 42:340-348, 1991.

54. Schneider J: Taprostene, a stable prostacyclin analogue, enhances the thrombolytic efficacy of saruplase (recombinant single-chain urokinase-type plasminogen activator) in rabbits with pulmonary embolized thrombi, *Prostaglandins* 41:595-606, 1991.

55. Yasuda T, Gold HK, Leinbach RC, et al: Kistin, a polypeptide platelet GPIIb/IIIa receptor antagonist, enhances and sustains coronary arterial thrombolysis with recombinant tissue-type plasminogen activator in a canine preparation, *Circulation* 83:1038-1047, 1991.

56. Terres W, Beythien C, Kupper W, et al: Effects of aspirin and prostaglandin E_1 on in vitro thrombolysis with urokinase: evidence for a possible role of inhibiting platelet activity in thrombolysis, *Circulation* 79:1309-1314, 1989.

57. Jang IK-K, Gold HK, Ziskind AA, et al: Differential sensitivity of erythrocyte-rich and platelet-rich arterial thrombi to lysis with recombinant tissue-type plasminogen activator: a possible explanation for resistance to coronary thrombolysis, *Circulation* 79:920-928, 1989.

58. Gertz SD, Kragel AH, Kalan JM, et al: Comparison of coronary and myocardial morphologic findings in patients with and without thrombolytic therapy during fatal first acute myocardial infarction, *Am J Cardiol* 66:904-909, 1990.

59. Kragel AH, Gertz SD, Roberts WC: Morphologic comparison of frequency and types of acute lesions in the major epicardial coronary arteries in unstable angina pectoris, sudden coronary death, and acute myocardial infarction, *J Am Coll Cardiol* 18:801-808, 1991.

60. Feldman RL, Rose B, Verbust KM: Hemodynamic and angiographic effects of prostaglandin E1 in coronary artery disease, *Am J Cardiol* 62:698-702, 1988.

61. Karinguian A, Legrand YJ, Caen JP: Prostaglandins: specific inhibition of platelet adhesion to collagen and relationship with cAMP level, *Prostaglandins* 23:437-457, 1982.

62. Ball G, Brereton GG, Fulwood M, et al: Effect of prostaglandin E1 alone and in combination with theophylline or aspirin on collagen-induced platelet aggregation and on platelet nucleotides including adenosine 3':5'-cyclic monophosphate, *Biochem J* 120:709-718, 1970.

63. Mills DCB, Smith JB: The influence of platelet aggregation on

drugs that affect the accumulation of adenosine 3':5'- cyclic monophosphate in platelets, *Biochem J* 121:185-196, 1971.

64. Golub M, Zia P, Matsuno M, et al: Metabolism of prostaglandins A$_1$ and E$_1$ in man, *J Clin Invest* 56:1404-1410, 1975.

65. Sharma B, Wyeth RP, Heinemann FM, et al: Addition of intracoronary prostaglandin E$_1$ to streptokinase improves thrombolysis and left ventricular function in acute myocardial infarction [abstract]. *J Am Coll Cardiol* II(suppl A)104A, 1988.

66. Harfenist EJ, Packham MA, Kinlough-Rathbone RL, et al: Inhibitors of ADP-induced platelet aggregation prevent fibrinogen binding to rabbit platelets and cause rapid deaggregation and dissociation of bound fibrinogen, *J Lab Clin Med* 97:680-688, 1981.

67. Swedberg K, Held P, Wadenvik H, et al: Central haemodynamic and antiplatelet effects of iloprost—a new prostacyclin analogue—in acute myocardial infarction in man, *Eur Heart J* 8:362-368, 1987.

68. Hackett D, Davies G, Maseri A: Effect of prostacyclin on coronary occlusion in acute myocardial infarction, *Int J Cardiol* 26:53-58, 1990.

69. Armstrong PW, Langevin LM, Watts DG: Randomized trial of prostacyclin infusion in acute myocardial infarction, *Am J Cardiol* 61:455-458, 1987.

69a. RISC Group: Risk of myocardial infarction and death during treatment with low dose aspirin and intravenous heparin in men with unstable coronary artery disease, *Lancet* 336:827-830, 1990.

70. Topol RJ, Ellis SG, Califf RM, et al: Combined tissue-type plasminogen activator and prostacyclin therapy for acute myocardial infarction, *J Am Coll Cardiol* 14:877-884, 1989.

71. Nicolini FA, Mehta JL, Nichols WW, et al: Prostacyclin analogue iloprost decreases thrombolytic potential of tissue-type plasminogen activator in canine coronary thrombosis, *Circulation* 81:1115-1122, 1990.

72. Kerins DM, Roy L, Kunitada S, et al: Pharmacokinetics of tissue-type plasminogen activator during acute myocardial infarction in men. Effect of a prostacyclin analogue, *Circulation* 85:526-532, 1992.

73. Darius H, Gorge G, Erbel R, et al: Platelet aggregation and coronary artery patency in patients with acute infarction treated with saruplase and Taprostene [abstract]. *J Am Coll Cardiol* 19:92A, 1992.

74. The RAPT Investigators: Randomized trial of Ridogrel, a combined thromboxane A$_2$/prostaglandin endoperoxide receptor antagonist, versus aspirin as adjunct to thrombolysis in patients with acute myocardial infarction, *Circulation* 89:588-595, 1994.

75. Lewis Jr HD, Davis JW, Archibald DG, et al: Protective effects of aspirin against acute myocardial infarction and death in men and unstable angina, *N Engl J Med* 309:396-403, 1983.

76. Cairns JA, Gent M, Singer J, et al: Aspirin, sulfinpyrazone, or both in unstable angina, *N Engl J Med* 313:1369-1375, 1985.

77. Roth GJ, Majerus PW: The mechanism of the effect of aspirin on human platelets: I. Acetylation of a particulate fraction protein, *J Clin Invest* 56:624-632, 1975.

78. Bates ER, McGillem MJ, Mickelson JK, et al: A monoclonal antibody against the platelet glycoprotein IIb/IIIa receptor complex prevents platelet aggregation and thrombosis in a canine model of coronary angioplasty, *Circulation* 84:2463-2469, 1991.

79. Pedersen AK, Fitzgerald GA: Dose-related kinetics of aspirin, *N Engl J Med* 311:1206-1211, 1984.

80. Bochner F, Siebert DM, Rodgers SE, et al: Measurement of aspirin concentrations in portal and systemic blood in pigs: effect on platelet aggregation, thromboxane and prostacyclin production, *Thromb Haemost* 61:211-216, 1989.

81. Patrignani P, Filabozzi P, Patrono C: Selective cumulative inhibition of platelet thromboxane production by low-dose aspirin in healthy subjects, *J Clin Invest* 69:1366-1372, 1982.

82. Weksler BB, Pett SB, Alonso D, et al: Differential inhibition by aspirin of vascular and platelet prostaglandin synthesis in atherosclerotic patients, *N Engl J Med* 308:800-805, 1983.

83. Kallmann R, Nieuwenhuis HK, Groot PGD, et al: Effects of low doses of aspirin, 10mg and 30mg daily, on bleeding time, thromboxane production and 6-keto-PGE1 excretion in healthy subjects, *Thromb Res* 45:355-361, 1987.

84. De Caterina R, Ginnessi D, Bernini W, et al: Selective inhibition of thromboxane-related platelet function by low-dose aspirin in patients after myocardial infarction, *Am J Cardiol* 55:589-590, 1985.

85. De Caterina R, Giannessi D, Bernini W, et al: Equal antiplatelet effects of aspirin 50 or 324 mg/day in patients after acute myocardial infarction, *Thromb Haemost* 54:528-532, 1985.

86. Rasmanis G, Vesterqvist O, Green K, et al: Effects of intermittent treatment with aspirin on thromboxane and prostacyclin formation in patients with acute myocardial infarction, *Lancet* 2:245-249, 1988.

87. Stampfer MJ, Jakubowski JA, Deykin D, et al: Effect of alternate-day regular and enteric-coated aspirin on platelet aggregation, bleeding time, and thromboxane A$_2$ levels in bleeding-time blood, *Am J Med* 81:400-404, 1986.

88. Clarke RJ, Mayo G, Price P, et al: Suppression of thromboxane A$_2$ but not of systemic prostacyclin by controlled-release aspirin, *N Engl J Med* 325:1137-1141, 1991.

89. Sullivan MHF, Zosmer A, Gleeson RP, et al: Equivalent inhibition of in vivo platelet function by low dose and high dose aspirin treatment, *Prostaglandins Leukotrienes Essential Fatty Acids* 39:319-321, 1990.

90. Ross-Lee LM, Elms MJ, Cham BE, et al: Plasma levels of aspirin following effervescent and enteric coated tablets, and their effect on platelet function, *Eur J Clin Phamacol* 23:545-551, 1982.

91. Hero CM, Rodgers SE, Lloyd JV, et al: A dose-ranging study of the antiplatelet effect of enteric coated aspirin in man, *Aust NZ J Med* 17:195-200, 1987.

92. Cerletti C, Marchi S, Lauri D, et al: Pharmacokinetics of enteric-coated aspirin and inhibition of platelet thromboxane A$_2$ and vascular prostacyclin generation in humans, *Clin Pharmacol Ther* 42:175-180, 1987.

92a. Jimenez AH, Stubbs ME, Tofler GH, et al: Rapidity and duration of platelet suppression by enteric-coated aspirin in healthy young men, *Am J Cardiol* 69:259-262, 1992.

93. Terres W, Schuster O, Kupper W, et al: Wirkunger neidrig dosierter acetylsalicysaure auf die thrombozyten von gesunden und patienten mit koronarer herzkrankheit, *Dsch Med Wschr* 114:1231-1236, 1989.

94. Patrono C: Aspirin as an antiplatelet drug, *N Engl J Med* 330:1287-1294, 1994.

95. Fitzgerald GA, Oates JA, Hawiger J, et al: Endogenous biosynthesis of prostacyclin and thromboxane and platelet function during chronic administration of aspirin in man, *J Clin Invest* 71:676-687, 1983.

96. Wallentin LC, and the Research Group on Instability In Coronary Artery Disease in Southeast Sweden: Aspirin (75 mg/day) after an episode of unstable coronary artery disease: long-term effects on the risk for myocardial infarction, occurrence of severe angina and the need for revascularization, *J Am Coll Cardiol* 18:1587-1593, 1991.

97. Dutch TIA Trial Study Group: A comparison of two doses of aspirin (30mg vs. 283mg a day) in patients after a transient ischemic attack or minor ischemic stroke, *N Engl J Med* 325:1261-1266, 1991.

98. Peto R, Warlow C, and the UK-TIA Study Group: United Kingdom transient ischemic attack (UK-TIA) aspirin trial: Interim results, *Br Med J (Clin Res)* 296:316-320, 1988.

99. Theroux P, Ouimet H, McCans J, et al: Aspirin, heparin, or both to treat acute unstable angina, *N Engl J Med* 319:1105-1111, 1988.

100. Wilson KM, Siebert DM, Duncan EM, et al: Effect of aspirin infusions on platelet function in humans, *Clin Sci* 79:37-42, 1990.

101. Cerletti C, Marchi S, Lauri D, et al: Pharmacokinetics of enteric-coated aspirin and inhibition of platelet thromboxane A_2 and vascular prostacyclin generation in humans, *Clin Pharmacol Ther* 42:175-180, 1987.

102. Dabaghi SF, Kamat SG, Payne J, et al: Effects of low dose aspirin on *in vitro* platelet aggregation in the early minutes after ingestion in normal subjects, *Am J Cardiol*, in press.

103. Lauri D, Zanetii A, Dejana E, et al: Effects of dipyridamole and low-dose aspirin therapy on platelet adhesion to vascular subendothelium, *Am J Cardiol* 58:1261-1264, 1986.

104. Reilly IAG, Fitzgerald GA: Inhibition of thromboxane formation in vivo and ex vivo: implications for therapy with platelet inhibitory drugs, *Blood* 69:180-186, 1987.

105. Reference deleted in proofs.

106. Mehta JL, Mehta P, Lopez L, et al: Platelet function and biosynthesis of prostacyclin and thromboxane A_2 in whole blood after aspirin administration in human subjects, *J Am Coll Cardiol* 4:806-811, 1984.

107. ISIS-2 (Second International Study of Infarct Survival) Collaborative Group: Randomized trial of intravenous streptokinase, oral aspirin, both, or neither among 17,187 cases of suspected acute myocardial infarction. ISIS 2, *Lancet* 2:349-360, 1988.

108. Robertson TL, Forman SA, Williams DO, et al: Aspirin, rt-PA, and reperfusion in AMI: a TIMI observational study [abstract]. *Circulation* 78(suppl II):II128, 1988.

109. Ohman EM, Califf RM, Topol EJ, et al: Consequences of reocclusion after successful reperfusion therapy in acute myocardial infarction. TAMI Study Group, *Circulation* 82:781-791, 1990.

110. Meijer A, Werter CJ, Verheugt FWA, et al: The APRICOT Study: aspirin versus coumadin in the prevention of recurrent ischemia and reocclusion after successful thrombolysis, a placebo-controlled angiographic follow-up study [abstract]. *J Am Coll Cardiol* 19:730-733, 1992.

110a. Folts JD, Stamler J, Loscalzo J: Intravenous nitroglycerin infusion inhibits cyclic blood flow responses caused by periodic platelet thrombus formation in stenosed canine coronary arteries, *Circulation* 83:2122-2127, 1991.

111. Hsia J, Hamilton WP, Kleiman N, et al: A comparison between heparin and low-dose aspirin as adjunctive therapy with tissue plasminogen activator for acute myocardial infarction, *N Engl J Med* 323:1433-1437, 1990.

112. Roux S, Christeller S, Ludin E: Effects of aspirin on coronary reocclusion and recurrent ischemia after thrombolysis: a meta-analysis, *J Am Coll Cardiol* 19:671-677, 1992.

113. TIMI Study Group: Comparison of invasive and conservative strategies after treatment with intravenous tissue plasminogen activator in acute myocardial infarction: results of the Thrombolysis in Myocardial Infarction (TIMI) Phase II Trial, *N Engl J Med* 320:618-627, 1989.

114. Ellis SG, Muller DW, Topol EJ: Possible survival benefit from concomitant beta-but not calcium-antagonist therapy during reperfusion for acute myocardial infarction, *Am J Cardiol* 66:125-128, 1990.

115. Steele PM, Chesbro JH, Stanson AW, et al: Balloon angioplasty: Natural history of the pathophysiologic response to injury in a pig model, *Circ Res* 57:105, 1985.

116. Barnathan ES, Schwartz JS, Taylor L, et al: Aspirin and dipyridamole in the prevention of acute coronary thrombosis complicating coronary angioplasty, *Circulation* 76:125-134, 1987.

117. Schwartz L, Bourassa MG, Lesperance J, et al: Aspirin and dipyridamole in the prevention of restenosis after percutaneous transluminal coronary angioplasty, *N Engl J Med* 318:1714-1719, 1988.

118. Phillips MD, Moake JL, Nolasco L, et al: Aurin tricarboxylic acid: a novel inhibitor of the association of von Willebrand factor and platelets, *Blood* 72:1898-1903, 1988.

119. Strony J, Phillips M, Brands D, et al: Aurin tricarboxylic acid in a canine model of coronary artery thrombosis, *Circulation* 81:1106-1113, 1990.

120. Weinstein M, Vosburgh E, Phillips M, et al: Isolation from commercial aurin tricarboxylic acid of the most effective polymeric inhibitors of von Willebrand factor interaction with platelet glycoprotein Ib. Comparison with other polyanionic and polyaromatic polymers, *Blood* 78:2291-2298, 1991.

121. Kleiman NS, Ohman EM, Califf RM, et al: Profound inhibition of platelet aggregation with monoclonal antibody 7E3 Fab after thrombolytic therapy. Results of the Thrombolysis and Angioplasty in Myocardial Infarction (TAMI) 8 Pilot Study, *J Am Coll Cardiol* 22:381-389, 1993.

122. Klimt CR, Knatterud GL, Stamler J, et al: Persantine-aspirin reinfarction study: II. Secondary coronary prevention with persantine and aspirin, *J Am Coll Cardiol* 7:251-269, 1986.

123. Elwood PC, Cochrane AL, Burr ML, et al: A randomized controlled trial of acetyl salicylic acid in the secondary prevention of mortality from myocardial infarction, *Br Med J (Clin Res)* 1:436-440, 1974.

124. Coronary Drug Project Research Group: Aspirin in coronary heart disease, *J Chronic Dis* 29:625-642, 1976.

125. Elwood PC, Sweetnam PM: Aspirin and secondary mortality after myocardial infarction, *Lancet* 2:1313-1315, 1979.

126. Aspirin Myocardial Infarction Study Research Group: A randomized, controlled trial of aspirin in persons recovered from myocardial infarction, *JAMA* 243:661-669, 1980.

127. Breddin K, Loew D, Lechner K, et al: The German-Austrian aspirin trial: a comparison of acetylsalicylic acid, placebo and phenprocoumon in secondary prevention of myocardial infarction, *Circulation* 62(suppl V):V63-V72, 1980.

128. Persantine-Aspirin Reinfarction Study Research Group: Persantine and aspirin in coronary heart disease, *Circulation* 62:449-461, 1980.

129. Antiplatelet Trialists' Collaboration: Secondary prevention of vascular disease by prolonged antiplatelet treatment, *Br Med J (Clin Res)* 296:320-331, 1981.

130. SALT Collaborative Group: Swedish aspirin low-dose trial (SALT) of 75mg aspirin as secondary prophylaxis after cerebrovascular ischaemic events, *Lancet* 338:1345-1349, 1991.

131. Settipane GA: Aspirin sensitivity and allergy, *Biomed Pharmacother* 42:493-498, 1988.

132. Ameisen JC: Aspirin-sensitive asthma, *Clin Exp Allergy* 20:127-129, 1990.

133. Rao GHR: Influence of anti-platelet drugs on platelet-vessel wall interactions, *Prostaglandins Leukotrienes Med* 30:133-145, 1987.

134. Cox SR, Vanderlugt JT, Gumbleton TJ, et al: Relationships between thromboxane production, platelet aggregability, and serum concentrations of ibuprofen or flurbiprofen, *Clin Pharmacol Ther* 41:510-521, 1987.

135. Evans AM, Nation RL, Sansom LN, et al: Effect of racemic ibuprofen dose on the magnitude and duration of platelet cyclo-oxygenase inhibition: relationship between inhibition of thromboxane production and the plasma unbound concentration of S(+)-ibuprofen, *Br J Clin Pharmacol* 31:131-138, 1991.

136. Lam JYT, Chesbro JH, Fuster V: Platelets, vasoconstriction, and nitroglycerin during arterial wall injury. A new antithrombotic role for an old drug, *Circulation* 78:712-716, 1988.

137. Loscalzo J: N-Acetylcysteine potentiates inhibition of platelet aggregation by nitroglycerin, *J Clin Invest* 76:703-708, 1985.

138. Stamler J, Cunningham M, Loscalzo J: Reduced thiols and the effect of intravenous nitroglycerin on platelet aggregation, *Am J Cardiol* 62:377-380, 1988.

139. Diodati J, Theroux P, Latour JG, et al: Effects of nitroglycerin at therapeutic doses on platelet aggregation in unstable angina pectoris and acute myocardial infarction, *Am J Cardiol* 66:683-688, 1990.

140. Gerzer R, Karrenbrock B, Siess W, et al: Direct comparision of the effects of nitroprusside, sin 1, and various nitrates on platelet aggregation and soluble guanylate cyclase activity, *Thromb Res* 52:11-21, 1988.

141. Stamler J, Mendelsohn ME, Amarante P, et al: *N*-Acetylcysteine potentiates platelet inhibition by endothelium-derived relaxing factor, *Circ Res* 65:789-795, 1989.

142. Benjamin N, Dutton JAE, Ritter JM: Human vascular smooth muscle cells inhibit platelet aggregation when incubated with glyceryl trinitrate: evidence for generation of nitric oxide, *Br J Pharmacol* 102:847-850, 1991.

143. Willis AL, Loveday M, Fulks J, et al: Selective anti-platelet aggregation synergism between prostacyclin-mimetic, RS93427 and the nitrodilators sodium nitroprusside and glyceryl trinitrate, *Br J Pharmacol* 98:1296-1302, 1989.

144. Jugdutt, BI, Warnica JW: Intravenous nitroglycerin therapy to limit myocardial infarct size, expansion, and complications: effect of timing, dosage, and infarct location, *Circulation* 78:906-919, 1988.

145. Yusuf S, Collins R, MacMahon S, et al: Effect of intravenous nitrates on mortality in acute myocardial infarction: an overview of the randomised trials, *Lancet* 1:1088-1092, 1988.

146. Becker RC, Corrao JM, Bovill EG, et al: Intravenous nitroglycerin-induced heparin resistance: a qualitative antithrombin III abnormality, *Am Heart J* 119:1254-1261, 1990.

147. Di Minno G, Cerbone AM, Mattioli PL, et al: Functionally thrombasthenic state in normal platelets following the administration of ticlopidine, *J Clin Invest* 75:328-338, 1985.

148. Gachet C, Cazenove JP, Ohlmann P, et al: The thienopyridine ticlopidine selectively prevents the inhibitory effects of ADP but not of adrenaline on cAMP levels raised by stimulation of the adenylate cyclose of human platelets by PGE, *Biochem Pharmacol* 40:2683-2687, 1990.

149. Hardisty RM, Powling MJ, Nokes TJC: The action of ticlopidine on human platelets. Studies on aggregation, secretion, calcium mobilization and membrane glycoproteins, *Thromb Haemost* 64:150-155, 1990.

150. Gent M, Easton JD, Hachinski VC, et al: The Canadian American ticlopidine study (CATS) in thromboembolic stroke, *Lancet* 1215-1220, 1989.

151. Hass WK, Easton JD, Adams HP, et al: A randomized trial comparing ticlopidine hydrochloride with aspirin for the prevention of strokes in high risk patients, *N Engl J Med* 321:501-507, 1989.

152. Balsano F, Rizzon P, Violi F, et al: Antiplatelet treatment with ticlopidine in unstable angina: a controlled multicenter clinical trial, *Circulation* 82:17-26, 1990.

153. Janzon L, Bergoqvist D, Boberg J, et al: Prevention of myocardial infarction and stroke in patients with intermittent claudication; effects of ticlopidine. Results from STIMS, the Swedish Ticlopidine Multicentre Study, *J Int Med* 227:301-308, 1990.

Chapter 30

ADJUNCTIVE AGENTS TO REDUCE ISCHEMIA, PRESERVE MYOCARDIAL FUNCTION, AND REDUCE MORTALITY

Steven E. Hearne
E. Magnus Ohman
Koon K. Teo

Complications following acute myocardial infarction (AMI) leading to death or major morbidity, such as angina, reinfarction, and heart failure, can occur either in the acute stage or during later follow-up. Although thrombolysis has become established as the major therapy for AMI, a number of other agents can be used adjunctively to reduce these serious complications, preserve ventricular function, and prolong survival. The specific goals of adjunctive therapy are to limit infarct size; improve left ventricular ejection fraction; prevent congestive heart failure, recurrent angina or infarction, and potentially fatal arrhythmias; and most importantly, to decrease mortality.

In this chapter the role of some of these adjunctive agents in MI will be discussed. There are large volumes of data from clinical trials and other studies evaluating the usefulness of beta blockers, calcium blockers, and nitrates in AMI. In addition to these established therapies, promising agents such as angiotensin-converting enzyme inhibitors and magnesium have been studied in the same setting.

For the busy clinician it can be confusing and frustrating to have to review the very large number of trials, the results of which often appear to be inconsistent. Yet it is important to know which data are reliable and applicable to clinical practice. In order to avoid selection or systematic biases, the data from all the trials should be examined. This is the approach taken in this chapter and the conclusions are drawn on the results of individual trials and published overviews of all the available randomized controlled trials of these agents.

BETA BLOCKERS

The principal mechanism of action of beta blockers is the competitive binding of these agents to the beta receptors in the appropriate effector tissues, resulting in blocking of the agonistic actions of circulating catecholamines. This action reduces myocardial oxygen demand by decreasing wall stress, heart rate, and contractility. Beta receptors are divided into two major subtypes: $beta_1$ and $beta_2$. The former receptors predominate in the heart, where they increase heart rate and contractility in response to stimulation by beta agonists such as norepinephrine and isoproterenol. The $beta_2$-receptors are located in the periphery, where they cause peripheral vasodilation as well as bronchial dilatation. Cardioselective beta blockers such as metoprolol and atenolol are those that preferentially bind to beta$_1$-receptors. Noncardioselective beta blockers include propranolol, timolol, and pindolol. Agents such as pindolol have intrinsic sympathomimetic activity, which confers partial agonist activity at low doses and antagonist activity at high doses.

Beta blockers can produce several beneficial effects by reducing heart rate, contractility, and blood pressure leading to decreased myocardial oxygen consumption and work load. During myocardial ischemia, administration of these agents results in favorable redistribution of blood flow from the epicardium to the endocardium. Administration of the agents before experimental infarction in animals also reduces infarct size and increases the threshold for ventricular fibrillation.

Clinically, beta blockers are beneficial in reducing mortality in the periinfarction setting as well as during late follow-up. They also have substantial impact on reducing infarct size, reinfarction, and ventricular fibrillation after MI. However, these agents are not without potential adverse effects. Their negative inotropic effect may cause congestive heart failure, hypotension, and high degrees of atrioventricular block, which may result in adverse hemodynamic side effects. Clinical trials of early intravenous and long-term beta blockade therapy have been conducted and will be described separately. However, in clinical practice the manner in which these agents are used should be considered a continuous process.

INTRAVENOUS BETA BLOCKERS

Over 30 trials[1-5] involving over 29,000 patients have been reported in which early intravenous treatment was started in AMI. The initial intravenous dose was either 10 to 15 mg of metoprolol, 5 to 10 mg of atenolol, or 5 to 10 mg of propranolol. The majority of these trials were conducted before the widespread use of thrombolytic therapy. Two of the largest trials of intravenous beta blockers early in AMI were the MIAMI[6] (Metoprolol In Acute Myocardial Infarction) trial, which evaluated metoprolol in 5778 patients, and the ISIS-1[4] (First International Study of Infarct Survival) trial, which evaluated atenolol in 16,105 patients. In the MIAMI trial the main endpoint was 14-day mortality. A statistically nonsignificant ($P = 0.29$) 13% mortality reduction was found in the metoprolol group. Seven-day mortality was the primary endpoint in the ISIS-1 trial, in which cardiovascular mortality was reduced by 14% during treatment (313 deaths in 8037 patients in the treated group compared with 365 deaths in 7990 patients treated with placebo, $P < 0.04$). In both trials most of the mortality reduction was observed within the first 48

hours (MIAMI trial: 41 deaths in control group and 29 deaths in treatment group; ISIS-1: 171 deaths in control group and 121 deaths in treatment group). Pooled data from 28 smaller trials of about 6000 patients showed beneficial effects throughout the 7 days of treatment post-MI. Mortality results from all trials show a 24% reduction during the first 48 hours, a 9% reduction in the next 48 hours, and little additional benefit thereafter. When the data from all the intravenous beta-blocker trials were pooled the overall mortality reduction in patients treated with intravenous beta blockers was about 13% ($P < 0.02$).

Several trials[7-9] have reported a lower incidence of ventricular fibrillation in patients treated with beta blockers. The data from 27 trials show a statistically significant 15% reduction in ventricular fibrillation ($P < 0.01$). A retrospective analysis of deaths in the ISIS-1 trial suggests that the early mortality benefit may be the result of a decrease in myocardial rupture and ventricular fibrillation in beta blocker-treated patients. A similar trend was observed in the trial by Hjalmarson et al.[10] and in the MIAMI trial.[6]

Beta blockers given intravenously have been documented to reduce the rate of reinfarction when data on about 29,000 patients were pooled and analyzed. The group treated with beta blockade had a reinfarction rate of 2.8% (308 of 11,021 patients) compared with 3.4% in the controls (371 of 11,070 patients) treated with placebo. This corresponds to a relative reductions of 18% ($P < 0.02$).

Coupled with the reduction in mortality and morbidity, evidence also exists that infarct size is reduced from 15% to 30% in patients treated with intravenous beta blockers within the first 12 hours of symptom onset. Several small trials have addressed this and are summarized in Table 30-1. In addition to preserving viable myocardial and ventricular function, this decrease in infarct size may indirectly lead to a decrease in myocardial rupture because of reduced transmural necrosis. Figure 30-1 summarizes the effects of early intravenous beta blockers on mortality, reinfarction, and ventricular fibrillation in AMI.

Beta blockers have also been shown to reduce ischemic pain[12,19-20] in the periinfarction setting. This effect appears to correlate well with the reductions of blood pressure, heart rate, and myocardial oxygen demand.

The TIMI-IIB[5] (Thrombolysis In Myocardial Infarction Phase IIB) study is the largest study of beta blockers in combination with thrombolytic therapy. In this study a subgroup of 1390 patients out of 3534 patients (39%) was randomly assigned to immediate intravenous metoprolol followed by oral metoprolol or to oral metoprolol begun on the sixth postinfarction day. Patients who were receiving beta blockers or calcium blockers at the time of admission were excluded (46%). The in-hospital and 42-day mortality rates were similar between the two groups. However, the immediate intravenous beta-blocker group experienced significantly fewer reinfarctions (16 of 696 in the active treatment group and 31 of 694 controls, $P < 0.05$) and recurrent ischemic events (107 of 696 active treatment vs. 147 of 694 placebo, $P < 0.005$). Those patients treated within 2 hours derived the greatest benefit in the reduction of cardiac events. Most important, a trend toward fewer intracranial hemorrhages with thrombolysis was observed in the group assigned to the immediate intravenous beta-blocker regimen. The TIMI-IIB data, in conjunction with the findings of the beneficial effects of immediate beta blockade, support the routine use of early intravenous beta blockade in patients with AMI in the absence of obvious contraindications.

Table 30-1. Reduction in infarction size with early IV treatment with beta blockers in AMI

Agent	Author	Number treated	Reduction (%)	*P*
Timolol	ICSG[11]	73	30	<.05
	TIARA[12]	102	24	<.01
Propranolol	MILIS†[13]	134	8	NS
	Norris[14]	33	25	<.05
	Peter[15]	47	10	NS
Metoprolol	MIAMI*[16]	1415	11	NS
	Herlitz[17]	461	17	<.01
	Boyle[18]	115	14	<.01
Atenolol	Yusuf[19]	244	30	<.001

*Trial entered patients up to 24 hours after onset of pain. Table includes only patients entered within 7 hours.
†Trial entered patients up to 18 hours after onset of pain. Table includes only patients entered within 8 hours.

LONG-TERM BETA BLOCKERS

The effects of long-term oral beta blockers started days to weeks after AMI have been examined in over 20,000 patients from at least 18 trials.[1,4,21] In eight other trials treatment was started early and continued over the long term. The endpoint of these trials was mortality; although most of these trials were too small to reliably detect a difference in mortality, favorable trends in mortality were present in most.

In the Beta Blocker Heart Attack Trial (BHAT) 138 (7.2%) of 1916 propranolol-treated patients and 188 (9.8%) of 1921 placebo-treated patients died during a median of 2 years of follow-up.[22] The difference in mortality was statistically significant ($P = 0.004$). In the trial by Hjalmarson et al.,[10] 22 of 680 patients treated with metoprolol versus 39 of 674 patients treated with placebo died ($P = 0.02$). In the trial by Salathia et al.,[23] 27 of 391 patients in the metoprolol group and 43 of 364 patients in the placebo group died ($P = 0.02$). In a follow-up of 1 to 3 years in the Norwegian Timolol Trial,[24] 98 of 945 patients receiving active treatment died compared to 152 of 934 placebo-treated patients ($P = 0.002$). The results of the pooled analysis of the 26 studies demonstrate a 23% reduction in risk of death (934 deaths in 12,438 or 7.6% of patients in the beta-blocker-treated group and 1124 deaths in 11,860 or 9.4% of patients not treated with beta blockers, $P < 0.0001$). Sudden death, in particular, has been significantly reduced by long-term beta blockade (data on 15,800 patients indicate a 32% reduction, $P < 0.0001$). Data available on reinfarction in about 20,000 patients[4] show a nonfatal reinfarction rate of 5.6% in patients treated with beta blockers and 7.5% in patients treated with placebo ($P < 0.0001$). Figure 30-2 summarizes the effects of long-term oral beta blockers on reinfarction, sudden death, and total mortality after MI.

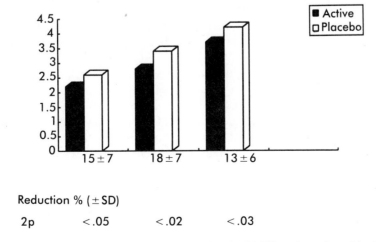

Fig. 30-1. Early intravenous beta blockade in MI: 29,000 patients from 31 trials.

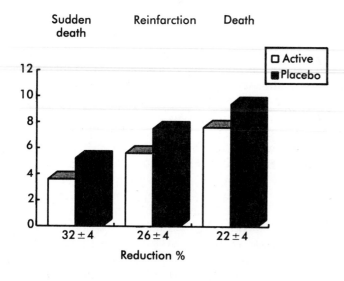

Fig. 30-2. Post MI beta-blocker patients: 25 pooled studies of 24,000 patients.

Mortality reduction during the postinfarction period was similar in trials in which therapy with beta blockers was started early and continued long term and in those trials in which treatment was started late. Patients on beta blockers did better regardless of age, sex, infarct location or size, or the presence or absence of heart failure. Therefore, benefit appears to be present across all subgroups of patients.

Although beta blockers have traditionally been thought to be contraindicated in congestive heart failure in AMI, there is good physiological evidence for a possible beneficial role in reducing the sympathetic drive in patients with chronic heart failure. A recent clinical trial of 383 patients with idiopathic dilated cardiomyopathy (ejection fraction <40%) randomized patients to receive 10 mg daily of metoprolol escalating weekly (15 mg, 30 mg, 50 mg, 75 mg, 100 mg) to a maximum dose of 150 mg/day vs. placebo.[25] The test dose of 10 mg/day was tolerated in 96% and the patients were followed for up to 18 months. At 12 months there was a significant improvement in the ejection fraction ($P < 0.0001$), a marginal reduction in the capillary wedge pressure ($P = 0.06$), and a significant improvement in exercise time ($P = 0.046$). Over the entire study duration the metoprolol-treated patients had a 34% reduction (95% confidence interval: -6% to 62%; $P = 0.058$) in primary endpoints (death or need for heart transplantation). Furthermore, the number of readmissions per patient for management of heart failure or arrhythmias was significantly reduced in metoprolol-treated patients (0.3 admissions) com-

pared with placebo-treated patients (0.5, $P < 0.04$). These findings are intriguing because they suggest that patients not ordinarily thought to be candidates for beta-blocker therapy may be candidates for low-dose therapy and that this may improve morbidity and, to a lesser extent, mortality. These findings await confirmation in patients with ischemic cardiomyopathy to further explore the use of beta blockers in patients with reduced left ventricular function.

In summary, beta blockers should be given intravenously to all patients with AMI who do not have contraindications to their use. These drugs have been shown unequivocally to decrease mortality, infarct size, recurrent angina, and reinfarction. The dose of intravenous beta blockers should be the equivalent of 5 to 15 mg metoprolol or 5 to 10 mg of atenolol followed immediately by oral loading. This should be continued through the postinfarction period. Absolute and relative contraindications to beta blockers are shown in Table 30-2.

Despite these very persuasive findings, a recent report from a thrombolytic registry of 100,000 patients in the United States with MI revealed that only 9% of patients receive intravenous beta blockers despite the overwhelming evidence of their benefits.[26] Similarly, a survey conducted in the United Kingdom noted that only 3% of physicians routinely use intravenous beta blockers and 31% use oral beta blockers as treatments in AMI. However, in the recently completed GUSTO-I trial intravenous atenolol was used in 42% of the patients and 74% of patients enrolled in the trial were discharged on atenolol. These observations suggest that the majority of patients with AMI eligible for thrombolysis could tolerate and potentially derive benefit from beta-blocker therapy. Wider use of this therapy would certainly have a favorable impact on a large number of patients with AMI.

CALCIUM-CHANNEL BLOCKERS

Calcium-channel blockers exhibit a number of effects that can theoretically be beneficial in AMI. They produce reductions in blood pressure and heart rate (verapamil and diltiazem), and myocardial contractility[27] (verapamil). They also enhance coronary blood flow to ischemic areas by relieving vasospasm and causing vasodilatation of collateral beds.[27] Also, calcium overload is implicated as the final common pathway in myocardial necrosis, and this has been shown to be inhibited by calcium-channel blockers in animals. As a result of calcium-channel blockade, mitochondrial structure and function are preserved and less intracellular calcium is available to stimulate proteases that induce myocardial cell damage.[28] In addition, some calcium-channel blockers have been shown to reduce platelet aggregation.[29] Despite these theoretical benefits in patients with MI and a demonstration

Table 30-2. Relative and absolute contraindications to IV beta blockers

Absolute	Relative
Type II second-degree AV block	History of bronchial asthma
Complete heart block	Bibasilar rales
Rales greater than half of lung fields	PR lengthening beyond 0.24 second
Cardiogenic shock	PCWP >20 mmHg
Heart rate below 50 per minute	
Systolic BP <95 mmHg	

of benefit in both animal and uncontrolled clinical studies, clinical trials with calcium-channel blockers in AMI have not been promising. The most commonly studied agents in this class are verapamil, diltiazem, and nifedipine.

Verapamil

There have been two major studies examining the role of verapamil in AMI. Patients receiving beta blockers were excluded in both of these trials. The DAVIT-I (First Danish Verapamil Infarction Trial)[30] researchers reported their results in 1984. This was a double-blind placebo-controlled trial of verapamil (0.2 mg/kg intravenously and 120 mg orally on admission, followed by 120 mg three times per day orally) or matched placebo for 6 months. Only patients with verified MI were included in the final study analysis. After 6 months, mortality was similar: 12.8% (92 of 717 patients) in the verapamil group and 13.9% (100 of 719 patients) in the placebo group. No significant difference in infarct size was found in a subgroup of 100 patients who were randomized within 4 hours of MI and treated with verapamil or placebo. Retrospective analyses of DAVIT-I showed that patients treated early with verapamil had increased mortality compared with placebo but that the patients who were alive on day 22 and treated with verapamil had a significant decrease in the incidence of death and reinfarction (P < 0.03). These retrospectively analyzed subgroup data formed the basis for the DAVIT-II trial.

In DAVIT-II[31] 1775 patients were randomized and treated with verapamil (120 mg three times per day) or matching placebo starting in the second week after MI (mean of 9 days). Treatment in this trial was for a mean follow-up period of 18 months. The total 18-month mortality in this trial was 11.1% in the verapamil group and 13.8% in the placebo group (P = 0.11). The mean rate of major clinical events (reinfarction and mortality) in this trial showed a trend favoring verapamil (16% in the verapamil group vs.

21% in the control group) but this did not reach a conventional level of significance (P = 0.07). In a subgroup analysis, patients without congestive heart failure had a slightly lower mortality in the verapamil-treated group (7% vs. 11% in the placebo group). There was no significant difference in mortality in patients with and without congestive heart failure in the group treated with verapamil.

When the DAVIT-I and DAVIT-II data are combined with previous trials[32] of verapamil in AMI, mortality in the active treatment group is 244 (9.2%) of 2644 patients and mortality in the placebo group is 266 (10%) out of 2649 patients (odds ratio = 0.91; 95% confidence intervals: 0.76 to 1.10). Data on reinfarction in the DAVIT I and II and other trials of verapamil in AMI show a trend toward less reinfarction in the group treated with verapamil, with 138 of 2606 patients treated with verapamil experiencing a recurrent MI and 171 of 2642 patients in the placebo group experiencing a recurrent MI (odds ratio = 0.80, 95% confidence interval: 0.63 to 1.01).

Diltiazem

The effect of diltiazem in MI has also been extensively studied. In the Multi-Center Diltiazem Post Infarction Trial (MDPIT)[33] 2466 patients with MI were randomized within 2 to 15 days to receive either diltiazem 60 mg four times per day orally or matching placebo. Follow-up was for a mean of 25 months. Primary endpoints were mortality and first cardiac event (cardiac death or nonfatal reinfarction). There were 166 deaths in the patients receiving diltiazem and 167 deaths in the patients receiving placebo. There were 222 total cardiac events in the placebo group and 202 cardiac events in the diltiazem group (P = NS). Subgroup analysis of this study revealed that in the 490 patients with pulmonary edema on chest x-ray diltiazem was associated with a significantly increased risk of recurrent cardiac events[33] (Cox hazard ratio = 1.85; 95% confidence interval: 1.24 to 2.75). In patients with an ejection fraction less than 40%, diltiazem was associated with a significantly increased risk of cardiac death (Cox hazard ratio = 1.67; 95% confidence interval: 1.04 to 2.71). In those 1909 patients without congestive heart failure on chest x-ray diltiazem was associated with a reduction of cardiac events (Cox hazard ratio = 0.77; 95% confidence interval: 0.61 to 0.98; P < 0.05) and in the 80% of patients with an ejection fraction greater than 40%[34] diltiazem was associated with a trend towards decreased incidence of cardiac death (Cox hazard ratio = 0.85; 95% confidence interval: 0.46 to 1.60). These data suggest that a differential effect of diltiazem may exist in different subgroups of patients although the effect on overall mortality did not differ from placebo. Whether or not these differential effects are real and therefore nullify the overall outcome can only be confirmed by other trial data. At present these subgroup analyses should be interpreted cautiously. Further retrospective subgroup analyses can be strongly influenced by selection and other biases and in general little reliance should be placed on them rather than on *a priori* primary endpoints.

When data from MDPIT were combined with the data from other trials[32] of diltiazem in AMI, the rate of cardiac death in the treated group was 11.4% (180 out of 1574 patients) and 11.5% (181 out of 1577 patients) in the placebo group (odds ratio = 0.99; 95% confidence interval: 0.80 to 1.24). Reinfarction occurred in 113 (7.3%) of 1557 patients treated with diltiazem and 142 (9.1%) of 1560 patients treated with placebo (odds ratio = 0.79; 95% confidence interval: 0.69 to 1.02), representing a nonsignificant trend toward decreased reinfarction in patients treated with diltiazem.

In the MDPIT study[35] 634 patients with non–Q-wave MI had a cumulative event rate (reinfarction or death) of 15% in 338 patients treated with placebo and of 9% in 296 patients treated with diltiazem (Cox hazard ratio = 0.65; 95% confidence interval: 0.43 to 0.96). The very limited data from this and the Multi-Center Diltiazem Reinfarction study appear to suggest a benefit in preventing reinfarction in the non–Q-wave infarction subgroup. The Multi-Center Diltiazem Reinfarction study,[36] which was undertaken to assess this hypothesis, randomized 576 patients to receive either diltiazem 90 mg QID orally or placebo for 14 days or until discharge from the hospital. The mean treatment period was 10 days and treatment was begun 24 to 72 hours after the onset of symptoms. Comparable numbers of patients in each group received beta blockers. The rate of reinfarction in the diltiazem group was 5.2%, and in the placebo group it was 9.4% ($P = 0.06$). Mortality at 14 days was similar in both groups, 3.1% in the placebo group and 3.8% in the diltiazem group, but post-MI angina was reduced by about 50% in the diltiazem group. The use of beta blockers was similar in the two groups, suggesting that diltiazem may have an added beneficial effect on reinfarction.

Nifedipine

Several trials have addressed the use of nifedipine in AMI. In the TRENT[37] study 4491 patients with suspected MI were treated for 1 month with nifedipine or placebo and 70% of the patients were entered within 8 hours after the onset of symptoms. The dose of nifedipine was 10 mg four times per day or matching placebo. In each group 64% of patients developed MI. Mortality was 6.3% in the placebo group and 6.7% in the nifedipine-treated group. The SPRINT-I study[38] randomly assigned 2276 patients to nifedipine or placebo at a dosage of 30 mg a day beginning between 7 and 22 days after MI. Treatment was continued for 10 months. Mortality rates were 6% in each group, indicating no treatment benefit and that only low-risk patients were randomized.

The SPRINT-II study group[39] recently reported the final results of the use of nifedipine 60 mg a day or placebo started as soon as possible after MI (usually less than 3 hours after the onset of symptoms). This study had to be stopped prematurely because of a trend toward a higher mortality in the treated group. Initially, 1358 patients were randomized, but 352 patients were excluded from the study because they either did not have MI or discontinued the medications on their own. In the 1006 patients treated, mortality was 18.7% among the nifedipine group and 16.6% in the placebo group. Early mortality, defined as during the first 6 days postinfarction, was 7.8% in the nifedipine group and 5.5% in the placebo group. In the 826 patients who continued treatment for up to 6 months mortality was 9.3% in the nifedipine group and 9.5% in the placebo group. There was also no difference in nonfatal MI or unstable angina between the two groups during the 6 months of follow-up.

There is no evidence that calcium-channel blockers have any beneficial effects during AMI and may indeed increase mortality when all the trials are summarized, as seen in Table 30-3. In patients who are intolerant of beta blockers, diltiazem and verapamil given days to weeks after infarction may reduce angina but will have no effect on mortality. Nifedipine can worsen outcome in the setting of AMI and should not be used at all in this setting.

In the GUSTO-I study approximately 20% of patients were treated with a calcium antagonist during the hospitalization. This may represent the use of calcium-channel antagonists in patients undergoing PCTA after MI to reduce vasospasm.

NITRATES

Nitrates have been used for many years in the treatment of symptomatic coronary artery disease. Their primary mode of action is to produce vascular smooth muscle relaxation, which results in vasodilatation. Nitrates dilate veins, arteries, and arterioles.[42] Venodilation results in the pooling of blood in the capacitance vessels. This latter action tends to decrease blood return to the heart and reduce left ventricular preload. In addition, nitrates tend to dilate the coronary artery bed. However, the primary mechanism of action of nitrates in reducing myocardial ischemia appears to be the result of a decrease in myocardial oxygen demand secondary to a decrease in blood pressure and a reduction in left ventricular systolic and diastolic volumes, with a resultant fall in ventricular filling pressure.[43]

Table 30-3. Effect of calcium-channel blockers in AMI

	Mortality		Reinfarction	
Study	Active	Control	Active	Control
Dihydropyridines				
Held et al.[32]	365/4731	330/4733	124/3646	111/3680
Lichtlen et al.[40]	12/214	2/211	—	—
Waters et al.[41]	2/192	3/191	14/192	8/191
TOTAL	379/5137	335/5135	138/3838	119/3871
	(7.4%)	(6.5%)	(3.5%)	(3.1%)
	Odds ratio = 1.16 (.99-1.35)		Odds ratio = 1.19 (.92-1.53)	
Verapamil				
DAVIT-II[31]	95/878	119/897	84/878	107/897
Held et al.[32]	149/1766	147/1752	54/1728	64/1727
TOTAL	244/2644	266/2649	138/2606	171/2624
	(9.2%)	(10.0%)	(5.3%)	(6.5%)
	Odds ratio = .91 (.76-1.1)		Odds ratio = .80 (.63-1.01)	
Diltiazem				
Held et al.[32]	180/1574	181/1577	113/1557	142/1560
	(11.4%)	(11.5%)	(7.3%)	(9.1%)
	Odds ratio = .99 (.80-1.24)		Odds ratio = .79 (.61-1.02)	

Table 30-4. Mortality in trials of intravenous nitroglycerin

	Deaths		
Study (follow-up)	Treated	Control	P
Bussman et al.[46] (18 months)	4/31 (13%)	12/28 (41%)	< .02
Nelson[55] (hospital)	0/14 (0%)	0/14 (0%)	NS
Jaffe[56] (hospital)	4/57 (7%)	2/57 (4%)	NS
Chihe[57] (hospital)	3/50 (6%)	8/45 (18%)	NS
Flaherty et al.[58] (3 months)	11/56 (20%)	11/48 (23%)	NS
Jugdutt et al.[45] (3 months)	24/154 (16%)	44/156 (28%)	< .01
Lis[59] (4 months)	5/64 (8%)	10/76 (13%)	NS
Overall	51/426 (12%)	87/425 (20.5%)	< .001

INTRAVENOUS NITROGLYCERIN

Seven randomized trials of intravenous nitroglycerin involving 851 patients have been reported.[44] In all these trials treatment was started within 24 hours of onset of symptoms. Exclusion criteria in most of these trials were chronic lung disease, pulmonary edema, cardiogenic shock, and systolic blood pressure less than 100 mm Hg.

The trials ranged in size from 28 to 310 patients. In the largest of these trials[45] a mortality rate of 15.6% in patients allocated to nitroglycerin and 28.2% in patients allocated to placebo ($P < 0.01$) was present at 3 months. In another trial[46] 60 patients were followed for 18 months. Observed mortality rates were 41.4% (12 of 29 patients) in the control group and 12.9% (4 of 31 patients) in the active group. The pooled mortality in these seven trials was 12% (51 of 426 patients) for the actively treated patients and 20.5% (87 of 425 patients) for those randomized to placebo ($P < 0.001$).

Early and late mortality were also analyzed separately. During the early period (7 days or hospital discharge) mortality was 4.9% (21 out of 426 patients) in the nitroglycerin group and 13.4% (57 of 425 patients) in the placebo group. After this period mortality rates in the four trials that continued to follow these patients was 10.3% (30 of 291 patients) in the treatment group and 11.5% (30 of 262 patients) the control group. These data suggest that the primary benefit of nitrates is early in the setting of AMI but that a further late trend in reducing mortality cannot be ruled out. Table 30-4 summarizes the trials of intravenous nitroglycerin in AMI.

INTRAVENOUS NITROPRUSSIDE

Three trials[47-49] of intravenous nitroprusside have also been conducted. Entry criteria in these trials were generally similar to those of the intravenous nitroglyc-

Table 30-5. Mortality in trials of oral nitrates in AMI

| Study (follow-up) | Deaths | | P Value |
	Treated	Control	
Mellen et al.[50] (Hospital)	11/108	10/89	NS
Newell et al.[51] (21 days)	25/181	24/165	NS
Oscharoff[52] (Hospital)	2/50	11/50	< .02
Ryan and Schnee[53] (Hospital)	9/54	12/54	NS
Fitzgerald and Bennett[54] (6 months)	21/184	14/176	NS
Overall	68/576 (11.9%)	71/534 (13.3%)	NS

erin trials. Only one trial[47] showed a significant mortality reduction at 1 month (6% mortality for the active treatment group vs. 12% in the placebo group, $P < 0.05$), whereas the other two trials showed trends toward mortality reduction in the active treatment group. Although the overall mortality reduction (14.3% for actively treated patients vs. 17.8% in controls, $P < 0.1$) was not statistically significant in the nitroprusside trials, these data are not significantly different from the results of the nitroglycerin trials.

ORAL NITRATES

In five smaller trials involving over 1000 patients[50-54] oral nitrates or placebo were started as soon as possible after MI was diagnosed. Nitrates were given for a range of 5 days to 6 months. Four trials[50-53] used pentaerythritol tetranitrate and one used isosorbide 5-mononitrate.[54] One of the trials[52] reported a convincingly significant reduction in mortality in nitrate-treated patients (4% in the treated group vs. 22% in the control group, $P < 0.02$). In three trials[50,52,53] in-hospital mortality and in one trial[51] 21-day mortality were reported. The overall mortality in the first few weeks after MI was 68 of 576 patients (11.9%) in the treated group and 71 of 534 (13.3%) in the control group (odds ratio-0.88; 95% confidence intervals: 0.53 to 1.88). Table 30-5 summarizes the trials of oral nitrates in AMI.

The pooled data from oral and intravenous nitroglycerin and nitroprusside therapy revealed that nitrate therapy was associated with a 31% relative reduction in mortality (95% confidence intervals, 16 to 44%, $P < 0.001$). Infarct size, assessed by serum creatine kinase, was reduced by 37% in the three intravenous nitroglycerin trials that reported such data.[45,46,56] Intravenous nitroglycerin has also been shown to improve regional and global left ventricular function[46,60] and to decrease the incidence of infarct expansion.[45] Figure 30-3 summarizes the data on trials of intravenous and oral nitrates in AMI. Based on the metaanalysis of nitrates previously described, the ISIS group in England and the GISSI study group in Italy decided to include an arm with nitrate therapy in a multifactorial design. The ISIS-4 study tested the hypothesis that oral nitrate therapy would reduce 30-day mortality after suspected AMI in the background of current beneficial therapy. Preliminary data on 58,000 patients enrolled in the ISIS-4 study were presented at the American Heart Association meeting in October of 1993. Oral nitrate use did not affect 30-day mortality in this study (7% vs. 7.2%). Similarly, the GISSI-3 study failed to document any reduction in 6-week mortality in 18,895 patients enrolled. These findings suggest that nitrate use for 30 days to 6 weeks after suspected infarction is not associated with an improvement in survival, but leaves the question regarding intravenous nitrates largely unanswered. The use of intravenous nitroglycerin therapy may still be associated with a significant improvement in survival and it remains the easiest therapy to use and titrate during the first 24 hours of AMI. These findings also suggest that nitrate use after MI should be limited to patients with recurrent angina or vasospasm or those in need of afterload reduction because of heart failure.

ANGIOTENSIN-CONVERTING ENZYME (ACE) INHIBITORS

Several studies have confirmed the progressive nature of left ventricular enlargement in the postinfarction period.[61-64] The use of ACE inhibitors post-MI has been shown to attenuate left ventricular enlargement and prevent further deterioration of left ventricular function.[65-67] These studies were done in either animals or patient groups but were too small to detect differences in long-term survival and clinical outcomes.

In the SAVE (Survival and Ventricular Enlargement) study[68] 2231 patients with ejection fractions of less than 40% and free of symptoms of congestive heart failure were randomized within 3 to 16 days after MI to receive either captopril or placebo. Patients were excluded if they had congestive heart failure, a creatinine greater than 2.5 mg/dL, other illnesses that would limit survival, or an unstable course post-MI. Captopril was

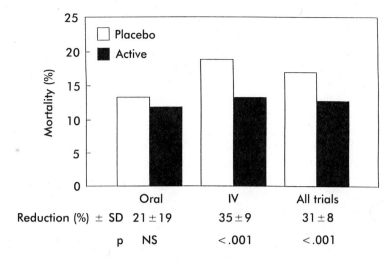

Fig. 30-3. Mortality from 15 trials of nitrates in AMI.

started with a test dose of 6.25 mg and increased to 50 mg three times daily as tolerated. The active and placebo groups did not differ in the use of beta blockers, calcium blockers, nitrates, or aspirin. Survivors were followed for an average of 42 months. Mortality in the placebo group was 275 of 1116 patients (25%), and in the treatment group mortality was 228 of 1115 patients (20%) ($P = 0.019$) Eighty-four percent of the deaths were from cardiovascular causes (234 patients or 21% in the placebo group and 188 patients or 16.9% in the captopril group, $P = 0.014$). The risk of recurrent fatal or nonfatal MI was also greatly reduced in the captopril group (170 patients in the placebo group and 133 in the captopril group, $P = 0.05$). There was also a reduction in mortality caused by congestive heart failure in the captopril group (38 deaths in the treated group vs. 58 deaths in the placebo group). Repeat hospitalizations for heart failure were 14% (154 of 1115 patients) in the treatment group and 17% (192 of 1116 patients) in the placebo group. Finally, the number of patients who either died from cardiac causes or had nonfatal events, such as recurrent infarction, congestive heart failure requiring ACE inhibitor treatment, or a repeat hospitalization for heart failure, was greatly reduced with captopril therapy (448 of 1116 patients or 40% in the placebo group and 359 of 1115 or 32% in the captopril group, $P < 0.001$). This represents a reduction of 24% for these combined events.

A second large trial of ACE inhibitors in AMI was the CONSENSUS-II trial.[69] In this trial 3046 patients were assigned to placebo and 3004 patients were assigned to receive intravenous enalapril within 24 hours of the onset of chest pain. This was followed by immediate oral treatment. Exclusion criteria were systolic blood pressure less than 105 mm Hg, MI requiring vasopressors, severe valvular stenosis, and allergy to or a clear indication for treatment with ACE inhibitors. This trial

was stopped early by the data and safety monitoring board because of a high likelihood that enalapril was no better than placebo. Follow-up ranged from 41 to 180 days. Mortality at the end of the trial was 286 in the placebo group and 312 in the enalapril group (9.4% vs. 10.2%, $P = 0.26$). The secondary endpoints of hospitalization for congestive heart failure and reinfarction were not statistically different between the two groups. However, the endpoint of change of therapy because of congestive heart failure was statistically significant in favor of enalapril (810 patients or 27% in the enalapril group and 908 patients or 30% in the placebo group, $P < 0.006$). The disappointing results of CONSENSUS-II may be explained by several factors. The dose of enalapril may have been inadequate. Angiotensin may be important early in the healing of MI,[70] and its inhibition may retard this process. Hypotension caused by infusion of intravenous enalapril may have increased the insult to the ischemic myocardium in the infarct region. Also, because the study was terminated prematurely the 95% confidence interval for mortality encompasses a *possible* 11% reduction in mortality.

Although not exclusively dealing with postinfarction patients, the data from the SOLVD[71] (Studies of Left Ventricular Dysfunction) Prevention trial should be discussed in the context of the antiischemic effects of enalapril shown in these trials. This is also relevant because the majority of patients had left ventricular dysfunction caused by ischemic heart disease. The SOLVD Prevention trial was designed to test the hypothesis that enalapril would reduce morbidity and mortality in patients who are not receiving drugs for congestive heart failure (diuretics, digoxin, or vasodilators). Patients were required to have an ejection fraction of less than 35%. Approximately 83% had a history of ischemic heart disease and 80% had a history of MI. The study enrolled 2117 patients in the placebo arm and 2111 patients in the enalapril arm. Overall mortality was 342 (15.8%) in the placebo group and 317 (14.8%) in the enalapril group ($P = 0.22$). Mortality from cardiovascular causes was 304 (14.1%) in the placebo group and 269 (12.6%) in the enalapril group ($P = 0.09$). This represents a strong trend towards reduced cardiovascular mortality in patients treated with enalapril. Interestingly, the diagnosis of congestive heart failure, treatment of congestive heart failure, or hospitalization for congestive heart failure were all significantly reduced by enalapril therapy ($P < 0.001$ for each of these endpoints). Finally, the combined endpoint of death or development of congestive heart failure occurred in 818 (38.6%) patients in the placebo arm and 630 (29.8%) patients in the enalapril arm ($P < 0.001$). The data from the SOLVD and SAVE trials clearly support the use of ACE inhibitors in patients with reduced ejection fraction regardless of cause.

The apparent discrepancy in the clinical benefit with ACE inhibitors in clinical trials of patients with reduced ejection fraction vs. studies evaluating patients with AMI was most recently addressed in the AIRE (Acute Infarction Ramipril Efficacy) study.[72] In this study 2006 patients with clinical evidence of heart failure occurring after an AMI were randomized to ramipril vs. placebo 3 to 10 days after infarction and followed for an average of 15 months. Mortality from all causes was significantly lower for patients randomized to ramipril (17%) vs. placebo (23%; 27% risk reduction, $P = 0.002$). Furthermore, there was a significant reduction in a composite clinical endpoint (death, reinfarction, stroke, and severe heart failure) in patients allocated to ramipril ($P = 0.008$). The treatment effect was also consistent across many subgroups including gender, older age, and whether intravenous thrombolytic therapy or beta blockers were used. This study thus confirms that ACE inhibition is associated with a significant reduction in mortality in patients with heart failure, including patients who develop it during MI.

During 1993 three large studies evaluating ACE inhibition in AMI were completed. Two of the studies evaluated captopril (ISIS-4 and Chinese study)[73,74] and one study (GISSI-3) examined lisinopril.[75] Preliminary data from these three trials were presented at the 1993 American Heart Association meeting. In the GISSI-3 study 18,895 patients were randomized to lisinopril vs. placebo. The 6-week mortality rate was significantly reduced in the actively treated patients (odds ratio = 0.88; 95% confidence interval: 0.79 to 0.99). On the other hand, captopril use in the ISIS-4 and Chinese studies was not associated with any significant reduction in mortality. When the three large-scale clinical trials were combined there was a statistically significant reduction in mortality with ACE inhibition in AMI (7.1% vs. 7.6%, $P = 0.004$). These trials are important in that they clearly document safety with the use of ACE inhibition. The findings suggest that there is a small survival benefit with ACE inhibition. This effect translates to approximately five lives saved per thousand patients treated during the early period after AMI.

The data from all the clinical trials of ACE inhibition in patients with AMI is consistent with the overall conclusion that this treatment is beneficial. Although the data from the long-term postinfarction trials are much more persuasive, the results of the short-term trials still suggest ACE inhibition can be beneficial, particularly for patients with heart failure or with large infarct size and considerable left ventricular damage. It is likely that the antiischemic effects of long-term ACE inhibition are obtained through mechanisms that affect early remodeling. Considerable work is ongoing in this area.

MAGNESIUM

The mechanisms by which magnesium produces beneficial effects in ischemic heart disease are not well understood. Some case control studies[76] suggest that magnesium concentration is lower and calcium concentration tends to be higher in patients who die of coronary artery disease when compared with patients who die from other causes.

In animals, low magnesium concentration appears to worsen catecholamine-induced myocardial necrosis.[77] This may be the result of an increased response to catecholamine-induced vasoconstriction associated with low magnesium concentrations.[78] Increasing magnesium concentration may also minimize myocardial necrosis by inhibiting calcium influx into cells or by reducing peripheral vascular resistance.[79-81] The antiplatelet effects of magnesium may also prevent propagation of coronary thrombus or reocclusion of a coronary artery after fibrinolytic treatment.[82] Magnesium infusion has also been shown in animals to increase the threshold for electrical excitation,[83] which has relevance for patients with low magnesium during an AMI because they more commonly also have ventricular arrhythmias.[79,84] Magnesium infusion has also been shown to reduce serious ventricular arrhythmias during the first 24 to 48 hours after MI. Magnesium has been used effectively in the treatment of torsades de pointes and other arrhythmias.[85,86]

Seven early randomized trials of intravenous magnesium in AMI have been recently reviewed.[87] Treatment was started within 12 hours of onset of chest pain. All studies excluded patients with high degrees of AV block, and in some trials an increased creatinine level, hypotension, cardiogenic shock, and age greater than 70 were exclusion criteria. Doses in trials varied between 30 and 90 millimoles of magnesium (8 to 22 g $MgSO_4$) and duration of infusion varied from 24 to 48 hours. Duration of follow-up varied from hospital discharge to 30 days. In

Table 30-6. Mortality in randomized trials of magnesium in AMI

Trial (follow-up)	Magnesium	Control	P Value
Rassmussen[88,89] (30 days)	9/135	23/135	<.01
Smith et al.[94] (hospital)	2/200	7/200	NS
Morton et al.[95-97] (hospital)	1/40	2/36	NS
Feldstedt et al.[91,92] (hospital)	10/150	8/148	NS
Ceremuzynski et al.[98] (hospital)	1/25	3/23	NS
Schecter et al.[90] (hospital)	1/59	9/56	<.01
Abraham et al.[99] (hospital)	1/48	1/46	NS
LIMIT-II[93] (28 days)	90/1150	118/1150	.04
Overall	115/1807 (6.5%)	171/1796 (9.5%)	<.001

six of the seven studies mortality was lower in magnesium-treated patients compared to controls and the difference was statistically significant in two of these trials.[88-90] Overall there was a 50% reduction of mortality, which was highly significant (25 deaths or 3.8% of 657 patients treated with magnesium and 53 or 8.2% of the 644 patients allocated to control, $P < 0.001$).

Long-term mortality data are available from two of the studies. In the study by Rassmussen et al.[88,89] 1-year mortality was 20% in the magnesium-treated group and 32% in the placebo group ($P < 0.02$), with most of the benefit being evident within the first month. The other study[91,92] showed no difference in either early or late deaths with 22 deaths in 150 patients in the magnesium group and 24 deaths in 148 patients in the control group during a median of 8 months of follow-up.

Information on serious ventricular arrhythmias is present from all trials as well. They were less common in the active treatment group in six of seven studies and this was statistically significant in two studies. The definition of serious ventricular arrhythmia varied among trials, but when taken together there was a significantly lower incidence of arrhythmias in the magnesium group ($P < .001$). Infarct size and recurrent angina were not systematically studied in these trials.

The LIMIT-II trial was until recently the largest prospective randomized trial of magnesium in AMI.[93] This was a randomized double-blind controlled study of 2316 patients with suspected AMI who received either placebo or magnesium sulfate intravenously over 24 hours [8 mmol bolus (2 g) and 65 mmol (15 g) continuous infusion]. The primary endpoint of this trial was 28-day mortality. Patients were similar in terms of cardiac risk factors, time to treatment, thrombolytic therapy, and type of infarct. For all patients in the trial mortality was 7.8% in the magnesium group and 10.3% in the placebo group ($P = 0.02$). The effect of magnesium on mortality was also studied in the 35% of patients who received thrombolytics and in those who did not have thrombolytic treatment. The odds ratio of death was 0.72 (95% confidence interval 0.49 to 0.99) in favor

of active magnesium treatment in those who had thrombolytic treatment. No significant interaction appeared to exist between treatments of magnesium and thrombolytic treatment on mortality. The major difference in mortality was noted in the first 2 days after MI. A lower incidence of left ventricular failure as assessed by clinical or radiographic methods was also present in the magnesium-treated group (11.2% of the magnesium group vs. 14.9% of the placebo group, $P = 0.009$, had clinical heart failure; 17.2% of magnesium-treated patients vs. 22% of placebo patients, $P = 0.004$, had radiographic evidence of heart failure).

Overall in over 3500 patients who were studied involving magnesium in AMI there was a total of 115 deaths in 1807 patients treated with magnesium and 171 deaths in 1796 patients treated with placebo. This corresponds to a relative reduction in risk of death of approximately 35%. The use of magnesium has not been found to be associated with significant serious adverse effects. Table 30-6 summarizes the trials of magnesium in AMI.

In the autumn of 1993 the ISIS study group presented the preliminary findings of the ISIS-4 study, in which half of the approximately 58,000 patients were randomized to receive a 24-hour infusion of intravenous magnesium vs. placebo in suspected AMI. Although these data are still preliminary and may undergo some final changes, there was a surprising trend towards a higher mortality in the patients allocated to magnesium (7.3% vs. 6.9%, $P = 0.1$). At this point it is unclear why there is a difference in outcome among the several trials performed, including the pooled analysis, and the most recent ISIS findings. Until the final analysis of ISIS-4 has been performed and can be put in perspective with the other trials evaluating magnesium therapy, no firm recommendation of its use can be made.

CONCLUSION

Several pharmacologic agents have been shown to be effective in reducing mortality and morbidity in the setting of AMI. It should be noted, however, that with a few exceptions practically all the trials of beta blockers, nitrates, and magnesium were conducted before the widespread use of thrombolytic therapy and the effects of these agents in the setting of thrombolysis have not been clearly demonstrated. However, the mechanisms of benefits of these agents are diverse and it is unlikely that thrombolysis will alter the mechanisms of action and nullify their effects even though the actual magnitudes of benefits may be attenuated. It should also be considered that 60% of patients presenting with an AMI do not receive thrombolytic therapy but remain eligible for the treatments shown to be beneficial and discussed in this chapter.

There is clear evidence from the information presented that beta blockers are an important treatment in patients with AMI. Available data suggest that this therapy should be started as soon as possible with intravenous administration followed by oral therapy for at least 3 months. This approach has been confirmed in multiple trials to reduce the mortality by approximately 15%. Although heart failure has been thought to be a relative contraindication to beta-blocker use, recent trials have refuted this. It is estimated that as many as 50% of all patients with AMI should be candidates for beta-blocker therapy during the hospitalization.

Angiotensin-converting enzyme inhibitors have been found to be associated with a marginal (approximately 3%) reduction in mortality in all patients with AMI. The clinical data suggest that the effect may be larger in those patients with congestive cardiac failure or large infarctions. Thus these patients should all receive oral ACE inhibition starting on day 3 after the onset of MI, unless a contraindication exists. The dose should be started low and titrated up to a maximal dose or as blood pressure or renal function tolerates. It is estimated that at least 60% of all patients with complicated AMI should be suitable for this therapy.

There is no evidence that oral nitrates or intravenous magnesium improves survival in patients with AMI. No study has confirmed or refuted the use of intravenous nitroglycerin. From a pathophysiological perspective there still remains some evidence that intravenous nitroglycerin may be beneficial to maximally dilate the coronary circulation to improve perfusion during AMI. For these reasons the use of intravenous nitrate could be recommended in most patients. On the other hand, intravenous magnesium has very little to add when all the other therapies are considered. Further examination of the ISIS-4 results will be important to consider the differences in the outcomes of several trials with intravenous magnesium.

When considering all possible adjunctive therapies in AMI one needs to develop a triage plan for therapies to maximize the dose of each agent. In uncomplicated small to moderate infarcts, beta blockers and sublingual nitroglycerin should be considered *sine qua non* in the absence of contraindications. In large infarcts or those complicated by heart failure, ACE inhibition and sublingual nitroglycerin should be the mainstays of therapy in the absence of contraindications. Oral beta blockade should be added after a test dose has been tolerated. In patients with low blood pressure beta blockers should be withheld. Furthermore, all MI patients on nitrates should have these tapered to allow the full therapeutic potential of beta blockade and/or ACE inhibition to be maximally applied. The use of nitrates or calcium antagonists should be reserved for those patients with recurrent angina or those undergoing angioplasty or other percutaneous interventions during MI.

Through the diligent work of clinical investigators examining outcomes in almost 200,000 patients, our treatment strategies for AMI have advanced considerably over the last two decades. The future treatments for management should concentrate on developing improved therapies for patients with cardiogenic shock, reinfarction, and secondary prevention protecting the coronary bed from further ischemic events.

REFERENCES

1. Yusuf S, Peto R, Lewis J, et al: Beta blockade during and after myocardial infarction: an overview of the randomized trials, *Prog Cardiovasc Dis* 17:335-371, 1985.
2. Åström M, Edhag O, Nyquist O, et al: Hemodynamic effects of intravenous sotalol in acute myocardial infarction, *Eur Heart J* 7:931-936, 1986.
3. Held PH, Hjalmarson A, Ryden L, et al: Central hemodynamic effects of metoprolol early in acute myocardial infarction. A placebo-controlled randomized study of patients with low heart rate, *Eur Heart J* 7:937-944, 1986.
4. ISIS-1 (First International Study of Infarct Survival) Collaborative Group: Randomized trial of intravenous atenolol among 16,027 cases of suspected acute myocardial infarction: ISIS-1, *Lancet* 2:57-65, 1986.
5. The TIMI Study Group: Comparison of invasive and conservative strategies after treatment with intravenous tissue plasminogen activator in acute myocardial infarction. Results of the Thrombolysis in Myocardial Infarction (TIMI) Phase II Trial, *New Engl J Med* 320:618-627, 1989.
6. The MIAMI trial research group: Metoprolol In Acute Myocardial Infarction (MIAMI). A randomized placebo-controlled international trial, *Eur Heart J* 6:199-226, 1985.
7. Norris RM, Barnaby P, Brown MA, et al: Prevention of ventricular fibrillation during acute myocardial infarction by intravenous propranolol, *Lancet* 2:883-886, 1984.
8. Ryden L, Arniego R, Arnman KI, et al: A double-blind trial of metoprolol in acute myocardial infarction: effects on ventricular tachycardia, *New Engl J Med* 308:614-618, 1983.
9. Yusuf S, Sleight P, Rossi PRF, et al: Reduction in infarct size, arrhythmias, chest pain, and morbidity by early intravenous beta blockade in suspected myocardial infarction, *Circulation* 67 (suppl I):32-41, 1983.
10. Hjalmarson A, Elmfeldt D, Herlitz J, et al: Effect on mortality of

metoprolol in acute myocardial infarction: a double-blind randomized trial, *Lancet* 2:823-827, 1981.

11. International Collaborative Study Group: Reduction of infarct size with the early use of timolol in acute myocardial infarction, *New Engl J Med* 310:9-15, 1984.

12. Roque R, Amuchastegui LM, Lopez Morillos MA, et al. and the TIARA study group: Beneficial effects of timolol on infarct size and late ventricular tachycardia in patients with acute myocardial infarction, *Circulation* 76:610-617, 1986.

13. Roberts R, Croft C, Gold HK, et al: Effect of propranolol on myocardial infarct size in a randomized blinded multi-center trial, *New Engl J Med* 311:218-255, 1984.

14. Norris RM, Sammel NL, Clarke ED, et al: Treatment of acute myocardial infarction with propranolol: further studies on enzyme appearance and subsequent left ventricular function in treated and control patients with developing infarcts, *Br Heart J* 43:617-622, 1980.

15. Peter T, Norris RM, Clarke ED, et al: Reduction of enzyme levels by propranolol after acute myocardial infarction, *Circulation* 57:1091-1095, 1978.

16. MIAMI Trial Research Group: Enzymatic estimation of infarct size, *Am J Cardiol* 56:27G-29G, 1985.

17. Herlitz J, Emanuelsson H, Swedberg K, et al: Goteborg Metoprolol Trial. Enzyme-estimated infarct size, *Am J Cardiol* 53:15D-21D, 1984.

18. Boyle DM, Barber JM, McIlmoyle EL, et al: Effect of very early intervention with metoprolol on acute myocardial infarct size, *Br Heart J* 49:229-233, 1983.

19. Richterova A, Herlitz J, Holmberg S, et al: Goteborg Metoprolol Trial: effects on chest pain, *Am J Cardiol* 53:32D-36D, 1984.

20. Ramsdale DR, Faragher EB, Bennett DH, et al: Ischemic pain relief in patients with acute myocardial infarction by intravenous atenolol, *Am Heart J* 103:459-467, 1982.

21. Boissel JP, Leizorovicz A, Picolet H, et al for the APSJ investigators: Secondary prevention after high-risk acute myocardial infarction with low-dose atebutolol, *Am J Cardiol* 66:251-260, 1990.

22. Beta-Blocker Heart Attack Research Group: A randomized trial of propranolol in patients with acute myocardial infarction: I. Mortality results. *JAMA* 247:1707-1714, 1982.

23. Salathia KS, Barber JM, McIlmoyle EL, et al: Very early intervention with metoprolol in suspected acute myocardial infarction, *Eur Heart J* 6:190-198, 1985.

24. Norwegian Multicenter Study Group: Timolol-induced reduction in mortality and reinfarction in patients surviving acute myocardial infarction, *New Engl J Med* 304:801-807,1981.

25. Waagstein F, Bristow MR, Swedberg K, et al: Beneficial effects of metoprolol in idiopathic dilated cardiomyopathy. Metoprolol in Dilated Cardiomyopathy (MDC) Trial, *Lancet* 342(8885):1441-1446, 1993.

26. Rogers WJ, Russel RO. Jr: National Registry of myocardial infarction's first 100,000 patients: what have we learned? *ACCEL* 25:5, 1993.

27. Braunwald E: Mechanism of action of calcium-channel blocking agents, *New Engl J Med* 307:1618-1627, 1982.

28. Reimer KA, Jennings RB: Effects of calcium channel blockers on myocardial preservation during experimental myocardial infarction, *Am J Cardiol* 55:107B-115B, 1985.

29. Johnson GJ, Leis LA, Francis GS: Disparate effects of the calcium channel blockers, nifedipine and verapamil on adrenergic receptors and thromboxane A_2-induced aggregation of human platelets, *Circulation* 73:847-854, 1986.

30. The Danish Study Group on Verapamil in Myocardial Infarction: Verapamil in acute myocardial infarction, *Eur Heart J* 5:516-528, 1984.

31. The Danish Study Group on Verapamil in Myocardial Infarction: Effect of verapamil on mortality and major events after acute myocardial infarction (The Danish Verapamil Infarction Trial II-DAVIT II), *Am J Cardiol* 66:779-785, 1990.

32. Held PH, Yusuf S, Furberg CD: Calcium channel blockers in acute myocardial infarction and unstable angina: an overview, *Br Med J* 299:1187-1192, 1989.

33. The Multicenter Diltiazem Postinfarction Trial Research Group: The effect of diltiazem on mortality and reinfarction after myocardial infarction, *New Engl J Med* 319:385-392, 1988.

34. Moss AJ, Oakes D, Benhorin J, et al: Effect of diltiazem on outcome in postinfarction patients with and without left ventricular dysfunction (abstract), *Circulation* 78(suppl II 2):II-97, 1988.

35. Boden WE, Krone RJ, Kleiger RE, et al: Diltiazem reduces long-term cardiac event rate after non–Q-wave infarction: Multicenter Diltiazem Post-Infarction Trial (MDPIT) (abstract), *Circulation* 78 (suppl II):II-96, 1988.

36. Gibson RS, Boden WE, Théroux P, et al: Diltiazem and reinfarction in patients with non–Q-wave myocardial infarction, *New Engl J Med* 315:423-429, 1986.

37. Wilcox RG, Hampton JR, Banks DC, et al: Trial of early nifedipine in acute myocardial infarction: the TRENT study, *Br Med J* 293:1204-1208, 1986.

38. The Israeli SPRINT Study Group: Secondary Prevention Reinfarction Israeli Nifedipine Trial (SPRINT). A randomized intervention trial of nifedipine in patients with acute myocardial infarction, *Eur Heart J* 9:354-364, 1988.

39. Goldbourt U, Solomon B, Reichter-Reiss H, et al. and the SPRINT Study Group: Early administration of nifedipine in suspected acute myocardial infarction: the Secondary Prevention of Reinfarction Israel Nifedipine Trial 2 Study, *Arch Intern Med* 153:345-353, 1993.

40. Lichtlen PR, Hugenholtz PG, Rafflenbeul W, et al. on behalf of the INTACT group: Retardation of angiographic progression of coronary artery disease by nifedipine. Results of the International Nifedipine Trial on Antiatherosclerotic Therapy (INTACT), *Lancet* 335:1109-1113, 1990.

41. Waters D, Lesperance J, Francetich M, et al: A controlled clinical trial to assess the effect of a calcium channel blocker upon the progression of coronary atherosclerosis. *Circulation* 82:1940-1953, 1990.

42. Imhof PR, Ott B, Frankhauser P, et al: Difference in nitroglycerin dose response in the venous and arterial beds, *Eur J Clin Pharmacol* 18:455-460, 1980.

43. McGregor M: Pathogenesis of angina pectoris and role of nitrates in relief of myocardial ischemia, *Am J Med* 74(suppl):21-27, 1983.

44. Yusuf S, Collins R, MacMahon S, et al: Effect on intravenous nitrates on mortality in acute myocardial infarction: an overview of the randomized trials, *Lancet* 1:1088-1092, 1988.

45. Jugdutt BI, Warnica JW: Intravenous nitroglycerin therapy to limit myocardial infarct size, expansion, and complications. Effect of timing, dosage, and infarct location, *Circulation* 78:906-919, 1988.

46. Bussman WD, Passek D, Seidel W, et al: Reduction of CK and CK-MB indexes of infarct size by intravenous nitroglycerin, *Circulation* 63:615-622, 1981.

47. Durrer JD, Lie KI, Van Capelle FJL, et al: Effect of sodium nitroprusside on mortality in acute myocardial infarction, *N Engl J Med* 306:1121-1128, 1982.

48. Cohn JN, Franciosa JA, Francis GS, et al: Effect of short-term infusion of sodium nitroprusside on mortality rate in acute myocardial infarction complicated by left ventricular failure. Results of a Veterans Administration Cooperative Study, *N Engl J Med* 306:1129-1135, 1982.

49. Hockings BEF, Cope GD, Clarke GM, et al: Randomized

controlled trial of vasodilator therapy after myocardial infarction, *Am J Cardiol* 48:345-352, 1981.

50. Mellen HS, Goldberg HS, Friedman HF: Therapeutic effects of pentaerythritol tetranitrate in the immediate postmyocardial infarction period, *N Engl J Med* 276:319-322, 1967.

51. Newell DJ and clinical collaborators: Pentaerythritol tetranitrate in acute myocardial infarction, *Br Heart J* 32:16-20, 1970.

52. Oscharoff A: Pentaerythritol tetranitrate as adjunctive therapy in the immediate postinfarction period, *Angiology* 15:505-514, 1964.

53. Ryan TJ, Schnee M: Pentaerythritol tetranitrate in acute myocardial infarction (abstract), *Circulation* 32 (suppl II):II-105, 1965.

54. Fitzgerald LJ, Bennett ED: The effects of oral isosorbide 5-mononitrate on mortality following acute myocardial infarction: a multicenter study, *Eur Heart J* 11:120-126, 1990.

55. Nelson GIC, Silke B, Ahuja RC, et al: Haemodynamic advantages of isosorbide dinitrate over furosemide in acute heart failure following myocardial infarction, *Lancet* i:730-733, 1983.

56. Jaffe AS, Geltman EM, Tiffenbrunn AJ, et al: Reduction of infarct size in patients with inferior infarctions with intravenous glyceryl trinitrate: a randomized study, *Br Heart J* 49:452-460, 1983.

57. Chiche P, Baligadoo SJ, Derrida JP: A randomized trial of prolonged nitroglycerin infusion in acute myocardial infarction, *Circulation* 59, 60 (suppl II):165, 1979. Abstract.

58. Flaherty JT, Becker LC, Bulkley BH, et al: A randomized prospective trial of IV nitroglycerin in patients with acute myocardial infarction, *Circulation* 68:576-588, 1983.

59. Lis Y, Bennett D, Lambert G, et al: A preliminary double-blind study of IV nitroglycerin in acute myocardial infarction, *Intens Care Med* 10:179-184, 1984.

60. Jugdutt BI, Sussex BA, Warnica JW, et al: Persistent reduction in left ventricular asynergy in patients with acute myocardial infarction by intravenous infusions of nitroglycerin, *Circulation* 68:1264-1273, 1983.

61. Eaton LW, Weiss JL, Bulkley BH, et al: Regional cardiac dilatations after acute myocardial infarction: recognition by two-dimensional echocardiography, *N Engl J Med* 300:57-62, 1979.

62. McKay RG, Pfeffer MA, Pasternak RC, et al: Left ventricular remodeling after myocardial infarction: a corollary to infarct expansion, *Circulation* 74:693-702, 1986.

63. Gaudron P, Eilles C, Ertl G, et al: Early remodeling of the left ventricle in patients with myocardial infarction, *Eur Heart J* 11(suppl B):139-146, 1990.

64. Pfeffer MA, Braunwald E: Ventricular remodeling after myocardial infarction: experimental observations and clinical implications, *Circulation* 81:1161-1172, 1990.

65. Pfeffer MA, Lammas GA, Vaughn DE, et al: Effect of captopril on progressive ventricular dilatation after anterior myocardial infarction, *N Engl J Med* 319:80-86, 1988.

66. Pfeffer JM, Pfeffer MA, Braunwald E: Influence of chronic captopril therapy on the infarcted left ventricle of a rat, *Circ Res* 57:84-95, 1985.

67. Pfeffer MA, Pfeffer JM, Steinberg C, et al: Survival after an experimental myocardial infarction: beneficial effects of long-term therapy with captopril, *Circulation* 72:406-412, 1985.

68. Pfeffer MA, Braunwald E, Moyé LA, et al. on the behalf of the SAVE Investigators: Effect of captopril on mortality and morbidity in patients with left ventricular dysfunction after myocardial infarction, *N Engl J Med* 327:669-677, 1992.

69. Swedberg K, Held P, Kjekshus J, et al. on behalf of the CONSENSUS II Study Group: Effects of the early administration of enalapril on mortality in patients with acute myocardial infarction, *N Engl J Med* 327:678-684, 1992.

70. Francis GS: Neuroendocrine activity in congestive heart failure, *Am J Cardiol* 60:33D-39D, 1990.

71. Yusuf S and the SOLVD Investigators: Effects of enalapril on mortality and the development of heart failure in asymptomatic patients with reduced ventricular ejection fractions, *N Engl J Med* 327:685-691, 1992.

72. Effect of ramipril on mortality and morbidity of survivors of acute myocardial infarction with clinical evidence of heart failure. The Acute Infarction Ramipril Efficacy (AIRE) Study investigators, *Lancet* 342(8875):821-828, 1993.

73. Flather M, Pipilis A, Collins R, et al: Randomized, controlled trial of oral captopril, of oral isorbide mononitrate and of intravenous magnesium sulphate started early in acute MI, *Eur Heart J* 15:585-588, 1994.

74. Preliminary results presented at American Heart Association meeting, October, 1993.

75. GISSI-3: Effects of lisinopril and transdermal glyceryl trinitrate after acute myocardial infarction, *Lancet* 343:1115-1122, 1994.

76. Elwood PC, Sweetnam PM, Beasley WH, et al: Magnesium and calcium in the myocardium cause of death and area differences, *Lancet* 2:720-722, 1980.

77. Mishra RK: Studies on experimental magnesium deficiencies in the albino rat. Functional and morphological changes associated with low intake of magnesium, *Rev Can Biol* 19:122-135, 1960.

78. Turlapaty PDMV, Altura BM: Magnesium deficiency produces spasm of coronary arteries: relationship to aetiology of sudden death in ischemic heart disease, *Science* 208:198-200, 1980.

79. Altura BM, Altura BT: Influence of magnesium on drug-induced contractions and ion content in rabbit aorta, *Am J Physiol* 220:938-944, 1971.

80. Turlapaty PD, Altura BM: Extracellular magnesium ions control calcium exchange and content of vascular smooth muscle, *Eur J Pharmacol* 52:421-423, 1978.

81. Shine KI: Myocardial effects of magnesium, *Am J Physiol* 237:H413-423, 1979.

82. Heptinstall S, Lyne S, Mitchell JRA, et al: Magnesium infusion in acute myocardial infarction, *Lancet* 1:552, 1986.

83. Ghani MF, Rabah M: Effect of magnesium chloride on electrical stability of the heart, *Am Heart J* 94:600-602, 1977.

84. Dyckner T, Wester PO: Ventricular extrasystoles and intracellular electrolytes before and after potassium and magnesium infusions in patients on diuretic treatment, *Am Heart J* 97:12-18, 1979.

85. Tzivoni D, Banai S, Schuger C, et al: Treatment of torsades de points with magnesium sulfate, *Circulation* 77:393-397, 1988.

86. Perticone F, Adinolfi L, Bonaduce D: Efficiency of magnesium sulfate in the treatment of torsades de pointes, *Am Heart J* 112:847-849, 1986.

87. Teo KK, Yusuf S, Collins R, et al: Effects of intravenous magnesium in suspected acute myocardial infarction: overview of randomized trials, *BMJ* 303:1499-1503, 1991.

88. Rasmussen HS, McNair P, Norregard P, et al: Intravenous magnesium in acute myocardial infarction, *Lancet* 1:234-236, 1986.

89. Rasmussen HS, Gronbaek M, Cintin C, et al: One-year death rate in 270 patients with suspected acute myocardial infarction, initially treated with intravenous magnesium or placebo, *Clin Cardiol* 11:377-381, 1988.

90. Schechter M, Hod H, Marks N, et al: Magnesium therapy and mortality in acute myocardial infarction, *Am J Cardiol* 66:271-274, 1990.

91. Feldstedt M, Bouchelouche P, Svenningsen A, et al: Magnesium substitution in acute ischemic heart syndromes, *Eur Heart J* 12:1215-1218, 1991.

92. Feldstedt M, Bouchelouche P, Svenningsen A, et al: Failing effect of magnesium-substitution in acute myocardial infarction, *Eur Heart J* 9:226, 1988.

93. Woods KL, Fletcher S, Roffe C, et al: Intravenous magnesium sulphate in suspected acute myocardial infarction: results of the second Leicester Intravenous Magnesium Intervention Trial (LIMIT-2), *Lancet* 339:1553-1558, 1992.

94. Smith LF, Heagerty AM, Bing RF, et al: Intravenous infusion of

magnesium sulfate after acute myocardial infarction: effects on arrhythmias and mortality, *Int J Cardiol* 12:175-180, 1986.

95. Morton BC, Smith FM, McKibbon TJ, et al: Magnesium therapy in acute myocardial infarction, *Magnesium* 1a:192-194, 1981.

96. Morton BC, Smith FM, McKibbon TJ, et al: The clinical effects of magnesium sulfate treatment in acute myocardial infarction, *Magnesium* 4:133-136, 1984.

97. Morton BC, Smith FM, McKibbon TJ, et al: Magnesium therapy

in acute myocardial infarction—a double-blind study, *Magnesium* 3:346-352, 1984.

98. Ceremuzynski L, Jurgiel R, Kulakoswski P, et al: Threatening arrhythmias in acute myocardial infarction are prevented by intravenous magnesium sulfate, *Am Heart J* 118:133-134, 1989.

99. Abraham AS, Rosenmann D, Kramer M, et al: Magnesium in the prevention of lethal arrhythmias in acute myocardial infarction, *Arch Intern Med* 147:753-755, 1987.

Chapter 31

ARRHYTHMIA PREVENTION IN THE HOSPITAL PHASE OF ACUTE MYOCARDIAL INFARCTION

Ronald W.F. Campbell

When coronary care units were established in the early 1960s their most important role was seen as the detection and speedy treatment of serious cardiac arrhythmias. The continuous real-time monitoring they provided revealed a remarkable range of cardiac rhythm disturbances, including ventricular fibrillation (VF), and it was hypothesized that VF might be predicted by antecedent ventricular arrhythmia patterns.[1] The concept was persuasive, but gradually it has been realized that primary VF (VF in the absence of shock or heart failure) cannot be anticipated by "warning arrhythmias."[2] Detailed ECG analysis has revealed an association of R-on-T ventricular ectopic beats with VF, but the relationship is merely temporal—both arrhythmias being "common" in the earliest hours of infarction—and the association is not of clinical predictive value.[2] Although the prognostic implications of VF complicating acute myocardial infarction (AMI) remain controversial,[3,4] quite obviously it has no advantageous features for patients. Therefore prevention would be desirable, if possible. However, with no method of predicting its occurrence, prevention of VF would require prescription of therapy to all at-risk patients. As VF complicates 5% to 10% of AMI cases,

the safety of such preventive therapy would be of paramount concern; for 90% to 95% of patients the drug will offer no benefit.

In recent years thrombolytic therapy has revolutionized the management of acute myocardial infarction.[5,6] Myocardial reperfusion dramatically alters cardiac electrophysiology and may be either arrhythmogenic (proarrhythmic) or antiarrhythmic. Arrhythmia protection during thrombolysis has been promoted by some, but as yet there are little data to encourage such an approach. In this chapter we will review the current options for prophylaxis of VF, examine the concept of reperfusion arrhythmias and the use of prophylaxis in that setting, and then briefly discuss the major public health problem of out-of-hospital cardiac arrest.

PROPHYLAXIS OF VENTRICULAR FIBRILLATION IN THE ACUTE PHASE OF MYOCARDIAL INFARCTION
Lidocaine

The arguments for and against lidocaine prophylaxis of VF have changed little since the advent of the thrombolytic era.[7] Lidocaine has been used extensively for the prophylaxis of VF,[8] although data supportive of efficacy and safety were scant until the publication by Koster and Dunning.[9] This paramedic- and ambulance-based study involved very early administration of pro-

Academic cardiology is supported by the British Heart Foundation.

371

Meta-analysis of lidocaine prophylaxis in AMI

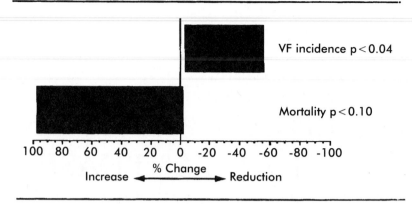

VF incidence p < 0.04

Mortality p < 0.10

Fig. 31-1. Meta-analysis of lidocaine prophylaxis in AMI. Based on data from 9155 patients randomized to lidocaine or placebo in 14 trials.[10]

phylactic intramuscular lidocaine (400 mg) vs. placebo to patients seen outside the hospital. Lidocaine significantly reduced the subsequent incidence of VF when compared with placebo (0.8% vs. 1.8%), but there was a significant excess of heart block and asystole (RR interval >6 seconds) in patients receiving lidocaine. Mortality was similar in the placebo- and the lidocaine-treated groups. The study demonstrates that lidocaine has prophylactic potential but that it offers this benefit at a substantial risk. The risk-benefit profile of lidocaine is such that it would be an unattractive intervention in hospitalized patients, for whom speedy defibrillation is probably most appropriate. Indeed, a recent meta-analysis suggested that prophylactic lidocaine may increase mortality,[10] although the difference was not statistically significant (Fig. 31-1). In some special circumstances, for example in rural practice, there may be an acceptable risk-benefit profile for lidocaine, but as yet this is only speculation. It is unclear whether current intravenous dosing regimens (see Chapter 31) along with careful monitoring of serum levels significantly improve the risk-benefit profile of prophylactic therapy relative to these earlier reports. Recent data from the GUSTO-I trial revealed that prophylactic lidocaine is currently used much more commonly in the United States than in other participating countries (25% vs. 4%, P <.001).[11] Among patients in the trial who did receive prophylactic lidocaine, the rate of asystole was slightly higher (6.4% vs. 5.6%, P = .02) but the overall 30-day mortality rate in this observational comparison was marginally lower (6.4% vs. 7.0%, P = .05).[11]

Beta blockers

Beta blockers are powerful antiarrhythmic agents although their potential in this regard is often overlooked. Beta blockers were one of the first interventions in acute-phase MI shown to modify the incidence of

VF,[12] and since that original publication others have provided supportive evidence.[13-15] In the study of Norris et al.[13] a significant reduction in so-called primary VF was noted in those patients who received a combination of intravenous and oral propranolol. In the Swedish metoprolol study, patients receiving intravenous and oral metoprolol had a significantly lower VF rate than their placebo-treated counterparts,[14] and in the ISIS-I study, which examined early atenolol use in AMI, patients receiving the beta blocker had significantly fewer incidents of acute-phase VF than their placebo-treated counterparts.[15] Thus there is compelling evidence that beta blockers can modify the expression of VF in early-phase MI. It is then difficult to understand why they are not used more widely, given that adverse effects in these studies were rare, and additional beneficial effects reported included reduced cardiac rupture, reduced pain, reduced infarct size, reduced complications, and an improved late prognosis.

The mechanism by which beta blockers may provide a benefit is not entirely clear. The benefit is probably a class effect in that it has been observed with both selective[14,15] and nonselective[12,13] beta-receptor antagonists. The explanation may be the direct blocking of the arrhythmogenic consequences of the sympathetic activation that occurs in AMI or conceivably might relate to stabilization of potassium concentrations. In one study patients pretreated with nonselective beta blockers had significantly higher plasma concentrations of potassium than patients not on beta blockers or those on only selective beta blockers.[16] Catecholamines increase peripheral potassium uptake and potassium concentrations fall. The muscle uptake of potassium is blocked by nonselective beta blockers but not by selective agents. Although there is a relationship between early-phase MI VF and plasma potassium concentrations, the fact that selective beta blockers protect against VF makes it unlikely that the effect is produced by electrolyte stabilization.

Magnesium

Magnesium has been advocated for the acute treatment of torsade de pointes.[17] Magnesium is also a vasodilator. Prophylactive administration of this agent has been investigated in acute-phase MI, and in three studies, a significant reduction in mortality was shown.[18-20] In two of these,[18,19] effects against arrhythmias were suggested although the term *arrhythmias* included a variety of events and was not restricted to the acute phase of MI. No specific effect against VF was identified. However, the LIMIT-2 study, a large double-blind randomized study of acute intravenous magnesium, suggested that magnesium did not affect either arrhythmias in general or VF in particular.[20] Mortality, however, was significantly reduced. Despite these encouraging smaller studies, in the recently completed ISIS-4 study intravenous magnesium had no significant effect on mortality after AMI.[21,22] Thus, in the absence of demonstrated magnesium deficiency (i.e., low serum levels), this agent currently has no role in the treatment of AMI.

Intravenous nitrates

Soon after the inception of Coronary Care Units there was controversy as to whether intravenous nitrate administration was good or bad in acute-phase MI. Some considered that nitrates would lower diastolic blood pressure and so would threaten already-critical flow in the coronary arteries. Perhaps occasionally patients may be so disadvantaged, but in a meta-analysis involving around 3000 patients from the prethrombolytic era, nitrates were associated with an improved prognosis.[23] There were also suggestions that nitrate therapy might reduce ventricular arrhythmias, principally ventricular ectopic beats,[24] but no large study has reported any beneficial effect of nitrates specifically on VF. Furthermore, the ISIS-4 (oral therapy)[22] and the GISSI-3 (IV and patch)[25] trials of 1 month of nitrate therapy in approximately 80,000 suspected AMI patients failed to show any benefit (or detriment) of therapy, making it unlikely that these agents have a significant antiarrhythmic effect in this setting.

Calcium antagonists

The evidence supporting the routine use of calcium antagonist therapy in the acute phase of MI is mixed at best.[26,27] Clinical studies have reported benefit,[28] detriment,[29] or have identified subgroups of patients who may benefit[30] although these patients may be difficult to identify prospectively. No antiarrhythmic benefits have been identified. The calcium antagonists are a complex group of drugs. Verapamil and diltiazem have important electrophysiological properties principally in the calcium-dependent structures such as the sinus and AV nodes, and there have been reports that they may control some rare forms of ventricular tachycardia.[31] There is, however, nothing to suggest that they might prevent VF by an electrophysiologic effect.

ACE inhibitors

Angiotensin-converting enzyme (ACE) inhibitors have rapidly become one of the most important classes of cardioactive agents. Their mortality benefits in patients with moderate and severe heart failure were first demonstrated in the CONSENSUS-I study, but a mechanical rather than an antiarrhythmic mechanism of benefit was observed.[32] VHeFT-2 revealed that sudden death rates, with or without warning, were reduced by enalapril therapy, particularly in those with lesser degrees of heart failure.[33] This has raised the possibility that either by a direct electrophysiological action or indirectly through altering wall tension, ACE inhibitors may be antiarrhythmic. There is a good rationale for examining ACE inhibitor therapy in acute-phase MI: for instance, it may prevent deleterious ventricular remodelling.[34] In the CONSENSUS-II study,[35] which involved very early intravenous administration of enalapril, recruitment was stopped prematurely because of increased mortality.[35] No antiarrhythmic effect was revealed. The recently completed ISIS-4 and GISSI-3 trials showed that early ACE inhibitor therapy in suspected AMI provided a modest, statistically significant reduction in 1-month mortality rates.[22,25] In ISIS-4 no effect on in-hospital VF or cardiac arrest was noted, but the ACE inhibitor group had a modest excess of second- and third-degree AV block relative to placebo.

REPERFUSION ARRHYTHMIAS

In 1935 Tennant and Wiggers reported a series of animal experiments in which the exposed left anterior descending coronary artery of a dog was first occluded and then released. In a proportion of animals coronary reperfusion was complicated by VF.[36] Subsequent animal experiments have confirmed the phenomenon of reperfusion arrhythmias,[37] but as yet, whether their primary mechanism is reentry or altered automaticity is unknown.[38,39] Ventricular tachycardia and VF are the common manifestations in animals. The window of their occurrence is relatively short (restricted to only a few minutes after reperfusion) and they may be modified by α-blocker therapy.[40]

On the basis of these animal studies it was widely believed that reperfusion ventricular arrhythmias would be a major problem in man, but reality has proved otherwise.[41] Reperfusion arrhythmias do occur in humans, but they are less "malignant" than in animals. Accelerated idioventricular rhythm is the most com-

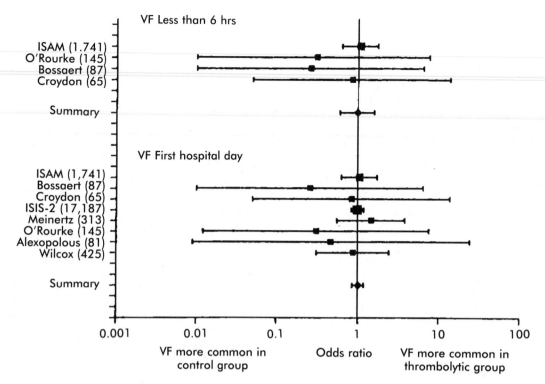

Fig. 31-2 Meta-analysis of trials of thrombolytic therapy vs. no thrombolytic therapy (control group) regarding incidence of VF during the first 6 hours of hospitalization and during the first hospital day. The odds ratios and 95% confidence limits for individual trials and for the pooled estimates are plotted on a logarithmic scale. The Y-axis lists the first author of the study and the total number of patients enrolled (in parentheses). The size of the symbol representing the odds ratio is proportional to the study sample size.[44]

mon[42]; it rarely causes symptoms and usually is self-limiting. It has been suggested that it might be a useful marker of successful reperfusion,[41] but although there unquestionably is an association, this is neither sensitive nor specific.[43] Reperfusion VF appears to be rare. A recent meta-analysis of 15 randomized trials of thrombolysis vs. no reperfusion therapy showed a similar incidence of VF in the first 6 hours and in the first 24 hours following treatment[44] (Fig. 31-2).

Maras et al. found that reperfusion VF occurred in 8.1% of treated patients and postulated that a less severe residual stenosis (80% or less) might be a predisposing factor,[45] possibly because of more abrupt reperfusion with clot lysis in arteries with less severe fixed stenosis. By contrast, Hackett et al.[46] observed no reperfusion VF in 32 successfully treated patients, but the small sample size could easily have missed the phenomenon.

In the recent Primary Angioplasty in Myocardial Infarction (PAMI) trial, patients randomized to direct angioplasty had a higher rate of VF than those in the t-PA group (6.7% vs. 2.0%, $P = .02$), which may have been an effect of the more abrupt reperfusion provided by the angioplasty procedure.[47]

Despite the relatively modest clinical problem posed by reperfusion arrhythmias, some have argued for routine prophylactic therapy in the setting of reperfusion therapy. There is no evidence that these arrhythmias can be reduced by beta blockers, and lidocaine does not prevent them.[48] In animal reperfusion arrhythmias, free radicals have been implicated as potentially arrhythmogenic factors with some evidence of an antiarrhythmic action of the free radical scavenger, superoxide dismutase.[49] In man this agent has also reduced "reperfusion" ventricular ectopic beats.[50] This is of scientific interest, but has little immediate clinical relevance. Further studies are needed to show that such intervention can prevent serious or life-threatening arrhythmias and that the benefit of the intervention outweighs its risks.

Serious reperfusion ventricular arrhythmias are uncommon in man, but the phenomenon is worthy of more attention. In animal experimentation it is easy to separate occlusion and reperfusion arrhythmias because coronary flow is under experimental control. In man relatively little is known of the dynamic behavior of the intravascular clot. Reperfusion may follow a different time course from that of animals and may stutter with repetitive phases of occlusion and reperfusion, each phase carrying an arrhythmogenic risk. Thus, some arrhythmias that appear to be reperfusion may in fact reflect reocclusion and vice versa. One study has reviewed acute-phase postocclusional VF in man to determine whether any might represent spontaneous reperfusion, but this seemed an unlikely explanation.[51]

OUT-OF-HOSPITAL ARRHYTHMIAS

In the last 10 years the hospital mortality of AMI cases has fallen remarkably and hospital survivors now have a good long-term prognosis.[52] Paramedic services are addressing out-of-hospital cardiac arrest. Success in this area is impressive, but the greatest mortality in cases of AMI occurs out of hospital, unattended by medical personnel and almost certainly arrhythmic. Prevention of this phenomenon represents a major public health challenge. Patients often have little or no warning. For many, the first manifestation is sudden death. Measures that effectively prevent sudden unexpected arrhythmic death in acute ischemic syndromes could have enormous impact, but for patients who suffer instantaneous arrhythmias, prophylactic pretreatment would be necessary. Currently prediction of patients who will have MI, far less those who will have MI complicated by VF, is insufficiently sensitive or specific to recommend prophylactic therapy to the enormous population that is potentially at risk. For patients who do have early symptoms of ischemia, there is the opportunity for self-administration of therapy if it could be shown to be effective and without significant risk. No such intervention is available at present. It is widely promulgated that patients who recognize the early stage of MI should chew aspirin for its antiplatelet action and thus perhaps prevent the formation or propagation of intravascular clot. There is no "field" evidence to support this approach although it has theoretic appeal. Whether it has a prophylactic antiarrhythmic effect is uncertain, although if an artery is kept open and perfusing, it would seem likely that electrophysiological disturbances might be minimized.

RECOMMENDATIONS

At the advent of the "thrombolytic era" it was widely considered that a variety of arrhythmogenic factors present in patients at the time of thrombolysis would require detailed attention and management.[7] The role of α-adrenergic tone and free radicals was anticipated to be important, and it was expected that thrombolytic therapy might be used in conjunction with a cocktail of antiarrhythmic agents to prevent these complications from undoing the benefit of thrombolysis. Reality has proved differently—thrombolysis is rarely complicated by serious arrhythmias.

The management of ventricular arrhythmias that manifest themselves in patients with acute-phase MI has been simplified (see Chapter 31). Those arrhythmias causing symptoms or hemodynamic instability deserve treatment, and there are now standardized protocols for this purpose. Hospital-based arrhythmia prophylaxis is

no longer seen as an important clinical need, although the use of early-phase beta blockade is still not as prevalent as it should be. Out-of-hospital arrhythmic death remains a major problem that has been little influenced by therapeutic advances. At present paramedic services provide the only salvage. Their modest success is determined by time and by bystander activities, and their availability is restricted to large population centers. Despite the advances of the last 20 years, too many potentially salvageable patients still die of ischemic arrhythmias.

REFERENCES

1. Lown B, Fakhro AM, Hood WB, et al: The coronary care unit. New perspectives and directions, *JAMA* 19:188-198, 1967.
2. Campbell RWF, Murray A, Julian DG: Ventricular arrhythmias in first 12 hours of acute myocardial infarction. Natural history study, *Br Heart J* 46:351-357, 1981.
3. Goldberg R, Szklo M, Kennedy H, et al: Short- and long-term prognosis of myocardial infarction complicated by ventricular fibrillation or cardiac arrest (abstract), *Circulation* 4 (suppl 2):89, 1978.
4. Schwartz PJ, Zaza A, Grazi S, et al: Effect of ventricular fibrillation complicating acute myocardial infarction on long-term prognosis. Influence of site of infarction, *Am J Cardiol* 57:384-389, 1985.
5. GISSI Study Group: Effectiveness of intravenous thrombolytic treatment in acute myocardial infarction, *Lancet* 1:397-401, 1986.
6. ISIS-2 Collaborative Group: Randomized trial of intravenous streptokinase, oral aspirin, both, or neither among 17,187 cases of suspected acute myocardial infarction: ISIS-2, *Lancet* 2:349-360, 1988.
7. Campbell RWF: Prophylactic antiarrhythmic therapy. In Califf RM, Mark DB, Wagner GS: *Acute coronary care in the thrombolytic era,* Chicago, 1988, Year Book Medical Publishers, Inc.
8. Wyman MG, Hammersmith L: Comprehensive treatment plan for the prevention of primary ventricular fibrillation in acute myocardial infarction, *Am J Cardiol* 33:661-667, 1974.
9. Koster RW, Dunning AJ: Intramuscular lidocaine for prevention of lethal arrhythmias in the prehospitalization phase of acute myocardial infarction, *N Engl J Med* 313:1105-1110, 1985.
10. MacMahon S, Collins R, Peto R, et al: Effects of prophylactic lidocaine in suspected acute myocardial infarction, *JAMA* 260:1910-1916, 1988.
11. Granger C, Sadowski Z, Pfisterer M, et al. for the GUSTO investigators: Prophylactic lidocaine was commonly used in the GUSTO trial, *J Am Coll Cardiol* Feb:315A, 1994 (suppl).
12. Snow PJD: Effect of propranolol in myocardial infarction, *Lancet* 2:551-553, 1965.
13. Norris RM, Barnaby PF, Brown MA, et al: Prevention of ventricular fibrillation during acute myocardial infarction by intravenous propranolol, *Lancet* 2:883-886, 1984.
14. Ryden L, Ariniego R, Arnman K, et al: A double-blind trial of metoprolol in acute myocardial infarction: effect on ventricular tachyarrhythmias, *N Engl J Med* 308:614-618, 1984.
15. ISIS-I (First International Study of Infarct Survival Collaborative Group): Randomised trial of intravenous atenolol among 16,027 cases of suspected acute myocardial infarction, *Lancet* 2:57-66, 1986.
16. Higham PD, Adams PC, Murray A, et al: Plasma potassium, serum magnesium and ventricular fibrillation: a prospective study, *Q J Med* 86:609-617, 1993.
17. Tzivoni D, Keren A, Cohen AM, et al: Magnesium therapy for torsade de pointes, *Am J Cardiol* 53:528-530, 1984.

18. Rasmussen HS, McNair P, Norregard P, et al: Intravenous magnesium in acute myocardial infarction, *Lancet* 1:234-236, 1986.

19. Shechter M, Hod H, Marks N: Beneficial effect of magnesium sulfate in acute myocardial infarction, *Am J Cardiol* 66:271-274, 1990.

20. Woods KL, Fletcher S, Roffe C, et al: Intravenous magnesium sulphate in suspected acute myocardial infarction: results of the second Leicester Intravenous Magnesium Intervention Trial (LIMIT-2), *Lancet* 339:1553-1558, 1992.

21. Seelig MS: Magnesium in acute myocardial infarction (International Study of Infarct Survival 4), *Am J Cardiol* 68:1221-1222, 1991.

22. Collins R: ISIS-4 results. Oral communication to the American Heart Association, Atlanta, Ga, Nov, 1993.

23. Jugdutt BI, Warnica JW: Intravenous nitroglycerin therapy to limit myocardial infarct size, expansion, and complications. Effect of timing, dosage, and infarct location, *Circulation* 78:906-919, 1988.

24. Bussman WD, Neuman K, Kaltenbach M: Effect of intravenous nitroglycerine on ventricular ectopic beats in acute myocardial infarction, *Am Heart J* 107:940-944, 1984.

25. GISSI-3 results: Oral communication to the American Heart Association, Atlanta, Ga, Nov 1993.

26. Ferrari R, Visioli O: Calcium channel blockers and ischemic heart disease: theoretical expectations and clinical experience, *Eur Heart J* 12 (suppl F):18-24, 1991.

27. Held PH, Yusuf S, Furberg CD: Calcium channel blockers in acute myocardial infarction and unstable angina: an overview, *Br Med J* 299:1187-1192, 1989.

28. Gibson RS, Boden WR, Theroux P, et al: Diltiazem and reinfarction in patients with non-Q wave myocardial infarction, *N Engl J Med* 315:423-429, 1986.

29. Wilcox RG, Hampton JR, Banks DC, et al: Trial of early nifedipine in acute myocardial infarction: the Trent Study, *Br Med J* 293:1204-1208, 1986.

30. Danish Study Group on Verapamil in Myocardial Infarction: Verapamil in acute myocardial infarction, *Eur Heart J* 5:516-528, 1984.

31. Klein GJ, Millman PJ, Yee R: Recurrent ventricular tachycardia responsive to verapamil, *PACE* 7:938-948, 1984.

32. The CONSENSUS Trial Study Group: Effects of enalapril on mortality in severe congestive heart failure: results of the Co-operative North Scandinavian Enalapril Survival Study (CONSENSUS), *N Engl J Med* 316:1429-1435, 1987.

33. Cohn JN, Johnson G, Ziesche RN, et al (V-HeFT II): A comparison of enalapril with hydralazine-isosorbide dinitrate in the treatment of chronic congestive heart failure, *N Engl J Med* 325(5):303-310, 1991.

34. Sharpe N, Smith H, Murphy J, et al: Treatment of patients with symptomless left ventricular dysfunction after myocardial infarction, *Lancet* 1:255-259, 1988.

35. Results of the Co-operative New Scandinavian Enalapril Survival Study II (CONSENSUS II): Effects of the early administration of enalapril on mortality in patients with acute myocardial infarction, *N Engl J Med* 327:678-684, 1992.

36. Tennant R, Wiggers C: The effect of coronary occlusion on myocardial contraction, *Am J Physiol* 112:351-362, 1935.

37. Hale S, Lange R, Alker K, et al: Correlates of reperfusion ventricular fibrillation in dogs, *Am J Cardiol* 53:1397-1400, 1984.

38. Corr P, Witkowski F: Potential electrophysiologic mechanisms responsible for dysrhythmias associated with reperfusion of ischemic myocardium, *Circulation* 68(suppl I):16-24, 1983.

39. Manning A, Hearse D: Reperfusion-induced arrhythmias: mechanisms and prevention, *J Mol Cell Cardiol* 16:497-516, 1984.

40. Corbalan R, Verrier R, Lown B: Differing mechanisms for ventricular vulnerability during coronary artery occlusion and release, *Am Heart J* 92:223-230, 1976.

41. Krunholz HM, Goldberger AL: Reperfusion arrhythmias after thrombolysis: electrophysiological tempest, or much ado about nothing, *Chest* 99 (suppl April):135S-140S, 1991.

42. Goldberg S, Greenspoon AJ, Urban PL, et al: Reperfusion arrhythmias: a marker of restoration of antegrade flow during intracoronary thrombolysis for acute myocardial infarction, *Am Heart J* 105:32-36, 1983.

43. Califf R, O'Neill W, Stack R, et al: Failure of simple clinical measurements to predict perfusion status after intravenous thrombolysis, *Ann Intern Med* 108:658-662, 1988.

44. Solomon SD, Ridker PM, Antman EM: Ventricular arrhythmias in trials of thrombolytic therapy for acute myocardial infarction. A meta-analysis, *Circulation* 88:2575-2581, 1993.

45. Maras P, Della Grazia E, Klugmann S, et al: Reperfusion ventricular arrhythmias during intracoronary thrombolysis, *Eur Heart J* 7(suppl A):23-30, 1986.

46. Hackett D, McKenna W, Davies G, et al: Reperfusion arrhythmias are rare during acute myocardial infarction and thrombolysis in man, *Int J Cardiol* 29:205-213, 1990.

47. Grines CL, Browne KF, Marco J, et al: A comparison of immediate angioplasty with thrombolytic therapy for acute myocardial infarction. The Primary Angioplasty in Myocardial Infarction Study Group, *N Engl J Med* 328:673-679, 1993.

48. Kuck KH, Schofer J, Schluter M, et al: Reperfusion arrhythmias in man—influence of intravenous lidocaine, *Eur Heart J* 6:163-167, 1985.

49. Mehta JL, Nichols WW, Saldeen TGP, et al: Superoxide dismutase decreases reperfusion arrhythmias and preserves myocardial function during thrombolysis with tissue plasminogen activator, *J Cardiovasc Pharmacol* 16:112-120, 1990.

50. Murohara Y, Yui Y, Hattori R, et al: Effects of superoxide dismutase on reperfusion arrhythmias and left ventricular function in patients undergoing thrombolysis for anterior wall acute myocardial infarction, *Am J Cardiol* 67:765-767, 1991.

51. Cowan JC, Been M, Gibb I: Lack of evidence of spontaneous reperfusion when ventricular fibrillation complicates early acute myocardial infarction, *Am J Cardiol* 59:1419-1420, 1987.

52. Pashos CL, Newhouse JP, McNeil BJ: Temporal changes in the care and outcomes of elderly patients with acute myocardial infarction, 1987 through 1990, *JAMA* 270:1832-1836, 1990.

Chapter 32

EFFORTS TO PREVENT REPERFUSION INJURY

William R. Herzog
Robert M. Califf

HISTORICAL BACKGROUND

The contemporary concept of reperfusion injury is rooted in 35 years of laboratory investigation, clinical observations, and clinical trials of reperfusion therapy. Researchers working with animal models in the early 1960s defined the ultrastructural and electrophysiological consequences of ischemia and reperfusion.[1,2] It was obvious that, depending on the duration of ischemia, reperfusion could salvage some myocardial cells. These investigators noted, however, that the time course of the structural changes associated with cell necrosis accelerated rapidly following reperfusion, raising the possibility that reperfusion was not a wholly benign process. Detailed biochemical and metabolic studies followed, leading to the concepts of calcium paradox and oxygen paradox. In isolated, perfused rat hearts, the reintroduction of Ca^{+2} into the perfusing solution after a brief Ca^{+2}-free period (3 to 4 minutes) caused extensive tissue damage and contracture.[3,4] Similar morphologic changes were seen when oxygen was returned to the perfusate after 40 to 50 minutes of anoxia. In each case, return of the missing element paradoxically caused even more harm.[5-7]

At the time, these phenomena had clinical relevance only for cardiac surgeons. Contractile dysfunction following cardiopulmonary bypass was (and still is) a clinical problem. The global ischemia produced by cardioplegic cardiac arrest was obviously of concern. Investigators began exploring ways of preserving as much myocardium as possible and returning contractile function as soon as possible by modifying the conditions of ischemia and reperfusion. As a result of a series of experiments, Rosenkranz and Buckberg articulated the general concept of reperfusion injury. They defined it as "those metabolic, functional, and structural consequences of restoring coronary arterial flow ... that can be avoided or reversed by modification of the conditions of reperfusion."[8] Over the years, improvements in cardioplegic solutions and technique have produced significant clinical benefit.[9] In addition, many investigators have found that reperfusion injury can be reduced.[10,11]

Cardiologists began thinking about the clinical relevance of reperfusion injury in the 1980s, when they began practicing reperfusion therapy for AMI. Braunwald and Kloner popularized the concept that reperfusion may have clinically significant deleterious effects on the myocardium in the short term in spite of its overall long-term benefit.[12,13] If those deleterious effects could be understood pathophysiologically, then it might be possible to prevent them and improve clinical outcomes. This goal stimulated considerable laboratory research, much of which focused on the phenomenon of myocardial stunning. *Stunning* may be defined as prolonged (but reversible) contractile dysfunction occurring after an episode of ischemia/reperfusion, which persists despite restoration of blood flow to normal resting levels. This phenomenon had been noted in animal models for years and generally considered one manifestation of reperfusion injury.[14]

Investigators recognized that concepts developed in models of global ischemia could have less relevance for regional ischemia, such as would occur in unstable angina or MI. These investigators[15-19] used models of in vivo regional ischemia to test various hypotheses about the pathophysiology of stunning as well as to test potential therapies. Also, using very sophisticated methodology, more and more was learned about the biochemical changes occurring on a cellular level during ischemia and reperfusion.[20-23] The efforts of these investigators have greatly advanced our understanding of stunning and of reperfusion injury in general, although significant uncertainties remain about their roles in routine clinical processes. Several potential therapies have shown promise in animal models, but early clinical trials involving efforts to ameliorate reperfusion injury have had disappointing outcomes. This may reflect the extreme difficulty of accurately modeling the clinical situation. Nonetheless this remains an area of active investigation, and more promising clinical trials are under way.

Although the benefits of reperfusion have been well documented in terms of reduction in mortality, lethal arrhythmias, and congestive heart failure, the improvement in left ventricular function has been less than expected. Most studies have shown no change or only a modest improvement in global left ventricular function, a modest improvement in infarct zone regional function, and a deterioration in noninfarct zone function from acute to follow-up studies. The demonstration of modest improvement in left ventricular function, coupled with a series of experiments in animal models demonstrating that reperfusion unleashes toxic metabolites on the myocardium, has led to the hope that the clinical outcomes of reperfusion could be improved by curbing reperfusion injury directly. This field of clinical investigation is complicated by a lack of general understanding of the determinants of left ventricular function during and after MI and the imprecision of the methods of measurement that must be used in human studies.

Lethal vs. nonlethal injury

Investigators typically categorize reperfusion injury as either *lethal* or *nonlethal,* terms that refer to the death of cells rather than to the death of the organism. It is easy to understand the potential clinical relevance of lethal reperfusion injury, which would depend on the number of affected cells; the evidence for nonlethal injury, however, is much stronger than the evidence for lethal injury. Nonlethal reperfusion injury is easier to demonstrate and may be a clinically significant problem because it can result in death of the organism if it causes malignant arrhythmias or prohibits adequate function of the myocardium to support the needed hemodynamic state.

Localization of reperfusion injury and potential clinical significance

Any cardiac tissue in the zone of ischemia/reperfusion is potentially vulnerable to reperfusion injury. Early

investigation focused primarily on the myocyte because a direct relationship can be shown between contractile function and clinical outcome. In recent years the coronary endothelium has become the major focus of investigation, although the intracellular matrix, vascular smooth muscle cells and cardiac conduction system are also affected by experimental reperfusion injury.[24]

The basic relationships between the duration of ischemia and death of the myocyte were elucidated using histopathologic techniques in a landmark series of experiments by Jennings et al.[25] They described the "wavefront" theory of myocardial necrosis to explain the time course of pathologic changes associated with ischemia and cell death: subendocardial cells die first, and as the duration of ischemia lengthens, the necrotic zone extends outward toward the epicardium in a progressive, wavefront fashion. They also noted that the pathologic changes associated with cell death occurred much more quickly following reperfusion than if the tissue simply remained ischemic (accelerated necrosis). These observations raised the question of whether reperfusion actually caused death of additional cells or merely accelerated the morphologic changes associated with cell death.

A central portion of their work and the experiments that followed was the demonstration that the ability to salvage myocardium by reperfusion is directly related to the presence and extent of collateral circulation to the infarct zone (see Chapter 11). In fact, species with different collateral blood flow complete the wavefront of myocardial necrosis in markedly different time frames. Because the pig has poor collateral circulation, the infarction is often complete within 45 minutes after coronary occlusion; the dog, with intermediate collateral flow, generally has surviving myocardium for up to 3 hours, whereas the rat has an even longer time period during which tissue can be salvaged by reperfusion.

This work led to experiments that monitored contractile function following an episode of ischemia/reperfusion, which showed that the contractile function of the remaining viable myocytes in reperfused myocardium returns slowly, over hours to days, despite the restoration of normal resting blood flow.[26] This reversible or nonlethal injury, called *myocardial stunning,* is observed even when the duration of ischemia is so brief that no necrosis occurs. The rate of return of function depends partly on the severity and duration of ischemia and partly on events that occur very early (within the first several minutes) in the reperfusion phase. Moreover, the kinetics of the return of the contractile function can be altered by interventions limited to the reperfusion phase. These observations form the basis for the concept that myocardial stunning is a manifestation of nonlethal reperfusion injury.[27]

The coronary endothelium is also vulnerable to the

effects of ischemia and reperfusion, but there is a relative disparity between microscopic and functional evidence of injury. Early ultrastructural studies showed that significant morphological changes in response to ischemia occurred later in endothelial cells than in myocytes.[28] This was interpreted to mean that endothelial cells were more resistant to ischemia than myocytes.

Subsequent studies have shown endothelial function in the coronary microcirculation to be very sensitive to the effects of ischemia and reperfusion.[29] In the dog model an ischemic episode that lasts for as little as 15 minutes produces two significant functional endothelial abnormalities: increased vascular permeability and compromised vasoregulatory ability.[30,31] The loss of vasoregulatory ability probably results from an impaired ability to generate nitric oxide (endothelium-derived relaxing factor). Analogous to myocytes, endothelial cells may be stunned—reversibly injured and dysfunctional—for a variable period of time following reperfusion.[32,33] Typically this would manifest itself as a zone of mild-to-moderate decrease in basal flow ("low reflow") and a loss of vasodilatory reserve.[34,35] Once again, these changes occur much faster with reperfusion than if ischemia continues. Although the endothelium has not yet been studied as extensively as myocytes, most investigators believe that endothelial stunning is also a manifestation of reperfusion injury.[36] In the setting of acute infarction, microvascular stunning would be most likely to have clinical relevance in cases of rapid reperfusion or in periinfarct zones.

Lethal and nonlethal reperfusion injuries overlap when vasoregulatory compromise causes diminished flow (low reflow) and predisposes to coronary spasm. Microvascular stunning may thus contribute to repeat episodes of myocyte stunning. It is conceivable that this postreperfusion blood flow compromise may result in the death of some myocytes that otherwise would have remained viable. In this way nonlethal reperfusion injury to the endothelial cell may be lethal to the myocyte via an indirect mechanism. Additionally, neutrophils in the reperfusing blood encounter the injured, dysfunctional endothelium. This interaction between neutrophils and endothelium is another way in which nonlethal injury to endothelial cells may contribute to cardiomyocyte injury.

Coronary microvascular stunning must be distinguished from the "no reflow" phenomenon, which is a severe reduction of flow to a certain vascular bed. Most clinicians are familiar with this phenomenon, which occurs relatively late—after 90 minutes of ischemia in the dog model.[28,37] It may be observed by coronary angiography soon after reperfusion and it has also been demonstrated by nuclear medicine techniques.[38] It always occurs in areas of irreversible myocyte injury. Microscopically, endothelial swelling and blebs are seen

in the precapillary and capillary beds. The zone of no reflow may worsen and extend during the several hours following reperfusion. This worsening seems to be associated with plugging of the capillaries with neutrophils. Some investigators believe that the worsening over time may represent a form of reperfusion injury, but this remains speculative.

Arrhythmias are another phenomenon frequently observed in animal models of ischemia/reperfusion. These arrhythmias typically originate from the ventricle (and may include ventricular fibrillation). The temporal association with reperfusion is unmistakable, making arrhythmia one of the most commonly acknowledged forms of reperfusion injury. In the usual sequence of events the arrhythmia occurs very quickly after reperfusion; the incidence is higher if flow returns abruptly to normal or supranormal levels. Lipid and protein components of the sarcolemma and the sacroplasmic reticulum are most likely the targets of this form of reperfusion injury, which can rapidly lead to arrhythmogenic disturbances of potassium and calcium homeostasis.

The injury required to produce arrhythmia is probably nonlethal to the individual cell, as evidenced by the finding that these arrhythmias are more frequent after brief ischemic episodes; in fact, reperfusion-induced arrhythmia is uncommon in most models after several hours of ischemia. One can speculate that some of the early, out-of-hospital mortality from MI may result from early spontaneous reperfusion and an associated arrhythmia. In the hospital setting reperfusion often occurs after several hours of ischemia and arrhythmias can be managed. Information from clinical trials on this topic has been complicated by the evidence that overall lethal arrhythmias are reduced by reperfusion[39]; however, more careful analysis indicates an early excess of serious arrhythmia[39] followed by a later and more substantial reduction. Although some cardiologists remain skeptical about the clinical relevance of this phenomenon, reperfusion-induced arrhythmia may take on more clinical significance as we strive to achieve reperfusion early.

BASIC MECHANISMS
Free radicals

Despite intense investigation the basic pathophysiology of reperfusion injury is still being elucidated. There are two leading hypotheses concerning the pathogenesis: the "oxyradical hypothesis" and the "calcium hypothesis."[40] These hypotheses developed from independent observations, but may be related. The "oxyradical hypothesis" maintains that a burst of oxygen-derived free radicals, produced at the time of reperfusion, inflicts damage on cellular components.[40,41] Membrane structures such as the sarcolemma and sarcoplasmic reticulum are believed to be particular sites of damage.

Endothelial cells, neutrophils, and myocytes all contain enzyme systems capable of producing and metabolizing free radicals. At the time of reperfusion the resident systems for scavenging free radicals are overwhelmed; the resultant cellular damage inflicted by free radicals could conceivably be either lethal or nonlethal.[42] In the case of stunning the injury falls short of cell death but causes resting contractile dysfunction that resolves over time (assuming maintenance of normal blood flow).[43]

Several lines of evidence support the oxyradical hypothesis. Free radical species appear in the effluent blood from transiently ischemic myocardium shortly after reperfusion.[44,45] The role of oxygen, available with reperfusion, as the chemical source of these radicals has been shown.[43] In these and other studies there is evidence of lipid peroxidation,[43,46] which may be a marker of damage (particularly to membranes) done by oxygen-derived radicals. Finally, many interventions designed to scavenge or rapidly metabolize free radicals have been shown to decrease reperfusion injury.[47-49] This effect occurs for infarction as well as stunning. Myocardial glutathione levels in particular have been related to the severity of stunning, with more severe stunning occurring in glutathione-depleted (thus having impaired free-radical defenses) isolated rat hearts.[50] Despite this evidence for a free-radical-mediated mechanism, the specific site of cellular injury resulting in stunning remains undefined.

The calcium hypothesis focuses on the critical role of Ca^{+2} as a second messenger in contractile function.[40,51] Clearly there is a defect in excitation-contraction coupling in stunned myocardium.[52] Impaired contractility may result from either an alteration in intracellular Ca^{+2} homeostasis or an alteration in myofibrillar sensitivity to intracellular Ca^{+2} transients.[52a] In either case one can postulate free radical damage as the primary event.

There are multiple proposed mechanisms for these effects, and this area of investigation remains controversial. In vitro studies show a rise in intracellular calcium concentration ($[Ca]_i$) after 10 minutes of global ischemia.[53] The $[Ca]_i$ remains elevated during the very early phase of reperfusion, 3 to 4 minutes, before returning toward normal.[20] Extracellular calcium probably enters the cell immediately following reperfusion; this may be because of increased $Na^+ - Ca^{+2}$ exchange as the cell reestablishes normal intracellular sodium concentration. Alternatively there could be free radical damage to membrane components involved in calcium hemostasis. It has been proposed that the relatively brief $[Ca]_i$ increase stimulates Ca^{+2}-dependent proteases, which may directly disrupt some myofibrils or cause a decreased affinity of troponin C for Ca^{+2}.

Other investigators have focused on the function of the sarcoplasmic Ca^{+2}, Mg^{+2}-ATPase in stunned myocardium. Normally Ca^{+2} is released from the sarcoplas-

mic reticulum (SR) during systole and pumped back into the SR during diastole. Krause et al. showed impaired function of the Ca^{+2}, Mg^{+2}-ATPase in stunned myocardium in one animal model.[54] It is conceivable that injury to the calcium pump might occur via free radicals.

Role of neutrophils

The role played by neutrophils has been the subject of considerable investigation in recent years. The reason for such interest is the evidence from animal models that limiting neutrophil accumulation and subsequent infiltration into reperfused myocardium can limit the degree of tissue damage.[55,56] Multiple investigators have observed this phenomenon when antineutrophil intervention precedes ischemia. In addition, Litt et al. have shown a beneficial effect in one animal model even when the neutrophil limitation occurs only during reperfusion.[56] This evidence strongly suggests that neutrophil-mediated myocardial injury is (at least partially) a form of reperfusion injury and is potentially preventable.

Studies in canine models show that neutrophils begin to accumulate in the reperfused coronary vasculature approximately 20 minutes following reperfusion.[57] They accumulate rapidly during the next 60 minutes and more slowly thereafter. In order to accumulate they must adhere to the endothelium; in a later phase they migrate through the endothelium into the myocardium. Although a great deal has been learned about endothelial-neutrophil interaction, the process is complicated by a multitude of contributing factors and it is not yet clear which factors are the most important when considering adhesion to endothelial cells injured and rendered dysfunctional by the process of reperfusion.

Most theories incorporate two major processes: failure of the endothelium to secrete normal vasodilatory substances and the activation and increased expression of various membrane-bound receptors and adhesion molecules. As mentioned earlier stunned endothelium loses the ability to generate nitric oxide (EDRF), adenosine, and PGI_2—substances that normally help to prevent the adherence of neutrophils and platelets as well as to decrease vascular resistance. The mechanism of this action is not fully understood, but neutrophil adherence is facilitated when the local concentration of these substances decreases.

Both neutrophils and endothelial cells contain adhesion molecules responsible for a variety of normal biologic functions. Neutrophils express a group of molecules known as the *integrins,* which form the CD18 complex. This complex is upregulated by the complement activation that occurs immediately following reperfusion. There is also a second group of adhesion molecules known as *LEC-CAMs.* The endothelial cell expresses ICAM-1 (intracellular adhesion molecule 1), which binds to the CD18 complex. Endothelial cells also express PAF (platelet-activating factor) and another molecule known as GMP-140, which also contributes to endothelial-neutrophil attachment (see Chapter 6).

POSSIBLE APPROACHES TO TREATMENT
Potential clinical consequences of reperfusion injury

When envisioning therapeutic approaches to reperfusion injury it is important to consider the clinical consequences that may occur as a result of alteration of the previously described pathophysiological mechanisms. In the early phases of reperfusion, arrhythmias, particularly ventricular fibrillation, may be prevented. During the early process of reperfusion the acceleration of necrosis that seems to occur might be delayed to allow additional therapies to salvage myocardium. The critical phase in which the noninfarcted myocardium must support the acutely damaged ventricle could be shortened with potential benefit if the severity and duration of myocardial stunning could be diminished. Finally, the long-term outlook could be enhanced by reducing the final size of the infarction through prevention of necrosis. Each of these clinical outcomes might be measured by a different set of endpoints, but the fundamental tenet of all is improved function of the left ventricle.

Analysis of large clinical trial data has indicated that an "early hazard" exists in the administration of thrombolytic therapy. Treated patients have a higher mortality in the first 24 hours than do untreated patients.[58] A systematic overview has indicated that in patients treated late (beyond 6 to 12 hours from symptom onset), the risk of myocardial rupture appears to be increased by thrombolytic therapy.[59] These findings have suggested that the process of reperfusion may be temporarily deleterious in the early period. More recent data from ASSET[60] and GUSTO-I[61] have not identified such an "early hazard" with the use of t-PA. Rather, early and sustained reperfusion has been associated with a lower mortality. These data suggest, but do not prove, that the early hazard is a function of streptokinase administration, perhaps because of the hypotension associated with it.

Human studies of left ventricular function

Three types of studies have evaluated myocardial salvage in humans. Studies comparing thrombolytic therapy with placebo or conservative care have shown only a two- to four-point difference in left ventricular function between the two groups (Fig. 32-1). Van de Werf[62] and Califf et al.[63] have pointed out the paradoxical nature of the relationship between left ventricular function improvement and mortality reduction in these trials. In general, studies demonstrating the greatest improvement in left ventricular function have not shown a mortality advantage, and studies with a mortality advantage generally do not show evidence of improvement in left ventricular function (Fig. 32-2). The most logical explanation for this paradox is that patients with markedly impaired acute left ventricular function are most likely to die in the control groups and to be salvaged in the thrombolytic therapy groups. Thus, patients with large infarctions are more likely to be alive for the follow-up measurement of left ventricular function.

Serial studies without a control group generally show

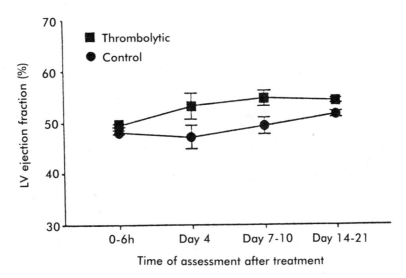

Fig. 32-1. Pooled analysis of left ventricular ejection fraction from randomized trials of thrombolytic therapy vs. control: thrombolytic therapy results in significantly higher ejection fraction ($P \leq 0.001$ for each time point), and the difference between thrombolytic and control does not increase after day 4. Includes 3066 ventriculographic observations. From Granger CB, Califf RM, Topol EJ: Thrombolytic therapy for acute myocardial infarction: a review, *Drugs* 44:293-325, 1992.

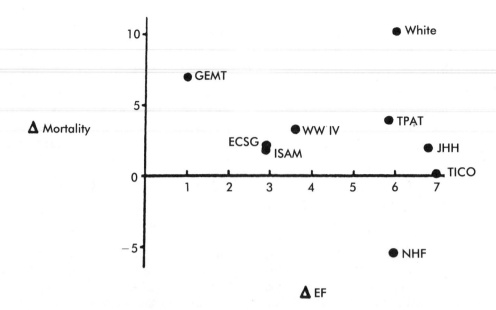

Fig. 32-2. Scatterplot showing relation of ejection fraction improvement vs. mortality reduction in 10 placebo-controlled intravenous thrombolytic therapy reperfusion trials. The graph demonstrates lack of any clear relation and, if anything, a paradoxical inverse one. Trials that have shown the most benefit in terms of ejection fraction improvement over placebo (ΔEF) have tended to exhibit the least mortality reduction. It is important to point out that these were trials of left ventricular ejection fraction and were not intended to detect differences of mortality. The trial abbreviations are as follows: ECSG = European Cooperative Study Group; TPAT = Tissue Plasminogen Activator – Toronto Trial; WWIV = Western Washington Intravenous Streptokinase Trial; GEMT = German Eminase Multicenter Trial; ISAM = Intravenous Streptokinase in Acute Myocardial Infarction; JHH = Johns Hopkins Hospital Trial; NHF = National Heart Foundation Trial; and TICO = Thrombolysis in Coronary Occlusion Trial. (From Harrison JK, Califf RM, Woodlief LH, et al: Systolic left ventricular function after reperfusion therapy for acute myocardial infarction: an analysis of determinants of improvement, *Circulation* 87:1531-1541, 1993.)

well-preserved left ventricular function throughout the course of the AMI, with little change from the first day to 1 week,[64,65] 6 weeks,[66] or 6 months.[67] Part of the explanation for this finding is that in the acute phase of the infarction the noninfarct zone is hyperkinetic ("compensatory hyperkinesis"). The major mechanism for this hyperkinesis is believed to be catecholamine-induced. Grines et al.[68] demonstrated that the function of the noninfarct zone is a critical determinant of survival and that the degree of hyperkinesis is predominantly a function of the degree of stenosis of epicardial vessels feeding the noninfarct zone. Relaxation of the noninfarct zone over the first week would be expected to cause a drop in the ejection fraction to at least partially offset any improvement that might be seen in the infarct zone. In a multivariable analysis Harrison et al.[64] demonstrated that the most important factor associated with improvement in global and infarct zone function was the degree of impairment at the acute study. All other factors were relatively minor compared with the degree of baseline impairment, but they included achievement of TIMI Grade 3 flow and relief of chest pain by 90 minutes (Table 32-1). Sur-

prisingly, time from symptom onset to treatment with thrombolytic therapy was not significantly associated with improvement in global or regional function, although the TIMI investigators have demonstrated a weak association in their population.

One of the most interesting and provocative findings of the GUSTO-I angiographic substudy was that the more rapid reperfusion associated with t-PA therapy led to better regional and global function by the time of the 90-minute angiogram, with little change beyond that point.[69] This finding implies that reperfusion may preserve function by preventing contractile loss in a wavefront fashion rather than salvaging severely ischemic (but not dead myocardial) cells that will regain function at a later date.

The third type of study has used technetium sestamibi (Tc-sestamibi) to measure the area at risk acutely and the amount of myocardium infarcted at follow-up. The special characteristics of Tc-sestamibi allow an accurate assessment of the area of perfusion of the infarct-related vessel if the agent can be injected before reperfusion is performed. The final infarct size is then calculated from a late image taken before the patient is discharged from

Table 32-1. Variables related to 7-day improvement

	Ejection fraction			Infarct zone function		
	B	**F**	**P**	**B**	**F**	**P**
Acute ejection fraction	−0.30	68.2	<0.001			NS
Acute infarct zone regional function			NS	−0.29	50.4	<0.001
Acute infarct-related artery patency*	1.92	7	0.009	−0.36	11	0.001
Resolution of chest pain	−1.23	5.4	0.02	−0.21	11.5	0.001
Acute noninfarct zone regional function	−0.70	7.7	0.006	−0.06	6.2	0.01
History of hypertension	1.92	6.9	0.009			NS
Inferior MI			NS	−0.19	4.6	0.03
Emergency bypass surgery			NS	0.44	4.3	0.04
R^2		0.23			0.16	

From Harrison JK, Califf RM, Woodlief LH, et al: Systolic left ventricular function after reperfusion therapy for acute myocardial infarction: an analysis of determinants of improvement, *Circulation* 87:1531-1541, 1993.
*Presence of Thrombolysis in Myocardial Infarction grade 3 flow—ejection fraction model; presence of Thrombolysis in Myocardial Infarction grade 0 flow—infarct zone regional function model.

the hospital. This technique has allowed a number of investigations that have essentially confirmed the work of Reimer and Jennings in a human model. The most important determinants of infarct size are area at risk, extent of collateral flow, and time to reperfusion, just as in the classic animal model. This method may allow a very sensitive estimate of the potential for clinical benefit in a small sample size.

These studies provide a mixed picture for the expectations of the clinical impact of therapies designed to prevent reperfusion injury. The methods of measurement of left ventricular function are complex and plagued by problems of bias about which patients return for follow-up studies. Multiple factors seem to affect the degree of infarct size and left ventricular functional return.

Clinical studies of therapeutic agents

Prostacyclin. Prostacyclin has a variety of effects on the vasculature and on constituents that may be important in the process of reperfusion injury. In animal models prostacyclin has been shown to reduce both infarct size and myocardial stunning, presumably through its demonstrated effects on free-radical formation or on neutrophil function. Other potentially beneficial effects of prostacyclin include its inhibition of platelet function, acceleration of thrombolysis, and reduction in preload and afterload.[70,71] After a series of promising animal experiments, we had the opportunity to investigate the effects of Iloprost, a prostacyclin analogue, in the setting of reperfusion with t-PA.

In the TAMI-4 pilot study 25 patients were treated with t-PA and Iloprost starting with a dose of 0.5 ng/kg/min and escalating to a stable dose of 2 ng/kg/min

for 48 hours. All of these patients were also treated with heparin, aspirin, lidocaine, and beta blocker if indicated. An additional 25 patients were treated with an identical regimen except that Iloprost was not given. Unfortunately, the Iloprost-treated patients had a lower 90-minute patency (44% vs. 60%) and a high rate of complications including flushing, headache, nausea, and hypotension. Although the study was too small to be definitive, not even a trend towards improvement in left ventricular function was observed. Interestingly, a trend towards a lower rate of reocclusion (7 vs. 25%) was observed with Iloprost, but the low patency combined with the side effect profile made this approach unsatisfactory for introduction into larger trials.

Superoxide dismutase. Superoxide dismutase (SOD) initially was an exciting potential approach to the clinical amelioration of reperfusion injury. This free-radical scavenger plays an essential role in normal cellular function by neutralizing the effects of free radicals produced within the cell. A recombinant form of this molecule has been produced, allowing for extensive animal and human experiments. Several experimental studies have also demonstrated a reduction in reperfusion arrhythmias.[72,73] Although the initially reported experiments were dramatically positive for reduction in infarct size, subsequent studies have yielded mixed results, perhaps because of the different experimental preparations.

The first moderate-sized clinical trial specifically designed to assess reperfusion injury was performed using SOD.[74] The design of the study called for the administration of intravenous SOD to patients undergoing direct coronary angioplasty or "rescue" coronary angioplasty so that certainty would exist that the drug

Table 32-2. Analysis of global ejection fraction (EF) and regional wall motion (RWM) for the primary efficacy population

	h-SOD	Placebo	P
Contrast ventriculogram			
Global EF (%)	n = 27	n = 28	
Baseline	51.6 ± 14.0	51.6 ± 13.4	NS
Change	+1.8 ± 8.7	±4.4 ± 8.8	NS
RWM-infarcted region (SD/C)	n = 27	n = 28	
Baseline	−2.98 ± 0.91	−3.10 ± 0.72	NS
Change	+0.44 ± 0.80	+0.92 ± 1.35	NS
RWM-Contralateral Wall (SD/C)	n = 27	n = 28	
Baseline	1.23 ± 1.90	0.90 ± 1.75	NS
Change	−0.07 ± 1.50	−0.38 ± 1.09	NS
Radionuclide ventriculogram			
Global EF (%)	n = 23	n = 17	
Baseline	46.7 ± 14.9	46.9 ± 12.7	NS
Change	+1.3 ± 9.8	+5.5 ± 9.7	NS
Regional EF-infarcted region (%)	n = 21	n = 15	
Baseline	24.2 ± 16.3	27.1 ± 13.5	NS
Change	+6.7 ± 12.9	+9.2 ± 13.9	NS
Regional EF-normal region (%)	n = 21	n = 15	
Baseline	60.1 ± 12.1	59.9 ± 13.3	NS
Change	+2.0 ± 14.3	+4.4 ± 12.3	NS

From Flaherty JT, Pitt B, Gruber JW, et al: Recombinant human superoxide dismutase (h-SOD) fails to improve recovery of ventricular function in patients undergoing coronary angioplasty for acute myocardial infarction, *Circulation* 89:1982-1991, 1994. *SD/C,* Standard deviations per chord.

was present at the time of reperfusion. The SOD was infused intravenously at a dose of 10 mg/kg as a bolus followed by 0.2 mg/kg/min for 60 minutes. The control group received a matching placebo.

Baseline characteristics were similar for the two groups, as would be expected by the process of randomization. Unfortunately, clinical outcomes were not different for the two groups. Furthermore, left ventricular ejection fraction and regional left ventricular function also were not different (Table 32-2). A difference was apparent in terms of ventricular arrhythmias occurring in the early hours of reperfusion, although no difference was found in the rate of ventricular fibrillation and no difference in resource use was observed.

Fluosol. Fluosol is a fluorohydrocarbon emulsion with a number of interesting biologic properties. The compound is capable of carrying much higher concentrations of oxygen than blood and therefore has been considered as a blood substitute. Its hydrocarbon properties allow it to flow in the microcirculation in areas not easily traversed by blood cells. Multiple animal studies have demonstrated that, in the models that have been studied, Fluosol given just before reperfusion can lead to reduction in infarct size as measured by staining techniques and to improvement in systolic left ventricular function.[17] The major mechanism for the improvement in these animal models remains unclear, although the predominant effect is thought to be through the

amelioration of the effects of reperfusion on the elaboration of toxic substances from white blood cells. As a postulated secondary effect, endothelial damage was also reduced by Fluosol administration, presumably because of inhibition of leukocyte adhesion. Long-term studies have shown no impairment of myocardial healing, a concern that had arisen from the recognition that the inflammatory response is an integral part of scar formation.

An initial pilot study of intravenous Fluosol in the setting of direct coronary angioplasty was markedly positive. In this study Forman et al.[17] randomized 26 patients with first anterior MI to intravenous Fluosol or placebo before angioplasty. Seven of 13 patients in the control group were excluded because of patency at the first coronary injection (4), referral to bypass surgery (1), or shock (2); 7 of 13 Fluosol patients were excluded because of patency at first injection (2), left main disease (2), and unsuccessful angioplasty (3), leaving only 12 patients for analysis. In these patients both global (54% vs. 42%) and regional (−1.6 vs. −2.9 standard deviations per chord) left ventricular function were better in the Fluosol group, and thallium infarct size (3.5% vs. 18% of left ventricle) was much smaller in Fluosol-treated patients.

TAMI-9 was designed specifically to determine whether these initially promising results could be replicated in the setting of thrombolytic agent administration.

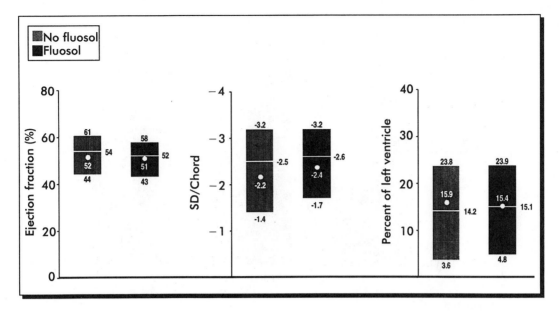

Fig. 32-3. This figure demonstrates the median and intraquartile ranges as well as the mean values for ejection fraction, infarct zone function, and thallium-estimated infarct size for patients who did and did not receive Fluosol. From Wall TC, Califf RM, Blankenship J, et al. and the TAMI-9 Research Group: Intravenous Fluosol in the treatment of acute myocardial infarction: results of the Thrombolysis and Angioplasty in Myocardial Infarction 9 Trial, *Circulation* 90:114-120, 1994.

The design of the study was to enroll patients with first infarction via telephone randomization, with a goal of treating as rapidly as possible. Only patients with first infarction were enrolled because infarct size and left ventricular function were used as primary endpoints. Based on calculations from previous studies it was determined that a sample size of just over 400 patients would be required to detect a difference of 3% to 4% in global left ventricular function.

The baseline characteristics of the patients were typical for thrombolytic trials with the majority of patients relatively young and otherwise healthy. The administration of the Fluosol and measurement of key endpoints were accomplished successfully.

The thallium infarct size, ejection fraction, and regional wall motion results are shown in Figure 32-3. No differences in any of these outcomes were observed. Table 32-3 shows the key clinical outcomes. An excess of pulmonary edema/heart failure was seen in the Fluosol-treated group, but these effects were only transient and did not lead to excess mortality. An interesting trend towards reduction of recurrent ischemia and reinfarction of borderline statistical significance was observed in the Fluosol group. These findings point more towards a role for Fluosol in the prevention of reocclusion rather than in a reduction in reperfusion injury.

ReothRx. Poloxamer 188 (ReothRx) is a substance that has a variety of properties that may be valuable in the treatment of acute ischemic heart disease, including

Table 32-3. Clinical outcomes in TAMI-9 patients

	No fluosol	Fluosol
Death (%)	3.7 (1.2, 6.2)	5.6 (2.6, 8.6)
Stroke (%)		
Hemorrhagic	0.9 (0.4, 2.2)	2.4 (0.3, 4.4)
Other		1.9 (0.1, 3.7)
Reinfarction (%)	4.2 (1.5, 6.9)	2.4 (0.4, 4.4)
CHF/pulmonary edema (%)	31 (24.8, 37.2)	45 (38.3, 51.7)*
Recurrent ischemia (%)	11 (6.8, 15.2)	6 (2.8, 9.2)†

From Wall TC, Califf RM, Blankenship J, et al. and the TAMI-9 Research Group: Intravenous Fluosol in the treatment of acute myocardial infarction: results of the Thrombolysis and Angioplasty in Myocardial Infarction 9 Trial, *Circulation* 90:114-120, 1994.
Numbers represent percentage of patients with event and 95% confidence intervals.
*$P = 0.004$.
†$P = 0.039$.

a potential for impacting on reperfusion injury. The unique structure of this compound provides it with both antithrombotic properties and properties that alter blood rheology. It is a nonionic copolymer that reduces surface tension and hydrophobic interactions of cellular constituents of blood, resulting in a reduction in blood viscosity and less strong red blood cell aggregation.[75,76] It has no effect on bleeding time, prothrombin time, or partial thromboplastin time[77] in the absence of

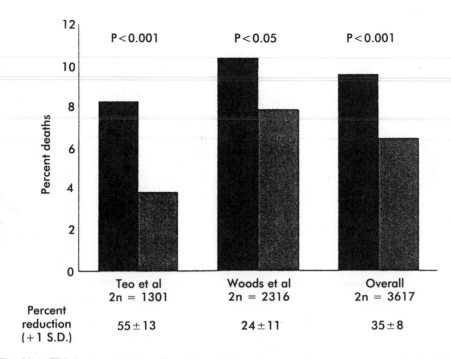

Fig. 32-4. This bar graph shows the effect of intravenous magnesium on mortality in AMI. Reductions in mortality are shown in the overview by Teo et al.,[90] in the LIMIT-2 study[85] and in the overall combined data from all trials. (From Yusuf S, Teo K, Woods K: Intravenous magnesium in acute myocardial infarction, *Circulation* 87:2043-2046, 1993.)

heparin. In animal models it speeds the time to thrombolysis and improves myocardial blood flow.[78]

Poloxamer 188 is a major constituent of the carrier solution for Fluosol. Accordingly, its effects on reperfusion injury have been intensively studied. In several experiments it appears to be equivalent to Fluosol in terms of reduction in myocardial infarct size.[79] Early clinical studies have shown promising results in the setting of thrombolysis, although in the setting of direct angioplasty the results have been less impressive. A large trial investigating the effects of this compound in patients with ST-segment elevation is currently underway.

Adenosine. Another approach to dealing with myocardial stunning is to replete the energy stores that are depleted in the process of reperfusion injury. An older approach with promising pilot results is the use of glucose, insulin, and potassium as a "cocktail" to improve the availability of myocardial energy stores. Despite promising results in the 1970s this approach has never become popular and remains seldom used, although interest in it is being rekindled. Newer approaches to this problem attempt to delve into the process of substrate provision to maintain myocardial ATP levels, which are critical for the mechanical functioning of the myocardium.

Adenosine is an endogenous purine nucleoside with a variety of potentially beneficial effects. It mediates coronary autoregulation, and this role appears to be especially important during ischemia or reperfusion. This agent has raised particular interest in the investigation of reperfusion injury because of its effects on inhibition of neutrophil adhesion and release of toxic substances during ischemia. Animal models have demonstrated an apparent reduction in infarct size when pretreated with adenosine.[80,81] Interestingly, one study found a reduction in infarct size only when lidocaine was coadministered with adenosine.[18] Other desirable properties of adenosine include vasodilation of coronary arterioles, direct inhibition of platelet aggregation and thromboxane release, and inhibition of sympathetic neurotransmission. Several pilot studies of adenosine are currently underway in humans.

White-cell mediators. Experimental studies have indicated that adhesive interaction between leukocytes and endothelial cells is essential for reperfusion injury to occur in the laboratory. Because these interactions are mediated by adhesion molecules, called *selectins*, inhibition of the actions of these adhesion molecules may be beneficial in the reduction of both myocardial and endothelial reperfusion injury. Experimental studies have now shown that interventions that block the selectins that are responsible for leukocyte adhesion both prevent adhesion and reduce experimental infarct size.[82] These agents are just entering early-phase clinical testing.

Magnesium. Intravenous magnesium supplementation has not traditionally been viewed as a treatment to prevent reperfusion injury, but this view may be changing. Magnesium has been used by some clinicians as part of the treatment for AMI for many years; its use has been more popular in Europe than in the United States. Initial small-scale clinical trials demonstrated decreased periinfarct arrhythmias, with a trend towards less periinfarct heart failure. Recent metaanalyses of the available data demonstrate a significant mortality benefit[83,84] (Fig. 32-4). These trials were conducted before the thrombolytic era. A recent randomized trial of magnesium in conjunction with thrombolytic therapy (reperfusion possibly achieved in the majority of cases) also shows a significant mortality benefit.[85] Mortality was reduced by 24% ($P = .03$) at 28 days (10.3% in the placebo group vs. 7.8% in magnesium-treated patients) and symptomatic left ventricular failure was substantially lower. Furthermore, 1-year mortality was reduced by 16% ($P = .04$).

Just as these promising results had been aggregated the ISIS-4 trial randomized over 50,000 patients to acute intravenous magnesium or standard care in the acute phase of MI. Contrary to the results of the systematic overview, no benefit was seen for magnesium, and an insignificant trend towards detriment was observed. Despite exhaustive review of subgroups, apparently no population could be found with a benefit from magnesium therapy.

The reasons for the discrepant results of these trials remain elusive. The proposed mechanism of benefit for magnesium was a reduction in stunning through mitigation of intracellular calcium overload,[86] although antiplatelet effects and improved collateral flow via coronary artery vasodilation have been proposed.[84,87] The ISIS-4 data, although convincingly large, predominately enrolled patients well past the time of administration of thrombolytic agents.[88] In the animal models that have been most convincing for magnesium, the reduction of stunning has been shown to occur only when magnesium levels are raised at the time of reperfusion.[89] The clinical and pathophysiological relevance of the discrepant trial results remains a topic of hot debate.

Despite years of basic investigation and a few clinical trials, prevention of reperfusion injury remains a research concept awaiting an effective clinical strategy. Continued pursuit of white-cell adhesion-mediating molecules appears to hold the most promise for clinical progress. Other methods of "rejuvenating" the myocardium to combat the negative aspects of stunning may enable patients to survive the critical period when compensatory mechanisms are not established. Finally, further information from completed clinical trials will be needed to resolve the magnesium controversy; for now, further basic research and pilot clinical studies must continue.

REFERENCES

1. Jennings RB, Sommers HM, Smyth GA, et al: Myocardial necrosis induced by temporary occlusion of a coronary artery in the dog, *Arch Pathol* 70:68-78, 1960.
2. Sommers HM, Jennings RB: Experimental acute myocardial infarction: histologic and histochemical studies of early myocardial infarcts induced by temporary or permanent occlusion of a coronary artery, *Lab Invest* 13:1491-1502, 1964.
3. Zimmerman ANE, Daems W, Hulsmann WC, et al: Morphologic changes of heart muscle caused by successive perfusion with calcium-free and calcium-containing solutions (calcium paradox), *Cardiovasc Res* 1:201-209, 1967.
4. Zimmerman ANE, Hulsmann WC: Paradoxical influence of calcium ions on the permeability of cell membranes in the isolated rat heart, *Nature* 211:646-647, 1966.
5. Feuvray D, De Leiris J: Ultrastructural modifications induced by reoxygenation in the anoxic isolated rat heart perfused with exogenous substrate, *J Mol Cell Cardiol* 7:307-314, 1975.
6. Hearse DJ, Humphrey SM, Nayler WG, et al: Ultrastructural damage associated with reoxygenation of the anoxic myocardium, *J Mol Cell Cardiol* 7:315-324, 1975.
7. Hearse DJ, Humphrey SM, Bullock GR: The oxygen paradox and the calcium paradox: two facets of the same problem? *J Mol Cell Cardiol* 10:641-668, 1978.
8. Rosenkranz ER, Buckberg GD: Myocardial protection during surgical coronary reperfusion, *J Am Coll Cardiol* 1:1235-1246, 1983.
9. Hearse DJ: Reperfusion of the ischemic myocardium, *J Mol Cell Cardiol* 69:605-616, 1977.
10. Haas GS, DeBoer LWV, O'Keefe DD, et al: Reduction of postischemic myocardial dysfunction by substrate repletion during reperfusion, *Circulation* 70(suppl I):I65-I74, 1983.
11. Stewart JR, Blackwell WH, Crute SL, et al: Inhibition of surgically induced ischemia/reperfusion injury by oxygen free radical scavengers, *J Thorac Cardiovasc Surg* 86:262-272, 1983.
12. Braunwald E, Kloner RA: The stunned myocardium: prolonged, postischemia ventricular dysfunction, *Circulation* 66:1146-1149, 1982.
13. Braunwald E, Kloner RA: Myocardial reperfusion: a double-edged sword? *J Clin Invest* 76:1713-1719, 1985.
14. Bolli R: Mechanism of myocardial "stunning", *Circulation* 82:723-738, 1990.
15. Bolli R, Zhu WX, Thronby JL, et al: Time-course and determinants of recovery of function after reversible ischemia in conscious dogs, *Am J Physiol* 254:H102-H114, 1988.
16. Kloner RA, Ellis SG, Lange R, et al: Studies of experimental coronary artery reperfusion: effects on infarct size, myocardial function, biochemistry, ultrastructure and microvascular damage, *Circulation* 68(suppl I):I8-I15, 1983.
17. Forman M, Bingham S, Kopelman H: Reduction of infarct size with intracoronary perfluorochemical in a canine preparation of reperfusion, *Circulation* 71:1060-1068, 1985.
18. Homeister JW, Hoff PT, Fletcher DD, et al: Combined adenosine and lidocaine administration limits myocardial reperfusion injury, *Circulation* 82:595-608, 1990.
19. Taylor AL, Golino P, Tckels R, et al: Differential enhancement of postischemic segmental systolic thickening by diltiazem, *J Am Coll Cardiol* 15:737-747, 1990.
20. Marban E, Kitakaze M, Kusuoka H, et al: Intracellular free calcium concentration measured with ^{19}FNMR spectroscopy in intact ferret hearts, *Proc Natl Acad Sci USA* 84:6005-6009, 1987.
21. Marban E, Kitakaze M, Doretsune Y, et al: Quantification of $[Ca^{2+}]$ in perfused hearts: critical evaluation of the 5F-BAPTA and nuclear magnetic resonance method as applied to the study of ischemia and reperfusion, *Circ Res* 66:1255-1267, 1990.

22. Hearse DJ: Ischemia, reperfusion and the determinants of tissue injury, *Cardiovasc Drug Ther* 4:767-776, 1990.

23. Schaper W, Schaper J: Problems associated with reperfusion of ischemic myocardium. In Piper HM (ed): *Pathophysiology of severe ischemic myocardial injury,* Dordrecht, 1990, Kluwer Academic Publishers.

24. Hearse DJ: Myocardial injury during ischemia and reperfusion. In Yellon DM, Jennings RB: *Myocardial protection: the pathophysiology of reperfusion and reperfusion injury,* New York, 1992, Raven Press.

25. Sommers HM, Jennings RB: Experimental acute myocardial infarction: histologic and histochemical studies of early myocardial infarcts induced by temporary or permanent occlusion of a coronary artery, *Lab Invest* 13:1491-1502, 1964.

26. Heyndrickx GR, Millard RW, McRitchie RJ, et al: Regional myocardial function and electrophysiological alterations after brief coronary artery occlusion in conscious dogs, *J Clin Invest* 56:978-985, 1975.

27. Bolli R: Post-ischemic myocardial stunning: pathogenesis, pathophysiology, and clinical relevance. In Yellon DM, Jennings RB: *Myocardial protection: the pathophysiology of reperfusion and reperfusion injury,* New York, 1992, Raven Press.

28. Kloner RA, Rude RE, Carlson N, et al: Ultrastructural evidence of microvascular damage and myocardial cell injury after coronary artery occlusion. Which comes first? *Circulation* 62:945-952, 1980.

29. Piper JM, Buderus S, Krutzfeldt A, et al: Sensitivity of the endothelium hypoxia and reoxygenation. In Piper HM (ed): *Pathophysiology of severe ischemic myocardial injury,* Dordrecht, 1990, Kluwer Academic Publishers.

30. Bolli R, Triana F, Jeroudi MO: Prolonged impairment of coronary vasodilation after reversible ischemia: evidence for microvascular "stunning," *Circ Res* 67:332-343, 1990.

31. Dauber IM, Van Benthuysen KM, McMurtry IF, et al: Functional coronary microvascular injury evident as increased permeability due to brief ischemia and reperfusion, *Circ Res* 66:986-998, 1990.

32. Van Benthuysen KM, McMurty IF, Horwitz LD: Reperfusion after acute coronary occlusion in dogs impairs endothelium-dependent relaxation to acetylcholine and augments contractile reactivity in vitro, *J Clin Invest* 79:265-274, 1987.

33. Tsao PS, Aoki N, Lefer DJ, et al: Time course of endothelial dysfunction and myocardial injury during myocardial ischemia and reperfusion in the cat, *Circulation* 82:1402-1412, 1990.

34. Vanhaecke J, Flameng W, Borgens M, et al: Evidence for decreased coronary flow reserve in viable postischemic myocardium, *Circ Res* 67:1201-1210, 1990.

35. Ku DD: Coronary vascular reactivity after myocardial ischemia, *Science* 218:576-578, 1982.

36. Kloner RM, Przyklenk K: Consequences of ischemic reperfusion on the coronary microvasculature. In Yellon DM, Jennings RB (eds): *Myocardial protection: the pathophysiology of reperfusion and reperfusion injury,* New York, 1992, Raven Press.

37. Ambrosio G, Weisman HF, Mannisi JA, et al: Progressive impairment of regional myocardial perfusion after initial restoration of postischemic blood flow, *Circulation* 80:1846-1861, 1989.

38. Schofer J, Montz R, Mathey DG: Scintigraphic evidence of the "no flow" phenomenon in human beings after coronary thrombolysis, *J Am Coll Cardiol* 5:593-598, 1985.

39. Volpi A, Cavalli A, Santoro E, et al: Incidence and prognosis of secondary ventricular fibrillation in acute myocardial infarction. Evidence for a protective effect of thrombolytic therapy—GISSI investigators, *Circulation* 82:1279-1288, 1990.

40. Bolli R: Myocardial stunning in man, *Circulation* 86:1671-1691, 1992.

41. Hammond B, Hess ML: The oxygen free radical system: potential mediator of myocardial injury, *J Am Coll Cardiol* 6:215-220, 1985.

42. Grisham MB, McCord JM: Chemistry and cytotoxicity of reactive oxygen metabolities. In Taylor AE, Matalon S, Ward PA (eds): *Physiology of oxygen radicals,* Bethesda, Md, 1986, American Physiological Society.

43. Bolli R, Jeroudi MO, Patel BS, et al: Direct evidence that oxygen-derived free radicals contribute to postischemic myocardial dysfunction in the intact dog, *Proc Natl Acad Sci USA* 86:4695-4699, 1989.

44. Bolli R, Patel B, Jeroudi M, et al: Demonstration of free radical generation in "stunned myocardium" of intact dogs with the use of the spin trap alpha-phenyl N-tert butyl nitrone, *J Clin Invest* 82:476-485, 1988.

45. Mergner G, Weglicki W, Kramer J: Postischemic free radical production in the venous blood of the regionally ischemia swine heart, *Circulation* 84:2079-2090, 1991.

46. Romaschin AD, Rebeya I, Wilson GJ, et al: Conjugated dienes in ischemic and reperfused myocardium: an in vivo chemical signature of oxygen free radical mediated injury, *J Mol Cell Cardiol* 19:289-302, 1987.

47. Jolly SR, Kane WJ, Balilie MB, et al: Canine myocardial reperfusion injury: its reduction by the combined administration or superoxide dismutase and catalase, *Circ Res* 54:277-285, 1984.

48. Myers ML, Bolli R, Lekich RF, et al: Enhancement of recovery of myocardial function by oxygen free-radical scavengers after reversible regional ischemia, *Circulation* 72:915-921, 1985.

49. Przyklenk K, Kloner RA: Superoxide dismutase plus catalase improve contractile function in the canine model of the "stunned myocardium," *Circ Res* 58:148-156, 1986.

50. Blaustein A, Deneke SM, Stolz RI, et al: Myocardial glutathione depletion impairs recovery after short periods of ischemia, *Circulation* 80:1449-1457, 1989.

51. Marban E, Koretsune YM, Correti M, et al: Calcium and its role in myocardial cell injury during ischemia and reperfusion, *Circulation* 80(suppl IV):17-22, 1989.

52. Kusuoka H, Koretsune Y, Chacko VP, et al: Excitation-contraction coupling in postischemic myocardium: does failure of activator Ca^{2+} transients underlie "stunning?" *Circ Res* 66:1268-1276, 1990.

52a. Soei LK, Sassen LMA, Fan DS, et al: Myofibrillar Ca^{2+} sensitization predominantly enhances function and mechanical efficiency of stunned myocardium, *Circulation* 90:959-969, 1994.

53. Steenbergen C, Murphy E, Levy L, et al: Elevation in cytosolic free calcium concentration early in myocardial ischemia in perfused rat heart, *Circ Res* 60:700-707, 1987.

54. Krause SM, Jacobus WE, Becker LC: Alterations in cardiac sarcoplasmic reticulum calcium transport in the postischemic "stunned" myocardium, *Circ Res* 65:526-530, 1989.

55. Mullane KM, Read N, Salmon JA, et al: Role of leukocytes in acute myocardial infarction in anesthetized dogs: relationship to myocardial salvage by anti-inflammatory drugs, *J Pharmacol Exp Ther* 228:510-522, 1984.

56. Litt MR, Jeremy RW, Weisman HF, et al: Neutrophil depletion limited to reperfusion reduces myocardial infarct size after 90 minutes of ischemia: evidence for neutrophil-mediated reperfusion injury, *Circulation* 80:1816-1827, 1989.

57. Dreyer WJ, Michael LH, West MS, et al: Neutrophil accumulation in ischemic canine myocardium: insights into time course, distribution, and mechanism of localization during early reperfusion, *Circulation* 84:400-411, 1991.

58. ISIS-3 Collaborative Group. ISIS-3: a randomised comparison of streptokinase vs. tissue plasminogen activator vs. anistreplase and of aspirin plus heparin vs. aspirin alone among 41,299 cases of suspected acute myocardial infarction, *Lancet* 339:753-770, 1992.

59. Honan MB, Harrell FE, Jr, Reimer KA, et al: Cardiac rupture, mortality and the timing of thrombolytic therapy: a meta-analysis, *J Am Coll Cardiol* 16:359-367, 1990.

60. Wilcox RG, von der Lippe G, Olsson CG, et al: Trial of tissue plasminogen activator for mortality reduction in acute myocardial

infarction: Anglo-Scandinavian Study of Early Thrombolysis (ASSET), *Lancet* 2:525-530, 1988.

61. Kleiman NS, White HD, Ohman EM, et al: for the GUSTO Investigators: Mortality 24 hours after thrombolysis in the GUSTO trial: corroborating evidence for the importance of early perfusion, *Circulation* 88(suppl I):I-17, 1993.

62. Van de Werf F, Arnold AE: Intravenous tissue plasminogen activator and size of infarct, left ventricular function, and survival in acute myocardial infarction, *Br Med J* 297:1374-1379, 1988.

63. Califf RM, Harrelson-Woodlief L, Topol EJ: Left ventricular ejection fraction may not be useful as an end point of thrombolytic therapy comparative trials, *Circulation* 82:1847-1853, 1990.

64. Harrison JK, Califf RM, Woodlief LH, et al: Systolic left ventricular function after reperfusion therapy for acute myocardial infarction: an analysis of determinants of improvement, *Circulation* 87:1531-1541, 1993.

65. Sheehan FH, Thery C, Durand P, et al: Early beneficial effect of streptokinase on left ventricular function in acute myocardial infarction, *Am J Cardiol* 67:555-558, 1991.

66. Sheehan FH, Braunwald E, Canner P, et al: The effect of intravenous thrombolytic therapy on left ventricular function: a report on tissue-type plasminogen activator and streptokinase from the Thrombolysis in Myocardial Infarction (TIMI Phase 1) Trial, *Circulation* 75:817-829, 1987.

67. Zaret BL, Wackers FJ, Terrin ML, et al: Assessment of global and regional left ventricular performance at rest and during exercise after thrombolytic therapy for acute myocardial infarction: results of the Thrombolysis in Myocardial Infarction (TIMI) II Study, *Am J Cardiol* 69:1-9, 1992.

68. Grines CL, Topol EJ, Califf RM, et al: Prognostic implications and predictors of enhanced regional wall motion of the noninfarct zone after thrombolysis and angioplasty therapy of acute myocardial infarction—the TAMI Study Groups, *Circulation* 80:245-253, 1989.

69. The GUSTO Investigators: An international randomized trial comparing four thrombolytic strategies for acute myocardial infarction, *N Engl J Med* 329:673-682, 1993.

70. Lefer AM, Ogletree ML, Smith JB, et al: Prostacyclin: a potentially valuable agent for preserving myocardial tissue in acute myocardial ischemia, *Science* 200:52-54, 1978.

71. Ribeiro LGT, Brandon TA, Hopkins DG, et al: Prostacyclin in experimental myocardial ischemia: effects on hemodynamics, regional myocardial blood flow, infarct size and mortality, *Am J Cardiol* 47:835-840, 1981.

72. Nejima J, Knight DR, Fallon JT, et al: Superoxide dismutase reduces reperfusion arrhythmias but fails to salvage regional function or myocardium at risk in conscious dogs, *Circulation* 79:143-153, 1989.

73. Kusama Y, Bernier M, Hearse DJ: Exacerbation of reperfusion arrhythmias by sudden oxidant stress, *Circ Res* 67:481-489, 1990.

74. Flaherty JT, Pitt B, Gruber JW, et al: Recombinant human superoxide dismutase (h-SOD) fails to improve recovery of ventricular function in patients undergoing coronary angioplasty for acute myocardial infarction, *Circulation* 89:1982-1991, 1994.

75. Grover FL, Kahn RS, Heron MW, et al: A nonionic surfactant and blood viscosity. Experimental observations, *Arch Surg* 106:307-310, 1973.

76. Smith CM, Hebbel RP, Turkey DP, et al: Pluronic F-68 reduces the endothelial adherence and improves the rheology of liganded sickle erythrocytes, *Blood* 69:1631-1636, 1987.

77. Robinson KA, Hunter RL, Stack JE, et al: Inhibition of coronary arterial thrombosis in swine by infusion of poloxamer 188, *J Inv Cardiol* 2:11-22, 1990.

78. Hunter RL, Bennett B, Check IJ: The effect of poloxamer 188 on the rate of in vitro thrombolysis mediated by t-PA and streptokinase, *Fibrinolysis* 4:117-123, 1990.

79. Justicz AG, Farnsworth WV, Soberman MS: Reduction of myocardial infarct size by poloxamer 188 and mannitol in a canine model, *Am Heart J* 122:671-680, 1991.

80. Olafsson B, Forman MB, Puett DW, et al: Reduction of reperfusion injury in the canine preparation by intracoronary adenosine: importance of the endothelium and the no-reflow phenomenon, *Circulation* 76:1135-1145, 1987.

81. Babbit DG, Bermani R, Forman MB: Intracoronary adenosine administered after reperfusion limits vascular injury after prolonged ischemia in the canine model, *Circulation* 80:1388-1399, 1989.

82. Polley MJ, Phillips ML, Wayner E, et al: CD62 and endothelial cell-leukocyte adhesion molecule 1 (ELAM-1) recognize the same carbohydrate ligand, sialyl-Lewis x, *Proc Natl Acad Sci* 88:6224-6228, 1991.

83. Horner SM: The efficacy of intravenous magnesium in acute myocardial infarction in reducing arrhythmias and mortality: meta-analysis of magnesium in acute myocardial infarction. *Circulation* 86:774-779, 1992.

84. Yusuf S, Teo K, Woods K: Intravenous magnesium in acute myocardial infarction, *Circulation* 87:2043-2046, 1993.

85. Woods KL, Fletcher S, Roffe C, et al: Intravenous magnesium sulphate in suspected acute myocardial infarction: results of the second Leicester Intravenous Magnesium Intervention Trial (LIMIT-2), *Lancet* 339:1553-1558, 1992.

86. Opie LH: Reperfusion injury and its pharmacologic modification, *Circulation* 80:1049-1062, 1989.

87. Herzog WR, Atar D, Gurbel PA, et al: The effect of magnesium supplementation on platelet aggregation in swine, *Magnesium Res* 6:349-353, 1993.

88. ISIS Collaborative Group: Randomised study of intravenous magnesium in over 50,000 patients with suspected acute myocardial infarction, *Circulation* 88(suppl I):I-292, 1993.

89. Atar D, Serebruany V, Poulton J, et al: Effects of magnesium supplementation in a porcine model of myocardial ischemia and reperfusion, *J Cardiovasc Pharmacol* vol 23, 1994 (in press).

90. Teo KK, Yusuf S, Furberg CD: Effects of prophylactic antiarrhythmic drug therapy in acute myocardial infarction: an overview of results from randomized controlled trials, *JAMA* 270:1589-1595, 1993.

Chapter 33

ROLE OF CORONARY ANGIOGRAPHY AFTER ACUTE MYOCARDIAL INFARCTION

Anthony C. De Franco
Joseph M. Sutton
Eric J. Topol

Risk stratification after myocardial infarction (MI) is an essential part of the patient's evaluation and care. Each year in the United States, more than 1 million individuals sustain an acute MI (AMI).[1] In the pre-thrombolytic era, approximately 80% of these patients survived to hospital discharge.[2] Mortality in the first 12 months was approximately 14%, with nearly three fourths of these deaths occurring within the first 5 months. Beginning in the second year, annual mortality persisted at 3% to 5%.[2] Although randomized, controlled trials of thrombolytic therapy for AMI have consistently demonstrated the unequivocal survival benefit of intravenous thrombolysis,[3-7] cumulative mortality at 1 year is in excess of 11%. Thus, the early and accurate identification of postinfarction patients at increased risk for complications and death remains an important clinical challenge. The optimal risk stratification strategy remains controversial; in particular, the appropriate use of diagnostic coronary angiography after AMI is an unresolved issue. In addition, the total cost of postinfarction and postthrombolytic care has significant implications for health care policy.

In this chapter, we evaluate several angiographic strategies in the context of the major reperfusion trials that incorporated early coronary angiography. We re-view the commonly accepted indications for coronary angiography during the acute phase of infarction, emphasizing the importance of uncoupling diagnostic angiography from dilation. We also examine the available data on the role of angiography in the uncomplicated patient that supports the use of either routine or selective angiography for risk stratification. Proponents of the selective approach claim that it is necessary to study only high-risk patient subsets and that such a strategy may prove to be most cost effective. Proponents of the routine approach argue that our current ability to detect reperfusion, reocclusion, or viable but ischemic myocardium noninvasively is limited and that the data supporting the prognostic value of noninvasive testing is especially limited for the postthrombolytic patient. Nevertheless, the currently available data can assist the physician in selecting the appropriate catheterization strategy for an individual patient.

EMERGENCY CORONARY ANGIOGRAPHY

Patients with AMI may undergo one of three broadly defined types of cardiac catheterization depending on the timing and principal purpose: emergency, urgent, or elective. Emergency coronary angiography, for the purposes of this review, is defined as the performance of the procedure as soon as possible after presentation, a priori, regardless of whether thrombolytic therapy has been initiated. For hospitals with 24-hour catheterization facilities, patients requiring emergency angiography must be immediately transferred from the emergency room or coronary care unit to the laboratory; for community hospitals without these resources, this strategy necessitates transfer to another institution.

There are three reasons to consider emergency coronary angiography. The first is *to confirm the diagnosis* of acute infarction when the clinical manifestation is ambiguous; the identity and status of the infarct artery and the extent of coronary disease can be determined simultaneously. For example, in patients with suggestive clinical symptoms but a nondiagnostic electrocardiogram (ECG) (e.g., those with left bundle branch block, prior infarction, or changes associated with left ventricular hypertrophy), confirmation of the diagnosis and documentation of the coronary anatomy can be especially useful. Patients with an acute occlusion of a distal segment of a single coronary artery require quite different therapeutic strategies than do those with advanced three-vessel disease or left main stenosis. If, on the other hand, the diagnosis of AMI is excluded, unnecessary empiric thrombolytic therapy and its associated risks can be avoided.

A second reason for emergency angiography is *to evaluate the need for and to perform mechanical revascularization* with direct balloon dilation of the infarct vessel. In select situations, direct or primary angioplasty is an effective alternative to intravenous thrombolytic therapy,[3,5,6,8-12] particularly for patients in whom thrombolysis is contraindicated, such as those who have had recent trauma, surgery, or stroke.[13] Patients who can be taken directly to the catheterization laboratory very soon after the onset of symptoms, such as hospitalized patients developing AMI while the catheterization laboratory is operational, are another group that can also benefit from direct percutaneous transluminal coronary angioplasty. Several randomized trials have recently shown comparable rates of reperfusion with direct angioplasty and intravenous thrombolysis.[14-18] In selected cases, mechanical reperfusion can avoid the delays and risks of thrombolysis and may afford a superior early patency rate (approximately 90%-95%) within 75 to 90 minutes after triage to direct angioplasty. However, until more data about the role of primary angioplasty are available, it is reasonable to conclude from the studies to date that primary coronary angioplasty is comparable to and may be superior to intravenous thrombolysis with respect to the endpoints of mortality reduction, reinfarction, and improvement of left ventricular function. Of course, for many patients with AMI, timely transfer to an open catheterization laboratory is not a viable option, and more rapid reperfusion can be achieved by means of

thrombolytic therapy, with 80% to 85% of patients achieving successful reperfusion within 60 to 90 minutes through the use of newer, accelerated regimens of intravenous tissue-type plasminogen activator (t-PA).[7,19,20]

The third and most common reason to recommend emergency coronary angiography is *to identify patients who have failed thrombolysis* within the first few hours of therapy. In approximately 5% to 8% of patients who have failed thrombolysis, selective contrast injection can actually facilitate clot dissolution by the transmission of hydrostatic pressure[1,21-24]; however, the primary role of emergency catheterization in this setting is *to identify candidates for rescue angioplasty* to recanalize the infarction-related vessel.[13,25]

Although the role of mechanical revascularization in MI is thoroughly reviewed in Chapters 34-36, several issues are pertinent to this discussion. Using emergency catheterization to identify candidates requiring rescue angioplasty (up to one fourth of patients, depending on the thrombolytic regimen) is an inefficient practice. An accurate, noninvasive assessment of the outcome of thrombolysis would be ideal, but current techniques, such as relief of chest discomfort, resolution of ECG ST-segment elevation, or ventricular dysrhythmias, all have proved unreliable.[26] In the Thrombolysis and Angioplasty in Acute Myocardial Infarction-I (TAMI-I) study, when chest pain improved after thrombolytic administration, the probability of a patent infarct artery was 71% and increased to 84% when pain completely resolved; unfortunately, these indices occurred in only 51% and 29% of patients, respectively, who had angiographically confirmed reperfusion. Similarly, an improvement in the initial ST-segment changes was associated with an 84% probability of a patent infarct vessel but occurred in only 38% of patients experiencing successful reperfusion. *Complete* normalization of the ST segments was associated with a patent infarct artery in 96% of cases, but this improvement occurred in only 6% of patients with an open artery at acute catheterization.[22] An analysis of reperfusion dysrhythmias,[26] the signal-averaged ECG,[27,28] and other methods have been similarly disappointing. In the future, if noninvasive methods such as analysis of creatinine kinase isoforms,[29,30] new radionuclide agents,[31-33] or digital, continuous 12-lead ECG ST-segment monitoring[34] are validated, they may allow for a much more efficient triage of patients with presumed failure of thrombolysis to emergency cardiac catheterization.

It is clear that patients who fail to reperfuse the infarction-related artery after thrombolysis have an especially poor prognosis.[35] The value of rescue angioplasty (see Chapter 27) was recently examined in the Randomized Evaluation of Salvage Angioplasty With Combined Utilization of Endpoints (RESCUE) trial.[25] In this international multicenter study, 150 patients with

Table 33-1. Some commonly accepted indications for emergent or urgent coronary angiography in acute myocardial infarction

1. To confirm the diagnosis before thrombolytic therapy.
2. To define the coronary anatomy and to assess candidacy for primary PTCA.*
3. To define the coronary anatomy and to assess candidacy for rescue PTCA for suspected failed thrombolysis or reocclusion.
4. Hypotension or hemodynamic collapse (unexplained or caused by ischemia).
5. Clinical or radiographic signs of congestive heart failure.
6. Clinical or echocardiographic signs of ventricular septal defect or new mitral insufficiency.

From De Franco A, Topol E: Invasive strategies in acute myocardial infarction in the elderly, *Cardiol Elderly* 2(3):274-289, 1994, with permission.
*PTCA, Percutaneous transluminal coronary angioplasty.

an anterior infarction who failed to reperfuse after any standard thrombolytic regimen underwent emergency catheterization. Those with Thrombolysis in Myocardial Infarction (TIMI) trial grade 0 or 1 flow within 8 hours of initial manifestation were randomized to receive either PTCA or medical therapy only. Rescue angioplasty, which was successful in 95% of patients, reduced the incidence of the combined endpoint of 30-day mortality and congestive heart failure (Killip class III or IV). However, there was no difference in the prespecified primary endpoint of resting ejection fraction. This result is in agreement with previous data combined from the TAMI trials, which suggested that patients who are thrombolysis failures can achieve the same low in-hospital and long-term mortality as patients in whom thrombolysis is successful if they are revascularized mechanically.[36] As in the RESCUE trial, this beneficial effect did not depend on improved myocardial salvage, because in this study patients who required angioplasty had worse initial and final ejection fraction measurements and less functional recovery of the infarct region. Thus, based on currently available data, emergency angiography and rescue angioplasty for thrombolysis failures may offer some patients an improvement in 30-day survival and functional status, albeit independent of resting left ventricular ejection fraction.

URGENT ANGIOGRAPHY

Urgent cardiac catheterization refers to an unplanned procedure done at any point from the first few hours after thrombolytic therapy to the time of hospital discharge and prompted by a clinical observation or event. There are several unequivocal indications for urgent coronary angiography in AMI (Table 33-1). *Hypotension* or *hemodynamic collapse,* with or without congestive heart failure, suggests severe ventricular

dysfunction and denotes either more extensive myocardial damage or ongoing myocardial ischemia with impending infarct extension. New auscultatory or echocardiographic findings that suggest *mitral valvular incompetence* or *ventricular septal defect* also mandate urgent angiography. *Reocclusion* after initially successful thrombolysis is another indication for urgent angiography (although readministration of a thrombolytic is an alternative when urgent angiography is unavailable) and may be suggested by the recurrence of chest discomfort with ECG changes. Ohman et al.[37] combined data from 810 patients enrolled in four of the TAMI trials. In the 733 patients in whom thrombolysis was initially successful, 91 (12.4%) experienced reocclusion during their hospitalization. Patients whose infarction-related vessel reoccluded had significantly higher rates of pulmonary edema (18.7% vs. 13.6%), sustained hypotension (25.3% vs. 16.5%), second- or third-degree heart block (25.3% vs. 12.8%), and a substantial increase in hospital mortality (11% vs. 4.5%). Although left ventricular ejection fraction was similar between the two groups at hospital discharge, patients with reocclusion had substantially worse function in the infarct zone and had lower overall ejection fractions at follow-up. Therefore, the relatively high incidence of recurrent ischemia and reinfarction (12%-20% of patients) after initially successful thrombolysis mandates vigilant clinical observation for residual ischemia and reocclusion.

In the GUSTO trial,[7] accelerated t-PA given with intravenous heparin resulted in a lower incidence of cardiogenic shock than the other three thrombolytic regimens tested (Table 33-2). Thus, for this indication, accelerated t-PA may decrease the need for emergency angiography. However, despite the overall improvement in 24-hour and 30-day mortality with accelerated t-PA, there were no differences in the need for emergency angiography, emergency PTCA, or emergency coronary artery hypass grafting (CABG) (Table 33-2).

Thus, urgent cardiac catheterization is performed to define the underlying anatomic defect and to triage the patient accordingly, either to urgent coronary angioplasty, urgent coronary bypass surgery, reconstructive valvular surgery, or ventricular septal defect repair. Relatively few data have been reported on this strategy, which appears to be widely accepted in centers where such triage is feasible. Some authorities suggest that routine early diagnostic catheterization is unnecessary after thrombolytic therapy for AMI. In this type of strategy, the role of urgent angiography may be particularly important. For example, the investigators of the large TIMI-II trial advocate "watchful waiting" after thrombolysis, with close surveillance for clinical indicators of recurrent ischemia. In this trial, 33% of patients assigned to this strategy required urgent or

Table 33-2. Incidence of various symptoms and results after treatment in the GUSTO trial*†

	SK (SQ)	SK (IV)	t-PA (accelerated regimen)	t-PA and SK	p Value: accelerated t-PA vs. both SK regimens
Cardiogenic shock	6.9	6.3	5.1	6.1	<0.001
Pulmonary edema	17.5	16.8	15.2	16.8	<0.001
Reinfarction	3.4	4.0	4.0	4.0	0.26
Recurrent ischemia	19.9	19.6	18.8	19.3	0.14
Emergency angiography	10.2	10.2	9.7	9.4	NS
Emergency PTCA	27.0	26.5	26.0	26.1	NS
Emergency CABG	8.5	8.8	9.5	9.5	NS

Data regarding symptoms adapted from GUSTO Investigators: *N Engl J Med* 329:673, 1993.
*Accelerated t-PA resulted in a lower incidence of cardiogenic shock than the other three regimens tested, which may decrease the requirement for emergency angiography. However, despite the overall improvement in 24-hr and 30-day mortality with accelerated t-PA, there were no differences in the need for emergency angiography, emergency PTCA, or emergency CABG.
†*SK*, Streptokinase; *t-PA*, tissue-type plasminogen activator; *PTCA*, percutaneous transluminal coronary angioplasty; *CABG*, coronary artery bypass grafting.

elective coronary angiography before hospital discharge.[38] In the TAMI-5 study, a relatively large proportion of patients treated conservatively after thrombolysis required urgent angiography.[39] Of the 288 patients randomly assigned to delayed catheterization, 75 (26%) crossed over to an urgent procedure within 5 days of admission for one or more of the following reasons: chest pain (82%), new ST-segment elevation (60%), or hypotension (35%). Patients who crossed over to urgent angiography had a poorer clinical outcome than patients who did not require this approach; the former group had a higher incidence of pulmonary edema (24% compared with 14%), lower predischarge ejection fractions (51.9% ± 11.3% compared with 54.2% ± 10.8%), and higher in-hospital mortality (7% compared with 3%). These results occurred despite an aggressive approach to myocardial revascularization with either emergency PTCA (49%) or CABG (15%). Unfortunately, clinical and hemodynamic variables on admission were poor predictors of which patients would subsequently require urgent angiography. Furthermore, one cannot assume that the *absence* of ischemia after thrombolytic therapy is due to significant myocardial salvage and the absence of any significant underlying residual stenosis. In such patients (who would not be recommended for catheterization with the TIMI-II strategy) *more* extensive myocardial necrosis despite thrombolytic therapy may be the cause of this clinical picture.[40]

In summary, urgent cardiac catheterization has an important role in the management of patients receiving thrombolytic therapy and for determining the optimal treatment strategy. Nevertheless, patients who require urgent angiography for persistent or recurrent ischemia are at a higher risk for immediate complications. Long term, these patients often have lower residual left ventricular function and suboptimal overall clinical outcomes despite the delivery of aggressive care. New

therapies are needed that increase the success of initial thrombolysis, further promote coronary artery stabilization, and prevent recurrent ischemia.

ELECTIVE ANGIOGRAPHY

Considerable controversy surrounds the role of elective angiography in the uncomplicated patient with presumed but unconfirmed reperfusion after the administration of a thrombolytic agent. Two approaches to planned, elective angiography have been proposed: *selective* and *routine*. In the selective approach, catheterization is performed for definite recurrent ischemia or an abnormal functional test that suggests inducible ischemia. In the routine approach, coronary angiography is a standard component of the postinfarction risk assessment. Although our preferred strategy in most patients is to recommend routine catheterization early in the hospital course, no definitive data mandate this approach. Cogent arguments support both strategies; currently we believe that either is acceptable.

Selective coronary angiography

Reserving cardiac catheterization in only selected cases can be supported for several reasons: The procedure is expensive, it is not available in most hospitals, and it has some risk. In addition, in the recent TIMI-II trial[38,41] and in the Should We Intervene Following Thrombolysis? (SWIFT) trial,[42] a "conservative" strategy of "watchful waiting" was equivalent to a late "invasive" strategy of empiric catheterization and angioplasty with respect to death, reinfarction, and ejection fraction. Furthermore, the conservative approach was considered more practical (Fig. 33-1).

Another argument for the restricted use of angiography is that defining the coronary anatomy may create a "reperfusion momentum,"[43] resulting in the premature or unnecessary triage to angioplasty or bypass

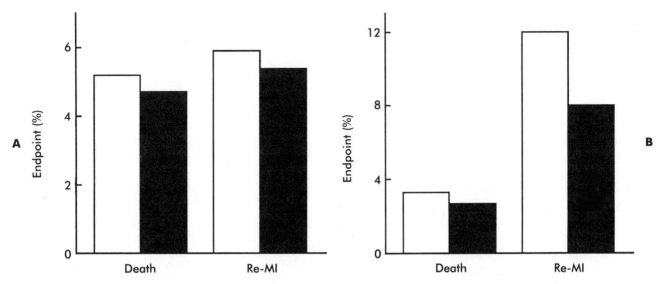

Fig. 33-1. Results of randomized trials comparing the prophylactic (□) and selective (■) strategies for cardiac catheterization and coronary angioplasty. **A,** Data for death or reinfarction *(Re-MI)* from 3262 patients in TIMI-2[38] who received tissue-type plasminogen activator. There was no difference in either endpoint for the two strategies. **B,** Data from 800 patients in the Should We Intervene Following Thrombolysis (SWIFT) trial[42] who received anistreplase show no difference in the death rate but do show a higher rate of reinfarction among patients who had prophylactic angioplasty. (From Topol E, Holmes D, Rogers W: Coronary angiography after thrombolytic therapy for acute myocardial infarction, *Ann Int Med* 114:877-885, 1991, with permission.)

surgery. The angiogram provides strictly *anatomic* data. In an asymptomatic patient after thrombolysis, for any documented residual stenosis in the infarction-related vessel that is associated with intact regional wall motion, the long-term outcome is likely to be favorable.[38,44-47] Long-term follow-up of patients managed with the conservative TIMI-II trial strategy showed that such patients are at particularly low risk for major events.[38] When lesions that are low risk based on clinical data are dilated solely because of their angiographic appearance (labeled the "oculostenotic" reflex), it seems likely that angiography was unnecessary. Of note, in the SWIFT trial,[42] prophylactic angioplasty in stable patients actually led to a significantly higher rate of reinfarction when compared with a conservative approach (see Fig. 33-1). Further, the potential exists for subsequent remodeling of the infarction-related vessel over time, precluding the need for dilation even on anatomic grounds.[48] In the TIMI and TAMI trials, 15% of patients were found to have a stenosis of less than 50% to 60% in an infarction-related vessel and thus did not require intervention.[38,43,49] This relatively low grade of narrowing presumably relates to continued lysis of thrombus and healing of the plaque rupture or fissure event.

In the United States, only 20% to 25% of the 6000 acute care hospital facilities have a cardiac catheterization laboratory.[50] Proponents of selective catheterization argue that restricted use of the procedure facilitates continuity of care in local community centers and avoids the need for interhospital transfer solely for predischarge angiography. Thus, a strategy of selective angiography may result in fewer unnecessary procedures, hospital transfers, and balloon angioplasty revascularizations, as well as a decrease in risk and possibly cost. Catheterization could be done electively in select patients if they had documented ischemia, particularly if such evidence suggested ischemia in multiple coronary artery territories.

Some advocates of this approach also recommend "selective" angiography in certain high-risk patients. In addition to postinfarction ischemia and congestive heart failure during the hospitalization period, a history of *prior* MI is clearly associated with increased late cardiac mortality. Complex or frequent *ventricular dysrhythmias* may be an indicator of residual ischemia and may correlate with an increased risk of late cardiac morbidity and mortality.[51-55] In all of these subgroups, the prognosis may improve with early catheterization, as well as with aggressive management of left ventricular dysfunction and dysrhythmias. Patients with an *ejection fraction less than 45%* and those spared from potentially large infarcts (e.g., a threatened anterior infarct successfully treated with thrombolytics) are also recommended for "selective" catheterization. However, the addition of many such "exceptions" to the "selective" approach ultimately leads to recommending coronary angiography in the majority of patients, thus effectively endorsing the "routine" catheterization strategy. As Kulick and Rahimtoola[56] have emphasized, up to 80% of patients whose risk was initially stratified by noninvasive methods will ultimately require angiography to accurately assess their postinfarction prognosis.

Routine coronary angiography

The predominant rationale for routine cardiac catheterization is to document the severity of the underlying coronary atherosclerotic disease; in particular, to define the coronary lesion responsible for the acute infarct, to evaluate the success of thrombolytic therapy, to identify patients with severe coronary artery disease, and, in selected cases, to facilitate early hospital discharge and return to work. The decision to perform angiography in the hemodynamically stable patient is often based in part on the clinician's assumption that the patient has been saved from an infarction but has moved back into the class of patients with unstable ischemic syndromes. This concept is supported by the observation from early placebo-controlled trials of thrombolytic therapy in which patients who received thrombolytics had a *higher* rate of reinfarction than conventionally managed patients.[3,57,58]

Defining the extent of coronary artery disease can be extremely valuable in planning therapeutic strategies that may promote long-term survival, free of infarction and angina. On the basis of data from the TIMI and TAMI trials, patients who undergo routine catheterization after intravenous thrombolysis can be separated into five discrete categories,* as shown in Fig. 33-2. Patients within these categories have different prognoses and require different management.

First, approximately 10% to 15% of patients have a minimal residual stenosis of the infarction-related vessel. These patients are more likely to be younger and female and are more likely to have single-vessel coronary disease with well-preserved ventricular function.[61] Routine angiography allows the physician to give these patients marked reassurance, because it provides precise definition of the coronary anatomy and because this diagnosis carries a better 1-year prognosis than that of the typical patient with a high-grade residual stenosis.[61]

Second, approximately 15% of patients will have an occluded infarction-related coronary artery and might benefit from delayed balloon angioplasty if late reperfusion proves to be clinically important. Experimental models[62,63] and observational studies[64-67] have suggested that a patent artery may be important in promoting infarct healing and preventing ventricular aneurysm formation and arrhythmias, even when there is

*References 21, 38, 41, 45, 49, 59, 60.

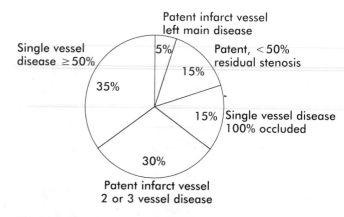

Fig. 33-2. Proportion of patients in each of the five anatomic subsets distinguished after thrombolytic therapy. (Adapted from Topol EJ, Califf RM, George BS, et al: *N Engl J Med* 317:581-588, 1987; TIMI Study Group: *N Engl J Med* 320:618-627, 1989; Topol E: Thrombolytic intervention. In Topol E (ed): *Textbook of interventional cardiology,* Philadelphia, 1989, WB Saunders, pp 76-120; Simoons ML, Betriu A, Col J, et al: *Lancet* 1:197-203, 1988; Topol E, Califf RM, George BS, et al: *Circulation* 77:1100-1107, 1988; Charles E, Rogers W, Reeder G, et al: *J Am Coll Cardiol* 13:152A, 1989.)

little or no opportunity for myocardial salvage. In both the TIMI-II and SWIFT trials,[38,42] patients with persistent total occlusions were categorically excluded from having coronary angioplasty. In the recent TAMI-6 trial,[68] patients seen 6 to 24 hours after pain onset were randomized to receive an intravenous thrombolytic or placebo. All patients underwent angiography within the next 24 hours; at that time, patients with a closed infarct vessel were again eligible for randomization to either late PTCA (34 patients) or no PTCA (37 patients). Late reperfusion with thrombolytic therapy resulted in a higher infarct vessel patency than did placebo (65% vs. 27%), as well as the avoidance of cavity expansion as reflected in the left ventricular end diastolic volume (127 vs. 159 ml). No specific benefit was observed in patients randomized to late PTCA. The authors speculate, however, that the numbers of patients in the late PTCA/no late PTCA arms might not have been large enough to detect clinically important differences between these two groups. In summary, the issue of performing routine catheterization as a possible prelude to late mechanical reperfusion for the failure of thrombolysis will require further study before final conclusions can be made.

Third, 5% of patients have left main stenosis or its equivalent and deserve consideration for prompt bypass surgery; correct diagnosis in this group of patients is thus essential. Although one would hope that noninvasive testing would identify these patients reliably, the limitations of current noninvasive methods (discussed later on) create the potential for such a critical anatomic subset to be missed.

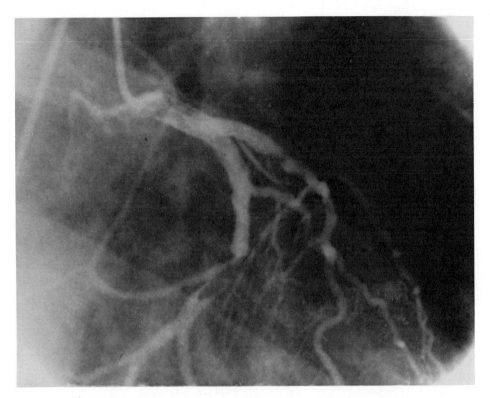

Fig. 33-3. Angiogram of the left coronary artery in the right anterior oblique view in a 44-year-old physician. This patient's first manifestation of coronary disease was an acute inferolateral infarct for which he was given tissue-type plasminogen activator. After complete resolution of his pain, he was transferred to our institution; catheterization revealed the severe stenosis with a large thrombus in the circumflex, as well as the (unexpected) severe stenosis in the proximal left anterior descending. Routine angiography can accurately identify those patients who are candidates for myocardial revascularization, such as this patient with severe multivessel coronary artery disease.

Fourth, approximately 30% of patients have two- or three-vessel coronary artery disease, defined as stenosis of more than 70% in a non–infarct-related vessel. Studies have indicated the serious prognostic implication of this finding[69]; an example of such a patient is illustrated in Fig. 33-3. In the TAMI trials, 236 of 855 patients (27.6%) had multivessel disease and their in-hospital mortality was 11.4% compared with only 4.2% in patients with single-vessel disease.[69] Although regression analysis confirmed that global left ventricular ejection fraction, TIMI-grade infarct vessel flow, and age all correlated with clinical outcome, the strongest independent predictor of in-hospital mortality was the number of diseased vessels. As a consequence, the authors concluded that coronary angiography is the procedure of choice for identifying the patients at highest risk. In a related study, Lee et al.[70] used a regression model based on the TAMI trials[21,23,60] to suggest that with respect to in-hospital mortality, each additional diseased, non–infarct-related vessel is equivalent in prognosis to a 16-year increase in age or a 13-point reduction in ejection fraction. Although uncovering two- or three-vessel dis-

ease does not, in itself, improve prognosis, it certainly may help to determine the patient's risk and lead to closer surveillance during follow-up and to lowering the threshold for recommending angioplasty or bypass surgery. The preferred type of coronary revascularization for such patients after thrombolysis is currently a focus of several randomized trials.[71]

In contrast, the fifth category of patients has an excellent overall prognosis (Fig. 33-2); this group includes the approximately 35% of patients who have single-vessel disease with a residual stenosis of more than 50%. Ellis et al.[72] have shown that the extent of residual stenosis after intravenous thrombolysis does not correlate with likelihood of recurrent ischemic events in the short term. A study by Little et al.[73] extends this observation to longer follow-up. Certainly, an important perspective gained from the TIMI-II and SWIFT trials is that a priori coronary angioplasty is unnecessary in asymptomatic patients with such an inherently low risk.[38,42]

Thus, coronary angiography can accurately identify the nearly 50% of patients who warrant consideration

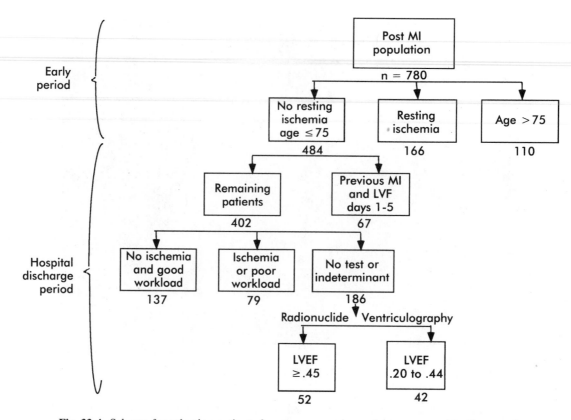

Fig. 33-4. Scheme for selecting patients for coronary angiography as proposed by Ross et al. According to this scheme, stratification during the early period is for patients surviving the first 5 days and eliminates patients 75 years of age or older while identifying patients with resting ischemic pain. Stratification at later times is for patients surviving to hospital discharge. Coronary angiography is recommended for selected groups *(heavy boxes)*. Numbers under the boxes show the distribution of patients in a test population on whom the scheme was applied. Although this strategy, if chosen, would reduce the number of angiograms performed after myocardial infarction *(MI)*, it is important to note that angiography would still be recommended for approximately 55% of patients. The sum of those recommended for catheterization (under the heavy boxes) is $186 + 67 + 79 + 42 = 374$; dividing this by 780 (the initial population) yields 55%. This scheme does not include patients with an ejection fraction of less than 20% or patients who had neither an exercise test nor left ventricular ejection fraction determination. *LVEF,* left ventricular ejection fraction, *LVF,* left ventricular failure. (Modified from Ross J, Gilpin E, Madsen E, et al: *J Am Coll Cardiol* 79:292, 1989. Used by permission.)

for revascularization; when coupled to functional testing, it can reassure both the physician and patient and, as discussed later, potentiate an early discharge and return to work. In addition, data from both the pre-thrombolytic era and recent trials identify clinical variables of patients at particularly high risk after MI. Ross et al.[52] used data from more than 1800 patients to derive a decision scheme for coronary angiography after MI to identify patients at increased risk of death within the first year. According to this analysis, patients less than age 75 years with a history of a prior MI, resting ischemia, left ventricular failure during the initial hospitalization, exercise-induced ischemia or a poor workload, or an ejection fraction of less than 44% all are at significantly increased risk of death in the first year (average mortality 16%). In these patients, the physician

should strongly consider catheterization. However, this scheme still predicts that approximately 55% to 60% of patients will require coronary angiography to complete their risk stratification and does not take into account the economic impact of the additional tests (e.g., radionuclide ventriculography) required in many patients. (Fig. 33-4).

Selective or routine catheterization?

Selective and routine catheterization appear to identify similar proportions of patients who are subsequently referred for bypass surgery. In the TIMI-II and SWIFT trials, 16% and 13%, respectively, of patients had bypass surgery in the conservative arms, whereas 15% in both trials were referred for bypass surgery after randomization to the invasive strategy. Thus, one could argue that

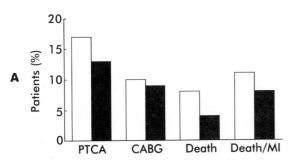
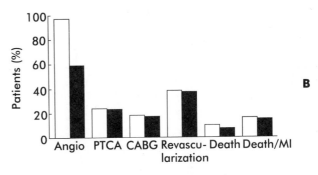

Fig. 33-5. A nonrandomized comparison of the routine (□; n = 197) and selective (■; n = 1461) cardiac catheterization strategies from the TIMI-II trials. **A,** Summary of in-hospital procedures and outcomes. The p values for each are as follows: coronary angioplasty *(PTCA),* p = 0.15; coronary artery bypass surgery *(CABG),* p > 0.2; death, p = 0.013; and death or reinfarction *(MI),* p > 0.2. **B,** Cumulative 1-year follow-up procedure utilization and outcomes. The only significant difference was for angiography *(Angio)* (97% compared with 59%, p > 0.001). *Revasc,* Revascularization. (From TIMI Study Group: *N Engl J Med* 320:618, 1989. Used by permission.)

clinical acumen and noninvasive tests may be sufficient for identifying patients with the most advanced or surgically remediable coronary artery disease.

Using retrospective TIMI-II data, Rogers et al.[38,41,74] compared selective and routine angiography and found that routine angiography provided no benefit. As shown in Fig. 33-5, the TIMI-IIA strategy of predischarge catheterization without angioplasty (197 patients) was compared with the conservative strategy of selective catheterization from TIMI-II (1461 patients). The higher in-hospital mortality of 8% for patients receiving catheterization with no angioplasty compared with 4% for patients receiving selective catheterization (p = 0.01) is difficult to explain given the lack of any clear-cut adverse outcomes associated with the procedure itself. Routine catheterization resulted in no reduction in either acute or 1-year adverse clinical outcomes. Nevertheless, it is noteworthy that the patients enrolled in the TIMI-II trial were a select group and had a considerably lower incidence of multivessel disease compared with patients in studies done in the prethrombolytic era. Patients with prior bypass surgery, severe hypertension, prior cerebrovascular disease, and lack of ST-segment elevation on the admission ECG all were excluded from the trial; these are precisely the groups that would be expected to have a high prevalence of multivessel coronary artery disease. Thus, the conclusions from the TIMI-II trial cannot be applied to these subsets of patients. Furthermore, the physician who recommends a selective approach should remember that 33% of patients in the "conservative" strategy required catheterization during the initial hospitalization and a total of 60% ultimately required catheterization within the year after the index infarction.

NONINVASIVE TESTING AFTER THROMBOLYSIS

The alternative to angiography for risk stratification is noninvasive testing to identify patients with residual ischemia, left ventricular dysfunction, or ventricular dysrhythmias. Angiography could then be performed only in patients selected on the basis of these studies. Whether or not exercise testing serves as the primary method of risk stratification, it can provide data on the physiologic significance of a known coronary stenosis, assess functional capacity, guide the prescription for exercise, and provide for patient reassurance.

Although the merit of stress tests after infarction has been widely recognized in the last decade,[75-77] nearly all reported data are derived from patients who did not have myocardial reperfusion therapy. Studies from the prethrombolytic era that confirm the value of noninvasive testing after completed MI are inapplicable to patients with threatened infarction who are successfully given thrombolytics. Furthermore, it is highly likely that interpretations of functional tests after intravenous thrombolytic therapy, especially when it is successful, will be extremely difficult. For example, a study of regional or global wall motion may give the false impression that function does not worsen during exercise because of the presence of viable but reversibly injured myocardium. Similarly, after successful thrombolysis, perfusion imaging with thallium may not allow reliable diagnosis of viable, noninfarcted tissue; studies to date have shown a poor sensitivity and specificity for noninfarct vessel anatomy.[78]

Recent studies of functional tests after intravenous thrombolysis are summarized in Table 33-3[78-82]; each of these studies has raised concerns about the value of functional testing in patients receiving reperfusion therapy, particularly when compared with the relatively high predictive accuracy of such testing in the prethrombolytic era.[75-77] Chaitman et al.[80] showed that abnormal results on a bicycle ergometry test done before discharge and at 6 weeks after discharge were not predictive of death or reinfarction at 6-month follow-up. Burns et al.[78] correlated the findings of quantitative single-photon

Table 33-3. Functional testing after thrombolysis*

Author	No. of patients	Study design	Test	Major finding
Simoons et al.[79]	533	Streptokinase compared with conventional therapy	Predischarge treadmill exercise	Functional test not predictive of reinfarction or death during 5-yr follow-up
Chaitman et al.[80]	1,958	t-PA, t-PA compared with catheterization and angioplasty (if suitable)	Predischarge and 6-week postdischarge supine bicycle ergometry and electrocardiogram	Functional test not predictive of reinfarction or death during 6-mo follow-up
Burns et al.[78]	47	t-PA compared with placebo	Exercise SPECT; thallium on day 8	Sensitivity of detecting substantial stenosis in the infarction-related vessel, 95%; specificity, 14%; for stenosis of a noninfarction-related vessel: sensitivity, 35%; specificity, 79%
Touchston et al.[81]	21	Streptokinase	Exercise thallium on day 10	Only 25% of patients with preserved regional wall motion have provocable ischemia
Weiss et al.[82]	37	Streptokinase	Exercise-gated blood pool scintigraphy at 7 weeks	46% of patients with early therapy and a significant residual stenosis had a negative test result, correlated with reduced evidence of salvage

From Topol E, Holmes D, Rogers W: Coronary angiography after thrombolytic therapy for acute myocardial infarction, *Ann Intern Med* 114:877-885, 1991.

*SPECT, Single photon emission computed tomography; *t-PA*, tissue-type plasminogen activator.

tomographic thallium scanning and coronary angiography after intravenous thrombolysis; the sensitivity of scintigraphy for diagnosing multivessel disease was only 35%, and specificity for infarction-related vessel disease (>50% stenosis) was 14%. Such levels of sensitivity are unacceptable when used for patient screening. Even if a test had a positive predictive accuracy of 95% for cardiac death within 5 years, such a level may be considered inadequate for an otherwise healthy 45-year-old.

The study with the most extensive follow-up was done by Simoons et al.[79] In 533 patients, event rates during the 5 years after reperfusion therapy were not predicted by a positive functional study. These investigators used a regression model to determine prognostic indices; five factors were key independent predictors of late prognosis: patient age, previous infarction, ejection fraction, the number of diseased coronary vessels, and the severity of residual stenosis in the infarction-related artery. Unlike the first three variables, the last two predictors can be derived only from cardiac catheterization. Furthermore, Sutton and Topol[40] have found that a negative post-thrombolytic exercise stress test correlates best with greater myocardial necrosis rather than with exercise time or hemodynamics, the time delay to reperfusion, or the severity of the infarct vessel stenosis. Paradoxically, inadequate myocardial salvage rather than optimal therapy with no residual ischemia may be the most likely explanation for this test result.

In addition to the fact that functional tests in the reperfusion era have not been adequately validated, many patients cannot perform an exercise test; this is a significant additional problem. In a series of patients treated conventionally during the last decade, the percentage of patients unable to do an exercise test has ranged from 20% to 45%.[75-77] These patients uniformly have a worse prognosis than those who can exercise, with mortality reaching 10% to 15% in the 2 years after infarction.[52,83-86] Furthermore, many studies of functional testing have excluded the elderly, a group with a substantially increased risk following infarction. These limitations of noninvasive testing are summarized in Table 33-4.

An important reason for the lack of validation of functional tests after thrombolysis is the relatively high rate at which coronary revascularization procedures are now done on the basis of provoked ischemia. These revascularization interventions were less widely applied 10 to 15 years ago when most predictive data on

Table 33-4. Some potential limitations of exercise testing/noninvasive risk assessment after myocardial infarction

1. Nearly all reported data are derived from patients who did not have myocardial reperfusion therapy; no study has correlated functional tests and long-term clinical outcome following pharmacologic reperfusion.
2. The testing may not allow diagnosis of viable, noninfarcted tissue.
3. Positive predictive accuracy and sensitivity in detecting multivessel coronary disease are lower than with angiography.
4. Reported series exclude certain subgroups (elderly, patients unable to exercise) that have a high long-term risk of recurrent ischemic events and mortality.
5. Follow-up duration is short in most reported studies; when follow-up is adequate, predictive value falls dramatically.
6. Submaximal testing may not attain sufficient workload to reliably exclude myocardial ischemia.
7. Simple exercise electrocardiographic markers are often difficult to interpret after thrombolysis because of persistent abnormalities.
8. Many patients will nevertheless require coronary angiography.

From De Franco A, Topol E: Invasive strategies in acute myocardial infarction in the elderly, *Cardiol Elderly* 2(3):274-289, 1994, with permission.

predischarge exercise testing were recorded.[73,75-77] In the absence of definitive data, proponents of stress testing conclude that this method of predischarge risk stratification (in combination with an assessment of left ventricular function and clinical evaluation) has been empirically validated based on the observation of an excellent 1-year outcome of "low-risk" patients (those < age 75 years without a history of prior infarction, etc.) in the conservative group of the TIMI-II trial. On the other hand, proponents of routine catheterization maintain that exercise testing is most useful *when coupled to angiography* to determine the physiologic significance of the coronary lesions present.

ECONOMIC CONSIDERATIONS: SELECTIVE VERSUS ROUTINE CATHETERIZATION

One of the major concerns about routine catheterization is cost and resource utilization. One analysis suggested that avoiding 50% of catheterizations and related unnecessary coronary revascularization procedures in the United States could provide a potential savings of more than $700 million yearly (Table 33-5).[49] Charles et al.[74] reported actual economic data from the TIMI-II trial in 310 patients. Although total hospital *charges* were higher for the invasive strategy compared with the conservative strategy ($15,918 compared to $12,588, respectively), the difference in actual hospital *costs* was considerably less ($10,496 compared with $8,826, respectively). Furthermore, follow-up data indi-

Table 33-5. Cost of angiography and coronary revascularization after thrombolysis in the TIMI-II trial*

Procedure	Cost per patient $	Patients No.	Cost $
Catheterization, no angioplasty	1,145	74	85,000
Catheterization, angioplasty	4,408	431	1,900,000
Coronary artery bypass grafts	24,119	5	362,000
TOTAL			2,347,000†

Adapted from Topol E: Mechanical intervention for acute myocardial infarction. In Topol E (ed): *Textbook of interventional cardiology*, Philadelphia; 1989, WB Saunders, p. 269. Used by permission.
*Based on projected excess cost per 1000 patients.
†Assuming that 300,000 patients with myocardial infarction receive intravenous thrombolytic therapy per year, calculations showed a projected annual savings of $704 million. If one did routine (all patients) catheterization and only selective revascularization, the cost would be 300,000 × $1145 = $343.5 million.

cated "a higher frequency of readmissions for angina pectoris during the first year after myocardial infarction, and during these hospitalizations, more than twice as many patients in the selective group underwent coronary arteriography as did patients in the routine catheterization group during the same time interval."[41] An adequate cost comparison of the two strategies would obviously have to include the cost of subsequent hospitalizations and, ideally, time lost from work.

Despite the cost of the procedure itself, a strategy of routine catheterization does not necessarily result in increased total cost; findings during angiography can result in a shortening of the hospital stay and thus in *decreased* cost. In a randomized trial comparing early (day 4) and conventional (day 7-10) hospital discharge, angiography combined with a functional test permitted 20% of patients with MI to be eligible for discharge at day 4.[87] The abbreviated stay was safe and resulted in a 30% reduction in hospital and professional charges ($5000 saved per patient). Translating these charges to costs and assuming a conservative estimate of 15% of patients eligible, the savings from day 4 discharge would be nearly $300 million per year. If one uncouples angiography from coronary angioplasty and performs all the angiograms but only the angioplasty procedures that are strictly indicated, the amount saved by early discharge would substantially offset the $343 million cost of this strategy (see Table 33-4) projected by the TIMI-II investigators.

Moreover, both third-party payers and employers view an early return to work as a desirable result of a complete anatomic and functional assessment and early discharge.[21] Patients with the minimal lesion syndrome or only single-vessel disease are excellent candidates for an early return to work. This pattern was noted in the early discharge trial.[21]

Other economic considerations include the small differences in *actual cost* as opposed to charge data between the invasive (incorporating prophylactic angioplasty) and conservative strategies in TIMI-II,[41,45] the fixed as opposed to variable costs of operating a cardiac catheterization laboratory, the costs of functional tests, and the costs of readmissions. Because of the difficulty in interpreting the ECG in the early days or weeks after MI, thallium scintigraphy is frequently used; in most centers the charge is in excess of $1000. If routine catheterization limits the need for thallium scintigraphy before discharge, at 6 weeks after discharge, or at both times, this may be a trade-off for a savings in cost. Finally, the cost of readmission for subsequent catheterization, particularly in facilities where the procedure is not done on an outpatient basis, is an important factor. As shown in Fig. 33-3, 59% of patients in TIMI-II who were managed using the conservative strategy ultimately underwent cardiac catheterization by 1-year follow-up.[74]

RESOLVING THE DILEMMA: SELECTIVE OR ROUTINE CATHETERIZATION?

No definitive data currently exist to recommend selective or routine cardiac catheterization. The guidelines published by the American College of Cardiology and American Heart Association[88] for managing patients with AMI after thrombolytic therapy do not specifically address this issue. It is essential to separate *diagnostic* angiography, which can be done safely, quickly, and relatively economically, from a *therapeutic* procedure such as coronary angioplasty. As we have discussed, the trials that have peripherally addressed this issue[38,42] compared a "package" of angiography and angioplasty with "no procedure" and analyzed the data using an intention-to-treat principle. Perhaps the best approach would be to use either selective or routine angiography if there is specific fundamental information that can be gained that cannot be determined from noninvasive tests and that may be of value for particular patient subsets. However, studies have not shown that routine predischarge coronary angiography leads to improved survival or lower reinfarction rates when compared with the selective strategy. Ideally, firm recommendations would be based on a randomized trial comparing "angiography with no prophylactic revascularization" with "no angiography"; unfortunately, such a trial is unlikely to be done.

Of note, in March 1990, Medicare disallowed reimbursement for routine cardiac catheterization after thrombolytic intervention in two states (Utah and Nevada). The decision not to support the use of angiography in asymptomatic patients is premature because the data are equivocal. Furthermore, we must emphasize the absolute proscription of revascularization

procedures in patients who undergo angiography but who do not have angina or inducible ischemia. No data support aggressive coronary intervention in these patients; therefore, at the very least, a "look, but don't touch" attitude should be adopted. There is marked geographic variability within the United States in the use of angiography after MI.[89] Such variability suggests that no current "standard of practice" exists. There may be proportionate use where facilities are available and much less utilization of angiography in hospitals without catheterization facilities. Assessment of long-term outcome for samples matched on the basis of demographic factors may provide some insight into the relative value of the liberal and the conservative uses of angiography.

MANAGEMENT OF PATIENTS EXCLUDED FROM THROMBOLYSIS

Despite the dramatic improvements in survival associated with thrombolytic therapy, only an estimated 20% to 30% of patients with AMI receive any thrombolytic regimen.[90-94] Although physicians withhold thrombolytics from many of these patients appropriately (e.g., those with prolonged cardiopulmonary resuscitation, recent major surgery, or stroke), for other unjustifiable and unfortunate reasons, many other patients are also excluded. For example, it is incorrect in routine practice to apply the same exclusionary criteria as in the major trials of thrombolytic therapy, such as age greater than 75 years, prior bypass surgery, previous MI, a remote history of cerebrovascular disease, a history of severe hypertension, and premenopausal status. These criteria were developed for the scientific analysis of the initial thrombolytic trials and should not be used to deny individual patients the benefits of thrombolytic therapy if a risk-benefit analysis is favorable. For example, although the elderly have an increased risk of thrombolytic complications, the potential benefit of therapy (given their otherwise significantly increased mortality) usually outweighs this risk. Retrospective studies suggest that, as a group, patients who are denied or appropriately excluded from thrombolytic therapy have as much as a fivefold increase in mortality in comparison with eligible patients.[95]

Patients undergoing angiography in the prethrombolytic era had a *higher* incidence of severe coronary disease than patients treated with thrombolytics. In three early angiographic studies,[96-98] the incidence of two- or three-vessel disease ranged from 59% to 74% (Fig. 33-6). In contrast, the frequency of two- or three-vessel disease in the TAMI and TIMI trials ranged from 27% to 49%. This difference may result from patient variability with respect to such factors as non–Q-wave infarction among patients in studies antedating thrombolysis, the greater likelihood of multivessel coronary disease in patients with severe hypertension, more advanced age, or any previous cerebrovascular

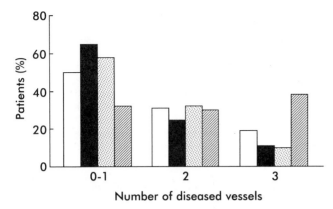

Fig. 33-6. Comparison of angiographic findings in recent reperfusion trials with those in studies done in the era before myocardial reperfusion. □, Mayo Clinic data (From Topol E, Holmes D, Rogers W: Coronary angiography after thrombolytic therapy for acute myocardial infarction, *Ann Intern Med* 114:877-885, 1991, with permission.); ■, the TIMI trial data[41]; ▨, TAMI trial data[46]; ▨, pooled data from studies[59-61] before the era of thrombolysis. The data suggest that when compared with historical controls, patients included in thrombolytic trials have less extensive multivessel coronary disease. (From Topol E, Holmes D, Rogers W: Coronary angiography after thrombolytic therapy for acute myocardial infarction, *Ann Intern Med* 114:877-885, 1991, with permission.)

disease (who would have been excluded from the thrombolytic trials), or the performance of angiography earlier during the natural history of coronary artery disease among patients receiving thrombolytic therapy. Given the higher incidence of multivessel coronary disease in patients ineligible for thrombolytic therapy, the physician should consider early angiography in the appropriate clinical context.

MANAGEMENT OF PATIENTS WITH PREVIOUS BYPASS SURGERY

Although patients with prior bypass surgery and a new, evolving MI are an increasingly common clinical problem, few data are available on the optimal treatment of these patients. In a review of 40 postbypass patients, Kavanaugh and Topol[99] cited several features of these patients that make their diagnosis more difficult and their treatment less likely to be successful. When the patients were first seen, the ECG was diagnostic in only 74% of patients. Overall, the ECG changes were less overt than in patients without prior bypass, with nearly one half lacking 2-mm ST elevation or more. These less dramatic changes may result from the more complex, interdependent collateral flow commonly seen in these patients. In these cases, emergency angiography may be required to confirm the diagnosis of AMI. Second, intravenous thrombolysis is less likely to be successful in this group of patients, perhaps because of the considerably larger clot burden present when the infarct is caused

by an acute occlusion of a vein graft. Thus, current thrombolytic regimens must clearly be improved to offer adequate acute treatment for these patients. Other investigators have suggested acute mechanical revascularization with PTCA[8] or with newer devices (e.g., the transluminal extraction catheter) capable of removing the volume of thrombus present in many acutely occluded vein grafts. Until these trials are complete, no definitive data mandate routine vs. selective catheterization in hemodynamically stable postbypass patients; our current practice is to perform routine catheterization in the absence of overt contraindications.

CONCLUSION

If a functional test could be developed that proved to be highly predictive of subsequent cardiac events, the need for cardiac catheterization described in this chapter would in large part be obviated. Unfortunately, developing such a test may be difficult. Reinfarction and recurrent ischemia after thrombolysis may well be *morphologic events* involving plaque fissuring or thrombosis; these events may not turn out to be predictable via physiologic assessment. Functional testing evaluates only the limitation of myocardial blood flow caused by a coronary lesion; instead, the more relevant question concerns the *stability* of the diseased coronary artery segment. Paradoxically, an even more direct coronary artery visualization with intravascular ultrasonography or angioscopy[100,101] rather than a noninvasive test may help select the patients at highest risk in the future. Furthermore, if newer agents (e.g., platelet fibrinogen receptor blockade and new antithrombin drugs) prove to be beneficial based on characteristics of the culprit lesion in the infarction-related vessel, the role of routine angiography may change significantly.

In the 1980s, thrombolytic therapy gained wide acceptance. Now, in the 1990s, we are confronted with developing the optimal follow-up and long-term care for this new population of patients. More clinical investigation and refinement of our current noninvasive techniques for diagnosing reperfusion or predicting recurrent ischemia will undoubtedly change the role of coronary angiography in the future.

REFERENCES

1. American Heart Association: *1990 heart facts,* Dallas, 1990, American Heart Association.
2. Dwyer E: After the myocardial infarction: a review and approach to risk stratification, *Cardiol Clin* 6:153-163, 1988.
3. Gruppo Italiano per lo Studio della Streptochinasi nell'Infarcto Miocardico: Effectiveness of intravenous thrombolytic treatment in acute myocardial infarction, *Lancet* 1:871-874, 1986.
4. ISIS-2 (Second International Study of Infarct Survival) Collaborative Study Group: Randomized trial of intravenous streptokinase, oral aspirin, both, or neither among 17,187 cases of suspected acute myocardial infarction: ISIS-2, *Lancet* 2:349-360, 1988.

5. AIMS Trial Study Group: Effect of intravenous APSAC on mortality after acute myocardial infarction: preliminary report of a placebo-controlled clinical trial, *Lancet* 85:545-549, 1988.

6. Wilcox RG, Olsson CG, Skene AM, et al: Trial of tissue plasminogen activator for mortality reduction in acute myocardial infarction. Anglo-Scandinavian study of early thrombolysis (AS-SET), *Lancet* 2:525-530, 1988.

7. GUSTO Investigators: An international randomized trial comparing four thrombolytic strategies for acute myocardial infarction, *N Engl J Med* 329:673-682, 1993.

8. O'Keefe JH, Rutherford BD, McConahay DR, et al: Early and late results of coronary angioplasty without antecedent thrombolytic therapy for acute myocardial infarction, *Am J Cardiol* 64:1221-1230, 1989.

9. Rothbaum DA, Linnemeier TJ, Landin RJ, et al: Emergency percutaneous transluminal coronary angioplasty in acute myocardial infarction: a 3 year experience, *J Am Coll Cardiol* 10:264-272, 1987.

10. Ellis SG, O'Neill WW, Bates ER, et al: Coronary angioplasty as primary therapy for acute myocardial infarction 6 to 48 hours after symptom onset: report of an initial experience, *J Am Coll Cardiol* 13:1122-1126, 1989.

11. Prida X, Holland J, Feldman R, et al: Percutaneous transluminal coronary angioplasty in evolving acute myocardial infarction, *Am J Cardiol* 57:1069-1074, 1986.

12. Miller P, Brodie B, Weintraub R, et al: Emergency coronary angioplasty for acute myocardial infarction. Results from a community hospital, *Arch Intern Med* 147:1565-1570, 1987.

13. Topol E: Coronary angioplasty for acute myocardial infarction, *Ann Intern Med* 109:970-980, 1988.

14. Zijlstra F, de Boer MJ, Hoorntje JC, et al: A comparison of immediate coronary angioplasty with intravenous streptokinase in acute myocardial infarction, *N Engl J Med* 328:680-684, 1993.

15. Ribeiro EE, Silva LA, Carneiro R, et al: Randomized trial of direct coronary angioplasty versus intravenous streptokinase in acute myocardial infarction, *J Am Coll Cardiol* 22:376-380, 1993.

16. Gibbons RJ, Holmes DR, Reeder GS, et al: Immediate angioplasty compared with the administration of a thrombolytic agent followed by conservative treatment for myocardial infarction. The Mayo Coronary Care Unit and Catheterization Laboratory Groups [see comments], *N Engl J Med* 328(10):685-691, 1993.

17. Grines CL, Browne KF, Marco J, et al: A comparison of immediate angioplasty with thrombolytic therapy for acute myocardial infarction. The Primary Angioplasty in Myocardial Infarction Study Group, *N Engl J Med* 328:673-679, 1993.

18. DeWood MA: Direct PTCA vs intravenous t-PA in acute myocardial infarction: Results from a prospective randomized trial, *Thrombolysis and Interventional Therapy in Acute Myocardial Infarction* VI George Washington University Pre-AHA Symposium:28-29, 1990.

19. Wall T, Califf R, George B, et al: Accelerated plasminogen activator dose regimens for coronary thrombolysis, *J Am Coll Cardiol* 19:482-489, 1992.

20. Neuhaus K, Feuerer W, Jeep-Teebe S, et al: Improved thrombolysis with a modified dose regimen of recombinant tissue-type plasminogen activator, *J Am Coll Cardiol* 14:1566-1569, 1989.

21. Topol EJ, Califf RM, George BS, et al: A randomized trial of immediate versus delayed elective angioplasty after intravenous tissue plasminogen activator in acute myocardial infarction, *N Engl J Med* 317:581-588, 1987.

22. Topol E, Califf R, Kereiakes D, et al: The Thrombolysis and Angioplasty in Myocardial Infarction (TAMI) trial, *J Am Coll Cardiol* 10:65B-74B, 1987.

23. Topol EJ, George BS, Kereiakes DJ, et al: A randomized controlled trial of intravenous tissue plasminogen activator and early intravenous heparin in acute myocardial infarction, *Circulation* 79:281-286, 1989.

24. Topol E, Califf R, George B, et al: Insights derived from the thrombolysis and angioplasty in myocardial infarction (TAMI) trials, *J Am Coll Cardiol* 12:24A-31A, 1989.

25. Ellis SG, Ribeiro da Silva E, Heyndrickx G, et al: For the RESCUE Investigators. Final results of the randomized RESCUE evaluating PTCA after failed thrombolysis for patients with anterior infarction (abstract), *Circulation* 88:2-106, 1993.

26. Califf RM, O'Neill W, Stack RS, et al: Failure of simple clinical measurements to predict perfusion status after intravenous thrombolysis, *Ann Intern Med* 108:658-662, 1988.

27. Tranchesi B, Verstraete M, Van de Werf F, et al: Usefulness of high-frequency analysis of signal-averaged surface electrocardiograms in acute myocardial infarction before and after coronary thrombolysis for assessing coronary reperfusion, *Am J Cardiol* 66:1196-1198, 1990.

28. Vatterott P, Hammill S, Bailey K, et al: Late potentials on signal-averaged electrocardiograms and patency of the infarct-related artery in survivors of acute myocardial infarction, *J Am Coll Cardiol* 17:330-337, 1991.

29. Seacord L, Abendschein D, Nohara R, et al: Detection of reperfusion within one hour after coronary recanalization by analysis of isoforms of the MM creatine kinase isoenzyme in plasma, *Fibrinolysis* 2:151-156, 1988.

30. Schofer J, Ress-Grigolo G, Voigt K, et al: Early detection of coronary artery patency after thrombolysis by determination of the MM creatine kinase isoforms in patients with acute myocardial infarction, *Am Heart J* 123:846-853, 1992.

31. Christian T, Clements I, Gibbons R: Noninvasive identification of myocardium at risk in patients with acute myocardial infarction and nondiagnostic electrocardiograms with technetium-99 Sestamibi, *Circulation* 83:1615-1620, 1991.

32. Gibbons R: Perfusion imaging with 99mTC-Sestamibi for the assessment of myocardial area at risk and the efficacy of acute treatment in myocardial infarction, *Circulation* 84(suppl 3): I37-I42, 1991.

33. Wackers F: Thrombolytic therapy for myocardial infarction: assessment of efficacy by myocardial perfusion imaging with technetium-99m sestamibi, *Am J Cardiol* 66:36E-41E, 1990.

34. Dellborg M, Riha M, Swedberg K: Dynamic QRS-complex and ST-segment monitoring in acute myocardial infarction during recombinant tissue-type plasminogen activator therapy. The TEAHAT Study Group, *Am J Cardiol* 67:343-349, 1991.

35. Califf R, Topol E, George B, et al: Characteristics and outcome of patients in whom reperfusion with intravenous tissue-type plasminogen activator fails: results of the Thrombolysis and Angioplasty in Myocardial Infarction (TAMI) I trial, *Circulation* 77:1090-1099, 1988.

36. Abbottsmith C, Topol E, George B, et al: Fate of patients with acute myocardial infarction with patency of the infarct-related vessel achieved with successful thrombolysis versus rescue angioplasty, *J Am Coll Cardiol* 16:770-778, 1990.

37. Ohman E, Califf R, Topol E, et al: Consequences of reocclusion after successful reperfusion therapy in acute myocardial infarction, *Circulation* 82:781-791, 1990.

38. TIMI Study Group: Comparison of invasive and conservative strategies after treatment with intravenous tissue plasminogen activator in acute myocardial infarction. Results of the thrombolysis in myocardial infarction (TIMI) phase II trial, *N Engl J Med* 320:618-627, 1989.

39. Muller D, Topol E, Ellis S, et al: Determinants of the need for early acute intervention in patients treated conservatively after thrombolytic therapy for acute myocardial infarction, *J Am Coll Cardiol* 18:1594-1601, 1991.

40. Sutton J, Topol E: The significance of a paradoxical negative

exercise tomographic thallium test in the presence of a critical residual stenosis after thrombolysis for evolving myocardial infarction, *Circulation* 83:1278-1286, 1991.

41. Rogers W, Babb J, Baim D, et al: Selective versus routine predischarge coronary arteriography after therapy with tissue-type plasminogen activator, heparin and aspirin for acute myocardial infarction, *J Am Coll Cardiol* 17:1007-1016, 1991.

42. SWIFT (Should We Intervene Following Thrombolysis?) Trial Study Group: The SWIFT trial of delayed elective intervention versus conservative treatment after thrombolysis with anistreplase in acute myocardial infarction, *Br Med J (Clin Res)* 302:555-560, 1991.

43. Holmes Jr D, Topol E: Reperfusion momentum: lessons from the randomized trials of immediate coronary angioplasty for myocardial infarction, *J Am Coll Cardiol* 14:1572-1578, 1989.

44. Baim DS, Diver DJ, Knatterud GL: PTCA "salvage" for thrombolytic failures—implications from TIMI II-A [abstract], *Circulation* 78:II112, 1988.

45. Rogers W, Babb J, Baim D, et al: Is pre-discharge coronary arteriography beneficial in patients with myocardial infarction treated with thrombolytic therapy? [abstract] *J Am Coll Cardiol* 15:64A, 1990.

46. Sleight P: Do we need to intervene after thrombolysis in acute myocardial infarction? [comment] *Circulation* 81:1707-1709, 1990.

47. Cheitlin M: The aggressive war on acute myocardial infarction: Is the blitzkrieg strategy changing? *JAMA* 260:2894-2896, 1988.

48. Schmidt W, Uebis R, von Essen R, et al: Residual coronary stenosis after thrombolysis with rt-PA or streptokinase: acute results and 3 weeks follow up, *Eur Heart J* 8:1182-1188, 1987.

49. Topol E: Thrombolytic intervention. In Topol E (ed): *Textbook of interventional cardiology,* Philadelphia, 1989, WB Saunders, pp 76-120.

50. Topol EJ, Bates ER, Walton JJ, et al: Community hospital administration of intravenous tissue plasminogen activator in acute myocardial infarction: improved timing, thrombolytic efficacy and ventricular function, *J Am Coll Cardiol* 10:1173-1177, 1987.

51. Dwyer E, McMaster P, Greenberg H, et al: Nonfatal cardiac events and recurrent infarction in the year after acute myocardial infarction, *J Am Coll Cardiol* 4:695-702, 1984.

52. Ross J, Gilpin E, Madsen E, et al: A decision scheme for coronary angiography after acute myocardial infarction, *J Am Coll Cardiol* 79:292-303, 1989.

53. Moss A, DeCamilla J, Davis H, et al: Clinical significance of ventricular ectopic beats in the early post-hospital phase of myocardial infarction, *Am J Cardiol* 39:635-640, 1977.

54. Bigger J, Fleiss J, Kleiger R, et al: The relationships among ventricular arrhythmias, left ventricular dysfunction, and mortality in the two years after myocardial infarction, *Circulation* 69:250-258, 1984.

55. Multicenter Post-Infarction Research Group: Risk stratification and survival after myocardial infarction, *N Engl J Med* 309:331-336, 1983.

56. Kulick D, Rahimtoola S: Is noninvasive risk stratification sufficient, or should all patients undergo cardiac catheterization and angiography after a myocardial infarction? In Cheitlin M (ed): *Dilemmas in clinical cardiology,* Philadelphia, 1990, FA Davis, vol 21, pp 3-25.

57. ISAM: A prospective trial of intravenous streptokinase in acute myocardial infarction (I.S.A.M.), *N Engl J Med* 314:1465-1471, 1986.

58. Gruppo Italiano per lo Studio della Streptochinasi nell'Infarcto Miocardico: Long-term effects of intravenous thrombolysis in acute myocardial infarction: final report of the GISSI study, *Lancet* 8564:871-874, 1987.

59. Simoons ML, Betriu A, Col J, et al: Thrombolysis with tissue plasminogen activator in acute myocardial infarction: no additional benefit from immediate percutaneous coronary angioplasty, *Lancet* 1:197-203, 1988.

60. Topol E, Califf RM, George BS, et al: Coronary arterial thrombolysis with combined infusion of recombinant tissue-type plasminogen activator and urokinase in patients with acute myocardial infarction, *Circulation* 77:1100-1107, 1988.

61. Kereiakes DJ, Topol EJ, George BS, et al: Myocardial infarction with minimal coronary atherosclerosis in the era of thrombolytic reperfusion, *J Am Coll Cardiol* 17:304-312, 1991.

62. Hochman JS, Choo H: Limitation of myocardial infarct expansion by reperfusion independent of myocardial salvage, *Circulation* 75:299-306, 1987.

63. Hale S, Kloner R: Left ventricular topographic alterations in the completely healed rat infarct caused by early and late coronary artery reperfusion, *Am Heart J* 116:1508-1513, 1988.

64. Kersschot IE, Brugada P, Ramentol M, et al: Effects of early reperfusion in acute myocardial infarction on arrhythmias induced by programmed stimulation: a prospective, randomized study, *J Am Coll Cardiol* 7:1234-1242, 1986.

65. Jeremy R, Allman K, Bautovitch G, et al: Patterns of left ventricular dilation during the six months after myocardial infarction, *J Am Coll Cardiol* 13:304-310, 1989.

66. Braunwald E: Myocardial reperfusion, limitation of infarct size, reduction of left ventricular dysfunction, and improved survival. Should the paradigm be expanded? *Circulation* 79:441-444, 1989.

67. Califf R, Topol E, Gersh B: From myocardial salvage to patient salvage in acute myocardial infarction: the role of reperfusion therapy, *J Am Coll Cardiol* 14:1382-1388, 1989.

68. Topol E, Califf R, Vandormael M, et al: A randomized trial of late reperfusion therapy for acute myocardial infarction, *Circulation* 85: 2090-2099, 1992.

69. Muller D, Topol E, Ellis S, et al: Multivessel coronary artery disease: a key predictor of short-term prognosis after reperfusion therapy for acute myocardial infarction, *Am Heart J* 121:1042-1049, 1991.

70. Lee K, Sigmon K, George B, et al: Early and complete reperfusion—a key predictor of survival after thrombolytic therapy [abstract]. *Circulation* 78:II500, 1988.

71. Gersh B, Robertson T: The efficacy of percutaneous transluminal coronary angioplasty (PTCA) in coronary artery disease. Why we need randomized trials. In Topol E (ed): *Textbook of interventional cardiology,* Philadelphia, 1989, WB Saunders, pp 240-253.

72. Ellis SG, Topol EJ, George BS, et al: Recurrent ischemia without warning. Analysis of risk factors for inhospital ischemic events following successful thrombolysis with intravenous tissue plasminogen activator, *Circulation* 80:1159-1165, 1989.

73. Little W, Constantinescu M, Applegate R, et al: Can coronary angiography predict the site of a subsequent myocardial infarction in patients with mild-to-moderate coronary artery disease? *Circulation* 78:1157-1166, 1988.

74. Charles E, Rogers W, Reeder G, et al: Economic advantages of a conservative strategy for acute myocardial infarction management: rt-PA without obligatory PTCA [abstract]. *J Am Coll Cardiol* 13:152A, 1989.

75. American College of Physicians: Evaluation of patients after recent acute myocardial infarction, *Ann Intern Med* 110:485-488, 1989.

76. Theroux P, Waters D, Halphen C, et al: Prognostic value of exercise testing soon after myocardial infarction, *N Engl J Med* 301:341-345, 1979.

77. Hamm L, Crow R, Stull G, et al: Safety and characteristics of exercise testing early after acute myocardial infarction, *Am J Cardiol* 63:1193-1197, 1989.

78. Burns R, Freeman M, Liu P, et al: Limitations of exercise thallium

single photon tomography early after myocardial infarction [abstract], *J Am Coll Cardiol* 13:125A, 1989.

79. Simoons ML, Vos J, Tijssen JG, et al: Long-term benefit of early thrombolytic therapy in patients with acute myocardial infarction: 5 year follow-up of a trial conducted by the Interuniversity Cardiology Institute of The Netherlands, *J Am Coll Cardiol* 14: 1609-1615, 1989.

80. Chaitman B, Younis L, Shaw L, et al: Exercise ECG test results in the TIMI II trial [abstract], *J Am Coll Cardiol* 15:251A, 1989.

81. Touchstone DA, Beller GA, Nygaard TW, et al: Functional significance of predischarge exercise thallium-201 findings following intravenous streptokinase therapy during acute myocardial infarction, *Am Heart J* 116:1500-1507, 1988.

82. Weiss AT, Maddahi J, Shah PK, et al: Exercise-induced ischemia in the streptokinase-reperfused myocardium: relationship to extent of salvaged myocardium and degree of residual coronary stenosis, *Am Heart J* 118:9-16, 1989.

83. Deckers J, Fioretti P, Brower R, et al: Prediction of one year outcome after complicated and uncomplicated myocardial infarction: bayesian analysis of predischarge exercise test results in 300 patients, *Am Heart J* 113:90-95, 1987.

84. Krone R, Gillespie J, Weld F, et al. and the Multicenter Post-Infarction Research Group. Low-level exercise testing after myocardial infarction: Usefulness in enhancing clinical risk stratification, *Circulation* 71: 80-89, 1985.

85. Gibson R, Beller G, Gheorghiade M, et al: The prevalence and clinical significance of residual myocardial ischemia two weeks after uncomplicated non-Q wave infarction: a prospective natural history study, *Circulation* 73:1186-1198, 1986.

86. Krone R, Dwyer E, Greenberg H, et al: Risk stratification in patients with first non-Q wave myocardial infarction: limited value of the early low level exercise test after uncomplicated infarcts, *J Am Coll Cardiol* 14:31-37, 1989.

87. Topol E, Burek K, O'Neill W, et al: A randomized controlled trial of hospital discharge three days after myocardial infarction in the era of reperfusion, *N Engl J Med* 318:1083-1088, 1988.

88. Guidelines for the early management of patients with acute myocardial infarction. A report of the American College of Cardiology/American Heart Association Task Force on Assessment of Diagnostic and Therapeutic Cardiovascular Procedures (Subcommittee to Develop Guidelines for the Early Management of Patients with Acute Myocardial Infarction), *J Am Coll Cardiol* 16:249-292, 1990.

89. Chassin M, Brook R, Park R, et al: Variations in the use of medical and surgical services by the Medicare population, *N Engl J Med* 314:285-290, 1986.

90. Lee T, Weisberg M, Brand D, et al: Candidates for thrombolysis among emergency room patients with acute chest pain, *Ann Intern Med* 110:957-962, 1989.

91. Jagger J, Murray R, Davies M, et al: Eligibility for thrombolytic therapy in acute myocardial infarction, *Lancet* 1:34-35, 1987.

92. Murray N, Lyons J, Layton C, et al: What proportion of patients with myocardial infarction are suitable for thrombolysis? *Br Heart J* 57:144-147, 1987.

93. Doorey A, Michelson E, Weber F, et al: Thrombolytic therapy of acute myocardial infarction: emerging challenges of implementation, *J Am Coll Cardiol* 10:1357-1360, 1987.

94. Hlatky M, Cotugno H, O'Connor C, et al: Adoption of thrombolytic therapy in the management of acute myocardial infarction, *Am J Cardiol* 61:510-514, 1988.

95. Cragg D, Friedman H, Bonema J, et al: Outcome of patients with acute myocardial infarction who are ineligible for thrombolytic therapy, *Ann Intern Med* 115:173-177, 1991.

96. Schulman S, Achuff S, Griffith L, et al: Prognostic cardiac catheterization variables in survivors of acute myocardial infarction: a five year prospective study, *J Am Coll Cardiol* 11:1164-1172, 1988.

97. Turner J, Rogers W, Mantle J, et al: Coronary angiography soon after myocardial infarction, *Chest* 77:58-64, 1980.

98. Betriu A, Castaner A, Sanz G, et al: Angiographic findings 1 month after myocardial infarction: a prospective study of 259 survivors, *Circulation* 65:1099-1105, 1982.

99. Kavanaugh K, Topol E: Acute intervention during myocardial infarction in patients with prior coronary bypass surgery, *Am J Cardiol* 65:924-927, 1991.

100. Siegel R, Ariani M, Fishbein M, et al: Histopathologic validation of angioscopy and intravascular ultrasound, *Circulation* 84:109-117, 1991.

101. Mizuno K, Satomura K, Miyamoto A: Angioscopic evaluation of coronary-artery thrombi in acute coronary syndromes, *N Engl J Med* 326:287-291, 1992.

102. Topol E: Mechanical intervention for acute myocardial infarction. In Topol E(ed): *Textbook of interventional cardiology,* Philadelphia, 1989, WB Saunders, pp 269-299.

Chapter 34

ROLE OF CORONARY ANGIOPLASTY IN ACUTE MYOCARDIAL INFARCTION

Robert D. Simari
Kirk N. Garratt
David R. Holmes, Jr.

The development of coronary angioplasty has revolutionized the care of patients with stable and unstable coronary syndromes. As described by Gruentzig et al.,[1] angioplasty was initially used in patients with stable angina and proximal subtotal coronary artery stenoses. With the development of steerable and lower profile systems and with increasing operator experience, the role of angioplasty has been expanded to include patients with unstable angina, multivessel disease, chronic total occlusions, and saphenous vein graft stenoses. Soon after its introduction, the potential role for coronary angioplasty in acute myocardial infarction (AMI) was considered.[2] The rationale for this was that coronary angioplasty would serve to disrupt the occluding thrombus responsible for the infarction as well as to dilate the underlying atherosclerotic stenosis. Achievement of the latter goal of decreasing the degree of luminal narrowing was thought to decrease the potential for recurrent ischemia.

The role for coronary angioplasty in AMI has evolved simultaneously with the development and use of thrombolytic agents. The optimal role of each of these reperfusion therapies continues to generate considerable controversy. The safety and efficacy of direct coronary angioplasty (without prior thrombolytic therapy) have been established in several large consecutive series by experienced operators.[3-5] Although these studies have typically been focused on the results of clinical practice, a few prospectively designed scientific studies have been completed. The results of a randomized trial of direct coronary angioplasty vs. intracoronary streptokinase have been published,[6] and results of four trials of direct angioplasty vs. intravenous lytic therapy have been reported.[7-10] These studies describe the outcome of a strategy of direct angioplasty in fewer than 1,000 patients. During this same period, more than 100,000 patients worldwide have been enrolled in scientifically controlled randomized trials of thrombolytic therapy for acute myocardial infarction.[11-13] Although controversy remains about the ideal thrombolytic agent and optimal adjunctive therapy, there is no question that thrombolytic therapy results in improved left ventricular function and decreased morbidity and mortality. The decision to proceed with either is often based on the apparent relative risks and benefits associated with the specific therapy. Equally important, the selection of either therapy often depends on the specific institution and physician the patient first chooses.

PATIENT MANAGEMENT IN HOSPITALS WITHOUT CATHETERIZATION FACILITIES

As of 1986,[14] only 19% of the hospitals in the United States had cardiac catheterization facilities. Of these

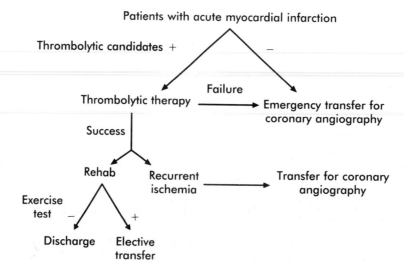

Fig. 34-1. Clinical strategy for the management of acute myocardial infarction in facilities without catheterization facilities.

hospitals, coronary angioplasty was available in two thirds. Because only a subset of these hospitals would have 24-hour capabilities with trained personnel available, the overwhelming majority of institutions lack 24-hour direct angioplasty capability. The clinical strategy for dealing with patients with AMI in these institutions is outlined in Fig. 34-1.

Because by definition these facilities do not have coronary angioplasty capability, for angioplasty to be considered, transfer is required. Emergent or urgent transfer for coronary angioplasty should be considered in four groups during the management of AMI: (1) in patients with contraindications to thrombolytic therapy or patients in whom thrombolysis is not going to be given (e.g., nondiagnostic electrocardiogram [ECG] but strong clinical suspicion of MI); (2) in patients in cardiogenic shock; (3) in patients who fail thrombolytic therapy; and (4) in patients with recurrent ischemia after thrombolytic therapy. Before transfer, patients in the first three categories should be given aspirin and intravenous (IV) heparin to stabilize and perhaps enhance the outcome of subsequent interventions.[15] β-Blockers should also be started if possible.

Transfer for direct coronary angioplasty

Large randomized studies have documented the efficacy and safety of thrombolytic therapy in patients with AMI.[11-13] Thus, given the universal availability of thrombolytic agents, early thrombolysis is essential in patients without contraindications to such therapy. However, depending on the exclusion criteria used, studies have suggested that 60% to 85% of patients with AMI might be excluded from receiving thrombolytic therapy.[16,17] Two large randomized trials using different selection criteria documented that only 37% of patients

met inclusion criteria for thrombolytic therapy.[11,18] Despite ever-expanding inclusion criteria (i.e., age > 75 years, time from onset of pain > 12 hours), a majority of patients will still not receive thrombolytic therapy.

The mortality rates in patients having AMI with clear contraindications to thrombolytic therapy or with non-diagnostic ECGs are five times higher than in eligible patients,[16] and these patients should be considered for emergent transfer to an institution with available catheterization facilities. Transfer should ideally be performed rapidly enough to permit catheterization and angioplasty in a time span 4 hours or less from the onset of chest pain. Air transfer may be necessary to achieve this goal. Patients who are hemodynamically or electrically unstable are ideal candidates for emergency transfer.

Transfer for thrombolytic failure

The identification of patients in whom thrombolytic therapy fails to achieve reperfusion within a time frame that allows for potential myocardial salvage is a major challenge in the management of AMI. Despite the promise of investigational techniques such as on-line ST-segment monitoring[19] and rapid creatine kinase (CK) isoform analysis,[20] simple clinical factors may not be capable of predicting accurately the patency status of the infarct-related artery.[21] Although defining a population that should be transferred to a tertiary hospital for "rescue" coronary angioplasty is difficult, certain guidelines may be applied. Unstable hemodynamics refractory to simple medical therapy should necessitate transfer. Complete resolution of ST-segment elevation is a fairly specific (96%), although infrequent, marker of successful reperfusion and identifies a population that may not require early transfer.[21] Any patient who is determined

Patients with acute myocardial infarctions

In hospital or transfers

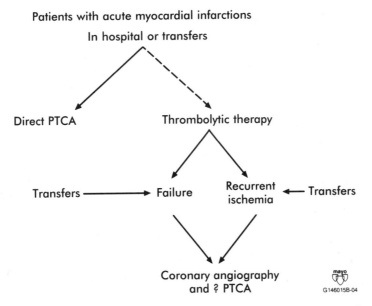

Fig. 34-2. Clinical strategy for the role of coronary angioplasty for acute transmural myocardial infarction in hospitals with 24-hour catheterization facilities.

to be of exceptionally high risk and who would not tolerate the 20% to 50% failure rate of thrombolytic therapy should be transferred. Such patients might include patients with known coronary anatomy and probable occlusion of a vessel supplying greater than two thirds of the viable myocardium.

Transfer for recurrent ischemia

Recurrent ischemia has been reported to occur in 18% to 32% of patients receiving successful thrombolytic therapy for AMI.[22] Although several small retrospective reviews have identified the degree of luminal stenosis as a predictor for early recurrent ischemia,[23-26] a large prospective study failed to correlate such events with angiographic findings.[22] Thus, recurrent ischemia, a common but unpredictable problem, must be dealt with as it occurs. Stabilization, followed by an appropriate method of transfer, is a reasonable strategy.

Submaximal exercise testing before discharge is recommended by recent American College of Cardiology–American Heart Association guidelines.[27] However, assessment of the prognostic power of postinfarction exercise testing was done in the prethrombolytic era.[28-31] Confirmation of the predictive power of postinfarction exercise testing after thrombolysis has not been easily obtained. The high rate of subsequent revascularization procedures and low rate of cardiac events after successful thrombolytic therapy may make prediction difficult.[32] In spite of this controversy, postinfarction exercise testing remains standard practice. Induced ischemia should be viewed as an indication for coronary angiography and possible angioplasty. The role of additional imaging techniques to standard exercise testing has been pre-

sented elsewhere (see Chapters 63 and 64). However, the location and size of the area involved by inducible ischemia may aid the angiographer in determining the suitability of interventional procedures.

PATIENT MANAGEMENT IN HOSPITALS WITH 24-HOUR CATHETERIZATION FACILITIES

The clinical strategy for the role of coronary angioplasty in the management of AMI in a hospital with 24-hour catheterization facilities is outlined in Fig. 34-2. The management of these patients begins in the emergency room. Initial use of aspirin, heparin, and β-blockade, if not contraindicated, is essential. In patients with contraindications to thrombolytic therapy, but also in potential thrombolytic candidates, direct angioplasty remains an important therapeutic option that can be widely applied in these institutions. The only strong contraindications to direct coronary angioplasty are patient unwillingness, an absolute lack of vascular access, or the inability to receive heparin anticoagulants; the latter is clearly a contraindication to thrombolytic therapy as well. Even patients with allergies to contrast media can be treated safely with direct angioplasty.

Direct angioplasty

There is a growing body of information regarding patients who are candidates for either thrombolytic therapy or direct coronary angioplasty. The evidence supporting the safety and efficacy of direct angioplasty originally came from large series by experienced operators[3-5] and has recently been supported by a multicenter registry[33] and small randomized trials.[7-9,11,34] Several series showed more than 90% success rates

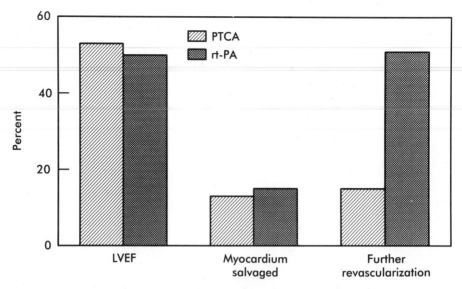

Fig. 34-3. Comparison of outcomes following direct coronary angioplasty or recombinant tissue-type plasminogen activator in acute myocardial infarction—Mayo Clinic trial. (Data from Gibbons RJ, Holmes DR, Reeder GS, et al: *N Engl J Med* 1993; 328:685.)

combined with less than 10% mortality for coronary angioplasty in AMI. In some cases, these series involved a majority of patients considered not to be candidates for thrombolysis.[4] Recently preliminary results from the multicenter Primary Angioplasty Revascularization (PAR) registry have confirmed the safety and efficacy of direct coronary angioplasty.[33] An early small randomized trial of direct coronary angioplasty vs. IV streptokinase by O'Neill et al.[6] showed decreased residual luminal stenoses (43% vs. 83%, P < 0.001) and greater improvement in global left ventricular function in the angioplasty group.

Emerging evidence suggests some benefits of direct coronary angioplasty over thrombolytic therapy. A study of direct coronary angioplasty vs. IV (rt-PA) recombinant tissue-type plasminogen activator in AMI recently completed at the Mayo Clinic demonstrated a similar degree of myocardial salvage and resulting global left ventricular function in each treatment arm (Fig. 34-3).[7] However, 50% of the patients who received thrombolytic therapy required additional mechanical revascularization before discharge compared with only 15% of patients receiving direct coronary angioplasty. Data from this trial also suggest that patency of the infarct-related artery may be achieved more quickly with direct angioplasty than is typically expected with IV thrombolysis.[35] Data from two similar trials of thrombolysis vs. direct coronary angioplasty[8,34] confirmed the impression that the latter is associated with less recurrent ischemia after infarction. The Netherlands trial demonstrated a higher subsequent left ventricular ejection fraction (51% vs. 44%) in patients undergoing direct coronary angioplasty rather than thrombolytic therapy. Thus, in a

hospital with available facilities, direct coronary angioplasty may have benefits over thrombolytic therapy. Because of the large number of patients not suitable for thrombolytic therapy, coronary angioplasty may be applied to a larger number of patients.

Several subgroups of patients may be ideally suited for direct coronary angioplasty. An important group is patients who develop cardiogenic shock in the setting of AMI.

Retrospective studies[36,37] have suggested a survival benefit among patients after successful coronary angioplasty compared with historical series of patients treated medically and in patients in whom angioplasty is unsuccessful.

The high mortality (20%-30%) of elderly patients in the treatment and placebo arms of thrombolytic trials[11,12] has led to the use of direct coronary angioplasty in elderly patients. A preliminary report of the PAR registry[33] has confirmed the safety and efficacy of direct coronary angioplasty in elderly patients found in smaller series.[38,39] Hospital mortality in patients more than 70 years old in the PAR registry was 8% compared with 4% in patients of all ages.

MI after coronary artery bypass grafting is associated with occlusion of a saphenous vein graft in approximately 70% of patients.[40] The success rate of thrombolytic therapy for these patients is not known, because they were excluded from major thrombolytic trials. A series reported by Kahn et al.[40] showed an 85% success rate in direct coronary angioplasty of saphenous vein graft occlusions and an overall hospital mortality of 10%. Because vein grafts are often larger and have lower flow rates than native coronary arteries, the burden of thrombus that they contain may be large.[41] Direct angioplasty with adjunctive intragraft administration of thrombolytic agents may be an effective strategy in this setting.

Patients seen relatively late in the development of AMI may be candidates for direct coronary angioplasty. Although benefits of thrombolytic therapy have been shown up to 24 hours after the onset of chest pain in AMI,[12] late coronary angioplasty may also decrease mortality if successful.[42] However, unsuccessful coronary angioplasty in this setting has been associated with a high hospital mortality: 43% mortality associated with unsuccessful angioplasty compared with 5.5% with successful angioplasty. These findings have not been confirmed in other series.

Patients seen with a clinical syndrome consistent with AMI but who do not have diagnostic ST-segment elevation may also benefit from early cardiac catheterization and coronary angioplasty if appropriate. A prospective[12] study and a retrospective[16] study have documented benefits from thrombolytic therapy in patients with left bundle branch block. Gruppo Italian per lo Studio della Streptochinasi nell'Infarcto Miocardico = 1 (GISSI-1)[11] showed no benefit of streptokinase in this group. Thus, early angiography may be diagnostic in cases of uncertainty and may lead to direct angioplasty.

Immediate angioplasty

Three large prospective randomized trials have compared the strategies of immediate coronary angiography and angioplasty after successful thrombolytic therapy vs. more conservative approaches.[43-45] In each case, immediate cardiac catheterization was associated with a greater risk of significant bleeding and need for bypass surgery and in one study increased mortality without a demonstrable improvement in left ventricular function. However, these were studies of routine cardiac catheterization and coronary angioplasty after thrombolytic therapy and not studies of a "rescue" strategy for failed thrombolytic therapy.

"Rescue" angioplasty

Data from major thrombolytic trials suggest that a large number of patients may have need for "rescue" angioplasty. Thrombolytic therapy has yielded variable rates of reperfusion ranging from 55% to 85%, depending on the agent and route used, the time to treatment, and the time of patency assessment. In patients in whom the infarct-related artery has failed to reperfuse, hospital mortality is increased.[46,47] These patients may benefit from rescue angioplasty. Unfortunately, as previously discussed, the identification of these patients is fraught with difficulty. A practical approach to this problem is based on two guidelines. First, one should not assume that an infarct-related artery has been reperfused in high-risk patients without clear clinical signs (resolution of ST-segment elevation, hemodynamic stability, and relief of chest pain). Second, urgent angiography should be performed in the patient with persisting signs or symptoms of myocardial ischemia as a diagnostic procedure without necessarily coupling it with coronary angioplasty.

Rescue angioplasty has been shown to be a safe and efficacious way to achieve reperfusion after failed thrombolysis.[48-50] Although the clinical outcomes after successful rescue angioplasty approximate those after successful thrombolytic therapy, unsuccessful rescue angioplasty is associated with increased mortality rates (39% vs. 6%).[48] Some have suggested that rescue angioplasty is more effective after combination lytic therapy (urokinase and rt-PA) rather than after treatment with rt-PA alone.[51]

The Thrombolysis and Angioplasty in Myocardial Infarction-V (TAMI-V) Trial[52] randomized patients to one of three thrombolytic regimens and to either immediate catheterization with coronary angioplasty for failed thrombolysis (Thrombolysis in Myocardial Infarction [TIMI] Trial grade flow 0 or 1) or predischarge catheterization. The aggressive strategy was associated with slightly higher predischarge patency rates (94 vs. 90%, $P = 0.065$) and improved wall motion in the infarct region. These benefits were obtained without significant increase in the use of blood products. However, TAMI-V was not a trial of rescue angioplasty because it did not randomize patients with failed thrombolysis to either angioplasty or conservative therapy. The ongoing Randomized Evaluation of Salvage Angioplasty with Combined Utilization of Endpoints (RESCUE) Trial will address this issue. Rescue angioplasty of right coronary artery occlusions has been associated with a greater incidence of adverse effects (heart block, bradycardia, etc.) than left coronary artery lesions.[48,53]

Elective angioplasty

Elective coronary angiography and angioplasty, if necessary, are indicated in the patient with recurrent ischemia after initially successful thrombolytic therapy. Because patients with clinically successful lytic therapy often still have severe residual coronary narrowings and unstable plaque morphologies, use of standard noninvasive tests to stratify patients after thrombolysis is reasonable. As mentioned, the full utility of exercise studies that use radionuclides or echocardiography to image the heart is uncertain in patients after MI and thrombolysis. It seems reasonable to use standard ECG evidence of ischemia during submaximal exercise testing to identify those patients who should undergo diagnostic angiography after an uncomplicated MI treated with lytic therapy. This approach would appear to have merit

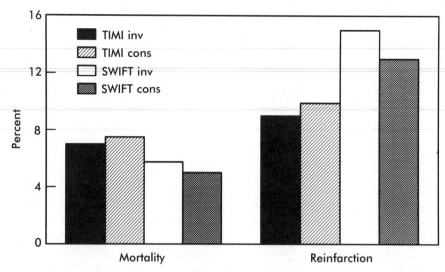

Fig. 34-4. Comparison of 1-year event rates after prophylactic coronary angioplasty after myocardial infarction—SWIFT vs. TIMI-II. (From SWIFT (Should We Intervene Following Thrombolysis) Trial Study Group: *Br Med J (Clin Res)* 302;555, 1991; Williams D, Braunwald E, Knatterud G, et al: *Circulation* 85:533, 1992.)

from a purely diagnostic and prognostic perspective, because the extent of coronary artery disease has important prognostic implications after MI. Ventriculography should also be performed, because definition of left ventricular function has great prognostic importance as well. The strategy of performing coronary angioplasty as a prophylactic measure to prevent subsequent ischemia after thrombolytic therapy has been tested in two large randomized trials.[54-56] Neither study demonstrated a benefit in left ventricular function, reinfarction, or mortality at 1 year with prophylactic coronary angioplasty (Fig. 34-4). However, both demonstrated a significant decrease in recurrent ischemia after infarction. Therefore, coronary angiography should be performed when there is spontaneous or exercise-induced ischemia after thrombolytic therapy, and angioplasty should be considered to minimize subsequent ischemic symptoms.

Evidence is emerging suggesting that ventricular function may improve with angioplasty after MI without evidence of ischemia. Montalescot et al.[57] demonstrated that successful angioplasty of the infarct-related artery in patients with Q-wave MI and without residual ischemia improved regional wall motion. Others[58] have shown that this improvement appears to be associated with the presence of collateral flow within the infarct zone. Although intriguing, these have been small studies, and this strategy has not been supported in larger-scale trials.

TECHNICAL CONSIDERATIONS (TABLE 34-1)

The goal of coronary angioplasty in AMI is rapid, safe reperfusion of the infarct-related artery. Angioplasty of other, even "significant" lesions should not be attempted unless dilation of the infarct-related artery and nonin-

Table 34-1. Adjuncts to coronary angioplasty for acute myocardial infarction

Always indicated
  Heparin
  Aspirin
When necessary
  Mechanical ventilation
  Mechanical cardiovascular support
    Intraaortic balloon counterpulsation
    Peripheral cardiopulmonary bypass
  Temporary pacemaker
  Pulmonary artery catheter
  Thrombolytic agents
  Antiplatelet agents (dextran, dipyridamole)
  Intracoronary devices (atherectomy, autoperfusion balloons)
Investigational
  Antiplatelet agents (IIB/IIIA receptor antibodies)
  Antithrombin agents (hirudin and analogues)
  Reperfusion pharmaceuticals (adenosine, perfluorochemicals, thromboxane inhibitors, superoxide dismutase)
  Mechanical devices (stents, lasers)

terventional support fail to stabilize the patient. The use of additional heparin, with an initial bolus of 10 to 15,000 units before dilation, and maintenance of an activated clotting time (ACT) of approximately 300 seconds are recommended. It is imperative to anticipate complications and take pre-emptive steps to ensure that the patient does not become unstable. If bradycardia or heart block are present, femoral venous access should be obtained and a transvenous pacemaker placed. Mechanical ventilatory support should be employed in patients with hypoxia, hypercarbia, or acidosis secondary to pulmonary edema before the patient has a chance to progress to the stage of respiratory arrest.

Arterial access should ideally be obtained via a femoral artery. If no femoral access is available, a brachial cutdown should be rapidly performed. In unstable patients, a contralateral femoral arterial sheath should be placed to facilitate rapid deployment of an intraaortic balloon pump if necessary. In our laboratory, routine monitoring of pulmonary artery wedge pressures is not performed. However, before initial coronary angiography, the left ventricular end diastolic pressure is measured. In the setting of relative systemic hypotension and elevated left ventricular filling pressures, an intraaortic balloon pump and Swan-Ganz catheter are placed even in a patient who appears stable.

Coronary angiography of the vessel least likely to be occluded is performed initially, followed by the other coronary arteries. Left ventriculography is usually delayed until after angioplasty to reduce the contrast load in patients who become hemodynamically unstable during the procedure (and may be at increased risk for acute tubular necrosis) and to prevent aggravation of hemodynamic instability. Occasionally ventriculography is used to help identify the infarct-related artery in the setting of multivessel disease. Confirming the early impression of Meyer et al.,[59] who suggested that coronary angioplasty for AMI was technically "much easier" than for patients with chronic stable angina, direct coronary angioplasty by experienced operators can be very successful. However, the management of intraluminal thrombus, reocclusion, and embolism can be challenging.

Before the patient leaves the catheterization laboratory, the arterial sheath is sewn into place after confirmation of therapeutic anticoagulation by activated clotting time (ACT). The patient is then transferred to the coronary care unit with a continuous IV infusion of heparin. Usually the heparin infusion is stopped 12 to 24 hours after the procedure and the ACT monitored until less than 180 seconds, at which time the sheath is removed with manual compression. The heparin may be restarted 4 hours later without a bolus or 8 hours later with an additional bolus. If at any time arterial hemorrhage or pseudoaneurysm is noted at the arterial puncture site, the heparin infusion should be reduced or stopped. Otherwise, heparin is usually continued an additional 24 to 48 hours after sheath removal. Because discontinuation of heparin may be temporally related to delayed vessel closure after coronary angioplasty, some operators advocate maintenance of IV heparin until the patient is fully ambulatory and then subcutaneous heparin until hospital discharge. Lifelong aspirin therapy is usually indicated, and some form of vasodilator therapy (e.g., nitroglycerin) should be used for at least 24 to 48 hours after dilation. The role of coumadin is still unsettled.

SPECIAL CHALLENGES
Reperfusion response

Coronary angioplasty for AMI is associated with unique challenges. Sudden coronary reperfusion and the thrombus burden involved are central to these challenges. Hemodynamic and electrical lability is common in myocardial MI. Although the differential characteristics of anterior and inferior wall infarction are well known, reperfusion of these zones can lead to additional hemodynamic or electrical compromise. This seems to be most significant with occlusions of the right coronary artery[40,48,50] in which reperfusion with either lytic therapy or balloon intervention can result in profound hemodynamic disturbances. Severe and occasionally prolonged hypotension occurs commonly on reperfusion of an infarcting inferior wall and may require the use of IV pressor agents or an intraaortic balloon pump. Both bradyarrhythmias and tachyarrhythmias occur frequently in this setting and may necessitate initiation of IV antiarrhythmic agents, atropine, temporary pacing, or defibrillation.

The underlying cause of these problems is not entirely clear. It seems to be at least partially related to the enriched parasympathetic innervation of the posterior left ventricular wall.[60] In addition, reperfusion of profoundly ischemic tissues may result in accelerated myocyte necrosis[61] or may be associated with a prolonged postischemic contraction abnormality labeled myocardial "stunning."[62,63] This apparent paradox has led to the concept that uncontrolled reperfusion of an acutely ischemic myocardial tissue bed may be deleterious, that is, may result in "reperfusion injury."

Reperfusion injury is currently believed to be the result of lipid peroxidation by oxygen-derived free radicals and calcium overload leading to cellular membrane damage and relative calcium insensitivity of the mechanisms of contraction.[61] Although some investigators have argued that little free oxygen is available during ischemia and that intrinsic free radical scavengers are abundant,[64] there is now a wealth of indirect and some direct evidence that oxygen radical formation occurs during ischemia. Electron paramagnetic resonance spectroscopy has demonstrated extremely short-lived oxygen radical formation with apparent binding to lipids and indicates that radical species are operative during the postischemic phase.[65,66] These oxygen radicals may be derived from neutrophils, which have been demonstrated to accumulate along the borders of ischemic tissues after reperfusion.[67] Oxygen radicals may also be the metabolic by-products of ischemic metabolism. In animal studies, treatment with free radical scavenger agents or drugs that block free radical generation has attenuated reperfusion injury.[68,69] This suggests that it may be possible to prevent necrosis of ischemic myocardium if reperfusion is accomplished in a manner that allows delivery of drugs before whole blood reperfusion to the ischemic zone. Currently this may be reliably accomplished only with acute bypass surgery and use of specialized cardioplegic solutions.[70] However, percutaneous methods for early drug delivery into profoundly ischemic myocardial beds may be developed in the future.

Persistent thrombus

It is now clear that intracoronary thrombus is responsible for the overwhelming majority of AMIs, and it is equally clear that the angiographic presence of thrombus is a risk factor for balloon angioplasty complications. Therefore, when one is undertaking balloon dilation in the setting of AMI, every effort should be made to minimize the tendency to further thrombosis. The use of high-dose heparin therapy and aspirin is now routine. The adjunctive use of additional platelet inhibitors, primarily dipyridamole and dextran 40, is routine in some laboratories, although few data are available to suggest these drugs have significant efficacy in this setting.

It is very likely that a new generation of superior thrombin inhibitors will be clinically available soon. Synthetic inhibitors are under study.[34,71,72] Although some appear to be highly effective in inhibiting thrombin, toxic side effects have been observed. Hirudin is a low-molecular-weight, naturally occurring inhibitor of thrombin found in the saliva of the European leech.[73] This agent can now be manufactured in large quantity by use of recombinant DNA technologies. In animal studies, hirudin has been significantly more effective than heparin plus aspirin in reducing fibrinogen and platelet deposition over arterial segments injured with balloon angioplasty[74] or into which stainless steel endovascular stents have been placed.[75] A comparison of IV hirudin with standard anticoagulant and antiplatelet therapies during balloon dilation is currently underway (TAMI-VII).

The complex process of thrombosis involves the interaction of plasma proteins, tissue elements, and platelets. Heparin is effective in interrupting thrombosis by inactivating serum proteinases required for conversion of coagulation factors from an inactive to an active form. Hirudin works by directly inhibiting the central activated clotting factor, thrombin. Other agents, such as ticlopidine[76] and antibodies to platelet receptors IIB/IIIA,[77] may be useful adjuncts in thrombus inhibition by reducing platelet adhesion or aggregation.

In addition to drug therapies, some mechanical approaches may be useful in overcoming persistent thrombus. A laser balloon catheter has been developed that can deliver laser energy in a diffuse manner over the arterial segment covered by the inflated balloon.[78] The local heat generated is highly effective in desiccating

thrombus and appears successful in restoring patency in occluded vessels. However, because of a very high rate of restenosis associated with this device, its development has been discontinued. Direct laser irradiation can ablate thrombus,[79] but continuous wave lasers create significant thermal injury to adjacent tissues.[80] Pulsed dye lasers are effective in thrombus ablation with minimal thermal injury.[81]

Prolonged balloon inflations may be useful in this setting,[82] although the mechanism of this approach is unclear. Prolonged balloon inflations are more likely to have an impact on vessel wall morphology than on intraluminal thrombus, and because some local blood stasis is probably attendant with any balloon inflation (including autoperfusion balloons), such an approach might be detrimental. Nonetheless, a recent review of therapies for abrupt closure after percutaneous transluminal coronary angioplasty indicated that prolonged balloon inflations were associated with a fourfold to fivefold increase in the probability of restoring normal blood flow.[83]

Direct extraction of thrombus from within occluded vessels may be useful in reducing the thrombus load to a sufficient degree that conventional techniques are then successful in treating the lesion. Mechanical thrombectomy by simple aspiration of thrombus has been reported[84] but may have limited utility because of the difficulty in extracting thrombus from any arterial segment other than the proximal coronary, the substantial amount of residual thrombus after the maneuver, and the risk of accidental release of the thrombus at the coronary ostium that could result in a catastrophic peripheral embolic event. Several new devices utilizing ultrasonic energy, microwave energy, and hydraulic energy are currently under study that may be useful in reducing intraluminal thrombus.

The use of directional atherectomy is attractive in the treatment of thrombotic lesions inasmuch as both the intraluminal thrombus and the underlying disruptive plaque may be removed, theoretically substantially reducing the risk of recurrent thrombus. Preliminary reports suggest that this approach may be effective.[85] Intravascular stents might be contraindicated in highly thrombotic segments except to the degree that they improve laminar flow through a disrupted segment and thereby reduce the propensity for thrombus generation. The use of adjunctive anticoagulant drugs and, perhaps, novel stent coatings or new stent materials may significantly reduce the thrombogenic potential of these devices.

No-reflow phenomenon

Occasionally an occlusive lesion is successfully dilated, but blood flow through the distal arterial segment appears to be persistently slow. This angiographic observation is sometimes referred to as the no-reflow phenomenon. This phenomenon has also been observed after the use of certain atherectomy devices.

The cause of the no-reflow phenomenon is unclear, but there are likely many contributing elements. As mentioned, prolonged ischemia apparently results in binding of oxygen radicals to lipids. This may result in membrane derangements which, on reperfusion, manifest as profound endothelial edema.[86] Although arteriographically not evident, edema in the capillary beds may be sufficient to reduce blood flow. In addition, the aggregation of circulating neutrophils in capillary beds may result in microvascular plugging.[87] In this regard, it is possible that administration of some antiinflammatory drugs may reduce the no-reflow phenomenon. For instance, prostaglandin E_1 can limit postischemic injury by many mechanisms, including inhibition of superoxide production by neutrophils and through cellular membrane stabilizing and cytoprotective mechanisms.[88] Adenosine also appears to have powerful inhibitory effects on oxygen free radical release and platelet aggregation, suggesting that exogenous adenosine administration may help preserve endothelial cell function and microvascular perfusion after ischemia.[89]

In the case of atherectomy devices, no reflow may be related to particulate embolization. The rotablator device is an atherectomy tool that can pulverize atheromatous lesions into extremely small particles.[90] If a large amount of atheroma is treated at one time with this device, the large volume of resulting particulate debris may cause microvascular plugging in the distal capillary beds. This complication might therefore be avoided by use of very small ablation burrs initially, with serial increases in burr size until a final desired lumen is achieved.

Complications related to use of thrombolytics

There is a well-documented risk of cerebrovascular accident with use of lytic therapy. Among patients who subsequently undergo emergent catheterization, it is often difficult to determine if a cerebrovascular accident is related to the drug or the catheterization procedure. In any case, there is clearly a risk of hemorrhagic stroke from a catheter-related cerebroembolic event when lytic agents have been used.

The femoral arterial sheath placed at the time of diagnostic angiography or balloon angioplasty must remain in place in patients who have received lytic therapy or who have been treated with high-dose anticoagulants until such time as their coagulation parameters permit safe removal of the sheath. This commonly requires patients to lie flat with an arterial sheath in place for 12 to 24 hours, and on occasion, the duration is much longer. Given the difficulty in the patient laying perfectly still, it should be apparent that

Table 34-2. Incidence of bleeding complications related to combined use of thrombolysis and immediate coronary angioplasty

	%
Total bleeding	40
Local	30
Intracranial	0.5-1.0
Gastrointestinal	3-5
Requiring transfusions	10-20

Adapted from Simoons M, Arnold AER, Betriu A, et al: *Lancet* 1:197-203, 1988; TIMI Study Group: *JAMA* 260:2849-2858, 1988; Topol E, Califf R, George B, et al: *N Engl J Med* 317:581-588, 1987.

this strategy carries a risk of significant femoral arterial bleeding even when the sheath is left in place. The risk of a significant bleed (i.e., one requiring blood transfusion or surgical intervention) is estimated at 10% to 20% (Table 34-2) among patients undergoing catheterization and concomitant lytic therapy. All patients requiring placement of a large-caliber arterial sheath during lytic therapy must be followed in an intensive care setting to optimize nursing care, must have frequent inspections made of the catheterization site, and should be evaluated by a vascular surgeon at the earliest sign of significant bleeding complications (see Chapter 56).

Recently a new therapy for the treatment of femoral pseudoaneurysms has emerged. Although ultrasound imaging has been widely used to identify pseudoaneurysms, several centers are now using ultrasound guided external compression of the "neck" of the pseudoaneurysm therapeutically. Small series have documented promising results.[91] Nonsurgical options for therapy of arterial complications might lead to significant decreases in the morbidity and mortality of interventional procedures.

CONCLUSION

The goal of reperfusion therapy in AMI is restoration of flow. By restoration of flow, there is the potential for the limitation of infarct size and salvage of myocardium; restoration of patency can also facilitate healing and remodeling, which has important long-term implications. In achievement of these goals, coronary angioplasty plays a number of valuable roles. Given that success rates for direct coronary angioplasty are high and there is documented myocardial salvage, dilation can be used as primary therapy if personnel and facilities are immediately available. This is particularly important in patients with hemodynamic compromise, those in whom contraindication to thrombolytic therapy exists, or those in whom thrombolytic therapy is not going to be administered. In addition, taking the patient for urgent *angiography* allows assessment of the severity and extent of coronary artery disease and may improve triage and selection of subsequent therapies such as coronary bypass graft surgery. Coronary angioplasty also plays an important role in the patient after thrombolytic therapy. It can be used when thrombolytic therapy fails, which occurs in up to 25% of patients. In this setting, success rates of rescue dilation are decreased. A successful procedure, however, results in improved short-term outcome. Finally, coronary angioplasty can be used to treat recurrent ischemia, a relatively common occurrence regardless of which specific thrombolytic agent is selected for use.

REFERENCES

1. Gruntzig AR, Senning A, Siegenthaler WE: Nonoperative dilatation of coronary artery stenosis: percutaneous transluminal coronary angioplasty, *N Engl J Med* 301:61-68, 1979.
2. Swan HJC: Thrombolysis in acute myocardial infarction: treatment of underlying coronary artery disease, *Circulation* 66:914-916, 1982.
3. Holmes D, Smith H, Vlietstra R, et al: Percutaneous transluminal coronary angioplasty, alone or in combination with streptokinase therapy, during acute myocardial infarction, *Mayo Clin Proc* 60:449-456, 1985.
4. O'Keefe JH, Rutherford BD, McConahay DR, et al: Early and late results of coronary angioplasty without antecedent thrombolytic therapy for acute myocardial infarction, *Am J Cardiol* 64:1221-1230, 1989.
5. Rothbaum DA, Linnemeier TJ, Landin RJ, et al: Emergency percutaneous transluminal coronary angioplasty in acute myocardial infarction: a 3 year experience, *J Am Coll Cardiol* 10:264-272, 1987.
6. O'Neill W, Timmis G, Bourdillon P, et al: A prospective randomized clinical trial of intracoronary streptokinase versus coronary angioplasty for acute myocardial infarction, *N Engl J Med* 314:812-818, 1986.
7. Gibbons RJ, Holmes DR, Reeder GS, et al: Immediate angioplasty compared with the administration of a thrombolytic agent followed by conservative treatment for myocardial infarction, *N Engl J Med* 328:685-691, 1993.
8. Grines CL, Browne KF, Marco J, et al: A comparison of immediate angioplasty with thrombolytic therapy for acute myocardial infarction. The Primary Angioplasty in Myocardial Infarction Study Group, *N Engl J Med* 328:673-679, 1993.
9. Ribiero A, Silva L, Carneiro R, et al: A randomized trial of direct PTCA vs intravenous streptokinase in acute myocardial infarction, *J Am Coll Cardiol* 17 (suppl A):152, 1991.
10. Zijlstra F, de Boer MJ, Hoorntje JC, et al: A comparison of immediate coronary angioplasty with intravenous streptokinase in acute myocardial infarction, *N Engl J Med* 328:680-684, 1993.
11. Gruppo Italiano per lo Studio della Streptochinasi nell'Infarto Miocardio: Effectiveness of intravenous thrombolytic treatment in acute myocardial infarction, *Lancet* 1:397-402, 1986.
12. ISIS-2 (Second International Study of Infarct Survival) Collaborative Group: Randomized trial of intravenous streptokinase, oral aspirin, both or neither among 17,187 cases of suspected acute myocardial infarction: ISIS-2, *Lancet* 2:349-360, 1988.
13. I.S.A.M. Study Group: A prospective trial of intravenous streptokinase in acute myocardial infarction (ISAM): mortality and infarct size at 21 days, *N Engl J Med* 314:1465-1471, 1986.
14. Topol EJ, Bates ER, Walton JA, et al: Community hospital administration of intravenous tissue plasminogen activator in acute myocardial infarction: improved timing, thrombolytic efficacy and ventricular function, *J Am Coll Cardiol* 10:1173-1177, 1987.
15. Douglas JS, Lutz JF, Clements SD, et al: Therapy of large intracoronary thrombi and candidates for percutaneous transluminal coronary angioplasty, *J Am Coll Cardiol* 11:238A, 1988.
16. Cragg DR, Friedman HZ, Bonema JD, et al: Outcome of patients with acute myocardial infarction who are ineligible for thrombolytic therapy, *Ann Intern Med* 115:173-177, 1991.
17. Lee TH, Weinberg MC, Brand DA, et al: Candidates for thrombolysis among emergency room patients with chest pain, *Ann Intern Med* 110:957-962, 1989.
18. Wilcox RG, von der Lippe G, Olson CG, et al: Trial of tPA for mortality reduction in acute myocardial infarction, *Lancet* 2:525-530, 1988.
19. Delborg M, Swedberg K: Dynamic QRS-complex and ST segment vectocardiographic monitoring in acute myocardial infarction, *Circulation* 80(suppl II):II355, 1989.
20. Seacord L, Abendschein D, Nohara R, et al: Detection of reperfusion within 1 hour after coronary recanalization by analysis of isoforms of the MM creatine kinase isoenzyme in plasma, *Fibrinolysis* 2:151-156, 1988.
21. Califf R, O'Neill W, Stack R, et al: Failure of simple clinical measurements to predict perfusion status after intravenous thrombolysis, *Ann Intern Med* 108:658-662, 1988.
22. Ellis SG, Topol EJ, George BS, et al: Recurrent ischemia without warning: analysis of risk factors for in-hospital ischemic events following successful thrombolysis with intravenous tissue plasminogen activator, *Circulation* 80:1159-1165, 1989.
23. Badger RS, Brown BG, Kennedy JW, et al: Usefulness of recanalization to luminal diameter of 0.6 mm or more with intracoronary streptokinase during acute myocardial infarction in predicting "normal" perfusion status, continued patency and survival at one year, *Am J Cardiol* 59:519-522, 1987.
24. Gash AK, Spann JF, Sherry S, et al: Factors influencing reocclusion after coronary thrombolysis for acute myocardial infarction, *Am J Cardiol* 57:175-177, 1986.
25. Harrison DG, Ferguson DW, Collins SM, et al: Rethrombosis after reperfusion with streptokinase: importance of geometry of residual lesions, *Circulation* 69:991-999, 1984.
26. Serruys PW, Wijns W, Van den Brand M, et al: Is transluminal coronary angioplasty mandatory after successful thrombolysis? Quantitative coronary angiographic study, *Br Heart J* 50:257-265, 1983.
27. Gunnar RM, Bourdillon PD, Divon DW, et al: Guidelines for the early management of patients with acute myocardial infarction, *J Am Coll Cardiol* 16:249-292, 1990.
28. American College of Physicians: Evaluation of patients after recent acute myocardial infarction, *Ann Intern Med* 110:485-488, 1989.
29. Cleempoel H, Vainsel H, Dramaix M, et al: Limitations on the prognostic value of predischarge data after myocardial infarction, *Br Heart J* 60:98-103, 1988.
30. Hamm LF, Crow RS, Stull GA, et al: Safety and characteristics of exercise testing early after acute myocardial infarction, *Am J Cardiol* 63:1193-1197, 1989.
31. Theroux P, Waters DD, Halphen C, et al: Prognostic value of exercise testing soon after myocardial infarction, *N Engl J Med* 301:341-345, 1979.
32. Topol EJ, Holmes DR, Rogers WJ: Coronary angiography after thrombolytic therapy for acute myocardial infarction, *Ann Intern Med* 114:877-885, 1991.
33. O'Neill W, Brodie B, Knopf W, et al: Initial report of the Primary Angioplasty Revascularization (PAR) registry. *Circulation* 84 (suppl II):II536, 1991.
34. Yasuda T, Gold HK, Yaoita H, et al: Comparative effects of aspirin, a synthetic thrombin inhibitor and a monoclonal antiplatelet glycoprotein-IIb/IIIa antibody on coronary artery reperfusion, reocclusion and bleeding with recombinant tissue-type plasmino-

gen activator in a canine preparation, *J Am Coll Cardiol* 16:714-722, 1990.

35. Berger PB, Bell MR, Holmes DR, et al: Comparison of time to therapy and reperfusion rates with direct PTCA and thrombolysis in acute myocardial infarction: results of the Mayo Clinic randomized trial of PTCA and rt-PA, *J Am Coll Cardiol* 19(suppl A):136A, 1992.

36. Hibbard MD, Holmes DR, Bailey KR, et al: Percutaneous transluminal coronary angioplasty in patients with cardiogenic shock, *J Am Coll Cardiol* 19:639-646, 1992.

37. Lee L, Erbel R, Brown T, et al: Multicenter registry of angioplasty therapy of cardiogenic shock: initial and long term survival, *J Am Coll Cardiol* 17:599-603, 1991.

38. Holland KJ, O'Neill WW, Bates ER, et al: Emergency percutaneous transluminal coronary angioplasty during acute myocardial infarction for patients more than 70 years of age, *Am J Cardiol* 63:399-403, 1989.

39. Lee TC, Laramee LA, Rutherford BD, et al: Emergency percutaneous transluminal coronary angioplasty for acute myocardial infarction in patients 70 years of age and older, *Am J Cardiol* 66:663-667, 1990.

40. Kahn J, Rutherford B, Conahay DM, et al: Usefulness of angioplasty during acute myocardial infarction in patients with prior coronary artery bypass grafting, *Am J Cardiol* 65:698-702, 1990.

41. Grines CL, Booth DC, Nissen SE, et al: Mechanism of acute myocardial infarction in patients with prior coronary artery bypass grafting and therapeutic implications, *Am J Cardiol* 65:1292-1296, 1990.

42. Ellis S, O'Neill W, Bates E, et al: Coronary angioplasty as primary therapy for acute myocardial infarction 6 to 48 hours after symptom onset: report of an initial experience, *J Am Coll Cardiol* 13:1122-1126, 1989.

43. Simoons M, Arnold AER, Betriu A, et al: Thrombolysis with tissue plasminogen activator in acute myocardial infarction: no additional benefit from immediate percutaneous coronary angioplasty, *Lancet* 1:197-203, 1988.

44. TIMI Study Group: Immediate versus delayed catheterization and angioplasty following thrombolytic therapy for acute myocardial infarction, *JAMA* 260:2849-2858, 1988.

45. Topol E, Califf R, George B, et al: A randomized trial of immediate versus delayed elective angioplasty after intravenous tissue plasminogen activator in acute myocardial infarction, *N Engl J Med* 317:581-588, 1987.

46. Dalin JE for the TIMI Investigators: Intravenous thrombolytic therapy in acute myocardial infarction—six month follow-up. NHLBI TIMI Trial, *J Am Coll Cardiol* 9:604, 1987.

47. Kennedy JW, Ritchie JL, et al: The Western Washington randomized trial of intracoronary streptokinase in acute myocardial infarction: a 12 month follow-up report, *N Engl J Med* 312:1073-1078, 1985.

48. Abbotsmith CW, Topol EJ, George BS, et al: Fate of patients with acute myocardial infarction with patency of the infarct related vessel achieved with successful thrombolysis versus rescue angioplasty, *J Am Coll Cardiol* 16:770-778, 1990.

49. Fung A, Lai P, Topol E, et al: Value of percutaneous transluminal coronary angioplasty after unsuccessful intravenous streptokinase therapy in acute myocardial infarction, *Am J Cardiol* 58:686-689, 1986.

50. Holmes D, Gersh B, Bailey K, et al: Emergency "rescue" percutaneous transluminal coronary angioplasty after failed thrombolysis with streptokinase: early and late results, *Circulation* 81(suppl IV):51-56, 1990.

51. Topol E, Califf R, George B, et al: Coronary arterial thrombolysis with combined infusion of recombinant tissue-type plasminogen activator and urokinase in patients with acute myocardial infarction, *Circulation* 77:1100-1107, 1988.

52. Califf R, Topol E, Stack R, et al: Evaluation of combination thrombolytic therapy and timing of cardiac catheterization in acute myocardial infarction: results of Thrombolysis and Angioplasty in Myocardial Infarction–Phase V randomized trial, *Circulation* 83:1543-1556, 1991.

53. Gacioch G, Topol E: Sudden paradoxic clinical deterioration during angioplasty of the occluded right coronary artery in acute myocardial infarction, *J Am Coll Cardiol* 14:1202-1209, 1989.

54. SWIFT (Should We Intervene Following Thrombolysis) Trial Study Group: SWIFT trial of delayed elective intervention with conservative treatment after thrombolysis with anistreplase in acute myocardial infarction, *Br Med J (Clin Res)* 302:555-560, 1991.

55. TIMI Study Group: Comparison of invasive and conservative strategies after treatment with intravenous tissue plasminogen activator in acute myocardial infarction: results of the Thrombolysis in Myocardial Infarction (TIMI) Phase II trial, *N Engl J Med* 320:618-627, 1989.

56. Williams D, Braunwald E, Knatterud G, et al: One year results of the Thrombolysis in Myocardial Infarction Investigation (TIMI) Phase II trial, *Circulation* 85:533-542, 1992.

57. Montalescot G, Faraggi M, Drobinski G, et al: Myocardial viability in patients with Q wave myocardial infarction and no residual ischemia, *Circulation* 86:47-55, 1992.

58. Sabia PJ, Powers ER, Ragosta M, et al: An association between collateral blood flow and myocardial viability in patients with recent myocardial infarction, *N Engl J Med* 327:1825-1831, 1992.

59. Meyer J, Merx W, Schmitz H, et al: Percutaneous transluminal coronary angioplasty immediately after intracoronary streptolysis of transluminal myocardial infarction, *Circulation* 66:905-913, 1982.

60. Thoren PN: Activation of left ventricular receptors with nonmedulated vagal afferent fibers during occlusion of a coronary artery in the cat, *Am J Cardiol* 37:1046, 1976.

61. Opie LH: Reperfusion injury and its pharmacologic modification, *Circulation* 80:1049-1062, 1989.

62. Braunwald E, Kloner RA: The stunned myocardium: prolonged ischemic ventricular dysfunction, *Circulation* 66:1146-1149, 1982.

63. Patel B, Kloner RA, Przyklenk K, et al: Postischemic myocardial "stunning": a clinically relevant phenomenon, *Ann Intern Med* 108:626-628, 1988.

64. Reimer KA, Jennings RB: Myocardial ischemia, hypoxia and infarction. In Fozzard HA, Haber E, Jennings RB, et al (eds): *The heart and cardiovascular system—scientific foundations,* New York, 1986, Raven Press, vol 2.

65. Bolli R, Jeroudi MO, Patel BS, et al: Direct evidence that oxygen derived free radicals contribute to postischemic myocardial dysfunction in the intact dog, *Proc Natl Acad Sci USA* 86:4695-4699, 1989.

66. Garlick PB, Davies MJ, Hearse DJ, et al: Direct detection of free radicals in the reperfused rat heart using electron spin spectroscopy, *Circ Res* 61:757-760, 1987.

67. Engler RL, Dahlgren MD, Peterson MA, et al: Accumulation of polymorphin nuclear cells during 3-H experimental myocardial ischemia, *Am J Phys* 251:H93-H100, 1986.

68. Bolli R: Oxygen derived free radicals in postischemic myocardial dysfunction ("stunned myocardium"), *J Am Coll Cardiol* 12:239-249, 1988.

69. Gross GJ, Farber ME, Hardman HF, et al: Beneficial actions of superoxide dismutase and catalase in stunned myocardium of dogs, *Am J Physiol* 58:148-156, 1986.

70. Wiatt DA, Ely SW, Lasley RD, et al: Appearing enriched asanguine cardioplegia provides superior myocardial protection, *Surg Forum* 38:265-267, 1987.

71. Hanson SR, Harker LA: Interruption of acute platelet dependent thrombosis by the synthetic antithrombin D-phenlalany-L-propyil-

L-arginyl chloromethyl ketone, *Proc Natl Acad Sci USA* 85:3184-3188, 1988.

72. Kaiser B, Markwardt F: Antithrombotic and hemorrhagic effects of synthetic and naturally occurring thrombin inhibitors, *Thromb Res* 43:613-620, 1986.

73. Markwardt F, Hauptmann J, Nowak G, et al: Pharmacological studies on the antithrombotic action of hirudin in experimental animals, *Thromb Haemost* 47:226-229, 1982.

74. Lam JY, Chesebro JH, Steele PM, et al: Antithrombotic therapy for deep arterial injury by angioplasty. Efficacy of common platelet inhibition compared with thrombin inhibition in pigs, *Circulation* 84:814-820, 1991.

75. Garratt KN, Heras M, Holmes Jr DR, et al: Platelet deposition and thrombosis in arterial stents: effect of hirudin compared with heparin plus antiplatelet therapy [abstract], *J Am Coll Cardiol* 15:209A, 1990.

76. Hardisty RM, Powling MJ, Nokes TJ: The action of triclopidine on human platelets. Studies on aggregation, secretion, calcium mobilization, and membrane glycoproteins, *Thromb Haemost* 64:150-155, 1990.

77. Bates ER, McGillem MJ, Mickelson JK, et al: A monoclonal antibody against the platelet glycoprotein IIb/IIIa receptor complex prevents platelet aggregation and thrombosis in a canine model of coronary angioplasty, *Circulation* 84:2463-2469, 1991.

78. Spears JR, James LM, Leonard BM, et al: Plaque media reweling with reversible tissue optical property changes during receptive CW Nd:YAG laser exposure, *Lasers Surg Med* 8:477-485, 1988.

79. Lee G, Ikeda RM, Stobbe D, et al: Effects of laser radiation on human thrombus: demonstration of a linear dissolution-dose relation between clot length and energy density, *Am J Cardiol* 52:876-877, 1983.

80. Isner JM, Steg PG, Clarke RH: Current status of cardiovascular laser therapy, *IEEE J Quantum Electr* 23:1756-1771, 1987.

81. Deckelbaum LI, Isner JM, Donaldson RF, et al: Reduction of laser induced pathologic tissue injury using pulsed energy delivery, *Am J Cardiol* 56:662-667, 1985.

82. King III S: Prediction of acute closure in percutaneous transluminal coronary angioplasty, *Circulation* 81(suppl III):IV5-IV8, 1990.

83. Lincoff AM, Popma JJ, Ellis SG, et al: Abrupt vessel closure complicating coronary angioplasty: clinical, angiographic, and therapeutic profile, *J Am Coll Cardiol* 19:926-935, 1992.

84. Holmes Jr DR, Lapeyre AC, Schwartz RS, et al: Thrombectomy of occluded coronary arteries: an initial clinical experience [abstract], *Circulation* 82:III623, 1990.

85. Holmes Jr DR, Ellis SG, Garratt KN: Directional atherectomy for thrombus containing lesions: improved outcome [abstract], *Circulation* 84(suppl II):II26, 1991.

86. Lefer AM, Tsao P, Lefer DJ, et al: Role of endothelial dysfunction in the pathogenesis of reperfusion injury after myocardial ischemia, *FASEB J* 5:2029-2034, 1991.

87. Engler RL, Schmid-Schonbein GW, Pavelac RS: Leukocyte capillary plugging in myocardial ischemia and reperfusion in the dog, *Am J Pathol* 111:98-111, 1983.

88. Farber NE, Gross GJ: Prostaglandin E1 attenuates postischemic contractile dysfunction after brief coronary occlusion and reperfusion, *Am Heart J* 118:17-24, 1989.

89. Ely SW, Berne RM: Protective effects of adenosine in myocardial ischemia, *Circulation* 85:893-904, 1992.

90. Bertrand ME, Fourrier JL, Auth DC, et al: Percutaneous coronary rotational angioplasty. In Topol EJ (ed): *Textbook of interventional cardiology*, Philadelphia, 1990, WB Saunders.

91. Fellmeth BD, Baron SB, Brown PR, et al: Repair of postcatheterization femoral pseudoaneurysms by color flow ultrasound guided compression, *Am Heart J* 123:547-551, 1992.

Chapter 35

EVOLVING ROLE OF CORONARY ARTERY BYPASS SURGERY IN THE TREATMENT OF ACUTE MYOCARDIAL INFARCTION

Dean J. Kereiakes
Robert H. Jones

The role of coronary bypass surgery in the treatment of patients with acute myocardial infarction (AMI) has undergone considerable evolution in the thrombolytic era. Bypass surgery has been performed as both a primary reperfusion procedure and delayed revascularization in sequential reperfusion strategies that employ intravenous (IV) thrombolytic therapy as initial treatment. The objectives, risks, and outcomes of bypass surgery may vary among the different indications for its use. This important topic is reviewed in the light of considerable new data on the use of coronary bypass surgery in the treatment of AMI.

SURGERY AS A PRIMARY REPERFUSION STRATEGY

Coronary bypass surgery was the first approach used to establish revascularization early during the course of an evolving AMI. Published reports summarizing data obtained for more than 1000 patients suggest an overall hospital mortality of approximately 5% and surgical reexploration for postoperative hemorrhage in less than 3% of patients not receiving thrombolytic therapy preoperatively.[2-10] Both experimental and clinical studies have stressed the importance of timing in primary

surgical reperfusion of AMI.[2,3,11-14] Emergency bypass surgery performed within 6 hours of infarct symptom onset has been associated with significantly greater preservation of left ventricular function and improved hospital and long-term (10-year) survival than surgery performed beyond 6 hours of chest pain onset.[2,3] Although emergency surgical revascularization does not appear to reduce the incidence of recurrent MI in long-term follow-up when compared with medical therapy alone, the mortality of recurrent infarction was significantly less in patients treated surgically.[2] The published experience with primary surgical reperfusion suggests low hospital (<5%) and long-term (2%-3%/year) mortality rates.[2,3,10,15,16] Both early and long-term mortality after primary surgical reperfusion was higher in patients with Q-wave MI vs. those with non–Q-wave infarction and in patients with multivessel coronary artery disease.[2,3] Only one trial has compared primary surgical reperfusion to medical therapy for AMI on a randomized basis. In this trial, the mortality in surgical patients (2.9%) was less than that observed in medically treated patients (20.6%), although small numbers of patients (34 patients in each group) were compared.[17] Nevertheless, these published data on primary surgical reperfusion

419

compared favorably with hospital (11%-24%) and long-term (8%-15% first year; 5%/year thereafter) mortality reported in unselected patients treated medically (no reperfusion strategy) for AMI.[15,18,19,20-23] Again, in the absence of appropriate control groups, we must caution attempts at comparison of outcomes as the selection process for surgical treatment may have biased results by including patients with more comorbidity in the comparison group. In the series reported by DeWood et al.,[2,3] 59% MI patients were in New York Heart Association class 1, 25% were in class 2, and only 10% were in class 4. Only 15% of these patients had a prior MI, and 29% had single-vessel coronary artery disease.

POTENTIAL ADVANTAGES OF PRIMARY SURGICAL REPERFUSION

Potential advantages offered by primary surgical revascularization relate to better control of the conditions under which myocardial reperfusion takes place. Both experimental and clinical experience with reperfusion of ischemic myocardium have suggested the importance of a normothermic, buffered reperfusate that is low in calcium and high in the Krebs cycle intermediates glutamate and aspartate in limiting adverse metabolic consequences of reperfusion.[24-28] In addition, a more gradual rate of reperfusion with lower perfusion pressures and a hyperosmotic reperfusate may limit adverse structural changes in cell membrane and capillary integrity. Controlled surgical reperfusion may facilitate administration of potentially important conjunctive agents such as calcium antagonists and antioxidants.[27]

Although clinical reports on primary surgical reperfusion for AMI have been promising, Spencer[29] has pointed out that the techniques for myocardial protection were in evolution during these studies and optimal methods for myocardial salvage were not used. It is possible that refinements in myocardial protection with controlled reperfusion may further expand the time window during which myocardial salvage can be achieved with primary surgical reperfusion.

The potential for greater reperfusion injury if initial perfusion of ischemic myocardium is accomplished with unmodified blood has led some investigators to recommend the saphenous vein graft conduit in preference to the internal mammary artery graft when emergency surgical revascularization is performed.[14,24] Greater technical demand and constraints of time may also influence the surgeon's choice of bypass conduit in favor of the saphenous vein graft despite recent observations of higher long-term graft patency rates and improved long-term survival in patients who have at least one internal mammary artery graft when compared with patients in whom only saphenous vein grafts are performed.[30-32] However, many surgeons place patients undergoing coronary artery bypass grafting (CABG) on cardiopulmonary bypass to cool and decompress the heart during harvest of internal mammary artery graft. This maneuver provides some myocardial protection for the short additional time required to prepare this conduit for grafting.

Despite concerns that myocyte swelling with consequent capillary obliteration would limit infarct artery runoff and result in early bypass graft closure in grafted infarct-related arteries,[33] graft patency rates appear high (>90%) and similar to rates observed for noninfarct arteries after elective bypass operations.[8,34] Although promising immediate and long-term results have been reported from a limited number of centers experienced with emergency primary surgical reperfusion for AMI, logistic and financial considerations will impede widespread use of this technique. Because approximately 12% of hospitals in the United States have both a catheterization laboratory and cardiothoracic surgical support,[35] primary surgical reperfusion therapy will continue to be restricted to very few centers.

Current treatment regimens for IV thrombolytic therapy followed by percutaneous (rescue) coronary angioplasty in patients who fail to reperfuse with thrombolysis alone may achieve successful infarct artery recanalization in 96% of patients with AMI.[36,37] In addition, at least 10% of patients with AMI will have no significant fixed atherosclerotic coronary obstruction after IV thrombolysis and heparin treatment.[38] These observations taken in the context of logistic and financial considerations suggest that coronary bypass surgery should serve an adjunctive rather than primary role in myocardial infarct reperfusion strategies.

Patients who develop cardiogenic shock early during the evolution of AMI may derive particular benefit from emergency surgical coronary revascularization. The aggregate experience of several centers using primary surgical reperfusion in patients with early cardiogenic shock complicating infarction has demonstrated a hospital mortality of 31% in 211 patients.[4,39-42] Historically this group of patients has had a particularly poor prognosis with conservative medical therapy (mortality > 80%) with or without intraaortic balloon pump counterpulsation if adjunctive coronary revascularization is not performed.[22] Whether surgery is better for these patients than emergency coronary angioplasty of the infarct vessel (see Chapters 26 and 46) remains unsettled.

ROLE OF CORONARY BYPASS SURGERY AFTER INTRAVENOUS THROMBOLYTIC THERAPY

The ease and rapidity of administration, as well as widespread availability, have made IV thrombolysis a logical first step in strategies aimed at myocardial reperfusion. However, intravenous thrombolysis fails to achieve infarct artery recanalization in 25% or more of treated patients,[43,44] and infarct artery reocclusion after initially successful thrombolysis occurs in another 10% to 20% of patients.[45-47] Coronary bypass surgery may play an important role in initiating or maintaining coronary perfusion that has not been established or sustained by pharmacologic or percutaneous balloon catheter techniques (or both).

BYPASS SURGERY AFTER RESCUE ANGIOPLASTY

Because the failure rate of percutaneous transluminal coronary angioplasty (PTCA) in the acute infarct setting appears to exceed that observed in elective PTCA cases, cardiothoracic surgical support should be available in centers practicing rescue or salvage PTCA in patients who fail to recanalize with IV thrombolysis alone.[48,49] Technical success of rescue PTCA may influence hospital and even long-term mortality.[36] An important recent observation has been the correlation of rescue PTCA success rates with the type of preceding thrombolytic regimen administered.[36,37,50] Coronary reocclusion after initially successful rescue PTCA is more frequent after tissue-type plasminogen activator (t-PA) monotherapy (29%) than after treatment with combination t-PA and urokinase (4%) or urokinase monotherapy (12%) (p = 0.045).[36] In addition, significantly higher rates of reocclusion have been observed after mechanical recanalization of the right coronary artery.[51] Patients who experience reocclusion have more regional (infarct zone) and global left ventricular dysfunction and a higher hospital mortality than patients with sustained infarct artery patency.[52] Recent data have suggested that successful mechanical "salvage" of pharmacologic failures may confer a survival advantage even in the absence of objective improvements in regional or global left ventricular function.[36]

We have previously reported improvement of left ventricular function after emergency coronary bypass surgery in patients with a failed attempt at rescue PTCA.[53] In patients with an initially successful rescue PTCA who have occlusive coronary dissection or refractory rethrombosis, we have recommended insertion of a perfusion catheter or balloon to maintain coronary flow enroute to surgery.[54,55] In this pharmacologic-mechanical-surgical sequential reperfusion strategy, bypass surgery is used to maintain perfusion that has been initiated by pharmacologic or balloon catheter techniques. When surgery is employed in this fashion, the timing of surgery (less than rather than greater than 6 hours after infarct symptom onset) does not appear to influence the degree of recovery in regional or global left ventricular function.[53] This observation is in contrast to reports of primary surgical reperfusion therapy for MI, which have observed significantly greater recovery in left ventricular function and improved survival when surgical revascularization is performed within 6 hours of infarct symptom onset.[3]

EMERGENCY SURGICAL REVASCULARIZATION AFTER IV THROMBOLYTIC THERAPY

We have recently evaluated indications for bypass surgery, associated changes in left ventricular function, and immediate and long-term outcomes in 36 patients operated on on an emergency basis (< 24 hours after IV thrombolytic therapy) from the 1387 total patients enrolled in the Thrombolysis and Angioplasty in Myocardial Infarction (TAMI) trials I to III and V.[56] The most frequent indications for emergency bypass surgery after IV thrombolysis were failure of immediate or attempted rescue PTCA (39%), left main or equivalent coronary artery disease (19%), and complex multivessel or high-risk coronary anatomy not amenable to PTCA. Emergency surgery was required more frequently in patients receiving t-PA monotherapy than in patients treated with t-PA/urokinase combination or urokinase monotherapy.[56,57] This finding may be related to the higher coronary reocclusion rates in t-PA monotherapy–treated patients after attempted rescue PTCA as noted previously.[36]

We have previously reported no hospital mortality in 16 patients undergoing emergency coronary bypass surgery who had stable prehospital hemodynamics and 3 hospital deaths among 8 patients with preoperative cardiogenic shock.[53] This observation is consistent with prior reports of primary surgical reperfusion therapy that have noted less than 5% hospital mortality in patients with stable preoperative hemodynamics and a 31% mortality in patients with cardiogenic shock complicating the early course of MI.[39-42] Patients in whom coronary bypass surgery is performed within 24 hours of receiving IV thrombolytic therapy require more red blood cell transfusions than patients in whom surgery is deferred more than 24 hours after thrombolysis (6.7 ± 4.5 vs. 2.6 ± 2.8 units of packed red blood cells; p = 0.001). Reoperation for postoperative hemorrhage occurred in 3 of 24 patients (12.5%) in our initial series of emergency surgery after IV thrombolytic therapy.[56,57]

The timing of surgery (less than vs. greater than 24 hours after thrombolysis) may also influence the surgeon's choice of bypass conduit (saphenous vein vs. internal mammary artery graft). For patients in whom the left anterior descending was the infarct-related artery, only 17% had an internal mammary artery graft placed to this vessel during emergency surgery vs. 68% of a similar group of patients operated on on a deferred (> 24-hour) basis. Greater technical complexity, constraints of time, and concerns for perioperative hemorrhage may influence the surgical preference for saphenous vein graft conduits in emergency situations. In addition, concerns regarding the potential for exacerbating reperfusion injury when revascularization is accomplished with unmodified blood using the internal mammary artery may be operative. These concerns appear less pertinent when surgery is employed as part of a sequential reperfusion strategy rather than a primary modality.

It is important to note that clinical factors in addition to coronary anatomic findings influence the decision to proceed with emergency vs. deferred coronary bypass surgery. For example, although left main or equivalent coronary artery disease was more frequently observed in the emergency surgical group (19% emergency vs. 8% deferred) it was possible to defer bypass surgery for 24 hours or more in the majority (75%) of patients with this coronary anatomic finding.[56] The presence of hemodynamic compromise, recurrent or protracted ischemic cardiac pain, complex ventricular ectopy, or ischemic myocardial dysfunction in noninfarct zones may influence the triage of patients to emergency vs. deferred surgical intervention.

Death in hospital occurred in 17% (6 of 36) patients having emergency bypass surgery after IV thrombolysis from the TAMI trial database.[56] Although this hospital mortality would on the surface appear higher than that noted in deferred patients (13 of 267; 5%), it must be viewed in the context of the critical clinical status present in many of these patients. Cardiogenic shock was present in 24%, and perioperative intraaortic balloon pump support was required in 22% of patients who underwent emergency surgery.[56]

DEFERRED (IN-HOSPITAL) CORONARY BYPASS SURGERY AFTER IV THROMBOLYSIS

The most frequent indications for deferred bypass surgery in 267 patients from the TAMI trial database were complex multivessel coronary disease (66%) and recurrent ischemic symptoms with coronary anatomy unsuitable for PTCA (13%).[56] Patients who had bypass surgery deferred 24 hours or more after IV thrombolytic therapy had less red blood cell transfusion and more frequently received an internal mammary artery bypass graft than did patients who had surgery on an emergency basis.[56,57]

Although death in hospital occurred in 13 of 267 deferred surgical patients (5%), it is important to note that deferred surgery was performed for refractory ischemic left ventricular pump dysfunction in 5 patients, papillary muscle dysfunction or rupture in 3 patients, and ventricular septal rupture in 3 patients.[56,57] These 11 patients would be expected to have a higher operative and hospital mortality even though surgery was performed on a "deferred" basis.

In a multivariate analysis involving 406 patients who had bypass surgery within 30 days of AMI, Applebaum et al.[58] found that only left ventricular ejection fraction

less than 30%, preoperative shock, and age greater than 70 years were associated with increased hospital death. In this study, the type and location of infarction, coronary anatomy, and time from infarction to operation were not associated with hospital mortality.

IMMEDIATE AND LONG-TERM OUTCOME AFTER CORONARY BYPASS SURGERY FOR AMI

Bypass surgery was performed during the initial hospitalization for AMI in 303 (22%) of 1387 patients enrolled into the TAMI trials I to III and V of IV thrombolytic therapy for AMI.[56,57] Surgery was emergent in 36 (12%) and deferred in 267 (88%) patients. The clinical and angiographic features of 303 surgical patients are compared in Table 35-1 with those of the other 1084 patients from the same trials who did not have bypass surgery performed during their initial hospitalization for AMI. Surgical patients were older (59.5 ± 9.8 vs. 56.0 ± 10.2; p < 0.0001), more often had diabetes mellitus (19% vs. 15%; p = 0.048), had prior MI (24% vs. 10%; p < 0.0001), and had cardiogenic shock more frequently early after thrombolytic therapy (8% vs. 5%; p = 0.059) than patients who did not have coronary bypass surgery performed. Surgically treated patients more often had multivessel coronary disease (79% vs. 38% had ≥ two-vessel disease; p = 0.0001). Despite the presence of multiple adverse clinical predictors in surgically treated patients, death in hospital was observed with similar frequency in surgical (6.6%) and nonsurgical (5.9%) patients. Clinical events in long-term follow-up (median 1092 days in surgical and 1099 days in nonsurgical patients) are shown in Table 35-2. The occurrence of death and nonfatal MI was similar in both groups, although the requirement for additional revascularization procedures (CABG and PTCA) was more frequent in patients who did not have bypass surgery during their initial hospitalization (18% nonsurgical vs. 7% surgical group). Within the surgically treated group, repeat revascularization procedures were more often required in those patients who had undergone emergency versus deferred surgical revascularization (20% emergency vs. 6% deferred).

Potentially important differences within the surgical group comparing emergency and deferred revascularization procedures included the more frequent requirement of packed red blood cell transfusions and less frequent use of internal mammary artery bypass conduits when surgery was performed on an emergency basis.[56,57] Lee, et al.[59] have also reported that when bypass surgery is performed after thrombolytic therapy, the risk of postoperative hemorrhage appears to be related to the interval between lytic treatment and operation. They observed no increase in postoperative bleeding in patients who had surgery 3 to 16 days after streptokinase infusion. However, patients who had surgery within 12

Table 35-1. Baseline characteristics of surgical and nonsurgical patients in the TAMI AMI registry*†

	Type of surgery			
	Emergency (n = 36)	Deferred (n = 267)	All (n = 303)	None (n = 1084)
Age, yr (1)	56.4 ± 11.1	60.0 ± 9.5	59.5 ± 9.8	56.0 ± 10.2
Male sex, %	72	83	82	78
Diabetes, % (2)	22	19	19	15
Prior MI, %	15	24	24	10
Smoking, %	58	78	76	79
Anterior MI location, % (3)	61	45	47	42
Cardiogenic shock, % (4)	24	6	8	5
Death in hospital, % (5)	17	5	7	6
Infarct artery				
Left anterior descending, %	56	40	42	36
Left circumflex, %	6	11	11	14
Right coronary, %	33	48	46	50
Left main coronary, %	6	0.4	1	0
No. of diseased vessels (>50% stenosis)				
0, %	0	1	1	7
1, %	22	20	20	56
2, %	42	31	32	27
3, %	36	47	46	11
Multivessel disease, % (≥2 vessels), % (6)	78	78	78	37
Acute coronary angioplasty, % (7)	39	8	18	32

*TAMI, Thrombolysis and Angioplasty in Myocardial Infarction; AMI, acute myocardial infarction.
†(1) $p < 0.001$ all vs. none; $p = 0.08$ emergency vs. deferred; (2) $p = 0.048$ all vs. none; (3) $p = 0.074$ emergency vs. deferred; (4) $p = 0.059$ all vs. none; $p = 0.002$ emergency vs. deferred; (5) $p = 0.016$ emergency vs. deferred; (6) $p < 0.0001$ all surgery vs. none; (7) $p < 0.0001$ all surgery vs. none; $p < 0.0001$ emergency vs. deferred surgery.

hours of thrombolysis had considerably greater requirements for blood and blood product transfusion.[59] Because the risk of transfusion-associated hepatitis and human immunodeficiency virus infection is influenced by the number of packed red blood cell units transfused,[60] deferral of bypass surgery by at least 12 to 24 hours appears preferable if waiting does not otherwise jeopardize patient outcome.

When surgical and nonsurgical patients from the TAMI series were asked to assess their general health status 1 year after hospital discharge, the majority of patients in both groups (74% surgical, 80% nonsurgical) considered themselves to be in excellent or good condition.[56] In addition, a similar percentage of surgical and nonsurgical patients were employed (3% and 1%, respectively) or disabled (10% and 8%, respectively). More patients in the surgical group were considered to be retired (46% vs. 30%), which likely reflects the higher mean age of patients in this group.[56]

INFLUENCE OF BYPASS SURGERY ON LEFT VENTRICULAR FUNCTION

Early clinical studies demonstrated improvement in left ventricular function if surgical reperfusion was achieved within 6 hours of infarct symptom onset.[3] As noted previously, these studies were performed early in the evolution of surgical myocardial preservation tech-

niques, and optimal myocardial salvage may not have been achieved. Using a sequential pharmacologic-mechanical-surgical (as required) reperfusion strategy, we have previously demonstrated substantial improvement in global left ventricular ejection fraction and regional (infarct zone) left ventricular function in patients undergoing emergency bypass surgery.[53] Because myocardial reperfusion had been initiated by pharmacologic or coronary angioplasty techniques (or both) in the majority (85%) of these patients, surgery was performed to sustain perfusion in patients in whom infarct artery patency could not be maintained by nonsurgical techniques.[53] In these patients, substantial recovery in left ventricular ejection fraction and regional infarct zone function was noted and was not dependent on timing (less than vs. greater than 6 hours from symptom onset) of the operation. In addition, improvement in noninfarct zone function of patients with multivessel coronary disease was observed and contributed to the overall improvement in global ejection fraction.

The impact of coronary bypass surgery after IV thrombolytic therapy on left ventricular function has been evaluated for both the emergency and deferred surgical groups, as well as nonsurgical patients from the TAMI trial database.[61] Analysis of immediate (90 minutes after thrombolysis) and late (predischarge)

Table 35-2. Clinical events in follow-up of TAMI AMI registry*

	No CABG	CABG	Emergency CABG	Deferred CABG
			%	
Death	6.2	7.2	3.7	7.7
Nonfatal MI	8.4	5.3	4.0	5.6
PTCA	10.2	4.2	12.0	3.1
CABG	7.7	3.2	8.0	2.5

*TAMI, Thrombolysis and Angioplasty in Myocardial Infarction; AMI, acute myocardial infarction; CABG, coronary artery bypass grafting; PTCA, percutaneous transluminal coronary angioplasty.

global ejection fraction and regional infarct zone function from paired contrast left ventriculograms is shown in Fig. 35-1. Surgically treated patients had more severe initial (preoperative) depression in global and regional infarct zone left ventricular function than did patients who did not undergo (preoperative) surgery. However, even after adjustment for immediate left ventricular function values, a greater degree of left ventricular functional recovery was observed in patients who had coronary bypass surgery. The results of immediate and predischarge evaluation of left ventricular function for patients having emergency vs. deferred bypass surgery are shown in Fig. 35-2. Improvement in global and regional infarct zone function was observed in both surgical groups, and no difference with respect to the degree or magnitude of functional recovery was noted between groups. Thus, the degree of recovery in both global and regional infarct zone function observed in patients who had bypass surgery as part of a sequential reperfusion strategy during their initial hospitalization for AMI exceeded the degree of functional recovery observed after IV thrombolytic therapy with or without coronary angioplasty (no surgery). Although some degree of enhancement in left ventricular function could be attributable to hormonal changes, most notably an increase in circulating catecholamines after bypass surgery,[62,63] the magnitude of such changes would appear small in comparison with the degree of functional improvement noted in our surgical series.[61] It is also likely that similar hormonal changes would occur secondary to AMI alone without bypass surgery.[64,65] Enhanced function of the noninfarct zone observed on early and predischarge left ventriculograms from the nonsurgical group supports this contention.[61] In contrast, dysfunction of the noninfarct zone observed in the majority of patients who underwent bypass surgery most likely reflects a higher incidence of multivessel coronary artery disease in these patients.[61] Postoperative improvement in noninfarct zone function reflecting alleviation of ischemia remote from the infarct zone

Table 35-3. Potential indications for emergency bypass surgery

1. After successful coronary thrombolysis
   a. ≥50% left main coronary artery stenosis with left anterior descending or circumflex infarct–related vessel and hemodynamic instability
   b. ≥75% left main coronary artery stenosis and right coronary infarct–related vessel
   c. Left main equivalent disease* with hemodynamic instability
   d. Multivessel disease with anatomy unsuitable for coronary angioplasty and ischemic dysfunction of noninfarct zones; hemodynamic and/or electrical instability
2. Unsuccessful angioplasty as a result of coronary dissection/rethrombosis with a large jeopardized myocardial region
3. Failure of or contraindications for thrombolytic or angioplasty infarct artery recanalization with infarction duration < 6 hr and a large jeopardized myocardial region
4. Cardiogenic shock in patients with multivessel disease unsuitable for coronary angioplasty

*90% stenosis of dominant circumflex coronary artery and left anterior descending infarct–related vessel or ≥90% anterior descending coronary artery stenosis with dominant circumflex infarct–related vessel.

contributed to the improvement in global left ventricular ejection fraction after coronary bypass surgery.[61]

CURRENT RECOMMENDATIONS FOR THE USE OF CORONARY BYPASS SURGERY IN THE TREATMENT OF AMI

Potential indications for the performance of emergency coronary bypass surgery during evolving AMI are shown in Table 35-3. After successful thrombolysis, complex or multivessel coronary disease particularly in the presence of persistent or recurrent ischemic chest pain, hemodynamic instability, or high-grade ventricular ectopy may be an indication for emergency coronary bypass surgery. If patient stability can be achieved with pharmacologic or intraaortic balloon pump support after successful infarct vessel recanalization, surgery can be deferred for 24 hours or more. This practice may afford the patient less blood product transfusion and a more optimal bypass conduit. Emergency surgery should be offered after failed PTCA (primary or rescue) if a large jeopardized myocardial region is present. Another group of patients who may benefit from emergency bypass surgery are those patients in whom thrombolytic therapy is contraindicated and in whom PTCA is either unsuccessful or cannot be performed. As noted previously, when surgery is used as a primary reperfusion modality, the best immediate and long-term results are achieved when revascularization is accomplished within 6 hours of infarct symptom onset.[2,3] Patients with multivessel coronary disease not suitable for PTCA and in whom cardiogenic shock evolves early in the course of MI may

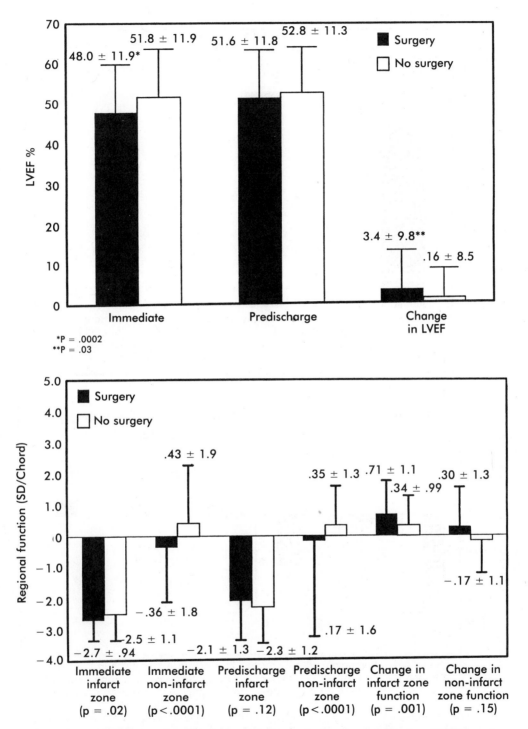

Fig. 35-1. A, Immediate and predischarge left ventricular ejection fraction *(LVEF)* and absolute change in LVEF between paired studies for patients with and without coronary bypass surgery. Surgical patients had more depressed immediate left ventricular function and a greater increment in LVEF before hospital discharge. **B,** Immediate and predischarge infarct zone regional left ventricular function in patients with and without coronary bypass surgery.

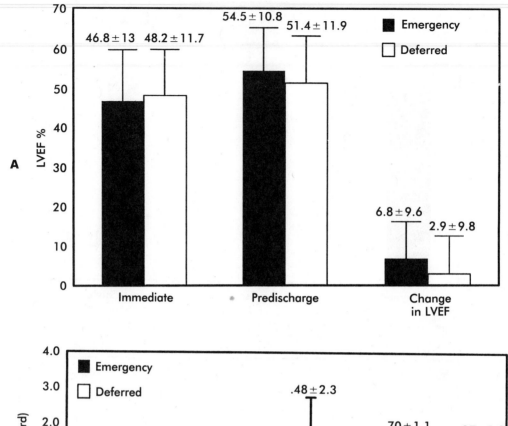

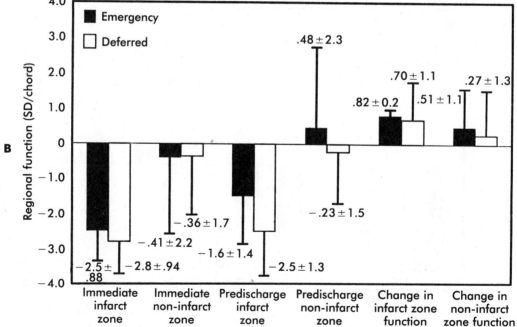

Fig. 35-2. A, Immediate and predischarge left ventricular ejection fraction *(LVEF)* for patients having emergency and deferred coronary bypass surgery. No significant differences in absolute LVEF or change in LVEF were observed. **B,** Immediate and predischarge infarct zone and noninfarct zone regional left ventricular function in patients with emergency and deferred coronary bypass surgery. No significant differences in absolute regional function or change in regional function were observed.

Table 35-4. Potential indications for deferred bypass surgery

1. Complex or multivessel coronary artery disease unsuitable for coronary angioplasty.
2. Left main coronary stenosis > 50% or left main equivalent coronary artery disease.
3. Recurrent myocardial ischemia refractory to medical therapy.
4. Mechanical complication of myocardial infarction (papillary muscle dysfunction or rupture; ventricular septal rupture).
5. Failure of percutaneous transluminal coronary angioplasty.

derive benefit from emergency surgical coronary revascularization.

Potential indications for the performance of deferred coronary bypass surgery after IV thrombolytic therapy are listed in Table 35-4. After successful thrombolysis, complex coronary anatomy not suitable for PTCA and particularly multivessel coronary artery disease are the most frequent indications for deferred surgery. We currently defer surgery for 5 to 7 days in the patient with a high-grade residual stenosis on the infarct vessel and multivessel coronary disease. These patients are operated on during their initial hospital admission for AMI and receive maximal medical therapy (intravenous nitroglycerine; heparin, aspirin) during the interval between infarction and surgical revascularization. Late developing mechanical complications of MI such as papillary muscle dysfunction or rupture and ventricular septal rupture may also require surgical intervention more than 24 hours after receiving IV thrombolytic therapy (see Chapter 53).

REFERENCES

1. Sustaita H, Chatterjee K, Matloff JM, et al: Emergency bypass surgery in impending and complicated acute myocardial infarction, *Arch Surg* 105:30-35, 1972.
2. DeWood MA, Notske RN, Berg R, et al: Medical and surgical management of early Q-wave myocardial infarction: I. Effects of surgical reperfusion on survival, recurrent myocardial infarction, sudden death in functional class at 10 or more years of follow up, *J Am Coll Cardiol* 14:65-77, 1989.
3. DeWood MA, Leonard J, Grunwald RP, et al: Medical and surgical management of early Q-wave myocardial infarction: II. Effects on mortality and global and regional left ventricular function at 10 or more years of follow up, *J Am Coll Cardiol* 14:78-90, 1989.
4. Phillips S, Zeff R, Skinner J: Reperfusion protocol and results in 738 patients with evolving myocardial infarction, *Ann Thorac Surg* 41:119-25, 1986.
5. Phillips S: Surgery in evolving acute myocardial infarction. In Roberts A, Conti CR (eds): *Current surgery of the heart,* Philadelphia, 1987, JB Lippincott, pp 247-256.
6. VanHecke J, Flameng W, Sergent P: Emergency bypass surgery: late effects on size of infarction and ventricular function, *Circulation* 72(suppl II):II179-II184, 1985.
7. Berg R, Selinger S, Leonard J: Immediate coronary bypass surgery for acute myocardial infarction, *J Cardiovasc Surg* 81:483-487, 1981.
8. Berg R, Selinger S, Leonard J, et al: Surgical management of acute myocardial infarction. In McGoon DC (ed): *Cardiac surgery,* Philadelphia, 1982, FA Davis, pp 61-74.
9. Katz N, Wallace R: Emergency coronary bypass surgery: indications and results. In Rackley CE (ed): *Advances in critical care cardiology,* Philadelphia, 1986, FA Davis, pp 67-72.
10. Athanasuleas CL, Geer DA, Araciniega JG, et al: A reappraisal of surgical intervention for acute myocardial infarction, *J Thorac Cardiovasc Surg* 93:405-414, 1987.
11. Maroko P, Libby P, Ginks W, et al: Coronary artery reperfusion: I. Early effects on local myocardial function in the extent of myocardial necrosis, *J Clin Invest* 51:2710-2718, 1972.
12. Costantini C, Corday E, Lang T, et al: Revascularization after three hours of coronary arterial occlusion: effects on regional cardiac metabolic function in infarct size, *Am J Cardiol* 36:368-384, 1975.
13. Allen BS, Okamoto F, Buckberg GD, et al: Studies of controlled reperfusion after ischemia: XV. Immediate functional recovery after six hours of regional ischemia by careful control of conditions of reperfusion and composition of reperfusate, *J Thorac Cardiovasc Surg* 82:621-635, 1986.
14. Allen BS, Buckberg GD, Schwaiger M, et al: Studies of controlled reperfusion after ischemia: XVI. Early recovery of regional wall motion in patients following surgical revascularization after eight hours of acute coronary occlusion, *J Thorac Cardiovasc Surg* 92:636-648, 1986.
15. DeWood M, Selinger S, Coleman W, et al: Surgical coronary reperfusion during acute myocardial infarction. In McGoon DC (ed): *Cardiac surgery,* ed 2, Philadelphia, 1987, FA Davis, pp 91-103.
16. Brower R, Fioretti P, Simoons M, et al: Surgical versus nonsurgical management of patients soon after myocardial infarction, *Br Heart J* 54:460-465, 1985.
17. Koshal A, Beanlands DS, Davies RA, et al: Urgent surgical reperfusion in acute evolving myocardial infarction: a randomized controlled study, *Circulation* 78:1171-1178, 1988.
18. DeWood M, Spores J, Notske R: Medical and surgical management of myocardial infarction, *Am J Cardiol* 44:1356-1364, 1979.
19. Kennedy H, Goldberg R, Szkol M: The prognosis of anterior myocardial infarction revisited: a community wide study, *Clin Cardiol* 2:455-464, 1979.
20. Henning H, Gilpen E, Covell J: Prognosis after acute myocardial infarction: a multivaried analysis of mortality and survival, *Circulation* 59:1124-1131, 1979.
21. Bonow K, Alpert J: The natural history and treatment of coronary artery disease, *Cardiovasc Med* 4:87-99, 1978.
22. Killip T, Kimball J: Treatment of myocardial infarction in a coronary care unit: a two year experience with 250 patients, *Am J Cardiol* 20:457-463, 1967.
23. Timmis G: *Cardiovascular review 1980,* Baltimore, 1980, Williams & Wilkins, p 53.
24. Vinten-Johansen J, Buckberg GD, Okamoto F, et al: Studies of controlled reperfusion after ischemia: V. Superiority of surgical versus medical reperfusion after regional ischemia, *J Thorac Cardiovasc Surg* 92:525-534, 1986.
25. Buckberg GD: Thoracic and cardiovascular surgery, *J Thorac Cardiovasc Surg* 92:43-47, 1986.
26. Vinten-Johansen J, Rosenkranz E, Buckberg GD, et al: Studies of controlled reperfusion after ischemia: VI. Metabolic and histochemical benefits of regional blood cardioplegic reperfusion without cardiopulmonary bypass, *J Thorac Cardiovasc Surg* 92:535-542, 1986.
27. Allen BS, Okomoto F, Buckberg GD, et al: Studies of controlled reperfusion after ischemia: IX. Reperfusate composition. Ben-

efits of marked hypocalcemia in diltiazem on regional recovery, *J Thorac Cardiovasc Surg* 92:564-572, 1986.

28. Allen BS, Okomoto F, Buckberg GD, et al: Studies in controlled reperfusion after ischemia: XIII. Reperfusion conditions: critical importance of total ventricular decompression during regional reperfusion, *J Thorac Cardiovasc Surg* 92:605-612, 1986.

29. Spencer FC: Emergency coronary artery bypass for acute infarction: an unproven clinical experiment, *Circulation* 68II:17-19, 1983.

30. Loop FL, Lytle PW, Cosgrove DM: Influence of the internal mammary artery graft on 10 year survival and other cardiac events, *N Engl J Med* 314:1-9, 1986.

31. Okies JE, Bag US, Biglow JC, et al: The internal mammary artery: the graft of choice, *Circulation* 70(suppl)I213-I217, 1984.

32. Tector AJ, Schmahl TM, Canino VR: The internal mammary artery graft: the best choice for bypass of the diseased left anterior descending coronary artery, *Circulation* 68(suppl II)II214-II219, 1983.

33. Mathey D, Rodewald G, Rentrop P, et al: Intracoronary streptokinase thrombolytic recanalization and subsequent surgical bypass of remaining atherosclerotic stenosis in acute myocardial infarction: complementary combined approach effecting reduced infarct size, preventing reinfarction and improving left ventricular function, *Am Heart J* 102:1194-1201, 1981.

34. Phillips S, Kongthaworn C, Zeff R, et al: Emergency artery revascularization: a possible therapy for acute myocardial infarction, *Circulation* 60:241-246, 1979.

35. Topol EJ, Bates ER, Walton JA, et al: Community hospital administration of intravenous tissue plasminogen activator in acute myocardial infarction: improved timing, thrombolytic efficacy and ventricular function, *J Am Coll Cardiol* 10:1173-1177, 1987.

36. Abbottsmith CW, Topol EJ, George BS, et al: Fate of patients with acute myocardial infarction with patency of the infarct related vessel achieved with successful thrombolysis versus rescue angioplasty, *J Am Coll Cardiol* 16:770-778, 1990.

37. Califf RM, Topol EJ, Stack RS, et al: Evaluation of combination thrombolytic therapy and timing of cardiac catheterization in acute myocardial infarction: results of Thrombolysis in Angioplasty of Myocardial Infarction–phase 5 randomized trial, *Circulation* 83:1543-1556, 1991.

38. Kereiakes DJ, Topol EJ, George BS, et al: Myocardial infarction with minimal coronary atherosclerosis in the era of thrombolytic reperfusion, *J Am Coll Cardiol* 17:304-312, 1991.

39. DeWood M, Spores J, Berg R: Acute myocardial infarction: a decade of experience with surgical reperfusion in 701 patients, *Circulation* 68:118-126, 1983.

40. Kirklin JK, Blackstone EH, Zorn GL, et al: Intermediate term results of coronary artery bypass grafting for acute myocardial infarction, *Circulation* 72(suppl II):II175-II178, 1985.

41. Nunley DL, Grunkemeier GL, Teply JF, et al: Coronary bypass operation following acute complicated myocardial infarction, *J Thorac Cardiovasc Surg* 85:485-491, 1983.

42. Laks H, Rosenkraz E, Buckberg G: Surgical treatment of cardiogenic shock after myocardial infarction, *Circulation* 74:11-16, 1986.

43. Topol EJ, Califf RM, Kereiakes DJ, et al: Thrombolysis and Angioplasty in Myocardial Infarction (TAMI) trial, *J Am Coll Cardiol* 10:65B-74B, 1987.

44. Califf RM, Topol EJ, George BS, et al: Characteristics and outcome of patients in whom reperfusion with intravenous tissue type plasminogen activator fails: results of the Thrombolysis and Angioplasty in Myocardial Infarction (TAMI) 1 trial, *Circulation* 77:1090-1099, 1988.

45. Harrison DG, Ferguson DW, Collins SH, et al: Rethrombosis after reperfusion with streptokinase: importance of geometry in residual lesions, *Circulation* 69:991-998, 1984.

46. Gold HK, Leinbach RC, Garabedian H, et al: Acute coronary reocclusion after thrombolysis with recombinant human tissue-type plasminogen activator: prevention by a maintenance infusion, *Circulation* 73:347-352, 1986.

47. Fung AY, Lai P, Topol EJ, et al: Value of percutaneous transluminal coronary angioplasty after unsuccessful intravenous streptokinase therapy in acute myocardial infarction, *Am J Cardiol* 58:686-691, 1986.

48. O'Neill WW, Kereiakes DJ, Stack RS, et al: Cardiothoracic surgical support is required during interventional therapy of myocardial infarction: results from the TAMI Study Group [abstract], *J Am Coll Cardiol* 9:124A, 1987.

49. Guidelines for percutaneous transluminal coronary angioplasty. A report of the American College of Cardiology/American Heart Association Task Force on Assessment of Diagnostic and Therapeutic Cardiovascular Procedures (Subcommittee on Percutaneous Transluminal Coronary Angioplasty), *J Am Coll Cardiol* 12:529-545, 1988.

50. Topol EJ, Califf RM, George BS, et al: Coronary arterial thrombolysis with combined infusion of recombinant tissue plasminogen activator and urokinase in patients with acute myocardial infarction, *Circulation* 5:1100-1107, 1988.

51. Gacioch GM, Topol EJ: Sudden paradoxic clinical deterioration during angioplasty of the occluded right coronary artery in acute myocardial infarction, *J Am Coll Cardiol* 14:1202-1209, 1989.

52. Ohman EM, Califf RM, Topol EJ, et al: Consequences of reocclusion after successful reperfusion therapy in acute myocardial infarction, *Circulation* 82:781-791, 1990.

53. Kereiakes DJ, Topol EJ, George BS, et al: Emergency coronary bypass surgery preserves global and regional left ventricular function after intravenous tissue plasminogen activator therapy for acute myocardial infarction, *J Am Coll Cardiol* 11:899-907, 1988.

54. Kereiakes DJ, Abbottsmith CW, Callard GM, et al: Emergent internal mammary artery grafting following failed percutaneous transluminal coronary angioplasty: use of transluminal catheter reperfusion, *Am Heart J* 113:1018-1020, 1987.

55. Hinohara T, Simpson JB, Phillips HR, et al: Transluminal catheter reperfusion: a new technique to reestablish blood flow after coronary occlusion during percutaneous transluminal coronary angioplasty, *Am J Cardiol* 57:684-688, 1986.

56. Kereiakes DJ, Topol EJ, Califf RM, et al: Favorable early and long-term prognosis following coronary bypass surgery therapy for myocardial infarction: results of a multicenter trial, *Am Heart J* 118:199-206, 1989.

57. Kereiakes DJ, Califf RM, George BS, et al: Comparison of immediate and long-term outcome of patients having emergent or deferred coronary bypass surgery following intravenous thrombolytic therapy for acute myocardial infarction, *J Am Coll Cardiol* 17:246A, 1991.

58. Applebaum R, House R, Rademaker A, et al: Coronary artery bypass grafting within thirty days of acute myocardial infarction. Early and late results in 406 patients, *J Thorac Cardiovasc Surg* 102:745-752, 1991.

59. Lee KF, Mandell J, Rankin JS, et al: Immediate versus delayed coronary grafting after streptokinase treatment: postoperative blood loss and clinical results, *J Thorac Cardiovasc Surg* 95:216-222, 1988.

60. Consensus conference: Perioperative red blood cell transfusion, *JAMA* 260:2700-2703, 1988.

61. Kereiakes DJ, Califf RM, George BS, et al: Coronary bypass surgery improves global and regional left ventricular function following thrombolytic therapy for acute myocardial infarction, *Am Heart J* 122:390-399, 1991.

62. Austin EH, Oldham HN, Sabastin DC, et al: Early assessment of rest and exercise on left ventricular function following coronary artery surgery, *Ann Thorac Surg* 35:159-169, 1983.

63. Floyd RD, Sabastin DC, Leekel R, et al: The effect of duration of hyperthermic cardioplegia on ventricular function, *J Cardiovasc Surg* 85:606-611, 1983.

64. Ceremuzynski L: Hormonal and metabolic reactions evoked by acute myocardial infarction, *Circ Res* 48:767-776, 1981.

65. Karlsberg RP, Cryer PE, Roberts R: Serial plasma catecholamine respond early in the course of clinical acute myocardial infarction: relationship to infarct extent and mortality, *Am Heart J* 102:24-31, 1981.

Chapter 36

THE USE OF NEW INTERVENTIONAL DEVICES IN EVOLVING ACUTE MYOCARDIAL INFARCTION

Harry R. Phillips
James E. Tcheng
Richard S. Stack

The GUSTO trial clearly established the relationship between the achievement of prompt TIMI grade 3 reperfusion and a reduction in mortality for patients with acute myocardial infarction (AMI) treated with thrombolytic therapy.[1,2] These results make mechanical reperfusion techniques seem especially appealing as a way to achieve prompt, unrestricted antegrade flow in the infarct vessel. Several recent prospective randomized studies have compared the use of immediate percutaneous transluminal coronary angioplasty (PTCA) versus intravenous thrombolytic therapy in patients with evolving AMI.[3-6] An overview of these studies indicates that primary angioplasty was more effective in achieving infarct vessel patency and preventing reocclusion (see Chapter 26). Patients treated with immediate angioplasty had a lower incidence of recurrent ischemia and mortality compared with patients treated with thrombolytic therapy. Hospital stays were shorter for patients treated with direct PTCA, and in-hospital costs were similar for the two treatment strategies.

In spite of these favorable results with primary PTCA, thrombolytic therapy is, and is likely to remain, the most commonly used treatment for AMI because of the logistical problems of transferring patients with infarcts to hospitals with catheterization laboratories. These studies show, however, that primary angioplasty may be the treatment of choice for patients with AMI who present to centers where immediate angioplasty can be performed with surgical backup. Moreover, these results imply that immediate angioplasty is the best treatment option for the large numbers of AMI patients in whom thrombolytic therapy is contraindicated. Immediate angiography and angioplasty may also be reasonable for patients in whom MI is suspected on clinical grounds, but in whom the diagnosis is unclear from the electrocardiogram (ECG).

Multiple observational studies suggest that patients presenting with cardiogenic shock in the setting of an AMI have poor outcomes when treated with thrombolytic therapy alone and that successful immediate angioplasty is associated with markedly enhanced survival[7-9] (see Chapter 46). Based on these data, immediate angiography and PTCA, if appropriate, is the treatment of choice for shock complicating AMI.

New interventional techniques including atherectomy, coronary stenting, and laser angioplasty are now used for coronary revascularization procedures in many interventional laboratories, either as primary interventions or as adjuncts to balloon angioplasty. Although the role of these devices is becoming better defined for patients in elective settings,[10] there has been little experience with them in the early stages of MI. This chapter will address the potential role of these devices in evolving MI in an era when an expanded role for immediate mechanical intervention is expected.[11] First the role of new devices in the management of abrupt closure after conventional PTCA will be considered; subsequently, each device will be briefly described and its potential role as primary intervention to achieve reperfusion in the patient with MI will be presented.

ABRUPT CLOSURE AFTER PTCA FOR EVOLVING MI

At present new interventional devices are most commonly used in the setting of evolving AMI when infarct vessel balloon angioplasty has failed or vessel reclosure is threatened. In the setting of AMI with intracoronary thrombus, angioplasty appears to be associated with a higher risk of vessel closure than in elective procedures.[12] Plaque instability with intraluminal thrombus,[13] poor distal runoff, and reduced cardiac output all contribute to vessel closure in this patient population. Prolonged dilatation with a perfusion balloon remains our preferred initial approach to management of inadequate angioplasty results in infarct patients. Adjunctive thrombolytic therapy has been used for patients with a large thrombus burden.[14] As shown in a recently completed randomized trial, intraaortic balloon pumping reduces the likelihood of vessel closure following infarct vessel angioplasty.[15]

Although the clinician typically focuses on the site of total occlusion in the infarct vessel, the state of the distal vascular bed may have an important effect on the success of the reperfusion strategy. The "no reflow" phenomenon first described by Kloner et al. refers to the paradox of relieving a coronary obstruction yet failing to achieve brisk antegrade flow in the infarct vessel.[16] This phenomenon has been documented in experimental models[17-19] and in humans by scintigraphy[20] and angiography.[21] It has been proposed that the "no reflow" phenomenon may occur more frequently after sudden reperfusion, as might occur with immediate infarct vessel angioplasty as opposed to more gradual reperfusion as might occur with thrombolytic therapy.[22] During direct infarct vessel angioplasty, distal clot embolization may play a role in slowing antegrade flow. Other potential mechanisms include microvascular damage,[23] neutrophil plugging of the capillary bed,[24] impaired coronary vasodilator reserve,[25] and small vessel spasm.[26,28]

The occurrence of the "no reflow" phenomenon appears to predict an increased mortality for patients with infarction undergoing angioplasty.[28] Currently there is no known strategy that will predictably prevent or reverse the "no reflow" phenomenon. Intracoronary nitroglycerine has been the traditional treatment. In

1992 Shani et al. presented preliminary data showing that intracoronary verapamil can reverse the phenomenon during angioplasty for AMI.[29]

If angioplasty is unsuccessful because of failure of the lesion to dilate, refractory recoil, or the presence of a limited dissection, directional atherectomy may be used to improve the angiographic result.[30] The technique of directional atherectomy is discussed further in the next section. Although directional atherectomy has been effective in the setting of intravascular thrombus,[31] there has been limited experience with the device in the setting of AMI. Nonetheless, directional atherectomy may be used to salvage patency when PTCA results are inadequate in patients with evolving MI (Fig. 36-1). Prolonged anticoagulation should be used to reduce the risk of abrupt closure when the device is used as a "salvage" strategy for failed infarct vessel angioplasty. This seems especially prudent in view of the increased out-of-lab abrupt closure rate that has been reported following the use of the device in patients who have recently received thrombolytic therapy for AMI.[32]

When vessel closure cannot be reversed with prolonged dilatation or directional atherectomy, coronary stenting may be considered. Coronary stents are also described in more detail in the next section. Stent thrombosis is the most serious complication of coronary stenting for failed angioplasty and is more common when there is preexistent intravascular thrombus, which is almost always the case in the setting of AMI.

The Gianturco-Roubin flexible stent (Cook Inc., Bloomington, Ind.) has recently been approved by the U.S. Food and Drug Administration for the treatment of failed PTCA. Iyer et al. reported the use of the Gianturco-Roubin stent in 46 patients with acute or threatened closure within 0 to 15 days after AMI.[33] Ten patients were considered to have evolving AMI; three of these ten patients (30%) had stent thrombosis, compared with 2 of 36 (6%) patients without evolving MI. All five patients with stent thrombosis had their stents successfully reopened. Prolonged intracoronary urokinase was administered prophylactically in seven patients after stent deployment and only one of these (14%) had stent thrombosis. The investigators concluded that "salvage" stenting in patients with evolving MI has a high risk of stent thrombosis and that prolonged intracoronary urokinase infusion should be considered for these patients.

There are no data available concerning use of other types of coronary stents to salvage failed PTCA in the setting of AMI. In addition to prolonged administration of intracoronary urokinase administered directly into the stented segment, it is critical to achieve ideal angiographic results and to pay meticulous attention to systemic anticoagulation. Patients in whom cardiogenic shock has been reversed by angioplasty and stent

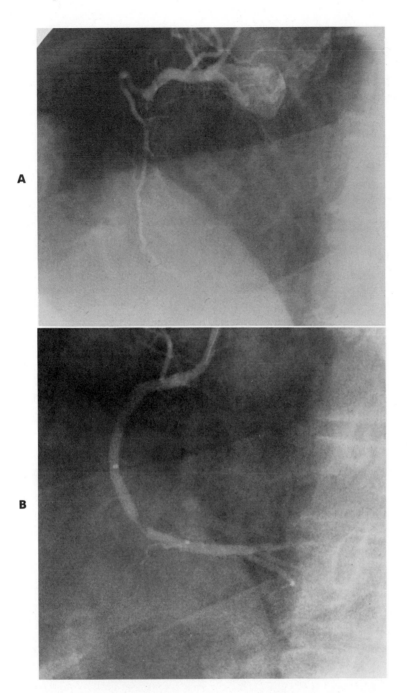

Fig. 36-1. Salvage of failed angioplasty using directional atherectomy in a patient with acute inferior wall myocardial infarction. **A,** Total occlusion of the right coronary artery. **B,** Perfusion balloon catheter in right coronary artery.   *Continued.*

deployment are at high risk if stent thrombosis occurs and should be considered for coronary bypass surgery. Surgery may be clearly indicated in such patients if angiographic results are not ideal after stenting.

New, more powerful antiplatelet agents, including monoclonal antibodies[34] and peptides[35] that are specific for the glycoprotein IIb/IIIa receptor of the platelet have been shown to reduce abrupt vessel closure after conventional coronary angioplasty. Compared with heparin, hirudin[36] and hirulog[37] are more specific thrombin antagonists, and clinical experience using these agents during coronary intervention is growing. More effective inhibition of thrombin and platelets has the potential to reduce the likelihood of thrombotic complications in the infarct patient in whom stent deployment is necessary.

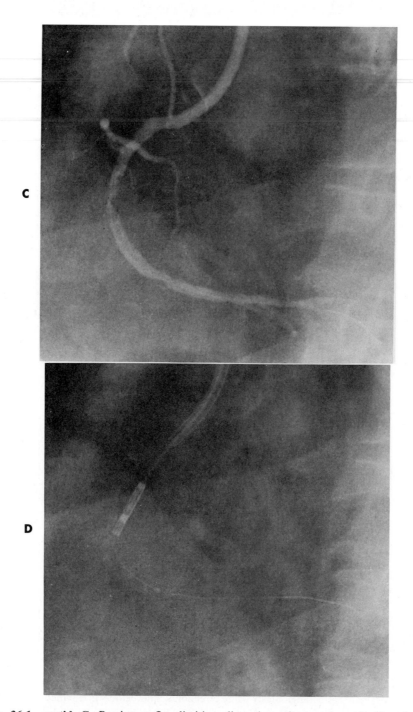

Fig. 36-1. cont'd. C, Persistent flow-limiting dissection after prolonged dilatation with perfusion balloon. **D,** 7 French directional atherectomy catheter across lesion in right coronary. *Continued.*

PRIMARY USE OF NEW INTERVENTIONAL TECHNOLOGY IN AMI

In spite of the enormous growth in the numbers of coronary angioplasty procedures performed annually, the effectiveness of the technique is limited by the problems of abrupt vessel closure and late restenosis, which occur in 5% to 8%[38] and 17% to 45%[39] of patients, respectively. New interventional devices have been developed in an attempt to overcome these problems. Although encouraging results have been reported using these devices for lesion morphologies that have not been ideally treated with conventional PTCA, little carefully controlled or randomized data are available to compare the use of these devices to one another or to PTCA.

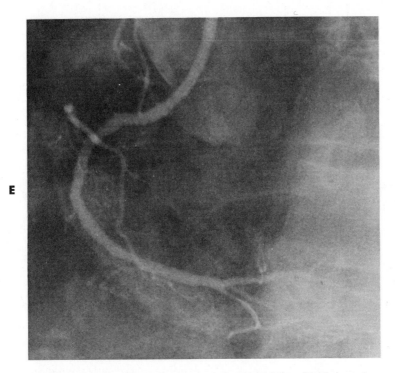

Fig. 36-1. cont'd. E, Final injection showing 25% residual stenosis.

Thus, the indication for the use of new devices in elective procedures has not yet been defined. Unfortunately, there are few reports of the use of new devices in the setting of AMI, and their efficacy in this clinical setting is even more uncertain. In view of the recent approval of several of these devices by the U.S. Food and Drug Administration and of their growing overall use, each device's potential role as a primary treatment for AMI will be reviewed.

Directional coronary atherectomy (DCA)

The directional coronary atherectomy catheter (Simpson Atherocath, Devices for Vascular Intervention, Redwood City, Calif.), which was the first new technology to be granted U.S. Food and Drug Administration approval for coronary revascularization, is shown in Figure 36-2. The device employs a cup-shaped cutter housed within a metal cylinder. An eccentric 5- or 9-mm longitudinal opening in the housing is opposed to the coronary plaque by a support balloon that is located on the opposite side of the housing. When the balloon is inflated, plaque is excised by advancement of the rotating cutter and trapped in the flexible nose cone of the catheter. The device may be used over any steerable 0.014-inch guidewire.

Based on observational data the DCA device appears to be especially useful for bulky, eccentric plaques,[40] bifurcation lesions,[41] and ostial lesions,[42] none of which are ideally suited for PTCA. Recently DCA was compared with conventional angioplasty in the CAVEAT randomized trial.[43] Patients who were treated with DCA had a trend toward a lower restenosis rate than patients treated with conventional angioplasty. However, the acute complication rate was greater, and there was no clinical benefit at 6 months in patients who were treated with DCA. Further randomized clinical trials are being designed in which a more extensive atherectomy technique is compared with conventional PTCA.

As noted previously, the presence of intraluminal thrombus has not adversely affected atherectomy results using the DCA catheter.[31] An increased risk of abrupt closure has been suggested, however, in patients who underwent DCA following treatment with thrombolytic therapy for AMI.[32] The New Approaches to Coronary Interventions (NACI) group compared the results of DCA in patients with recent MI versus patients without MI.[44] The clinical success rate in 147 patients with recent AMI was 83% compared with 88.4% in the 438 patients without recent MI (P = ns). In the group with recent MI, the clinical success rate increased from 77% for DCA performed 1 to 9 days after AMI to 90% for DCA performed 10 to 19 days after AMI and to 95% for DCA performed 20 to 30 days after AMI. The authors concluded that the results of DCA are less favorable in patients with recent MI than in those without MI. They postulated that there was a trend towards an improved success rate with an increasing time interval after MI.

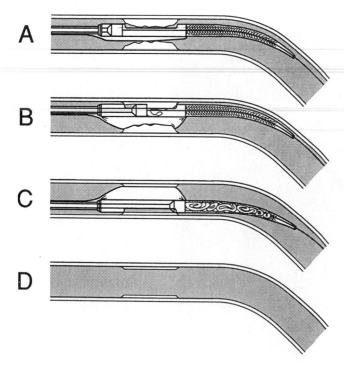

Fig. 36-2. Directional coronary atherectomy procedure. **A,** Atherectomy catheter is placed across the stenotic lesion. **B,** The inflated balloon pushes the housing against the lesion. The portion of the plaque that protrudes into the housing through the opening is excised by a rotating cup-shaped cutter. **C,** The catheter is rotated, and multiple cuts are made. The excised tissue is stored in the distal collecting chamber. **D,** After atherectomy. (With permission from Holmes DR, Garratt KN: *Atherectomy,* Boston, Mass., 1992, Blackwell Scientific Publications.)

There are no data concerning the use of DCA during evolving AMI, but extrapolating from the above results, it seems likely that the clinical success rate would be even lower than in patients with recent events. Accordingly, DCA should not be used preferentially in patients with AMI unless there is an unusual anatomic situation for which PTCA is unsuited. As noted previously, however, DCA may have a role in salvaging failed angioplasty in carefully selected patients.

Extraction atherectomy

The transluminal extraction catheter (TEC, Interventional Technologies Inc., San Diego, Calif.) has recently been approved by the U.S. Food and Drug Administration for general use in the United States. As shown in Figure 36-3 it is a hollow torque tube with two conical front-cutting blades that follow a dedicated steerable guidewire. A unique design feature of this atherectomy catheter is its ability to constantly aspirate during cutting. Observational studies have suggested that the device may have a role in treating degenerated vein grafts that contain friable plaque and thrombus.[45]

The aspiration feature of the TEC may also allow the device to remove intravascular thrombus. Larkin et al. reported using the transluminal extraction catheter in 19 patients with AMI who either had contraindications to or failed thrombolytic therapy.[46] All patients were treated within 12 hours of the onset of MI. Use of the TEC device was technically possible in 17 patients, and complication-free success was achieved in 16 of the 17 patients. There was one acute reocclusion in the hospital.

Thus, preliminary experience suggests that the transluminal extraction catheter may be effective in patients with AMI. The precise role of the TEC relative to PTCA in the treatment of these patients is not yet clear, but it may prove to have special utility in patients who have a large thrombus burden.

Rotational ablation

The high-speed rotational ablation catheter (Rotablator, Heart Technology, Seattle, Wash.) was also recently approved by the U.S. Food and Drug Administration. High-speed rotational ablation is performed using an olive-shaped burr, the leading edge of which is impregnated with small diamond chips. The burr follows a dedicated steerable guide wire and is rotated at approximately 200,000 rpm by an air-driven turbine. This device appears to have special utility in treating stenoses in calcified coronary arteries including ostial lesions.[47] Lesions that have not yielded to balloon dilatation have been successfully treated with high-speed rotational ablation.[48] The ERBAC study was a randomized trial in which patients with complex lesion morphology were randomized to conventional angioplasty, rotational extraction, or excimer laser angioplasty. Preliminary results indicate that overall procedural success was superior with rotational ablation.[49]

There are no reports on the use of rotational ablation in the setting of AMI. The mechanism of action of the Rotablator catheter is to pulverize plaque into microparticulate matter, which is not removed by the catheter but is instead absorbed by the microcirculation. If passed through a vessel segment containing thrombus, the catheter may cause distal embolism of clot, and use of the device is not recommended when thrombus is present.[50] Nonetheless, the Rotablator may prove to be a useful adjunct to direct angioplasty in carefully selected patients whose lesions are heavily calcified or fail to dilate with PTCA.

Coronary stents

Vascular stents are thin metallic scaffolds that mechanically support the vessel wall. Stents are delivered in a collapsed state and are deployed either by self-expansion or by inflation of a delivery balloon. Coronary stents were designed to solve the dual problems of abrupt closure and late restenosis.

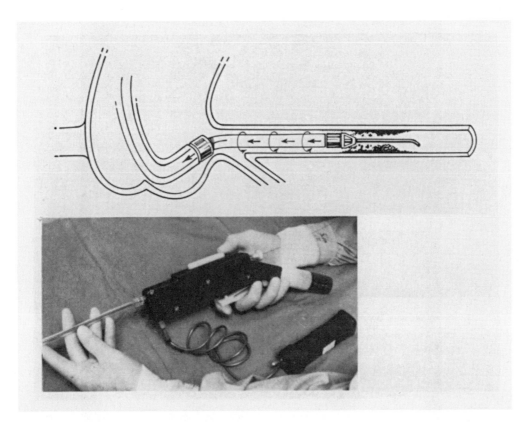

Fig. 36-3. Diagrammatic representation of the transluminal extraction catheter being advanced across an atherosclerotic plaque over a 0.014-inch guidewire. The excised fragments are removed by continuous suction through the central lumen of the catheter. (With permission from Stack RS: *Am J Cardiol* 62:3F-24F, 1988.)

The Gianturco-Roubin stent (Cook Inc., Bloomington, Ind.) has been reported to be effective in reversing abrupt closure after angioplasty.[51] With the recent U.S. Food and Drug Administration approval of the Gianturco-Roubin stent for failed PTCA, the use of intracoronary stenting is likely to increase. In addition, interim results of the Benestent[52] and Stress[53] randomized trials indicate that deployment of the Palmaz-Schatz stent (Johnson & Johnson Interventional Systems, Warren, N.J.) in primary lesions reduces restenosis compared with conventional angioplasty. If these data are confirmed in the final analyses, there will be further impetus to use coronary stents. The Gianturco-Roubin stent is shown in Figure 36-4.

Intracoronary stents have been used in patients with evolving MI only in the setting of failed infarct vessel angioplasty, as discussed previously. The problem of intraluminal thrombus and the predisposition to stent thrombosis make it unlikely that currently available metallic stents will be deployed as a primary intervention in AMI. The development of a metallic stent with an antithrombotic coating has reduced stent thrombosis in an experimental model.[54] Biodegradable polymeric stents

have been under development at several centers.[55-57] Zidar et al. have shown that a stent constructed from poly L-lactide may be less thrombogenic than metallic stents.[58] In addition, heparin coating of the polymer stent may further reduce adherence of platelets and fibrin to the stent. Polymeric stents may also allow sustained delivery of antiproliferative drugs to further reduce restenosis. Ultimately the development of stents with drug delivery capability may expand the role of stenting in AMI.

Ablative laser angioplasty

Two different wavelengths of light are currently being used to ablate tissue as adjuncts to the performance of balloon angioplasty. These include the excimer laser wavelength of 308 nm and the holmium:YAG wavelength of 2100 nm. Excimer laser angioplasty systems manufactured by Advanced Interventional Systems (Irvine, Calif.) and Spectranetics (Colorado Springs, Colo.) received U.S. Food and Drug Administration approval for coronary use in 1992 and 1993 respectively.

Excimer laser ablation occurs at a wavelength that is transparent to water, modestly absorbed by hemoglobin,

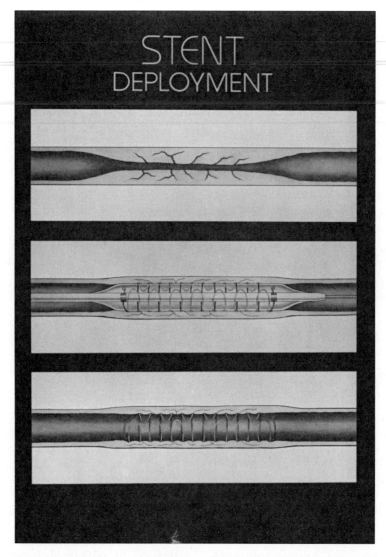

Fig. 36-4. Diagrammatic representation of Gianturo-Roubin coil stent supporting dissected segment of coronary plaque.   (Courtesy of Cook Cardiology, a division of Cook Inc, Bloomington, Ind.)

and strongly absorbed by plaque. Observational data suggest that excimer laser angioplasty can produce superior results compared with conventional balloon angioplasty in certain complex plaque morphologies, including long lesions, aortoostial stenoses, saphenous vein graft disease in grafts ≤3 mm in diameter, lesions resistant to balloon crossing and/or dilation, and total occlusions.[59] In comparison, the experience with thrombus ablation is considerably more limited. Rosenfield et al.[60] reported dissolution of clot in a series of six patients with angiographically visible filling defects; in all cases, however, the clot was at least 3 days old and the mean estimated age was 33 days. Less satisfactory outcomes were observed in 12 patients with lesions containing thrombus as reported by Estella et al.[61]; in this study, the clinical success rate was only 58%, and the presence of

thrombus was the most important predictor of poor outcome. Recent work has also clearly documented that exposure of blood to 308 nm radiation results in pressure shock wave formation that might predispose a vessel to dissection.[62]

The strong absorption of 2100 nm holmium:YAG radiation by matter containing water has led to investigation of this device in the setting of thrombosis. In an initial experience, Topaz et al.[63] reported a high rate of successful thrombolysis in a small number of patients with intracoronary thrombus or AMI involving grafts and native coronary arteries. Although this report seems promising, the problem of blood (and the water contained therein) in the field between the treatment catheter tip and the target thrombus remains to be overcome.

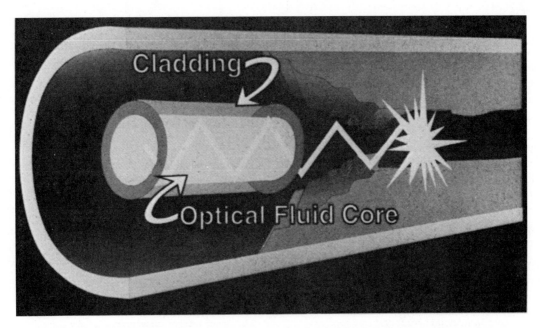

Fig. 36-5. Diagrammatic representation of selective laser thrombolysis. The unique catheter has an optical fluid core that delivers laser energy to the thrombus. (With permission from Gregory KW: A session-specific approach to new-device angioplasty. In Topol EJ (editor): *Textbook of Interventional Cardiology,* Philadelphia, 1993, WB Saunders.)

These limited data do not support the utilization of either the excimer or the holmium laser in the treatment of acutely occluded infarct vessels. Neither device is particularly selective of thrombus over other elements, particularly plaque or water. Although further investigation is continuing, more appropriate wavelengths (featuring selective and preferential absorption of energy by thrombus compared with water and plaque) seem to be a better potential approach.

Selective laser thrombolysis

Theoretically the ideal wavelength of light to treat fresh thrombus would be highly absorbed by clot while being poorly absorbed or transparent to other surrounding media, particularly water, atherosclerotic plaque, and the endothelium and other tissue components of the vascular wall. The wavelengths of visible light that conform most closely to these characteristics are at approximately 480 nm. One laser, the pulsed dye laser, can be "tuned" to this approximate frequency by proper selection of the lasing medium. In addition, this wavelength is readily transmitted through contrast. By taking advantage of the refractive index of contrast, a virtual "fluid core" optical channel can be used to transmit the energy through short distances in the coronary vasculature to the level of a thrombus, even when contact between the tip of the catheter and the target thrombus is not achieved (Fig. 36-5).

Preliminary investigation of this device has proven encouraging. den Heijer, et al. reported on 18 patients with AMI and infarct arteries approached with selective laser thrombolysis because of contraindications to thrombolytic drugs or failure to reperfuse.[64] With the first prototype system, 12 of these patients were treated, with qualitative thrombus ablation and improvement in TIMI flow in 10 patients (83%). Two patients, both considered high risk, ultimately died because of left ventricular failure and one patient died after bypass surgery. There were no perforations or dissections.

Gregory et al. have also reported on initial results, including a series of 16 patients who were either not treatable with thrombolytic agents or who had failed to reperfuse.[65,66] All patients had angiographically identifiable thrombus. Laser thrombolysis was believed to be effective in removing thrombus in 15 of the 16 patients. The mean TIMI coronary flow grade increased from 0.7 to 2.4. Subsequently all patients were treated with adjunctive angioplasty or atherectomy. Angiographic success was obtained in 15 of 16 patients (94%). There were no cases of perforation, abrupt closure, recurrent infarction, or death during the hospitalizations.

Selective laser thrombolysis is an intriguing approach to the interventional treatment of the patient with AMI. Theoretically, use of wavelengths around 480 nm may selectively ablate thrombus without other local effects. However, clinical data regarding its use have been extremely limited and its role remains to be defined.

CONCLUSIONS

Significant numbers of patients with evolving MI will be treated with mechanical interventions in the 1990s. Primary angioplasty without preceding thrombolytic therapy has achieved remarkably good results in restoring perfusion in patients with AMI; however, in an important subgroup of patients, angioplasty achieves suboptimal results because of complex plaque morphology or excessive thrombus. So far, new interventional technologies have played a minor role in overcoming these problems. As improvements are made in devices, operative techniques, and adjunctive pharmacologic interventions, these devices may make an important contribution in achieving rapid and sustained infarct vessel patency.

REFERENCES

1. The GUSTO Angiographic Investigators: The effects of tissue plasminogen activator, streptokinase, or both on coronary artery patency, ventricular function, and survival after acute myocardial infarction, *N Engl J Med* 329:1615-1622, 1993.
2. The Gusto Investigators: An international randomized trial comparing four thrombolytic strategies for acute myocardial infarction, *N Engl J Med* 329:673-682, 1993.
3. Grines CL, Browne KF, Marco J, et al: A comparison of immediate angioplasty with thrombolytic therapy for acute myocardial infarction, *N Engl J Med* 328:673, 1993.
4. Zijlstra F, de Boer MJ, Hoorntje JC, et al: A comparison of immediate coronary angioplasty with intravenous streptokinase in acute myocardial infarction, *N Engl J Med* 328:680, 1993.
5. Gibbons RJ, Holmes DR, Reeder GS, et al: Immediate angioplasty compared with the administration of a thrombolytic agent followed by conservative treatment for myocardial infarction, *N Engl J Med* 328:685, 1993.
6. Ribeiro EE, Silva LA, Carneiro R, et al: Randomized trial of direct coronary angioplasty vs. intravenous streptokinase in acute myocardial infarction, *J Am Coll Cardiol* 22:376-80, 1993.
7. O'Neill WW, et al: Coronary angioplasty therapy of cardiogenic shock complicating acute myocardial infarction (abstract), *Circulation* 72:III-309, 1985.
8. Moosvi AR, Khaja F, Villanueva L, et al: Early revascularization improves survival in cardiogenic shock complicating acute myocardial infarction, *J Am Coll Cardiol* 19:907, 1992.
9. Lee L, Bates ER, Pitt B, et al: Percutaneous transluminal coronary angioplasty improves survival in acute myocardial infarction complicated by cardiogenic shock, *Circulation* 78:1345, 1988.
10. Popma JJ, Leon MB: A lesion-specific approach to new-device angioplasty. In Topol EI (ed: *Textbook of interventional cardiology,* Philadelphia, 1993, WB Saunders.
11. Lange RA, Hillis LD: Immediate angioplasty for acute myocardial infarction, *N Engl J Med* 328:726, 1993.
12. Tenaglia AN, Fortin DF, Frid DS, et al: A simple scoring system to predict PTCA abrupt closure, *J Am Coll Cardiol* 19:139, 1992
13. Fuster V, Badimon L, Badimon JJ, et al: The pathogenesis of coronary artery disease and the acute coronary syndrome, *N Engl J Med* 326:242-250, 1992.
14. Grines CL: Angioplasty in the patient with acute myocardial infarction. In Roubin GS, Califf RM, O'Neill WW, et al. *Interventional cardiovascular medicine principles and practice,* New York, 1993, Churchill Livingstone.
15. Ohman EM, George BS, White CJ, et al: The use of aortic counterpulsation to improve sustained coronary artery patency during acute myocardial infarction: results of a randomized trial, *J Am Coll Cardiol* 21:397A, 1993.
16. Kloner RA, Ganote CE, Jennings RB, et al: The "no-reflow" phenomenon following temporary coronary occlusion in the dog, *J Clin Invest* 54:1496-1508, 1974.
17. Kloner RA, Rude RE, Carlson N, et al: Ultrastructural evidence of micravascular damage and myocardial cell injury after coronary artery occlusion: which comes first? *Circulation* 62:5:945-952, 1980.
18. VanHaecke J, et al: Evidence for decreased coronary flow reserve in viable postischemic myocardium, *Circ Res* 67:1201-1210, 1990.
19. Ambrosio G, Weistian HF, Mannisi JA, et al: Progressive impairment of regional myocardial perfusion after initial restoration of postischemic blood flow, *Circulation* 80:1846-1861, 1989.
20. Schofer J, Montz R, Mathey DG, et al: Scintigraphic evidence of the "no reflow" phenomenon in human beings after coronary thrombolysis, *J Am Coll Cardiol* 5:593-598, 1985.
21. Feld H, Lichstein E, Schachter J, et al: Early and late angiographic findings of the "no-reflow" phenomenon following direct angioplasty as primary treatment for acute myocardial infarction, *Am Heart J* 123(3):782-784, 1992.
22. Yamazaki S, Fujibayashi Y, Rajagopalan R, et al: Effects of staged versus sudden reperfusion after acute coronary occlusion in the dog, *J Am Coll Cardiol* 7:564-572, 1986.
23. Kloner RA: No reflow revisited, *J Am Coll Cardiol* 7:1814-5, 1989.
24. Dreyer WJ, Michael LH, West MS, et al: Neutrophil accumulation in ischemic canine myocardium. Insights into time course, distribution, and mechanism of localization during early reperfusion, *Circulation* 84:400-411, 1991.
25. Mehta JL, Nichols WW, Donnelly WH, et al: Impaired canine coronary vasodilator response to acetylcholine and bradykinin after occlusion-reperfusion, *Circ Res* 64:43-54, 1989.
26. VanBenthuysen KM, McMurtry IF, Horwitz LD, et al: Reperfusion after acute coronary occlusion in dogs impairs endothelium-dependent relaxation to acetylcholine and augments contractile reactivity in vitro, *J Clin Invest* 79:265-274, 1987.
27. Ku DD: Coronary vascular reactivity after acute myocardial ischemia, *Science* 218:576-578, 1982.
28. Feld H, Schulhoff N, Lichstein E, et al: Direct angioplasty as primary treatment for acute myocardial infarction resulting in the "no-reflow" phenomenon predicts a high mortality rate, *Circulation* 86:I-135, 1992.
29. Shani J, Feld H, Frankel R, et al: Reversal of the no reflow phenomenon with intracoronary verapamil during coronary angioplasty for acute myocardial infarction, *Circulation* 86:I-852, 1992.
30. Vetter JW, Robertson GC, Selmon MR, et al: Use of directional coronary atherectomy for failed PTCA, *Circulation* 86:I-249, 1992.
31. Ellis SG, De Cesare NB, Pinkerton CA, et al: Relation of stenosis morphology and clinical presentation to the procedural results of directional coronary atherectomy, *Circulation* 84(2):644-653, 1991.
32. Potkin BN, Mintz GS, Pichard AD, et al: Late, out-of-laboratory, abrupt closure after angiographically successful directional coronary atherectomy, *Am J Cardiol* 69:263, 1992.
33. Iyer SS, Bilodeau L, Cannon AD, et al: Stenting the infarct related artery within 15 days of the acute event: immediate and long term outcome using the flexible metallic coil stent, *J Am Coll Cardiol* 21:291A, 1993.
34. Tcheng JE, Topol EJ, Kleiman NS, et al: Improvement in clinical outcomes of coronary angioplasty by treatment with the GPIIb/IIIa inhibitor chimeric 7E3:multivariable analysis of the EPIC study, *Circulation* 88:I-506, 1993.
35. Tcheng JE, Ellis SG, Kleiman NS, et al: Outcome of patients treated with the GPIIb/IIIa inhibitor integrelin during coronary angioplasty: results of the Impact study, *Circulation* 88:I-595, 1993.
36. van den Bos AA, Deckers JW, Heyndrickx GR, et al: Safety and

efficacy of recombinant hirudin (CGP 393) versus heparin in patients with stable angina undergoing coronary angioplasty, *Circulation* 88(I):2058-2066, 1993.

37. Topol EJ, Bonan R, Jewitt D, et al: Use of a direct antithrombin, hirulog, in place of heparin during coronary angioplasty, *Circulation* 87:1622-1629, 1993.

38. Detre KM, Holmes DR Jr, Holubkov R, et al: Incidence and consequences of periprocedural occlusion. The 1985-1986 National Heart, Lung, and Blood Institute percutaneous transluminal coronary angioplasty registry, *Circulation* 82(3):739-750, 1990.

39. Califf RM, Fortin DF, Frid DS, et al: Restenosis after coronary angioplasty: an overview, *J Am Coll Cardiol* 17(suppl):2B-1313, 1991.

40. Hinohara T, Vetter JW, Selmon MR, et al: Directional coronary atherectomy is effective treatment for extremely eccentric lesions, *Circulation* 84:II-520, 1991.

41. Monsour M, et al: Feasibility of directional atherectomy for the treatment of bifurcation lesions, *Coronary Artery Disease* 3:761, 1992.

42. Robertson GC, et al: Directional coronary atherectomy for ostial lesions, *Circulation* 84 (supplIII):II-521, 1991.

43. Topol EJ, Leya F, Pinkerton CA, et al: A comparison of directional atherectomy with coronary angioplasty in patients with coronary artery disease, *N Engl J Med* 329:221-227, 1993.

44. Ghazzal ZMB, Hinohara T, Scott N, et al: Directional coronary atherectomy in patients with recent myocardial infarction: a NACI registry report, *J Am Coll Cardiol* 21:32A, 1993.

45. O'Neill WW, Kramer BL, Sketch MH Jr, et al: Mechanical extraction atherectomy: report of the U.S. transluminal extraction catheter investigation, *Circulation* 86:I-779, 1992.

46. Larkin TJ, Niemyski PR, Parker MA, et al: Primary and rescue extraction atherectomy in patients with acute myocardial infarction, *Circulation* 84:II-537, 1991.

47. Buchbinder M, O'Neill W, Warth D, et al: Percutaneous coronary rotational ablation using the Rotablator: results of a multicenter study (abstract), *Circulation* 82(suppl III):III-309, 1990.

48. O'Neill WW: Mechanical rotational atherectomy. In Roubin GS, Califf RM, O'Neill WW, et al: *Interventional cardiovascular medicine: principles and practice,* New York, 1993, Churchill Livingstone.

49. Reifart N, et al: Comparison of Excimer laser, Rotablator, and balloon angioplasty for the treatment of complex coronary lesions: a randomized trial (abstract), *Circulation* (suppl I)86:I-1489, 1992.

50. Bertrand ME, Bauters C, Lablanche JM: Percutaneous coronary rotational angioplasty with the Rotablator. In Topol EJ (ed): *Textbook of interventional cardiology,* Philadelphia, 1993, WB Saunders.

51. Roubin GS, Cannon AD, Agrawal SK, et al: Intracoronary stenting for acute and threatened closure complicating percutaneous transluminal coronary angioplasty, *Circulation* 85(3):916-927, 1992.

52. Serruys PW, Macaya C, de Jaegere P, et al: Interim analysis of the Benestent trial, *Circulation* 88:I-594, 1993.

53. Schatz RA, Penn IM, Baim DS, et al: STent REStenosis Study (STRESS): analysis of in-hospital results, *Circulation* 88:I-594, 1993.

54. Bailey SR, et al: Heparin coating of endovascular stents decreases subacute thrombosis in a rabbit model, *Circulation* 86:I-186, 1992.

55. Lincoff AM, van der Gressen WJ, Schwartz RS, et al: Biodegradable and biostable polymers may both cause vigorous inflammatory responses when implanted in porcine coronary arteries (abstract) *J Am Coll Cardiol* (suppl) 21:179A, 1993.

56. Zidar JP, Gammon RS, Chapman CD, et al: Short and long-term vascular tissue response in the Duke bioabsorbable stent (abstract), *J Am Coll Cardiol* (suppl) 21:439A, 1993.

57. Suswa T, Shiraki K, Shimizu Y: Biodegradable intracoronary stents in adult dogs (abstract) *J Am Coll Cardiol* (suppl) 21:484A, 1993.

58. Zidar JP, Mohammad SF, Culp SC, et al: In vitro thrombogenicity analysis of a new bioabsorbable balloon-expandable, endovascular stent, *J Am Coll Cardiol* 21:483A, 1993.

59. Bittl JA, et al: Clinical success, complications and restenosis rates with excimer laser coronary angioplasty. The Percutaneous Excimer Laser Coronary Angioplasty Registry, *J Am Coll Cardiol* 70(20):1533-1539, 1992.

60. Rosenfield, K, Pieczek A, Losordo DW, et al: Excimer laser thrombolysis for rapid clot dissolution in lesions at high risk for embolization: a potentially useful new application for excimer laser, *J Am Coll Cardiol,* 19 (suppl A):104A, 1992.

61. Estella P, Ryan TJ Jr, Landzberg JS, et al: Excimer laser-assisted coronary angioplasty for lesions containing thrombus, *J Am Coll Cardiol* 21(7):1550-1556, 1993.

62. Tcheng JE, Phillips HR, Wells LD, et al: A new technique for reducing pressure pulse phenomena during coronary excimer laser angioplasty, *J Am Coll Cardiol* 21:386A, 1993.

63. Topaz O, Rozenbaum EA, Battista S, et al: Laser facilitated angioplasty and thrombolysis in acute myocardial infarction complicated by prolonged or recurrent chest pain, *Cathet Cardiovasc Diagn* 28:7-16, 1993.

64. den Heijer P, van Dijk RB, Pentinga ML, et al: Laser thrombolysis—first clinical results, *Circulation* 86:I-651, 1992.

65. Gregory KW, Block PC, Knopf LA, et al: Laser thrombolysis in acute myocardial infarction, *J Am Coll Cardiol* 21:289A, 1993.

66. Gregory KW, Prince MR, LaMuraglia GM, et al: Effect of blood upon the selective ablation of atherosclerotic plaque with a pulsed dye laser, *Lasers Surg Med* 10:533, 1990.

Chapter 37

NONINVASIVE DEFINITION OF FAILED REPERFUSION AT THE BEDSIDE: LOOKING BEYOND THE TIP OF THE CATHETER

Mitchell W. Krucoff
E. Magnus Ohman
Kathleen M. Trollinger
Robert Christensen
Sharon T. Sawchak
Akbar Shah
James E. Pope
Robert M. Califf

Few clinical scenarios are as striking as that of a classical AMI. Similarly, few medical therapies are as dramatic as successful thrombolysis. Although textbook coronary reperfusion is occasionally seen at the bedside with complete relief of chest pain, normalization of the ECG, and a burst of accelerated idioventricular rhythm, more frequently patients show only marginal improvement following therapy, or may stabilize briefly only to deteriorate again. Pain relief that gives a clinical impression of apparent improvement may result from the nonspecific effects of narcotics rather than from thrombus dissolution. Although the classical successes of thrombolytic therapy provide memorable examples for practitioners, in many cases the bedside evaluation of thrombolytic efficacy remains a difficult dilemma. This dilemma is compounded by the knowledge that time spent observing or testing patients with failed reperfu-

sion will allow additional cell death, reducing the potential benefit of any subsequent interventions. Conversely, premature or inaccurate assumption of failed thrombolysis may lead to risky and expensive procedures in patients who may be likely to do at least as well without them.

In this chapter we will review objective and subjective noninvasive tools for the bedside identification of patients with failed or inadequate reperfusion following thrombolytic therapy. As will be discussed, in the 1990s we have two distinct goals: to develop a rapid and accurate noninvasive means of detecting changes in coronary patency as a surrogate for angiography and to quantify the ongoing, cumulative, and dynamic insult of infarction before, during, and after any single angiographic "snapshot." The next section of this chapter will review briefly the history of reperfusion therapy and the angiographic definition of reperfusion. Following this, we will examine the individual noninvasive "tools" that have been proposed for use in defining reperfusion. Finally, we will consider strategies for the future.

"FAILED" REPERFUSION: TIP OF THE CATHETER OR TIP OF THE ICEBERG?

The rationale for the use of thrombolytic therapy in AMI was provided in the late 1970s by the pioneering studies of DeWood et al.[1] These investigators performed acute angiography in a series of MI patients and provided unequivocal documentation of the relatively ubiquitous role of thrombus in AMI presentations in humans.[1] These observations led to the early intervention studies by Rentrop et al., the Western Washington group, and Simoons et al. using intracoronary streptokinase.[2-4]

Reperfusion defined angiographically was initially viewed as something that either happened or failed to happen.[5-7] Angiographic reperfusion was presumed to define interruption of the infarction. Based on early animal lab experiments showing that cell death moved as a time-dependent "wavefront" through the distribution of the occluded artery,[8] angiographic reperfusion (either spontaneous or pharmacologic) was presumed to produce salvage of the myocardium that was not yet irreversibly injured. Such myocardial salvage was intuitively expected to be measurable as improved left ventricular function and improved survival. Despite case reports demonstrating dramatic improvements in left ventricular function with reperfusion, data correlating angiographic reperfusion with recovery of ventricular function or improved mortality showed substantially more modest benefits, particularly in randomized trials of intracoronary thrombolytic therapy.[3-7,9] Post hoc explanations of why angiographic reperfusion produced only small measurable differences were many. The relatively small patient numbers in these trials resulted in inadequate statistical power to detect small differences attributable to treatment. The time delay imposed by the logistics of urgent catheterization combined with delays in patient presentation and diagnosis might leave little myocardium to salvage.[10-12] But other observations of cyclic changes in coronary flow,[13] of variability in the briskness of restored coronary flow,[14,15] and of collateralization of occluded infarct vessels[16,17] pointed to ambiguous areas of the angiographic "gold standard" on which the "definition" of reperfusion was based. Whether restored blood flow occurred early enough, was stable or brisk enough, whether nutrient blood was able to perfuse tissue at a microvascular level or was impeded, with "no reflow" beyond the epicardial vessel,[18-20] whether oxygenated blood restored deranged myocardial metabolic machinery or caused further injury with reperfusion[21-23] are questions about the ongoing pathophysiology of infarction that remain unanswerable using angiographic parameters. The definition of these areas literally lies beyond the tip of the angiographic catheter.

The advent of intravenous delivery of thrombolytics substantially reduced time to treatment, and large randomized trials reported unequivocal mortality benefits in the treated groups compared to placebo.[10,24] These benefits were presumed to be the result of reperfusion of the infarct artery, but only one trial to date has definitively shown this to be the case for patients with TIMI-3 flow at 90 minutes after drug administration.[25] In this study angiographic TIMI-3 flow was achieved in only about 50% of patients given thrombolytic therapy. The "open artery hypothesis," targeting early and sustained patency of the infarct artery as the goal of AMI intervention continues to be supported by data suggesting that patients who fail to achieve arterial patency suffer more in-hospital complications and have a higher rate of early mortality.[26-30] However, angiographically-defined reperfusion continues to be ambiguous in patients with cyclic flow, TIMI-2 flow, collateralized occlusions, no reflow, or reperfusion injury.[15-23] The potential for noninvasive physiologic markers to better define this spectrum of "failed" reperfusion and to clarify the relationship between angiographic flow and functional outcome remains a substantial challenge that is the focus of much current work.

REPLACING THE CATHETER'S TIP

Despite efforts to maximize the efficacy of intravenous thrombolytic therapy,[25,31-36] around 50% of treated patients fail to achieve sustained TIMI-3 flow and experience suboptimal outcomes as a result. Preliminary data suggest that more aggressive reperfusion strategies in such patients may improve outcomes[32,37] (see Chapter 27). The dilemma remains how to identify these patients quickly and accurately enough to treat them more aggressively without subjecting many patients with TIMI-3 flow to unnecessary procedures.

Defining patients with failed or suboptimal reperfusion in real time is the primary goal for noninvasive markers for the 1990s. Clinicians frequently interpret the relief of chest pain as their primary evidence of reperfusion. In a field experience of over 250 AMI presentations, physicians were convinced they knew the patency status of their patients in over 95% of bedside evaluations 90 minutes after administration of thrombolytic therapy.[38] As discussed in the next section, actual data on their accuracy has confirmed earlier reports that routine descriptors of clinical evaluation at the bedside are both nonspecific and insensitive predictors of angiographic patency.[38-40]

Having administered thrombolytic therapy to a patient with an AMI, the opportunity for the practitioner to discriminate calmly between a classical reperfusion response and some other of the array of responses to thrombolytic therapy is instantly sacrificed to the pressure to "do" something—to make a decision, to administer further therapy, to head for the catheterization laboratory, or to put the patient to bed. Timeliness and practicality are as primary for noninvasive markers of failed reperfusion as they are for the bedside examination. Markers that delay therapy, interfere with therapy, or that cannot produce reperfusion-related information rapidly or, ideally, in "real time" are not likely to play an important role in acute decision making as angiographic surrogates.

Bedside descriptors that can be assessed as markers of reperfusion in this time framework are generally subjective, most notably the severity of residual chest pain. However, chest pain is a problematic outcome measure. The natural anxiety that patients with AMI feel may make the pain seem worse than it otherwise might. On the other hand, standard clinical care, which includes sedation and narcotics, may relieve symptoms without affecting underlying pathophysiology. Consequently, the inaccuracy of the bedside assessment in determining infarct artery reperfusion is not surprising. The potential benefits of objective markers of reperfusion in this setting are self-evident. To realize this benefit, noninvasive markers must provide practical, timely, objective information that can be assessed as repeatedly as necessary.

The final theoretic requirement for noninvasive markers is adequate accuracy defining failed reperfusion. As discussed earlier, developing a surrogate for angiography may not be the proper goal, particularly in cases where the angiographic images are themselves ambiguous. Ideally, the noninvasive definition of failed reperfusion would use markers that strongly and independently correlate with adverse clinical outcomes. As a platform from which appropriate decisions about further or more aggressive therapy could be made, noninvasive markers achieving this end could not only serve as a surrogate for angiographic assessment but could be even more useful than angiography for ongoing patient management.

THE TOOLS
Reversal of ischemia and interruption of infarction

The restoration of antegrade blood flow by thrombolysis initiates a complex cascade of cellular events. These events may be broadly, if somewhat simplistically, grouped into three categories: the reversal of ischemia, the interruption of infarction, and the acceleration of necrosis in cells destined to die. Reversal of ischemia provides the familiar clinical changes, such as relief of chest pain, reduction of ST-segment deviation on the ECG, and sometimes improvement of ventricular function with hemodynamic stabilization. The interruption of infarction halts the process of cell death and cellular enzyme leakage, allowing healing to begin. At the bedside, most of the "classical" response to reperfusion results from the reversal of ischemia in still viable tissue, whereas the longer-term clinical patient outcome is more likely to be related to the successful interruption of the infarction per se. Although generally related, over the dynamic course of an MI recurrent ischemia may occur with or without further cellular necrosis. Similarly, massive cellular necrosis and/or cellular injury from reperfusion may produce clinical deterioration with chest pain, dysrhythmias, and pump failure in the absence of further ischemia. The conjunction and disjunction of these two broad components of the clinical infarction syndrome may help to explain conceptually the relative independent and combined information conveyed by specific noninvasive markers of reperfusion and their ability to define patients with failed reperfusion. This same understanding helps to highlight the enormous potential of combined application of noninvasive markers for patency prediction, risk stratification, and as a measure of response to therapy in the definition of optimal patient care.

Specific noninvasive reperfusion markers

Five main markers have been reported, either individually or in concert, to provide information about the reperfusion status of the infarct vessel: clinical assessment, dysrhythmias, ventricular perfusion and function imaging, serum enzymatic and other biochemical markers, and ECG changes.

Clinical assessment. Bedside clinical evaluation of a patient's ischemic symptom status provides readily available data that can be dynamically reassessed on an ongoing basis. It provides important adjunctive information for patient evaluation, care, and prognosis. However, multiple studies have now shown that clinical symptoms are both nonspecific and insensitive as a means of predicting reperfusion[39,40] (Table 37-1). Despite the "memorable" cases, the overall inaccuracy of the bedside evaluation as currently practiced should discourage the use of clinical evaluation *alone* as a technique for the noninvasive determination of infarct artery patency.

Dysrhythmias. Dysrhythmias attributed to reperfusion include accelerated idioventricular rhythms, ventricular fibrillation, ventricular tachycardia, and profound bradycardia, among others[41-43] (see Chapter 31). Unfortunately all these dysrhythmias are uncommon following reperfusion and are also observed in patients with completed infarction in the absence of reperfusion. Data currently available suggest that dysrhythmias are neither sensitive nor specific enough to identify reperfusion for clinical purposes.[39,44-48] Newer approaches linking the onset and characteristics of dysrhythmias to

Table 37-1. Relation of traditional predictors of reperfusion to observed patency of infarct-related artery

Descriptor	Proportion of sample (n = 386)	Observed patency	95% confidence intervals
ST segment			
Unchanged	0.56	0.63	0.56, 0.70
Improved	0.38	0.84	0.76, 0.90
Resolved	0.06	0.96	0.79, 1.0
Chest pain			
Unchanged or worsened	0.20	0.60	0.48, 0.71
Improved	0.51	0.71	0.64, 0.78
Resolved	0.29	0.84	0.75, 0.90
Arrhythmia			
None	0.64	0.72	0.65, 0.78
Ventricular tachycardia >100	0.06	0.67	0.45, 0.84
Ventricular tachycardia <100	0.07	0.75	0.55, 0.89
Ventricular fibrillation	0.08	0.77	0.58, 0.90
2° atrioventricular block	0.03	0.64	0.31, 0.89
3° atrioventricular block	0.05	0.74	0.49, 0.91
Severe sinus bradycardia	0.16	0.72	0.59, 0.83

From Califf RM, O'Neil W, Stack RS, et al and the TAMI Study Group: Failure of simple clinical measurements to predict perfusion status after intravenous thrombolysis, *Ann Int Med* 108:658-662, 1988.

the timing of other events, as will be mentioned at the end of this chapter, may improve the accuracy and utility of dysrhythmias as noninvasive markers of reperfusion.[45-47]

Ventricular function and perfusion. The use of radioisotopes for noninvasive assessment of reperfusion has undergone considerable investigation in recent years. Early studies used thallium-201 scintigraphy for assessment of myocardial salvage, but this technique has several important limitations. To assess accurately the area of myocardium at risk during coronary occlusion and reperfusion, serial images have to be obtained *before* and 6 hours to 6 days *after* administration of thrombolytic therapy.[49] Patients with successful reperfusion are distinguished by more thallium-201 redistribution and a smaller defect in the infarct zone compared with baseline images. However, the requirement for pretherapy images creates an unacceptable delay in the administration of thrombolytic therapy. In addition, delayed redistribution may be hard to separate from persistent ischemia and scar tissue in the myocardium.[50]

Imaging with technetium-99m stannous pyrophosphate has also been used to detect reperfusion. This

Table 37-2. Plasma markers of myocardial necrosis

Constituent	Molecular weight*	Cardio-specific	Commercial rapid assay†
Myoglobin	17,800	No	Yes
Total creatine kinase	85,000	No	No
CK-MM subforms	85,000	No	No
Creatine kinase MB	85,000	Yes	Yes
CK-MB subforms	85,000	Yes	No
Troponin T	37,000	Yes	No
Myosin light chains	26,000	Yes	No

*Dalton
†Assay time <20 minutes

infarct-avid isotope has been noted to create a strongly positive image in patients with early peak in CK-MB suggestive of successful reperfusion.[51,52] In contrast to the thallium studies, in this type of study intravenous radiolabeled stannous pyrophosphate is injected soon after completion of thrombolytic therapy and imaging is performed 2 hours later, on average. Thus results from pyrophosphate scanning cannot be used for early decision making after administration of thrombolysis.

To address the limitations of thallium-201 and pyrophosphate scanning, newer perfusion agents have been developed.[53] Technetium-99m sestamibi is a newer perfusion agent that, like thallium, is taken up in the myocardium in proportion to blood flow.[54] The half-life of sestamibi is very brief (2.2 minutes), but there is minimal redistribution over time. Imaging of the area at risk, as detected by preintervention injection of sestamibi, can therefore be performed 1 to 5 hours after injection, but repeat injections to detect reperfusion can only be performed 24 to 48 hours after thrombolysis.[55] Although technetium-99m sestamibi imaging is an important tool for assessment of infarct size and myocardium at risk,[56] it is not helpful for early detection of reperfusion.[53] Development of radioisotopes with shorter half-lives, which are predominantly flow tracers, or use of nuclear magnetic resonance spectroscopy[57] may eventually provide a more practical imaging method for noninvasive detection of reperfusion. At present, such applications remain experimental.

Serum markers of reperfusion. A variety of intracellular components arising from the myocardium have been used to diagnose AMI[58] (Table 37-2). These markers have also been used to assess reperfusion noninvasively after thrombolytic therapy. The pattern of appearance in blood depends on several factors that include (1) the intracellular location, particularly cytosolic vs. membrane bound, (2) molecular weight (smaller soluble molecules are cleared more quickly), (3) local perfusion and lymph flow, and (4) the rate of elimination

Table 37-3. Noninvasive detection of reperfusion using CK-MB levels

Study	N	Acute angiography	Measure	Percentage with criteria	Sensitivity (%)	Specificity (%)
Kondo	29	Yes	Time to peak CK-MB	79	69	57
Katus	36	No	Time to peak CK-MB	58	77	94
Lewis	50	Yes	Rate of CK-MB rise	82	100	100
Garabedian	69	Yes	Rate of CK-MB rise	66	83	100
Abendschein	32	No	Rate of CK-MB rise	N/A	92	20
Ong	26	No	Curve fitting	77	95	83
Grande	77	No	Curve fitting	N/A	86	100

from the blood.[59] As the process of cellular death progresses, the cytosolic-located markers are washed out into the blood early, whereas membrane-bound molecules appear at a later stage. Reperfusion of infarcting myocardium accelerates the rate of appearance of both types of intracellular constituents in plasma by increasing local perfusion and consequent washout. For such data to be useful in detection of reperfusion at the bedside, three conditions must be met: (1) the profile of reperfusion must be sufficiently distinct from that of continued occlusion for clinical decision making, (2) adequate diagnostic certainty for clinical decision making must be attainable rapidly (ideally within 30 to 60 minutes), and (3) the test results must be rapidly available to the clinical team.

Measurement of serum myoglobin has been used to assess reperfusion after thrombolysis. Ellis et al. reported that a sharp early peak occurs as early as 48 minutes after successful reperfusion.[60] The early release of myoglobin is characterized by a discontinuous "staccato" pattern.[61] Thus, frequent (30-minute) sampling is required during the first hours after thrombolysis to delineate patients with successful reperfusion clearly. To date, the diagnostic utility of serum myoglobin for noninvasive detection of reperfusion has been studied in fewer than 200 patients. Reported sensitivities range from 36% to 85%, with specificities from 83% to 100%.[62-65] Although newer rapid assays are available, these have not been tested for assessment of reperfusion.[66]

Other cardiospecific markers for noninvasive assessment include myosin light chains[67] and Troponin T.[68] Both are structural proteins with relatively small cytosolic pools, indicating that their detection will be delayed. Furthermore, there are no commercially available assays that can be performed quickly enough for clinical decision making, relegating these markers to only retrospective assessment of reperfusion. A rapid assay for Troponin T is currently being tested and is expected to be available in the near future.

Several studies have examined total creatine kinase release after thrombolysis. Early studies found that peak total CK activity occurred earlier in patients with successful reperfusion.[69] Subsequent studies found that time-to-peak of total CK was highly sensitive for detection of reperfusion.[48,65,70-71] However, the time-to-peak measure requires sampling over the first 24 hours, which precludes its use for acute decision making. The use of total creatine kinase has been superseded by measuring MM or the more cardiospecific creatine kinase MB subunits.

Creatine kinase MM exists in three subforms (MM-3, MM-2, and MM-1). When CK-MM is released from dying cells it is in the form of MM-3 (tissue form); it subsequently undergoes conversion to MM-2 and MM-1 by successive enzymatic cleavage of the terminal lysine from each M subunit. As the MM-3 subform is the first to appear in blood after myocardial necrosis, it has been the primary focus of efforts to develop a noninvasive marker of reperfusion.[72] Aspects of the profile of MM-3 release that have been studied have included the rate of increase,[63,73] rate of decrease,[74] and changes in the ratio of MM-3 to MM-1.[63,73,75] All these measures have been observed to be relatively sensitive and specific in small numbers of patients. The major limitation of MM isoform use is that electrophoresis is required for the assay, resulting in long analytical times. In addition, MM isoforms lack cardiospecificity.[72]

The results of studies examining creatine kinase MB for noninvasive detection of reperfusion are summarized in Table 37-3.[52,76-80,84] The majority of these have used techniques that require repeated sampling during the first 24 hours of MI so that curve fitting methods can be used to define the peak of CK-MB. All three studies examining the rate of CK-MB release have been in small cohorts[77,78,80] and only one study examined a rapid assay.[77] Nevertheless, these studies are suggestive that the release pattern of CK-MB may be useful to detect reperfusion. There is an approximately 30-minute delay between the rapid increases of myoglobin and CK-MB. For earlier delineation of CK-MB release after thrombolysis, newer quantitative assays for CK-MB subforms have been developed.[81] Creatine kinase MB-2 represents the tissue form that undergoes conversion in blood to MB-1, similar to the MM subforms. Using high-voltage electrophoresis to separate MB-2 and MB-1, it has been suggested that the ratio of MB-2 to MB-1 reflects coronary artery patency within 2 hours of thrombolytic therapy.[82] However, as the release of MB and MM subforms and CK-MB is simultaneous after reperfusion in man,[83,84] assessment of these subunits adds little over measuring CK-MB for noninvasive detection.[85] Thus, assessment of MB subunits does not provide any higher diagnostic sensitivity and is complicated by long assay times.

The TAMI study group has assessed a rapid CK-MB assay to identify patients who failed to restore patency after thrombolytic therapy.[86] The rapid assay is commercially available (ICON QSR CK-MB, Hybritech Inc.) and is based on dual monoclonal technique. This assay requires 10 minutes to complete and is therefore potentially suitable for noninvasive detection of reperfusion. Of 232 patients enrolled in the TAMI-7 study, 100 had CK-MB values obtained within 10 minutes of acute angiography.[86] The slope of CK-MB release, rather than absolute CK levels, was the enzyme variable most closely associated with reperfusion ($P < 0.0001$). The sensitivity and specificity of this variable alone was enhanced by the use of clinical descriptors, as is discussed later in this chapter.

ECG monitoring. One of the earliest noninvasive correlates of reperfusion described was sudden alteration of the ECG.[87-89] Rapid changes in ST-segment levels and accelerated changes in QRS morphology have both been evaluated as indicators of reperfusion. The necrosis of myocytes and their replacement by inert scar tissue is generally considered the pathophysiology behind the loss of R-wave forces and the development of Q waves in MI.[90] The pathophysiology underlying the accelerated development of Q waves observed in some patients following reperfusion is less clear. Some investigators have proposed that rapid Q-wave evolution is a marker of reperfusion injury. Others have considered these changes to be evidence of accelerated healing or at least electrical neutralization by ion washout of the necrotic area, similar to the enzymatic washout with reperfusion described earlier. "Regrowth" of R waves following reperfusion of an apparent Q-wave MI has been hypothesized to represent ECG evidence of myocardial salvage.[89] No convincing data exist to determine which if any of these theories is correct.

The development of new computer-assisted ECG monitoring devices with continuous, real-time capabilities has renewed interest in quantifying accelerated QRS changes following reperfusion. Continuous recordings of the absolute vector differences summated over QRS waveforms from Frank leads X, Y, and Z have shown how much more rapidly QRS changes can occur in the setting of reperfusion than in the setting of completed infarction, as illustrated in Figure 37-1.[91,92] With the interruption of infarction by reperfusion, an accelerated formation of Q waves and reduction of R waves are frequently observed; that is, the interruption of infarction by reperfusion primarily affects the initial QRS forces. On the other hand, with the reversal of ischemia it is primarily the terminal S-wave forces that change with restoration of R-wave amplitude,[93-95] as illustrated in Figure 37-2. Thus, the QRS vector difference combines both the initial and the terminal QRS forces into a single absolute measurement, making discrimination between completed infarction, recurrent ischemia, or combinations of the two as a result of reperfusion essentially impossible using QRS vector difference as measured by current devices. The refinement of this marker, however, remains an active area of investigation.

It is noteworthy that ST-segment elevation, the pathognomonic finding that has identified patients with AMI as candidates for thrombolytic or interventional trials over the past decade, is not, in fact, a marker of infarction but of ischemia.[96] As shown in Figure 37-3, ST-segment elevation, classically called *injury current*, will occur within seconds of a coronary flow interruption, even in the complete absence of myocardial necrosis. Partial reduction in flow sufficient to generate ischemia in the same coronary site in the same individual will not generate such focal ST-segment elevation, but rather nonfocal ST-segment depression (Fig. 37-4). Because total coronary flow interruption clinically is most likely to be caused by abrupt thrombotic occlusion at the site of an atheroma, with persistence of such occlusion leading fairly rapidly to frank myocardial necrosis, ST-segment elevation in patients presenting with persistent chest pain has and continues to serve as the most objective single identifier of patients likely to benefit from reperfusion therapies. As an objective noninvasive parameter that can be relatively easily measured on a continuous basis, this intimate relationship between coronary patency and the presence of ST-segment elevation makes ST-segment recovery analysis the single most accurate and most useful noninvasive surrogate for angiography.

Early attempts to quantify sudden ST recovery associated with reperfusion used serial static ECGs to measure percentage recovery. Generally, the first ECG acquired after patient presentation was compared with a second ECG taken at either a fixed time interval after the initial ECG, at the onset of therapy (e.g., 90 minutes, 3 hours), or at a specified event, such as at the moment of an angiographic contrast injection.[39,87-89,97-102] The use of different time intervals and different lead sets for analysis led to a variety of different recovery thresholds purported to identify successful reperfusion, as shown in Table 37-4.

Continuous ST-segment monitoring before, during,

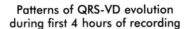

Patterns of QRS-VD evolution
during first 4 hours of recording

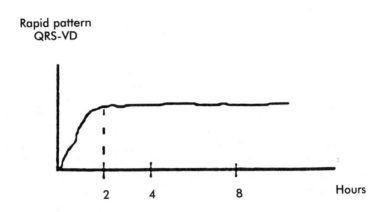

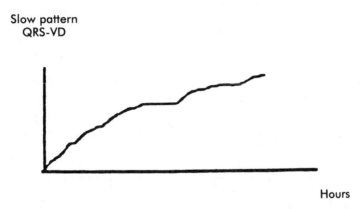

Fig. 37-1. Patterns of QRS vector difference (QRS-VD) over early hours of MI. "Rapid pattern" associated with reperfusion, "slow pattern" associated with failed reperfusion. (Modified from Dellborg et al: Increased rate of evolution of QRS changes in patients with AMI: results from the Vermut Study, *J Electrocardiol* 26:244-248, 1993).

and after thrombolytic therapy revealed significant shortcomings of these static approaches,* largely because of undersampling in the midst of a highly dynamic MI, one version of which is illustrated in Figures 37-5A and B. In a series of independent studies, rapid and profound ST-segment changes, confirmed angiographically to represent cyclic changes in coronary flow, were observed in 25% to 35% of all AMI patients.[13,40,106-110] Thus ST-segment levels on the first diagnostic ECG frequently do not capture the true peak injury current. This

may affect either the detection of late episodes of lesser reelevation, suggesting reocclusion, or the timing of predicted reperfusion, if compared only to the presenting ECG levels,[103,108] as illustrated in Figure 37-5C.

With the advent of digital computer-assisted ECG monitors that could record and analyze ECGs in real time,[105,107,110] new methods of ST-segment recovery analysis were developed.[106,107,110,111] Previously used terms like "normalization" or "return of ST segments to baseline," although descriptive, were impossible to translate into quantifiable parameters. Even with reperfusion, ST-segment levels rarely return to isoelectric levels or any level that could be described as "normal."

*References 13, 38, 40, 91, 92, 103-110.

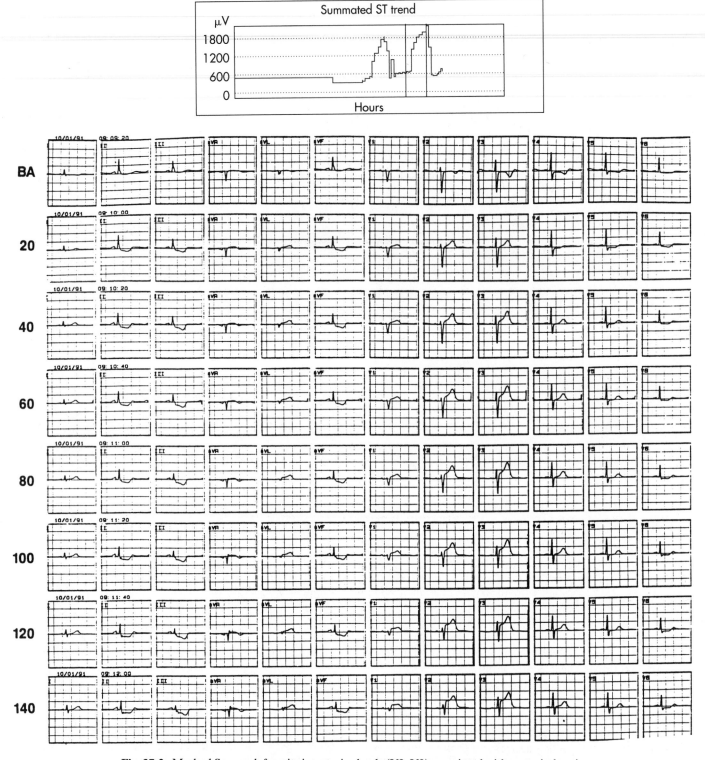

Fig. 37-2. Marked S-wave deformity in anterior leads (V2, V3) associated with acute ischemic changes, no myocardial necrosis, during 140-second elective angioplasty occlusion of the left anterior descending artery. (Modified from Krucoff MW, Sawchak ST, Pope JE, et al: Rethinking classical ECG patterns of ischemia and infarction: insights from investigations with continuous ECG monitoring, *The Newspaper of Cardiology* 12:8-17, 1992.)

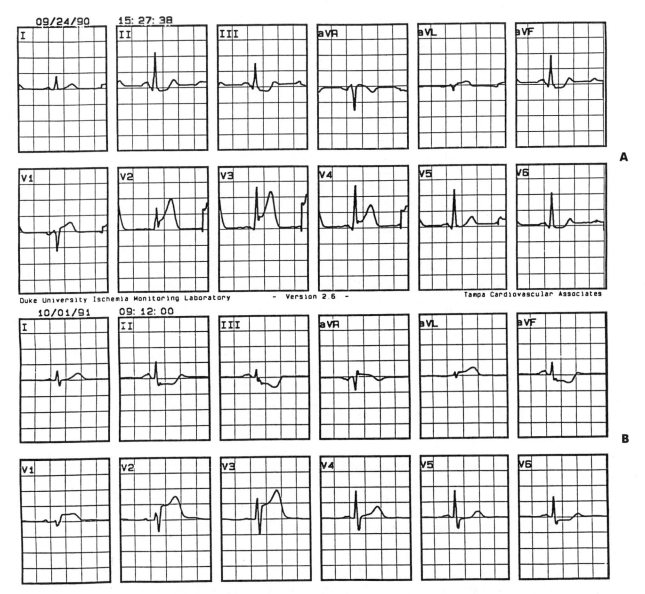

Fig. 37-3. Two patients with acute ischemic ST-segment elevation. **A,** Patient with 2 hours of chest pain, enzymatic evidence of necrosis, and occluded right coronary artery shows ischemic pattern superimposed on clinical MI. **B,** Patient with 140-second elective angioplasty occlusion (from Fig. 37-2), with acute ischemia but no infarction. (Modified from Krucoff MW, Sawchak ST, Pope JE, et al: Rethinking classical ECG patterns of ischemia and infarction: insights from investigations with continuous ECG monitoring, *The Newspaper of Cardiology* 12:8-17, 1992.)

Patients presenting with AMI rarely have previous baseline ECGs for comparison, and by definition present with ST abnormalities. Rapidly achieving a "steady-state" ST level—defined only as the absence of any further >100 uV change over a period of time—provided a sensitive and specific marker of reperfusion, as shown in Figure 37-6, but required retrospective analysis.[104] In addition, however, this marker was intrinsically dependent on a shift from static comparisons to continuous assessment. This shift had many implications for the assessment of ST-segment levels during the acute phases of infarction. For example, using static data, two ECGs showing 5 mm of anterior ST elevation

were taken as evidence of persistent occlusion, as illustrated in Figures 37-7A and B. Using continuously updated data, an ECG showing 5 mm of ST elevation was evidence of occlusion if the earlier ST levels were 5 mm or lower, but was considered evidence of reperfusion if the ST levels were 10 mm or higher earlier. Conversely, using static references, ECGs with borderline changes left the clinician dependent on other tests or assessments to judge the efficacy of thrombolytic therapy. Using continuously updated ECG assessment, borderline changes are usually just an intermediate phase of recovery or reelevation. Improved definition is provided over a period of a few minutes

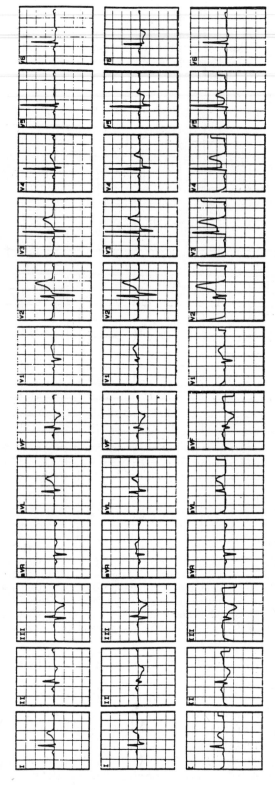

Fig. 37-4. ECG patterns at baseline (BA), ischemia during exercise testing (ETT), and during elective balloon occlusion (PTA) in patient with single vessel 95% disease of left anterior descending artery. In the same individual with the same coronary anatomy, demand-related ischemia with ETT shows ST depression in V4-6. With ischemia, no necrosis, from brief total occlusion of left anterior descending artery, anterior ST elevation is seen in leads V2-5. (Modified from Krucoff MW, Sawchak ST, Pope JE, et al: Rethinking classical ECG patterns of ischemia and infarction: insights from investigations with continuous ECG monitoring, *The Newspaper of Cardiology* 12:8-17, 1992.)

Table 37-4. Description of each of the static electrocardiogram recovery analysis methods*

Method	Author	Leads	↑ / ↓	Measured	ST-Red. (%)	Time (min)
I	von Essen	I, II, III	↑ and ↓	J + 60 ms	>55	60
II	Hogg	Worst lead	↑	J point	≥50	180
III	Saran	Worst lead	↑	J point	>25	180
IV	Hackworthy	12 leads	↑	J + 40 ms	>40	60, 120
V	Clemmensen	11 leads	↑	J point	≥20	90

*Leads used to calculate the amount of ST recovery, measurement of only elevation or both elevation and depression, measurement point, percent recovery required for patent prediction, and time from onset of treatment to the stipulated moment of the patency assessment.

↑ = ST elevation: ↓ = ST depression.

Red. = reduction.

(Modified from Veldkamp RF, Green CL, Wilkins ML, et al for the Thrombolysis and Angioplasty in Myocardial Infarction (TAMI) 7 Study Group: Comparison of continuous ST-segment recovery analysis with methods using static electrocardiograms for noninvasive patency assessment during acute myocardial infarction. *Am J Cardiol* 73:1069-1074, 1994.

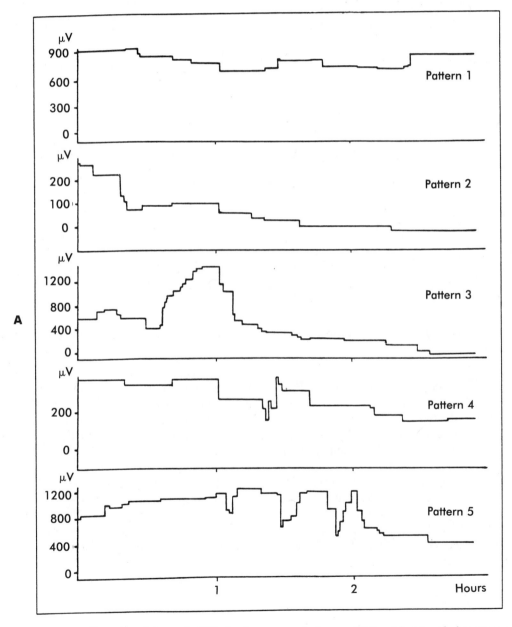

Fig. 37-5. Patterns of dynamic ST behavior over early hours of MI, subject to mischaracterization by static sampling. **A,** Patterns from most active lead in 12-lead continuous ECG recordings. (Modified from Veldkamp RF, Green CL, Wilkins ML, et al for the Thrombolysis and Angioplasty in Myocardial Infarction (TAMI) 7 Study Group: Comparison of continuous ST-segment recovery analysis with methods using static electrocardiograms for noninvasive patency assessment during acute myocardial infarction, *Am J Cardiol* 73:1069-1074, 1994.)

Continued.

Patterns of ST-VM variability
during first 4 hours of recording

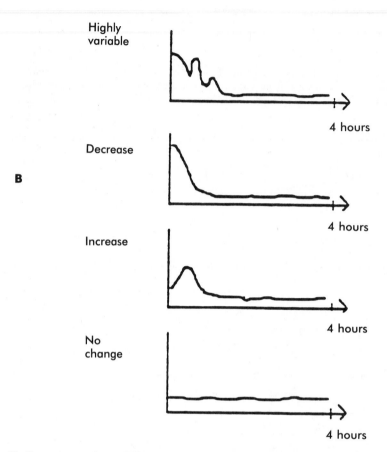

Fig. 37-5. cont'd. B, Similar patterns from ST-vector magnitude (ST-VM) continuous recordings.   (Modified from Dellborg et al, 1993.)

Continued.

as the pattern develops more clearly, as shown in Figure 37-8.

To maximize the potential of ST-segment change information to provide accurate indication of the patency status of the infarct artery, the continuously updated 12-lead ST-segment recovery analysis method was developed based on quantitative, self-referenced ST recovery or reelevation thresholds and defined lead sets.[107] As illustrated in Figure 37-9, this method relies on the identification of "peaks" and "troughs" within a trend of ST-segment activity over time. These points represent transition periods, where quantified ST-segment worsening changes to recovery ("peaks") or recovery changes to reelevation ("troughs"). The specific thresholds, which include rules for the selection of the leads measured, the time periods over which changes can be assessed, and the ST deviation amplitudes defining reelevation and recovery, were derived from an unblinded field experience with patients undergoing acute angiographic definition during infarction and are reproduced in the box on p. 462.[107] This method was subsequently tested in a blinded, angiographically correlated 144-patient substudy of the TAMI 7 trial.[40] Continuous ST-segment recovery analysis in TAMI 7 had a positive predictive accuracy of 81% for identifying patients with coronary occlusion on the first contrast injection at 90 minutes, out of a population with an angiographic pretest probability of occlusion of 23%. The absence of criteria-based ST recovery on blinded analysis correlated far more powerfully with angiographic occlusion than did clinical descriptors such as chest pain relief. In a multivariable statistical model whose results are shown in Table 37-5 and both ST-segment recovery analysis and chest pain descriptors, the chest pain information did not contribute at all to the predictive information. In the overall model, blinded

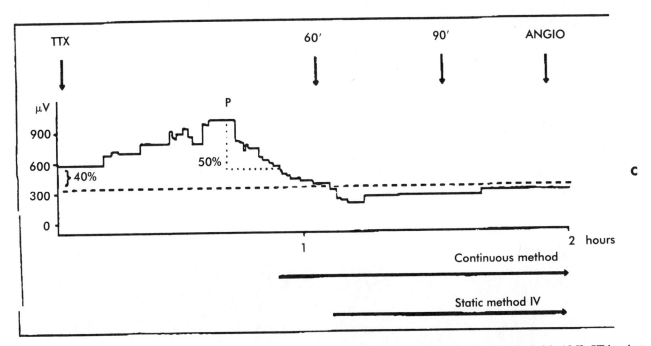

Fig. 37-5. cont'd. C, Trend of peak lead ST-segment level (Y-axis) vs. time (X-axis) in a patient presenting with AMI. ST level at presentation, at 600 µV elevation, increases later to peak level *(P)* of 950 µV elevation. 50% recovery, as evidence of reperfusion, is taken as 60 minutes after therapy *(TTX)* if only the presenting level is used, but actually occurs at 45 minutes if the continuously documented peak level is recorded. (Modified from Veldkamp RF, Green CL, Wilkins ML, et al for the Thrombolysis and Angioplasty in Myocardial Infarction (TAMI) 7 Study Group: comparison of continuous ST-segment recovery analysis with methods using static electrocardiograms for noninvasive patency assessment during acute myocardial infarction, *Am J Cardiol* 73:1069-1074, 1994.)

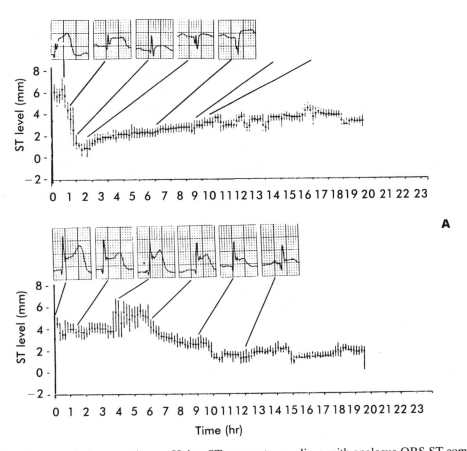

Fig. 37-6. A, ST level vs. time trends from continuous Holter ST-segment recordings, with analogue QRS-ST complexes displayed above, from two patients treated with intracoronary lytics. In patient above, with anterior infarction and successful reperfusion, rapid ST recovery to "steady-state" level is noted in the first 2 hours from presentation. In patient below, with inferior infarction and failed reperfusion, ST recovery to steady state occurs but gradually and over a 10 to 12 hour period. (Modified from Krucoff MW, Green CE, Satler LF, et al: Noninvasive detection of coronary artery patency using continuous ST-segment monitoring, *Am J Cardiol* 57:916-923, 1986.)

Continued.

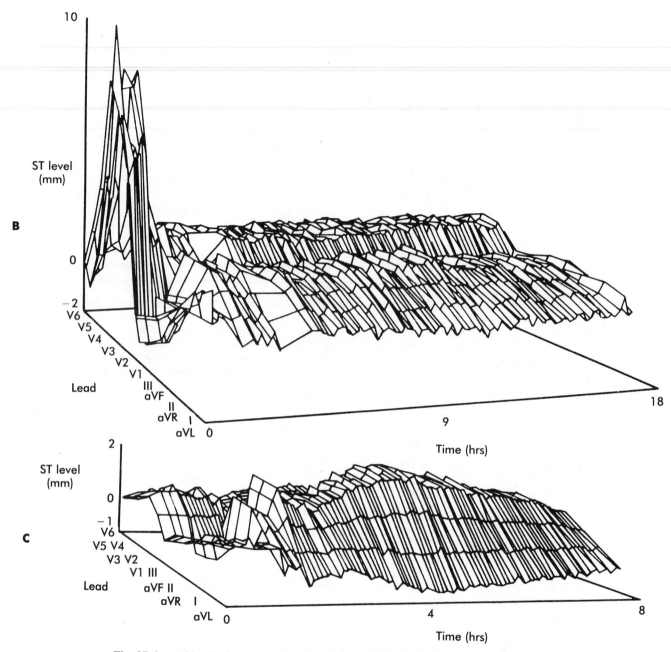

Fig. 37-6. cont'd.   B, Continuous trend of 12-lead ST levels over time in anterior infarction shows rapid recovery from reperfusion, similar to Holter trend. (Modified from Krucoff et al, 1990.) **C,** Continuous 12-lead ST levels over time in inferior infarction show gradual worsening and gradual recovery with failed reperfusion, similar to Holter trend. (Modified from Krucoff MW, Wagner NB, Pope JE, et al: The portable programmable microprocessor-driven real-time 12-lead electrocardiographic monitor: a preliminary report of a new device for the noninvasive detection of successful reperfusion or silent coronary reocclusion, *Am J Cardiol* 65:143-148, 1990.)

ST-segment recovery analysis alone contributed over two thirds of the available predictive information.

Because many emergency departments or smaller hospitals administer thrombolytic therapy but may not have quick access to personal computers or cardiologists familiar with the continuously updated ST-recovery method, the salient principles defining transition points were translated into logistic algorithms and incorporated into the bedside 12-lead ST-segment monitor (Mortara ST-100, Mortara Instrument, Milwaukee) as an automated "patency assessment" program.[112] This program requires the clinician to reject noisy ECGs when displayed but otherwise operates at the push of a button. In a field experience using this program, physicians were asked to log on paper their clinical assessment of infarct artery patency 90 minutes after thrombolytic

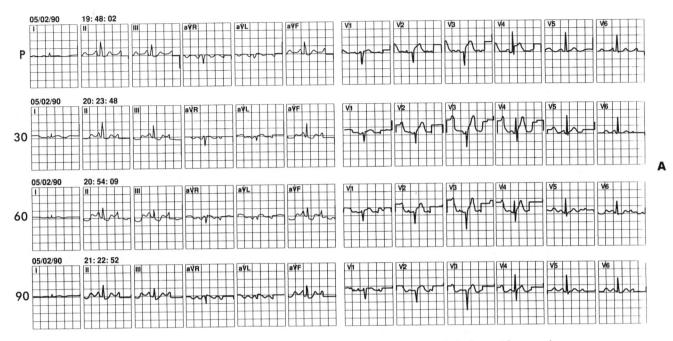

Fig. 37-7. A, Standard 12-lead ECGs at 30-minute intervals following lytic therapy for anterior infarction. ST elevation of 6-7 mm in the anterior leads appears to persist, suggesting failed reperfusion, over the first 60 minutes, with >50% recovery suggesting reperfusion seen on the ECG at 90 minutes.   *Continued.*

therapy or just before angiographic contrast injection. The automated program was immediately run in parallel, and the resultant assessments were compared in 262 patients, 62 of whom had simultaneous angiography at the moment of assessment. Notably, when either the physician or the ST monitor concluded that the infarct artery was occluded, the other disagreed in over 50% of cases. Using an angiographic "referee," the clinical assessment had an overall accuracy of 65%, whereas the stand-alone automated ST-segment recovery program had an overall accuracy of 87%.[38]

As with all noninvasive markers, examination of current limitations provides the clearest insight into future needs and directions. Whereas ST-segment elevation and recovery in the setting of reperfusion largely represents the onset and reversal of ischemia, it is also affected by the interruption of infarction. As shown in Figure 37-6A, nonischemic repolarization abnormalities associated with the rapid formation of Q waves frequently cause late ST-segment reelevation. Over a 24-hour period such ST-segment levels may elevate by 200 to 400 uV (2 to 4 mm). When reperfusion is a singular event, as in this example, this late reelevation is easily distinguished from ischemic reelevation caused by reocclusion of the infarct artery, the former occurring over many hours and the latter occurring over minutes, as shown in Figures 37-9 and 37-10. However, in late presentations where Q waves are already established, the extent to which ST elevation represents active ischemia from viable tissue vs. repolarization changes

from completed infarction may be ambiguous. A patient who presents after 8 hours of chest pain with deep anterior Q waves and 4 mm of anterior ST elevation that does not change over 30 minutes of continuous monitoring may have a persistently occluded infarct artery or may have had 12 mm of ST elevation 6 hours ago and now has only the abnormal residual of his postreperfusion scar. Fortunately the ST-segment recovery technique is most accurate where patients have the most ischemic territory at risk and the most to gain from accurate information on the success of reperfusion.

There are other important limitations to current ST-segment recovery analysis. Although the practice of applying a 12-lead ECG to patients during AMI is widespread, the skin preparation necessary for high-quality ST-segment analysis of a low-noise ECG signal is not. Inadequate skin preparation may introduce excessive noise into the ECG recordings and result in reduced discriminatory value of the technique. The difference is no more complex, and no less important, than the difference in techniques used to hook a patient up for a treadmill test compared to those used to hook a patient up for a single ECG. In addition to the skin preparation and lead anchoring, the band-pass filters and other signal/noise smoothing techniques of the devices themselves vary substantially across devices. Noise levels can still be bothersome, even in the very best devices. In bedside monitoring systems originally designed to provide arrhythmia monitoring, ST-segment software "add ons" are rendered virtually useless by noise infiltration in

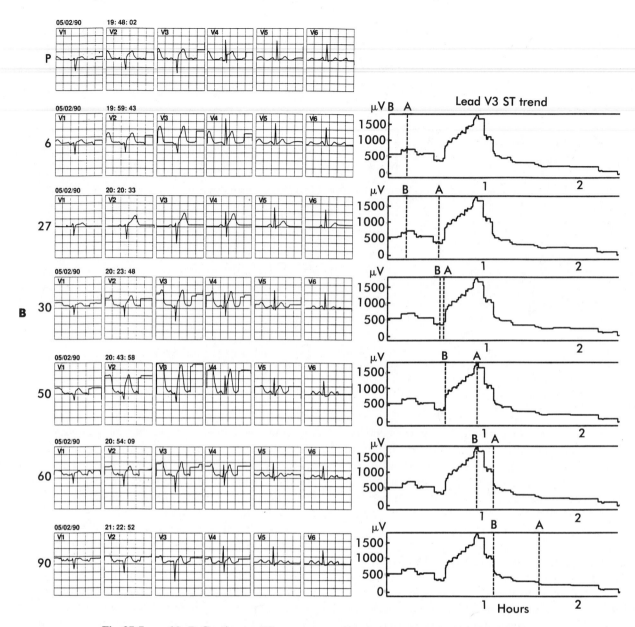

Fig. 37-7. cont'd. B, Continuous ST-segment monitor shows early peak of 8 mm 6 minutes after onset of lytics, with recovery suggesting reperfusion at 27 minutes, then reelevation to a peak of 19 mm of ST elevation from 30 to 50 minutes after therapy. At 60 minutes, 6 mm of ST elevation represents >50% recovery from the preceding 19-mm level, suggesting stable reperfusion at 60- rather than 90-minute documentation achieved with static sampling. (Modified from Krucoff MW, Croll MA, Pope JE, et al for the TAMI 7 Study Group: Continuous 12-lead ST-segment recovery analysis in the TAMI 7 study: performance of a noninvasive method for real-time detection of failed myocardial reperfusion, *Circulation* 88:437-446, 1993.)

the ST measurements. Patients with nondiagnostic ECGs or bundle branch blocks have not been included in previous investigations, and it is unclear how well the current systems would work in such patients. Finally, although ST-segment recovery analysis represents the best single noninvasive marker for real-time definition of patency, it seems likely that the predictive information can be further enhanced by integrating other markers into the final interpretations.

The continuous 12-lead characterization of ST recovery and reelevation provides an alternative conceptual model of the state of coronary blood flow distal to an unstable coronary plaque. As illustrated in Figure 37-9, identification of transition points over time allows even the most dynamic clinical course to be characterized as a series of periods of recovery and worsening, with a consistent and predictable relationship to the degree of nutritive coronary flow. Nutritive flow in this sense refers

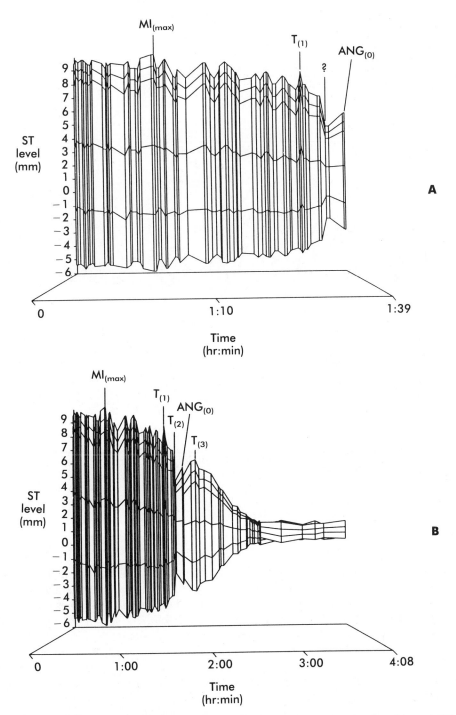

Fig. 37-8. A, Continuous 12-lead ST-segment monitoring in a patient with AMI, with peak ST deviation (MImax) of 10-mm elevation, acute transition (T1) point preceding to 5-mm level. This abrupt 50% recovery suggests reperfusion; however, reelevation of .8 to 1 millimeter rapidly follows, suggesting possible reocclusion at "?" The "?" of whether or not reperfusion or reocclusion occurred remains indeterminate at the moment of TAMI 7 protocol angiography, based on 1 hour 39 minutes of monitoring. **B,** In this same patient, continued monitoring over the next 20 minutes shows definite reelevation from reocclusion and, subsequently, from the last transition (T3) 30 minutes after the moment of "?" (now definite T2); stable >50% ST recovery shows persistent reperfusion. (Modified from Krucoff MW, Croll MA, Pope JE, et al for the TAMI 7 Study Group: Continuous 12-lead ST-segment recovery analysis in the TAMI 7 study: performance of a noninvasive method for real-time detection of failed myocardial reperfusion, *Circulation* 88:437-446, 1993.)

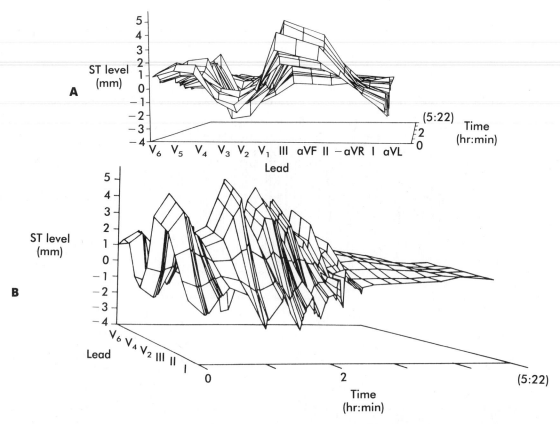

Fig. 37-9. Continuous 12-lead ST-segment monitoring during inferior AMI. **A,** Three-dimensional graphic displays ST-segment level (Y-axis) for each of 12 leads (Cabrerra sequence, X-axis) over time (Z-axis). In this 10-degree rotation the repeated precordial pattern of inferior ST elevation and anterior ST depression is appreciated. **B,** Same patient and graphic display, rotated to 60 degrees to better display time axis, showing dynamic, repeated periods of ST-segment recovery and reelevation noninvasively representing cyclic flow changes of patency in the infarct artery.   *Continued.*

to adequate coronary perfusion with relief of ischemia; the typical definition of reperfusion in terms of angiographic flow does not include any indication of whether the flow is adequate to meet the needs of the remaining viable myocardial cells in that vascular bed. The timing and duration of periods of recovery, as well as the severity and duration of periods of ST elevation, provide quantitative noninvasive descriptors of the speed and stability of nutritive reperfusion.[107,114] Faster, more complete, more stable reperfusion defined by quantitative ST-segment recovery has been associated with reduced infarct size and/or improved mortality in four independent reports to date.[110,113-116]

In addition to defining reperfusion more physiologically as the restoration of nutritive flow to the infarct zone, ST-recovery analysis may provide information about the status of distant areas of myocardium that are supplied by partially obstructed coronary arteries. Despite more than a decade of research, controversy persists as to whether ST-segment depression in leads oriented away from the primary infarct zone, or "reciprocal" ST-segment depression, represents an electrical

"mirror image" of the infarct, or a marker of a high-risk group with distant ischemia or larger infarctions. Defined by a static ECG, these two subgroups are indistinguishable. As shown in Figure 37-11, however, when patients with reciprocal ST depression are analyzed continuously and ST depression recovery literally "mirrors" ST elevation recovery over time, patients with benign clinical outcomes are identified.[117,118] When ST elevation recovers but ST depression persists, however, significantly larger infarctions and higher mortality have been reported.[117,118]

In summary, angiographically defined TIMI-3 flow has been correlated with improved left ventricular function and improved survival, as well as with ST-segment recovery in over 90% of patients.[25] Other angiographic categories, such as TIMI-2 flow or collateralized, occluded infarct arteries appear to be more ambiguous. In addition, angiography provides only a "snapshot" of a very dynamic coronary pathophysiology. ST-segment recovery analysis provides a more physiologically based continuous assessment of the nutritive adequacy of coronary flow, which has independently

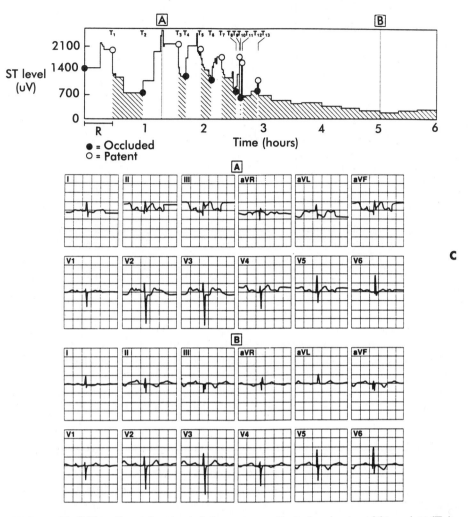

Fig. 37-9. cont'd C, Two-dimensional trend, from same patient, showing transition points (Tn) where elevation becomes >50% recovery or recovery becomes reelevation, suggesting reperfusion and reocclusion, using continuously updated "peak" and "trough" levels of the continuously updated ST-segment recovery analysis method. Analogue ECGs are stored for quality control of all measurements. (Modified from Krucoff MW, Croll MA, Pope JE, et al: Continuously updated 12-lead ST-segment recovery analysis for myocardial infarct artery patency assessment and its correlation with multiple simultaneous early angiographic observations, *Am J Cardiol* 71:145-151, 1993.)

been correlated with infarct size and mortality. Although there are still important limitations in the application of the technique, ST-segment analysis is the most powerful, clinically usable tool for evaluating the speed, stability, and adequacy of reperfusion noninvasively and in real time.

INTEGRATION OF NONINVASIVE PREDICTORS: THE "INSTRUMENT" OF THE FUTURE

During an AMI the clinician assesses and weighs symptoms, signs, and test results to reach an adequate level of certainty about the patient's diagnosis, possible natural history, and likely benefits from available therapies.

Although clinicians usually perform such analyses nonquantitatively, in such complex situations multivariable statistical models may assist clinical judgement by ordering the importance of descriptors based on the strength with which they predict the outcome of interest. By detecting where information is additive as additional descriptors are included in a model, ambiguities latent in one parameter may be offset by the "simultaneous" inclusion of other relevant parameters.

In patients who present with AMI, there are many situations where a multivariable approach would be expected to improve predictions of outcome. For example, the patient with persistent 4 mm anterior ST-segment elevation might be either regarded as a probable LAD occlusion or as a probable reperfusion or completed anterior infarction if the initial QRS forces, simultaneously tracked, showed active change vs. persistent static Q waves, respectively. The patient with rising inferior ST segments who suddenly develops a bundle branch block might be either regarded as having

Summary of ST measurement and parameter definitions

I. *ST measurement matrix* (trend):
    A. The most abnormal single lead from the maximally abnormal ECG (default)
    B. Summated deviation (sum of absolute differences per lead) if:
        1. Single most abnormal lead designation changes across 2 or more leads, or
        2. Two or more precordial zones show ST elevation

II. Transition points:
    A. *Transition "peak"*: the most abnormal ECG immediately preceding a period of ≥50% ST-segment recovery
    B. *Transition "trough"*: the most normalized ECG immediately preceding a period of ST reelevation

III. ST-segment "recovery" and "reelevation":
    A. *ST-segment "recovery"*:
        1. developing over a <3-hour period
        2. Resolution of:
            a. ≥50% of the immediately previous most abnormal matrix level (transition peak), or
            b. 35%-49% of the immediately previous transition peak and ≥50% of the most abnormal matrix level over the entire recording period up to the current ECG
    B. *ST-segment "reelevation"*:
        1. developing over a <1-hour period
        2. lasting >60 seconds
        3. lead or leads in matched "fingerprint" zone
        4. ≥150 uV in two/leads, or
        5. ≥200 uV *or* ≥ST level of immediately previous transition peak, whichever occurs first, in a single lead
    C. *ST recovery interval*: time from first ECG achieving ST-segment recovery to time of first ECG achieving ST-segment reelevation

IV. Trend parameters:
    A. *Time to first evidence of reperfusion*: time from onset of lytic therapy to onset of first ST-segment recovery interval
    B. *Patent Physiology Index (PPI)*: sum of the duration of all ST-recovery intervals divided by the duration of the total recording period × 100.
    C. *Number of transitions*: total number of transition peaks and troughs over the recording period

V. *ST patency assessment score*:

+5	+4	+3	+2	+1	0	−1	−2	−3	−4	−5
DEFINITE		POSSIBLE			INDETERMINATE		POSSIBLE		DEFINITE	
	PATENT								OCCLUDED	

From Krucoff MW, Croll MA, Pope JE, et al: Continuously updated 12-lead ST-segment recovery analysis for myocardial infarct artery patency assessment and its correlation with multiple simultaneous early angiographic observations, *Am J Cardiol* 71:145-151, 1993.

persistent right coronary occlusion if CPK enzymes rose slowly and chest pain persisted, or as having right coronary reperfusion if CPK enzymes rose rapidly and chest pain resolved.

These intuitive presumptions are supported by data from existing multivariable models. In Figure 37-12 the receiver operating characteristics (ROC) curves are shown from the TAMI-7 study[40] for clinical descriptors alone, ST-segment recovery analysis alone, and a best model combining the two as predictors of failed reperfusion. As was described earlier, ST-segment analysis alone was far more predictive than clinical descriptors alone. From the curve it is observed, however, that although ST recovery alone is highly specific, its ROC curve has a flattened or "plateau" to its sensitivity for detecting occlusion. When combined in an optimized statistical model, even though the vast majority of the predictive information originates from the ST-recovery analysis, there is clear enhancement of the sensitivity portion of the curve when the clinical descriptors are also taken into consideration—the overall diagnostic content of the model increased significantly.

The use of serum CK-MB changes to detect persistent occlusion in TAMI-7 was also enhanced by selected clinical variables.[86] The combined CK-MB and clinical model had a significantly better diagnostic yield than CK-MB analysis or clinical assessment alone.

Ventricular arrhythmias assessed in isolation have shown little or no predictive value for detecting reperfusion. When correlated with additional information, such as the timing of the arrhythmia relative to therapy onset or relative to the R-R intervals as an index of prematurity (R-on-T vs. late ectopics, etc.) the information content of arrhythmias for predicting reperfusion improved.[45-47] Current work correlating the timing of dysrhythmias to continuous ST-segment recovery may provide even further enhancement.[47]

In a retrospective analysis, combined analysis of ST recovery, CPK enzyme curves, and dysrhythmias were

Table 37-5. Best clinical models for noninvasive patency assessment

Variable	All clinical variables and ST monitoring ($n = 138$)		
	Coefficient	χ^2	P
ST recovery	−0.367	39.91	< .0001
Time to treatment	−0.011	5.62	.018
Age	−0.172	6.95	.0084
Time to catheterization	−0.0040	3.41	.064
Total model χ^2		58.35	

Modified from Krucoff MW, Croll MA, Pope JE, et al for the TAMI 7 Study Group: Continuous 12-lead ST-segment recovery analysis in the TAMI 7 study: performance of a noninvasive method for real-time detection of failed myocardial reperfusion, *Circulation* 88:437-446, 1993.

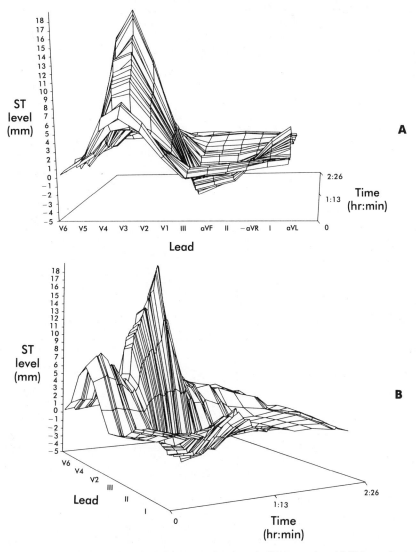

Fig. 37-10. Continuous 12-lead ST-segment monitoring during anterior AMI in patient discussed in Figure 37-7. **A,** Ten-degree rotation shows anterolateral and high lateral ST elevation with inferior ST depression. **B,** Seventy-degree rotation shows cyclic changes, recovering from 6-mm millimeter ST peak at presentation to 3-mm millimeter level only to reelevate to 19-mm elevation before final stable reperfusion around 60 minutes after onset of therapy. (Modified from Krucoff MW, Croll MA, Pope JE, et al for the TAMI 7 Study Group: Continuous 12-lead ST-segment recovery analysis in the TAMI 7 study: performance of a noninvasive method for real-time detection of failed myocardial reperfusion, *Circulation* 88:437-446, 1993.)

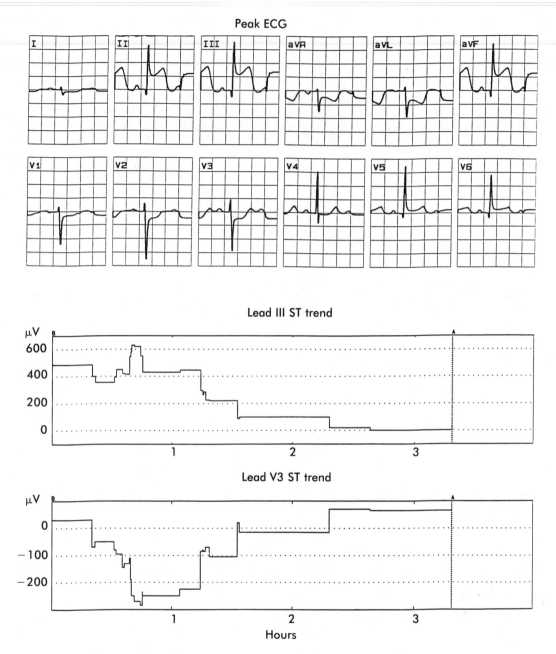

Fig. 37-11. Continuous trend of ST-segment level vs. time showing most elevated lead (above) and most depressed lead (below) defines a "mirror image" of continuous recovery over time, associated with benign prognosis. Persistent ST depression despite recovery of ST elevation defines a very high-risk prognosis. See text for detail. (Modified from Shah A, Green CL, Trollinger KM, et al: Differentiation of "benign mirror image" from high-risk reciprocal ST depression using continuous 12-lead ST-segment recovery analysis, *J Am Coll Cardiol* Special Issue:895-898, 1994.)

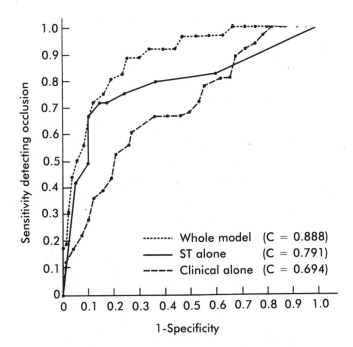

Fig. 37-12. Receiver operating characteristic (ROC) curves plotting sensitivity vs. 1-specificity of blinded prediction of coronary patency 90 minutes after lytic therapy in TAMI 7 trial. Performance of clinical descriptors, ST-segment recovery analysis, and a combined statistical model are plotted. See text for detail. (From Krucoff MW, Croll MA, Pope JE, et al for the TAMI 7 Study Group: Continuous 12-lead ST-segment recovery analysis in the TAMI 7 study: performance of a noninvasive method for real-time detection of failed myocardial reperfusion, *Circulation* 88:437-446, 1993.)

reported to yield almost perfect emulation of angiographic findings.[48] Although the methods are not readily translated into the real-time world of acute care and some other questions about these data persist, including whether a "perfect" match to angiographic appearance is good or bad, the fundamental message is clear. Statistically guided combination of multiple rapidly obtained and reassessable noninvasive markers will, in the future, provide the best possible way to define reperfusion.

And when all the predictive power of combined markers does not simply emulate angiographic findings, the clinician must consider the role of nutritive flow on myocardial physiology and reflect further on how best to define, or to redefine, our concepts of reperfusion beyond the tip of a catheter.

REFERENCES

1. DeWood MA, Spores J, Notske R, et al: Prevalence of total coronary occlusion during the early hours of transmural myocardial infarction, *N Engl J Med* 303:897-902, 1980.
2. Rentrop P, Blanke H, Karsch KR, et al: Selective intracoronary thrombolysis in acute myocardial infarction and unstable angina pectoris, *Circulation* 63:489-497, 1981.
3. Kennedy JW, Ritchie J, Davis K, et al: Western Washington Randomized Trial of intracoronary streptokinase in acute myocardial infarction, *N Engl J Med* 309(24):1477-1482, 1983.
4. Simoons ML, Serruys PW, van den Brand M, et al for the Working Group on Thrombolytic Therapy in Acute Myocardial Infarction of the Netherlands Interuniversity Cardiology Institute: Early thrombolysis in acute myocardial infarction: limitation of infarct size and improved survival, *J Am Coll Cardiol* 7:717-728, 1986.
5. Mathey DG, Kuck KH, Tilsner V, et al: Nonsurgical coronary artery recanalization in acute transmural myocardial infarction, *Circulation* 63:489-497, 1981.
6. Leiboff R, Katz R, Wasserman A, et al: Randomized, angiographically controlled trial of intracoronary streptokinase in acute myocardial infarction, *Am J Cardiol* 53:404-407, 1984.
7. Valentine R, Pitts D, Brooks-Brunn J, et al: Effect of thrombolysis (streptokinase) on left ventricular function during acute myocardial infarction, *Am J Cardiol* 58:896-899, 1986.
8. Jennings R, Reimer K: Factors involved in salvaging ischemic myocardium: effect of reperfusion of arterial blood, *Circulation* (suppl I):I25-I36, 1983.
9. Raizner A, Tortoledo F, Verani M, et al: Intracoronary thrombolytic therapy in acute myocardial infarction: a prospective, randomized, controlled trial, *Am J Cardiol* 55:301-308, 1985.
10. Gruppo Italiano Per Lo Studio Della Streptochinasi Nell'infarcto Miocardio (GISSI): Effectiveness of intravenous thrombolytic treatment in acute myocardial infarction, *Lancet* 1:397-401, 1986.
11. Sheehan FH, Mathey DG, Scholfer J, et al: Factors that determine recovery of left ventricular function after thrombolysis in patients with acute myocardial infarction, *Circulation* 71:1121-1128, 1985.
12. Tiefenbrunn A, Sobel B: Timing of coronary recanalization, paradigms, paradoxes, and pertinence, *Circulation* 85:2311-2315, 1992.
13. Hackett D, Davies G, Chierchia S, et al: Intermittent coronary occlusion in acute myocardial infarction: value of combined thrombolytic and vasodilator therapy, *N Engl J Med* 317:1055-1059, 1987.
14. The Thrombolysis In Myocardial Infarction (TIMI) Study Group: The Thrombolysis in Myocardial Infarction (TIMI) trial: Phase 1 findings, *N Engl J Med* 312:932-936, 1985.
15. Karagounis L, Sorensen SG, Memlove RL, et al: Does Thrombolysis in Myocardial Infarction (TIMI) perfusion grade 2 represent a mostly patent artery or a mostly occluded artery? Enzymatic and electrocardiographic evidence from the TEAM-2 study, *J Am Coll Cardiol* 19:1-10, 1992.
16. Habib GB, Heibig J, Forman SA, et al: Influence of coronary collateral vessels on myocardial infarct size in humans. Results of phase I Thrombolysis in Myocardial Infarction (TIMI) trial. The TIMI Investigators, *Circulation* 83:739-746, 1991.
17. Boehrer J, Lange R, Willard J, et al: Influence of collateral filling of the occluded infarct-related coronary artery on prognosis after acute myocardial infarction, *Am J Cardiol* 68:10-12, 1992.
18. Feld H, Lichstein E, Schachter J, et al: Early and late angiographic findings of the "no-reflow" phenomenon following direct angioplasty as primary treatment for acute myocardial infarction, *Am Heart J* 123:782-786, 1992.
19. Dreyer W, Michael L, West S, et al: Neutrophil accumulation in ischemic canine myocardium: insights into time course, distribution, mechanism of localization during early reperfusion, *Circulation* 84:400-411, 1991.
20. Marsh J, Smith T: Calcium overload and ischemic myocardial injury, *Circulation* 83:709-712, 1991.
21. Kloner R, Giacomelli F, Alker K, et al: Influx of neutrophils into the walls of large epicardial coronary arteries in response to ischemia/reperfusion, *Circulation* 84:1758-1772, 1991.
22. Nayler W, Elz J: Reperfusion injury: laboratory artifact or clinical dilemma, *Circulation* 74:215-221, 1986.

23. Kolodgie F, Virmani R, Farb A: Limitation of no-reflow injury by blood-free reperfusion with oxygenated perfluorochemical (Fluosol-DA 20%), *J Am Coll Cardiol* 18:215-225, 1991.

24. ISIS-2 Collaborative Group: Randomized trial of intravenous streptokinase, oral aspirin, both, or neither among 17,187 cases of suspected acute myocardial infarction: ISIS-2, *Lancet* ii:349-360, 1988.

25. The GUSTO Angiographic Investigators: The effects of tissue plasminogen activator, streptokinase, or both on coronary artery patency, ventricular function, and survival after acute myocardial infarction, *N Engl J Med* 329:1615-1622, 1993.

26. Fortin DF, Califf RM: Long-term survival from acute myocardial infarction: salutary effect of an open coronary vessel, *Am J Med* 88:9-15, 1990.

27. Ohman EM, Califf RM, Topol EJ, et al and the TAMI Study Group: Consequences of reocclusion after successful reperfusion therapy in acute myocardial infarction, *Circulation* 82:781-791, 1990.

28. Aguirre FV, Kern MJ, Hsia J, et al: Importance of myocardial infarct artery patency on the prevalence of ventricular arrhythmia and late potentials after thrombolysis in acute myocardial infarction, *Am J Cardiol* 68:1410-1416, 1991.

29. Galvani M, Ottani F, Ferrini D, et al: Patency of the infarct-related artery and left ventricular function as the major determinants of survival after Q-wave acute myocardial infarction, *Am J Cardiol* 71:1-7, 1993.

30. Lamas GA, Pfeffer MA, Braunwald E: Patency of the infarct-related coronary artery and ventricular geometry, *Am J Cardiol* 68:41D-51D, 1991.

31. Collen D: Synergism of thrombolytic agents: investigational procedures and clinical potential, *Circulation* 77(4):145-149, 1988.

32. Califf RM, Topol EJ, Stack RS, et al: Evaluation of combination thrombolytic therapy and timing of cardiac catheterization in acute myocardial infarction: the TAMI 5 randomized trial, *Circulation* 83:1543-1556, 1991.

33. Neuhaus KL, Tebbe U, Gottwik M, et al: Intravenous recombinant tissue plasminogen activator (rt-PA) and urokinase in acute myocardial infarction: results of the German Activator Urokinase Study (GAUS), *J Am Coll Cardiol* 12:581-587, 1988.

34. Wall TC, Califf RM, George BS, et al and the TAMI 7 Study Group: Accelerated plasminogen activator dose regimens for coronary thrombolysis, *J Am Coll Cardiol* 19:482-489, 1992.

35. de Bono DP, Simoons ML, Tijssen J, et al: Effect of early intravenous heparin on coronary patency, infarct size, and bleeding complications after alteplase thrombolysis: results of a randomized double blind European Cooperative Study Group Trial, *Br Heart J* 67:122-128, 1992.

36. Topol EJ for the GUSTO Investigators: An international randomized trial comparing four thrombolytic strategies for acute myocardial infarction, *N Engl J Med* 329:673, 1993.

37. Ellis S, Van de Werf F, Ribeiro-DeSilva E, et al: Present status of rescue coronary angioplasty: current polarization of opinion and randomized trials, *J Am Coll Cardiol* 19:681-686, 1992.

38. Krucoff MW, Crater SW, Veldkamp RF, et al: Duke University Medical Center Ischemia Monitoring Laboratory. Automation and implementation of the Duke ST-segment recovery patency assessment method in a portable computerized electrocardiographic monitor, *Computers In Cardiol* 51, 1992.

39. Califf RM, O'Neil W, Stack RS, et al and the TAMI Study Group: Failure of simple clinical measurements to predict perfusion status after intravenous thrombolysis, *Ann Int Med* 108:658-662, 1988.

40. Krucoff MW, Croll MA, Pope JE, et al for the TAMI 7 Study Group: Continuous 12-lead ST-segment recovery analysis in the TAMI 7 study: performance of a noninvasive method for real-time detection of failed myocardial reperfusion, *Circulation* 88:437-446, 1993.

41. Pogwizd S, Corr P: Electrophysiologic mechanisms underlying arrhythmias due to reperfusion of ischemic myocardium, *Circulation* 76:404-426, 1987.

42. Gore JM, Ball SP, Corrao JM, et al: Arrhythmias in the assessment of coronary artery reperfusion following thrombolytic therapy, *Chest* 94:727-730, 1988.

43. Cercek B, Lew AS, Laramee P, et al: Time course and characteristics of ventricular arrhythmias after reperfusion in acute myocardial infarction, *Am J Cardiol* 60:214-218, 1987.

44. Miller F, Krucoff M, Satler L, et al: Ventricular arrhythmias during reperfusion, *Am Heart J* 112:928-932, 1986.

45. Gorgels AP, Vos MA, Letsch IS, et al: Usefulness of the accelerated idioventricular rhythm as a marker for myocardial necrosis and reperfusion during thrombolytic therapy in acute myocardial infarction, *Am J Cardiol* 61:231-235, 1988.

46. Gressin V, Louvard Y, Pezzano M, et al: Holter recording of ventricular arrhythmias during intravenous thrombolysis for acute myocardial infarction, *Am J Cardiol* 69:152-159, 1992.

47. Zehender M, Ulzolino S, Furtwangler A, et al: Time course and interrelation of reperfusion-induced ST changes and ventricular arrhythmias in acute myocardial infarction, *Am J Cardiol* 68:1138-1142, 1991.

48. Hohnloser SH, Zabel M, Kasper W, et al: Assessment of coronary artery patency after thrombolytic therapy: accurate prediction utilizing the combined analysis of three noninvasive markers, *J Am Coll Cardiol* 18:44-49, 1991.

49. Beller GA: Role of myocardial perfusion imaging in evaluating thrombolytic therapy for acute myocardial infarction, *J Am Coll Cardiol* 9:661-668, 1987.

50. Beller GA: Noninvasive assessment of myocardial salvage after coronary reperfusion: a perpetual quest of nuclear cardiology, *J Am Coll Cardiol* 14:874-876, 1989.

51. Wheelan K, Wolfe C, Corbett J, et al: Early positive technetium-99m stannous pyrophosphate images as a marker of reperfusion after thrombolytic therapy for acute myocardial infarction, *Am J Cardiol* 56:252-256, 1985.

52. Kondo M, Yuzuki Y, Arai H, et al: Comparison of early myocardial technetium-99m pyrophosphate uptake to early peaking of creatine kinase and creatine kinase-MB as indicators of early reperfusion in acute myocardial infarction, *Am J Cardiol* 60:762-765, 1987.

53. Christian TF, Gibbons RJ: Detection of recanalization with the use of radioisotope techniques, *Cor Art Dis* 3:481-488, 1992.

54. Gibbons RJ: Technetium 99m sestamibi in the assessment of acute myocardial infarction, *Semin Nucl Med* XXI:213-222, 1991.

55. Wackers FJTh: Thrombolytic therapy for myocardial infarction: assessment of efficacy by myocardial perfusion imaging with technetium-99m sestamibi, *Am J Cardiol* 66:36E-41E, 1990.

56. Christian TF, Schwartz RS, Gibbons RJ: Determinants of infarct size in reperfusion therapy for acute myocardial infarction, *Circulation* 86:81-90, 1992.

57. Rehr RB, Fuhs BE, Lee F, et al: Differentiation of reperfused-viable (stunned) from reperfused-infarcted myocardium at 1 to 3 days postreperfusion by in vivo phosphorus-31 nuclear magnetic resonance spectroscopy, *Am Heart J* 122:1571-1582, 1991.

58. Califf RM, Ohman EM: The diagnosis of acute myocardial infarction, *Chest* 101(suppl):106S-115S, 1992.

59. Ellis AK: Serum protein measurements and the diagnosis of acute myocardial infarction, *Circulation* 83:1107-1110, 1991.

60. Ellis AK, Little T, Masud AR, et al: Patterns of myoglobin release after reperfusion of injured myocardium, *Circulation* 72:639-647, 1985.

61. Ellis AK, Saran BR: Kinetics of myoglobin release and prediction

of myocardial myoglobin depletion after coronary artery reperfusion, *Circulation* 80:676-683, 1989.

62. Ellis AK, Little T, Masud AR, et al: Early noninvasive detection of successful reperfusion in patients with acute myocardial infarction, *Circulation* 78:1352-1357, 1988.

63. Laperche T, Steg PG, Benessiano J, et al: Patterns of myoglobin and MM creatine kinase isoforms release early after intravenous thrombolysis or direct percutaneous transluminal coronary angioplasty for acute myocardial infarction, and implications for the early noninvasive diagnosis of reperfusion, *Am J Cardiol* 70:1129-1134, 1992.

64. Clemmensen P, Jurlander B, Grande P, et al: Monitoring peak serum-myoglobin for noninvasive prediction of coronary reperfusion in patients (abstract), *Circulation* 84(suppl II):II-116, 1991.

65. Katus HA, Diedrich KW, Scheffold T, et al: Noninvasive assessment of infarct reperfusion: the predictive power of the time to peak value of myoglobin, CKMB, and CK in serum, *Eur Heart J* 9:619-624, 1988.

66. Ellis AK: Detection of coronary recanalization with the use of plasma myoglobin determinations, *Cor Art Dis* 3:475-480, 1992.

67. Katus HA, Diedrich KW, Schwarz F,et al: Influence of reperfusion on serum concentrations of cytosolic creatine kinase and structural myosin light chains in acute myocardial infarction, *Am J Cardiol* 60:440-445, 1987.

68. Katus HA, Remppis A, Scheffold T, et al: Intracellular compartmentation of cardiac troponin T and its release kinetics in patients with reperfused and nonreperfused myocardial infarction, *Am J Cardiol* 67:1360-1367, 1991.

69. Blanke H, von Hardenberg D, Cohen M, et al: Patterns of creatine kinase release during acute myocardial infarction after nonsurgical reperfusion: comparison with conventional treatment and correlation with infarct size, *J Am Coll Cardiol* 3:675-680, 1984.

70. Gore JM, Roberts R, Ball SP, et al: Peak creatine kinase as a measure of effectiveness of thrombolytic therapy in acute myocardial infarction, *Am J Cardiol* 59:1234-1238, 1987.

71. Bosker HA, van der Laarse A, Cats VM, et al: Are enzymatic tests good indicators of coronary reperfusion? *Br Heart J* 67:150-154, 1992.

72. Abendschein DR: Detection of recanalization with the use of creatine kinase-MM subforms, *Cor Art Dis* 3:461-467, 1992.

73. Schofer J, Ress-Grigolo G, Voigt KD, et al: Early detection of coronary artery patency after thrombolysis by determination of the MM creatine kinase isoforms in patients with acute myocardial infarction, *Am Heart J* 123:846-853, 1992.

74. Puleo PR, Perryman MB, Bresser MA, et al: Creatine kinase isoform analysis in the detection and assessment of thrombolysis in man, *Circulation* 75:1162-1169, 1987.

75. Abendschein D, Seacord LM, Nohara R, et al: Prompt detection of myocardial injury by assay of creatine kinase isoforms in initial plasma samples, *Clin Cardiol* 11:661-664, 1988.

76. Lewis BS, Ganz W, Laramee P, et al: Usefulness of a rapid initial increase in plasma creatine kinase activity as a marker of reperfusion during thrombolytic therapy for acute myocardial infarction, *Am J Cardiol* 62:20-24, 1988.

77. Garabedian HD, Gold HK, Yasuda T, et al: Detection of coronary artery reperfusion with creatine kinase-MB determinations during thrombolytic therapy: correlation with acute angiography, *J Am Coll Cardiol* 11:729-734, 1988.

78. Ong L, Coromilas J, Zimmerman JM, et al: A physiologically based model of creatine kinase-MB release in reperfusion of acute myocardial infarction, *Am J Cardiol* 64:11-15, 1989.

79. Grande P, Granborg J, Clemmensen P, et al: Indices of reperfusion in patients with acute myocardial infarction using characteristics of the CK-MB time-activity curve, *Am Heart J* 122:400-408, 1991.

80. Abendschein DR, Ellis AK, Eisenberg PR, et al: Prompt detection of coronary recanalization by analysis of rates of change of concentrations of macromolecular markers in plasma, *Cor Art Dis* 2:201-212, 1991.

81. Puleo PR: Detection of coronary artery patency after thrombolytic therapy of acute myocardial infarction using creatine kinase-MB subforms, *Cor Art Dis* 3:468-474, 1992.

82. Puleo PR, Perryman MB: Noninvasive detection of reperfusion in acute myocardial infarction based on plasma activity of creatine kinase MB subforms, *J Am Coll Cardiol* 17:1047-1052, 1991.

83. Christenson RH, Ohman EM, Vollmer RT, et al: Serum release of the creatine kinase tissue-specific isoforms MM2 and MB2 is simultaneous during myocardial reperfusion, *Clin Chim Acta* 200:23-34, 1991.

84. Christenson RH, Ohman EM, Clemmensen P, et al: Characteristics of creatine kinase-MB and MB isoforms in serum after reperfusion in acute myocardial infarction, *Clin chem* 35:2179-2185, 1989.

85. Christenson RH, Ohman EM, Wall TC, et al: Relationship between infarct-related coronary artery flow after thrombolytic therapy and release of tissue-specific isoforms of creatine kinase, *J Am Coll Cardiol* (abstract), 19(suppl A):303A, 1992.

86. Ohman EM, Christenson RH, Califf RM, et al: Noninvasive detection of reperfusion after thrombolysis based on serum creatine kinase MB changes and clinical variables, *Am Heart J* 126:819-826, 1993.

87. Ganz W, Geft I, Shah PK, et al: Intravenous streptokinase in evolving acute myocardial infarction, *Am J Cardiol* 53:1209-1216, 1984.

88. Blanke H, Scherff F, Karsch KR, et al: Electrocardiographic changes after streptokinase-induced recanalization in patients with acute left anterior descending artery obstruction, *Circulation* 68:406-412, 1983.

89. Goldberg S, Urban P, Greenspon A, et al: Limitation of infarct size with thrombolytic agents—electrocardiographic indexes, *Circulation* 68 (suppl I):I-77-I-82, 1983.

90. Startt-Selvester RH, Wagner GS, Ideker RE: Myocardial infarction. In *Comprehensive electrocardiology: theory and practice in health and disease,* Elmsford, NY, Pergamon Press, 1989.

91. Dellborg M: Dynamic vectorcardiographic monitoring of patients during myocardial ischemia and infarction, doctoral dissertation, 1991, University of Goteborg.

92. Dellborg M, Steg PG, Simoons M, et al: Increased rate of evolution of QRS changes in patients with acute myocardial infarction: results from the Vermut Study, *J Electrocardiol* 26:244-248, 1993.

93. Glazier JJ, Chierchia S, Margonato A, et al: Increase in S-wave amplitude during ischemic ST-segment depression in stable angina pectoris, *Am J Cardiol* 59(15):1295-1299, 1987.

94. Wagner NB, Sevilla DC, Krucoff MW, et al: Transient alterations of the QRS complex and ST segment during percutaneous transluminal balloon angioplasty of the left anterior descending coronary artery, *Am J Cardiol* 62(16):1038-1042, 1988.

95. Wagner NB, Sevilla DC, Krucoff MW, et al: Transient alterations of the QRS complex and ST segment during percutaneous transluminal balloon angioplasty of the right and left circumflex coronary arteries, *Am J Cardiol* 63(17):1208-1213, 1989.

96. Krucoff MW, Sawchak ST, Pope JE, et al: Rethinking classical ECG patterns of ischemia and infarction: insights from investigations with continuous ECG monitoring, *The Newspaper of Cardiology* 12:8-17, 1992.

97. Hogg KJ, Hornung RS, Howie CA, et al. Electrocardiographic prediction of coronary artery patency after thrombolytic therapy

after AMI: use of the ST-segment as a non-invasive marker, *Br Heart J* 60:275-280, 1988.

98. Hackworthy RA, Vogel MB, Harris PJ: Relationship between changes in ST segment elevation and patency of the infarct-related coronary artery in acute myocardial infarction, *Am Heart J* 112:279-284, 1986.

99. Von Essen R, Schmidt W, Uebis R, et al: Myocardial infarction and thrombolysis: electrocardiographic short-term and long-term results using precordial mapping, *Br Heart J* 54:6-10, 1985.

100. Saran RK, Been M, Furniss SS, et al: Reduction in ST-segment elevation after thrombolysis predicts either coronary reperfusion or preservation of left ventricular function, *Br Heart J* 64:113-117, 1990.

101. Clemmensen P, Ohman EM, Sevilla DC, et al: Changes in standard electrocardiographic ST-segment elevation predictive of successful reperfusion in acute myocardial infarction, *Am J Cardiol* 66:1407-1411, 1990.

102. Ross AM for the TIMI Investigators: Electrocardiographic and angiographic correlations in myocardial infarction patients treated with thrombolytic agents: a report from the NHLBI Thrombolysis in Myocardial Infarction (TIMI) trial, *J Am Coll Cardiol* 2:495-501, 1985.

103. Veldkamp RF, Green CL, Wilkins ML, et al for the Thrombolysis and Angioplasty in Myocardial Infarction (TAMI) 7 Study Group: Comparison of continuous ST-segment recovery analysis with methods using static electrocardiograms for noninvasive patency assessment during acute myocardial infarction, *Am J Cardiol* 73:1069-1074, 1994.

104. Krucoff MW, Green CE, Satler LF, et al: Noninvasive detection of coronary artery patency using continuous ST-segment monitoring, *Am J Cardiol* 57:916-923, 1986.

105. Krucoff MW, Wagner NB, Pope JE, et al: The portable programmable microprocessor-driven real-time 12-lead electrocardiographic monitor: a preliminary report of a new device for the noninvasive detection of successful reperfusion or silent coronary reocclusion, *Am J Cardiol* 65:143-148, 1990.

106. Kwon K, Freedman B, Wilcox I, et al: The unstable ST segment early after thrombolysis for acute infarction and its usefulness as a marker of recurrent coronary occlusion, *Am J Cardiol* 67:109-115, 1991.

107. Krucoff MW, Croll MA, Pope JE, et al: Continuously updated 12-lead ST-segment recovery analysis for myocardial infarct artery patency assessment and its correlation with multiple simultaneous early angiographic observations, *Am J Cardiol* 71:145-151, 1993.

108. Shah PK, Cercek B, Lew AS, et al: Angiographic validation of bedside markers of reperfusion, *J Am Coll Cardiol* 21:55, 1993.

109. Col J, Pirenne B, Decoster O, et al: Basic components and patterns of acute ischemia recovery assessed from continuous ST monitoring in acute myocardial infarction treated by thrombolytic therapy, *J Electro Cardiol* 2:23, 1994.

110. Dellborg M, Riha M, Swedberg K: Dynamic QRS-complex and ST-segment monitoring in acute myocardial infarction during recombinant tissue-type plasminogen activator therapy, *Am J Cardiol* 67:343-349, 1991.

111. Dellborg M, Topol EJ, Swedberg K: Dynamic QRS complex and ST-segment vectorcardiographic monitoring can identify vessel patency in patients with acute myocardial infarction treated with reperfusion therapy, *Am Heart J* 122:943-948, 1991.

112. Veldkamp RF, Bengtson JR, Sawchak ST, et al: Evolution of an automated ST-segment analysis program for dynamic real-time, noninvasive detection of coronary occlusion and reperfusion, *J Electro Cardiol* 25 (suppl):182-187, 1992.

113. Krucoff MW: Electrocardiographic monitoring and coronary occlusion: fingerprint pattern analysis in dimensions of space, time, and mind, *J Electro Cardiol* 22:232-237, 1989.

114. Barbash GI, Roth A, Hod H, et al: Rapid resolution of ST elevation and prediction of clinical outcome in patients undergoing thrombolysis with alteplase (recombinant tissue-type plasminogen activator): results of the Israeli Study of Early Intervention in Myocardial Infarction, *Br Heart J* 64:241-247, 1990.

115. Mauri F, Gasparini M, Barbonaglia L, et al: Prognostic significance of the extent of myocardial injury in acute myocardial infarction treated by streptokinase (the GISSI Trial), *Am J Cardiol* 63:1291-1295, 1989.

116. Krucoff MW, Trollinger KM, Veldkamp RF, et al for the TAMI 9 Study Group: Detection of recurrent ischemia with continuous electrocardiographic monitoring: early risk stratification following thrombolytic therapy, *Circulation* 86(suppl):4, 1992.

117. Wong CK, Freedman SB: Usefulness of continuous ST monitoring in inferior wall acute myocardial infarction for describing the relation between precordial ST depression and inferior ST elevation, *Am J Cardiol* 72:532-537, 1993.

118. Shah A, Green CL, Trollinger KM, et al: Differentiation of "benign mirror image" from high-risk reciprocal ST depression using continuous 12-lead ST-segment recovery analysis, *J Am Coll Cardiol* Special Issue:895-898, 1994.

Chapter 38

MONITORING THE COAGULATION SYSTEM AFTER THROMBOLYTIC THERAPY

Robert A. Harrington
B. Gail Macik

The first goal in delivering thrombolytic therapy to the patient with an acute myocardial infarction (AMI) is to achieve rapid patency of the infarct-related artery. After successful reperfusion occurs, the clinician strives to maintain vessel patency and prevent reocclusion with the use of various antithrombotic regimens. Throughout these treatment periods, the competing goal is to avoid the major complication of thrombolytic and antithrombotic agents: hemorrhage.

Monitoring the initial and sustained effects of thrombolytic therapy is complicated by the paucity of clinical outcome data. Clinical assessment of the acute infarct patient, with a reliance on history and physical signs, has not proved to be reliable.[1] Bedside monitoring using standard 12-lead electrocardiograms (ECGs), continuous ST-segment monitoring, or cardiac enzymes has proved to be more successful in predicting initial reperfusion.[2,3] Studies have also shown that reocclusion after thrombolytic therapy occurs commonly and that the consequences may be severe[4]; reinfarction is the second most common cause of early mortality in the thrombolytic treated patient.[5] Finally, hemorrhagic complications of thrombolytic therapy are significant, with intracranial hemorrhage, the most feared complication of thrombolytic therapy, occurring in 0.3% to 1.0% of treated patients.[6]

By monitoring the coagulation system after administration of thrombolytic therapy and subsequently during the phase of conjunctive antithrombotic therapy, the clinician gains information that may improve the care of the patient. Coagulation laboratory testing offers insight into the reperfusion process and may allow the clinician to lessen the reocclusion risk while minimizing hemorrhagic complications. Although several commonly available laboratory assays are believed to be useful in the management of the thrombolytic treated patient, many of the assays to be discussed are primarily research tools at this time. Some of these may prove valuable in the future care of the acute infarct patient.

In this chapter, we briefly review the hemostatic and fibrinolytic mechanisms. We discuss the use of simple laboratory testing after thrombolytic therapy, focusing on the clinical usefulness and practical limitations of each test. We discuss several biochemical markers that may prove useful at identifying subsets of patients who fail to reperfuse, who are at an increased risk of reocclusion, or who have a greater propensity toward hemorrhage. In addition to their diagnostic utility, markers of the hemostatic system may be used to guide transfusion therapy in the actively bleeding patient.

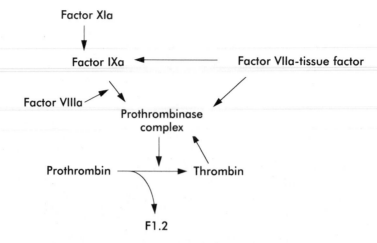

Fig. 38-1. Generation of thrombin. *F1.2,* Fragment 1.2.

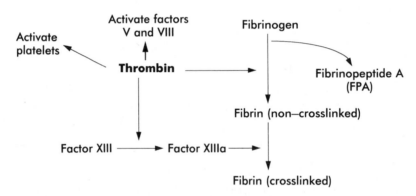

Fig. 38-2. Role of thrombin.

OVERVIEW OF COAGULATION AND FIBRINOLYSIS

Coagulation involves a complex series of enzymatic reactions ending with the formation of a fibrin mesh in and around a primary platelet plug, producing a stable hemostatic clot. The generation of thrombin, a serine proteinase, is a pivotal step in the coagulation process (Fig. 38-1). Although thrombin plays several vital roles in coagulation (Fig. 38-2), a primary function is the enzymatic cleavage of fibrinopeptides A and B from fibrinogen to form fibrin. Thrombin's feedback activation of factors V and VIII, pivotal catalysts of the enzymatic reactions comprising the coagulation process, accelerates the generation of more thrombin and serves to accelerate the entire coagulation process. In addition, thrombin activates factor XIII, which cross-links and stabilizes fibrin polymers. Thrombin's role as a potent activator of platelets aids primary hemostasis as well. Paradoxically, thrombin also indirectly initiates its own regulation. Thrombin, when bound to thrombomodulin, a protein expressed on unperturbed endothelium, will activate the protein C pathway. Protein C catabolizes

factors V and VIII and stops further thrombin generation. Lack of thrombin regulation or inactivation may mediate the reocclusion that follows successful reperfusion.

Fibrinolysis involves the enzymatic dissolution of the fibrin clot (Fig. 38-3). Plasminogen, the principal enzyme of the fibrinolytic system, binds to fibrin during thrombus formation. Endothelial cells release the physiologic activator of plasminogen, tissue-type plasminogen activator (t-PA), when stimulated by the formation of fibrin strands on their surface. The plasminogen is activated to plasmin, which then enzymatically degrades fibrin. The smallest fibrin degradation products are the crossed-linked segments commonly known as D-dimers. In excess, plasmin may dissociate from fibrin and also may degrade circulating fibrinogen. Because fibrinogen, unlike fibrin, is not cross-linked, no D-dimer degradation products are released. The clinically available thrombolytic agents urokinase (UK), streptokinase (SK), anistreplase (APSAC), and t-PA all act as either direct or indirect plasminogen activators in the conversion of plasminogen to enzymatically active plasmin. Plasmin, in

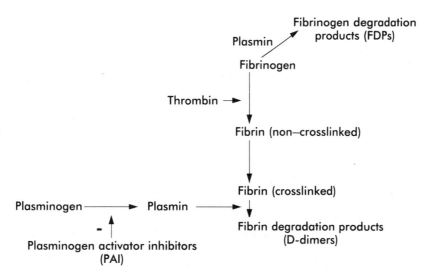

Fig. 38-3. Fibrinolytic system.

addition to its action on fibrin and fibrinogen, can also degrade factors V and VIII, thus interfering with further fibrin production and contributing to creation of the systemic lytic state.

HEMATOLOGIC PARAMETERS AFTER THROMBOLYTIC THERAPY

After administration of thrombolytic therapy (Table 38-1), fibrinogen levels decrease and fibrin(ogen) degradation products increase, reflecting the depletion of fibrinogen and the degradation of fibrin. Plasminogen levels also decrease as the available circulating zymogen is converted to the active enzyme plasmin. The use of SK or UK, which are not fibrin specific, results in a greater degree of fibrinogen depletion than does t-PA because they act on freely circulating plasminogen. t-PA must bind to fibrin before activating similarly bound plasminogen, thus limiting the production of freely circulating plasmin. Apart from agent specificity, there may be individual differences in the hematologic response to thrombolytic therapy.

Stump et al. have reported that, following t-PA administration, older women with lower body weight have more intense systemic fibrinogenolysis than do other patient groups.[7] This is reflected by lower nadir fibrinogen levels, a greater change in fibrinogen from baseline, and higher levels of fibrinogen degradation products. Because lower fibrinogen levels are associated with bleeding,[8] and because more bleeding occurs in older, lighter women, it may be that weight- and sex-adjusted dosing protocols are necessary to reduce bleeding complications in certain patient groups.[7]

Investigators have shown that blacks, treated with t-PA, have more intense fibrinogenolysis than do whites treated in a comparable fashion, as reflected in lower

fibrinogen levels, a greater change in fibrinogen levels from baseline, higher levels of fibrin(ogen) degradation products, and higher t-PA levels at the end of a maintenance infusion.[9] In this study, these hemostatic differences were accompanied by a trend toward improved 90-minute patency of the infarct-related artery in the black population (91% vs. 72%, $P = 0.051$) and a significantly higher transfusion rate for blacks compared with whites. This finding suggests that there may be an increased sensitivity to fibrinolysis with t-PA in certain populations. Whether this will translate into improved clinical outcomes awaits larger validation studies. For now, dosing regimens for t-PA should be kept constant across different racial populations.

MONITORING THROMBOLYTIC THERAPY: ROUTINE LABORATORY TESTING

After administration of thrombolytic therapy, several readily available clinical laboratory tests are useful in monitoring the patient's response to therapy, ensuring adequate anticoagulation and minimizing the risk of hemorrhagic complications (Table 38-2). These tests include the activated partial thromboplastin time (aPTT), the activated clotting time (ACT), the bleeding time (BT), and the platelet count. Although various studies have highlighted the utility of each of these tests, each has significant limitations, which must be understood by the clinician to interpret the tests appropriately.

aPTT

The aPTT is the most readily available test for detecting perturbations in the intrinsic and common coagulation pathways (Fig. 38-4). The test is typically performed by incubating citrated plasma with phospholipid emulsion and an activator (kaolin or celite),

Table 38-1. Hematologic parameters after thrombolytic therapy*

Parameters		Comments
Fibrinogen	Decrease	Depletion is marker of lytic state
D-Dimers	Increase	
FDPs	Increase	
Plasminogen	Decrease	
Factor V	Decrease	Depletion is marker of lytic state
Factor VIII	Decrease	Depletion is marker of lytic state
FPA	Increase	Persistent elevation may be marker of failed reperfusion; recurrent elevation may be marker of reocclusion.
TAT	Increase	Same as FPA
PAI		Elevated baseline levels may correlate with persistent reocclusion

*FDPs, Fibrinogen degradation products; FPA, fibrinopeptide A; TAT, thrombin–antithrombin III; PAI, plasminogen activator inhibitor.

Table 38-2. Value of coagulation laboratory tests in the individual patient*

Assays	Reperfusion	Reocclusion	Hemorrhage
aPTT	No	Yes	Yes
ACT	No	No	No
Fibrinogen	No	No	Yes (guide therapy)
D-Dimers	No	No	No
Platelet count	No	No	Yes
Bleeding time	No	No	Yes (guide therapy)
Factor V	No	No	No
Factor VIII	No	No	No
Plasminogen	No	No	No
FPA	?	?	No
TAT	?	?	No
PAI	?	No	No

*aPTT, Activated partial thromboplastin time; ACT, activated clotting time; FPA, fibrinopeptide A; TAT, tyrosine aminotransferase; PAI, plasminogen activator inhibitor.

initiating the reaction by the addition of calcium chloride and measuring the time to clot formation.[10] The normal range varies widely from reagent to reagent, mostly because of the differing responsiveness of the various phospholipids. Each clinical laboratory should establish a normal and therapeutic (heparin) range for the aPTT based on the reagent in use. This range should be reestablished with each change in reagent lot. Patient

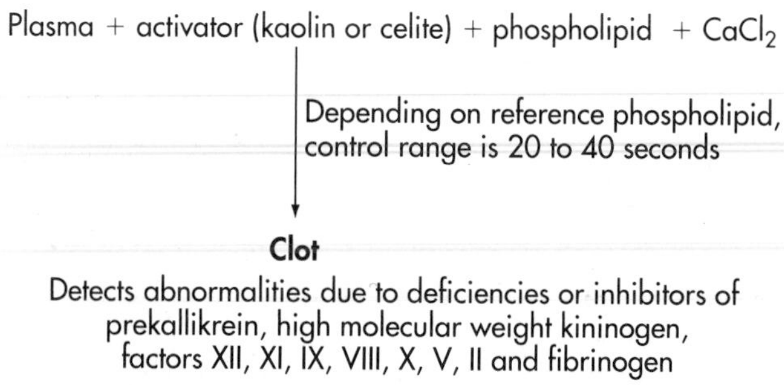

Plasma + activator (kaolin or celite) + phospholipid + $CaCl_2$

Depending on reference phospholipid, control range is 20 to 40 seconds

Clot

Detects abnormalities due to deficiencies or inhibitors of prekallikrein, high molecular weight kininogen, factors XII, XI, IX, VIII, X, V, II and fibrinogen

Fig. 38-4. Activated partial thromboplastin time.

management must be based on the aPTT reference parameters established by the laboratory performing the test.

Protamine titration, anti-Xa levels, and anti-IIa levels all have been used to try to validate the therapeutic aPTT range for heparin therapy.[11] These validating reference levels, however, are derived from experience with experimental models of venous thrombosis[12] and not from studies of patients with acute arterial occlusion. No true gold standard assay for determining a therapeutic heparin effect exists at this time, although for 25 years the aPTT has been the standard method of assessing the effects of heparin therapy.[13]

The use of the aPTT to monitor heparin effect is limited both by problems inherent to the assay itself and by variation in an individual patient's response to heparin. The baseline aPTT may be influenced by inappropriate sample collection, especially resulting in undercitration or overcitration of the sample, shortening of the aPTT by elevated factor VIII or fibrinogen levels, or interference with the assay by inhibitors of the test reaction, including specific clotting factor inhibitors or nonspecific phospholipid antibodies (lupus anticoagulant). Different brands of aPTT reagent have varying responsiveness to heparin,[14,15] resulting in differing aPTTs obtained on the same heparinized plasma sample. The method of collection,[16] as well as the instrumentation used to perform the assay,[17] can affect the aPTT. Cohen et al.[18] have recently shown that measurement of the aPTT varies, depending on the delay to sample assay. The obvious implication is that the ex vivo measurement may not accurately reflect the in vivo anticoagulation status if delays occur in sample measurement.

The differing response to heparin among patients independent of the aPTT assay itself may, in part, result from variation in available heparin-binding proteins.[11] In the thrombolytic treated patient, platelets activated by plasmin release platelet factor 4,[19] a heparin-neutralizing protein. Plasmin also activates vitronectin, another potent heparin-binding protein.[20] Some investigators have suggested that intravenous (IV) nitroglycerin can induce heparin resistance, perhaps through a qualitative antithrombin III abnormality,[21] although this observation is still being investigated.[22]

Significant laboratory delays in receiving, processing, and reporting aPTT results may result in suboptimal heparin dosing. Bedside monitoring of the aPTT from a finger stick or venous sample of whole blood is now being evaluated clinically in many hospitals. Recent studies have shown that a good correlation with the standard laboratory aPTT is achievable.[23] Becker et al.[24] have recently reported that the time from sample acquisition to result reporting is 143 minutes for the standard aPTT and 3 minutes for the bedside aPTT. The time to achievement of a therapeutic aPTT was significantly less with the bedside monitor than with standard laboratory testing.

Current limitations of the whole blood bedside instruments include lack of established whole blood clotting parameters, comparison of whole blood values to plasma-based parameters, a different assay system that may not be identical, moderate correlation coefficients ($R = 0.8$) between whole blood aPTTs and plasma aPTTs, and confounding of accuracy problems by singlet testing while most plasma determinations are still performed in duplicate to control for errors intrinsic to the assay conditions. Despite these early limitations, the whole blood aPTT instruments are appealing, especially if they are used to establish a therapeutic threshold and not a tight therapeutic range. Newer generations of these instruments may overcome the initial shortcomings. Whether patients will benefit from rapid reporting of results, which more closely reflect the rapidly changing anticoagulation status, awaits larger clinical outcome studies. Initial results from the Global Utilization of Streptokinase and Tissue Plasminogen Activator for Occluded Coronary Arteries (GUSTO) trial provide evidence that these bedside devices are at least equivalent to standard laboratory testing as they relate to patient outcome.

Measurement of the aPTT is helpful in the patient with active bleeding after thrombolytic therapy, because knowledge of the extent of the coagulopathy may help in delineating treatment options, including the decision to administer blood products. In the actively bleeding patient, an aPTT should be the first laboratory test performed; it provides a rapid assessment of the integrity of the patient's hemostatic capabilities. Because the fibrinogen depletion that follows thrombolytic therapy will increase the aPTT, rapid determination of the aPTT allows identification of the persistent lytic state. Because heparin also contributes to the prolongation of the aPTT, the reptilase time, which is not affected by heparin, can be performed to determine the relative contribution of the lytic state to the increased aPTT. For practical purposes this is unnecessary. The

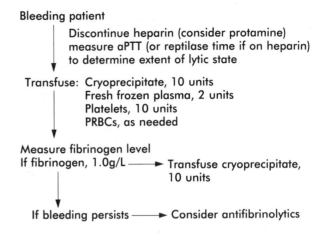

Fig. 38-5. Using the laboratory in managing the bleeding patient. *aPTT,* Activated partial thromboplastin time; *PRBCs,* packed red blood cells. (Modified from Sane DC, Califf RM, Topol EJ, et al: *Ann Intern Med* 111:1010, 1989. Used by permission.)

aPTT should provide sufficient information to aid in the acute treatment of the bleeding patient. Sane et al.[25] have devised a helpful algorithim using readily available laboratory tests to aid in the management of the bleeding patient after thrombolytic administration (Fig. 38-5). After transfusion therapy, the aPTT should be followed at regular intervals (every 6-12 hours) to ensure that replacement therapy has been adequate and that the lytic and anticoagulant effects are diminishing.

RECOMMENDATIONS FOR THE MANAGEMENT OF HEPARIN THERAPY

Although Topol et al.[26] have shown that early administration of heparin does not dramatically affect 90-minute patency after t-PA, other investigators have shown higher patency rates at 18,[27] 48,[28] and 81[29] hours after thrombolytic administration when heparin is given concomitantly with the thrombolytic agent. Early results from the GUSTO trial using a standard heparin regimen of a 5000-unit bolus, followed by a 1000 unit/hour IV drip, reveal that the degree to which the aPTT reflects a heparin effect correlated with body weight, age, and sex, with large, younger men having the lowest aPTTs at 24 hours after thrombolytic administration.[30]

We currently recommend weight adjustment for heparin, giving a 60 unit/kg IV bolus, followed by a 15 unit/kg/hour maintenance infusion. In all patients, the aPTT should be measured at 6, 12, and 24 hours after administration of thrombolytic therapy (Fig. 38-6). If the aPTT is less than two times the baseline aPTT (or the control if baseline is not available), additional heparin should be given and a repeat aPTT sent 6 hours later after a new steady state has been reached.

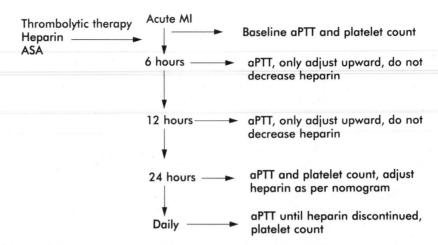

Fig. 38-6. Role of the coagulation laboratory in the care of the stable MI patient. *MI*, Myocardial infarction; *aPTT*, activated partial thromboplastin time; *ASA*, aspirin.

Early after the administration of thrombolytic therapy there is depletion of circulating fibrinogen, as well as factors V and VIII, leading to an increase in the measured aPTT, and reflecting the systemic lytic state. Heparin should not be decreased in the first 24 hours after thrombolytic administration, because even a markedly elevated aPTT may reflect primarily the lytic state and not the anticoagulant effects of heparin.[31] After 24 hours, heparin therapy may be adjusted using a standard heparin nomogram, constructed in individual laboratories, and based on reference aPTTs obtained using the local aPTT reagent.[32] An example of such a nomogram based on a control aPTT of 26 to 36 seconds is shown in Table 38-3.

Achievement of a therapeutic aPTT, defined as two times the baseline, is crucial. Data from the Heparin Aspirin Reperfusion Trial (HART) investigators demonstrates that patency at 18 hours is correlated with the aPTT.[33] In this study only 45% of patients with an aPTT less than 1.5 times baseline had infarct artery patency at an 18-hour catheterization, whereas 95% of patients who had an aPTT greater than 2 times baseline at 8 and 12 hours after thrombolytic administration had infarct artery patency at an 18-hour catheterization. Patients with early recurrent ischemia after thrombolysis have a poorer outcome even without progression to infarction.[34] These patients represent a special challenge with regard to anticoagulation, because the aggressive use of heparin carries with it a corresponding increase in hemorrhagic risk. For these patients, achieving and maintaining an aPTT 2.5 to 3 times baseline aPTT is reasonable until the patient stabilizes or an intervention is performed.

Careful attention to the aPTT may be beneficial in minimizing hemorrhagic complications of heparin therapy. Although a low aPTT may put the patient at risk from reocclusion, an exceptionally high aPTT may put

Table 38-3. Heparin nomogram for control aPTT of 26 to 36 seconds

aPTT (sec)	Bolus dose (units)	Stop infusion (min)	Rate change (units/hr)	Repeat aPTT (hr)
<50	5000	0	Increase (150)	6
50-59	0	0	Increase (100)	6
60-85	0	0	No change	Next A.M.
86-95	0	0	Decrease (50)	Next A.M.
96-120	0	30	Decrease (100)	6
>120	0	60	Decrease (150)	6

Modified from Cruickshank MK, Levine MN, Hirsh J, et al: *Arch Intern Med* 151:333-337; 1991.
aPTT, Activated thromboplastin time.

the patient at an increased hemorrhagic risk. Though not including any thrombolytic or AMI patients in their analysis, Landefeld et al.[35] have found that the intensity of heparin therapy, as measured by the aPTT, strongly correlates with the risk of bleeding. In their series, an aPTT more than 3.0 times control was associated with an eightfold increase in major bleeding risk. An analysis of hemorrhagic events in the Thrombolysis in Myocardial Infarction-II trial (TIMI-II) population found that patients with an aPTT greater than 90 seconds during early hospitalization was associated with significant increase in both major and minor hemorrhagic events.[36] For most patients who do not have any evidence of recurrent ischemia, it is preferable to minimize the hemorrhagic risks and maintain the aPTT in a range of 2 to 2.5 times baseline aPTT. When there is clinical evidence of recurrent ischemia, a higher risk of bleeding is acceptable to improve the clinical outcome, and an aPTT range of 2.5 to 3 times baseline is a reasonable goal.

ACTIVATED CLOTTING TIME

The activated clotting time (ACT) is a simply performed, readily available test of whole blood coagulation useful for the monitoring of heparin therapy. First described by Hattersley[37] in 1966, the automated ACT is the standard method of assessing adequacy of anticoagulation during cardiopulmonary bypass[38] and coronary angioplasty.[39] Whole blood is obtained and mixed in a tube containing diatomaceous earth or glass particles that activate the clotting process, and time to clot formation is determined by an automated device.

The benefits of the ACT include the ease of performance, the rapidity of results that allow immediate clinical action, and the ability to perform the test at the bedside. A major limitation is that the two most widely used automated devices, HemoTec ACT monitor (Medtronic Hemotec, Inc., Englewood, Colo.) and Hemochron 800 ACT monitor (HCH, International Technidyne, Edison, N.J.) are not interchangeable. There is considerable variation between the two devices in assessing the adequacy of anticoagulation.[40] As with the aPTT, the ACT depends on the reagents used, with one study showing that ACT's obtained using diatomaceous earth may be 20% higher than those determined using glass particles.[41] In addition, handling of the specimen rapidly and as outlined in the manufacturer's instructions is crucial to obtaining reproducible results.

Most clinical studies concerning the use of the ACT to monitor heparin anticoagulation have focused on the patient undergoing cardiopulmonary bypass (CPB) for cardiac surgery. Traditional practice has been to give 300 units of heparin/kg and to initiate CPB when the ACT is more than 400 seconds.[42] Additional heparin is given to maintain a similar ACT until CPB is discontinued, at which time protamine is administered to neutralize heparin. It should be noted that the so-called therapeutic ACT was determined arbitrarily and is used in settings where very high heparin levels are desirable. At very high doses of heparin, like those used during CPB or PTCA, it is likely that the ACT is a more accurate assessment of the patient's anticoagulation status. No study that correlates the ACT with more conventional levels of heparin has been done.

Animal studies have supported the suspected importance of heparin in preventing thrombotic complications during angioplasty.[43] Initially heparin was given empirically (10,000-unit bolus, then 3000 units/hour) during coronary angioplasty until Ogliby et al.[39] showed that such empiric heparin administration resulted in 11% of patients having an ACT of less than 300 seconds. Dougherty et al.[44] subsequently reported that major periangioplasty complications correlate with the procedural ACT; an ACT greater than 300 seconds is associated with fewer periprocedural complications than an ACT less than 250 seconds, suggesting that an ACT greater than 300 seconds is desirable for performing coronary angioplasty. Despite the attractiveness of this readily available test, no data are available to document the usefulness of monitoring the ACT during or after thrombolytic therapy. Its routine use as an instrument to monitor an individual's anticoagulation status in the postthrombolytic period cannot be recommended.

FIBRINOGEN, FIBRINOGEN DEGRADATION PRODUCTS, AND D-DIMERS

Most clinical laboratories have the capability to readily measure fibrinogen, fibrinogen degradation products (FDPs), and D-dimers. At present there are no data to support the routine measurement of these hemostatic markers in the uncomplicated thrombolytic treated patient. Early thrombolytic investigators questioned whether the degree of fibrinogenolysis, as determined by a drop in plasma fibrinogen level, correlated with infarct vessel patency. Collen et al.[45] in 1986, reported that a greater decrease in fibrinogen was associated with a higher incidence of vessel patency, as determined by early angiography. In the TIMI-I experience, Rao et al.[8] reported that administration of SK resulted in a significantly greater degree of fibrinogenolysis than did t-PA. The effectiveness of SK to open occluded vessels likely depends on the creation of such an intense lytic state. Although t-PA causes much more systemic fibrinogenlysis than was originally conceptualized, its success is not predicated on the achievement of systemic lytic effects.[7] Routine measurement of fibrinogen after thrombolytic administration does not allow prediction of infarct vessel patency. After t-PA and initial successful reperfusion, a greater change in fibrinogen level (baseline-nadir) may be associated with a decreased incidence of reocclusion.[7] Stump et al.[7] suggest that this may result from the anticoagulant and antiplatelet effects of fibrinogen degradation products, though this is unconfirmed. We do not recommend the routine measurement of fibrinogen after thrombolytic therapy.

FDPs are elevated after both fibrinogenolysis and fibrinolysis and do not adequately reflect fibrin specific degradation. The development of antibodies that recognize the double bond present in fibrin but not fibrinogen has allowed the accurate measurement of specific fibrin degradation products (D-dimers) and are better markers of fibrin dissolution and effective lytic therapy.[46,47] Lew et al.[48] first reported the elevation of plasma D-dimers after administration of streptokinase. The appearance of D-dimers in the blood after thrombolytic therapy does seem to predict coronary clot lysis[47,49] and not just nonspecific soluble fibrin dissolution.[50,51] Unfortunately, although the number of FDPs, including specific assays for D-dimers, do increase after therapy with all thrombolytic agents, no study has shown any significant correlation between extent of the increase and early vessel patency.[52-54]

Despite careful investigation, researchers[8,25,36,55] have been able to demonstrate only a weak relationship between the extent of fibrinogen depletion and bleeding complications. An analysis of the TIMI-I data did show a correlation between the incidence of bleeding events and lower 5-hour fibrinogen levels and higher FDP levels.[8] Interestingly, despite the achievement of a more intense systemic lytic effect with SK, there was no significant difference in hemorrhagic complications between SK and t-PA. Califf et al.,[55] in reporting the TAMI experience of patients treated with t-PA, showed that, as a group, only nadir fibrinogen levels correlated significantly with blood loss; however, they believed that there was little role for the routine monitoring of fibrinogen and FDP because of the weak relationship with hemorrhage in the individual patient. Recent results from the TIMI-II trial confirm these earlier impressions that changes in fibrinogen and FDP are not predictive of individual clinical hemorrhagic events.[36] Gore et al.[56] have shown no significant differences in fibrinogen depletion or in FDP in patients with central nervous system hemorrhagic events and those without such events treated with t-PA in the TIMI-II trial.

Knowledge of the fibrinogen level is important when the patient with hemorrhage after thrombolytic therapy is evaluated. In the patient who is actively bleeding after thrombolytic therapy, a fibrinogen level should be sent immediately, because its depletion defines the extent of the lytic state. Fibrinogen levels can help guide therapy with cryoprecipitate to ensure adequate fibrinogen replacement for hemostasis, but in the actively bleeding patient, initial therapy with 10 units of cryoprecipitate should not be delayed by waiting for the return of laboratory results. Cryoprecipitate contains 200 to 250 mg of fibrinogen and 80 units of factor VIII/unit.[25] This dose of cryoprecipitate should be sufficient for hemostasis, but after infusion of the 10 units, a repeat fibrinogen level should be determined and an additional 10 units transfused if the fibrinogen level remains less than 1.0 g/L.[25] Laboratory guidance of transfusion therapy is essential not only to maximize hemostatic potential but to minimize the infectious complications of indiscriminate transfusions.[57]

PLATELETS

Monitoring of platelet number and function plays an important role in patient care after administration of thrombolytic therapy.[58] Both the TIMI and TAMI groups have observed thrombocytopenia to be a potent predictor of major hemorrhage after thrombolytic therapy. In an analysis of patients assigned to a conservative strategy in the TIMI-II study, Bovill et al.[36] found that a platelet count of less than 100,000/μl,

occurring during the first 5 days after thrombolytic administration, was strongly associated with major and minor bleeding. In fact, thrombocytopenia was one of the most significant predictors of in-hospital hemorrhage after thrombolysis.

In a separate study of patients enrolled in the TAMI trials II, III, and V and the UK trial, Harrington et al.[59] defined thrombocytopenia as either a nadir platelet count of less than 100,000/μl or a change of more than one half from baseline. Patients with thrombocytopenia had substantially more blood loss and a higher in-hospital mortality than patients without thrombocytopenia. Linear regression models demonstrated thrombocytopenia to be an independent variable significantly associated with both hemorrhage and mortality in surgical and nonsurgical patients even when other important prognostic factors (including age, acute ejection fraction, number of diseased vessels, and need for intraaortic balloon counter pulsation) were considered.

Platelet counts should be measured daily after administration of thrombolytic therapy, because the appearance of thrombocytopenia identifies a subset of patients at increased risk of hemorrhage and death. The appearance of thrombocytopenia should prompt a search for reversible causes of the thrombocytopenia, but there is no evidence to support platelet transfusions in these patients based on platelet count alone. The etiology of thrombocytopenia after thrombolytic therapy is likely multifactorial, but a significant percentage may be caused by heparin-induced thrombocytopenia (HIT), an unusual but potentially catastrophic complication of heparin therapy.[60] The diagnosis of HIT is typically one of exclusion, but the laboratory measurement of heparin-associated platelet aggregation may confirm the suspected diagnosis.[61]

Platelet dysfunction typically occurs after thrombolytic therapy for several reasons, including use of aspirin, the disruption of platelet aggregation through lysis of fibrinogen bound to platelets,[62] the cleavage of membrane receptor glycoprotein Ib, and the creation of fibrinogen degradation products that inhibit aggregation.[63] Clinically platelet function has most frequently been assessed by the template bleeding time (BT); and, as such, it has been proposed as a method of predicting hemorrhagic risk after thrombolytic therapy. Gimple et al.[64] have reported that a BT of more than 9 minutes, when performed 90 minutes after thrombolytic delivery, correlates poorly with hemorrhage (sensitivity 69%; specificity 69%). The BT has not been shown to be a reliable baseline predictor of thrombolytic associated bleeding, because as a predictive test it suffers from problems of reproducibility and an overall lack of precision.[65] The BT may be useful as an assay of platelet function to determine if the bleeding patient would benefit from platelet transfusion therapy when postthrombolytic hemorrhage continues despite administration of cryoprecipitate and fresh frozen plasma.[25] A bleeding time of more than 9 minutes suggests significant platelet dysfunction and can be used as an indication to transfuse platelets in these patients. In the severely bleeding patient, the BT should be used only to monitor the effectiveness of therapy, and initiation of therapy should not be delayed. In cases of severe and life-threatening hemorrhage, we recommend immediate transfusion of 10 units of platelets.

SPECIAL LABORATORY TESTING

Special laboratory testing may eventually be useful in monitoring the thrombolytic patient, although these tests are currently research tools. A discussion of the assays is warranted because the available data provide insight into the reperfusion and reocclusion processes. Molecular markers of the lytic state, by providing an assessment of the extent of fibrin dissolution, could indirectly provide an assessment of vessel patency. These markers would be clinically beneficial if they could be used to predict patients at risk for hemorrhagic events before or after thrombolytic therapy. In the patient with active bleeding after thrombolytic therapy, special laboratory testing may also be useful in guiding management decisions, particularly regarding transfusion therapy. Finally, it is likely that in the future we will use these sensitive markers of thrombin generation and activity to more accurately monitor antithrombotic therapy. A substudy of the GUSTO trial should provide valuable insight into the ability of these assays to correlate not only with the level of anticoagulation but with clinical outcomes as well.

Although promising, these assays do have limitations,[25] the most immediate being availability. In addition, because these tests are quite time consuming to perform, the delay in reporting may not allow adequate monitoring of rapidly changing hemostatic parameters. If not properly collected, artificial ex vivo activation of the fibrinolytic system may lead to inaccurate results. Finally, there is variability in the test results depending on the methodology used. Despite these problems, in the following sections we examine the available data on FPA, thrombin–antithrombin III (TAT) complex, Fragment 1.2 (F1.2), and plasminogen activator inhibitor-1 (PAI-1) to provide insight into the reperfusion and reocclusion processes, to allow some assessment of hemorrhagic risk, and to contemplate what the future of coagulation monitoring after thrombolytic therapy may hold.

Fibrinopeptide A

During the thrombin-mediated conversion of fibrinogen to fibrin, fibrinopeptide A (FPA) is enzymatically cleaved from fibrinogen and thus serves as a sensitive marker of thrombin activity. Eisenberg et al.[66] in 1986 first noted the paradoxical increase in FPA levels after SK administration. Other investigators[67,68] have shown that FPA levels are elevated after t-PA administration as well. This transient increase in thrombin activity, as reflected by the increase in FPA levels, may be secondary to release of thrombin sequestered in the clot, reexposure of the subendothelium providing a new thrombogenic stimulus, further activation of thrombin by the lytic state, and new thrombogenic surfaces produced by ischemic damage to the endothelium.[69]

The creation of a transient procoagulant state after thrombolytic administration may help explain why reocclusion occurs despite the intensity of the lytic state and concomitant anticoagulation. Animal models have suggested that reocclusion after thrombolysis is a thrombin-mediated phenomenon[70-75]; markers of thrombin generation and activity may be useful in assessing the efficacy of therapy and allowing some prediction of the reocclusion process.

Eisenberg et al.[76] have reported that patients with persistent clinical occlusion after thrombolytic administration may have markedly elevated levels of FPA that do not decline until IV heparin is administered. They also observed that the continued presence of thrombin activity, as determined by serial measurements of FPA levels, may be a marker of reocclusion after initially successful thrombolytic therapy. Although Ring et al.[77] were unable to demonstrate that monitoring of FPA levels allowed prediction of reocclusion, Rapold et al.[78] have shown that an increasing or persistently elevated FPA level, occurring despite IV heparin therapy, correlates well with clinical evidence of reocclusion. Although FPA is a very sensitive method of assessing thrombin activity, methodologic problems involving sampling artifact limit its current usefulness to the research arena.

TAT complex

Circulating thrombin binds with antithrombin III to form the TAT complex. Once bound to antithrombin III, thrombin is no longer enzmatically active. The measurement of these complexes is possible and reflects the generation and subsequent inactivation of thrombin. Gulba et al.[79] have examined changes in the TAT complex as a predictor of thrombolytic induced patency. In a series of 55 patients treated with preactivated prourokinase or t-PA and who had vessel patency demonstrated at 90-minute angiography, TAT consistently increased in cases of early reocclusion. Although the early results are intriguing, whether FPA or TAT will be useful in helping the clinician predict the patient at risk for early reocclusion awaits the results of larger clinical trials.

F1.2

F1.2, a small peptide cleaved from prothrombin during its enzymatic conversion to thrombin, is a sensitive marker of ongoing thrombin generation.[80] Its measurement could be useful in the thrombolytic treated patient, because its appearance in the blood reflects continued prothrombinase complex activity and procoagulant potential. Its usefulness has been demonstrated in studies of patients receiving chronic warfarin therapy, where it has been shown to be more sensitive of suppression of thrombin generation than the standard prothrombin time.[81] Eisenberg et al.[82] have recently shown that F1.2 increases after administration of t-PA, indicating that the thrombin generation that follows thrombolysis occurs, at least in part, because of prothrombin activation. This suggests that an effective approach to thrombolysis and adjunctive antithrombotic therapy could include agents that have inhibitory effects earlier in the coagulation cascade (i.e., anti–factor Xa agents).[82] No study to date has shown F1.2 to be useful in predicting clinical efficacy or safety events.

PAI-1

Because natural inhibitors of the fibrinolytic system may adversely affect thrombolytic efficacy, investigators have measured PAI-1 and attempted to correlate it with vessel patency. Barbash et al.[83] have shown that PAI-1 activity is significantly higher in patients with occluded infarct vessels, as determined at a day 3 catheterization. Using a 90-minute angiogram for patency assessment, Sane et al.[84] have shown that PAI-1 levels do correlate, albeit weakly, with vessel patency. The antifibrinolytic role of PAI-1 needs further study to appropriately assess its clinical utility.

SUMMARY

The coagulation system involves a complex series of enzymatic reactions designed to maintain a balance between fibrin clot formation and degradation. The challenges in managing the AMI patient after the administration of thrombolytic are immense. Knowledge of the mechanisms of the coagulation system and the ability to monitor these changes in the individual patient greatly aids in the care during the periinfarct period. Standard laboratory assays such as the aPTT, the platelet count, and the fibrinogen level help in the management of these patients. Understanding the limitations of these assays is crucial to maximizing their use. More work needs to be done before assays such as FPA, TAT, F1.2, and PAI-1 levels are useful to the practicing clinician. For now, understanding these assays allows the clinician better insight into the mechanisms of reperfusion, reocclusion, and hemorrhage after thrombolytic therapy.

REFERENCES

1. Califf RM, O'Neil W, Stack RS, et al: Failure of simple clinical measurements to predict perfusion status after intravenous thrombolysis, *Ann Intern Med* 108:658-662, 1988.
2. Krucoff MW, Wagner NB, Pope JE, et al: The portable programmable microprocessor-driven real-time 12-lead electrocardiographic monitor: a preliminary report of a new device for the noninvasive detection of successful reperfusion or silent coronary reocclusion, *Am J Cardiol* 65:143-148, 1990.
3. Ohman EM, Christenson RH, Sigmon KN, et al: Non-invasive detection of reperfusion after thrombolysis using rapid CK-MB analysis [abstract], *Circulation* 82:281, 1990.
4. Ohman EM, Califf RM, Topol EJ, et al: Consequences of reocclusion after successful reperfusion therapy in acute myocardial infarction, *Circulation* 82:781-791, 1990.
5. Ohman EM, Sigmon K, Wall TC, et al: Why do people die after thrombolytic therapy? *Circulation* 80(suppl II):II349, 1989.
6. Levine MN, Goldhaber SZ, Califf RM, et al: Hemorrhagic complications of thrombolytic therapy in the treatment of myocardial infarction and venous thromboembolism, *Chest* 102:364S-373S, 1992.
7. Stump DC, Califf RM, Topol EJ, et al: Pharmacodynamics of thrombolysis with recombinant tissue-type plasminogen activator. Correlation with characteristics of and clinical outcomes in patients with acute myocardial infarction, *Circulation* 80:1222-1230, 1989.
8. Rao AK, Pratt C, Berke A, et al: Thrombolysis in Myocardial Infarction (TIMI I) trial–phase I: hemorrhagic manifestations and changes in plasma fibrinogen and the fibrinolytic system in patients treated with recombinant tissue plasminogen activator and streptokinase, *J Am Coll Cardiol* 11:1-11, 1988.
9. Sane DC, Stump DC, Topol EJ, et al: Racial differences in responses to thrombolytic therapy with recombinant tissue-type plasminogen activator. Increased fibrin(ogen)olysis in blacks, *Circulation* 83:170-175, 1991.
10. Houge C: Partial thromboplastin time (PTT) and activated partial thromboplastin time tests. In Williams WJ, Beutler E, Ersley AJ, et al (eds): *Hematology,* ed 4, New York. 1990, McGraw-Hill, pp 1766-1768.
11. Hirsh J: Heparin, *N Engl J Med* 324:1565-1574, 1991.
12. Chiu HM, Hirsh J, Yung WL, et al: Relationship between the anticoagulant and antithrombotic effects of heparin in experimental venous thrombosis, *Blood* 49:171-184, 1977.
13. Spector I, Corn M: Control of heparin therapy with activated partial thromboplastin times, *JAMA* 201:75-77, 1967.
14. Bain B, Forster T, Sleigh B: Heparin and the activated partial thromboplastin time – a difference between the in-vitro and in-vivo effects and implications for the therapeutic range, *Am J Clin Pathol* 74:668-673, 1980.
15. Shojania AM, Tetreault J, Turnbull G: The variations between heparin sensitivity of different lots of activated partial thromboplastin time reagent produced by the same manufacturer, *Am J Clin Pathol* 89:19-23, 1988.
16. Peterson P, Gottfried E: The effects of inaccurate blood sample volume on prothrombin time and activated partial thromboplastin time, *Thromb Haemost* 47:101-103, 1982.
17. Brandt JT, Triplett DA: Laboratory monitoring of heparin. Effects of reagents and instruments on the activated partial thromboplastin time, *Am J Clin Pathol* 76(suppl):530-537, 1981.
18. Cohen JA, Charles L, Wason TD, et al: Delay in sample processing may significantly decrease whole blood and plasma aPTTs obtained from heparinized patients resulting in establishment of erroneous therapeutic whole blood aPTT ranges, *Blood* 80(suppl 1):488a, 1992.
19. Holt JC, Niewiarowski S: Biochemistry of α-granule proteins, *Semin Hematol* 22:151-163, 1985.
20. Preissner KT, Muller-Berghaus G: Neutralization and binding of heparin by S-protein/vitronectin in the inhibition of factor Xa by antithrombin III, *J Biol Chem* 262:12247-12253, 1987.
21. Becker RC, Corrao JM, Bovill EG, et al: Intravenous nitroglycerin-

induced heparin resistance: a qualitative antithrombin III abnormality, *Am Heart J* 119:1254-1261, 1990.

22. Bode V, Welzel D, Franz G, et al: Absence of drug interaction between heparin and nitroglycerin: randomized placebo-controlled cross-over study, *Arch Intern Med* 150:2117-2119, 1990.

23. Ansell J, Tiarks C, Hirsh J, et al: Measurement of the activated partial thromboplastin time from a capillary (fingerstick) sample of whole blood. A new method for monitoring heparin therapy, *Am J Clin Pathol* 95:222-227, 1991.

24. Becker R, Cyr J, Corraro J, et al: Bedside aPTT monitoring: a convenient, rapid and accurate assessment of systemic anticoagulation in heparinized patients, *J Am Coll Cardiol* 21(suppl A):219A, 1993.

25. Sane DC, Califf RM, Topol EJ, et al: Bleeding during thrombolytic therapy for acute myocardial infarction: mechanisms and management, *Ann Intern Med* 3:1010-1022, 1989.

26. Topol EJ, George BS, Kereiakes DJ, et al: A randomized controlled trial of intravenous tissue plasminogen activator and early intravenous heparin in acute myocardial infarction, *Circulation* 79:281-286, 1989.

27. Hsia J, Hamilton WP, Kleiman N, et al: A comparison between heparin and low-dose aspirin as adjunctive therapy with tissue plasminogen activator for acute myocardial infarction, *N Engl J Med* 323:1433-1437, 1990.

28. Bleich SD, Nichols T, Schumacher R, et al: The role of heparin following coronary thrombolysis with tissue plasminogen activator (t-PA), *Circulation* 80(suppl II):II113, 1989.

29. de Bono DP, Simoons ML, Tijssen J, et al: Effect of early intravenous heparin on coronary patency, infarct size, and bleeding complications after alteplase thrombolysis: results of a randomised double blind European Cooperative Study Group trial, *Br Heart J* 67:122-128, 1992.

30. Granger CB, Califf RM, Hirsh J, et al: APTTs after thrombolysis and standard intravenous heparin are often low and correlate with body weight, age and sex: experience from the GUSTO trial, *Circulation* 86(suppl I):I258, 1992.

31. Bovill EG, Granger CB, Ross A, et al: Thrombin inhibition is more closely related to PTT than to heparin level after thrombolysis and heparin therapy, *J Am Coll Cardiol* 21(suppl A):137A, 1993.

32. Cruickshank MK, Levine MN, Hirsh J, et al: A standard heparin nomogram for the management of heparin therapy, *Arch Intern Med* 151:333-337, 1991.

33. Hsia J, Kleiman N, Aguirre F, et al: Heparin-induced prolongation of partial thromboplastin time after thrombolysis: relation to coronary artery patency. HART Investigators, *J Am Coll Cardiol* 20:31-35, 1992.

34. Califf RM, Topol EJ, Ohman EM, et al: Isolated ischemia after thrombolytic therapy is a frequent, important and expensive adverse clinical outcome, *J Am Coll Cardiol* 19:301A, 1992.

35. Landefeld CS, Cook EF, Flatley M, et al: Identification and preliminary validation of predictors of major bleeding in hospitalized patients starting anticoagulant therapy, *Am J Med* 82:703-713, 1987.

36. Bovill EG, Terrin ML, Stump DC, et al: Hemorrhagic events during therapy with recombinant tissue-type plasminogen activator, heparin, and aspirin for myocardial infarction. Results of the Thrombolysis in Myocardial Infarction (TIMI), phase II trial, *Ann Intern Med* 115:256-265, 1991.

37. Hattersley PG: Activated coagulation time of whole blood, *JAMA* 196:150-154, 1966.

38. Ponari O, Corsi M, Manotti C, et al: Predictive value of preoperative in-vitro and in-vivo studies for correct individual heparinization in cardiac surgery, *J Thorac Cardiovasc Surg* 78:87-94, 1979.

39. Ogilby JD, Kopelman HA, Klein LW, et al: Adequate heparinization during PTCA: assessment using activated clotting times, *Cathet Cardiovasc Diagn* 18:296-209, 1989.

40. Reich DL, Zahl K, Perucho MH, et al: An evaluation of two activated clotting time monitors during cardiac surgery, *J Clin Monitor* 8:33-36, 1992.

41. Weiner BH, Voyce S, Heller LI, et al: What is the right activated clotting time? *Circulation* 86(suppl I):I250, 1992.

42. Edmunds LH, Addonizio VP: Extracorporeal circulation. In Colman RW, Hirsh J, Marder VJ, et al (eds): *Hemostasis and thrombosis. Basic principles and clinical practice,* ed 2, Philadelphia, 1987, JB Lippincott, pp 901-912.

43. Heras M, Chesebro JH, Penny WJ, et al: Importance of adequate heparin dosage in arterial angioplasty in a porcine model, *Circulation* 78:654-660, 1988.

44. Dougherty KG, Marsh KC, Edelman SK, et al: Relationship between procedural activated clotting time and in-hospital post-PTCA outcome, *Circulation* (suppl III):III189, 1990.

45. Collen D, Bounameaux H, DeCock F, et al: Analysis of coagulation and fibrinolysis during intravenous infusion of recombinant human tissue-type plasminogen activator in patients with acute myocardial infarction, *Circulation* 73:511-517, 1986.

46. Prisco D, Paniccia R, Bonechi F, et al: Evaluation of new methods for the selective measurement of fibrin and fibrinogen degradation products, *Thromb Res* 56:547-551, 1989.

47. Eisenberg PR, Jaffe AS: Detection of coronary clot lysis with an improved ELISA for cross-linked fibrin degradation products, *J Am Coll Cardiol* 17:144A, 1991.

48. Lew AS, Berberian L, Cercek B, et al: Elevated serum D dimer: a degradation product of cross-linked fibrin (XDP) after intravenous streptokinase during acute myocardial infarction, *J Am Coll Cardiol* 7:1320-1324, 1986.

49. Eisenberg PR, Jaffe AS, Stump DC, et al: Validity of enzyme-linked immunosorbent assays of cross-linked fibrin degradation products as a measure of clot lysis, *Circulation* 82:1159-1168, 1990.

50. Francis CW, Doughney K, Brenner B, et al: Increased immunoreactivity of plasma after fibrinolytic activation in an anti-DD ELISA system. Role of soluble crosslinked fibrin polymers, *Circulation* 79:666-673, 1989.

51. Brenner B, Francis CW, Totterman S, et al: Quantitation of venous clot lysis with the D-dimer immunoassay during fibrinolytic therapy requires correction for soluble fibrin degradation, *Circulation* 81:1881-1825, 1990.

52. Arnold AER, Brower RW, Collen D, et al: Increased serum levels of fibrinogen degradation products due to treatment with recombinant tissue-type plasminogen activator for acute myocardial infarction are related to bleeding complications but not to coronary patency, *J Am Coll Cardiol* 14:581-588, 1989.

53. Simank HG, Simon M, Bode C, et al: Clinical usefulness of D-dimer: evaluation during fibrinolytic treatment of venous thrombosis or myocardial infarction, *Thromb Res* 56:541-546, 1989.

54. Brenner B, Francis CW, Fitzpatrick PG, et al: Relation of plasma D-dimer concentrations to coronary artery reperfusion before and after thrombolytic treatment in patients with acute myocardial infarction, *Am J Cardiol* 63:1179-1184, 1989.

55. Califf RM, Topol EJ George BS, et al: Hemorrhagic complications associated with the use of intravenous tissue plasminogen activator in treatment of acute myocardial infarction, *Am J Med* 85:353-359, 1988.

56. Gore JM, Sloan M, Price TR, et al: Intracerebral hemorrhage, cerebral infarction, and subdural hematoma after acute myocardial infarction and thrombolytic therapy in the Thrombolysis in Myocardial Infarction Study. Thrombolysis in Myocardial Infarction, Phase II, pilot and clinical trial, *Circulation* 83:448-459, 1991.

57. Langdale LA: Infectious complications of blood transfusions, *Infect Dis Clin North Am* 6:731-744, 1992.

58. Coller BS: Platelets and thrombolytic therapy, *N Engl J Med* 322:33-42, 1990.

59. Harrington RA, Sane DC, Califf RM, et al: Clinical importance of thrombocytopenia occurring in the hospital phase after administration of thrombolytic therapy for acute myocardial infarction, *J Am Coll Cardiol* 23:891-898, 1994.

60. Warkentin TE, Kelton JG: Heparin-induced thrombocytopenia, *Annu Rev Med* 40:31-44, 1989.

61. Miller ML: Heparin-induced thrombocytopenia, *Clev Clin J Med* 56:483-490, 1989.

62. Loscalzo J, Vaughan DE: Tissue plasminogen activator promotes platelet disaggregation in plasmin, *J Clin Invest* 79:1749-1755, 1987.

63. Adelman B, Michelson AD, Loscalzo J, et al: Plasmin effect on platelet glycoprotein IB–von Willebrand factor interactions, *Blood* 65:32-40, 1985.

64. Gimple LW, Gold HK, Leinbach RC, et al: Correlation between template times and spontaneous bleeding during treatment of acute myocardial infarction with recombinant tissue-type plasminogen activator, *Circulation* 80:581-588, 1989.

65. Hirsch DR, Goldhaber SZ: The bleeding time: its potential utility among patients receiving thrombolytic therapy, *Am Heart J* 119:158-167, 1990.

66. Eisenberg PR, Sherman L, Rich M, et al: Importance of continued activation of thrombin reflected by fibrinopeptide A to the efficacy of thrombolysis, *J Am Coll Cardiol* 7:1255-1262, 1986.

67. Owen J, Friedman KD, Grossman BA, et al: Thrombolytic therapy with tissue plasminogen activator or streptokinase induces transient thrombin activity, *Blood* 72:616-620, 1988.

68. Rapold HJ: Promotion of thrombin activity by thrombolytic therapy without simultaneous anticoagulation, *Lancet* 335:481-482, 1990.

69. Eisenberg PR: Role of new anticoagulants as adjunctive therapy during thrombolysis, *Am J Cardiol* 67:19A-24A, 1991.

70. Fitzgerald DJ, Fitzgerald GA: Role of thrombin and thromboxane A2 in reocclusion following coronary thrombolysis with tissue-type plasminogen activator, *Proc Natl Acad Sci USA* 86:7585, 1989.

71. Mellott MJ, Connolly TM, York SJ, et al: Prevention of reocclusion by MCI-9038, a thrombin inhibitor, following t-PA-induced thrombolysis in a canine model of femoral arterial thrombosis, *Thromb Haemost* 64:526, 1990.

72. Yasuda T, Gold HK, Yaoita H, et al: Comparative effects of aspirin, a synthetic thrombin inhibitor and a monoclonal antiplatelet glycoprotein IIb/IIIa antibody on coronary artery reperfusion, reocclusion and bleeding with tissue-type plasminogen activator in a canine preparation, *J Am Coll Cardiol* 16:714, 1990.

73. Chesebro JH, Fuster V: Reperfusion, specific thrombin inhibition and reocclusion after thrombolysis, *J Am Coll Cardiol* 16:723, 1990.

74. Heras M, Chesebro JH, Webster MWI, et al: Hirudin, heparin, and placebo during deep arterial injury in the pig. The in vivo role of thrombin in platelet-mediated thrombosis, *Circulation* 82:1476, 1990.

75. Haskel EJ, Prager NA, Sobel BE, et al: Relative efficacy of antithrombin compared with antiplatelet agents in accelerating coronary thrombolysis and preventing early reocclusion, *Circulation* 83:1048, 1991.

76. Eisenberg PR, Sherman LA, Jaffe AS: Paradoxic elevation of fibrinopeptide A after streptokinase: evidence for continued thrombosis despite intense fibrinolysis, *J Am Coll Cardiol* 10:527-529, 1987.

77. Ring ME, Butman SM, Bruck DC, et al: Fibrin metabolism in patients with acute myocardial infarction during and after treatment with tissue-type plasminogen activator, *Thromb Haemost* 60:428-433, 1988.

78. Rapold HJ, Kuemmerli H, Weiss M, et al: Monitoring of fibrin generation during thrombolytic therapy of acute myocardial infarction with recombinant tissue-type plasminogen, *Circulation* 79:980-989, 1989.

79. Gulba DC, Barthels M, Westhoff-Bleck M: Increased thrombin levels during thrombolytic therapy in acute myocardial infarction. Relevance for the success of therapy, *Circulation* 83:937-944, 1991.

80. Lau HK, Rosenberg JS, Beeler DL, et al: The isolation and characterization of a specific antibody population directed against the prothrombin activation fragments F2 and F1 + 2, *J Biol Chem* 254:8751-8761, 1979.

81. Millenson MM, Bauer KA, Kistler JP, et al: Monitoring "mini-intensity" anticoagulation with warfarin: comparison of the prothrombin time using a sensitive thromboplastin with prothrombin fragment F1 + 2 levels, *Blood* 79:2034-2038, 1992.

82. Eisenberg PR, Sobel BE, Jaffe AS: Activation of prothrombin accompanying thrombolysis with recombinant tissue-type plasminogen activator, *J Am Coll Cardiol* 19:1065-1069, 1992.

83. Barbash GI, Hod H, Roth A, et al: Correlation of baseline plasminogen activator inhibitor activity with patency of the infarct artery after thrombolytic therapy in acute myocardial infarction, *Am J Cardiol* 64:1231-1235, 1989.

84. Sane DC, Stump DC, Topol EJ, et al: Correlation between baseline plasminogen activator inhibitor levels and clinical outcome during therapy with tissue plasminogen activator for acute myocardial infarction, *Thromb Haemost* 65:275-279, 1991.

Chapter 39

THERAPEUTIC DRUG MONITORING IN THE ACUTELY ILL PATIENT

Daniel B. Mark
Gary Dunham

The physician caring for the patient with an acute myocardial infarction (AMI) has to contend with an ever-expanding array of available medicines. Most of these agents can provide significant benefit but can also induce serious harm if used improperly, especially in a critically ill postinfarction patient. The decision regarding which drug to use (and when) for a given MI patient is the subject of other chapters in this volume and is not discussed here. The purpose of this chapter is to review the current status of therapeutic drug monitoring in the setting of an AMI. Because monitoring of thrombolytic therapy is described in detail elsewhere, this specific issue is not considered here. This chapter covers three topics. First, we review the basic concepts of pharmacokinetics needed to appreciate the full potential of therapeutic drug monitoring. Second, we discuss the principles, indications, and appropriate timing of measuring drug levels. Finally, we review the agents most commonly monitored with serum drug levels in the coronary care unit (CCU) setting and describe how to use levels most effectively.

BASIC CONCEPTS

To understand serum drug levels, one must appreciate how the drug enters the bloodstream, how it is distributed in the tissues, and how it leaves the body. Several key terms applied to these processes include absorption, distribution, metabolism, excretion, and elimination.

Absorption refers to the movement of drug into the systemic circulation from the site of administration. For an intravenous (IV) drug, absorption is (with rare exceptions) 100%. Oral administration may provide much less drug to the systemic circulation of the AMI patient because of decreased gastrointestinal blood flow, vomiting, irreversible binding of the drug to another drug (e.g., antacids) present in the intestinal tract, and destruction by gastric acid or intestinal microorganisms. For this reason, in the acutely ill cardiac patient, we always prefer to give IV drugs whenever possible. Note that when the patient is converted from IV to oral drug administration, serum drug levels may fall because of incomplete absorption and lead to an apparent "relapse."

After being absorbed into the portal blood, several cardiac drugs given by the oral route are also subject to a significant "first-pass" metabolism by the liver, which further reduces the amount reaching the systemic circulation. For example, the oral dose of propranolol (40-80 mg) is eight times the IV dose (5-10 mg), largely because of hepatic first-pass metabolism.

Distribution refers to the pattern of dissemination of drug throughout the tissues of the body. After a drug enters the bloodstream, some becomes bound to plasma proteins (particularly albumin and α_1-acid glycoprotein). The remainder of the drug is distributed into the blood volume and those tissues with an extensive vascular supply. From there, the drug moves at a slower rate into other tissues and extravascular spaces. Drug distribution is often described with a conceptual model that can be useful in understanding drug levels, even though it has no physiologic basis per se. Initial distribution of drug in the vascular system defines the central volume of distribution, whereas subsequent distribution to the less vascular tissues and extravascular spaces defines the peripheral volume of distribution. The "apparent volume of distribution" is composed of both the central and peripheral components (or compartments) and refers to the hypothetical volume (in liters per kilogram body weight) that the total drug in the body would occupy if it were uniformly distributed at the steady-state serum level. A high volume of distribution indicates that most of the drug in the body is concentrated in the peripheral compartment. For example, digoxin has a high volume of distribution (average 5-7 L/kg) and is concentrated in skeletal muscle (10- to 20-fold greater than serum levels) and in cardiac muscle (30- to 60-fold greater). In contrast, a small volume of distribution indicates that most of the drug remains in the central compartment (i.e., blood pool). Furosemide, with a volume of distribution of 0.1 L/kg, is a good example. One practical consequence of a large volume of distribution is that most of the drug in the body is extravascular and not readily available for excretion, whereas a drug with a small volume of distribution is contained primarily in the vascular system and is readily excreted.

An important determinant of a drug's volume of distribution is the extent to which the drug is reversibly bound to plasma proteins. Only the unbound fraction of a drug is available for distribution to the peripheral compartment (and target tissues) and for renal excretion, and only the unbound fraction is thought to be pharmacologically active. The greater the amount of drug bound to plasma proteins, the lower the volume of distribution. Also, if a drug is highly protein bound (e.g., >90%), there may be important consequences if it is given concurrently with another drug that competes for the same binding sites. If the free (unbound) circulating drug is only a small percentage of total circulation drug, even if only 1% or 2% is displaced from protein-binding sites by another drug, there may be a substantial rise in the free (pharmacologically active) drug concentration. For example, warfarin is more than 99% protein bound. When a patient on warfarin therapy with a therapeutic prothrombin time is started on phenytoin therapy, warfarin is displaced from protein-binding sites, and the free (active) serum levels may rise twofold to fourfold. The net result is that the patient's prothrombin time will become markedly prolonged despite the fact that no change was made in the warfarin dose.

Elimination refers to removal of active drug from the body. A drug may be eliminated by either excretion or metabolism to an inactive form. The major organs of drug elimination are the liver and the kidneys. Drug elimination by each of these organs is measured by the drug clearance (i.e., the volume of blood made drug-free per unit time by the eliminating organ). The maximum clearance of a drug by the liver or kidneys is limited by the blood flow to these organs: An organ cannot clear blood that never reaches it. In addition, the efficiency with which each organ clears its blood of a given drug is determined by the extent to which the drug is bound to protein (and thus unavailable for excretion and, to a lesser extent, metabolism).

Metabolism refers to chemical (enzymatic) alteration of the drug molecule, usually as a prelude to excretion. The liver is the predominant organ of drug metabolism, and hepatic enzyme activity is an important determinant of the ability of the liver to clear a drug. Metabolites are usually inactive, but some may have pharmacologic activity (e.g., *N*-acetylprocainamide, or NAPA).

Propranolol, verapamil, and lidocaine are examples of drugs that are highly extracted and metabolized by the liver. The liver is so efficient at removing these drugs from the blood that their clearance is essentially equal to the hepatic blood flow. A clinically important corollary is that the clearance of these drugs is reduced in patients with congestive heart failure and a decreased cardiac output. In contrast, quinidine, phenytoin, and theophylline are drugs that are cleared by the liver but are poorly extracted. Clearance of these agents depends predominantly on hepatic enzyme activity rather than hepatic blood flow.

Excretion by the kidney usually occurs by a combination of passive filtration by the glomerulus and active secretion by the tubules. Digoxin and procainamide (about 50%) are examples of drugs excreted predominantly by the kidney.

The rate of elimination of a drug from the body is often expressed as the drug's half-life ($t_{1/2}$). The half-life is simply the time interval during which half of the drug present in the body at the beginning of the interval is eliminated. Most drugs are eliminated from the body in such a way that in each $t_{1/2}$ interval, 50% of the drug remaining in the body is eliminated (regardless of what quantity of drug this actually represents). The half-life of a drug is directly proportional to its volume of distribution and inversely proportional to its total body clearance rate. Thus, a drug with a large volume of distribution (highly concentrated in peripheral tissues) or a slow clearance rate by liver and kidneys will have a relatively long $t_{1/2}$.

THERAPEUTIC DRUG MONITORING
Drug levels

The goal of measuring serum drug levels is to provide information that allows the clinician to maximize therapeutic efficacy while minimizing toxicity. In a critically ill patient in the CCU, rapidly achieving and maintaining

Table 39-1. Drugs currently monitored in the Duke University Coronary Care Unit

---

Digoxin
Disopyramide
Flecainide
Lidocaine
Phenytoin (Dilantin)
Procainamide/NAPA*
Quinidine
Theophylline

---

*NAPA, N-Acetylprocainamide.

therapeutic drug levels are often of paramount importance. For selected drugs, measuring serum levels can provide early and continued guidance to the physician seeking to avoid making therapeutic errors. We have had a therapeutic drug-monitoring laboratory located in our CCU for the past 13 years. Data on drug levels are available around the clock. The drugs we are currently able to monitor with serum levels are listed in Table 39-1.

Use of drug levels is based on several important assumptions. First, it is assumed that the therapeutic efficacy of a drug is dependent on achieving a certain concentration of drug (the "therapeutic level") in the serum. Second, it is assumed that drug at the site of pharmacologic action (tissue receptors) is in equilibrium with drug in the plasma, so that the latter is a measure (albeit indirect) of the former. Finally, it is assumed that levels outside the therapeutic level correlate reasonably well with toxic effects (high levels) or subtherapeutic effects (low levels) of the drug.

Factors affecting drug levels

Certain characteristics of the patient, including the patient's physiologic makeup, the presence of certain disease states, and other pharmacologic therapy, can affect drug levels and drug-dosing decisions (Table 39-2). As a patient grows older, there is a gradual decline in the capacity of organs to eliminate drugs from the body (especially the liver and kidneys). Thus, a drug dose that is barely adequate for a healthy 35-year-old person may be excessive for a healthy 75-year-old. Although it is reasonable to anticipate a lower clearance of most drugs (and thus a longer $t_{1/2}$) in the elderly patient, there is enough individual variation to make a steady-state serum level the best way to adjust for this decreased clearance properly.

When drug dose is calculated on a milligram per kilogram of body weight basis, most drugs are properly dosed using the patient's total body weight. Certain drugs, such as digoxin and theophylline, however, do not distribute significantly to adipose tissue, and their dosage should be based on estimated lean body weight (LBW).

For men:

$$LBW = 50 \text{ kg} + (2.3 \times \text{inches} > 5 \text{ ft})$$

For women:

$$LBW = 45.5 \text{ kg} + (2.3 \times \text{inches} > 5 \text{ ft})$$

In some cases, a genetically determined variation in drug metabolism can affect clearance. The best known cardiac example is procainamide, which is metabolized by the liver to NAPA. Approximately 50% of white and 90% of black persons are fast acetylators (i.e., they convert procainamide to NAPA more rapidly). Because NAPA, which is excreted almost entirely by the kidneys, may cause significant toxicity if levels get too high, fast acetylators with renal impairment are harder to manage successfully on procainamide than slow acetylators.

Disease states generally produce an exaggeration of the diminished drug clearance seen in older patients (see Table 39-2). Serum creatinine levels are a good gauge of the kidneys' abilities to clear a drug, but it must be recognized that, as the patient ages, for any creatinine value, the corresponding creatinine clearance decreases. Creatinine clearance can be estimated from the serum creatinine and the patient's age and height with the formula:

$$\text{Estimated creatinine clearance} = \frac{(140 - \text{age}) \times \text{lean body weight (kg)}}{72 \times \text{serum creatinine}}$$

If the patient is a woman, the value obtained should be multiplied by 0.85. Serum protein levels (clotting factor activity; reflected in prothrombin time and serum transferrin levels) can give an indication of hepatic synthetic function in the case of severe hepatic disease, although the activity of the hepatic drug-clearing systems cannot be measured directly in the clinical setting. In most patients seen in our CCU, decreased hepatic drug clearance is the result of diminished cardiac systolic function, with consequent decreased hepatic blood flow. For example, we have found that when a patient with AMI on a 1 to 2 mg/min lidocaine infusion has a normal or low serum lidocaine level, the cardiac output measured with a Swan-Ganz catheter is virtually always normal. On the other hand, a patient who becomes toxic on a 2 mg/min infusion almost always has a severely depressed cardiac output.

Drug level indications and timing

The proper time to obtain a drug level depends on the reason for obtaining the level (Table 39-3). A few simple principles suffice for the majority of problems seen in practice. For routine monitoring (e.g., to ensure that the patient is "therapeutic" at the current dosage regimen), the patient should be at steady state and the level obtained should be the trough concentration (i.e., just be-

Table 39-2. Factors affecting drug levels (examples)

Factor	Major effects
Patient characteristics	
Age	Decreases hepatic metabolism with increasing age
	Decreases renal excretion with increasing age
	Most drugs distribute to total weight
Body weight	Digoxin and theophylline distribute to lean weight
Genetics	Rapid acetylators metabolize procainamide faster
Habits	Smoking increases theophylline clearance
Diseases	
Impaired renal function	Reduces clearance of drugs by kidneys (e.g., digoxin, procainamide)
Impaired hepatic function	Reduces clearance by liver (e.g., lidocaine, theophylline)
Impaired cardiac function	Decreases blood flow to liver and kidneys with decreased drug clearance
Malabsorption	Decreases absorption of oral medications
Malnutrition (severe)	Decreases protein binding and increases free (unbound) drug
Drug interactions	
Decreased absorption	Psyllium (Metamucil) decreases absorption of digoxin
Reduced metabolism	Cimetidine decreases metabolism of theophylline
Decreased renal excretion	Quinidine reduces renal excretion of digoxin

Table 39-3. Indications for and timing of serum drug levels

Indication	When to obtain level
Document "therapeutic levels"	After steady state (four-five half-lives): anytime for IV,* just before next dose for oral drugs†
Suspected toxicity on clinical grounds	At time of suspected toxicity
Suspected therapeutic failure	For emergent situations, immediately; otherwise, after steady state: anytime for IV, just before next dose for oral drugs
Establish serum level in patient already taken agent in question	Before initiation of therapy in acute cardiac unit or emergency room, as indicated by therapeutic plan
Document that a loading dose has brought serum level into the therapeutic range	After distribution into tissues: 30-60 min after completion of loading dose for most drugs

*IV, Intravenous.
†The longer the drug's half-life ($t_{1/2}$), the less important timing the sample in relation to doses given becomes; however, the level should not be obtained until the drug has fully distributed into tissues.

fore the next dose of drug is given). "Steady state" is clinically defined as no changes in drug dosage and no physiologic and metabolic changes in the patient for a period equal to five half-lives of the drug. Physiologically, steady state exists when the amount of drug entering the body is exactly balanced by the amount eliminated from the body, and the drug in the blood is in equilibrium with the drug in the tissues. If the drug is being given by continuous IV infusion, the level may be obtained any time steady state has been reached. When a toxic drug reaction is suspected, the level should be obtained while the patient is experiencing symptoms. When a therapeutic failure is suspected, the dosing regimen should be examined to see if the patient received enough of the drug and has had time to reach steady state. In an acute situation (e.g., a patient receiving IV lidocaine who begins having episodes of ventricular tachycardia), a level can be obtained immediately if the dosing regimen appears reasonable. Otherwise a trough level should be obtained. When a patient is seen in the emergency department or intensive care unit for the first time and is already taking a medication such as digoxin or theophylline but has not achieved the therapeutic goal (e.g., patients with rapid atrial fibrillation or acute bronchospasm), it is quite helpful to document the patient's pretreatment level as a guide to future therapy. Finally, after one gives an IV loading dose and waits about 1 hour for the drug to distribute into the tissues, it is sometimes reasonable (but frequently not necessary) to obtain a drug level to establish that the loading dose given has placed the patient appropriately in the therapeutic range.

Dosing regimens and drug levels

In the CCU, most drugs are administered with an initial loading dose, followed by a maintenance dose. From time to time the dosing regimen may place the patient's drug levels outside of the therapeutic range, and dose adjustments must be made. There are a few simple relationships between drug dosing and serum levels that are worth remembering. First, without a loading dose it takes about five half-lives for a maintenance dose to bring the patient to steady-state levels. Because such delay is usually unacceptable in the AMI patient, we typically administer a loading dose for the drugs in Table 39-1. (The exceptions are quinidine, disopyramide, and flecanide.) The goal of the loading dose is to place the patient promptly in the therapeutic range and to keep the serum level therapeutic until maintenance therapy can bring the patient to a steady state. The blood level achieved by a given loading dose is related principally to the patient's weight and the drug's volume of distribution.

Second, during maintenance therapy, the steady-state blood level of the drug depends on the dose administered (including extent of absorption) or infusion rate and drug clearance. The $t_{1/2}$ of a drug is a useful guide to how frequently (i.e., at what interval) an intermittently dosed drug should be given to maintain adequate steady-state serum levels. Note that the relationship between dosing interval and $t_{1/2}$ works best for rapidly absorbed agents. Drugs that are slowly absorbed (e.g., many of the newer sustained-release formulations) are often given at intervals greater than their $t_{1/2}$. For example, the $t_{1/2}$ of procainamide is about 3 hours in a patient with normal renal and hepatic function, and once therapeutic steady-state levels are achieved, the drug must be given every 3 to 4 hours to maintain those levels. With a sustained-release procainamide formulation, however, a double dose of the drug is given every 6 hours. (Note that a sustained-release formulation generally does not alter the total daily dose of the drug but the intervals over which that dose is given.)

Finally, to increase steady-state serum levels rapidly, it is necessary to give a partial loading dose and increase the maintenance dose. Otherwise, the five half-lives rule will determine when the new level is achieved. When a drug level must be adjusted downward, one can estimate how long to hold the drug before instituting a new lower dose from a knowledge of the drug's $t_{1/2}$ (during one $t_{1/2}$, 50% of the drug in the body will be eliminated).

MONITORING CARDIAC DRUGS
Lidocaine

Lidocaine is the standard drug for treatment of life-threatening ventricular arrhythmias. The drug is rapidly and efficiently cleared by the liver, with hepatic clearance approximately equal to hepatic blood flow. It is not significantly cleared by the kidneys. Thus, the major determinants of lidocaine blood levels are the infusion rate, hepatic blood flow (reduced by older age, heart failure, and concomitant therapy with β-blockers or cimetidine) and hepatic microsomal enzyme activity. Congestive heart failure not only decreases hepatic clearance but also lowers the volume of distribution for lidocaine. In heart failure, both the loading dose and the maintenance infusion rate must therefore be decreased. In primary hepatic disease (e.g., cirrhosis), the maintenance infusion rate may need to be decreased; the need for this should be judged with serum levels.

Our standard loading and maintenance doses in the CCU are shown in Table 39-4. The therapeutic range in our laboratory is 2.0 to 5.0 μg/ml. The $t_{1/2}$ for lidocaine is normally 1.5 hours; it may be prolonged to 13 hours in a patient in cardiogenic shock. The average Duke University CCU $t_{1/2}$ of lidocaine is 5.5 hours.

If plasma lidocaine levels are low and the patient experiences an unacceptable ventricular arrhythmia, the level can be rapidly raised by a 50-mg IV bolus (over 2-5 minutes) with an increase in the infusion rate by 1 mg/min. Note that an increased infusion rate without a bolus would require about 8 hours (assuming a normal $t_{1/2}$) to reach the new steady-state level. In our experience with the CCU population, infusion rates of 3 mg/min or greater are commonly associated with toxicity and are not advisable.

Procainamide

There are several important determinants of serum procainamide levels. About half of the parent compound and all of the pharmacologically active metabolite NAPA are excreted by the kidney, so any reduction in renal function decreases procainamide and NAPA clearance and increases their $t_{1/2}$. Toxicity can be avoided in this situation by lengthening the interval between oral doses to approximate the new $t_{1/2}$. Although about 40% of procainamide is converted by liver enzymes to NAPA, the effect of hepatic disease in procainamide clearance is not well characterized. With severe liver disease, the dosing interval may need to be lengthened. Serum levels should be used to monitor therapy in this setting. Similarly, in heart failure the clearance of procainamide is probably decreased, and the dosing interval may need to be lengthened.

As mentioned previously, the acetylator phenotype is important because fast acetylators generate a higher concentration of NAPA and are more likely to become toxic in the setting of renal insufficiency. As a rule of thumb, if the NAPA level 1 hour after an appropriate IV loading dose is more than 1.5 μg/ml, the patient is likely to be a fast acetylator. Because of the high prevalence of the fast acetylator phenotype, we avoid using procain-

Table 39-4. Antiarrhythmic IV regimens*

Drug	Loading dose	Maintenance infusion
Lidocaine		
No CHF	75 mg IV initial dose (over 2 min) then 50 mg IV (over 1 min) every 5 min	2 mg/min
Mild CHF	75 mg, 50 mg, 50 mg	1-2 mg/min
Moderate CHF	75 mg, 50 mg	1 mg/min
Cardiogenic shock	75 mg	0.5 mg/min
Procainamide		
No renal insufficiency	17 mg/kg IV over 30-60 min as tolerated by blood pressure	3 mg/kg/hr (range 2-6 mg/min)
Mild-moderate renal insufficiency	15 mg/kg	2 mg/kg/hr (range 1.5-4 mg/min)
Severe renal insufficiency	13 mg/kg	1 mg/kg/hr (range 0.8-1.8 mg/min)
Renal failure	Do not use	
Quinidine†		
300 mg IV quinidine gluconate over 30-60 min	—	Repeat dose every 6-12 hr *or* 1-2 mg/min

*CHF, Congestive heart failure; *IV*, intravenous.
†No loading dose of quinidine is given because of an increased prevalence of excessive vasodilation and consequent hypotension.

amide in black patients with severe renal impairment. Although the pharmacologic activity of NAPA is only 15% to 20% of the parent compound, its toxic potential appears cumulative with that of procainamide.

Our procainamide IV dosing regimen is based on the patient's renal function (see Table 39-4). Without renal insufficiency, the $t_{1/2}$ for procainamide is 3 to 4 hours and that for NAPA is 8 to 10 hours; with moderate to severe renal insufficiency, $t_{1/2}$ for procainamide is prolonged to 8 to 24 hours and that for NAPA is 12 to 70 hours. The longer $t_{1/2}$ of NAPA relative to procainamide explains why this drug can be so difficult to manage in patients with renal insufficiency; a dosing regimen that will replace the procainamide lost from the body every procainamide $t_{1/2}$ (thus keeping procainamide levels at steady state) will cause a significant accumulation of NAPA.

The therapeutic range of procainamide is 4 to 10 μg/ml. Although maximal therapeutic efficacy may require higher levels, toxicity also becomes more frequent at those levels. In our laboratory, NAPA levels greater than 30 μg/ml are considered potentially toxic.

To increase plasma procainamide levels upward, we choose a target serum level and calculate the percentage of desired serum level our target increment represents. For example, if a patient arrives in the CCU with a steady-state procainamide level of 4 μg/ml and we wish to raise the serum level to 8 μg/ml, the percentage increment in level desired is (8-4)/8 = 50%. We thus need to give 50% of the loading dose appropriate to the patient's renal function to achieve the desired new level. For a 50-kg woman with normal kidneys, this would be

425 mg of procainamide. To convert from a continuous IV infusion to an oral regimen, we calculate the total 24-hour IV dose once steady-state therapeutic serum levels have been achieved; we then give one fourth of this daily dose every 6 hours (if the patient has good renal function) using one of the sustained-release formulations. The IV infusion is stopped 4 hours after the first oral dose has been given.

Quinidine

Quinidine is eliminated predominantly by hepatic metabolism. Because of the tremendous reserve capacity of the liver enzyme systems, hepatic clearance of quinidine does not appear significantly altered until the very end stage of liver disease. At the other end of the spectrum, drugs that induce the hepatic enzymes (e.g., phenytoin or phenobarbital) may increase the clearance of quinidine and reduce its half-life. Renal impairment has less impact on the clearance, although in severe renal dysfunction it appears that the dose of quinidine needs to be decreased. There are few data on the effects of heart failure, but absorption from the gastrointestinal tract may be slowed and the volume of distribution may be reduced. Although quinidine may have a dramatic effect on digoxin levels (see the section on digoxin presented later), the converse is not true.

Many clinicians avoid giving IV quinidine because of concern about inducing hypotension. Based on our experience, we believe that the hypotensive properties of IV quinidine are probably equivalent to those of IV phenytoin. We use IV quinidine as an alternative to IV procainamide in appropriate patients (e.g., those without hypotension or volume depletion) unable to tolerate the latter drug (see Table 39-4). Just as with phenytoin, we have a nurse in the room during the infusion to monitor blood pressure every 5 to 10 minutes. We do not administer a loading dose with IV quinidine because that usually produces excessive vasodilation.

Because there are several formulations of quinidine available, dosage is in part dependent on the form used. For uncoated tablets of quinidine sulfate, the dosing interval is every 6 hours, and we give 400 to 600 mg in each dose if the patient is younger than 65 years and 300 mg if the patient is age 65 years or more. For the sustained-release form of quinidine sulfate (Quinidex), the dose is 600 mg every 8 hours for age 65 years or less and 300 mg every 8 hours for those age 65 years or more. In severe renal impairment, the dose is 50% less, and the dosing interval is extended to every 12 hours. A sustained-release 324-mg tablet of quinidine gluconate (Quinaglute) is approximately equal to a 300-mg dose of the sustained-release form of quinidine sulfate.

The therapeutic range for quinidine is 1.5 to 5 μg/ml. The normal $t_{1/2}$ is 6 to 7 hours.

Theophylline

Theophylline is eliminated almost completely by hepatic metabolism. Thus, factors that affect hepatic enzyme activity have important effects on serum theophylline levels. In severe liver disease and in congestive heart failure, theophylline clearance is reduced (causing its $t_{1/2}$ to be prolonged). Drugs that induce hepatic enzyme activity, such as phenytoin, will increase theophylline clearance. In addition, smoking dramatically increases theophylline clearance. The other major drug interaction is with cimetidine, which decreases theophylline clearance. It is important to recognize that there is a large interpatient variability in theophylline clearance and that dosing guidelines must be adjusted to the individual using serum levels.

Because theophylline is not water soluble, it must be administered in IV form as aminophylline. In the body, aminophylline (which is 80% theophylline) is rapidly converted to theophylline. We calculate the IV loading dose for theophylline from the desired serum concentration (SC), the LBW, and the drug's volume of distribution (which averages about 0.5 L/kg). Thus:

$$\text{Loading dose (mg)} = \text{desired SC} \times \text{LBW} \times 0.5$$

Because the therapeutic range for theophylline is 10 to 20 μg/ml, we generally aim for an initial level of 12 to 15 μg/ml. For example, for a lean 70-kg man, the loading dose would be $15 \times 70 \times 0.5 = 525$ mg.

The maintenance IV dose for the majority of patients is 0.2 to 1.0 mg/kg/hr. Patients with a normal theophylline $t_{1/2}$ (6-8 hours) should be started on 0.4 to 0.6 mg/kg/hr. Patients who generally need a lower dose ($t_{1/2}$ = 12-24 hours) include those with advanced age, heart failure, or severe hepatic dysfunction. Patients who need higher doses ($t_{1/2}$ = 3-4 hours) include young, relatively healthy individuals and heavy smokers; we usually start them on 0.8 to 0.9 mg/kg/hr.

When a patient comes to the emergency room who is already on theophylline and the clinician desires to establish and maintain a therapeutic theophylline level, an immediate level should be obtained before any theophylline is given. If the situation is so critical that the patient cannot wait for the serum theophylline level, a miniloading dose of 2.5 mg/kg can be given as long as the patient is not clinically theophylline toxic. If the situation is not that urgent, the clinician can use the patient's current SC and the desired serum level to calculate the additional loading dose the patient should receive before starting on a maintenance infusion:

$$\text{Additional loading dose (mg)} = (\text{desired SC} - \text{current SC}) \times \text{LBW} \times 0.5$$

For example, if the level in the emergency room is 5 μg/ml and we wish to get a lean 70-kg patient to 15 μg/ml, we should give $(15 - 5) \times 70 \times 0.5 = 350$ mg. If the patient is critically ill, it may be useful to obtain a serum level 30 to 60 minutes after completion of the loading dose to determine the need for an additional loading dose.

To convert from maintenance IV aminophylline to maintenance oral theophylline, we calculate the total daily IV drug dose with steady-state therapeutic levels, adjust for the conversion from aminophylline to theophylline, and then pick an oral dosing interval (e.g., every 8 hours) and dose. For example, if the patient is receiving 40 mg/hr of IV aminophylline, he or she is receiving $40 \times 24 = 900$ mg/day. Because aminophylline is 80% theophylline, this is equal to 768 mg/day of theophylline. If we plan to give the patient TheoDur every 8 hours, we need to give 200 mg every 8 hours. In general, we stop the IV infusion about 4 hours after the first oral dose has been given.

Digoxin

Almost 50% of the serum levels run in our laboratory are digoxin levels. At least 60% of these are inappropriate (e.g., level unnecessary or drawn at the wrong time). Although digoxin has been used therapeutically much longer than any of the other drugs discussed in this section, it still causes more confusion than any other agent we deal with.

Digoxin is excreted primarily by the kidneys, and there is a close correlation between renal digoxin clearance and the creatinine clearance (see the section on factors affecting drug levels). Thus, as the serum creatinine rises or the patient ages, creatinine (and digoxin) clearance fall. The relationship between crea-

Table 39-5. Digoxin clearance

Creatinine clearance (ml/min)	Approximate digoxin $t_{1/2}$ (days)	Time required to achieve steady state (days)
≥ 60	1.5	7
30	2	10
15	3	15
≤ 10	4-5	20-25

tinine clearance (estimated from the formula given previously), digoxin $t_{1/2}$, and time required to achieve steady state after initiation of therapy or a dose change are shown in Table 39-5. Note that even with normal renal function, digoxin has a $t_{1/2}$ of 1.5 days; it therefore requires 7 days for digoxin therapy to reach steady state. For a patient with end-stage renal disease, steady-state levels may take up to 3 weeks to achieve.

The interaction between quinidine and digoxin is well known. Quinidine decreases the renal excretion of digoxin and may cause a 50% to 100% rise in serum digoxin levels. When a patient already receiving digoxin begins taking quinidine, it is important to keep the long $t_{1/2}$ of digoxin in mind: After every dose change in either quinidine or digoxin, it will take about 1 week (with normal renal function) before a steady-state digoxin level can be obtained. Thus, serum levels and dose changes of digoxin should never be performed on a daily basis. A similar interaction is seen between digoxin and amiodanone, and great caution should be exercised when using these two agents together.

To load with digoxin, we give 0.012 to 0.015 mg/kg of lean body weight (rounded to nearest 0.125-mg dose). Because the volume of distribution of digoxin is reduced in severe renal insufficiency, we reduce the loading dose for such patients to 0.01 mg/kg of LBW. The loading dose can be given intravenously or by mouth, depending on the clinical situation; we usually give half of the load initially, one fourth 6 hours later, and the final fourth after another 6 hours.

Maintenance digoxin dose is calculated as the percentage of the total loading dose that is eliminated each day. The percentage lost each day can be estimated as:

$$\frac{\text{Estimated creatinine clearance}}{5} + 14$$

The maintenance dose then is (loading dose) × (% lost each day). Therapeutic levels for digoxin are 0.8 to 2.0 mg/ml. Note that it takes about 8 hours after a dose is given for the drug to distribute into the tissues fully. Thus, it makes no sense to see if the patient's level of digoxin is "therapeutic" by checking a level 2 hours after the morning digoxin dose; the level should be drawn at trough (i.e., just before the next dose).

If a patient has a "toxic" digoxin level (but does not require emergency treatment with digoxin Fab fragments [Digibind]), the drug should be held long enough for the level to fall back into the therapeutic range. The creatinine clearance will determine how long it takes for the level to fall by half (i.e., one half-life). The maintenance dose must also be reduced accordingly.

BIBLIOGRAPHY

Abernethy DR, Greenblatt DJ: Drug disposition in obese humans. An update, *Clin Pharmacokinet* 11:199-213, 1986.

Brown JE, Sand DG: Therapeutic drug monitoring of antiarrhythmic agents, *Clin Pharmacokinet* 7:125-186, 1982.

Burton ME, Vasko MR, Brater DC: Comparison of drug dosing methods, *Clin Pharmacokinet* 10:1-37, 1985.

Dunham GD, Allen WM, Bellinger RL: *Duke University Heart Center Cardiovascular clinical pharmacology design guide,* Durham, NC, 1991, Duke University Press.

Holford NHG, Sheiner LB: Understanding the dose-effect relationship: clinical application of pharmacokinetic-pharmacodynamic models, *Clin Pharmacokinet* 6:429-453, 1981.

Kates RE: Plasma level monitoring of antiarrhythmic drugs, *Am J Cardiol* 52:8C-13C, 1983.

Levy RH, Bauer LA: Basic pharmacokinetics. A review, *Ther Drug Monit* 8:47-58, 1986.

Pentel P, Benowitz N: Pharmacokinetic and pharmacodynamic considerations in drug therapy of cardiac emergencies, *Clin Pharmacokinet* 9:273-308, 1984.

Woosley RL, Echt DS, Rosen DM: Effects of congestive heart failure on the pharmacokinetics and pharmacodynamics of antiarrhythmic agents, *Am J Cardiol* 57:25B, 1986.

Chapter 40

ECHOCARDIOGRAPHIC ASSESSMENT AND MONITORING OF THE PATIENT WITH ACUTE MYOCARDIAL INFARCTION: PROSPECTS FOR THE THROMBOLYTIC ERA

Frank D. Tice
Joseph Kisslo

The evolution of invasive and noninvasive cardiac imaging has greatly facilitated the care of patients with acute myocardial infarction (AMI). Available imaging modalities now include echocardiography, radionuclide angiography and perfusion imaging, left ventricular contrast and coronary angiography, positron emission tomography, nuclear magnetic resonance imaging, and ultrafast cine computed tomography.

Echocardiography has a unique ability to image the moving cardiac chamber, walls, and valves (Fig. 40-1). It continues to offer distinct advantages over other techniques. First, it is portable, which means that information can be obtained quickly and without moving a critically ill patient from the cardiac care unit to a remote laboratory. Second, information is available immediately, with no need for time-consuming processing of the data. Third, the technique is more widely available and far less expensive than other available technologies.

Finally, there is no known risk to echocardiographic assessment.

With the currently available equipment, our experience demonstrates that approximately 90% of patients can be adequately imaged from the transthoracic approach. With the advent of transesophageal echocardiography, nearly all patients can now be studied successfully. The addition of continuous-wave, pulsed-wave, and color Doppler techniques to two-dimensional (2-D) echocardiography has made it possible to obtain not only an assessment of ventricular function but also hemodynamic and valvular data. Most important, echocardiography offers information that often cannot be acquired from clinical assessment alone. Even in today's environment of cost containment, echocardiography provides marked benefit to patients in the earliest stages of AMI.

The purpose of this chapter is to review the utility of echocardiography in the precardiac and cardiac care unit

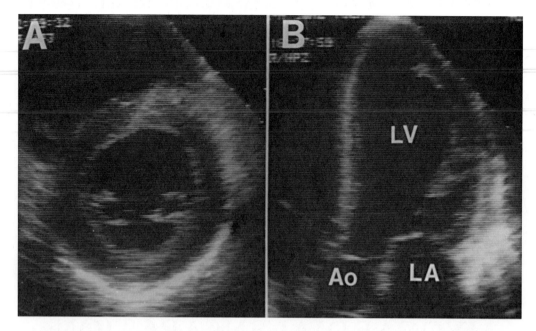

Fig. 40-1. Echocardiographic short axis of the left ventricle **(A)** at the level of the papillary muscles. Long axis of the left ventricle **(B)** from the ventricular apex. Echocardiography is unique in its ability to image the chambers, walls, and valves in real time. *LV,* Left ventricle; *LA,* left atrium; *Ao,* aortic root.

phases of AMI, periods now characterized by aggressive therapy as the standard of care.

DIAGNOSIS OF MI

Almost immediately after occlusion of a coronary artery, the dependent myocardium ceases to contract.[2] This regional asynergy precedes development of electrocardiographic (ECG) abnormalities and chest pain.[3,4] Two-dimensional echocardiography accurately identifies segmental wall motion abnormalities[5] and therefore can be of value in the early recognition of MI.

Echo in infarction

Many investigators have evaluated the sensitivity of 2-D echocardiography in the diagnosis of MI.[6-11] In a recent study, Sabia et al.[6] found regional wall motion abnormalities at the time of emergency room (ER) evaluation in 27 of 29 patients with enzymatically proven MI.[6] Gibson et al.[10] evaluated 75 consecutive patients with AMI 7.9 ± 3.1 hours after admission to the coronary care unit. Regional akinesia or dyskinesia was identified in all patients. Visser et al.[8] found regional asynergy within 12 hours of symptom onset in 64 of 66 patients with enzymatically proven MI. These studies and others have convincingly demonstrated that 2-D echocardiography can identify segmental wall motion abnormalities in greater than 90% of patients with early MI.

Role of echo in the ER

Less than one third of patients seen in the ER with chest pain will subsequently prove to have AMI.[12] It would be of obvious benefit to identify low-risk patients that could either be safely discharged or admitted to non–cardiac care unit beds. Echocardiography may be useful in this risk stratification.

One way by which echocardiographic assessment can be helpful is identification of conditions other than MI that can cause severe or prolonged chest pain. Such findings might include pericardial effusion (suggestive of acute pericarditis), aortic stenosis, hypertrophic cardiomyopathy, elevated right heart pressures or right atrial thrombi (suggestive of pulmonary embolism), and aortic dissection.[13] This latter condition can be identified with a high degree of sensitivity and specificity by transesophageal echocardiography, as discussed later.

An additional use of echocardiography in the ER has been recently proposed by Sabia et al.,[6] based on the high sensitivity of wall motion abnormalities for AMI. They studied 180 patients being evaluated for suspected infarction with 2-D echocardiography at the time of manifestation. Management decisions were made by ER physicians without knowledge of echocardiography results. An alternative management algorithm was then constructed and analyzed. Briefly, patients without diagnostic ST elevation on ECG would be studied with 2-D echocardiography at the time of manifestation.

Those with regional wall motion abnormalities would be admitted, whereas those with normal wall motion or global dysfunction would be discharged. With this strategy, Sabia et al.[6] concluded that only 2 patients of the 30 ultimately proved to have MI would have been discharged. Both of these patients had small, uncomplicated infarcts. Hospital admissions would have been reduced by 32% and total costs decreased by 24%.

Before this management strategy can be recommended, however, a prospective study confirming safety and cost savings needs to be performed. The medical and legal consequences of discharging even small numbers of patients with AMI are potentially serious. In addition, it should be recognized that many patients with unstable ischemic syndromes without infarction may not have wall motion abnormalities.[13] Nevertheless, most physicians would advocate admission for such individuals.

Selecting patients for acute reperfusion

The high sensitivity of echocardiography in detecting AMI has also prompted interest in its use for selecting patients for reperfusion therapy.[14] Many large-scale studies have convincingly established the life-saving benefit of prompt thrombolytic therapy in MI with progressive benefit from earlier treatment.[15-17] In patients with a history highly suggestive of ischemia and classic ST-segment elevation on ECG, 2-D echocardiography is superfluous for diagnosis. Unfortunately, more than one half of patients with AMI will not have diagnostic ECG changes.[18,19] Such patients would obviously benefit from an alternative technique for identifying AMI so that reperfusion therapy could be promptly administered.

Unfortunately, the ability of 2-D echocardiography to fill this role is limited by its poor *specificity* in diagnosing AMI. It is not possible at present to reliably differentiate segmental wall motion abnormalities attributable to old infarction, AMI, or ischemia without infarction.

In the study of Sabia et al.,[6] regional wall motion abnormalities were identified in 87 out of 169 patients successfully imaged on admittance to the ER with symptoms suggestive of AMI. Only 27 of these patients (31%) subsequently proved to have infarction by enzyme assays. Peels et al.[7] found regional asynergy in 26 of 43 patients admitted to the ER with chest pain, of which only 12 (46%) subsequently had enzymatically documented infarction. Subsequent cardiac catheterization, however, demonstrated 22 of these 26 patients (85%) to have significant coronary artery disease. These studies and others emphasize that administration of reperfusion therapy on the basis of 2-D echocardiography findings would result in substantial overtreatment.

The major utility of 2-D echocardiography in patients with symptoms suggestive of MI but without diagnostic ECG changes may be in the identification of patients *not* requiring reperfusion therapy. The high sensitivity of regional wall motion abnormalities in AMI means that patients with normal wall motion by echocardiography are unlikely to be experiencing myonecrosis. The negative predictive value of absent wall motion abnormalities by 2-D echocardiography has been reported to be 94% to 97% in patients being evaluated for possible AMI.[6,7] Patients who have an MI despite normal wall motion by echocardiography tend to have small infarcts and a good in-hospital prognosis even without reperfusion therapy.[1,6,10]

EARLY ASSESSMENT IN MI

Despite the limitations of echocardiography in the diagnosis of AMI, its use in the early assessment of patients with recognized infarction can be invaluable. Because the equipment is portable, echocardiography is ideal for use in the coronary care unit. Echocardiographic evaluation in this setting provides important information about left ventricular function, infarct size, and in-hospital prognosis.

Evaluation of left ventricular function

Much of the information provided by early echocardiographic assessment of patients with AMI is derived from analysis of global and regional left ventricular function. Global left ventricular function is usually assessed by calculating ejection fraction. Such a calculation involves estimating end-systolic and end-diastolic left ventricular volumes, which can be done using a variety of geometric models.[20-22]

The American Society of Echocardiography recently reviewed available algorithms for quantitating left ventricular volume and proposed the disc summation method (modified Simpson's rule) as the preferable approach.[22] This method uses two nearly orthogonal apical views of the left ventricle to divide it into multiple "discs," as illustrated in Figure 40-2. The volume of the ventricle is then calculated at both end-systole and end-diastole by summing the volumes of individual discs using the formula outlined in Figure 40-2. Although the optimal number of discs for this method of analysis has not been determined, many laboratories use 20. Ejection fraction can be reported as (end-diastolic volume − end-systolic volume)/end-diastolic volume.

Most commercially available ultrasound machines have software packages that facilitate calculation of ejection fraction by a variety of methods, including the disc summation method. Nevertheless, it can be appreciated from this discussion that quantitation of ejection fraction can be cumbersome and time consuming. In addition, accurate measurements require that echocardiographic images be carefully optimized so that the

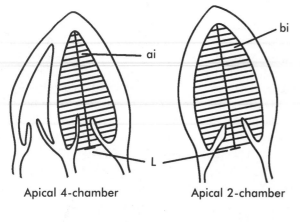

$$V = \frac{\pi}{4} \sum_{i=1}^{n} ai \cdot bi \cdot \frac{L}{n}$$

ai = Septal-lateral diameter of left ventricle
bi = Anterior-inferior diameter of left ventricle
n = Number of discs

Fig. 40-2. Disc summation method for the calculation of left ventricular volume.

entire left ventricular endocardium is visualized. As such, many echocardiographers prefer to visually estimate ejection fraction using all available views to construct a mental image of left ventricular function. Although some experienced echocardiographers are undoubtedly quite accurate with such an approach, it invariably introduces considerable interobserver variability and, in most instances, suffers from a lack of validation with other techniques. In contrast, although subject to mathematical magnification of measurement errors and limitations imposed by the nongeometric shape of the human left ventricle, quantitative echocardiographic estimation of ejection fraction has been shown to be reproducible and accurate.[20,23]

A limitation to the utility of calculating ejection fraction in the setting of acute infarction is compensatory hyperkinesis of nonischemic walls, with resultant preservation of global systolic function.[24,25] Concomitant assessment of regional wall motion is therefore essential. Regional left ventricular function is most commonly evaluated by dividing the left ventricle into multiple segments and examining each in several echocardiographic views. After visual inspection of wall motion and thickening, a numeric score is assigned to each segment and a wall motion index calculated. The localization of wall motion abnormalities with this type of analysis has been demonstrated to correlate remarkably well with angiographic asynergy.[5]

The clinical use of echocardiography in assessing regional left ventricular function has been hindered by the lack of a common scoring system among reported studies. In an effort to address this problem, the American Society of Echocardiography recently proposed a 16-segment model of the left ventricle, along with suggested nomenclature for each segment and a standardized scoring scale.[22]

We have adopted the American Society of Echocardiography system at our institution. Figure 40-3 illustrates the utilized views and segmental division of the left ventricle. Normally contracting or hyperkinetic segments are assigned a score of 1, hypokinetic segments 2, akinetic segments 3, dyskinetic segments 4, and aneurysmal segments 5. The sum of all assigned scores is divided by the number of visualized segments to yield a wall motion index. Therefore, an index of 1 would indicate normal function, whereas progressively higher scores would reflect an increasing degree of ventricular dysfunction.

Estimation of infarct size

It is generally appreciated that the extent of myocardial necrosis is of paramount importance in determining outcome after AMI.[26-28] As noted, 2-D echocardiography can effectively localize left ventricular dysfunction in the AMI period. Therefore, attempts have been made to quantitate infarct size with echocardiography.

Although the echocardiographic extent of regional left ventricular dysfunction in AMI has been shown to correlate with peak creatinine phosphokinase MB-isoenzyme level, scintigraphic assessment of infarct size, and postmortem measurement of myocardial necrosis, there is nearly universal agreement that wall motion abnormalities overestimate anatomic infarct size.[8,29-32] A variety of factors likely account for this, including ischemic dysfunction in the peri infarct zone, "tethering" of normal myocardium by adjacent infarcted muscle, concomitant ischemia in areas distant from the infarction territory, a nonlinear relationship between transmural extent of necrosis and wall motion abnormalities, and areas of fibrosis consequent to previous infarction.[31-33]

The advent of aggressive reperfusion strategies, including thrombolytic therapy, has further complicated early quantification of infarct size, because salvage of abnormally contracting myocardium can be achieved.[34,35] Recovery of function may be delayed after reestablishment of perfusion as a result of myocardial "stunning."[36] It is therefore more appropriate to consider the extent of regional dysfunction detected acutely as an indicator of the "risk area" in evolving MI rather than an estimate of infarct size.[25] Nevertheless, analysis of regional wall motion abnormalities can provide useful prognostic information in patients with AMI.

Assessment of prognosis

Early echocardiographic assessment of left ventricular function has been used to predict in-hospital com-

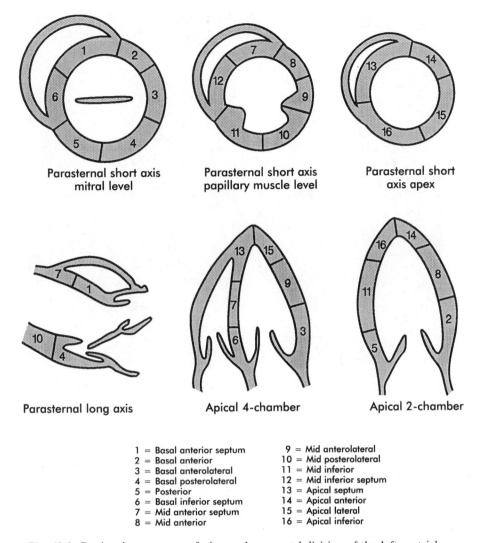

Parasternal short axis
mitral level

Parasternal short axis
papillary muscle level

Parasternal short
axis apex

Parasternal long axis

Apical 4-chamber

Apical 2-chamber

1 = Basal anterior septum	9 = Mid anterolateral
2 = Basal anterior	10 = Mid posterolateral
3 = Basal anterolateral	11 = Mid inferior
4 = Basal posterolateral	12 = Mid inferior septum
5 = Posterior	13 = Apical septum
6 = Basal inferior septum	14 = Apical anterior
7 = Mid anterior septum	15 = Apical lateral
8 = Mid anterior	16 = Apical inferior

Fig. 40-3. Regional coronary perfusion and segmental division of the left ventricle.

plications after AMI. This can be of great importance when one is deciding which patients can be safely discharged from the cardiac care unit. At our institution, patients with AMI judged to be at low risk for subsequent complications are moved from the coronary care unit to a less intensive (and less costly) stepdown unit after 24 hours.

Most clinical studies investigating the utility of echocardiography in risk stratification after MI have utilized analysis of regional wall motion with a semi-quantitative scoring system such as that outlined previously. Using their own scoring system, Nishimura et al.[33] evaluated 61 consecutive MI patients with echocardiography within 12 hours of manifestation. Congestive heart failure, malignant ventricular arrhythmia, or death developed in 24 of 27 patients with a wall motion index of 2.0 or more but in only 6 of 34 patients with an index of less than 2.0. Most important these complications developed in 79% of Killip class I patients with a wall

motion index of 2.0 or more. Thus, echocardiography was especially valuable for risk stratification of patients judged to be stable on the basis of clinical variables.

In a more recent study, Berning and Steensgaard-Hansen[37] prospectively evaluated 201 consecutive MI patients with echocardiography 12 to 72 hours after manifestation. Using a different regional wall motion scoring system, they identified a close relationship between the degree of left ventricular dysfunction as assessed by wall motion index and in-hospital mortality. The superiority of wall motion index assessment to risk stratification by Killip class was also noted. Several other studies have also demonstrated the relationship between echocardiographic extent of acute left ventricular dysfunction and the in-hospital development of serious complications.[6,10,38,39]

The ability of echocardiographic wall motion analysis to predict early complications after MI is not surprising, given the recognized relationship between left ventricu-

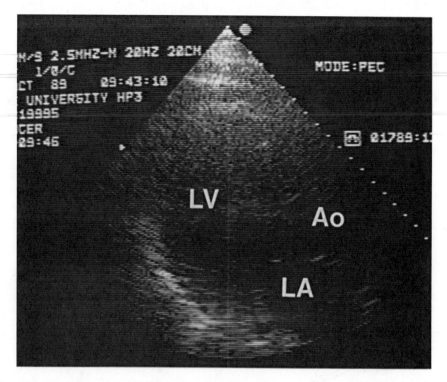

Fig. 40-4. Low parasternal long axis of the left ventricle in a patient difficult to image. No adequate target information is present. *LV,* Left ventricle; *LA,* left atrium; *Ao,* aortic root.

lar function and prognosis. It must be noted, however, that all of the available studies were performed before the widespread use of aggressive reperfusion strategies. There is an evolving consensus that the salutary effects of reperfusion on mortality are more substantial than can be explained on the basis of myocardial salvage alone.[40,41] Whether reperfusion therapy in AMI alters the prognostic information obtained with early echocardiographic assessment of left ventricular function is uncertain. Presently we use early echocardiography frequently in MI patients because our experience would suggest the obtained information continues to add importantly to the clinical assessment.

LIMITATIONS OF ECHOCARDIOGRAPHY IN AMI

It is apparent from the previous discussion that the utility of echocardiography in early MI relies heavily on careful analysis of segmental wall motion. An obvious limitation to a useful study is suboptimal image quality, which can make wall motion analysis more difficult (Fig. 40-4). It is of paramount importance to make sure that the endocardium for a wall segment is clearly visualized before making an assessment of function. Fortunately, even when one adheres to this restriction, the use of multiple acoustic windows in each patient enables successful wall motion analysis in approximately 90% of individuals.

A potentially greater limitation to the appropriate use of echocardiography in AMI is inadequate experience of the interpreting physician. Most expert echocardiographers would agree that wall motion analysis is one of the most difficult aspects of echocardiographic evaluation. Some insight into this potential limitation can be inferred from experience with stress echocardiography, which obviously requires accurate segmental wall motion analysis. In a recent investigation, Picano et al.[42] evaluated the importance of expertise in the interpretation of dipyridamole echocardiography tests. Interpreters were divided into "experts," individuals who had performed and interpreted 100 or more stress echocardiographic studies, and "beginners," individuals who had performed and interpreted less than 20 stress echocardiographic evaluations. It should be emphasized that the interpreters labeled as beginners were cardiologists who had completed a full training program in echocardiography. Using cardiac catheterization showing more than 70% stenosis in at least one major coronary artery as the reference standard, the diagnostic accuracy ([true positive plus true negative]/total number of tests) of beginners was 62% compared with 85% for experienced observers. The beginners then underwent a supervised training program involving performance and interpretation of an additional 100 stress echocardiographic studies. Subsequent evaluation showed that the

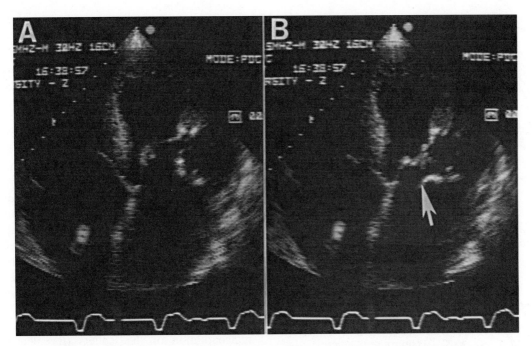

Fig. 40-5. Apical four-chamber views from a patient with a ruptured papillary muscle head. **A,** Diastole with the mitral leaflets in the left ventricle. **B,** With systole the posterior mitral leaflet is thrown into the left atrium because of the rupture of the head of the papillary *(arrow).*

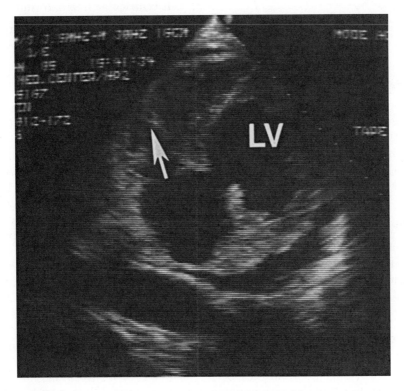

Fig. 40-6. Short axis of the left ventricle *(LV)* from a patient with a pseudoaneurysm of the left ventricle. The pseudoaneurysm is posterior and to the left of the LV, and it has ruptured into the right ventricle *(arrow).*

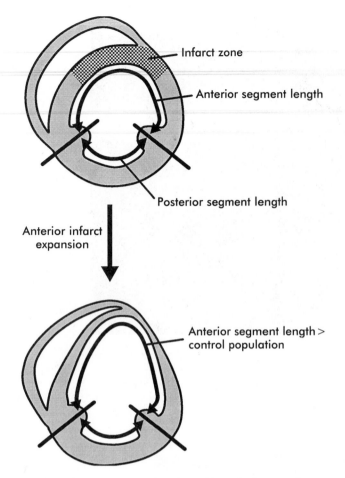

Fig. 40-7. Infarct expansion after transmural anterior myocardial infarction.

diagnostic accuracy of the beginners had increased to a level equal that of the experts.

Therefore, the proper use of echocardiography in the AMI setting requires the availability of an interpreter experienced in segmental wall motion analysis. The absence of such an individual invites erroneous diagnosis and prognostication, with potentially adverse consequences.

COMPLICATIONS OF AMI

Echocardiography plays an invaluable role in the assessment of complications of MI. Again, the ability to bring the imaging hardware to the bedside of an often critically ill patient makes echocardiography a superior choice relative to other imaging modalities.

Ventricular septal defect

Rupture of the interventricular septum complicates 1% to 3% of MIs and carries a poor prognosis if unrepaired.[43] Outcome can be improved with prompt recognition and early surgical intervention.[44] Although 2-D echocardiography alone is relatively insensitive in detecting ventricular septal rupture, the addition of

pulsed-wave and color Doppler techniques allows accurate diagnosis and localization in nearly all patients.[45,46] In addition, 2-D and Doppler assessment can characterize right ventricular function and accurately estimate right ventricular pressure in these patients, both of which have prognostic significance.[46]

Papillary muscle rupture

Papillary muscle rupture is a rare but serious complication of AMI, resulting in severe mitral regurgitation and pulmonary edema. The mortality rate without surgical therapy is 90% by 1 week.[43] Remarkably, a significant murmur is absent in most patients.[47] Even if present, it is often difficult to distinguish from the murmur of a ventricular septal defect. 2-D and Doppler echocardiographic imaging is the diagnostic test of choice when papillary muscle rupture is suspected. Though it is occasionally difficult to distinguish from ischemic mitral regurgitation without papillary muscle rupture, careful inspection of the mitral apparatus for malcoaptation of the leaflets (flail leaflet) and the presence of a torn papillary muscle attached to mobile chordae usually allows the diagnosis to be made (Fig. 40-5).[25] Like ventricular septal defect, evidence is accumulating that prompt recognition and early surgical intervention improves prognosis.[48]

Left ventricular free wall rupture

Rupture of the left ventricular free wall usually results in massive hemopericardium with subsequent hemodynamic deterioration and rapid death.[25,43] Occasionally, patients survive, however, and prompt recognition may allow lifesaving surgery. Echocardiographic assessment invariably demonstrates pericardial effusion, with features of tamponade. Location of the rupture is usually not visualized.[25]

In rare cases, cardiac rupture may be confined by adherent pericardium and thrombus to a localized area, resulting in a pseudoaneurysm. Left ventricular pseudoaneurysm can be easily recognized echocardiographically by the presence of systolic bulging, a narrow neck with pulsed-wave and color Doppler evidence of bidirectional flow between the left ventricle and pseudoaneurysm cavitary, and a saccular shape (Fig. 40-6).[49,50] Prompt surgical repair is indicated because of the propensity for rupture.[51]

Infarct expansion

Infarct expansion refers to progressive thinning and disproportionate dilation of an infarct area not attributable to new myocardial injury.[52] It should be distinguished from infarct extension, which results from new myocardial necrosis. It is most often seen after large, transmural anterior MI and generally begins within the first 24 hours.[52] The mechanism is thought to be

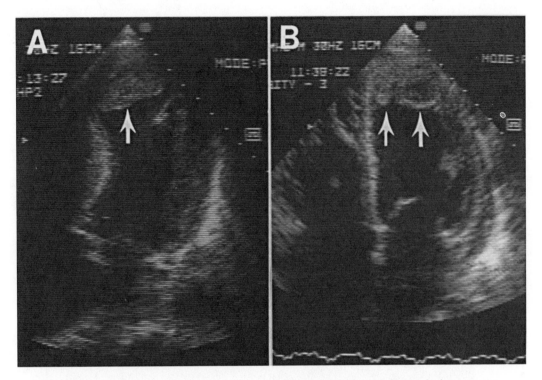

Fig. 40-8. A, apical four-chamber view in a patient with an evolving left ventricular aneurysm and layered mural thrombus at the apex *(arrow).* **B,** Similar view in another patient with multiple apical mural thrombi *(arrows).*

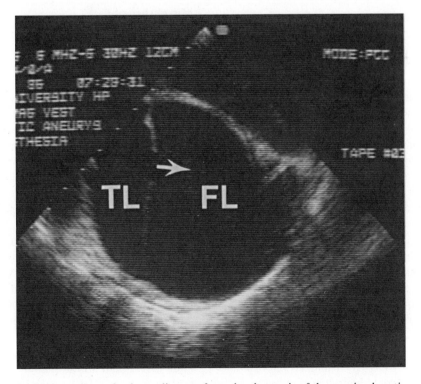

Fig. 40-9. Transesophageal echocardiogram from the short axis of the proximal aortic root in a patient with dissection of the proximal aorta. The arrow shows the communications between the true lumen *(TL)* and false lumen *(FL).*

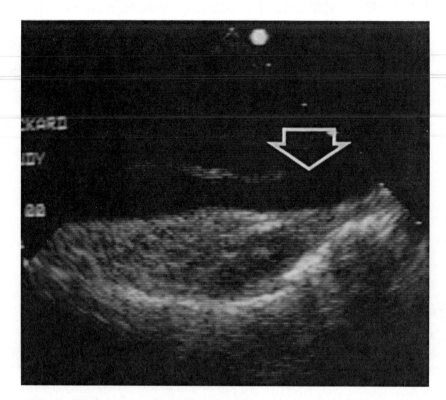

Fig. 40-10. Transesophageal echocardiogram of the descending aorta in the longitudinal plane. The arrow shows the communication between the true lumen and false lumen with the intimal flap between. Posterior is a large thrombus.

primarily slippage between myocyte bundles, resulting in a decrease in the number of myocytes across the infarct wall.[53] Infarct expansion is not only a risk factor for myocardial rupture, aneurysm formation, and late ventricular remodeling but also portends higher short-term mortality.[54] Reperfusion therapy has been reported to reduce infarct expansion, and animal experiments suggest even late reperfusion beyond the period of possible myocardial salvage may be beneficial.[55,56]

2-D echocardiography can readily detect infarct expansion. The heart is imaged in the parasternal short-axis view at the level of the papillary muscles and divided into anterior and posterior segments using the papillary muscles as landmarks (Fig. 40-7). The lengths of these segments are then measured. If the length of the infarct-containing segment exceeds that for an age- and sex-matched control group, infarct expansion is said to be present (Fig. 40-7).[57] Serial echocardiographic studies, however, are often required to establish the diagnosis.[52]

Although serial echocardiographic examination is certainly feasible in nearly all infarct patients, cost considerations suggest that only the highest risk patients be followed—those with large transmural anterior infarcts. Early recognition could be followed by aggressive afterload reduction therapy, which may limit infarct expansion.[58]

Mural thrombi

Stroke complicates approximately 6% of anterior MIs, usually as a result of embolization of a left ventricular thrombus.[59,60] The incidence of left ventricular thrombi after anterior MI is estimated to be 30% to 40%, with the majority forming within the first week and the bulk of the remainder during the second week.[59-61] Left ventricular thrombus formation after inferior MI is rare.[60] Fibrinolytic therapy during AMI has not clearly altered the incidence of left ventricular thrombus formation.[59] 2-D echocardiography remains the diagnostic test of choice for detecting mural thrombi, with a sensitivity of 77% to 92% and a specificity of 84% to 94% (Fig. 40-8).[60,62]

Although anticoagulation likely reduces the incidence of left ventricular thrombus formation and subsequent embolization,[60] controversy exists about whether to treat all patients with anterior infarction or only those with thrombi identified on echocardiographic assessment. An additional question is when to perform the echocardiogram. Examination within the first 48 hours may be too soon to detect many left ventricular thrombi, whereas later assessment would postdate embolization in some patients.

These questions have not been adequately addressed with randomized trials, but Weintraub and Ba'albaki[61] have created a decision analysis model based on a review of the available literature. They concluded that the risk of embolic stroke in anterior MI would be reduced from 4.5% to 1.1% if all patients were anticoagulated and to 1.6% if echocardiographic assessment was used to guide therapy. The slight reduction in embolic events achieved by anticoagulating all patients would be offset by a nearly threefold increase in the incidence of major bleeding complications. They proposed a strategy of empiric anticoagulation on admission for all patients with anterior infarction, with echocardiographic evaluation at 7 days or the time of discharge. Only patients with visible left ventricular thrombi would be anticoagulated with warfarin sodium (Coumadin), whereas those without thrombi would be reexamined at the time of office follow-up.

Whether or not this is a safe and effective strategy remains to be proved. In the absence of a large prospective trial addressing these issues, the recent American College of Chest Physicians' Conference on Antithrombotic Therapy strongly recommended anticoagulation for all patients with anterior Q-wave infarction for a 3-month period.[60]

Right ventricular infarction

Right ventricular necrosis is recognized as a frequent complication of inferior AMI, occurring in 25% to 53% of cases.[63] In the majority of patients, right ventricular involvement is of no hemodynamic significance. Occasionally, however, a characteristic clinical syndrome results with hypotension, elevated jugular venous pressure, and clear lung fields.[64] Recognition is important because of the need to avoid excessive preload reduction and administer adequate volume.

2-D echocardiography can accurately identify right ventricular infarction.[25] The usual findings include a dilated, globally hypocontractile right ventricle with concomitant contractile abnormalities of the inferior left ventricle. In many patients, the diagnosis can be made solely on the basis of clinical and ECG findings. Echocardiography is usually unnecessary unless differentiation from pericardial effusion with tamponade or simultaneous assessment of left ventricular function is required.

TRANSESOPHAGEAL ECHOCARDIOGRAPHY

Transesophageal echocardiography (TEE) is an exciting new technology that has added rapidly to the quality of patient care. Its role in the management of patients with AMI is still being defined, but we have found it to often be of significant utility at our institution. Of note, TEE retains the benefit of portability, which is an obvious advantage over competing imaging technologies such as ultrafast cine computed tomography and nuclear magnetic resonance imaging when managing acutely ill patients.

One area where TEE has gained widespread acceptance is in the initial assessment of patients with unexplained chest pain in whom aortic dissection is a consideration (Figs. 40-9 and 40-10). TEE has been reported to be more accurate than computed tomography or angiography in the diagnosis of aortic dissection.[65] Aortic dissection can occasionally involve the coronary arteries and cause concomitant MI.[66] TEE can be of great benefit in diagnosing such patients and thereby facilitate avoidance of potentially disastrous thrombolytic therapy.

TEE can also be useful in assessing ventricular function and diagnosing complications of MI, including ventricular septal defect, papillary muscle rupture, and left ventricular free wall rupture.[67-69] In the majority of cases, transthoracic echocardiography will provide the necessary information, but occasionally patients cannot be adequately assessed as a result of poor acoustic transmission. This is particularly a problem in patients whose airways are being mechanically ventilated. Such individuals can be safely evaluated with TEE, even if they are critically ill.[70]

SUMMARY

Echocardiography continues to play the predominant role among noninvasive imaging techniques in the assessment of patients with AMI. The information provided from early echocardiographic evaluation greatly enhances the management of these patients and in particular gives information often inapparent from clinical assessment.

It is likely that the role of echocardiography in AMI will continue to grow. Future areas of interest include the use of digital storage and display of echocardiographic images, which enables side-by-side comparison of serial studies[62]; the improvement and expanded use of contrast echocardiography, which allows investigation of myocardial perfusion after intravenous injection of special contrast agents capable of crossing the pulmonary circulation[71]; and the continued development of invasive echocardiographic modalities, including intracoronary and intracardiac imaging.

REFERENCES

1. Kloner RA, Parisi AF: Acute myocardial infarction: diagnostic and prognostic application of two-dimensional echocardiography, *Circulation* 75:521-524, 1987.
2. Tennant R, Wiggers CJ: The effect of coronary occlusion on myocardial infarction, *Am J Physiol* 112:351-361, 1935.
3. Battler A, Froelicher VF, Gallagher KP, et al: Dissociation between regional myocardial dysfunction and ECG changes during ischemia in the conscious dog, *Circulation* 62:735-744, 1980.
4. Hauser AM, Gangadharan V, Ramos RG, et al: Sequence of mechanical, electrocardiographic, and clinical effects of repeated coronary artery occlusion in human beings: echocardiographic observations during coronary angioplasty, *J Am Coll Cardiol* 5:193-197, 1985.

5. Kisslo JA, Robertson D, Gilbert BW, et al: A comparison of real-time, two-dimensional echocardiography and cineangiography in detecting left ventricular asynergy, *Circulation* 55:134-141, 1977.

6. Sabia P, Afrookleh A, Touchstone DA, et al: Value of regional wall motion abnormality in the emergency room diagnosis of acute myocardial infarction: a prospective study using two-dimensional echocardiography, *Circulation* 84 (suppl I):I85-I92, 1991.

7. Peels CH, Visser CA, Kupper AJ, et al: Usefulness of two-dimensional echocardiography for immediate detection of myocardial ischemia in the emergency room, *Am J Cardiol* 65:687-691, 1990.

8. Visser CA, Lie KI, Kan G, et al: Detection and quantification of acute, isolated myocardial infarction by two-dimensional echocardiography, *Am J Cardiol* 47:1020-1025, 1981.

9. Loh IK, Charuzi Y, Beeder C, et al: Early diagnosis of nontransmural myocardial infarction by two-dimensional echocardiography, *Am Heart J* 104:963-968, 1982.

10. Gibson RS, Bishop HL, Stamm RB, et al: Value of early two-dimensional echocardiography in patients with acute myocardial infarction, *Am J Cardiol* 49:1110-1119, 1982.

11. Horowitz RS, Morganroth J, Parrotto C, et al: Immediate diagnosis of acute myocardial infarction by two-dimensional echocardiography, *Circulation* 65:323-329, 1982.

12. Lee TH, Cook EF, Weisberg MG, et al: Acute chest pain in the emergency room: identification of low risk patients, *Arch Intern Med* 145:65-69, 1985.

13. Gersh BJ: Noninvasive imaging in acute coronary disease: a clinical perspective, *Circulation* 84(suppl I):I140-I147, 1991.

14. Oh JK, Miller FA, Shub C, et al: Evaluation of acute chest pain syndromes by two-dimensional echocardiography: its potential application in the selection of patients for acute reperfusion therapy, *Mayo Clin Proc* 62:59-66, 1987.

15. Gruppo Italiano per lo Studio Della Streptochinasi Nell'Infarrto Miocardio (GISSI): Effectiveness of intravenous thrombolytic treatment in acute myocardial infarction, *Lancet* 1:397-401, 1986.

16. ISIS-2 Collaborative Group: Randomized trial of IV streptokinase, oral aspirin, both or neither among 17, 187 cases of suspected acute myocardial infarction, *Lancet* 2:349-360, 1988.

17. Yusuf S: Overview of results of randomized clinical trials in heart disease: I. Treatments following myocardial infarction, *JAMA* 260:2088-2093, 1988.

18. McGuinness JB, Begg TB, Semple T: First electrocardiogram in recent myocardial infarction, *Br Med J (Clin Res)* 2:449-451, 1976.

19. Lee TH, Rouan GW, Weisberg MC, et al: Sensitivity of routine clinical criteria for diagnosing myocardial infarction within 24 hours of hospitalization, *Ann Intern Med* 106:181-186, 1987.

20. Quinones MA, Waggoner AD, Reduto LA, et al: A new, simplified and accurate method for determining ejection fraction with two-dimensional echocardiography, *Circulation* 64:744-753, 1981.

21. Carr KW, Engler RL, Forsythe JR, et al: Measurement of left ventricular ejection fraction by mechanical cross-sectional echocardiography, *Circulation* 59:1196-1206, 1979.

22. Schiller NB, Shah PM, Crawford M, et al: Recommendations for quantification of the left ventricle by two-dimensional echocardiography, *J Am Soc Echo* 5:358-367, 1989.

23. Gordon EP, Schnittger I, Fitzgerald PJ, et al: Reproducibility of left ventricular volumes by two-dimensional echocardiography, *J Am Coll Cardiol* 2:506-513, 1983.

24. Stack RS, Phillips HR, Grierson DS, et al: Functional improvement of jeopardized myocardium following intracoronary streptokinase infusion in acute myocardial infarction, *J Clin Invest* 72:84-95, 1983.

25. Kaul S: Echocardiography in coronary artery disease, *Curr Probl Cardiol* 15:233-298, 1990.

26. Page DL, Caulfield JB, Kastor JA, et al: Myocardial changes associated with cardiogenic shock, *N Engl J Med* 285:133-137, 1971.

27. Harnarayan C, Bennett MA, Pentecost BL, et al: Quantitative study of infarcted myocardium in cardiogenic shock, *Br Heart J* 32:728-732, 1970.

28. Multicenter Postinfarction Research Group: Risk stratification and survival after myocardial infarction, *N Engl J Med* 309:331-336, 1983.

29. Nixon JV, Narahara KA, Smitherman TC: Estimation of myocardial involvement in patients with acute myocardial infarction by two-dimensional echocardiography, *Circulation* 62:1248-1253, 1982.

30. Weiss JL, Bulkley BH, Hutchins GM, et al: Two-dimensional echocardiographic recognition of myocardial injury in man: comparison with postmortem studies, *Circulation* 63:401-408, 1981.

31. Lieberman AN, Weiss JL, Jugdutt BI, et al: Two-dimensional echocardiography and infarct size: Relationship of regional wall motion and thickening to the extent of myocardial infarction in the dog, *Circulation* 63:739-746, 1981.

32. Nieminen M, Parisi AF, O'Boyle JE, et al: Serial evaluation of myocardial thickening and thinning in acute myocardial infarction: Identification and quantification using two-dimensional echocardiography, *Circulation* 66:174-180, 1982.

33. Nishimura RA, Tajik AJ, Shub C, et al: Role of two-dimensional echocardiography in the prediction of in-hospital complications after acute myocardial infarction, *J Am Coll Cardiol* 4:1080-1087, 1984.

34. Lavallee M, Cox D, Patrick TA, et al: Salvage of myocardial function by coronary artery reperfusion 1, 2, and 3 hours after occlusion in conscious dogs, *Circ Res* 53:235-247, 1983.

35. Braunwald E: The path to myocardial salvage by thrombolytic therapy, *Circulation* 76(suppl II):II2-II7, 1987.

36. Braunwald E, Kloner RA: The stunned myocardium: prolonged, postischemic ventricular dysfunction, *Circulation* 66:1146-1149, 1982.

37. Berning J, Steensgaard-Hansen F: Early estimation of risk by echocardiographic determination of wall motion index in an unselected population with acute myocardial infarction, *Am J Cardiol* 65:567-576, 1990.

38. Heger JJ, Weyman AE, Wann LS, et al: Cross-sectional echocardiographic analysis of the extent of left ventricular asynergy in acute myocardial infarction, *Circulation* 61:1113-1118, 1980.

39. Horowitz RS, Morganroth J: Immediate detection of early high-risk patients with acute myocardial infarction using two-dimensional echocardiographic evaluation of left ventricular regional wall motion abnormalities, *Am Heart J* 103:814-822, 1982.

40. Braunwald E: Myocardial reperfusion, limitation of infarct size, reduction of left ventricular dysfunction, and improved survival: Should the paradigm be expanded? *Circulation* 79:441-444, 1989.

41. Califf RM, Topol EJ, Gersh BJ: From myocardial salvage to patient salvage in acute myocardial infarction: the role of reperfusion therapy, *J Am Coll Cardiol* 14:1382-1388, 1989.

42. Picano E, Lattanzi F, Orlandini A, et al: Stress echocardiography and the human factor: the importance of being expert, *J Am Coll Cardiol* 17:666-669, 1991.

43. Buda AJ: The role of echocardiography in the evaluation of mechanical complications of acute myocardial infarction, *Circulation* 84(suppl I):I109-I121, 1991.

44. Scanlon PJ, Montoya A, Johnson SA, et al: Urgent surgery for ventricular septal rupture complicating acute myocardial infarction, *Circulation* 72(suppl II):II185-II190, 1985.

45. Fortin DF, Sheikh KH, Kisslo J: The utility of echocardiography in the diagnostic strategy of postinfarction ventricular septal rupture: a comparison of two-dimensional echocardiography versus Doppler color flow imaging, *Am Heart J* 121:25-32, 1991.

46. Helmcke F, Mahan EF, Nanda NC, et al: Two-dimensional echocardiography and Doppler color flow mapping in the diagnosis of ventricular septal rupture, *Circulation* 81:1775-1783, 1991.

47. Nishimura RA, Schaff HV, Shado C, et al: Papillary muscle rupture complicating acute myocardial infarction: analysis of 17 patients, *Am J Cardiol* 51:373-377, 1983.

48. Replogle RL, Campbell CD: Surgery for mitral regurgitation associated with ischemic heart disease: results and strategies, *Circulation* 79(suppl I):I122-I125, 1989.

49. Catherwood E, Mintz GS, Kotler MN, et al: Two-dimensional echocardiographic recognition of left ventricular pseudoaneurysm, *Circulation* 62:294-303, 1980.

50. Roelandt JRTC, Sutherland GR, Yoshida K, et al: Improved diagnosis and characterization of left ventricular pseudoaneurysm by Doppler color flow imaging, *J Am Coll Cardiol* 12:807-811, 1988.

51. Vlodaver Z, Coe JI, Edwards JE: True and false left ventricular aneurysms: propensity of the latter to rupture, *Circulation* 51:567-572, 1975.

52. Weiss JL, Marino PN, Shapiro EP: Myocardial infarct expansion: recognition, significance and pathology, *Am J Cardiol* 68:35D-44D, 1991.

53. Weisman HF, Bush DE, Mannisi JA, et al: Cellular mechanisms of myocardial infarct expansion, *Circulation* 78:186-201, 1988.

54. Eaton LW, Weiss JL, Bulkley BH, et al: Regional cardiac dilatation after acute myocardial infarction, *N Engl J Med* 300:57-62, 1979.

55. Touchstone DA, Beller GA, Nygaard TW, et al: Effects of successful intravenous reperfusion therapy on regional myocardial function and geometry in humans: a tomographic assessment using two-dimensional echocardiography, *J Am Coll Cardiol* 13:1506-1513, 1989.

56. Hochman JS, Choo H: Limitation of myocardial infarct expansion by reperfusion independent of myocardial salvage, *Circulation* 75:299-306, 1987.

57. Pfeffer MA, Braunwald E: Ventricular remodeling after myocardial infarction: experimental observations and clinical implications, *Circulation* 81:1161-1172, 1990.

58. Oldroyd KG, Pye MP, Ray SG, et al: Effects of early captopril administration on infarct expansion, left ventricular remodeling, and exercise capacity after acute myocardial infarction, *Am J Cardiol* 68:713-718, 1991.

59. Cerebral Embolism Task Force: Cardiogenic brain embolism: the second report of the Cerebral Embolism Task Force, *Arch Neurol* 46:727-743, 1989.

60. Cairns JA, Hirsh J, Lewis HD, et al: Antithrombotic agents in coronary artery disease, *Chest* 102:456S-481S, 1992.

61. Weintraub WS, Ba'albaki HA: Decision analysis concerning the application of echocardiography to the diagnosis and treatment of mural thrombi after anterior wall acute myocardial infarction, *Am J Cardiol* 64:708-716, 1989.

62. Feigenbaum H: Role of echocardiography in acute myocardial infarction, *Am J Cardiol* 66:17H-22H, 1990.

63. Rodrigues EA, Dewhurst NG, Smart LM, et al: Diagnosis and prognosis of right ventricular infarction, *Br Heart J* 56:19-26, 1986.

64. Cohn JN, Guiha NH, Broder MI, et al: Right ventricular infarction: clinical and hemodynamic features, *Am J Cardiol* 33:209-214, 1974.

65. Erbel R, Daniel W, Visser C, et al: Echocardiography in diagnosis of aortic dissection, *Lancet* 1:457-461, 1989.

66. Ballal RS, Nanda NC, Gatewood R, et al: Usefulness of transesophageal echocardiography in the assessment of aortic dissection, *Circulation* 84:1903-1914, 1991.

67. Patel AM, Miller FA, Khanderia BK, et al: Role of transesophageal echocardiography in the diagnosis of papillary muscle rupture secondary to myocardial infarction, *Am Heart J* 118:1330-1333, 1989.

68. Koenig K, Kasper W, Hofman T, et al: Transesophageal echocardiography for diagnosis of rupture of the ventricular septum or left papillary muscle during acute myocardial infarction, *Am J Cardiol* 59:362, 1987.

69. Maeta H, Imawaki S, Shiraishi Y, et al: Repair of both papillary and free wall rupture following acute myocardial infarction, *J Cardiovasc Surg* 32:828-832, 1991.

70. Pearson AC, Castello R, Labovitz AJ: Safety and utility of transesophageal echocardiography in the critically ill patient, *Am Heart J* 119:1083-1089, 1990.

71. Feinstein SB: Myocardial perfusion: contrast echocardiography perspectives, *Am J Cardiol* 69:36H-41H, 1992.

Chapter 41

THE NATIONAL CLINICAL PRACTICE GUIDELINES FOR UNSTABLE ANGINA

Daniel B. Mark
Robert H. Jones

Practice guidelines are "systematically developed statements to assist practitioners and patient decisions about appropriate health care for specific clinical circumstances."[1] The need for such guidelines has been stimulated by repeated demonstrations of dramatic variations in the clinical practice among clinicians and by research showing that there is a significant underuse of therapies shown conclusively to be effective (e.g., aspirin and beta blockers for AMI). Guidelines have also been advocated by those who believe that they will provide a means of cost containment, although this has never been definitively demonstrated. In the act that created the Agency for Health Care Policy and Research (AHCPR) in 1989, Congress specifically charged the new agency with the responsibility for creating national practice guidelines. The first cardiovascular guideline sponsored by AHCPR was for congestive heart failure; the second was for unstable angina.[2] Additional guidelines currently under preparation include cardiac rehabilitation and AMI.

There are two important features of the AHCPR guideline process that distinguish it from many of the guidelines previously created by specialty societies. First, the guidelines are explicitly evidence based, meaning that all recommendations must be tied to some level of scientific evidence, and the strength of the recommendations made has to be clearly linked to the quantity and quality of scientific evidence available on that subject. Second, the panels creating the guidelines are broadly constituted to be representative both of health care professionals (specialists and generalists) and health care consumers. Each guideline is created by a contractor to AHCPR charged with the responsibility for producing the guideline documents and an independent (nonfederal) panel of experts nominated to their position by relevant professional societies and other organizations.

The purpose of this chapter is to review briefly the process used to create the Unstable Angina Guideline and to provide an overview of the Guideline's content. Because the guideline is in the public domain, we have reproduced (with slight modifications) major portions of the text without specific attribution. Guideline recommendations are presented in bold text. In some places, the text from the Quick Reference Guide has been substituted for the longer text of the parent guideline. Although much of the key content is therefore summarized in this chapter, we still recommend that individuals managing unstable angina patients obtain and review copies of the original guideline documents (which can be obtained free from AHCPR by calling 1-800-358-9295).

BACKGROUND

The Clinical Practice Guideline for Unstable Angina represents an attempt to standardize the diagnosis and management of this important clinical syndrome as well as to identify areas in need of further research. The principal goals of the Unstable Angina Guideline were

Table 41-1. Grading of evidence

	Strength of evidence = A	Strength of evidence = B	Strength of evidence = C
Primary evidence	Randomized controlled trials	Well-designed clinical studies	Panel consensus
Secondary evidence	Other clinical studies	Clinical studies related to topic but not in an unstable angina population	Clinical studies related to topic but not in an unstable angina population

to produce a clinically workable definition for the syndrome and to define diagnostic and therapeutic strategies that were likely to maximize medical benefits for unstable angina patients. The guideline specifically indicates that recommendations are expected to be flexibly applied by physicians using clinical judgment and are not meant to serve as a "cookbook" of unthinking medical practice. The Unstable Angina Guidelines were created over a period of approximately 18 months by a collaborative effort of a Duke University Medical Center team (led by Dr. Robert H. Jones) and an expert panel (led by Dr. Eugene Braunwald). The panel included, in addition to Dr. Braunwald, eight other cardiologists, two cardiac surgeons, two internists, one family medicine physician, one emergency medicine physician, two nurses, one public health specialist, and one consumer representative. The process of creating the guideline involved three full panel meetings, an extensive literature review relative to unstable angina, and five major drafts of the guideline documents. In the literature review 5000 potentially relevant abstracts were identified, of which 2500 were reviewed. All studies were graded: there were 130 randomized trials, 319 excellent clinical studies, and 1351 good clinical studies. These data form the backbone of the guideline. In November 1993 the prefinal guideline draft was then reviewed by 75 separate peer reviewers representing the broad spectrum of disciplines involved in the care and management of unstable angina. Additional revisions were undertaken after the comments from the peer reviewers were received, and the final guideline was published in March 1994.

One of the signal features of this guideline process was the use of evidence-based recommendations. Table 41-1 shows the grading of evidence scheme used in the guideline. A "strength of evidence = A" recommendation was based on at least one major randomized clinical trial, whereas a "strength of evidence = C" recommendation was based on panel consensus because of the absence of sufficient high-quality data to provide firmer justification. One of the revealing features of creating this guideline was the relative infrequency with which recommendations received the "A" rating. This relates both to the absence of adequate clinical studies in many areas as well as the fact that many clinical practices have now become so ingrained into current practice that it

would be virtually impossible to test their utility in a randomized trial setting.

DEFINITION AND EPIDEMIOLOGY

One of the major challenges in creating the unstable angina guideline was to come up with an acceptable definition for this syndrome.[3] Review of previous research revealed scores of different definitions that tended to be of two basic types: some defined unstable angina prospectively, based on the clinical presentation of the patient at the point of entry into the medical care system; others defined unstable angina retrospectively, usually after cardiac enzymes had been used to rule out MI. These latter definitions were recognized to be useful for some forms of clinical research but not appropriate for a clinical practice guideline. Definitions also varied according to whether they required objective ECG findings to be part of the diagnosis. To reach an acceptable definition the panel recognized, first, that unstable angina was a clinical syndrome (meaning that there was no gold standard or definitive test for its presence) and that, second, it fell between stable angina and AMI in the spectrum of coronary disease presentations. Because much of the management of unstable angina is critically tied to the first hours of presentation, a definition was selected that could be used prospectively, based on data available at presentation. When other diagnoses become evident (e.g., non–Q-wave MI, noncoronary chest pain), patients exit from this guideline and are managed as appropriate to their updated diagnosis.

The guideline recognized three principle presentations of unstable angina:
- **rest angina** — defined as angina occurring at rest and usually prolonged greater than 20 minutes, occurring within a week of presentation
- **new onset angina** — angina of at least Canadian Cardiovascular Society class (CCSC) III severity, with onset within 2 months of initial presentation
- **increasing angina** — previously diagnosed angina that is distinctly more frequent, longer in duration, or lower in threshold (i.e., increased by at least one CCSC class within 2 months of initial presentation to at least CCSC III severity).

By design, this operational definition includes patients who will subsequently be found to have had an

Table 41-2. Grading of angina pectoris by the Canadian Cardiovascular Society classification system

Class	Description of stage
Class I	Ordinary physical activity such as walking, climbing stairs, does not cause angina. Angina (occurs) with strenuous, rapid, or prolonged exertion at work or recreation.
Class II	Slight limitation of ordinary activity. Angina occurs on walking or climbing stairs rapidly, walking up-hill, walking or stair climbing after meals, or in cold, or in wind, or under emotional stress, or only during the few hours after awakening. Walking more than two blocks on the level and climbing more than one flight of ordinary stairs at a normal pace and in normal condition.
Class III	Marked limitations of ordinary physical activity. Angina occurs on walking one to two blocks on the level and climbing one flight of stairs in normal conditions and at a normal pace.
Class IV	Inability to carry on any physical activity without discomfort—anginal symptoms may be present at rest.

From Campeau L: Grading of angina pectoris (Utter), *Circulation* 54(3):522-523, 1976.

AMI, as well as patients who will subsequently be found not to have significant coronary disease. The Canadian Cardiovascular Society classification system upon which parts of this diagnosis are based is shown in Table 41-2.[4]

Only about 10% of patients with CAD have unstable angina as their initial presentation if patients who experience MI are retrospectively excluded. However, patients with established CAD (either chronic stable angina or prior MI) commonly cycle through unstable phases. As a clinical syndrome, unstable angina shares ill-defined borders with chronic stable angina (presentation with lower risk) and AMI (presentation with higher risk). Unstable angina occurs in a variety of clinical scenarios, including in patients with known CAD, with prior stable CAD, soon after MI, and following myocardial revascularization by either CABG or PTCA. Patients presenting with unstable angina may undergo any of the diagnostic and therapeutic procedures used for other CAD patients, therefore recommendations for the management of patients with unstable angina of necessity address questions pertinent to patients with any mode of presentation of CAD.

Unstable angina presents as a constellation of clinical symptoms and can be defined in many different ways. The strictness of the definition of unstable angina used in the method of assigning death to this cause vs. other ischemic heart disease diagnoses can greatly influence reported mortality rates. Moreover, published series of patients with unstable angina commonly begin with the definitive diagnosis of the condition and not at the onset of symptoms. Therefore, the mortality observed in any series of carefully defined patients with unstable angina will tend to understate the risk in comparison with the mortality rate expected for those patients at the time of initial presentation for acute chest pain. The diagnosis of unstable angina at the time of hospital admission carries a risk of death that is intermediate between the diagnosis of stable angina and AMI. This fact is well illustrated by data from the Duke Cardiovascular Databank, which describes the rate of cardiac death in 21,761 patients

treated for CAD at Duke between 1985 and 1992 (Fig. 41-1). The three patient groups were defined by the diagnoses of stable angina, unstable angina, or AMI at the time of admission. All three groups of patients have the highest risk of cardiac death at the time of presentation, and the risk declines so that by 2 months, mortality rates were indistinguishable in all three populations.

INITIAL EVALUATION AND TREATMENT
Telephone presentation

Recommendation: Because both clinical examination and ECG are critical to early risk assessment, the initial evaluation of the patient with symptoms suggesting possible unstable angina should be done by a medical practitioner in a facility equipped to perform an ECG and not over the telephone (strength of evidence = B).

Appropriate triage of the patient who presents to a clinician over the telephone can be difficult, and both the patient and the practitioner often have difficulty knowing which symptoms can be ignored or explored as a nonemergent problem and which should receive more immediate attention. In general, patients with known CAD who call to report exacerbation or recurrence of symptoms should, for the most part, be encouraged to seek direct medical care. The main exception is for patients who are calling for advice regarding modification of medication as part of an ongoing treatment plan. Most patients without known CAD should be referred to a medical facility for a clinical evaluation and a 12-lead ECG. The rationale for this derives in part from the critical importance of the ECG in the early evaluation and triage of unstable angina.[5-9]

Ultimately patients must retain the responsibility of deciding whether they will seek medical attention and, if so, in what environment. The guideline specifically recognizes that a medical practitioner cannot be expected to assume responsibility for a patient with a potentially severe cardiac condition who does not present for direct evaluation. However, practitioners

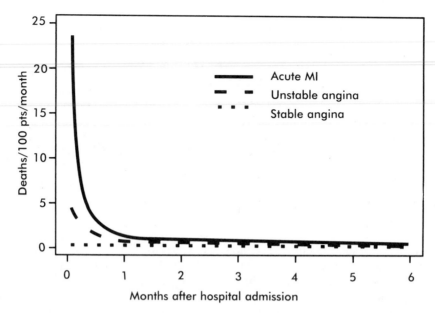

Fig. 41-1. Outcomes of 21,761 medically treated patients at Duke University Medical Center (1985-1992), grouped by admission ischemic heart disease diagnosis.

should be cautious not to provide inappropriate reassurance to patients who are reluctant to seek further medical attention. If the patient declines to come in for evaluation, it would be prudent for the clinician to create a record of the conversation with the patient for his or her office files, as suggested in Chapter 70.

Outpatient facility vs. emergency department presentation

Recommendation: Patients with suspected unstable angina who have a symptom duration greater than 20 minutes, hemodynamic instability, or recent loss of consciousness should generally be referred to an emergency department (ED). Other patients with suspected unstable angina may be seen initially either in an ED or in an outpatient facility at the discretion of the attending physician (strength of evidence = C).

The decision about where to perform the initial patient evaluation must be based on the individual patient's presenting complaint and circumstances, the options for transportation, and the local facilities available. Obviously high-risk patients, such as those referred to in the preceding recommendation, should go directly to an ED. Others may be seen at an outpatient facility.

Initial evaluation

The first 10 to 20 minutes of the initial encounter with the patient should include a brief assessment of the urgency with which evaluation must be done and treatment started. The urgency of evaluation for patients with ongoing pain at rest upon presentation is substantially greater than for patients whose symptoms have already resolved. If the patient is hemodynamically

stable and does not appear to be in great distress, the initial evaluation can precede treatment decisions; otherwise, both must be done simultaneously. Diagnosis of hemodynamic instability is based on the patient's systolic blood pressure (i.e., ≤ 90 mm Hg), respiratory status (i.e., acutely dyspneic), mental state (i.e., confused or obtunded), and peripheral circulation (i.e., vasoconstricted, diaphoretic).

In patients with symptoms suggesting unstable angina, there are two complementary and equally important components to the initial assessment: (1) assessment of the likelihood of CAD (Table 41-3), and (2) assessment of the likelihood of adverse outcomes (Table 41-4). At the conclusion of the initial evaluation it should be possible to assign the patient to one of four diagnostic categories: not CAD, stable angina, AMI, or unstable angina.

Low- and intermediate-risk patients. Initial evaluation of low- and intermediate-risk patients who arrive at a medical facility in a pain-free state, have unchanged or normal ECGs, and are hemodynamically stable represents a diagnostic rather than an urgent therapeutic challenge. Among these, patients meeting criteria for unstable angina should receive an aspirin (160 to 324 mg) unless definite contraindications are present. Patients without pain but with definite ischemic ECG changes should be treated during this initial phase as if they have ongoing pain. Low-risk patients can usually be managed further on an outpatient basis, as can patients who are found to have another cause of their symptoms that is nonthreatening (e.g., anxiety, musculoskeletal pain). A few low-risk patients may require hospitalization, such as those who have other diseases that might

Table 41-3. Likelihood of significant coronary artery disease in patients with symptoms suggesting unstable angina*

High likelihood (e.g., 0.85-0.99)	Intermediate likelihood (e.g., 0.15-0.84)	Low likelihood (e.g., 0.01-0.14)
Any of the following features:	Absence of high likelihood features and any of the following:	Absence of high or intermediate likelihood features but may have:
History of prior MI or sudden death or other known history of CAD	Definite angina: males < 60 or females < 70 years of age	Chest pain classified as probably not angina
Definite angina: males ≥ 60 or females ≥ 70 years of age	Probable angina: males ≥ 60 or females ≥ 70 years of age	One risk factor other than diabetes
Transient hemodynamic or ECG changes during pain	Chest pain probably not angina in patients with diabetes	T-wave flattening or inversion < 1 mm in leads with dominant R-waves
Variant angina (pain with reversible ST-segment elevation)	Chest pain probably not angina and two or three risk factors other than diabetes†	Normal ECG
ST segment elevation or depression ≥ 1 mm	Extracardiac vascular disease	
Marked symmetrical T-wave inversion in multiple precordial leads	ST depression 0.05 to 1 mm	
	T-wave inversion ≥ 1 mm in leads with dominant R-waves	

*Note: Estimation of the likelihood of significant coronary artery disease is a complex, multivariable problem that cannot be fully specified in a table such as this; therefore, the table is meant to illustrate major relationships rather than offer rigid algorithms.
†Coronary artery disease risk factors include diabetes, smoking, hypertension, and elevated cholesterol.

Table 41-4. Short-term risk of death or nonfatal MI in patients with unstable angina*

High risk	Intermediate risk	Low risk
At least one of the following features must be present:	No high-risk feature but must have any of the following:	No high- or intermediate-risk feature but may have any of the following features:
Prolonged ongoing (>20 min) rest pain	Prolonged (>20 min) rest angina, now resolved, with moderate or high likelihood of CAD	Increased angina frequency, severity, or duration
Pulmonary edema, most likely related to ischemia	Rest angina (>20 min or relieved with rest or sublingual nitroglycerin)	Angina provoked at a lower threshold
Angina at rest with dynamic ST changes ≥1 mm	Nocturnal angina	New onset angina with onset 2 weeks to 2 months before presentation
Angina with new or worsening MR murmur	Angina with dynamic T-wave changes	Normal or unchanged ECG
Angina with S3 or new/worsening rales	New onset CCSC† III or IV angina in the past 2 weeks with moderate or high likelihood of CAD	
Angina with hypotension	Pathologic Q waves or resting ST depression ≤1 mm in multiple lead groups (anterior, inferior, lateral) Age > 65 years	

*Note: Estimation of the short-term risks of death and nonfatal MI in unstable angina is a complex, multivariate problem that cannot be fully specified in a table such as this. Therefore, the table is meant to offer general guidelines and illustration rather than rigid algorithms.
†CCSC = Canadian Cardiovascular System Classification.

make outpatient management more difficult or patients who live in areas remote from an appropriate health care facility.

High-risk patients

Recommendation: The initial assessment of the high-risk patient with possible unstable angina must start with a rapid evaluation of the probability of immediate adverse outcomes and the need for emergency diagnostic and therapeutic interventions. Patients with ongoing symptoms, hemodynamic instability, or recent loss of consciousness should have a directed history, physical examination, and 12-lead ECG completed within 20 minutes of arrival to a medical facility (strength of evidence = B). Specific diagnoses that must be explicitly considered are AMI meeting criteria for reperfusion therapy, aortic dissection, leaking or ruptured thoracic aneurysm, pericarditis with tamponade, pneumothorax, and pulmonary embolism. Other non-cardiovascular diagnoses may need to be considered as well, depending on initial findings (strength of evidence = B).

Intensive medical treatment should begin immediately in the ED in patients with ongoing rest pain or definite ECG ischemia and should continue as the patient is transported to the definitive care environment. Ongoing rest pain despite initial treatment should drive initial evaluation at a more urgent pace; therapy for such patients should be more aggressive than is required for patients with pain that resolves rapidly as treatment is begun. Patients who appear unstable should have simultaneous evaluation and treatment. Intravenous access can be obtained while a brief cardiovascular history and physical examination are performed and an ECG is taken. When initial blood work is obtained, samples should be sent for determination of creatine kinase (CK). Medical personnel trained in cardiopulmonary resuscitation should remain in close attendance during the period of initial stabilization. Oxygen should be administered by mask or nasal cannula.

Initial treatment and triage

Recommendation: Patients with unstable angina and ongoing rest pain should be placed at bed rest during the initial phase of medical stabilization (strength of evidence = C).

Recommendation: Patients with obvious cyanosis, respiratory distress, or high-risk features (see Table 41-3) should receive supplemental oxygen. A finger pulse oximetry or arterial blood gas determination should be used to confirm adequate arterial oxygen saturation and continued need for supplemental oxygen (strength of evidence = C).

Recommendation: As soon as the diagnosis of unstable angina is made, patients should be placed on continuous ECG monitoring for ischemia and arrhythmia detection (strength of evidence = C).

Drugs to be considered for use at the time of initial evaluation and treatment of patients with symptoms suggestive of unstable angina include aspirin, heparin, nitrates, and beta blockers. Certainty of diagnosis, severity of symptoms, hemodynamic state, and medication history will determine the choice and timing of drugs used in individual patients. Treatment with an indicated drug should begin in the ED; it should not be delayed until hospital admission. Aggressiveness of drug dosage will depend on the severity of symptoms and, for many drugs, will require modification throughout the subsequent hospital course. A summary of the drugs com-

monly used in the ED in unstable angina is provided in Table 41-5.

Recommendation: Intravenous thrombolytic therapy is not indicated in patients who do not have evidence of acute ST-segment elevation or left bundle branch block (LBBB) on their 12-lead ECG (strength of evidence = A).

The failure of IV thrombolytic therapy to improve clinical outcomes in the absence of AMI with ST-segment elevation or left bundle branch block has now been clearly demonstrated.[10-12] A metaanalysis of recent studies of thrombolytic therapy in unstable angina patients shows no benefit of thrombolysis vs. standard therapy for reduction of AMI. Thrombolytic agents may actually increase the risk of MI by 1.7% (95% confidence interval −2.4 to +5.8%) (Fig. 41-2).

The distinction between unstable angina and AMI often cannot be definitively made during the initial evaluation. Patients with ECG changes diagnostic of epicardial injury (i.e., ≥1 mm ST elevation in two or more contiguous leads, or ST depression in V1 through V3) or left bundle branch block with a consistent history should be managed as if they have an AMI, including prompt administration of aspirin, beta blockers, and reperfusion therapy. In most large trials of reperfusion therapy, such patients have a ≥95% prevalence of AMI.[13]

Recommendation: All patients with the diagnosis of unstable angina should receive regular aspirin 160 to 324 mg as soon as possible after presentation unless a definite contraindication is present, such as evidence of ongoing major or life-threatening hemorrhage, a significant predisposition to such hemorrhage (e.g., recent bleeding peptic ulcer), or a clear history of severe hypersensitivity to aspirin (strength of evidence = A).

The recommendation for an initial aspirin to be given in the ED is based on the efficacy of this therapy in independently reducing mortality in AMI patients enrolled in the ISIS-2 trial.[14] These data, combined with the recognition that a definitive distinction between AMI and unstable angina is frequently not possible at the time of acute presentation, led to the recommendation to initiate aspirin immediately in appropriate patients. No randomized trials or other studies compare immediate with a more delayed initiation of aspirin in unstable angina. The efficacy of aspirin in reducing the relative risk of death or MI in patients with unstable angina patients is summarized in Figure 41-3.[15-19] This metaanalysis suggests that aspirin reduces the risk of MI by 48% and the risk of death by 51%, with a 47% reduction in the combined risk of death and MI. No data directly compare the efficacy of different doses of aspirin in patients presenting with unstable angina. However, an overview of different doses in the long-term treatment of patients with CAD suggest equal efficacy of doses in the

Table 41-5. Summary of drugs commonly used in the emergency department to treat patients with symptoms suggestive of unstable angina

Drug category	Clinical condition	When to avoid*	Usual dose (low-high)
Aspirin	Diagnosis of unstable angina or AMI	Hypersensitivity, active bleeding, severe bleeding risk	324 mg (160 mg-324 mg)
Heparin	Unstable angina in high-risk category and some intermediate-risk patients	Active bleeding, history of heparin-induced thrombo-cytopenia, severe bleeding risk, recent stroke	80 units/kg IV bolus with constant IV infusion at 18 units/kg/hr titrated to maintain aPTT between 46 and 70 seconds†
Nitrates	Ongoing pain or ischemia	Hypotension	Sublingual (1-3 tablets)‡ IV (5-100 mg/min)
Beta blockers	Diagnosis of unstable angina	PR ECG segment > 0.24 seconds, second- or third-degree AV block, heart rate < 60, systolic blood pressure < 90 mmHg, shock, left ventricular failure with CHF, severe reactive airway disease	Oral dose appropriate for specific drug IV metoprolol 1-5 mg slow IV every 5 minutes to 15 mg total IV propranolol 0.5-1.0 mg IV atenolol 5 mg every 5 minutes to 10 mg total
Narcotics	Persistent pain following initial therapy with nitrates and beta blockers	Hypotension, respiratory depression, confusion, obtundation	Morphine sulfate 2-5 mg IV

*Allergy or prior intolerance contraindication for all.
†Dose regimen assumes a mean control aPTT of 30 seconds and a therapeutic goal of 1.5 to 2.5 times control.
‡Patients with symptoms suggestive of unstable angina and ongoing pain should be given sublingual NTG 0.3 to 0.4 every 5 minutes until discomfort is relieved, three tablets have been given, or limiting symptoms or signs develop. If discomfort is still present after three tablets, IV NTG should be started promptly at a dose of 5 μg/min and titrated up to 75 to 100 μg/min for limiting side effects.

range of 75 to 324 mg per day.[20] It appears reasonable to initiate aspirin treatment in patients with unstable angina with a dose of at least 160 mg, as used in the ISIS-2 trial.[14] Thereafter, an aspirin dose of 80 to 324 mg can be used for long-term therapy.

Recommendation: IV heparin should be started as soon as a diagnosis of intermediate- or high-risk unstable angina is made (strength of evidence = A). The initial dose is 80 units/kg by IV bolus followed by a constant infusion of 18 units/kg/hr, maintaining the activated partial thromboplastin time at 1.5 to 2.5 times control.

There is clear and compelling evidence that IV heparin started early in the course of unstable angina reduces the risk of subsequent MI and recurrent unstable angina.[15,16,18] The efficacy of aspirin and heparin in combination is suggested by their complementary mechanisms of action and demonstrated value in different phases of the disease, but this benefit has not been unequivocally demonstrated relative to monotherapy. Aspirin has been shown to provide benefits with an initial ED dose in patients who are later confirmed to have AMI.[14] Aspirin may also prevent reactivation of acute ischemic heart disease when heparin therapy is discontinued later in the hospital course.[21] Finally, aspirin has demonstrated efficacy in long-term secondary prevention.[20] Heparin, on the other hand, is the most

efficacious agent available to reduce early in-hospital ischemic events.[15] Thus, the combination of the two agents for initial therapy in unstable angina is strongly recommended.

Recommendation: High-risk unstable angina patients should be admitted to an ICU whenever possible (strength of evidence = B). Intermediate-risk unstable angina patients should be admitted to an ICU or a monitored cardiac bed (strength of evidence = C). Low-risk unstable angina patients may be managed as outpatients with planned early follow-up evaluations (strength of evidence = C).

OUTPATIENT CARE

Patients with unstable angina who are judged in the initial evaluation and treatment phase to be at low risk for adverse outcomes can, in many cases, be safely evaluated further as outpatients. Typically, these are patients who have experienced new-onset or worsening symptoms that may be caused by ischemia, but they have not had severe, prolonged, or rest episodes in the preceding 2 weeks. Follow-up from the initial evaluation should occur as soon as possible but generally within 72 hours. In patients without known CAD, the three goals of outpatient care are to assess the cause of the patient's symptoms further, to evaluate the risk of future adverse cardiac events, and to provide adequate symptom relief.

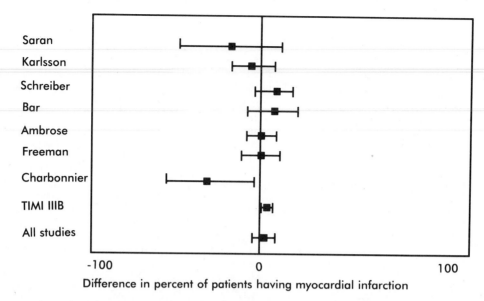

Difference in percent of patients having myocardial infarction

Fig. 41-2. Overview of effect of thrombolytic agents on progression to AMI in patients presenting with unstable angina. (Data from Saran, Bhandari, Narain et al, 1990; Karlsson, Berglund, Bjorkholm et al, 1992; Screiber, Rizik, White et al, 1992; Bar, Verheught, Col et al, 1992; Ambrose, Torre, Sharma et al, 1992; Freeman, Langer, Wilson et al, 1992; Charbonnier, Bernadet, Schiele et al, 1992; TIMI-IIIB [in press].)

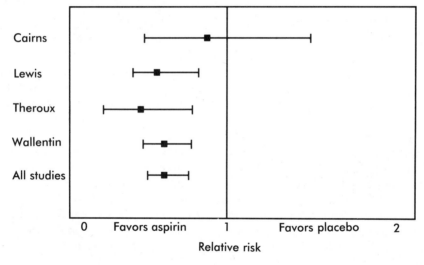

Relative risk

Fig. 41-3. Overview of effect of aspirin vs. placebo on relative risk of death or MI in unstable angina.

In patients with known CAD, the primary concern is whether to intensify medical therapy or to consider PTCA or CABG.

All patients should have a history, physical examination, and ECG. Any evidence of a worsening symptom pattern may necessitate hospital admission for control and further diagnostic workup. Evaluation should also include a search for factors that might precipitate or exacerbate unstable angina, such as fever, tachyarrhythmias, hyperthyroidism, severe anemia, cocaine use, noncompliance with medical therapy, environmental

temperature extremes, severe psychosocial stress, and changes in the level of physical exertion or life-style.

Recommendation: Exercise or pharmacologic stress testing generally should be part of the detailed outpatient workup. However, patients found to have high-risk features (see Table 41-4), such as evidence of significant LV dysfunction or an interval acceleration or worsening of symptoms while on appropriate levels of medical therapy, should be considered for direct referral to cardiac catheterization. In addition, patients who have symptoms that are very unlikely to be caused by CAD or

those who are felt to be at very low risk for cardiac events can be managed conservatively, with stress testing reserved for recurrent or worsening symptoms (strength of evidence = C).

Patients who have a low likelihood of CAD and are at low risk may benefit by further evaluation that may include a trial of nitrates and/or beta blockers. Use of noninvasive testing in this population should be delayed until the clinical presentation is more clear, to avoid the anxiety and cost associated with the false-positive test results that are common in this low-risk population. In general, intermediate-risk patients and low-risk patients with an intermediate or high likelihood of CAD benefit from noninvasive testing.

Recommendation: Medical therapy for presumed CAD usually begins with sublingual nitroglycerin, followed by oral beta blockers. Long-acting topical or oral nitrates may be added, but care should be taken to use regimens that reduce the likelihood of tolerance. In general, for low-risk outpatients, therapy with aspirin and one antianginal medication is sufficient initial treatment unless patients have additional indications for multiagent therapy (e.g., hypertension, supraventricular arrhythmia; strength of evidence = C). Long-acting forms of antianginal drugs are preferable to enhance patient compliance (strength of evidence = C).

Recommendation: Patients with established CAD who are already on medical therapy should have their medical regimen reviewed and dosages increased as appropriate and as tolerated (strength of evidence = C).

Recommendation: Patients who continue to report symptoms that they think reflect cardiac disease and are not reassured that they do not have CAD by appropriate noninvasive tests, counseling, and rehabilitation may be candidates for cardiac catheterization to confirm the absence of CAD (strength of evidence = C).

Recommendation: Patients with established CAD or those who are judged to be at intermediate- or high-risk for CAD should be maintained on aspirin at 80 to 324 mg per day unless contraindications are present (strength of evidence = A).

Generally one clinic visit should be sufficient to establish a working diagnosis, assess risk, and develop a management plan. Serial outpatient evaluation and noninvasive testing may be required, depending on the patient's specific findings and response to treatment. Patients with specific indications may be referred for outpatient or inpatient cardiac catheterization.

INTENSIVE MEDICAL MANAGEMENT
Medical therapy

Intensive medical treatment should begin immediately in the emergency department for patients at high or intermediate risk of death or nonfatal MI (See Table 41-4). For high-risk patients, such as those with ongoing

angina at rest and/or those who appear unstable, simultaneous evaluation and treatment assume an urgency greater than for intermediate-risk patients, such as those with prior discomfort who are asymptomatic during the initial evaluation period. Two of the major goals of this phase of care are to relieve pain and ischemia and to plan a definitive treatment strategy for the underlying disease process. A few patients will require prompt triage to emergency or urgent cardiac catheterization and/or placement of an IABP. However, most patients usually stabilize after a brief period of intensive pharmacologic management.

Recommendation: Patients whose symptoms are not fully relieved with three sublingual nitroglycerin tablets and initiation of beta-blocker therapy (when possible), as well as all nonhypertensive high-risk unstable angina patients, may benefit from IV nitroglycerin, and such therapy is recommended in the absence of contraindications. Intravenous nitroglycerin should be started at a dose of 5 to 10 μg/min by continuous infusion and titrated up by 10 μg/min every 5 to 10 minutes until relief of symptoms or limiting side effects (headache or hypotension with SBP < 90 mm Hg or more than 30% below starting mean arterial pressure levels if significant hypertension is present; strength of evidence = B). Topical, oral, or buccal nitrates are acceptable alternatives for patients without ongoing or refractory symptoms (strength of evidence = B).

Recommendation: Patients on IV nitroglycerin should be started on oral or topical nitrate therapy once they have been free of symptoms for 24 hours (strength of evidence = C). Tolerance to nitrates is dose- and duration-dependent and typically becomes significant only after 24 hours of continuous therapy. Responsiveness to nitrates can be restored by increasing the dose or switching the patient to a nonparenteral form of therapy and using a nitrate-free interval. As long as the patient's symptoms are not adequately controlled, the former option should be selected. Topical, oral, or buccal nitrates should be given with a 6- to 8-hour nitrate-free interval (strength of evidence = C).

Most studies of IV nitroglycerin in unstable angina have been small and uncontrolled. There are no randomized placebo-controlled trials that address either the efficacy of the drug in symptom relief or reduction of cardiac events for unstable angina. Pooled analysis of studies of nitroglycerin in patients with AMI from the prethrombolytic era suggested a 35% reduction in mortality.[22] However, the recently completed ISIS-4 and GISSI-3 trials in AMI patients receiving thrombolytic therapy failed to confirm this benefit.[23] Thus, the rationale for the use of this agent in unstable angina is extrapolated from pathophysiologic principles, uncontrolled studies of efficacy, and clinical experience.[24-26] There are no data that define the proper timing of initiation of therapy or its useful duration.

Recommendation: IV (for high-risk patients) or oral (for intermediate- and low-risk patients) beta blockers should be started in the absence of contraindications (strength of evidence = B).

Recommendation: Choice of the specific beta-blocking agent is not as important as ensuring that appropriate candidates receive this therapy. If there are concerns about patient intolerance because of existing pulmonary disease, especially asthma, LV dysfunction, or risk of hypotension or severe bradycardia, initial selection should favor a short-acting agent, such as propranolol or metoprolol, or the ultra-short-acting agent, esmolol. Mild wheezing or a history of COPD should prompt a trial of a short-acting agent at a reduced dose (e.g., 2.5 mg IV metoprolol, 12.5 mg oral metoprolol, or 25 μg/kg/min esmolol as initial doses) rather than complete avoidance of beta-blocker therapy (strength of evidence = C).

Initial studies of beta-blocker benefits in acute ischemic heart disease were small and uncontrolled. Metaanalysis of the available trials indicates a 13% reduction in risk of progression to AMI.[27] No clear effects on mortality in unstable angina have been shown to date. However, randomized trials in AMI, recent MI, and stable angina with silent ischemia have all shown a mortality benefit for beta blockers.[28] Thus, the overall rationale for the use of beta blockers is compelling enough to make them a routine part of care for patients with unstable angina in the absence of contraindications. The choice of beta blocker for an individual patient is based primarily on pharmacokinetic and side-effect criteria. There is no evidence that any member of this class of agents is more effective in producing beneficial effects in unstable angina than any other. The duration of benefits with long-term oral therapy is uncertain but appears, according to the AMI literature, to last for at least 5 years.

Recommendation: Calcium channel blockers may be used to control ongoing or recurrent ischemic symptoms in patients already on adequate doses of nitrates and beta blockers, in patients unable to tolerate adequate doses of one or both of these agents, or in patients with variant angina (strength of evidence = B). Calcium channel blockers should be avoided in patients with pulmonary edema or evidence of LV dysfunction (strength of evidence = B). Nifedipine should not be used in the absence of concurrent beta blockade (strength of evidence = A).

There are several small randomized trials involving the use of a calcium-channel blocker in unstable angina.[29-31] Generally, their efficacy in relieving symptoms appears to be equivalent to that of beta blockers.[32] A metaanalysis of the effects of calcium channel blockers on death or nonfatal MI in unstable angina showed no

effect.[33] Thus, evidence for the beneficial effects of calcium channel blockers in unstable angina is predominantly limited to control of symptoms.

Recommendation: Aspirin, once per day at a dose of 80 to 324 mg, should be continued indefinitely following presentation with unstable angina (strength of evidence = A).

The benefits of aspirin appear to be sustained when therapy is continued for 1 to 2 years following the initial presentation with unstable angina. Longer-term follow-up data in this particular population are lacking, but given the relatively short-term prognostic impact of unstable angina in coronary disease patients, long-term efficacy can be extrapolated from other studies of aspirin therapy in coronary disease.

Recommendation: Heparin infusion should be continued for 2 to 5 days or until revascularization is performed (strength of evidence = C).

Initial heparin dosage is 80 units/kg bolus and IV infusion of 18 units/kg/hr.[34] An aPTT is obtained 6 hours after beginning infusion, with the goal of keeping the aPTT between 46 and 70 seconds or approximately 1.5 to 2.5 times control. For hospitals with a mean control aPTT value of about 30 seconds, heparin dosage can be adjusted as shown in Table 41-6. An aPTT should be obtained 6 hours after any dosage change and used to adjust heparin infusion until the aPTT is therapeutic (1.5 to 2.5 times control). When two consecutive aPTTs are therapeutic, an aPTT may be ordered and heparin adjusted every 24 hours. In addition, significant change in the patient's clinical condition (e.g., recurrent definite ischemia, bleeding, hypotension) should prompt an immediate aPTT determination.

Serial hemoglobin/hematocrit and platelet measurements are recommended at least daily for the first 3 days of heparin therapy. In addition, any clinically significant bleeding, recurrent symptoms, or hemodynamic instability should prompt an immediate determination. Serial platelet counts are necessary to monitor for heparin-induced thrombocytopenia. Mild thrombocytopenia may occur in 10% to 20% of patients receiving heparin and usually appears in the first 1 to 3 days of therapy; severe thrombocytopenia (platelet count < 100,000) occurs in 1% to 2% of patients and typically appears after 3 to 5 days of therapy. A rare complication (probably less than 0.2% incidence) is heparin-induced thrombocytopenia with thrombosis. A high clinical suspicion for this syndrome mandates immediate cessation of all heparin therapy (including that used to flush IV lines) pending further evaluation.

Most of the trials evaluating the use of heparin in unstable angina have continued therapy for ≥5 days. The efficacy of shorter infusion regimens thus remains undefined. Evaluation of data from the Montreal Heart Institute randomized trial of heparin and aspirin showed a significantly increased reactivation rate after with-

Table 41-6. Heparin dose adjustment algorithm

For an:	Make the following dose adjustment:
aPTT <35	80 unit/kg bolus, increase drip 4 units/kg/hour
aPTT 35-45	40 unit/kg bolus, increase drip 2 units/kg/hour
aPTT 46-70	no change
aPTT 71-90	reduce drip 2 units/kg/hour
aPTT >90	hold heparin for 1 hour, reduce drip 3 units/kg/hour

drawal of the study drug with heparin alone.[21] The combination of heparin and aspirin appears to mitigate this increase, although even with aspirin there is hematologic evidence of increased thrombin activity after cessation of IV heparin.

Laboratory testing

Recommendation: Total CK and CK-MB should be measured every 6 to 8 hours for the first 24 hours after admission (strength of evidence = B).

Standard criteria for diagnosis of AMI are based on demonstrating elevation and subsequent decline of creatine kinase (CK) levels, along with evolutionary changes on serial 12-lead ECGs. CK-MB, the most sensitive and specific diagnostic marker for AMI, begins to rise within 6 hours of myocardial injury and levels peak at 10 to 18 hours. Total CK begins to rise at about 12 hours after symptom onset and peaks at 12 to 24 hours. Because of the rapid rise and clearance of CK-MB and total CK, timing of blood sampling is crucial in achieving maximal detection of AMI.[35] The literature is mixed, however, on the optimal sampling interval. After the admission sample, recommendations range from every 6 to every 12 hours for the first 24 hours. A sampling interval of every 6 to 8 hours is recommended to maximize sensitivity. Patients presenting more than 24 hours after symptom onset who have negative serial CK-MBs should have serial LDH isoenzyme determinations. Elevation of LDH_1 is usually seen within 12 to 24 hours of myocardial necrosis and may fall to nondiagnostic levels by 72 hours. Although there are several new and encouraging laboratory tests for myocardial injury on the horizon (e.g., troponin T, myoglobin), so far none have documented sufficient efficacy to be included in the guideline.

Recommendation: A follow-up ECG should be obtained 24 hours after admission and whenever the patient has recurrent symptoms or a change in clinical status (strength of evidence = C).

Serial ECGs are performed in unstable angina to detect the evolutionary changes of AMI, transient and persistent ischemic complications, and disturbances of rhythm or conduction. In the absence of specific clinical indications the optimal sampling interval for ECGs is uncertain. New data from continuous ST-segment monitoring show much more dynamic activity of the ST segment in unstable angina patients than had been previously appreciated (see Chapter 37). Such patients may be in a tenuous equilibrium between coronary thrombus propagation and thrombolysis with resulting intermittent transient coronary occlusion, often in the absence of symptoms. The therapeutic implications of these findings are still unclear. Furthermore, continuous ST segment monitoring is not widely available at present. Thus the panel recommends that after the admission ECG, repeat ECGs should be obtained at 24 hours and then at 48 hours. In addition, a repeat ECG should be obtained whenever the patient's clinical condition changes (e.g., recurrent symptoms, hypotension, arrhythmia, pulmonary edema).

Assessment of efficacy of initial medical therapy

Recommendation: The goal of intensive medical therapy for unstable angina is to institute a regimen in which patients receive daily aspirin (80 to 324 mg) and IV heparin (adjusted to maintain an aPTT value of 1.5 to 2.5 times control) plus nitrates and beta blockers (with a resting heart rate ≤ 60 beats per minute). Calcium channel blockers may be added in the subset of patients with significant hypertension (systolic blood pressure ≥ 150 mm Hg), patients who have refractory ischemia on beta blockers, and in patients with variant angina. Recurrent symptoms after the initial hemodynamic goals of therapy have been achieved may be regarded as a failure of medical therapy and should prompt consideration of urgent cardiac catheterization (strength of evidence = C).

During the early treatment of unstable angina, patients are started on an initial medical regimen, with serial reassessments to determine the success of therapy and the occurrence of significant complications. During the initial hours of therapy, medications are titrated up to their target doses as permitted by the patient's hemodynamic state and general medical condition. Before the target regimen is achieved, the patient may have recurrent symptoms requiring the physician to consider whether a change in course (such as emergency catheterization) would be appropriate. In addition, once a desired level of medical therapy has been reached, recurrent symptoms may indicate a need for a still more intensive regimen or for triage to early cardiac catheterization.

The optimal level of medical therapy for the unstable angina patient has not yet been established. Two general approaches have been proposed to define adequate medical therapy. The first defines adequate medical therapy as maximally tolerated doses of nitrates, beta blockers, and calcium-channel blockers plus aspirin and heparin. The implication of this definition is that failure of medical therapy cannot be declared until each drug has been increased up to the limiting levels so that any further increment would cause hemodynamic deterioration or toxicity. The second approach is to define adequate medical therapy by arbitrary levels of each of the key therapeutic agents. This is the approach that has been adopted in the above recommendation.

Because achievement of steady-state medication effects may require 24 hours or more even with parenteral administration, some criteria for adequate medical therapy also specify a minimum duration such therapy should be continued before the patient is referred for invasive study. Intensive medical treatment for unstable angina is usually very effective. In one recent study only 2% of patients admitted with unstable angina were found to be truly refractory to medical therapy.[36] For this guideline a patient will not be said to have failed (or to be "refractory") to medical therapy until he or she is receiving aspirin (≥ 80 mg/day) and IV heparin with an aPTT of 1.5 to 2.5 times control. In addition, in the absence of limiting symptoms, IV NTG should be infused at ≥ 50 μg/min (or topical NTG at ≥ 1 inch of ointment every 6 hours for three doses, followed by a 6 to 8 hour nitrate-free interval or an equivalent regimen of oral or buccal nitrates). Beta blockers should be used to keep the resting heart rate at an average of ≤ 60 beats/minute. Significant hypertension (i.e., resting SBP ≥ 150 mm Hg) resistant to first-line medical therapy is an indication for addition of calcium-channel blockers. Although it is theoretically desirable to have this regimen in place for ≥ 24 hours before declaring any patient a failure of medical therapy, to do so in all cases may be inappropriate or even dangerous. In particular, patients who have one or more recurrent, severe, prolonged (>20 minutes) ischemic episodes, particularly when accompanied by pulmonary edema, a new or worsening MR murmur, hypotension, or new ST- or T-wave changes should be considered high risk, regardless of the level of medical therapy, and triaged to early cardiac catheterization. Patients with shorter, less severe ischemic episodes without accompanying hemodynamic or ECG changes are at substantially lower risk and should be continued on medical therapy to the prespecified targets.

Evaluation and management of early ischemic complications

The major ischemic complications seen in unstable angina are AMI, recurrent unstable angina, acute ischemic pulmonary edema, new or worsening MR, cardiogenic shock, malignant ventricular arrhythmias, and advanced AV block. Aside from maximizing the medical regimen described in the previous section and instituting appropriate adjunctive therapy (e.g., pulmonary artery pressure monitoring and inotropic therapy for shock, antiarrhythmic therapy for malignant ventricular arrhythmias, pacemaker therapy for symptomatic high-grade block), the clinician should consider insertion of an intraaortic balloon pump (IABP), cardiac catheterization, or both in a patient who develops major ischemic complications.

Intraaortic balloon pumping

Recommendation: An IABP should be considered in unstable angina patients who have symptoms refractory to aggressive medical management or hemodynamic instability if emergency cardiac catheterization is not possible or as a bridge to stabilize the patient on the way to the catheterization laboratory or the operating room (strength of evidence = B). Exceptions to this recommendation are made for patients with severe peripheral vascular disease, significant aortic insufficiency, or known severe aortal-iliac disease, including aortic aneurysm (strength of evidence = C). Placement of an IABP for stabilization may precede or follow diagnostic catheterization depending on specific circumstances, such as the anticipated delay for alternate approaches and level of expertise available in the immediate care environment (strength of evidence = C).

Recommendation: Patients not stabilized after placement of an IABP should be reevaluated to ensure proper functioning of the device and to reaffirm that the most likely diagnosis remains unstable angina. If so, emergency catheterization should be considered (strength of evidence = B).

Intraaortic balloon pump counterpulsation is a method of providing temporary circulatory assistance in the form of reduced afterload and increased coronary perfusion pressure. A balloon catheter is placed percutaneously via the femoral artery and positioned in the descending thoracic aorta with the tip of the catheter several centimeters distal to the left subclavian artery. The device is synchronized with the ECG or arterial pulse tracing so that the balloon is rapidly inflated during diastole (after closure of the aortic valve) with an inert gas (helium) and rapidly deflated just before the onset of systole (and opening of the aortic valve). The IABP produces a significant reduction in afterload, with a consequent reduction in myocardial work and oxygen demand. It also increases the cardiac output by a modest amount (usually 10% to 20%, depending on the extent of LV dysfunction). Finally, the IABP increases thoracic aortic diastolic pressure, with a consequent increase in coronary perfusion pressure. Whether this latter effect increases coronary blood flow distal to a critical coronary stenosis or decreases the likelihood of early progression to complete coronary occlusion remains controversial.

Because patients entering the initial intensive management phase of unstable angina represent the highest risk subgroup, the need for IABP in this subgroup is anticipated to be in the range of 3%. The IABP almost always stabilizes patients with severe myocardial ischemia and causes an almost immediate and dramatic relief of pain and ECG changes.[37] Therefore the persistence of continued symptoms after introduction of the IABP suggests that unstable angina is not solely responsible for the presenting condition; the patient should be evaluated further as mandated by signs or symptoms of other primary or associated diagnoses.

There are no randomized trials of IABP use in unstable angina. Uncontrolled series suggest that it is a very effective short-term method of stabilizing a patient with the unstable angina.[38] In experienced centers approximately 10% to 15% of patients will develop vascular complications with prolonged use of balloon pumps, often compromising distal limb blood flow.[39] For this reason patients receiving an IABP should be maintained on full-dose IV heparin with serial monitoring of aPTT unless contraindications to heparin therapy exist. About half of all ischemic leg complications are reversed by pump removal; many of the remainder require an embolectomy procedure. Because of the complications associated with the use of IABP, it should be attempted only in centers that have clinicians who are experienced in the placement of the device and have access to emergency vascular surgery support should it be required.

Emergency/urgent cardiac catheterization

Recommendation: If chest discomfort with objective evidence of ischemia persists for ≥ 1 hour after aggressive medical therapy, triage to emergency cardiac catheterization should be strongly considered (strength of evidence = B).

Recommendation: Urgent cardiac catheterization should be considered in patients with unstable angina who have recurrent ischemic episodes despite appropriate medical therapy or those who have high-risk unstable angina (strength of evidence = B).

Recommendation: Acute revascularization is indicated for patients with refractory pain (≥ 1 hour on aggressive medical therapy) who are found at catheterization to have an acutely occluded major coronary vessel, severe subtotal occlusion of a culprit vessel, or severe multivessel disease with impaired LV function (strength of evidence = B).

In this guideline emergency cardiac catheterization refers to a diagnostic catheterization study that is performed immediately or as soon as possible (i.e., < 6 hours) after the precipitating event. Urgent catheterization is performed because of less severe precipitating events or because the patient exhibits features of high-risk unstable angina (see Table 41-4). Urgent cardiac catheterization is usually performed within 24 hours of presentation of the precipitating event. Elective catheterization, which is discussed later in this chapter, is used to describe all diagnostic catheterization procedures that do not meet the above criteria.

Because catheterization is a diagnostic procedure, it provides health benefits only when it yields information that can be used to plan and execute effective therapies. Thus its utility is closely related to subsequent decisions about triage for revascularization.

Preparation for nonintensive phase

Recommendation: Patients who become asymptomatic should be progressively mobilized and instructed to notify their health care team if mobilization causes recurrent symptoms (strength of evidence = C).

Recommendation: If parenteral nitrate and beta-blocker therapy was required initially, such regimens can be converted to nonparenteral regimens after the patient has been stable and painfree for at least 24 hours (strength of evidence = C).

The large majority of patients with unstable angina will stabilize and become painfree with appropriate intensive medical therapy. Transfer from intensive to nonintensive medical management is undertaken when the patient is hemodynamically stable (including no uncompensated CHF) and ischemia has been successfully suppressed for ≥ 24 hours. Once these criteria are satisfied, any parenteral medicines can be converted to nonparenteral regimens in preparation for this transfer. Heparin use should be reassessed after 24 hours and may be discontinued in selected patients, such as those who are found to have a clearly identified secondary cause for unstable angina (e.g., anemia). Aspirin is continued without interruption. Typically, most high-risk unstable angina patients can be stabilized within 24 to 48 hours of admission to the ICU. Some unstable patients will progress to AMI, and others will require urgent cardiac catheterization, PTCA, or CABG. However, the majority of patients will rapidly become asymptomatic on aggressive medical therapy.

NONINTENSIVE MEDICAL MANAGEMENT

All high-risk and some intermediate-risk unstable angina patients will be moved to the nonintensive phase of management after 1 or more days of intensive management and stabilization. Some of these latter patients will have undergone cardiac catheterization, and some will also have had one or more revascularization procedures. Other intermediate-risk unstable angina patients initially may be admitted to a monitored intermediate care unit until the diagnosis of MI can be excluded and it is clear that the patients' symptoms are adequately controlled on medical therapy. These patients then enter the nonintensive phase of management. Still other intermediate-risk and some low-risk patients may be admitted directly to a regular hospital bed with telemetry capabilities, thereby proceeding directly to the nonintensive phase.

Transfer out of the intensive care phase is an important indicator that the patient has progressed to a lower risk state. At this point emphasis shifts from acute stabilization to design of a maintenance medical regimen that will suppress reactivation of acute disease activity. In addition, a major focus is placed on risk stratification with primary goals of assessing the future risk of adverse cardiac events, the sufficiency of medical therapy in controlling symptoms, and the need for diagnostic cardiac catheterization and revascularization. By this point in the hospital course, most patients with AMI have been identified; their subsequent management is outside the scope of the Unstable Angina Guideline, but is discussed in other sections of this book.

Continuous ECG monitoring at this phase is generally unnecessary. All patients should be instructed to notify nursing personnel immediately if chest discomfort recurs. Recurrent ischemic episodes should prompt a brief nursing assessment, an emergency ECG, and generally should be brought to the attention of a physician. The patient's medical regimen should be reevaluated, and doses of antiischemic agents should be increased as tolerated. Patients who have pain or ECG evidence of ischemia increasing in severity for greater than 20 minutes and unresponsive to NTG should be transferred to the intensive management phase protocol. Patients who respond to sublingual NTG do not need to be transferred. However, a second recurrence of chest pain of at least 20 minutes duration in the setting of appropriate medical therapy should prompt the return of the patient to a monitored environment and the initiation of the management steps outlined in the intensive management phase (p. 511).

In general, patients reaching this phase would be referred within 1 to 2 days either for noninvasive functional testing or for cardiac catheterization. Patients can be considered ready for discharge from the hospital when their evaluation is complete and an appropriate outpatient therapeutic regimen has been established.

Steps to move the patient toward readiness for hospital discharge should be initiated during this phase. These steps include instruction on home diet and exercise, physical activity, resumption of sexual relations, return to work, and resumption of driving and other usual activities. In addition, detailed discussion should be conducted with the patient, his or her family, and the patient's advocate to review the events since presentation and their significance, the patient's current status, the major diagnostic and therapeutic options, and the patient's general prognosis. The slower pace of this phase of the patient's hospitalization, in contrast to the early stabilization and intensive care phases, offers the most appropriate time for CAD education.

Recommendation: In this phase, the patient and his or her family should begin to work toward risk-factor modification goals (strength of evidence = C).

NONINVASIVE TESTING

The entire process of managing patients with unstable angina requires ongoing risk stratification. Much prognostic information of value can be derived from the initial assessment and the patient's subsequent course over the first few days of management. In many cases noninvasive stress testing provides a useful supplement to these clinically based risk assessments.

However, some patients, such as those with rest angina and ECG-documented ischemia, have such a high likelihood of CAD and high risk of adverse events that noninvasive risk stratification would not be likely to identify a subgroup with sufficiently low risk to merit noninterventional strategies. Other patients are not willing to consider interventional treatment because they have severe complicating illnesses or are of advanced age so that referral for cardiac catheterization would not be reasonable. Still other patients may be felt to have a very low likelihood of CAD after their initial complete evaluation, with an associated risk of cardiac events so low that even a positive test would not merit referral for catheterization. Any patients who do not fall into one of the above exception categories are reasonable candidates for risk stratification by noninvasive testing.

The goals of noninvasive testing in a patient with unstable angina who has recently been stabilized are to estimate the subsequent prognosis, especially for the next 3 to 6 months, to decide what additional testing and adjustments in therapy are required based on this prognosis, and to provide the patient with the information and reassurances necessary to return to a life-style that is as full and productive as possible.

Selection of noninvasive tests

Recommendation: Exercise or pharmacologic stress testing should generally be an integral part of the outpatient evaluation of low-risk patients with unstable angina. In most cases testing should be done within 72 hours of presentation (strength of evidence = B).

Recommendation: Unless cardiac catheterization is indicated, noninvasive exercise or pharmacologic stress testing should be performed in low- or intermediate-risk patients (see Table 41-3) hospitalized with unstable angina who have been free of angina and CHF for a minimum of 48 hours (strength of evidence = B).

Recommendation: Choice of initial stress testing modality should be based on an evaluation of the patient's resting ECG, his or her physical ability to perform exercise, and on the local expertise and technologies available. In general, the exercise treadmill test should be the standard mode of stress testing used in patients with a normal ECG who are not taking digoxin. Patients with widespread resting ST depression (≥ 1 mm), ST changes secondary to digoxin, LV hypertrophy, LBBB/significant intraventricular conduction deficit (IVCD), or preexcitation usually should be tested using an imaging modality. Patients unable to exercise because of physical limitations (e.g., arthritis, amputation, severe peripheral vascular disease, severe COPD, general

debility) should undergo pharmacologic stress testing in combination with an imaging modality (strength of evidence = B).

Recommendation: Choice among the different imaging modalities that can be used with exercise or pharmacologic stress testing should be based primarily on the local expertise available to perform and interpret the study (strength of evidence = C).

Noninvasive "functional" testing or stress testing refers to a series of provocative tests that use either exercise or pharmacologic means to detect ischemia or inhomogeneity in myocardial blood flow because of obstructive CAD. The exercise tests are based on the principle of using a progressive physiologic stress (usually treadmill or bicycle exercise) to increase myocardial work and oxygen demand while using some method (ECG, function, perfusion) to document objective evidence of ischemia. Provocation of ischemia at a low workload (e.g., <5 to 6 metabolic equivalents [METS]) signifies a high-risk patient who would generally merit referral to cardiac catheterization. On the other hand, attainment of a higher workload (e.g., ≥5 to 6 METS) without ischemia is associated with a better prognosis, and many such patients can be safely managed conservatively. Other patients, including those who tolerate only a low workload but have no evident ischemia or those who develop ischemia at a high workload, represent an intermediate-risk group for whom several reasonable strategies can be proposed.

In low-risk patients it is unclear whether an imaging modality adds importantly to a standard treadmill test. Thus, the selection of which test to use with an individual patient should be based primarily on patient characteristics, knowledge of local availability, and interpretation expertise. Because of simplicity, lower costs, and widespread familiarity with performance and interpretation, the standard ECG treadmill is the most reasonable test to select in patients able to exercise who have a normal resting ECG. Patients with an abnormal baseline ECG that would interfere with interpretation of the exercise results should have an imaging modality added to their test; patients unable to exercise should have a pharmacologic stress test.

The optimal testing strategy in women remains less well defined than in men. All major forms of exercise testing have been reported to be less accurate for diagnosis in women. At least a portion of the lower reported accuracy derives from a lower pretest likelihood of CAD in populations of women compared with men. The relative accuracy of noninvasive testing for prognosis in women and men has not been studied adequately. Until data are reported to clarify this issue, it is reasonable to use noninvasive testing for prognosis in women as freely as in men, with proper consideration of the influence of gender on the pretest likelihood of CAD.

Use of noninvasive test results in patient management

Recommendation: Patients with a low-risk exercise test result (predicted average annual cardiac mortality <1%/year) can be managed medically without need for referral to cardiac catheterization (strength of evidence = B).

Recommendation: Patients with a high-risk exercise test result (predicted average annual cardiac mortality ≥4%/year) should be referred for prompt cardiac catheterization (strength of evidence = B).

Recommendation: Patients with intermediate-risk exercise test results (predicted average annual cardiac mortality 2% to 3%/year) should be referred for additional testing, either cardiac catheterization or an (alternative) exercise imaging study (strength of evidence = C).

Recommendation: A stress test result of intermediate risk combined with evidence of LV dysfunction should prompt referral to cardiac catheterization (strength of evidence = C).

Noninvasive tests are most useful in patient management decisions when risk can be stated in terms of the probability of adverse cardiac events over time. A large population of patients must be studied to derive and test equations needed to predict risks for individual patients accurately. No noninvasive study has been reported in a sufficient number of patients after stabilization of unstable angina to develop and test the accuracy of a multivariable equation to report test results in terms of absolute risk. Therefore, data borrowed from studies of patients with stable angina must be used if risk is to be reported as events over time. Although the pathologic process evoking ischemia may be different in the two subgroups, it is likely that the use of prognostic nomograms derived on groups of patients with stable angina would also be predictive of risk in patients with recent unstable angina after stabilization. Using this untested assumption, the much larger literature derived from populations that include patients with both stable and unstable angina provides equations for risk stratification that converts physiologic changes observed during noninvasive testing into statements of risk expressed as events over time. One such nomogram, developed on a predominantly stable angina population, was included in the Unstable Angina Guidelines[40] (Fig. 41-4).

CARDIAC CATHETERIZATION AND MYOCARDIAL REVASCULARIZATION

The goal of cardiac catheterization in patients with unstable angina is to provide detailed structural information necessary to assess prognosis and to select an appropriate long-term management strategy. The procedure is usually helpful in choosing between medical therapy, percutaneous transluminal coronary angio-

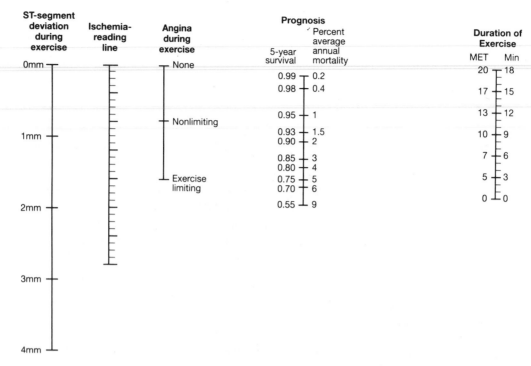

Fig. 41-4. Prognostic exercise treadmill score. Determination of prognosis proceeds in five steps. First, the observed amount of exercise-induced ST-segment deviation (the largest elevation or depression after resting changes have been subtracted) is marked on the line for ST-segment deviation during exercise. Second, the observed degree of angina during exercise is marked on the line for angina. Third, the marks for the ST-segment deviation and degree of angina are connected with a straight edge. The point where this line intersects the ischemia-reading line is noted. Fourth, the total number of minutes of exercise in treadmill testing according to the Bruce protocol (or equivalent in multiples of resting oxygen consumption [METs] from an alternative protocol) is marked on the exercise-duration line. Fifth, the mark for ischemia is connected with that for exercise duration. The point at which this line intersects the line for prognosis indicates the 5-year survival rate and the average annual mortality with these characteristics. (From Mark DB, Shaw L, Harrell FE et al, Prognostic value of a treadmill exercise score in outpatients with suspected coronary artery disease, *N Engl J Med* 325:849-853, 1991.)

plasty (PTCA), and coronary artery bypass graft surgery (CABG) in patients at significant risk for future events.

Patients come to cardiac catheterization for several indications that may develop at any time during the initial hospitalization for unstable angina. Cardiac catheterization is usually indicated in patients who fail to stabilize with medical therapy or who have breakthrough symptoms despite adequate medical therapy and high-risk patients categorized by other clinical findings or noninvasive testing. Other possible indications for catheterization include significant CHF, malignant ventricular arrythmias, significant LV dysfunction or a large perfusion detected by noninvasive study, or physical examination or echocardiographic evidence of significant MR, aortic stenosis, or hypertrophic cardiomyopathy. Finally, patients in an intermediate- or high-risk category with previous PTCA or CABG should generally be considered for cardiac catheterization, unless prior catheterization data indicate that no further revascularization is likely to be technically possible.

In all cases the general indications for catheterization and revascularization are tempered by individual patient characteristics and preferences. In the very frail elderly and those with serious comorbid conditions, patient and physician judgments about risks and benefits are particularly important.

Cardiac catheterization

This guideline proposes two alternative definitive treatment strategies termed *early invasive* and *early conservative*. Randomized trial data did not support the inherent superiority of either strategy based on medical outcomes.[11] The decision about which strategy to pursue for given patients should be based on the patient's estimated risk (See Table 41-4), available facilities, and patient preference. These strategies are defined below.

Recommendation: In the early invasive strategy, cardiac catheterization is performed routinely in all hospitalized patients who have no contraindications,

usually within 48 hours of presentation (strength of evidence = A).

Recommendation: In the early conservative strategy, cardiac catheterization is performed routinely in patients admitted to the hospital with unstable angina who are candidates for a revascularization procedure and have one or more of the following high-risk indicators: prior revascularization (PTCA or CABG), associated CHF or depressed LV function (EF < 0.50) by noninvasive study, malignant ventricular arrhythmia, persistent or recurrent pain/ischemia, and/or a functional study indicating high risk (strength of evidence = A).

Recommendation: Diagnostic catheterization should not be performed on patients with extensive comorbidity in whom the likely benefits of revascularization in terms of length and quality of life would not outweigh the risk (strength of evidence = B).

The proper role and timing of cardiac catheterization in unstable angina remains controversial. Diagnostic catheterization benefits patients primarily by enhancing the accuracy of prognostic stratification, which can be used to adjust medical therapy as well as to plan specific revascularization therapy. The population of patients with unstable angina admitted to the hospital includes a subgroup that should routinely receive catheterization and another subgroup for whom invasive study is optional and can be deferred pending further clinical developments. The group that should routinely receive catheterization consists of all high-risk patients (see Table 41-4) and intermediate-risk patients with a prior PTCA or CABG, patients with CHF or depressed LV function (i.e., EF < 0.50) by noninvasive study, and patients recognized to be high risk by noninvasive exercise or pharmacologic stress testing.

The principal data upon which these recommendations are based are the TIMI 3B results.[11] This study randomized 1473 patients with unstable angina requiring hospital admission for early (18 to 48 hours) invasive or early conservative strategies. At 42 days 15.5% of the early invasive patients had died, had a nonfatal MI, or had a positive 6-week exercise test vs. 17.7% of the early conservative patients ($P = .26$). Of the invasive group 97.7% of patients underwent diagnostic catheterization (as assigned) compared with 64% of the conservative group ($P < .001$). Revascularization by 42 days had been performed in 61% of the invasive group and 49% of the conservative group ($P < .001$). In addition, conservatively treated patients had a significantly higher use of antianginal medicines and more hospital readmissions by the 6-week follow-up.

Revascularization

Recommendation: Patients found at catheterization to have significant left main disease (≥50%) or significant (≥70%) three-vessel disease with depressed LV function (EF < 0.50) should be referred promptly for CABG surgery (strength of evidence = A).

Recommendation: Patients with two-vessel disease with proximal severe subtotal stenosis (≥95%) of the LAD and depressed LV function should be referred promptly for revascularization (strength of evidence = B for CABG; strength of evidence = C for PTCA).

Recommendation: Patients with significant CAD should be considered for prompt revascularization (PTCA or CABG) if they have any of the following: failure to stabilize with medical treatment; recurrent angina/ischemia at rest or with low-level activity; and/or ischemia accompanied by CHF symptoms, an S3 gallop, new or worsening MR, or definite ECG changes (strength of evidence = B).

Recommendation: For patients with significant CAD not included in the above recommendations, two strategies are possible: early invasive and early conservative. In the early invasive strategy, CABG or PTCA is performed. In the early conservative strategy, revascularization is performed only on patients who meet the criteria for failure of initial therapy necessitating cardiac catheterization. Medical therapy without revascularization is continued for patients without criteria for failure of therapy (strength of evidence = A).

Revascularization is used to improve prognosis, relieve symptoms, and improve functional capacity in patients with obstructive CAD. In general, the indications for revascularization in the patient with unstable angina who has been stabilized are the same as for the patient with stable angina, but the impetus for some form of revascularization is stronger than in the latter patient. Moreover, long-term survival rates after CABG are similar for unstable angina patients who present with rest angina, increasing angina, new-onset angina, or post-MI angina.[41]

CABG and PTCA are the two revascularization strategies available. Implicit in this guideline is the understanding that the initial selection of the revascularization mode will be modified or supplemented when necessitated by changes in the patient's condition. Thus, subsequent referrals of a PTCA patient to CABG surgery or of a CABG patient to PTCA (i.e., therapeutic crossovers) are integral parts of the initial treatment strategy. However, excessive crossover rates suggest inappropriate treatment selection, inadequate technical results, or both. In addition, although the percutaneous intervention strategy is referred to in this guideline as PTCA, it should be recognized that this term refers to a family of techniques including standard balloon angioplasty, perfusion balloon (prolonged dilation) angioplasty, atherectomy, laser angioplasty, and intracoronary stenting.

The TIMI 3B results comparing early invasive vs.

early conservative catheterization and revascularization have been described in the previous section. Two randomized trials compared medical and surgical therapy in unstable angina. The National Cooperative Study Group randomized 288 patients between 1972 and 1976 at nine academic centers.[42] The Veterans Administration Cooperative Study Group randomized 468 patients between 1976 and 1982 at 12 VA hospitals.[43-45] Both studies included patients with progressive or rest angina accompanied by ST and T-wave changes. Patients over age 70 or with a recent MI were excluded. The VA study included only men.

In the National Cooperative Study, hospital mortality was 3% for medicine and 5% for CABG ($P = NS$). Follow-up to 30 months failed to show any differences in survival between the therapies. In the VA study, survival to 2 years was the same for medicine and CABG overall and in subgroups defined by number of disease vessels. A post hoc analysis of patients with depressed LV function, however, showed a significant survival advantage with CABG surgery. All randomized trials of CABG vs. medicine (including those in stable angina) have found improved symptom relief and functional capacity with CABG. Long-term follow-up in these trials has suggested that by 10 years there is a significant attenuation of both symptom relief and survival benefits from CABG surgery. However, all these randomized trials reflect an earlier technical era for both CABG surgery and medicine. Improvements in anesthesia and surgical techniques, including internal mammary artery grafting to the LAD artery and improved intraoperative myocardial protection with cold potassium cardioplegia, are not reflected in these trials. Also, the routine use of heparin and aspirin in the acute phase and the range of therapeutic agents available represent significant differences in current practice from the era in which these trials were performed.

Three published and two unpublished randomized trials of PTCA have now been reported. The VA Angioplasty Compared With Medicine (ACME) trial tested PTCA vs. medicine in single-vessel disease and found improved functional status and quality of life at 6 months in the PTCA arm.[46] The RITA trial enrolled 1011 patients in the United Kingdom with one-, two-, or three-vessel disease that had equal chance of revascularization success with either PTCA or CABG.[47] Approximately 60% of the enrolled patients were reported to have angina at rest prior to randomization. An interim analysis at 2.5 years of follow-up show an equivalent rate of hard cardiac events (death, MI) and a much higher repeat revascularization rate in the PTCA arm. The German Angioplasty Bypass Surgery Investigation (GABI), which randomized 358 patients with multivessel CAD and ≥ class 2 angina to CABG or multivessel PTCA, recently reported that at 6-month follow-up the primary endpoint (angina rates) was similar and there was no significant difference in the rates of hard cardiac events (death, MI) between the CABG and PTCA groups. Initial results have recently been presented for the Coronary Artery Bypass Revascularization Investigation (CABRI) trial, involving 1054 CAD patients randomized to PTCA or CABG. The Emory Angioplasty vs. Surgery Trial (EAST) also reported outcomes in 392 patients with multivessel disease randomized between PTCA and CABG. The results of these two unpublished trials did not differ substantially from the results of the RITA trial.[48]

One large registry compared 5-year survival with medicine, PTCA, and CABG in 9263 CAD patients treated between 1984 and 1990.[49] In this nonrandomized comparison, extensive statistical adjustments were used to control for prognostically important baseline differences created by treatment selection. For patients with three-vessel disease or two-vessel disease with a proximal severe (≥ 95%) LAD stenosis, surgical survival at 5 years was significantly better than medicine, and a similar trend in favor of CABG was found in comparison with PTCA. In less severe two-vessel disease, revascularization improved survival relative to medicine, and there was a trend for PTCA to provide better survival results (because of lower procedural mortality) than CABG. In one-vessel disease all therapies were associated with high 5-year survival rates with very small differences among groups.

The available data can be used to formulate some general principles about the role of revascularization in unstable angina. The first general principle is that the more extensive the CAD, the larger the benefit in survival realized from revascularization.[50] In the most severe forms of CAD (e.g., left main disease, three-vessel disease), CABG provides the best long-term survival results. In intermediate forms of CAD (e.g., two-vessel disease), revascularization provides improved survival relative to medicine, although the absolute survival benefit is smaller than in three-vessel disease. In general, the patient with high-risk two-vessel disease (as defined by impaired LV function, older age, or coexisting vascular disease) will have improved survival with CABG surgery. For other two-vessel disease patients, PTCA may provide modest survival benefits relative to medicine. In the least severe CAD patients (i.e., one-vessel disease), observational data have shown good survival associated with medical therapy, PTCA, and CABG. The primary treatment choice is usually between medicine and PTCA, with CABG reserved for those patients with large areas of myocardium at risk, those who fail medical therapy, or those who are technically unsuitable for PTCA.

The second general principle is that survival benefits of revascularization are magnified on the absolute scale by factors that increase overall medical risk, especially LV dysfunction and advanced age. In particular, multivessel CAD benefits from CABG are substantially larger on an absolute scale in patients with depressed LV function. These factors also tend to increase the procedural risks of revascularization so that patients who have the most to gain from revascularization in the long run are also the ones who have the highest short-term risk from the procedure itself.[50,51]

HOSPITAL DISCHARGE AND POSTDISCHARGE CARE

The natural history of unstable angina is typically characterized by either progression to nonfatal MI or death on the one hand, or resumption of the more quiescent clinical course of chronic stable angina on the other. The acute phase of unstable angina is usually over within 8 weeks. The need for continued hospitalization of the unstable angina patient is determined by whether the in-patient objectives of that hospitalization have been achieved.

Patients who have undergone successful revascularization will usually have the remainder of their hospitalization defined by the standard protocol for the given procedure (e.g., 1 to 2 days for PTCA, 5 to 7 days for CABG). Patients electing medical treatment after a cardiac catheterization or functional study include both a low-risk group that can be discharged rapidly (e.g., 1 to 2 days after testing) and a high-risk group unsuitable for or unwilling to have coronary revascularization. These latter patients may require prolonged hospitalization to establish adequate (or as adequate as possible) symptom control and to ensure that the risk of cardiac events in the next 4 to 6 weeks has fallen to an acceptably low level.

The goal during the hospital discharge phase of care is to prepare the patient for normal activities outside the hospital, to the extent possible. The goal of the postdischarge outpatient-care phase is to make adjustments in the discharge regimen that appear most appropriate after an initial period away from direct patient care. The long-term management of the unstable angina patient ends as the patient reenters the stable phase of coronary artery disease.

Discharge medical regimen

Recommendation: Patients should continue on ASA, 80 to 324 mg per day, indefinitely after discharge (strength of evidence = B).

Recommendation: In general, the classes of medications necessary to achieve adequate symptom control should be continued after discharge. Patients with successful revascularization without recurrent ischemia do not require postdischarge antianginal therapy. Patients with unsuccessful revascularization or with recurrent symptoms following revascularization should be continued on the regimen required in hospital to control their symptoms (strength of evidence = C).

Recommendation: All patients with signs or symptoms suggesting ongoing ischemia should be given sublingual nitroglycerin and instructed in its use (strength of evidence = C).

In most cases the in-patient medical regimen used in the nonintensive phase of the illness will be continued postdischarge. The need for continued medical therapy after discharge relates to potential prognostic benefits (primarily shown for aspirin and beta blockers), control of symptoms (nitrates and calcium antagonists), and treatment of major risk factors such as hypertension, hyperlipidemia, and diabetes mellitus. Thus, selection of a medical regimen will be individualized to the specific needs of each patient and the events that have occurred in hospital.

Postdischarge follow-up

Recommendation: The plan for follow-up medical care should be made, whenever possible, at the time of discharge (strength of evidence = C). In general, low-risk patients and patients with successful CABG or PTCA should be seen in an outpatient facility at 2 to 6 weeks, and higher-risk patients should return in 1 to 2 weeks (strength of evidence = C).

Recommendation: Patients who have stable or no anginal symptoms at the follow-up outpatient visit should be managed further as for stable coronary artery disease (strength of evidence = C).

Recommendation: Specific instructions should be given on smoking cessation, daily exercise, and diet (strength of evidence = B). Where possible and appropriate, consideration should be given to referral to a smoking-cessation program or clinic and/or an outpatient cardiac rehabilitation program (strength of evidence = C).

Recommendation: Health care providers should initiate a conversation with the patient to discuss the safety and timing of the resumption of sexual activity (e.g., 2 weeks for low-risk patients to 4 weeks for post-CABG patients) (strength of evidence = C).

Recommendation: Beyond the instructions for daily exercise, patients require specific instruction on activities that are permissible and those that should be avoided (e.g., heavy lifting, climbing stairs, yard work, household activities). Specific mention should be made of resumption of driving and return to work (strength of evidence = C).

Recommendation: Because the hospital stay for unstable angina patients is often very short, it has been found that one way to increase patient compliance with the treatment regimen and risk factor modification program is to provide telephone follow-up (strength of evidence = B).

Where personnel and budget resources allow, the health care team may consider establishing a follow-up system in which nurses telephone patients approximately once a week for the first 4 weeks after discharge. This structured program would gauge the progress of the patient's recovery, reinforce the CAD education taught in hospital and in the postdischarge visit, address patient questions and concerns, and monitor progress in meeting risk factor behavior modification goals.

It is presently unclear whether patients who come through an episode of unstable angina without complications are at increased risk for future episodes of unstable angina, but the overall risk for death or MI is similar to that of other CAD patients with their characteristics who have not had unstable angina. The last element in the management of unstable angina therefore is the follow-up clinic visit at the point where the patient's disease activity has returned to the baseline level.

REFERENCES

1. Field MJ, Lohr KN (eds): Institute of Medicine—clinical practice guidelines: directions for a new program, Washington, DC, 1990, National Academy Press.
2. Braunwald E, Mark DB, Jones RH, et al: Unstable angina: diagnosis and management, *Clinical Practice Guideline Number 10, AHCPR Publication No. 94-0602*, Rockville, Md, March 1994, Agency for Health Care Policy and Research and the National Heart, Lung, and Blood Institute, Public Health Service, US Department of Health and Human Services.
3. Braunwald E: Unstable angina: a classification, *Circulation* 80(2): 410-414, 1989.
4. Campeau L: Grading of angina pectoris (letter), *Circulation* 54(3):522-523, 1976.
5. Goldman L, Cook EF, Brand DA, et al: A computer protocol to predict myocardial infarction in emergency department patients with chest pain, *N Engl J Med* 307:588-596, 1988.
6. Goldman L, Weinberg M, Weisberg M, et al: A computer-derived protocol to aid in the diagnosis of emergency room patients with acute chest pain, *N Engl J Med* 307:588-596, 1982.
7. Selker HP, Griffith JL, D'Agostino RB: A tool for judging coronary care unit admission appropriateness, valid for both real-time and retrospective use. A time-sensitive predictive instrument (TIPI) for acute cardiac ischemia: a multicenter study, *Med Care* 29:610-627, 1991.
8. Pozen MW, D'Agostino RB, Selker RP, et al: A predictive instrument to improve coronary-care-unit admission practices in acute ischemic heart disease. A prospective multicenter clinical trial, *N Engl J Med* 310(20):1273-1278, 1984.
9. Nyman I, Areskog M, Areskog NH, et al: Very early risk stratification by electrocardiogram at rest in men with suspected unstable coronary heart disease, *J Intern Med* 234:293-301, 1993.
10. TIMI IIIA Investigators: Early effects of tissue-type plasmogen activator added to conventional therapy on the culprit coronary lesion in patients presenting with ischemic cardiac pain at rest, *Circulation* 87:38-52, 1993.
11. The TIMI IIIB Investigators: Effects of tissue plasminogen activator and a comparison of early invasive and conservative strategies in unstable angina and non-Q-wave myocardial infarction. Results of the TIMI IIIB trial, *Circulation* 89(4):1545-1556, 1994.
12. Bar FW, Verheugt FW, Col J, et al: Thrombolysis in patients with unstable angina improves the angiographic but not the clinical outcome. Results of UNASEM, a multicenter, randomized, placebo-controlled, clinical trial with anistreplase, *Circulation* 86:131-137, 1992.
13. The GUSTO Investigators: An international randomized trial comparing four thrombolytic strategies for acute myocardial infarction, *N Engl J Med* 329:673-682, 1993.
14. ISIS-2 (Second International Study of Infarct Survival): Randomised trial of intravenous streptokinase, oral aspirin, both, or neither among 17,187 cases of suspected acute myocardial infarction: ISIS-2, *Lancet* 2:349-360, 1988.
15. Theroux P, Waters D, Qiu S, et al: Aspirin versus heparin to prevent myocardial infarction during the acute phase of unstable angina, *Circulation* 88(1):2045-2048, 1993.
16. Theroux P, Ouimet H, McCans J, et al: Aspirin, heparin, or both to treat acute unstable angina, *N Engl J Med* 319:1105-1111, 1988.
17. Wallentin LC: Aspirin (75 mg/day) after an episode of unstable coronary artery disease: long-term effects on the risk for myocardial infarction, occurrence of severe angina and the need for revascularization. Research Group on Instability in Coronary Artery Disease in Southeast Sweden, *J Am Coll Cardiol* 18(7): 1587-1593, 1991.
18. RISC Group: Risk of myocardial infarction and death during treatment with low-dose aspirin and intravenous heparin in men with unstable coronary artery disease, *Lancet* 336(8719):827-830, 1990.
19. Lewis HD Jr, Davis JW, Archibald DG, et al: Protective effects of aspirin against acute myocardial infarction and death in men with unstable angina. Results of a Veterans Administration Cooperative Study, *N Engl J Med* 309(7):396-403, 1983.
20. Antiplatelet Trialist's Collaboration: Collaborative overview of randomized trials of antiplatelet therapy. I. Prevention of death, myocardial infarction, and stroke by prolonged antiplatelet therapy in various categories of patients, *Br Med J* 308:81-106, 1994.
21. Theroux P, Waters D, Lam J, et al: Reactivation of unstable angina after the discontinuation of heparin, *N Engl J Med* 327:141-145, 1992.
22. Yusuf S, MacMahon S, Collins R, et al: Effect of intravenous nitrates on mortality in acute myocardial infarction: an overview of the randomised trials, *Lancet* 1:1088-1092, 1988.
23. Gruppo Italiano per lo Studio della Sopravvivenza nell'Infarto Miocardico: GISSI-3: effects of lisinopril and transdermal glyceryl trinitrate singly and together on 6-week mortality and ventricular function after acute myocardial infarction, *Lancet* 343:1115-1122, 1994.
24. Dellborg M, Gustafsson G, Swedberg K: Buccal versus intravenous nitroglycerin in unstable angina pectoris, *Eur J Clin Pharmacol* 41(1):5-9, 1991.
25. Kaplan K, Davison R, Parker M, et al: Intravenous nitroglycerin for the treatment of angina at rest unresponsive to standard nitrate therapy, *Am J Cardiol* 51(5):694-698, 1983.
26. Roubin GS, Harris PJ, Eckhardt I, et al: Intravenous nitroglycerine in refractory unstable angina pectoris, *Aust N Z J Med* 12(6):598-602, 1982.
27. Yusuf S, Wittes J, Friedman L: Overview of results of randomized clinical trials in heart disease: II. Unstable angina, heart failure, primary prevention with aspirin, and risk factor modification, *JAMA* 260:2259-2263, 1988.
28. Yusuf S, Wittes J, Friedman L: Overview of results of randomized clinical trials in heart disease. I. Treatments following myocardial infarction, *JAMA* 260:2088-2093, 1988.
29. Gerstenblith G, Ouyang P, Achuff SC, et al: Nifedipine in unstable angina: a double-blind randomized trial, *N Engl J Med* 306(15): 885-889, 1982.

30. Lubsen J, Tijssen JG: Efficacy of nifedipine and metoprolol in the early treatment of unstable angina in the coronary care unit: findings from the Holland Interuniversity Nifedipine/metoprolol Trial (HINT), *Am J Cardiol* 60(2):18A-25A, 1987.

31. Muller JE, Turi ZG, Pearle DL, et al: Nifedipine and conventional therapy for unstable angina pectoris: a randomized double-blind comparison, *Circulation* 69:728-739, 1984.

32. Theroux P, Taeymans Y, Morissette D, et al: A randomized study comparing propranolol and diltiazem in the treatment of unstable angina, *J Am Coll Cardiol* 5(3):717-722, 1985.

33. Held PH, Yusuf S, Furberg CD: Calcium channel blockers in acute myocardial infarction and unstable angina: an overview, *Br Med J* 299:1187-1192, 1989.

34. Raschke RA, Reilly BM, Guidry JR, et al: The weight-based heparin dosing nomogram compared with a "standard care" nomogram, *Ann Intern Med* 119:874-881, 1993.

35. Lee TH, Goldman L: Serum enzyme assays in the diagnosis of acute myocardial infarction, *Ann Intern Med* 105:221-223, 1986.

36. Grambow DW, Topol EJ: Effect of maximal medical therapy on refractoriness of unstable angina pectoris, *Am J Cardiol* 70:577-581, 1992.

37. Rankin JS, Newton JR Jr, Califf RM, et al: Clinical characteristics and current management of medically refractory unstable angina, *Ann Surg* 200:457-465, 1986.

38. Aroesty JM, Weintraub RM, Paulin S, et al: Medically refractory unstable angina pectoris. II. Hemodynamic and angiographic effects of intraaortic balloon counterpulsation, *Am J Cardiol* 43(5):883-888, 1979.

39. Makhoul RG, Cole CW, McCann RL: Vascular complications of the intraaortic balloon pump: an analysis of 436 patients, *Am Surg* 59:564-568, 1993.

40. Mark DB, Shaw L, Harrell FE, et al: Prognostic value of a treadmill exercise score in outpatients with suspected coronary artery disease, *N Engl J Med* 325:849-853, 1991.

41. Rahimtoola SH, Nunley D, Grunkemeier G, et al: Ten-year survival after coronary bypass surgery for unstable angina, *N Engl J Med* 308(12):676-681, 1983.

42. Russell RO, Moraski RE, Kouchoukos N, et al: Unstable angina pectoris: National Cooperative Study Group to compare surgical and medical therapy, *Int J Cardiol* 28(2):209-213, 1978.

43. Luchi RJ, Scott SM, Deupree RH: Comparison of medical and surgical treatment for unstable angina pectoris. Results of a Veterans Administration Cooperative Study, *N Engl J Med* 316(16):977-984, 1987.

44. Scott SM, Luchi RJ, Deupree RH: Veterans Administration Cooperative Study for treatment of patients with unstable angina. Results in patients with abnormal left ventricular function, *Circulation* 78(3 Pt 2):I113-I1121, 1988.

45. Sharma GV, Deupree RH, Khuri SF, et al: Coronary bypass surgery improves survival in high-risk unstable angina. Results of a Veterans Administration Cooperative study with an 8-year follow-up. Veterans Administration Unstable Angina Cooperative Study Group, *Circulation* 84(Suppl 5):III260-III267, 1991.

46. Parisi AF, Folland ED, Hartigan P: A comparison of angioplasty with medical therapy in the treatment of single-vessel coronary artery disease, *N Engl J Med* 326:10-16, 1992.

47. RITA Trial Participants: Coronary angioplasty versus coronary artery bypass surgery: the Randomised Intervention Treatment of Angina (RITA) trial, *Lancet* 341:573-580, 1993.

48. King SB III, Lembo NJ, Weintraub WS, et al. for the East Investigators: A randomized trial comparing coronary angioplasty with coronary bypass surgery: the Emory Angioplasty versus Surgery Trial, *N Engl J Med,* 1994 (in press).

49. Mark DB, Nelson CL, Califf RM, et al: The continuing evolution of therapy for coronary artery disease: initial results from the era of coronary angioplasty, *Circulation* 89(5):2015-2025, 1994.

50. Califf RM, Harrell FE Jr, Lee KL, et al: The evolution of medical and surgical therapy for coronary artery disease: a 15-year perspective, *JAMA* 261:2077-2086, 1989.

51. Califf RM, Harrell FE Jr, Lee KL, et al: Changing efficacy of coronary revascularization: implications for patient selection, *Circulation* 78 (suppl I):185-191, 1988.

Chapter 42

STABILIZING THE UNSTABLE ARTERY

Christopher B. Granger
Robert M. Califf

Acute ischemic heart disease, which includes both unstable angina and AMI, is initiated in most cases by fissuring or rupture of an atherosclerotic plaque, with development of an associated platelet/fibrin thrombus (see Chapter 1). The majority of early adverse events following this plaque rupture result directly from unfavorable shifts in the dynamic equilibrium of factors promoting continued thrombus formation and vessel occlusion on the one hand, and factors opposing vessel occlusion through thrombus dissolution or other mechanisms on the other. Enhanced understanding of the factors leading to thrombus formation and propagation and of the therapies most effective in controlling these factors forms the basis for the effective treatment of the patient with acute ischemic heart disease, regardless of whether the eventual diagnosis is AMI or unstable angina. The treatment of this syndrome has two major goals: first to ensure that myocardial perfusion is present and then to stabilize the unstable artery.

The old concepts of acute ischemic heart disease are reflected in a clinical nomenclature that distinguished among unstable angina, non–Q-wave MI and Q-wave MI. This nomenclature, although partially justified from the perspective of pathophysiology, is largely irrelevant to the clinician seeing a patient in the emergency setting. In the early acute phase it is often not possible to distinguish between unstable angina and MI because the clinical presentations, physical findings, and electrocardiographic manifestations may be identical. Furthermore, unstable angina may progress to MI, which may be followed by unstable angina. This diagnostic dilemma necessitates management strategies that take into account the spectrum and continuum of acute coronary syndromes.[1-3] Although a great deal has been learned about the effective management of patients presenting with ST-segment elevation who are eligible for thrombolytic or other reperfusion therapy, much less attention has been paid to patients who do not have ST-segment elevation on the admitting electrocardiogram. Even though non–Q-wave infarction has traditionally been thought to have an intermediate early prognosis between unstable angina and Q-wave infarction, recent studies have shown that patients with AMI without ST elevation are a heterogeneous group, with worse prognosis strongly related to the presence of ST-segment shift. Part of the misconception about the prognosis of patients without ST elevation may stem from the lack of a commonly used nomenclature to distinguish between patients with and without ST-segment shift.[4] Because most patients with acute ischemic syndromes fall into the category of no ST elevation and/or are not eligible for thrombolytic therapy, and the majority of deaths and nonfatal major complications occur in this group[5,6] (Table 42-1), the development of effective management strategies in this group should receive a high priority.

Figure 41-1 demonstrates the instantaneous risk of death (hazard) as a function of time and presenting clinical syndrome in patients undergoing coronary angiography and found to have significant coronary artery disease.[7] The risk of death is markedly higher in the first few days and declines substantially beyond that point. After approximately 2 months of follow-up the risk to the

Table 42-1. Proportion of patients and outcome according to presence or absence of ST elevation at presentation and by treatment or no treatment with thrombolytic therapy.

Patient group	% of total	Mortality rate	% of total deaths
ST ↑/LBBB and thrombolytic treated	31%	7%	16%
ST ↑/LBBB and not thrombolytic treated	28%	19%	42%
No ST ↑/LBBB	40%	13%	42%

Data from 637 patients with acute myocardial infarction from 106 hospitals participating in the GUSTO MI log.

patient who had unstable angina at baseline is essentially indistinguishable from that of the patient who had stable angina. This time course provides a basis for the concept that more rapid stabilization of the artery may more rapidly lower the risk to the level of risk of the patient with stable angina.

All this information makes a compelling argument that clinicians evaluating patients with acute ischemic syndromes should be armed with a new nomenclature for classifying patients and that, as treatment decisions are made, they should have a firm mental image of the forces at play on the endothelial surface of the culprit artery. Until rapid tests to diagnose ongoing myocardial necrosis, such as the troponin-T[8] test currently being evaluated in the GUSTO II trial, are available, the primary classification of patients with acute coronary syndromes should be those with and those without ST-segment elevation. In the former group rapid reperfusion is essential, whereas in both groups medical stabilization of coronary perfusion is essential to maximize the chance of a favorable long-term outcome. A secondary classification of patients without ST elevation should be based on the presence or absence of ST depression, because of the prognostic importance of this finding.

The findings concerning the duration of risk associated with the unstable syndrome suggest that if progression of the lesion-associated thrombus can be retarded so that acute coronary occlusion is prevented, medical therapy to stabilize the plaque itself could return the patient to the same chronic risk level as before the event.

This chapter is primarily concerned with interventions that might be effective in preventing further ischemic events in the short term and the midterm by modulating the factors critical to the unstable syndrome. The major focus is on the coagulation system, including platelet function and thrombin activation. Control of

coronary vasomotor tone is also critical, and mechanical approaches obviously play a crucial role in situations in which the likelihood of success with purely medical therapy is too low. As the biologic substrate becomes better understood, stabilizing the unstable atherosclerotic plaque will become a major area of medicine.

MANAGEMENT GOALS

The clinical course of patients who present with acute ischemic heart disease without ST-segment elevation typically involves approximately a 10% risk of either early mortality or nonfatal MI. In the United States approximately two thirds of these patients undergo cardiac catheterization and most go on to revascularization with angioplasty or bypass surgery.[9] The principal goals in management of these patients can be divided into two broad categories: prevention of death and prevention of other adverse events, including recurrent ischemia, (re)infarction, congestive heart failure, or stroke, which are primarily the result of ongoing or recurrent thrombosis.

MANAGEMENT APPROACH

The primary pathophysiologic processes that must be modified in the early management of acute coronary syndromes are plaque rupture and resultant thrombosis, spasm, and humoral alterations that contribute to inadequate coronary blood flow and adverse outcomes (Fig. 42-1). Revascularization is important to successfully treat the underlying occlusive disease in certain patients. In patients with refractory ischemia or shock, intraaortic balloon pumping support may be indicated to stabilize both the hemodynamics and coronary flow.

The initial assessment and institution of therapy for acute ischemic heart disease should occur rapidly upon the patient's arrival in the emergency department. In patients with symptoms of acute myocardial ischemia an ECG should be obtained within 15 minutes of their arrival in the emergency department. This initial ECG provides crucial information about whether to consider thrombolytic therapy.

A summary of the effects of major treatments for unstable angina, obtained from pooling results from randomized clinical trials, is shown in Figure 42-2.

Thrombolytic therapy

In the absence of ST-segment elevation or bundle branch block, thrombolytic therapy has not been shown to be beneficial, even if MI is suspected.[10] A pooled analysis of randomized trials of thrombolytic therapy vs. control for patients without ST elevation demonstrates a trend towards a detrimental effect with thrombolytic therapy, although the number of patients treated is small enough to fail to exclude the possibility of a small treatment benefit[11-21] (Table 42-2). This analysis is

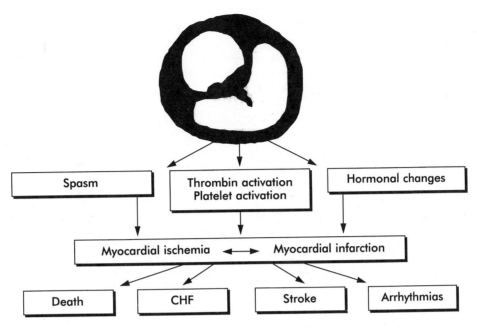

Fig. 42-1. Pathophysiology of unstable angina and subsequent adverse events.

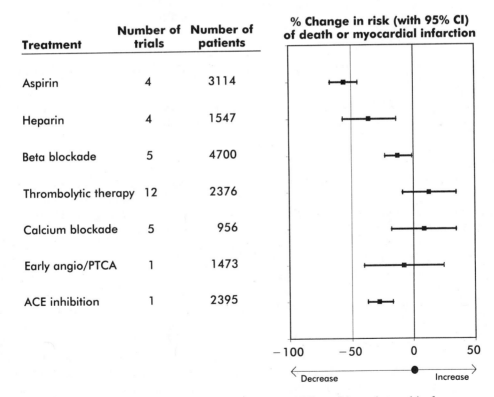

Treatment	Number of trials	Number of patients
Aspirin	4	3114
Heparin	4	1547
Beta blockade	5	4700
Thrombolytic therapy	12	2376
Calcium blockade	5	956
Early angio/PTCA	1	1473
ACE inhibition	1	2395

Fig. 42-2. Percent change in risk of death or MI (with 95% confidence intervals) of common therapies for unstable angina, determined by pooling data from randomized clinical trials. Data for each therapy are from: thrombolytic therapy, Table 42-2; aspirin, Table 42-3; heparin, Table 42-4; beta blockade,[94] 1988; calcium channel blockade, Table 42-5; early angiography and PTCA, Braunwald et al.[7]; ACE inhibition, Yusuf et al.[93]

Table 42-2. Randomized trials of thrombolysis in unstable angina

First author	Journal	Thrombolytic			No thrombolytic			Lytic	F/U
		N	Death	Death or MI	N	Death	Death or MI		
Nicklas	*JACC*	20	2	2	20	0	2	t-PA	in-hospital
Lawrence	*Thromb Res*	20	1	1	20	4	8	SK	6 mo
Saran	*Int J Cardiol*	24	2	4	24	4	7	SK	6 mo
Williams	*Circulation*	45	0	3	22	0	1	t-PA	48 hrs
Freeman	*Circulation*	35	1	3	35	1	2	t-PA	in-hospital
Bar	*Circulation*	80	3	13	79	1	6	APSAC	in-hospital
Schreiber	*Circulation*	96	0	8	53	0	2	UK	96 hrs
Karlsson	*Am Heart J*	105	3	11	100	2	12	t-PA	45 days
Serneri	*Lancet*	20	1	1	19	0	0	t-PA	7 days
van den Brand	*EHJ*	19	1	5	17	0	3	t-PA	24 hrs
Chaudhary	*Am J Cardiol*	26	1	4	24	2	5	t-PA	72 hrs/2 wks
TIMI-IIIB	*Circulation*	729	17	65	744	19	51	t-PA	42 days
Pooled		1219	2.6%	9.8%	1157	2.9%	8.6%		
95% CI for death or MI				8.2%-11.5%			6.9%-10.2%		

Lytic = thrombolytic agent; SK = streptokinase; APSAC = anistreplase; UK = urokinase; CI = confidence interval.

Table 42-3. Randomized trials of aspirin in unstable angina

First author	Journal	Aspirin			No aspirin			F/U
		N	Death	Death or MI	N	Death	Death or MI	
Theroux	*N Engl J Med*, 1988	243	0	6	236	2	15	6 days
RISC	*Lancet*, 1990	399	6	26	397	10	68	3 months
Lewis	*N Engl J Med*, 1983	625	10	31	641	21	65	12 weeks
Cairns	*N Engl J Med*, 1985	276	6	17	279	22	36	18 months
Pooled		1543	1.4%	5.2%	1571	3.5%	11.7%	
95% CI for death or MI				4.1%-6.3%			10.1%-13.3%	

heavily influenced by the largest trial, the TIMI-IIIB trial, which contributed almost two thirds of the overall sample. There was a strong trend towards a higher risk of subsequent MI in these patients after thrombolytic therapy (7%, 95% CI 5.6% to 8.4%) compared with placebo (5.5%, 95% CI 4.2% to 6.8%).

The reasons for the apparently worse outcome with thrombolytic therapy are unclear but may be because these drugs have a benefit only in the presence of total coronary occlusion. When the absence of benefit is added to the risk that accompanies thrombolytic therapy, the net result would generally be negative. In addition, intralesional bleeding associated with use of thrombolytic therapy may further destabilize a non-occlusive plaque.[23] It is also possible that in the absence of a totally occluded artery before treatment the creation of a prothrombotic effect through exposure of clot-bound thrombin to the circulating blood as the fibrin is lysed[24-26] may actually be more likely to produce coronary occlusion than to prevent it. Patho-

logic findings of platelet aggregates in the distal coronary bed[27] and angioscopic findings of more "white thrombi"[28] suggest that in unstable angina, thrombi are platelet rich and relatively fibrin poor and therefore may not be as susceptible to thrombolytic therapy.[29,30]

Antiplatelet therapy

Aspirin. Aspirin irreversibly acetylates platelet cyclooxygenase, blocking the formation of prostaglandins, including thromboxane A_2, and thereby decreasing platelet aggregation.[31] Because of the important role of platelets in thrombosis at the site of plaque rupture and the circulating and urinary metobolites of platelet activation in patients with unstable angina,[32-34] the use of aspirin has a strong pathophysiologic rationale.

A large body of data from clinical trials has established aspirin as one of the most important aspects of medical treatment for the broad spectrum of coronary artery disease and for acute coronary syndromes in

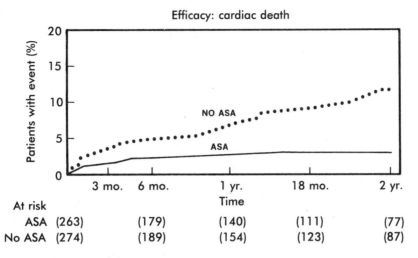

Fig. 42-3. Cumulative cardiac mortality of patients assigned to aspirin vs. placebo. (Reproduced from Cairns JA et al: Aspirin, sulfinpyrazone, or both in unstable angina. Results of a Canadian multicenter trial, *N Engl J Med* 313:1369-1375, 1985.)

particular. For AMI the early administration of aspirin (325 mg/day) was shown to result in a 23% reduction in 6-week vascular deaths in the ISIS-2 trial.[35] There have been four major randomized trials of aspirin for patients with unstable angina, three of which were stopped early because of the unequivocal benefit of aspirin in reducing death and MI (Table 42-3).

Two randomized trials[36,37] have established the usefulness of aspirin in reducing early morbidity during the early in-hospital phase in patients with unstable angina. Theroux et al.[36] studied 479 patients enrolled within 24 hours of symptoms, who were randomized to aspirin 325 mg twice a day vs. placebo, as well as to heparin 1000 U/hr vs. placebo, in a 2 × 2 factorial design. The primary endpoints were refractory ischemia, infarction, and death during study-drug administration. The trial was terminated early, at the first interim analysis, because of a strongly positive finding that, compared with placebo, both aspirin and heparin were associated with a significant reduction in MI.

The RISC group enrolled 945 men in the subacute phase, up to 72 hours after admission to coronary care units for unstable coronary symptoms (non–Q-wave MI or unstable angina). Patients were randomized in a 2 × 2 factorial design to aspirin (75 mg a day) vs. placebo, and to heparin (15,000 to 20,000 units divided into 6 intravenous doses per day for 5 days) vs. placebo. Because of the occurrence of anterior Q-wave infarction or a normal exercise treadmill test, 149 patients were excluded, leaving 796 patients for analysis. Endpoints were death and MI for 1 year of follow-up, which was modified to 3 months when the ISIS-2 results forced the follow-up phase to be abbreviated. The results showed a dramatic benefit from aspirin, with over a 50% reduction of death plus nonfatal MI at 5 days, 30 days, and 90 days.

Two additional randomized trials evaluated the use of aspirin for unstable angina, beginning in the later hospital phase. In the Veterans Administration study[38] 1338 men with presumed unstable angina admitted to the hospital within 48 hours were randomized to aspirin 324 mg per day or placebo; 72 were withdrawn from the analysis because of the subsequent diagnosis of AMI at admission. The trial was stopped before the target enrollment was reached because of a highly positive result: the primary endpoint of death or nonfatal MI at 12 weeks was 51% lower in the aspirin group (5% vs. 10.1% in the placebo group, *P* < 0.0005). One-year mortality was also lower in the aspirin group (5.5 vs. 9.6%, *P* = 0.008), even though the study drug was stopped after 12 weeks. The Canadian trial[39] compared aspirin 325 mg four times a day vs. placebo, and sulfinpyrazone vs. placebo, in a 2 × 2 factorial design, for patients within 8 days of hospitalization. Patients in the aspirin group experienced a similar 51% reduction in mortality and nonfatal MI during the 18-month follow-up (*P* = 0.008) (Fig. 42-3).

Taken together, these four trials establish aspirin in a dose of at least 75 mg per day as the cornerstone of medical treatment for unstable angina, with more than a 50% reduction in death and in nonfatal MI.

What remains unknown is which dose of aspirin is most effective. In a variety of atherosclerotic states, doses ranging from 30 mg[40] to 325 mg per day have been found to reduce the risk of vascular events,[41] but inadequate comparative data exist to make a statement about differences in clinical outcome. However, a direct relationship has been demonstrated between doses of oral aspirin and risk of gastrointestinal complications. Accordingly we recommend a dose of 80 to 160 mg per day as a "middle ground" until comparative studies are available. Furthermore, because of the observation that the highest risk of ischemic events occurs shortly after diagnosis, we recommend a nonenteric-coated aspirin for the first dose to ensure that absorption problems do not hinder the achievement of the desired antiplatelet effect.

Ticlopidine. For the small percentage of patients who are unable to tolerate aspirin because of hypersensitivity an alternative antiplatelet agent is ticlopidine, which appears to interfere with ADP-mediated platelet aggregation and the platelet glycoprotein IIb/IIIa receptor.[42] The delay in full antiplatelet effect of at least 3 days, however, may limit the effectiveness of ticlopidine in the acute phase. In one quarter of all coronary care units in Italy, Balsano et al.[43] randomized 652 patients within 48 hours of hospital admission for unstable angina to routine care plus ticlopidine (250 mg twice daily) vs. routine care alone, in an unblinded design. No patients received aspirin. The trial was stopped early for undisclosed reasons. The ticlopidine group had a significantly ($P < 0.009$) reduced primary endpoint of death and nonfatal MI at 6 months of 7.3% compared with 13.6% without ticlopidine. In one trial comparing ticlopidine with aspirin in patients with cerebrovascular disease, ticlopidine was associated with a superior reduction in vascular events compared with aspirin.[44]

Although we generally recommend ticlopidine for aspirin-allergic patients, several characteristics of the drug have prevented it from supplanting aspirin as the first-line antiplatelet therapy. Ticlopidine is much more expensive than aspirin. Additionally, approximately 2% of patients develop a reversible neutropenia and 1% develop severe neutropenia or agranulocytosis, and therefore complete blood counts and white blood cell count differentials should be checked every 2 weeks for the first 3 months of therapy. A second-generation drug, clopidogrel, is an analogue of ticlopidine with similar antiplatelet properties but without the risk of neutropenia. It is currently being compared to aspirin for patients at risk for coronary, cerebral, or peripheral vascular ischemia in a large CAPRIE trial.

Glycoprotein IIb/IIIa antagonists. Although aspirin reduces the risk of coronary events in patients with acute ischemic syndromes, its antiplatelet effects are relatively weak. This observation leads to the question of whether even more profound platelet inhibition would further improve patient outcome. The glycoprotein IIb/IIIa receptor, found in the platelet membrane, is a member of the integrin family of receptors involved with cellular interactions and cellular adhesion. A variety of stimuli to platelet aggregation cause externalization of this receptor on the surface of the platelet. Platelet aggregation is then caused by binding of fibrinogen to a receptor on each of two platelets. Recent advances in biologic

methods have yielded both antibodies and small peptides that can successfully block the receptor.

c7E3 is a chimeric monoclonal antibody to the IIb/IIIa receptor and has been tested in the setting of angioplasty for unstable angina. In two independent studies, intravenous administration of the antibody reduced the risk of acute ischemic events in patients undergoing angioplasty. The larger trial, EPIC I, evaluated 2099 patients with either acute ischemic syndrome or complex lesion morphology. The 30-day rate of death, nonfatal MI coronary surgery, and angioplasty was 28% less in patients treated with high-dose c7E3.[45] These benefits have been shown to extend and to widen out to 6 months of follow-up.[46] However, patients on high-dose 7E3 also had doubling of the major bleeding rate. The EPILOGUE trial is evaluating the impact of various nonpharmacologic management strategies to reduce the risk of groin bleeding and of lower heparin dosing in conjunction with c7E3, with hopes of maintaining the same enhanced efficacy while reducing the bleeding risk.

A second approach to the IIb/IIIa receptor using integrelin, a small peptide with great specificity for the receptor, has been promising in early studies. The potential advantage of integrelin is its short half-life, thereby potentially enhancing the ability of the health providers to manage bleeding complications when they occur. In the setting of angioplasty, integrelin appears to have efficacy similar to that of c7E3.[47]

If more profound platelet inhibition proves to be clinically effective and to have an acceptable bleeding risk, it is possible that such therapy could markedly reduce the need for mechanical intervention during the acute phase of the syndrome, thereby reducing risk and saving money, because many of these patients might stabilize and never need a procedure. Alternatively, IIb/IIIa blockade could improve the risk-to-benefit profile of percutaneous intervention to the extent that earlier procedures could be done safely, thus reducing the need for prolonged hospitalization and multiple noninvasive tests.

Antithrombin therapy

Heparin. There is clear evidence that heparin reduces the incidence of refractory ischemia and reinfarction when used early in the course of unstable angina. Heparin exerts its anticoagulant effect primarily through the action of antithrombin III, a proteolytic enzyme that inactivates thrombin, factor Xa, and other activated clotting factors.[48] Heparin forms a complex with antithrombin III that markedly accelerates its inhibition of thrombin. The antithrombin effect, with subsequent reduction of clot formation because of reduced fibrin formation and less platelet activation, forms the pathophysiologic rationale for the use of heparin to stabilize the unstable artery.

Table 42-4. Randomized trials of heparin in unstable angina

First author	Journal	Heparin			No heparin			F/U
		N	Death	Death or MI	N	Death	Death or MI	
Theroux[36]	*NEJM*, 1988	240	0	3	239	2	18	6 days
RISC[37]	*Lancet*, 1990	408	NA	45	388	NA	49	3 months
Serneri[19]	*Lancet*, 1990	39	0	0	19	0	1	7 days
Cohen[62]	*Circulation*, 1994	105	NA	4	109	NA	9	5 days
Pooled		792	0	6.6%	755	0.8%	10.2%	
95% CI for death or MI				4.8%-8.3%			8.0%-12.4%	

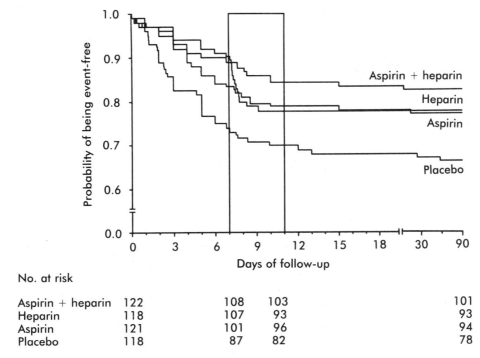

Fig. 42-4. Probability of being free from death, MI, or recurrent unstable angina. (From Theroux P, Waters D, Lam J, et al. Reactivation of unstable angina after the discontinuation of heparin, *New Engl J Med* 327:141-145, 1992.)

There have been a series of studies evaluating heparin in the treatment of unstable angina (Table 42-4), the two most important of which are the Montreal Heart and RISC studies. As reviewed earlier, Theroux[49] studied 479 patients randomized to heparin 5000 unit bolus, followed by 1000 units/hr adjusted to a PTT 1.5 to 2 times that of control for a mean of 6 days, aspirin, both, or neither in a factorial design. Heparin therapy was associated with significant reductions in death, MI, and refractory ischemia (Fig. 42-4). After the placebo arm in this study was discontinued, the heparin vs. aspirin randomization continued to a total of 484 patients in those two groups.[49] Compared to aspirin, heparin was associated with a significant reduction in MI during study drug administration, at 3.7% and 0.8% respectively, (*P* = 0.035).

The RISC group studied heparin dosed as an intravenous injection every 6 hours for a total of 15,000 to 20,000 units per day for 5 days vs. placebo, and aspirin vs. placebo. The intermittent heparin therapy resulted in a trend towards lower death or MI, but only during the drug administration period. The lack of a more pronounced effect of heparin may have been the result of a delay in starting heparin (averaging 2 days after last symptoms), and/or the particular dosing regimen used.

There are no data that directly address which is the best dosing of heparin for unstable angina. However, the deep venous thrombosis/pulmonary embolism literature suggests that intermittent dosing is associated with a higher bleeding rate. Therefore we feel that continuous intravenous heparin should be used, and a rational target for degree of anticoagulation is an aPTT that is two to three times that of the control, which has been shown to result in less reocclusion after thrombolysis compared to lesser degrees of anticoagulation.[50] Although the available data show that 5 days of heparin therapy is effective, the optimal duration of heparin therapy is not known. Until further data are available, administration of intravenous heparin for at least 3 days in patients who have true unstable angina is recommended.

Coumadin. A patient with an acute ischemic syndrome remains at increased risk of recurrence during the initial several months after hospital discharge. A second ischemic event is likely to involve further plaque disruption and extension of the thrombus. Meade et al.[51] have demonstrated that factor VIIa plays a key role in the genesis of these events in patients without a previous cardiac event, and our current understanding of the coagulation system points to inhibition of this process as a critical avenue of secondary prevention. From this perspective the administration of low-dose coumadin, in an amount sufficient to keep factor VIIa levels suppressed, may prevent recurrent events. An overview of studies of coumadin in the postinfarction period reveals an effect comparable and perhaps superior to aspirin in terms of prevention of reinfarction and death. Low-dose aspirin added to Coumadin has been shown to reduce mortality significantly, as well as embolic events, in patients with mechanical heart valves, at the expense of a moderate increase in bleeding.[52] Several trials, including the Coumadin Aspirin Reinfarction Study (CARS), are currently evaluating low-dose coumadin as preventive therapy after discharge from ischemic syndromes. In this study 6000 patients 3 to 21 days after MI are being randomized to aspirin (160 mg), aspirin (80 mg) plus coumadin (1 mg), or aspirin (80 mg) plus coumadin (3 mg). The primary endpoint is a composite of cardiovascular death, ischemic stroke, and nonfatal MI, with follow-up planned for 4 years. Until these results are available, aspirin without Coumadin should be considered the standard treatment for unstable angina. However, for patients with unstable angina and other borderline indications for anticoagulation, such as severe left ventricular dysfunction, low-dose Coumadin (2 to 3 mg) combined with low-dose aspirin (80 mg) may be considered.

New direct thrombin inhibitors. The direct thrombin inhibitors bind to the thrombin catalytic site (PPACK, argatroban), the substrate recognition site (hirugen), or both (hirudin, hirulog) (Fig. 42-5). Unlike heparin, which can be inactivated by platelet factor 4 and heparinases and which requires the cofactor antithrombin III, these potent compounds directly attach to thrombin and have no circulating inhibitors. Furthermore, and perhaps most importantly, hirudin and related compounds can inactivate clot-bound thrombin,[53] along

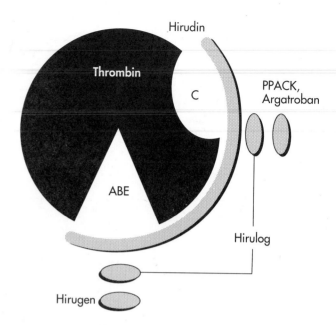

Fig. 42-5. Direct thrombin inhibitors and their binding to the catalytic site *(C)* and the anionic binding exosite *(ABE)*.

with circulating thrombin; however, this is not true with heparin because of the large size of the active heparin antithrombin III complex.[54] Preclinical studies have reinforced the biochemical and in vivo superiority of hirudin.[55-58] These potential advantages of hirudin over heparin have stimulated several large randomized clinical trials in unstable angina, AMI, and with angioplasty.

The initial results of a recombinant hirudin and of hirulog in Phase II trials have been encouraging. Topol et al. reported results of a trial designed to evaluate angiographic effects of hirudin vs. heparin in patients with unstable angina.[59] A total of 166 patients were randomized to a 3-day infusion of varying doses of hirudin (weight adjusted) vs. heparin. Treatment with hirudin resulted in a more stable and predictable effect on the aPTT, with 71% of hirudin-treated patients maintained in a 40-second aPTT target range, as opposed to only 16% of heparin-treated patients ($P < 0.001$). Paired angiography (baseline and at follow-up, conducted before any coronary intervention) demonstrated greater improvement in culprit-vessel diameter for hirudin, reflecting better thrombus resolution. Bleeding complications were not found to be increased with hirudin, and there was a nonstatistically significant decrease in rates of MI and recurrent angina. Lidon et al. showed that administration of hirulog resulted in effective inhibition of markers of thrombin activity and favorable clinical outcomes in 55 patients with unstable angina.[60]

The TIMI 5 trial evaluated hirudin as an adjunct to thrombolytic therapy for AMI. Preliminary results[61] demonstrated improved angiographic and clinical out-

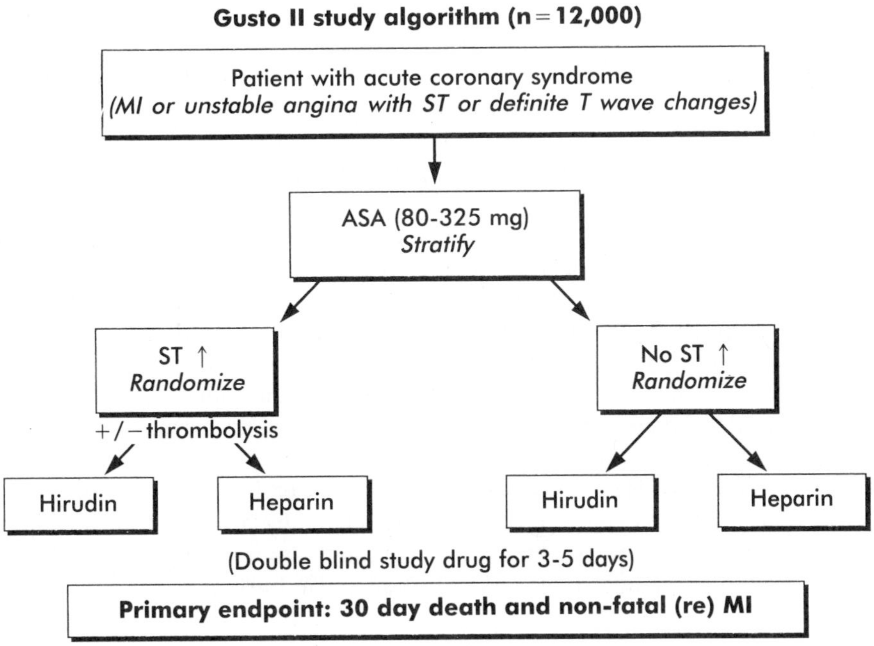

Gusto II study algorithm (n = 12,000)

```
┌─────────────────────────────────────────────────────────┐
│           Patient with acute coronary syndrome            │
│ (MI or unstable angina with ST or definite T wave changes)│
└─────────────────────────────────────────────────────────┘
                            │
                            ▼
                  ┌──────────────────┐
                  │  ASA (80-325 mg)  │
                  │     Stratify      │
                  └──────────────────┘
                   ↙                ↘
          ┌──────────┐          ┌──────────┐
          │   ST ↑   │          │  No ST ↑ │
          │ Randomize│          │ Randomize│
          └──────────┘          └──────────┘
        +/- thrombolysis
        ↙         ↘              ↙          ↘
  ┌────────┐ ┌────────┐   ┌────────┐  ┌────────┐
  │ Hirudin│ │ Heparin│   │ Hirudin│  │ Heparin│
  └────────┘ └────────┘   └────────┘  └────────┘

        (Double blind study drug for 3-5 days)
┌─────────────────────────────────────────────────────────┐
│  Primary endpoint: 30 day death and non-fatal (re) MI     │
└─────────────────────────────────────────────────────────┘
```

Fig. 42-6. GUSTO II algorithm.

come with hirudin compared with heparin after t-PA, and this trial also found no increase in bleeding complications. Thus, there is some mechanistic evidence that hirudin is more effective than heparin, as measured by improvement in coronary artery thrombus dissolution or prevention of accumulation, as well as some evidence to suggest overall clinical benefit. The TIMI 6 trial evaluated hirudin as an adjunct to streptokinase, and the results of this study are also consistent with a better outcome with hirudin, with no higher bleeding risk. TIMI 7 and 8 are evaluating hirulog in unstable angina.

The GUSTO IIb trial is an international, multicenter trial comparing hirudin (at a maintenance infusion dose of .1 mg/kg/hour for 3 to 5 days) with heparin for patients with the broad spectrum of acute coronary syndromes (Fig. 42-6). The GUSTO IIa trial was prematurely discontinued because of higher than expected rates of hemorrhagic stroke, prompting a reduction in the dosage of both hirudin and heparin.[61b] Eligible patients are those who have had symptoms of ischemia at rest within 12 hours, and who have ST-segment or definite T-wave changes. The primary endpoint is 30-day mortality or nonfatal (re)infarction. In addition, the trial will collect information and analyze the effects of practice patterns, use of noninvasive testing, cardiac catheterization, revascularization, and international differences in the management of acute coronary syndromes. The TIMI 9 trial has a design that is similar to GUSTO II, with the exception of studying only patients with AMI receiving thrombolytic therapy. Results of both these studies should be available in late 1995.

Combination of aspirin and heparin: possible prevention of heparin rebound. The use of aspirin and heparin in combination is a logical approach towards stabilizing the unstable coronary plaque because each inhibits a different aspect of the clotting process. Neither Theroux nor RISC had adequate power to address whether the combination is better than either agent alone. The Antithrombotic Therapy in Acute Coronary Syndromes Research Group randomized 214 patients with unstable angina or non–Q-wave MI to heparin plus aspirin (for 3 to 4 days, followed by aspirin plus Coumadin) vs. aspirin alone.[62] At 14 days there was a significant reduction in ischemic events of recurrent ischemia, (re)infarction, or death in the combination group compared to aspirin alone (10.5% vs. 27%, $P < 0.004$). The combined evidence supports the use of both aspirin and heparin in the acute phase of unstable angina, particularly in the absence of high bleeding risk.

There is also evidence that the combination of aspirin and heparin at least partially protects against a reactivation of thrombotic events upon discontinuing heparin, as reported by Theroux et al.[63] (see Fig. 42-4). Clinical events of death, MI, or recurrence of angina occurred in 13% of patients at a median of 9.5 hours after discontinuation of heparin. On the other hand the combination of heparin *and* aspirin was not associated with this reactivation phenomenon, with recurrence in only 5% of patients, which was the same as aspirin alone or double placebo. In another study,[64] after discontinuing intravenous heparin in a group of 35 patients with recent unstable coronary syndromes, all of whom were on aspirin, we demonstrated a consistent and significant rise in three markers of thrombin activity: fibrinopeptide A, prothrombin fragment 1.2, and activated protein C. Each marker peaked 3 to 6 hours after heparin discontinuation, and four patients developed recurrent ischemia within 12 hours of stopping heparin. This phenomenon after stopping antithrombin therapy is not restricted to heparin, as illustrated by Gold et al.[65] who showed an increase in thrombin activity and clinical thrombotic events after stopping the direct thrombin inhibitor argatroban. After stopping a 4-hour infusion of argatroban in 43 patients with unstable angina, fibrinopeptide A and thrombin antithrombin complex levels increased, and nine patients developed recurrent unstable angina at a mean of 5.8 hours. These studies together provide hematologic and clinical evidence for a rebound increase in thrombotic tendency after discontinuing antithrombotic therapy and call for the clinician to be vigilant for a temporary destabilization upon stopping antithrombin therapy.

Fuster has recently proposed tapering heparin to prevent this rebound phenomenon by switching to a progressively decreasing subcutaneous regimen. However, this regimen has yet to receive formal clinical testing.

Nitrates

Nitroglycerin exerts beneficial effects in acute ischemic heart disease both by decreasing preload and consequently reducing myocardial oxygen demand, and by relieving the coronary vasospasm, "cyclic flow," and intermittent ischemia as demonstrated both angiographically[66] and with continuous monitoring of the ST segment.[67] Intravenous nitroglycerin has also been shown to have anti-platelet activity,[68] although the clinical significance of this is not known.

Although there have been no large randomized clinical trials evaluating intravenous nitrates for unstable angina, a series of small studies[69-71] provide information that intravenous nitroglycerin is beneficial for relief of ischemia. In spite of an overview of early studies showing a substantial benefit from intravenous nitrates in AMI,[72] the preliminary results of the GISSI-3 trial (intravenous nitroglycerin) and the ISIS-4 trial (oral nitroglycerin) showed no statistically significant benefit to nitroglycerin following AMI. Preliminary results[73,74] were a 35-day mortality in GISSI-3 of 6.5% for nitroglycerin vs. 6.9% for placebo, and in ISIS-4 of 7% for nitroglycerin vs. 7.2% for placebo. In GISSI-3, higher-risk patients and patients treated with ACE inhibitors appeared to benefit more from intravenous nitroglycerin. The final results and the details of GISSI-3 may enable a more accurate determination of whether and when intravenous nitroglycerin is indicated for AMI. Based on the currently available clinical trial results and the pathophsysiology,

we recommend the use of intravenous nitroglycerin in the acute setting of ongoing ischemia for the entire spectrum of acute coronary syndromes.

Although partial hemodynamic tolerance with intravenous nitroglycerin may occur in as many as 50% of patients within 12 to 24 hours,[75,76] some effect usually persists for at least 48 hours.[77] Therefore although the development of tolerance may differ substantially from patient to patient, intravenous nitroglycerin should generally be changed to intermittent transdermal or oral dosing after 24 to 48 hours, as long as ischemia does not recur. Alternatively, if ischemia recurs, increasing the dose of intravenous nitroglycerin will generally at least partially and transiently overcome the effect of tolerance.[77]

Whether intravenous nitroglycerin can be abruptly replaced by transdermal preparations or should be gradually tapered as transdermal therapy is initiated is unknown. Furthermore the appropriate dose and duration of nitrate therapy remain unclear. No studies comparing the effects of different dosing regimens on primary clinical event rates are available. In our practice we start intravenous nitroglycerin at a dose of 5 to 10 mcg/min and increase it to a dose of at least 50 to 100 mcg/min as tolerated by the blood pressure, using volume administration if needed to support the blood pressure. Others advocate simply increasing the nitroglycerin until the mean arterial pressure drops by 10%.

In most patients with acute ischemic syndromes who do not undergo revascularization, oral nitrates have been used as part of the discharge medical regimen. The major goal of therapy in this phase is to prevent recurrent coronary ischemia caused by either increased cardiac work or to coronary vasospasm, which might precipitate another plaque event. Although the effect of nitrates in patients with unstable angina without ongoing angina in this phase of the ischemic syndrome has not been tested specifically, extrapolation of the ISIS-4 results to the entire spectrum of acute coronary syndromes would suggest that although oral nitrates may have a small beneficial effect, *routine* use in the absence of ongoing ischemia is of lower priority than other proven therapies.

Beta blockers

Beta-blocking agents are competitive antagonists of catecholamines that act by blocking the beta adrenergic receptors at the cell membrane. The primary benefit of beta blockers in relieving the symptoms of myocardial ischemia stems from the blockade of the myocardial beta$_1$ receptors, with consequent decreased heart rate and contractility, which in turn reduce myocardial work load and oxygen demand. In addition, the reduction in progression to infarction in unstable angina, the long-term highly significant reduction in reinfarction in postinfarction trials,[78] and the blunting of the circadian morning increase in thrombotic events[79] suggest that beta blockade may have a stabilizing effect on the unstable or potentially unstable atherosclerotic plaque.

Along with early, small, uncontrolled studies there have been several randomized trials of beta blockade vs. placebo for patients with unstable angina. Three trials showed a trend toward reduction in nonfatal MI and death.[80-82] A metaanalysis of trials of patients with "impending myocardial infarction"[83,84] suggests that beta blockers result in a significant reduction in progression to infarction, and specifically that initial intravenous beta blockade followed by oral beta blockade for 1 week results in a 13% reduction in the risk of developing MI (29% in the beta-blocker groups, 32% in the control groups, $P < 0.04$).[85] Although there have not been adequate numbers of patients with unstable angina studied to demonstrate a significant reduction in mortality with beta blockers, randomized trials in AMI[86] and recent infarction[87-90] have all shown reduced mortality; the totality of evidence thus strongly supports the use of beta blockers for patients with unstable angina who are able to tolerate them.

When a rapid effect of beta blockade is desired to control acute ongoing ischemia, intravenous dosing is preferable, in part because of hepatic "first pass" metabolism, particularly with the lipid-soluble agents such as propranolol and metoprolol. Esmolol has been reported to be safe and effective,[91] although it is quite expensive. Extrapolation from AMI trials suggests that a number of beta blockers, including atenolol and metoprolol, would be safe and effective when given intravenously. We therefore reserve esmolol for patients with relative contraindications to beta blockers as a class (reduced left ventricular function, conduction system abnormality, lung disease) in whom the short half-life would allow for rapid reversal of any adverse effects.

At the time of discharge we strongly believe that beta-blocking agents should be prescribed unless a significant contraindication is present. Because of the combined antiischemic, antiarrhythmic, and possible antiplaque rupture effect, this class of drugs can accomplish multiple goals. Every effort should be made to use dosages that have been found to be effective in clinical trials (atenolol, 100 mg/day; propranolol 60 to 80 mg tid; timolol 10 mg bid; metoprolol 100 mg bid).

Calcium blockers

By blocking the inward flux of calcium through cell membranes, calcium channel blockers reduce myocardial contractility, block AV conduction, and relax vascular smooth muscle cells. Various classes have different relative effects: dihydropyridines (nifedipine, nicardipine, nimodipine, amlodipine, felodipine) cause more vasodilation and less negative inotropic and atrioven-

tricular conduction blocking effects than diltiazem and verapamil. Calcium blockers might be beneficial as a result of decreased oxygen demand by decreasing afterload and contractility and by improving myocardial blood supply through coronary vasodilation.

The largest trial of calcium blockers for unstable angina was the HINT trial,[92] which tested nifedipine and metoprolol in a 2×2 factorial design. Nifedipine alone increased the risk of death and nonfatal MI by 16%, metoprolol decreased the risk by 24%, and the combination decreased the risk by 20%. None of these differences was statistically significant. A metaanalysis, both of nifedipine alone and of all calcium blockers,[93] showed no effect on mortality or infarction (Table 42-5). Moving along the spectrum into non–Q-wave MI without significant ventricular dysfunction, diltiazem appears to decrease recurrent ischemia and reinfarction[94] but has not been demonstrated to lower mortality. For patients with left ventricular dysfunction and heart failure,[95,96] as well as for the overall group of patients with AMI,[93] calcium channel blockers, and in particular nifedipine, appear to cause harm.

The NAMIS trial randomized patients not on beta blockers to nifedipine or metoprolol and patients with recurrent symptoms on beta blockers to nifedipine or placebo.[97] Nifedipine appeared to be detrimental in patients without beta blockers, but in those on adequate beta-blocking doses, nifedipine significantly reduced recurrent ischemic episodes; however, the study was too small to provide definite information on death or nonfatal infarction.

These data suggest that calcium blockers may have a role in treating patients with unstable angina in the absence of heart failure but that they should generally be reserved for patients who have been treated with nitrates and beta blockers (or who do not tolerate beta blockers) and who need an additional antianginal agent.

Angiotensin converting enzyme (ACE) inhibitors

In addition to improving survival in patients with left ventricular dysfunction (see Chapter 30), treatment with ACE inhibitors also appears to prevent the development of unstable angina and MI. In the SOLVD trials patients randomized to enalapril had a 23% reduction in follow-up MI and a 20% reduction in follow-up unstable angina ($P < 0.001$ for both).[98] Patients who had angina at the time of trial enrollment had a 28% (95% confidence interval, 17% to 37%) reduction in MI or hospitalization for angina ($P = 0.01$). In the SAVE trial of patients with left ventricular dysfunction following AMI, captopril compared with placebo was associated with a 25% reduction in recurrent infarction, 12% vs. 15% respectively, ($P = 0.015$).[99] It has been postulated that the reduction in ischemic events is in part caused by effects

Table 42-5. Randomized trials of calcium blocker therapy in unstable angina

First author	Journal	Calcium blocker			No calcium blocker			F/U
		N	Death	Death or MI	N	Death	Death or MI	
Gerstenblith[111]	*NEJM*	68	7	15	70	5	15	4 months
Muller[97]	*Circulation*	68	4	9	65	0	9	14 days
HINT[92]	*BHJ*	271	1	50	244	2	42	48 hours
Andre-Fouet[112]	*EHJ*	34	0	3	36	0	1	< 10 days
Theroux[113]	*Circulation*	50	2	5	50	2	4	5.1 months
Pooled 95% CI for death or MI		491	2.9%	16.7% 13.4%-20%	465	1.9%	15.3% 12%-18.5%	

Table 42-6. Complications of coronary angioplasty as a function of time from unstable angina presentation

	< 1 week	1-2 weeks	> 2 weeks	P < 1 week vs. > 2 weeks
Number	310	220	227	
Success rate	79.1%	84.8%	86.3%	
Q wave MI	6.5%	6.6%	1.6%	< 0.05
Emergency CABG	9.4%	6.1%	4.8%	< 0.05
Follow-up mortality	8%	2.5%	2.4%	

Adapted from Myler RK, Shaw RE, Stertzer SH, et al: Unstable angina and coronary angioplasty, *Circulation* 82(suppl II):II-88 – II-95, 1990.

at the cellular level, inhibiting the growth and proliferation of vascular smooth muscle cells or having beneficial effects on endothelial function. Because the effect of preventing acute coronary syndromes was not seen until after 6 months of treatment, the effect is not an acute one but may in part be the result of a long-term effect of stabilizing the plaque. These findings support the need to use ACE inhibitors in patients with depressed left ventricular function (left ventricular ejection fraction < 35%); additional data from clinical trials in patients with preserved left ventricular function are needed before these agents can be routinely recommended for other ischemic heart disease patients.

Intraaortic balloon pumping

Percutaneous intraaortic balloon pumping is a means of temporary cardiovascular support that both decreases cardiac afterload and increases coronary perfusion pressure. The net effect is to improve cardiac output while creating a beneficial effect on the balance of myocardial oxygen supply and demand. Uncontrolled series suggest that this may be a highly effective method to stabilize the patient with refractory unstable angina.[100] There is also evidence that intraaortic balloon pumping for 48 hours may help preserve coronary patency after angioplasty in the setting of AMI,[101] perhaps because of brisker or higher pressure flow through the unstable lesion while healing begins. Although there is an approximately 12% risk of vascular complication (usually reversible) with prolonged balloon

pumping in experienced centers, balloon pumping should be considered for all patients with refractory ischemia and/or cardiogenic shock.

Early cardiac catheterization and revascularization

Urgent or emergency cardiac catheterization is indicated for patients who have refractory ischemia. However, patients in the early acute phase of unstable angina are at higher risk for thrombotic complications of angioplasty, including MI, abrupt closure, and need for emergency bypass surgery than patients with stable symptoms.[102] Table 42-6 illustrates the higher risk of complications in patients who undergo coronary angioplasty early after presentation with unstable angina. More recent data indicate that patients undergoing angioplasty with unstable ischemic syndromes appear to have a higher rate of restenosis.[103,104]

Although it has been shown that after thrombolytic therapy for AMI, a delay of 5 days in performing nonemergency angioplasty is associated with a better outcome,[105] it is not known whether a delay in the performance of angioplasty for acute coronary syndromes not treated with thrombolytic therapy will result in a better overall outcome. Angiographically visible coronary thrombus is associated with higher rates of abrupt closure after angioplasty,[106,107] and therefore it has been postulated that treatment to reduce the thrombus might lower the subsequent risk of complications associated with angioplasty. Uncontrolled studies have observed that patients with unstable angina who are treated with 3 to 6 days of heparin have lower rates of abrupt closure.[108,109] As previously described, the use of c7E3 reduces the rate of acute ischemic complications and the risk of late unstable angina. Because the acute phase is associated with active coronary thrombosis and an unstable coronary plaque, treating patients whose ischemia is medically controlled with antithrombotic therapy for at least 24 to 48 hours before coronary intervention seems prudent.

The issue of whether to perform routine cardiac catheterization and revascularization when anatomically appropriate was addressed by the TIMI IIIB trial,[9] in which 1473 patients with unstable angina/non–Q-wave infarction were randomly assigned to "early invasive" vs. "early conservative" strategies, as well as t-PA vs. placebo, in a 2×2 factorial design. All patients were treated with aspirin and intravenous heparin for 72 hours. The early invasive strategy called for catheterization 18 to 48 hours after enrollment and revascularization when technically feasible and appropriate in the view of the angiographer. The early conservative strategy called for catheterization only for spontaneous or provocable ischemia. In the early invasive arm, 38% underwent angioplasty and 25% underwent bypass surgery within 6 weeks, for a total revascularization rate of 61%; in the early conservative arm, 26% underwent angioplasty and 24% underwent bypass surgery, for a total revascularization rate of 49%. Although there was no detectable difference in 42-day mortality and nonfatal MI (2.4% and 5.1% for the invasive group vs. 2.5% and 5.7% for the conservative group), there were advantages to the invasive strategy for several "soft" endpoints. The invasive group had fewer readmissions (54 vs. 86, $P = 0.004$), less nitrate use (33% vs. 43%, $P = 0.001$), and less angina. Based on these results, early routine catheterization is a reasonable but not essential strategy, as it appears to improve coronary perfusion, decrease ischemia, and decrease subsequent hospitalization and medication needs, at the cost of earlier intervention. More effective antithrombotic and antiplatelet therapy may make this strategy even more effective.

FUTURE GOALS IN ACUTE-PHASE AND LONG-TERM MANAGEMENT
Acute-phase management

Although current management directed at stabilizing the unstable plaque improves outcome, our ability to modify the process of plaque fissure and accurately and specifically inhibit the various components of the thrombotic process is limited. The wide array of new potent antiplatelet agents, direct thrombin inhibitors, and agents to specifically inhibit other aspects of the clotting system that are currently being developed need to be tested in clinical trials. Development of the ideal combination of antithrombotic agents that will arrest and prevent further coronary thrombosis without causing unacceptable bleeding risk is a major goal.

Resource use and allocation

Optimal use of resources to practice high-quality, cost-effective care will depend on determining the necessary duration of intensive medical therapy and the best timing and method of percutaneous intervention. Currently, acute management of patients with suspected acute coronary syndromes is often limited by diagnostic uncertainty. Better methods to determine whether there is active thrombosis, an unstable plaque, and/or myocardial necrosis at the time of presentation in patients with nondiagnostic ECGs will enable earlier, directed management of these patients.

Long-term stabilization and atherosclerosis regression

Once the patient has survived the in-hospital phase without a recurrent ischemic event, attention must be turned to maintaining stability of the infarct-related lesion because of the heightened risk over the next 6 to 8 months. Continuation of antiplatelet and beta-blocking agents are the most proven approaches, but as previously discussed, continuing antithrombin therapy and ACE inhibition have a sound empirical basis for secondary prevention in this setting. Other potential approaches include modification of lipid metabolism and endothelial cell function and, eventually, suppression of inflammatory cell function and smooth cell growth.

Angioplasty itself may be a method of converting a lipid-rich lesion with associated thrombus into a fibrotic plaque with much lower risk of plaque disruption. Follow-up studies after angioplasty consistently demonstrate a low risk of sudden MI as a manifestation of restenosis, probably because the fibrous lesion is physically resistant to disruption. The potential benefits of the mechanical approach must always be weighed against the immediate risk.

In postmenopausal women the administration of estrogen has been associated with a marked reduction in ischemic heart disease events. Estrogen appears to be essential for the maintenance of endothelial function, particularly normal vasomotor responses of the coronary arteries. In addition, estrogen administration raises HDL cholesterol and lowers LDL cholesterol. The counterbalancing effects of increased risk of breast and uterine cancer remain to be quantified adequately by randomized clinical trials, such as the Heart & Estrogen/progestin Replacement Study (HERS).

An overview of studies of atherosclerosis "regression" using lipid-lowering strategies consistently show more of an effect on acute ischemic events than on the degree of stenosis of epicardial vessels. It has been theorized that the major reason for this finding is that plaque vulnerability is largely a function of the size of the lipid pool and the inflammatory reaction at the level of the fibrous cap of the plaque to oxidized low-density lipoprotein. Although the prerequisite further clinical trials are in progress, both aggressive lipid lowering and administration of antioxidant vitamins may offer a substantial reduction in secondary events.

In summary a variety of methods will be used to attempt to keep the culprit lesion quiescent during the recovery period from an acute ischemic event. Currently, aspirin and beta blockers as well as ACE inhibitors are recommended, especially for patients with reduced left ventricular function; in the near future low-dose anticoagulation, aggressive lipid lowering, antioxidant vitamins, and estrogen in women may become routine therapy. In the more distant future specific methods of preventing plaque rupture though control of macrophage function and lipid metabolism, combined with specific growth factor inhibition, may become part of the therapeutic program.

REFERENCES

1. Mark DB: Assessment of paronosis in patients with coronary artery disease. In Roubin GS, Califf RM, O'Neill WW et al (eds): *Interventional cardiovascular medicine,* Churchill Livingstone, New York, 1994, Churchill Livingstone.
2. Fuster V, Badimon L, Badimon JJ, et al: The pathogenesis of coronary artery disease and the acute coronary syndromes (1), *N Engl J Med* 326:242-250, 1992.
3. Fuster V, Badimon L, Badimon JJ, et al: The pathogenesis of coronary artery disease and the acute coronary syndromes (2), *N Engl J Med* 326:310-318, 1992.
4. Sgarbossa EB, Topol EJ: Semantic ambiguity, the "non-" nosology and myocardial infarction, *J Clin Epidemiol,* 1994 (in press).
5. Cragg DR, Friedman HZ, Bonema JD, et al: Outcome of patients with acute myocardial infarction who are ineligible for thrombolytic therapy, *Ann Int Med* 115:173-177, 1991.
6. Muller DW, Topol EJ: Selection of patients with acute myocardial infarction for thrombolytic therapy, *Ann Int Med* 113:949-960, 1990.
7. Braunwald E, Mark DB, Jones RH, et al: *Unstable angina: diagnosis and management*—Clinical Practice Guideline Number X—AHCPR Publication No. 94-0682, Rockville, Md: Agency for Health Care Policy and Research and the National Heart, Lung, and Blood Institute, Public Health Service, US Department of Health and Human Services, March, 1994.
8. Hamm CW, Ravkilde J, Gerhardt W, et al: The prognostic value of serum troponin T in unstable angina, *N Engl J Med* 327:146-150, 1992.
9. TIMI IIIB Investigators: Effects of tissue plasminogen activator and a comparison of early invasive and conservative strategies in unstable angina and non-Q-wave infarction: results of the TIMI IIIB trial, *Circulation* 89(4):1545-1556, 1994.
10. Fibrinolytic Therapy Trialists' (FTT) Collaborative Group: Indications for fibrinolytic therapy in suspected acute myocardial infarction: collaborative overview of early mortality and major morbidity results from all randomized trials of more than 1000 patients, *Lancet* 343(8893):311-322, 1994.
11. Nicklas J, Topol EJ, Kander N, et al: Randomized, double-blind, placebo-controlled trial of tissue plasminogen activator in unstable angina, *J Am Coll Cardiol* 13:434-441, 1989.
12. Lawrence JR, Shepherd JT, Bone I, et al: Fibrinolytic therapy in unstable angina pectoris, a controlled clinical trial, *Thromb Res* 17:767-777, 1980.
13. Saran RK, Bhandari K, Narani VS, et al: Intravenous streptokinase in a subset of patients with unstable angina: a randomized controlled trial, *Int J Cardiol* 28:209-213, 1990.
14. Williams DO, Topol EJ, Califf RM, et al and Coinvestigators: Intravenous recombinant tissue-type plasminogen activator in patients with unstable angina pectoris, *Circulation* 82:376-383, 1990.
15. Freeman MR, Langer A, Wilson RF, et al: Thrombolysis in unstable angina: randomized double-blind trial of t-PA and placebo, *Circulation* 85:150-157, 1992.
16. Bär FW, Verheugt FW, Col J, et al: Thrombolysis in patients with unstable angina improves the angiographic but not the clinical outcome, *Circulation* 86:131-177, 1992.
17. Schreiber TL, Rizik D, White C, et al: Randomized trial of thrombolysis versus heparin in unstable angina, *Circulation* 86:1407-1414, 1992.
18. Karlsson JE, Berglund U, Bjorkholm A, et al for the TRIC Study Group: Thrombolysis with recombinant human tissue-type plasminogen activator during instability in coronary artery disease: effect on myocardial ischemia and need for coronary revascularization, *Am Heart J* 124:1419-1426, 1992.
19. Serneri GG, Gensini GF, Poggesi L, et al: Effect of heparin, aspirin, or alteplase in reduction of myocardial ischaemia in refractory unstable angina, *Lancet* 335:615-618, 1990.
20. van den Brand M, van Zijl A, Geuskens R, et al: Tissue plasminogen activator in refractory unstable angina. A randomized double-blind placebo-controlled treal in patients with refractory unstable angina and subsequent angioplasty, *Eur Heart J* 12:1208-1214, 1991.
21. Chaudhary H, Crozier I, Hamer A, et al: Tissue plasminogen activator using a rapid-infusion low-dose regimen for unstable angina, *Am J Cardiol* 69:173-175, 1992.
22. Reference deleted in proofs.
23. Waller BF, Rothbaum DA, Pinkerton CA, et al: Status of the myocardium and infarct-related coronary artery in 19 necropsy patients with acute recanalization using pharmacologic (streptokinase, r-tissue plasminogen activator), mechanical (percutaneous transluminal coronary angioplasty) or combined types of reperfusion therapy, *J Am Coll Cardiol* 9(4):785-801, 1987.
24. Eisenberg PR, Sherman LA, Jaffe AS: Paradoxic elevation of fibrin peptide A after streptokinase: evidence for intense thrombosis despite intense fibrinolysis, *J Am Coll Cardiol* 10:527-529, 1987.
25. Rapold HJ: Promotion of thrombin activity by thrombolytic therapy without simultaneous anticoagulation, *Lancet* 1:481-482, 1990.
26. Rapold HJ, de Bono D, Arnold AER, et al for the European Cooperative Study Group: Plasma fibrinopeptide A levels in patients with acute myocardial infarction treated with alteplase, *Circulation* 85:928-934, 1992.
27. Davies MJ, Thomas AC, Knapman PA, et al: Intramyocardial platelet aggregation in patients with unstable angina suffering sudden ischemic cardiac death, *Circulation* 73(3):418-427, 1986.
28. Mizuno K, Satomura K, Miyamoto A, et al: Angioscopic evaluation of coronary artery thrombi in acute coronary syndromes, *N Engl J Medicine* 326(5):287-291, 1992.
29. Jang IK, Golk HK, Ziskind AA, et al: Differential sensitivity of erythrocyte-rich and platelet-rich arterial thrombi to lysis with recombinant tissue-type plasminogen activator: a possible explanation for resistance to coronary thrombolysis, *Circulation* 79:920-928, 1989.

30. Ambrose J: Plaque disruption and the acute coronary syndromes of unstable angina and myocardial infarction: if the substrate is similar, why is the clinical presentation different? *Am J Cardiol* 19(7):1653-1658, 1992.

31. Willard JE, Lange RA, Hillis LD: The use of aspirin in ischemic heart disease, *N Engl J Med* 327:175-281, 1992.

32. Sobel M, Salzman EW, Daview GC, et al: Circulating platelet products in unstable angina pectoris, *Circulation* 63:300-306, 1981.

33. Fitzgerald DJ, Roy L, Catella F, et al: Platelet activation in unstable coronary disease, *N Engl J Med* 315:983-989, 1986.

34. Willerson JT, Golino P, Eidt J, et al: Platelet mediators and unstable coronary artery lesions: experimental evidence and potential clinical implications, *Circulation* 75:156-162, 1989.

35. ISIS-2 (Second International Study of Infarct Survival) Collaborative Group: Randomised trial of intravenous streptokinase, oral aspirin, both, or neither among 17,187 cases of suspected acute myocardial infarctions: ISIS-2, *Lancet* 2(8607):349-360, 1988.

36. Theroux P, Ouimet H, McCans J, et al: Aspirin, heparin, or both to treat unstable angina, *N Engl J Med* 319:1105-1111, 1988.

37. RISC Group: Risk of myocardial infarction and death during treatment with low-dose aspirin and intravenous heparin in men with unstable coronary artery disease, *Lancet* 336:827-830, 1990.

38. Lewis HD Jr, Davis JW, Archibald DG, et al: Protective effects of aspirin against acute myocardial infarction and death in men with unstable angina: results of a Veterans' Administration Cooperative Study, *N Engl J Med* 309:396-403, 1983.

39. Cairns JA, Gent M, Singer J, et al: Aspirin, sulfinpyrazone, or both in unstable angina. Results of a Canadian multicenter trial, *N Engl J Med* 313:1369-1375, 1985.

40. The Dutch TIA Trial Study Group: A comparision of two doses of aspirin (30 mg vs. 283 mg a day) in patients after a transient ischemic attack or minor ischemic stroke, *N Engl J Med* 325(18):1261-1266, 1991.

41. Antiplatelet Trialists' Collaboration: Secondary prevention of vascular disease by prolonged antiplatelet treatment, *Br Med J* 296:320-331, 1988.

42. McTavish D, Faulds D, Goa KL: Ticlopidine. An updated review of its pharmacology and therapeutic use in platelet-dependent disorders, *Drugs* 40:238-259, 1990.

43. Balsano F, Rizzon P, Violi F, et al: Antiplatelet treatment with ticlopidine in unstable angina. A controlled multicenter clinical trial, *Circulation* 82:17-26, 1990.

44. Hass WK, Easton JD, Adams HP Jr, et al for the Ticlopidine Aspirin Stroke Group: A randomized trial comparing ticlopidine hydrochloride with aspirin for the prevention of stroke in high-risk patients, *N Engl J Medicine* 321(8):501-507, 1989.

45. The EPIC Investigation: Use of monoclonal antibody directed against the platelet glycoprotein IIb/IIIa receptor in high-risk coronary angioplasty, *N Eng J Med* 330(14):956-961, 1994.

46. Topol EJ, Califf RM, Weisman HS, et al for the EPIC Investigators: Reduction of clinical restenosis following coronary intervention with early administration of platelet IIb/IIIa integrin blocking antibody, *Lancet* 343(8902):881-886, 1994.

47. Tcheng JE, Kleiman NS, Harrington RA, et al: Outcome of patients treated with the GPIIb/IIIa inhibitor Integrelin during coronary angioplasty: results of the IMPACT study, *Circulation* 88(suppl I):I-595, 1993.

48. Hirsh J: Heparin, *N Engl J Med* 324:1565-1574, 1991.

49. Theroux P, Waters D, Qiu S, et al: Aspirin versus heparin to prevent myocardial infarction during the acute phase of unstable angina, *Circulation* 88:2045-2048, 1993.

50. Arnout J, Simoons M, de Bono D, et al: Correlation between level of heparinization and patency of the infarct-related coronary artery after treatment of acute myocardial infarction with alteplase (rt-PA), *J Am Coll Cardiol* 20:513-519, 1992.

51. Meade TW, Mellows S, Brozovic M, et al: Haemostatic function and ischaemic heart disease: principle results of the Northwick Park Heart Study, *Lancet* 2:533-537, 1986.

52. Turpie AG, Gent M, Laupacis A, et al: A comparison of aspirin with placebo in patients treated with warfarin after heart valve replacement, *New Engl J Med* 329:524-529, 1993.

53. Talbot MD, Ambler J, Butler KD, et al: Recombinant desulfatohirudin (CGP 39393) anticoagulant and antithrombotic properties in vivo, *Thromb Haemost* 61:77-80, 1989.

54. Weitz JI, Hudoba M, Massel D, et al: Clot-bound thrombin is protected from inhibition by heparin-anti-thrombin III but is susceptible to inactivation by antithrombin III-independent inhibitors, *J Clin Invest* 86:385-391, 1990.

55. Heras M, Chesebro JH, Webster MWI, et al: Hirudin, heparin, and placebo during deep arterial injury in the pig. The in vivo role of thrombin in platelet mediated thrombosis, *Circulation* 82:1476-1484, 1990.

56. Heras M, Chesebro JH, Penny WJ, et al: Effects of thrombin inhibition on the development of acute platelet-thrombus deposition during angioplasty in pigs: heparin versus recombinant hirudin, a specific thrombin inhibitor, *Circulation* 79:657-665, 1989.

57. Badimon L, Merino A, Badimon J, et al: Hirudin and other thrombin inhibitors: experimental results and potential clinical applications, *Trends Cardiovasc Med* 1:261-267, 1991.

58. Lam JYT, Chesebro JH, Steele PM, et al: Antithrombotic therapy for deep arterial injury by angioplasty, *Circulation* 84:814-820, 1991.

59. Topol EJ, Fuster V, Harrington RA, et al: Recombinant hirudin for unstable angina pectoris: a multicenter, randomized angiographic trial, *Circulation* 89(4):1557-1566, 1994.

60. Lidon RM, Theroux P, Juneau M, et al: Initial experience with a direct antithrombin, hirulog, in unstable angina, *Circulation* 88:1495-1501, 1993.

61. TIMI 5 Trial: Preliminary results presented at the 42nd Annual Scientific Session of the American College of Cardiology, Atlanta, March, 1993.

61b. The Global Use of Strategies to Open Occluded Coronary Arteries (GUSTO) IIa Investigators: Randomized trial of recombinant hirudin for acute coronary syndromes, *Circulation* (in press).

62. Cohen M, Adams PC, Parry G, et al and the Antithromotic Therapy in Acute Coronary Syndromes Research Group: Combination antithrombotic therapy in unstable rest angina and non-Q-wave infarction in nonprior aspirin users, *Circulation* 89:81-88, 1994.

63. Theroux P, Waters D, Lam J, et al: Reactivation of unstable angina after the discontinuation of heparin, *N Engl J Med* 327:141-145, 1992.

64. Granger CB, Miller J, Bovill EG, et al: Rebound increase in thrombin generation and activity after cessation of intravenous heparin in patient with acute coronary syndromes, Manuscript submitted for publication, 1994.

65. Gold HK, Torres F, Garabedian H, et al: Evidence for a rebound coagulation phenomenon after cessation of a 4-hour infusion of a specific thrombin inhibitor in patients with unstable angina pectoris, *J Am Coll Cardiol* 21:1039-1047, 1993.

66. Hackett D, Davies G, Chierchia S, et al: Intermittent coronary occlusion in acute myocardial infarction. Value of combined thrombolytic and vasodilator therapy, *New Engl J Med* 317:1055-1059, 1987.

67. Krucoff MW, Croll MA, Pope JE, et al: Continuously updated 12-lead ST-segment recovery analysis for myocardial infarct artery patency assessment and its correlation with multiple

simultaneous early angiographic observations, *Am J Cardiol* 71:145-151, 1993.

68. Diodati J, Theroux P, Latour JG, et al: Effects of nitroglycerin at therapeutic doses on platelet aggregation in unstable angina pectoris and acute myocardial infarction, *Am J Cardiol* 59:683-688, 1990.

69. Curfman GD, Heinsimer JA, Lozner EC, et al: Intravenous nitroglycerin in the treatment of spontaneous angina pectoris: a prospective, randomized trial, *Circulation* 67:276-282, 1983.

70. Kaplan K, Davison R, Parker M, et al: Intravenous nitroglycerin for the treatment of angina at rest unresponsive to standard nitrate therapy, *Am J Cardiol* 51:694-698, 1983.

71. Lin S, Flaherty JT: Crossover from intravenous to transdermal nitroglycerin therapy in unstable angina pectoris, *Am J Cardiol* 56:742-748, 1985.

72. Yusuf S, Collins R, MacMahon S, et al: Effect of intravenous nitrates on mortality in acute myocardial infarction: an overview of the randomised trials, *Lancet* 1:1088-1092, 1988.

73. GISSI-3 preliminary results presentation, 66th Scientific Sessions of the American Heart Association, November, 1993.

74. ISIS-4 preliminary results presentation, 66th Scientific Sessions of the American Heart Association, November, 1993.

75. Elkayam U, Kulick D, McIntosh N, et al: Incidence of early tolerance to the hemodynamic effects of continuous infusion of nitroglycerin in patients with coronary heart disease and heart failure, *Circulation* 76:577-584, 1987.

76. May DC, Popma JJ, Black WH, et al: In vivo induction and reversal of nitroglycerin tolerance in human coronary arteries, *N Engl J Med* 317:805, 1987.

77. Jugdutt BI, Warnica JW: Tolerance with low-dose intravenous nitroglycerin therapy in acute myocardial infarction, *Am J Cardiol* 64:581, 1989.

78. Yusuf S, Peto R, Lewis J, et al: Beta blockade during and after myocardial infarction, *Prog Cardiovasc Dis* 27:335-371, 1985.

79. Willich SN, Linderer T, Wegscheider K, et al: Increasing morning incidence of myocardial infarction in the ISAM study: absence with prior beta-adrenergic blockade, *Circulation* 80:853, 1989.

80. Lusben J, Tijssen JGP for the HINT Research Group: Efficacy of nifedipine and metoprolol in the early treatment of unstable angina in the coronary care unit: findings from the Holland Interuniversity Nifedipine/Metoprolol Trial (HINT), *Am J Cardiol* 60:18A-25A, 1987.

81. Telford AM, Wilson C: Trial of heparin versus atenolol in prevention of myocardial infarction in intermediate coronary syndrome, *Lancet* 1:1225-1228, 1981.

82. Gottlieb S, Weisfeldt M, Ouyang P, et al: Effect of the addition of propranolol to therapy with nifedipine for unstable angina pectoris: a randomized, double-blind, placebo-controlled trial, *Circulation* 73:331-337, 1987.

83. Yusuf S, Wittes J, Fiedman L: Overview of results of randomized clinical trials in heart disease. II. Unstable angina, heart failure, primary prevention with aspirin, and risk factor modification, *JAMA* 260:2259-2263, 1988.

84. Yusuf S, Wittes J, Friedman L: Overview of results of randomized clinical trials in heart disease. I. Treatments following myocardial infarction, *JAMA* 260:2088-2093, 1988.

85. Yusuf S: The use of beta-blockers in the acute phase of myocardial infarction. In Califf RM, Wagner GS (eds): *Acute coronary care,* Boston, 1986, Martinus Nijhoff.

86. ISIS-1 Collaborative Group: A randomized trial of intravenous atenolol among 16,027 cases of suspected acute myocardial infarction, *Lancet* 2:57-66, 1986.

87. Yusuf S, Peto R, Lewis J, et al: Beta blockade during and after myocardial infarction, *Prog Cardiovasc Dis* 27:335-371, 1985.

88. Beta-blocker Heart Attack Trial Research Group: A randomized trial of propranolol in patients with acute myocardial infarction: I. Mortality results, *JAMA* 247:1707-1714, 1982.

89. Multicenter International Study: Supplementary report: reduction in mortality after myocardial infarction with long-term beta-adrenergic receptor blockade, *Br Med J* 2:419-421, 1977.

90. Norwegian Multicenter Study Group: Timolol-induced reduction in mortality and reinfarction in patients surviving acute myocardial infarction, *N Engl J Med* 304:801-807, 1981.

91. Wallis DE, Pope C, Littman WJ, et al: Safety and efficacy of esmolol for unstable angina pectoris, *Am J Cardiol* 62:1033-1037, 1988.

92. Holland Interuniversity Nifedipine/metoprolol Trial (HINT) Research Group: Early treatment of unstable angina in the coronary care unit. A randomised double-blind, placebo-controlled comparison of recurrent ischemia in patients treated with nifedipine or metoprolol or both, *Br Heart J* 56:400-413, 1986.

93. Yusuf S, Held P, Furberg C: Update of effects of calcium antagonists in myocardial infarction or angina in light of the second Danish verapamil infarction trial (DAVIT-II) and other recent studies, *Am J Cardiol* 67(15):1295-1297, 1991.

94. Gibson RS, Boden WE, Theroux P, et al: Diltiazem and reinfarction in patients with non Q-wave myocardial infarction. Results of a double-blind, randomized, multicenter trial, *N Engl J Med* 315:423-429, 1986.

95. The Multicenter Diltiazem Postinfarction Trial Research Group: The effect of diltiazem on mortality and reinfarction after myocardial infarction, *N Engl J Med* 319:385-392, 1988.

96. Goldstein RE, Boccussi SJ, Cruess D, et al: Diltiazem increases late-onset congestive heart failure in postinfarction patients with early reduction in ejection fraction, *Circulation* 83:52-60, 1991.

97. Muller JE, Turi ZG, Pearle DL, et al: Nifedipine and conventional therapy for unstable angina pectoris: a randomized, double-blind comparison, *Circulation* 69:728-739, 1984.

98. Yusuf S, Pepine CJ, Garces C, et al: Effect of enalapril on myocardial infarction and unstable angina in patients with low ejection fractions, *Lancet* 340:1173-1178, 1992.

99. Pfeffer MA, Braunwald E, Moye LA, et al, on behalf of the SAVE (Survival and Ventricular Enlargement Trial) Investigators: Effect of captopril on mortality and morbidity in patients with left ventricular dysfunction after myocardial infarction: results of the Survival and Ventricular Enlargement Trial, *N Engl J Med* 327(10):669-677, 1992.

100. Aroesty JM, Weintraub RM, Paulin S, et al: Medically refractory unstable angina pectoris. II. Hemodynamic and angiographic effects of intraaortic balloon counterpulsation, *Am J Cardiol* 43:883-888, 1979.

101. Ohman EM, George BS, White CJ, et al: The use of aortic counterpulsation to improve sustained coronary artery patency during acute myocardial infarction: results of a randomized trial, *Circulation* 90:792-799, 1994.

102. Myler RK, Shaw RE, Stertzer SH, et al: Unstable angina and coronary angioplasty, *Circulation* 82 (suppl II):88-95, 1990.

103. Harrington RA, Holmes DR, Berdan LG, et al for the CAVEAT Investigators: Clinical characteristics and outcomes of patients with unstable angina undergoing percutaneous coronary intervention in CAVEAT (abstract), *J Am Coll Cardiol* 1994 (in press).

104. Frid DJ, Fortin DF, Lam LC, et al. Effects of unstable symptoms on restenosis (abstract), *Circulation* 82:III-427, 1990.

105. Topol EJ, Califf RM, George BS, et al and the Thrombolysis and Angioplasty in Myocardial Infarction Study Group: A randomized trial of immediate versus delayed elective angioplasty after intravenous tissue plasminogen activator in acute myocardial infarction, *N Engl J Med* 317:581-588, 1987.

106. Ellis SG, Roubin GS, King SB III, et al: Angiographic and clinical

predictors of acute closure after native vessel coronary angioplasty, *Circulation* 77:372-379, 1988.

107. Cowley MJ, Kelsey SF, Holubkov R, et al and participating investigators: Factors influencing outcome with coronary angioplasty: 1985-1986 NHLBI PTCA Registry, *Circulation* 11:148A, 1988.

108. Topol EJ: Integration of anticoagulation, thrombolysis and coronary angioplasty for unstable angina pectoris, *Am J Cardiol* 68:136B-141B, 1991.

109. Hettleman BD, Aplin RA, Sullivan PR, et al. Three days of heparin pretreatment reduces major complications of coronary angioplasty in patients with unstable angina (abstract), *J Am Coll Cardiol* 15:154, 1990.

110. Gerstenblith F, Ouyang P, Achuff SC, et al: Nifedipine in unstable angina. A double-blind, randomized trial, *New Engl J Med* 306:885-889, 1982.

111. Andre-Foulet X, Usdin JP, Gayet C, et al: Comparison of short-term efficacy of diltiazem and propranolol in unstable angina at rest—a randomized trial in 70 patients, *Eur Heart* 4:691-698, 1983.

112. Theroux P, Taeymans Y, Morissette D, et al: A randomized study comparing propranolol and diltiazem in the treatment of unstable angina, *J Am Coll Cardiol* 5:717-722, 1985.

Chapter 43

CURRENT APPROACHES TO THE UNSTABLE CORONARY ARTERY: UNSTABLE ANGINA AND NON–Q-WAVE MI THROMBOLYTIC THERAPY

Craig E. Hjemdahl-Monsen
John A. Ambrose

Unstable angina and non–Q-wave myocardial infarction (MI) are common clinical manifestations for patients with an unstable coronary plaque. These patients are at risk for recurrent ischemia, MI, and the need for coronary revascularization. Treatment strategies focus on reducing ischemic episodes and the need for revascularization.

The rationale for using a thrombolytic agent in the treatment of the unstable plaque stems from our current understanding of the pathophysiology of the acute coronary syndromes of unstable angina, MI and sudden cardiac death, and the effectiveness of thrombolytic agents in the treatment of AMI manifesting with ST-segment elevation. Platelet activation leading to aggregation and thrombus formation plays an integral part in the pathogenesis of unstable angina and non–Q-wave infarction and might also be amenable to the use of thrombolytic agents.

The modest improvements seen in clinical and angiographic studies of thrombolytic therapy for unstable angina and non–Q-wave MI may be related to small but important differences in the pathophysiologic substrate compared with acute Q-wave MI.

PATHOGENESIS OF THE UNSTABLE PLAQUE

The natural history of coronary atherosclerosis begins with a raised fatty streak in the lumen of the artery typically adjacent to branch points in the vessel. Progression to the development of the fibrous plaque is related to the continued incorporation of lipid into the plaque associated with smooth muscle proliferation and the synthesis of extracellular matrix. Organization of thrombus secondary to clinically asymptomatic bouts of plaque fissuring may also be responsible for the slow progression of coronary artery disease. Patients with known risk factors for coronary artery disease accelerate this progression to more advanced stages of atherosclerosis.[1] The fibrous plaque is characterized pathologically by the proliferation of smooth muscle cells, foam cells consisting of intracellular accumulations of cholesterol, as well as extracellular cholesterol deposits. The lipid deposits may result in a soft core beneath a thin fibrous cap.

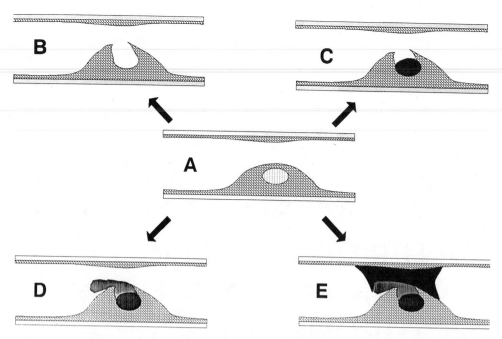

Fig. 43-1. Schematic representation of an atherosclerotic plaque (*A*) that may undergo disruption of the fibrous cap, exposing the underlying plaque material and leading to an irregularly shaped plaque with no thrombus (*B*), small amount of thrombus (*C*), moderate amount of layered thrombus (*D*), or occlusive thrombus (*E*) superimposed on the atherosclerotic plaque.

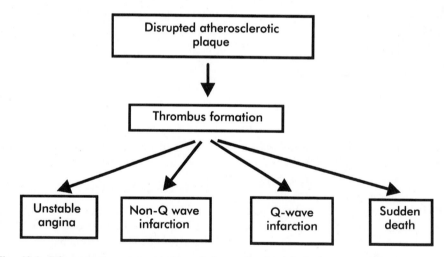

Fig. 43-2. Diagramatic representation of the pathophysiologic steps leading to the acute coronary syndromes.

At some point in the natural history of certain atherosclerotic plaques, particularly those with a lipid core underlying the fibrous cap, disruption or fissuring of the thin fibrous cap may occur, exposing the underlying plaque material to the flowing blood.[2,3] The exposure of the deep vessel wall material becomes a trigger for platelet adhesion, aggregation, and fibrin formation.[4] This rapid progression of the plaque with its resultant thrombus may lead to alterations in blood flow, as well as the release of various vasoactive substances (Fig. 43-1). Partial or complete occlusion of the coronary artery may result, leading to either unstable angina, non–Q-wave MI, Q-wave MI, or sudden death. The resulting clinical syndrome is multifactorial but is dependent on the amount of obstruction before and after plaque disruption, the rate of progression of the occlusion, the duration of total occlusion, and the presence or absence of recruitable collaterals (Fig. 43-2).[5] Because these syndromes usually share a common pathophysiology, as described earlier, unstable angina, MI, and sudden death are usually categorized as the acute coronary syndromes. The pathophysiologic

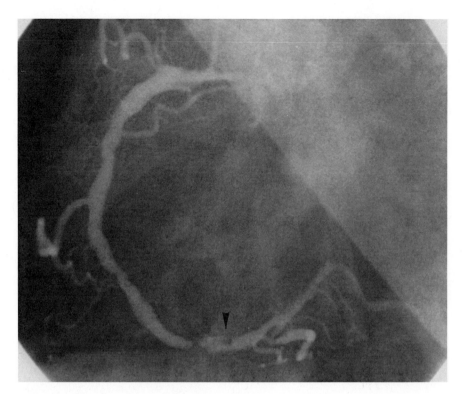

Fig. 43-3. Angiographic image of the right coronary artery in a patient with unstable angina demonstrating an intracoronary filling defect (*arrow*).

link that joins these syndromes is the development of a disrupted atherosclerotic plaque with resulting thrombus formation.[6]

ROLE OF THROMBUS

Before considering the utility of thrombolytic therapy in unstable angina and non–Q-wave infarction, one should examine the evidence for the role of thrombus in these syndromes. Pathologic data obtained by careful, serial sectioning of the coronary arteries indicate the presence of thrombus superimposed on a disrupted atherosclerotic plaque in patients dying soon after a bout of unstable angina.[3,7]

In addition to pathologic data implicating thrombus in the acute coronary syndromes, there is much angiographic validation for the role of thrombus in these syndromes. Intracoronary thrombus has been described commonly in patients with unstable angina. Intracoronary filling defects that are believed to represent intraluminal thrombus are seen in 1% to 85% of patients with unstable angina (Fig. 43-3).[8-11] A specific morphology or shape to the plaque has also been reported in patients with unstable angina. There is likely much overlap between the definitions of intracoronary thrombus and complex plaque. These complex plaques (eccentric or concentric with irregular borders or overhanging edges) are seen in most ischemia-producing lesions responsible for unstable angina and non–Q-wave MI in

which the culprit vessel is less than 100% occluded and likely represent the pathologic description of plaque disruption with thrombus formation.[12,13]

Angioscopy, which allows direct in vivo visualization of the coronary plaque, has been shown to demonstrate visible thrombus in most patients with unstable coronary syndromes but not in stable angina.[14,15] This technique appears more sensitive than angiography for the detection of thrombus.[16]

Biochemical markers indicating activation of platelets or the clotting system are found commonly in the acute coronary syndromes. Platelet-related metabolites of thromboxane are elevated in the urine of patients with unstable angina after episodes of rest pain.[17] Evidence for fibrin formation or activation of the fibrinolytic system has also been demonstrated in some patients with unstable angina, as shown by elevated levels of fibrinopeptide A, D-dimer, or other related factors,[18-20] although there are conflicting data.[21]

The role of thrombus in the unstable plaque is also supported by the clinical response of patients to antithrombotic therapy. Antiplatelet therapy with either aspirin, ticlopidine, or anticoagulation with intravenous (IV) heparin significantly decreases the incidence of cardiac events during and after hospitalization in patients with unstable angina.[22-26]

Given our understanding of the pathophysiology of the acute coronary syndromes and the role of thrombus

Table 43-1. Thrombolytic trials in unstable angina*

Study	No. of patients	Regimen	Angiographic result	Clinical result
Uncontrolled				
Rentrop et al.[27]	5	SK IC	No change	No improvement
Mandelkorn et al.[11]	17	SK IC	Improved	—
Vetrovec et al.[28]	12	SK IC	Improved	Improved
Ambrose et al.[29]	37	SK IC	No change	—
Gotoh et al.[30]	37	UK IC	Improved	Worsened
De Zwaan et al.[31]	41	SK IC, t-PA IV	Improved	No improvement
Bar et al.[33]	126	APSAC	Improved	No improvement
Gulba et al.[33]	10	SK, t-PA, or UK + proUK IV	—	Improved
DiSciascio et al.[34]	7	t-PA IC	Mixed	—
Brochier et al.[35]	16	SK, APSAC, t-PA, or UK	No change	—
Controlled				
Lawrence et al.[36]	40	SK IV + warfarin vs. warfarin	—	Improved
Topol et al.[37]	40	t-PA IV	No change	No improvement
Gold et al.[38]	24	t-PA IV	Improved	Improved
Nicklas et al.[39]	40	t-PA IV	No change	No improvement
Schreiber et al.[40]	25	UK + heparin vs. heparin	No change	Improved
Freeman et al.[41]	70	t-PA IV	No change	No improvement
Williams et al.[42]	67	t-PA IV	Improved	—
Saran et al.[43]	48	SK IV	—	Improved
Neri-Serneri et al.[44]	97	t-PA IV	—	No improvement
Schreiber et al.[45]	149	UK IV	—	No improvement
Ardissino et al.[46]	24	t-PA	No change	Improved

*SK, Streptokinase; IC, intracoronary; UK, urokinase; IV, intravenous; t-PA, tissue-type plasminogen activator; APSAC, anisoylated plasminogen streptokinase complex; proUK, prourokinase.

in unstable angina and non-Q infarction, it would be anticipated that thrombolytic therapy would have a possible use in these syndromes.

ANGIOGRAPHIC AND CLINICAL TRIALS OF THROMBOLYTIC THERAPY

The utility of thrombolysis in unstable angina and non–Q-wave MI has been assessed in a growing number of studies. These studies have focused on the angiographic and clinical responses to therapy with an assortment of thrombolytic agents given either intravenously or directly into the coronary arteries. A number of the studies have been uncontrolled. Until recently, the number of patients in each study has been limited, and only a minority of patients have had non–Q-wave infarction. The results of these studies in large part have been mixed. There appears to be at best only a modest benefit from thrombolysis, particularly in the setting of unstable angina. A summary of the findings of these studies is represented in Table 43-1.

Angiographic results

Mixed angiographic results have been seen in coronary artery stenosis severity in patients with unstable angina who received thrombolytic therapy. Some of the variables that seem to influence the response to throm-

bolytic therapy include angiographic evidence of thrombus, the presence of total coronary occlusion before thrombolysis, and the timing of thrombolysis from the last episode of ischemic pain.

Several studies have shown the absence of angiographic improvement after thrombolytic therapy. In a study examining the role of intracoronary streptokinase, Rentrop et al.[27] administered intracoronary streptokinase to five patients with unstable angina and noted no angiographic improvement in lesion severity. In a larger study, Ambrose et al.[29] reported no angiographic improvement in a group of 37 patients with less than totally occluded arteries who were given intracoronary streptokinase for unstable angina or non–Q-wave infarction. This study incorporated quantitative digital angiographic techniques to measure the response to therapy. Only five of the patients showed angiographic improvement, and most of the improvement in stenosis severity was minimal. In a study involving seven patients with unstable angina and intracoronary thrombus, DiSciascio et al.[34] found two patients improved, whereas five worsened or did not change angiographically post thrombolysis. Brochier et al.[35] found no change in stenosis severity in 16 patients given one of several thrombolytic agents in an uncontrolled trial. Of the controlled studies using thrombolytic therapy for unstable angina, several studies failed to find angiographic improvement after thrombolysis.[37,39-41,46] Freeman et al.[41] did, however, note a reduction in intracoronary thrombus after thrombolysis. Morphologic severity of the culprit coronary lesion was also not improved by the use of urokinase infusion plus heparin vs. heparin alone in a study of 25 patients performed by Schreiber et al.[40]

Conversely, angiographic improvement was seen in 10 of 13 infusions of intracoronary streptokinase in 12 patients with unstable angina in a study from Vetrovec et al.[28] Eleven of 13 lesions had preinfusion evidence of intraluminal thrombus. In six lesions, the artery was totally occluded. Mandelkorn et al.[11] showed angiographic improvement in 7 of 17 patients given intracoronary streptokinase for unstable angina or non–Q-wave infarction. Intracoronary filling defects were reported by Gold et al.[38] to be less common in those patients with refractory unstable angina receiving infusions of IV tissue-type plasminogen activator (t-PA) compared with control patients not receiving thrombolysis. In a study of 41 patients, De Zwaan et al.[31] found angiographic improvement in 22 patients who received either intracoronary streptokinase or IV t-PA, particularly in patients with total coronary occlusion. Gotoh et al.[30] found lesion improvement in 20 of 21 patients who had angiographic evidence of thrombus out of a group of 37 patients with unstable angina who received intracoronary urokinase. UNASEM,[32] a multicenter trial of 126 patients randomized to IV anistreplase (APSAC) or placebo, reported a significant improvement of mean diameter stenosis from 70% to 59% in the group of patients receiving thrombolysis for unstable angina, although there was no improvement if initially occluded vessels were excluded. In a randomized study by Williams et al.,[42] there was angiographic improvement in the group of patients who received low-dose t-PA and heparin but not in the group who received higher-dose t-PA or placebo. However, the improvement was small (from 75% diameter reduction to 71%), although it was statistically significant. Analysis of the individual responses in each group indicated that one or two patients showed marked angiographic improvement on follow-up whether they received heparin alone or either low- or high-dose t-PA with heparin.

Clinical results

Regarding the clinical efficacy of thrombolysis in unstable angina and non–Q-wave MI, the results have also been mixed. The endpoints for these studies have included recurrent ischemia, the need for revascularization, and progression or extension of MI.

In uncontrolled studies, several investigators[27,30-32] have found no improvement in the clinical course of patients after thrombolysis for unstable angina. Gotoh et al.[30] found that although patients with thrombus im-

proved angiographically after thrombolysis, these patients faired worse clinically. Seventy-one percent showed recurrent ischemia, and 24% developed MI within 1 month of thrombolysis. Several controlled studies have shown no clinical improvement[37,39,41,44,45] after thrombolysis. Of these studies, Nicklas et al.[39] reported an improvement in pacing thresholds to inducement of ischemia after thrombolysis. However, there was no improvement in subsequent clinical course.

Clinical improvement was noted in several uncontrolled trials involving small numbers of patients.[28,33] Lawrence et al.[36] found IV streptokinase, followed by warfarin, to be clinically superior to warfarin alone in patients with unstable angina who were followed for 6 months. Other studies have noted clinical improvement as well.[38,40,43,46] Schreiber et al.[40] noted less ischemia for 24 hours after infusion of urokinase for unstable angina. However, there were no clinical differences between treated and control patients at 7 days. In patients with "refractory" symptoms, Neri-Seneri et al.[44] found clinical improvement that was apparent for only the first day after thrombolysis. In a study of similarly "refractory" patients by Ardissino et al.,[46] none of the 11 patients receiving t-PA had recurrent ischemic symptoms during the 72 hours of study follow-up. However, 10 of these 11 patients had recurrent symptoms after this 72-hour period.

The variability of clinical outcome after thrombolysis in unstable angina may depend on the balance of thrombotic and thrombolytic forces at work on the culprit lesion. It is known that thrombolytic therapy increases thrombin formation probably by release of active thrombin from partially lysed thrombi and by new formation of thrombin. Thrombolytic therapy also activates platelets.[47,48] These thrombotic processes may result in a paradoxical increase in thrombotic events in some patients.[49]

Thrombolysis in Myocardial Infarction-III trial

Perhaps the most ambitious attempt to define the role of thrombolytic therapy is the recently completed Thrombolysis in Myocardial Infarction (TIMI-III) trial.[50] This study focused on the angiographic and clinical results of t-PA plus IV heparin and aspirin compared with heparin and aspirin alone in a large group of patients with unstable angina or non–Q-wave MI. The structure of the trial involved a smaller trial consisting of 306 patients randomized to t-PA and heparin vs. heparin alone and studied angiographically before and after therapy (IIIA), as well as a larger trial of 1392 patients additionally assessing the value of early angiography and revascularization therapy (IIIB) vs. a conservative strategy consisting of continued medical therapy with catheterization for recurrent ischemia. The inclusion criteria for this trial included the presence of at least 5 minutes but less than 6 hours of rest pain within 12 hours of enrollment. Patient requirements were documented evidence of coronary artery disease by either electrocardiographic (ECG) changes associated with pain, a prior history MI, or prior angiographic evidence of coronary disease. Patients with recent MI or coronary angioplasty were excluded from the trial.

In the angiographic arm of the study, 306 patients were randomized to t-PA or placebo. t-PA was infused intravenously at a dose of 0.8 mg/kg over 90 minutes, with one third of the dose given as a bolus. A maximum dose of 80 mg was used. The patients were then treated with heparin and maximal medical therapy. Angiograms were obtained at baseline and at follow-up 18 to 48 hours later. Approximately two thirds of patients in each group had unstable angina, and one third had a diagnosis of non–Q-wave infarction. The baseline angiographic data revealed an 84% mean diameter stenosis of the culprit lesion. Eighteen percent of the patients had totally occluded culprit lesions. Apparent or possible thrombus was identified in 75% of patients. Twenty-five percent of the treated group showed an improvement in stenosis severity of greater than 10% or an improvement of antegrade flow of at least two TIMI grades compared with only 15% improvement in the placebo group. This was not statistically significant. However, an improvement greater than 20% in diameter stenosis or improvement of two TIMI grade flows was seen in 15% of the treated group compared with only 5% of the placebo group. This difference was highly significant. Clinical and angiographic variables indicating improvement in a multivariate model included non–Q-wave infarction, apparent thrombus, and t-PA administration.

The results of the clinical arm of the TIMI trial (IIIB) have yet to be reported in the literature. Preliminary results based on the primary endpoints of death or MI within 42 days after treatment have failed to show a benefit of thrombolytic therapy. The death rate at the end of 1 year was also unrelated to thrombolytic therapy.

In summary, angiographic trials of thrombolytic therapy indicate some benefit in the presence of total occlusion or visible thrombus before therapy. However, angiographic improvement does not correlate with clinical improvement. Clinical benefits have been described but overall are very modest. Recent reports also suggest an increase in thrombotic endpoints after thrombolysis in unstable angina. Other than TIMI-III, only a small percentage of patients had non–Q-wave infarction in these studies. Because the final results of TIMI-IIIB have yet to be published, the role of thrombolytic therapy in this later syndrome has yet to be determined.

COMPARISON WITH TRIALS IN MI

To gain an appreciation of the difficulty in duplicating the favorable results of thrombolysis in MI in patients with unstable angina and non–Q-wave MI, we must consider the differences in clinical endpoints and pathophysiologic substrates between syndromes. These differences require that large studies be performed to achieve the statistical power necessary to demonstrate a difference in treatment modalities.

Clinical definition

In contrast to acute myocardial infarction (AMI) manifesting with ST-segment elevation, unstable angina is a clinical condition that is somewhat heterogeneous. The recent onset of low workload or resting chest pain associated with transient ST-T changes on ECG, a sudden change in the frequency or severity of prior stable angina, or rest chest pain after MI without a significant rise in the creatine phosphokinase level are useful definitions for unstable angina. Patients with this history might be expected to have a disrupted atherosclerotic plaque with superimposed thrombus. However, there are other clinical manifestations considered in the classification of unstable angina[51] that may have different mechanisms for precipitation of angina. These patients might not be responsive to thrombolytic therapy.

Clinical endpoints

Trials of thrombolysis in MI have focused on the reduction in mortality and preservation of left ventricular function after thrombolysis. Clinical endpoints for thrombolysis in unstable angina have a low incidence. MI or refractory angina occurs in 2% and 10%, respectively, in the first week after onset in patients treated with anticoagulant therapy.[24,25] To achieve a significant reduction in these clinical events, a study would have to randomize thousands of patients.[52]

Pathophysiologic substrate

It is now generally accepted that the acute coronary syndromes of unstable angina, MI, and sudden cardiac death share a common pathophysiologic substrate. However, there are probably important differences in the disrupted atherosclerotic plaque responsible for these syndromes that account for their different clinical manifestations, as well as explain their response to thrombolytic therapy.

Patients who have AMI with ST-segment elevation are found to have totally occluded infarct-related arteries in 70% to 90% of cases. Although somewhat fewer patients have totally occluded infarct-related arteries in non–Q-wave infarction, 80% to 90% of patients with unstable angina have patent ischemia-related arteries.[13] Therefore, using recanalization of a totally occluded artery as an endpoint is not applicable in all patients with unstable angina. Because fewer culprit lesions are totally occluded in unstable angina, the amount of acute thrombus may be less compared with patients with MI.[53] We have postulated that one of the main pathophysiologic differences between AMI and unstable angina may be the amount of plaque-associated thrombus. In unstable angina the amount of thrombus, specifically the fibrin component of the thrombus, may be less than in AMI, and therefore the benefit of thrombolytic therapy would only be marginal.[54]

There may also be other differences in the relative composition of the thrombotic material between MI and unstable angina. Thrombus forming in the presence of flowing blood as is usually the case in unstable angina is platelet-rich. This is opposed to the "red thrombus" seen in patients with AMI and total coronary occlusion. This would account for the differences in presumed color of the thrombus seen angioscopically by Mizuno et al.[15] If thrombus in unstable angina were more platelet-rich, conventional thrombolytic agents would not be beneficial and might even be detrimental because of the procoagulant and proplatelet-activating properties of these drugs.[48]

The age of the thrombus may also influence the response to thrombolytic agents. Thrombus formation in unstable angina may occur slowly over days to weeks. After plaque disruption, thrombus forming in unstable angina can occur in layers.[7] These layers may build up over a period before the symptoms of unstable angina begin. The occlusive thrombus in patients with MI is only hours old at the time of manifestation. Thrombus that is relatively old and organized may not be as amenable to thrombolysis as fresh thrombus seen in AMI. The possibility of achieving more effective thrombolysis by means of a prolonged infusion of a thrombolytic agent has been recently demonstrated by Lopez-Sendon et al.[55] in a preliminary communication. In a group of 60 patients randomized to receive a 24-hour infusion of urokinase, followed by heparin vs. heparin alone, thrombolysis was shown to decrease the incidence and duration of ischemic episodes compared with heparin. Longer infusion of thrombolytic therapy may therefore enable more of the plaque-associated thrombus to be lysed. However, the risks of such prolonged therapy may outweigh the potential benefits.

Finally, it is not entirely clear that the cause of refractory angina in patients with unstable angina is thrombus alone. It may be that coronary vasoconstriction from platelet-related factors or platelet aggregates may be more important as a cause of recurrent ischemia in these patients. Although antiplatelet agents have thus far not had a dramatic effect on subsequent episodes of angina in patients with unstable angina, agents that are potent enough to block other important pathways of platelet aggregation (e.g., thrombin) have not as yet been evaluated.

SUMMARY

It is generally accepted that the acute coronary syndromes of unstable angina, MI, and sudden death share a common pathophysiology. Thrombus plays an important role in these syndromes. Despite the utility of thrombolytic therapy in AMI manifesting with ST elevations in achieving vessel patency and decreasing mortality, the benefits of thrombolytic therapy for unstable angina and non–Q-wave infarction are more modest. Reasons for the limitations of thrombolytic therapy in these syndromes include differences in endpoints and qualitative and quantitative differences in the thrombotic material compared with Q-wave MI. Given all the data at the present time, we believe that the routine use of thrombolytic therapy in the acute management of unstable angina cannot be recommended.

REFERENCES

1. Fuster V, Steele PM, Chesebro JH: Role of platelets and thrombosis in coronary atherosclerotic disease and sudden death, *J Am Coll Cardiol* 5:175B-184B, 1985.
2. Falk E: Plaque rupture with severe pre-existing stenosis precipitating coronary thrombosis. Characteristic of coronary atherosclerotic plaques underlying fatal occlusive thrombi, *Br Heart J* 50:127-134, 1983.
3. Davies MJ, Thomas AC: Plaque fissuring—the cause of acute myocardial infarction, sudden ischaemic death, and crescendo angina, *Br Heart J* 53:363-373, 1985.
4. Fuster V, Steele PM, Chesebro JH: Role of platelets and thrombosis in coronary atherosclerotic disease and sudden death, *J Am Coll Cardiol* 5:175B-184B, 1985.
5. Ambrose JA, Hjemdahl-Monsen CE: Acute ischemic syndromes: coronary pathophysiology and angiographic correlations. In Rahimtoola S (ed): *Acute myocardial infarction,* 1991, New York, Elsevier Science Publishing, pp 64-77.
6. Gorlin R, Fuster V, Ambrose JA: Anatomic-physiologic links between acute coronary syndromes, *Circulation* 74:6-9, 1986.
7. Falk E: Unstable angina with fatal outcome: dynamic coronary thrombosis leading to infarction and/or sudden death, *Circulation* 71:699-708, 1985.
8. Bresnahan DR, Davis DR, Holmes Jr DR, et al: Angiographic occurrence and clinical correlates of intraluminal coronary artery thrombus: role of unstable angina, *J Am Coll Cardiol* 6:285-289, 1985.
9. Vetrovec GW, Cowley MJ, Overton H, et al: Intracoronary thrombus in syndromes of unstable myocardial ischemia, *Am Heart J* 102:1202-1208, 1981.
10. Capone G, Wolf NM, Meyer B, et al: Frequency of intracoronary filling defects by angiography in angina pectoris at rest, *Am J Cardiol* 56:403-406, 1985.
11. Mandelkorn JB, Wolf NM, Sing S, et al: Intracoronary thrombus in nontransmural myocardial infarction and in unstable angina pectoris, *Am J Cardiol* 52:1-6, 1983.
12. Ambrose JA, Winters SL, Stern A, et al: Angiographic morphology and the pathogenesis of unstable angina pectoris, *J Am Coll Cardiol* 5:609-616, 1985.
13. Ambrose JA, Hjemdahl-Monsen CE, Borrico S, et al: Angiographic demonstration of a common link between unstable angina pectoris and non-Q wave acute myocardial infarction, *Am J Cardiol* 61:244-247, 1988.
14. Sherman CT, Litvack F, Grundfest W, et al: Coronary angioscopy in patients with unstable angina pectoris, *N Engl J Med* 315:913-919, 1986.

15. Mizuno K, Satomura K, Miyamoto A, et al: Angioscopic evaluation of coronary-artery thrombi in acute coronary syndromes, *N Engl J Med* 326:287-291, 1992.

16. Ramee SR, White CJ, Collins TJ, et al: Percutaneous angioscopy during coronary angioplasty using a steerable microangioscope, *J Am Coll Cardiol* 17:100-105, 1991.

17. Fitzgerald DJ, Roy L, Catella F, et al: Platelet activation in unstable coronary disease, *N Engl J Med* 315:983-989, 1986.

18. Theroux P, Latour JG, Leger-Gauthier C: Fibrinopeptide A and platelet factor levels in unstable angina pectoris, *Circulation* 75:156-162, 1987.

19. Kruskal JB, Commerford PJ, Franks JJ, et al: Fibrin and fibrinogen-related antigens in patients with stable and unstable coronary artery disease, *N Engl J Med* 317:1361-1365, 1987.

20. Eisenberg PR, Kenzora JL, Sobel BE, et al: Relation between ST shifts and thrombin activity in patients with unstable angina, *J Am Coll Cardiol* 18:898-903, 1991.

21. Alexopoulos D, Ambrose JA, Stump D, et al: Thrombosis-related markers in unstable angina pectoris, *J Am Coll Cardiol* 17:866-871, 1991.

22. Cairns JA, Gent M, Singer J, et al: Aspirin, sulfinpyrazone, or both in unstable angina, *N Engl J Med* 313:1369-1375, 1985.

23. Lewis HD, Davis JW, Archibald DG, et al: Protective effects of aspirin against acute myocardial infarction and death in men with unstable angina. Results of a Veterans Administration cooperative study, *N Engl J Med* 309:396-403, 1983.

24. Telford AM, Wilson C: Trial of heparin versus atenolol in prevention of myocardial infarction in intermediate coronary syndrome, *Lancet* 1:1225-1228, 1981.

25. Theroux P, Ouimet H, McCans J, et al: Aspirin, heparin, or both to treat acute unstable angina, *N Engl J Med* 319:1105-1111, 1988.

26. Wallentin LC, and Research Group on Instability in Coronary Artery Disease in Southwest Sweden: Aspirin (75 mg/day) after an episode of unstable coronary artery disease: long-term effects on the risk for myocardial infarction, occurrence of severe angina and the need for revascularization, *J Am Coll Cardiol* 18:1587-1593, 1991.

27. Rentrop P, Blanke H, Karsch KR, et al: Selective intracoronary thrombolysis in acute myocardial infarction and unstable angina pectoris, *Circulation* 63:307-317, 1981.

28. Vetrovec GW, Leinbach RC, Gold HK, et al: Intracoronary thrombolysis in syndromes of unstable ischemia: angiographic and clinical results, *Am Heart J* 104:946-952, 1982.

29. Ambrose JA, Hjemdahl-Monsen C, Borrico S, et al: Quantitative and qualitative effects of intracoronary streptokinase in unstable angina and non-Q wave infarction, *J Am Coll Cardiol* 9:1156-1165, 1987.

30. Gotoh K, Minamino T, Katoh O, et al: The role of intracoronary thrombus in unstable angina: angiographic assessment and thrombolytic therapy during ongoing anginal attacks, *Circulation* 77:526-534, 1988.

31. De Zwaan C, Bar FW, Janssen JHA, et al: Effects of thrombolytic therapy in unstable angina: clinical and angiographic results, *J Am Coll Cardiol* 12:301-309, 1988.

32. Bar FW, Verheugt FW, Col J, et al: Thrombolysis in patients with unstable angina improves the angiographic but not the clinical outcome. Results of UNASEM, a multicenter, randomized, placebo-controlled, clinical trial with anistreplase, *Circulation* 86:131-137, 1992.

33. Gulba D, Jost S, Zwicky P, Lichtlen P: Thrombolytic therapy in unstable angina, *J Am Coll Cardiol* 11:49A, 1988.

34. DiSciascio G, Kohli RS, Goudreau E, et al: Intracoronary recombinant tissue-type plasminogen activator in unstable angina: a pilot angiographic study, *Am Heart J* 122:1-6, 1991.

35. Brochier ML, Raynaud P, Rioux P, et al: Thrombosis and thrombolysis in unstable angina, *Am J Cardiol* 68:105B-109B, 1991.

36. Lawrence JR, Shepherd JT, Bone I, et al: Fibrinolytic therapy in unstable angina pectoris; a controlled clinical trial, *Thromb Res* 17:767-777, 1980.

37. Topol EJ, Nicklas JM, Kander NH, et al: Coronary revascularization after intravenous tissue plasminogen activator for unstable angina pectoris: results of a randomized, double-blind, placebo-controlled trial, *Am J Cardiol* 62:368-371, 1988.

38. Gold HK, Johns JA, Leinbach RC, et al: A randomized, blinded, placebo-controlled trial of recombinant human tissue-type plasminogen activator in patients with unstable angina pectoris, *Circulation* 75:1192-1199, 1987.

39. Nicklas J, Topol EJ, Kander N, et al: Randomized, double-blind, placebo-controlled trial of tissue plasminogen activator in unstable angina, *J Am Coll Cardiol* 13:434-441, 1989.

40. Schreiber TL, Macina G, McNulty A, et al: Thrombolytic therapy in unstable angina and non-Q wave myocardial infarction: a randomized trial of urokinase vs aspirin, *Am J Cardiol* 64:840-844, 1989.

41. Freeman MR, Langer A, Wilson RF, et al: Thrombolysis in unstable angina; randomized double-blind trial of t-PA and placebo, *Circulation* 85:150-157, 1992.

42. Williams DO, Topol EJ, Califf RM, et al: Intravenous recombinant tissue-type plasminogen activator in patients with unstable angina pectoris, *Circulation* 82:376-383, 1990.

43. Saran RK, Bhandari K, Narain VS, et al: Intravenous streptokinase in the management of a subset of patients with unstable angina: a randomized controlled trial, *Int J Cardiol* 28:209-213, 1990.

44. Neri-Serneri GGN, Gensini GF, Poggesi L, et al: Effect of heparin, aspirin, or alteplase in reduction of myocardial ischaemia in refractory unstable angina, *Lancet* 335:615-618, 1990.

45. Schreiber T, Rizik D, White C, et al: Randomized trial of thrombolysis versus heparin in unstable angina, *Circulation* 84(suppl II):II346, 1991.

46. Ardissino D, Barberis P, DeServi S, et al: Recombinant tissue-type plasminogen activator followed by heparin compared with heparin alone for refractory unstable angina pectoris, *Am J Cardiol* 66:910-914, 1990.

47. Chesebro JH, Zoldhelyi P, Fuster V: Pathogenesis of thrombosis in unstable angina, *Am J Cardiol* 68:2B-10B, 1991.

48. Coller BS: Platelets and thrombolytic therapy, *N Engl J Med* 322:33-42, 1990.

49. Waters D, Lam JYT: Is thrombolytic therapy striking out in unstable angina? *Circulation* 86:1642-1644, 1992.

50. TIMI IIIA Investigators: Early effects of tissue-type plasminogen activator added to conventional therapy on the culprit coronary lesion in patients presenting with ischemic cardiac pain at rest: results of the thrombolysis in myocardial ischemia (TIMI IIIA) trial, *Circulation* 87:38-52, 1993.

51. Braunwald E: Unstable angina. A classification, *Circulation* 80:410-414, 1989.

52. Ambrose JA, Alexopoulos D: Thrombolysis in unstable angina: Will the beneficial effects of thrombolytic therapy in myocardial infarction apply to patients with unstable angina? *J Am Coll Cardiol* 13:1666-1671, 1989.

53. Brown BG, Gallery CA, Badger RS, et al: Incomplete lysis of thrombus in the moderate underlying atherosclerotic lesion during intracoronary infusion of streptokinase for acute myocardial infarction: quantitative angiographic observations, *Circulation* 73:653-661, 1986.

54. Ambrose JA: Plaque disruption and the acute coronary syndromes of unstable angina and myocardial infarction: If the substrate is similar, why is the clinical presentation different? *J Am Coll Cardiol* 19:1653-1658, 1992.

55. Lopez-Sendon J, Coma-Canella I, Peinado R, et al: Prolonged i.v. infusion of urokinase in recent onset unstable angina. A randomized study, *Circulation* 86:I387, 1992.

Chapter 44

PERCUTANEOUS CORONARY REVASCULARIZATION IN PATIENTS WITH UNSTABLE ANGINA

Robert M. Califf
Harry R. Phillips

The growing realization that unstable angina results from a disrupted atherosclerotic plaque with attendant production of thrombosis and vasoconstriction provides a fascinating venue for consideration of the current and future role of percutaneous revascularization methods in the treatment of unstable angina. Multiple clinical[1] and pathophysiologic[2,3] studies have demonstrated that a "culprit" lesion responsible for the acute event can usually be identified in patients with unstable angina. This culprit lesion is similar to the lesion of AMI in that the involved plaque has a fissure on the surface, but it differs in that the amount of disruption of the plaque is generally less, the lumen is seldom totally occluded, and the adherent thrombus is often more rich in platelets.

Several important aspects of the classification and natural history of unstable angina are worthy of careful consideration when placing percutaneous intervention in perspective. Unstable angina is a clinical diagnosis with a wide spectrum of presentations and prognoses. In the unstable angina guideline recently published by the Agency for Health Care Policy and Research,[4] unstable angina includes angina at rest, new onset exertional angina (for <2 months) of Canadian Class III or greater, or recent (for <2 months) acceleration of angina

causing progression of at least one Canadian Class in severity and at least Class III symptoms (with less than usual exertion). Thus the broad classification ranges from the patient who has one bout of rest angina to the patient with repetitive bouts of ischemia associated with ST-segment changes on maximal medical therapy. Furthermore, because definitive evidence of myocardial necrosis cannot be obtained until enough time has passed for cardiac enzymes to appear in the serum and to be sampled and measured, often patients will be classified initially as having unstable angina but later, when the cardiac enzymes return, as having non–Q-wave MI. The inclusion in a single classification of patients with different criteria for diagnosis and consequently with different prognoses has led to considerable confusion in the literature.

The varying acute prognoses conferred by these different clinical presentations is further confounded by the variable time course of the instability once the diagnosis is made. In most cases the negative prognosis associated with unstable angina declines exponentially upon diagnosis, reaching the same risk as that of stable angina after approximately 1 year of treatment (Fig. 44-1). However, the bulk of the risk is seen in the first

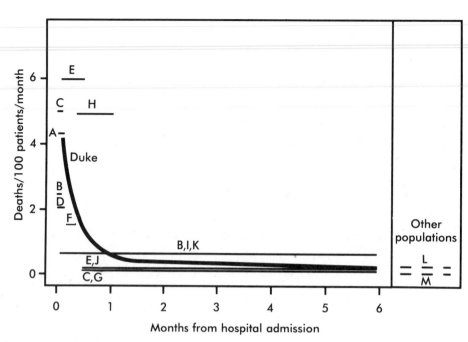

Source: Published data as shown in Table 5 and unpublished data, Duke Cardiovascular Databank.

Fig. 44-1. Outcomes of medically treated patients with unstable angina. (From Braunwald E et al: Unstable angina: diagnosis and management, 1994, US Department of Health and Human Services.)

several months. Thus, patients diagnosed early in the course of the disease would have a much worse prognosis than that seen in a series in which the majority of patients had already "cooled off" before enrollment.

PATHOPHYSIOLOGIC ISSUES

The disrupted atherosclerotic plaque is the focus for understanding the relevant therapeutic targets when specific therapies need to be identified. Factors leading to plaque disruption include the location of the lesion (areas of greater shear stress are at higher risk), the size of the lipid pool (larger lipid pools are more likely to be associated with plaque disruption), and the infiltration of the plaque with macrophages, which are thought to weaken the integrity of the fibrous cap of the plaque, making it more susceptible to fissuring. In addition, the same ischemic "triggers" (see Chapter 2) responsible for creating plaque disruption as the initial inciting event also can perpetuate the process in the acute phase of instability. Thus, swings in blood pressure, high pulse pressure, and sympathetic tone are likely to be important therapeutic targets. Once the plaque is disrupted, the amount of thrombus that occludes the artery depends on many systemic and local factors, including the degree of platelet activation, the balance of the intrinsic fibrinolytic and thrombin formation systems, and the flow patterns in the artery. Medical therapy is thus aimed at antagonizing platelet activation, thrombin and fibrin formation, and at combating neurohumoral substances that lead to vessel constriction.

This environment increases the risk of abrupt vessel closure during a revascularization procedure and initial hospitalization in patients with unstable angina, compared with stable angina patients. Abrupt vessel closure is presumed to result either from the creation of an intimal "flap" that falls upon the vessel in an unfortunate manner or from progressive thrombosis. There is increasing evidence that the usual abrupt closure has elements of both processes: vessels with more disruption and longer dissections are more thrombogenic and likely to have platelet-rich thrombus, which is difficult to combat with antithrombin therapy.

For similar reasons, the risk of recurrent stenosis after initially successful percutaneous intervention could be higher in patients with unstable angina than in patients with stable angina. The major pathophysiologic causes of late recurrence of stenosis include vessel architecture, including recoil and remodeling, as well as cellular proliferation; both these areas could be affected negatively by the unstable atherosclerotic plaque at the time of intervention. A major method of encroachment of a plaque upon the lumen of a vessel after coronary intervention could be through the incorporation of thrombus into the plaque.[5] Thus, a vessel that was disrupted by plaque fissuring or rupture before the procedure could create a more thrombogenic environment, leading to more abundant mural thrombus after the procedure. In addition to the obvious effects of such a process on plaque mass, the presence of activated platelets and other humoral factors associated with clotting leads to the elaboration of a variety of growth factors that have been demonstrated to produce cellular proliferation.

CLINICAL OUTCOMES

In terms of presentation and time course, the heterogeneity of the populations reported upon in the literature makes comparisons across different reports treacherous. The problem is compounded by the fact that mortality rates are low, creating a situation in which the most important outcomes are very definition-dependent, such as nonfatal MI; subjective, such as functional status; or subject to investigator bias, such as angioplasty "success." Nonfatal MI will be underreported by as much as 50% if the clinician caring for the patient is making the decision on classification. Furthermore, reported event rates can substantially differ, depending upon the threshold for classifying an enzyme elevation as an MI. New Q waves on the ECG are rare with percutaneous intervention, but two- to threefold elevations of CK-MB isoenzymes are common. Whether these enzyme "bumps" should be counted as MIs in the same sense as enzyme elevations in medically treated patients remains uncertain. Clinical "success" rates also depend upon the visual reading of the angiogram, which can differ from that of a core laboratory by as much as 20%; the clinician performing the procedure is almost always overly optimistic.

Despite these problems, several themes are clear. First, complications of all kinds are more frequent in patients with unstable angina than in patients with stable angina during and after percutaneous intervention. Second, these complications can be reduced by careful pharmacologic therapy designed to reduce the thrombogenicity of the environment at the time of the intervention. Finally, the relative risks and benefits of percutaneous intervention compared with medical or surgical therapy in this setting and the specific strategy of percutaneous intervention that would yield the best results remain unclear.

A variety of studies (Table 44-1) have demonstrated that the rates of death, nonfatal MI, and need for emergency surgery are greater in patients with unstable angina than in patients with stable angina. In a review of studies reported by de Feyter and Serruys,[6] the angiographic success rate was 92% in patients with stable angina, compared with 89% in medically stabilized

Table 44-1. Outcomes of patients with stable and unstable angina

			Major complication rate		
	Patients	**Success rate (%)**	**Death (%)**	**MI (%)**	**Acute surgery (%)**
Stable angina	10,129	92	0.7	1.6	2.5
Unstable angina					
Stabilized	1036	89	0.3	5.1	5.8
Refractory	1438	85	1.3	6.3	6.8
Post-MI	634	88	1.1	6.3	6.5

From deFeyter PJ, Serruys PW: Percutaneous transluminal coronary angioplasty for unstable angina. In Topol EJ, (ed): *Textbook of interventional cardiology*, ed. 2, Philadelphia, 1994, WB Saunders.

unstable angina, 88% in post-MI angina, and 85% in medically refractory unstable angina. In concert with these lower success rates, the risk of death, nonfatal MI, and surgery increases with the increasing severity of unstable angina.

A detailed analysis of the CAVEAT I trial provides considerable insight into the importance of classification of unstable angina when attempting to understand risk. Overall, 65% of patients were classified as having unstable angina on enrollment into the trial. On initial review of the outcome data, unstable angina per se did not appear to be a potent predictor of outcomes. However, when the attributes leading to the diagnosis were evaluated, patients with angina at rest associated with ST-segment changes on the ECG were found to be at substantially increased risk of negative outcomes, including both nonfatal MI and the need for emergency bypass surgery (Table 44-2). Thus, the high-risk group comprised patients with truly active unstable angina. Furthermore, these patients with "hot" unstable angina were particularly at risk for negative outcomes if treated with directional atherectomy rather than standard angioplasty.

An important issue guiding clinical management is whether the degree of medical stabilization is sufficient before proceeding with percutaneous intervention. The most intriguing single experience was reported by Myler et al.,[7] in which the rates of MI were 6.5%, 6.6%, and 1.6% in patients undergoing intervention following medical stabilization of less than 1 week, 1 to 2 weeks, or more than 2 weeks, respectively, after an initial diagnosis of unstable angina. Corresponding emergency surgery rates were 9.4%, 6.1%, and 4.8%. These data make a strong case for considerable medical stabilization before percutaneous intervention. However, they do not account for the possibility that the lower event rates in patients with later procedures could be the result of the attrition of high-risk patients through death or clinically

Table 44-2. CAVEAT results

	30-day outcomes			6-month outcomes			
	Death	MI	CABG	Death	MI	CABG	Repeat PTCA
Stable angina							
DCA (N = 174)	0	6.3	1.7	1.2	6.9	3.4	24.7
PTCA (N = 149)	1.0	3.4	1.3	1.0	4.0	4.0	27.5
Accelerating angina							
DCA (N = 111)	0	4.5	0.9	1.0	6.3	9.0	26.1
PTCA (N = 125)	0	2.4	0.8	0	3.2	7.2	32.0
Rest pain, ECG changes, or post-MI pain							
DCA (N = 223)	0	9.0	6.7	2.2	10.8	11.7	34.1
PTCA (N = 223)	0.5	3.6	3.6	1.0	4.9	9.0	31.8

required procedures before the 2-week waiting time. Furthermore, no difference in mortality was observed among the three time periods.

Despite substantial data about the risks of percutaneous procedures in patients with unstable angina, there is little information about the potential benefits relative to other forms of therapy. This situation, of course, simply reflects the lack of comparative clinical trials on percutaneous revascularization in general. Recently, however, the Angioplasty Compared to Medicine (ACME) trial reported that angioplasty resulted in improved exercise time and better quality of life compared with medical therapy in patients with stable angina.[8] Several studies have compared angioplasty with bypass surgery in the setting of multivessel disease,[9-11] and short-term survival rates were comparable; many patients in these trials had unstable angina, but the results have not yet provided detailed information about this subgroup.

In a large observational study by Mark et al. from Duke[12] that compared approaches to the treatment of coronary disease, approximately 35% of 7710 patients had unstable angina. Patients with mild disease did equally well with medical therapy, angioplasty, or surgery, and patients with severe three-vessel disease had better survival with surgery. Patients with high-grade proximal single-vessel disease or moderate two-vessel disease had at least equivalent survival with angioplasty and surgery. When the patients with unstable angina were evaluated separately, the results were no different from the population as a whole; the relative benefit of different forms of revascularization as a function of anatomy was the same in the unstable angina patients as in the entire population.

Only one randomized trial has specifically addressed the issue of the timing of percutaneous intervention. The TIMI IIIB trial[13] randomly allocated 696 patients with

unstable angina or small non–Q-wave infarctions to a strategy of early invasive therapy and allocated 696 similar patients to a conservative strategy. The early invasive strategy included aspirin and heparin therapy for 18 to 48 hours, with half of these patients also randomized to t-PA in a factorial design. At the 18- to 48-hour time point this strategy called for coronary angiography and revascularization of patients with suitable coronary anatomy. In comparison the patients randomized to the conservative strategy were similarly treated with aspirin and heparin, and one half the group received t-PA, but coronary angiography was not performed unless there was evidence of recurrent ischemia or pump failure. Indications for angiography included recurrent angina with ECG changes, more than 20 minutes of ischemic ECG changes on ambulatory monitoring, definite ischemia on predischarge functional testing, or Canadian Class III or IV angina after discharge. After 42 days (Table 44-3) and 1 year of follow-up no differences were seen in death and only a slight nonsignificant trend was seen in the combined endpoint of death and nonfatal infarction. Although the patients assigned to the early invasive strategy had more revascularization procedures even at 1 year, the patients assigned to the early conservative strategy had more readmissions and a need for more intensive medical therapy during the 1-year follow-up. From the perspective of the total health care budget the early, aggressive approach appeared slightly favored, although the detailed analysis needed to provide a confident perspective on cost is not available.

The lack of previous solid information and the apparent lack of difference in 1-year outcome and cost in the TIMI IIIB study have led to a recommendation for either of two general strategies of revascularization in patients with unstable angina. In the early aggressive strategy an angiogram is planned for all patients except

Table 44-3. TIMI-IIIB outcomes (42 days)

	Early invasive strategy (N = 696)	Early conservative strategy (N = 696)	P
Death (%)	2.4	2.5	
Nonfatal MI (%)	5.1	5.7	
Positive ETT (%)	8.6	10.0	
Σ of above (%)	16.2	18.1	.33
Length of stay (days)	10.2	10.9	.01
Rehospitalization (%)	7.8	14.1	< .001

those in whom it is medically contraindicated. In the early conservative strategy, angiography is used only for the following conditions, unless a contraindication is present: (1) patients with prior angioplasty, surgery, or MI; (2) patients who fail to stabilize on medical therapy; (3) patients who strongly prefer aggressive therapy; (4) patients with high-risk clinical findings or noninvasive test results; and (5) patients with significant heart failure or known left ventricular dysfunction. Thus, the conservative strategy calls for left ventricular function measurement through noninvasive imaging methods and provocative testing for ischemia in all patients not requiring an early catheterization because of failure of medical therapy. The aggressive strategy can be expected to lead to a higher rate of early complications and more early expenses in return for fewer complications and hospitalizations and less cost later.

SPECIFICS OF THERAPY

The general medical therapy of patients undergoing percutaneous intervention in the setting of unstable angina should emphasize the same elements as in all treatment of unstable angina. Antiplatelet therapy is mandatory, and aspirin is the current standard therapy at a dosage of 160 to 325 mg per day. Antithrombin therapy with heparin is considered routine and is recommended by the Unstable Angina Clinical Practice Guideline.[4] Concern remains about "rebound" or reactivation of the thrombogenic propensity of the culprit lesion[14,15] when heparin is discontinued, but the clinical efficacy of heparin has been demonstrated in several clinical trials. Beta blockers are routinely recommended to reduce the likelihood of severe sympathetic surges with concomitant platelet activation and enhanced shear forces on the culprit lesion. Definitive evidence exists concerning the efficacy of nitrates in preventing recurrent ischemic episodes in patients with unstable angina,[16] but no evidence is available concerning their effect on coronary events (death and MI). Because of this documented symptomatic benefit we attempt to achieve high levels of nitrates early with rapid conversion to oral or topical

forms on an irregular schedule to combat nitrate tolerance. The choice of intensive care unit, step-down facility, or general hospital service is determined by risk stratification as outlined in the Unstable Angina Clinical Practice Guideline.

Antiplatelet therapy

The specifics of antiplatelet therapy are worthy of careful consideration when percutaneous intervention is being planned for the patient with unstable angina. The importance of aspirin in the prevention of abrupt closure and its attendant complications of death, nonfatal MI, and emergency surgery has been established in carefully controlled clinical trials.[14-19] Particularly in the setting of unstable angina with the enhanced risk of vessel closure and the primacy of platelet-rich thrombi in the pathophysiology, adequate platelet coverage is requisite. Accordingly, we initiate aspirin with 160 mg in a chewable form, as in ISIS-2[20], in case a patient rapidly develops refractory ischemia that requires emergency intervention.

More potent platelet inhibition will soon be available for clinical practitioners. Aspirin inactivates platelets through irreversible inhibition of the cyclooxygenase pathway. As discussed in Chapter 29, however, much more potent platelet inhibition can be achieved through the blockade of the glycoprotein IIb/IIIa receptor on the platelet surface. The Evaluation of Platelet Inhibition to prevent ischemic Complications (EPIC) trial focused on patients with unstable angina in the evaluation of c7E3 Fab, a chimeric monoclonal antibody to the IIb/IIIa receptor.[21] A bolus of 0.25 mg/kg, followed by an infusion of 10 mg/min for 12 hours, produced a 35% reduction in the composite endpoint of death, MI, and need for emergency percutaneous procedures during the first 30 days after treatment. This benefit was achieved at the cost of a doubling of transfusions. In the unstable angina population, rigidly defined as patients with at least two bouts of rest angina associated with ECG changes, the beneficial effects of c7E3 Fab were substantial. Importantly, the initial benefits were sustained and perhaps even enhanced at the 6-month followup (Table 44-4). Further analysis of the data indicated that modification of the heparin dose to give a lower amount when profound platelet inhibition is achieved may significantly reduce the bleeding complications. Additionally, the large amount of variation in transfusions from site to site in the EPIC trial points out the need for uniform application of transfusion criteria and better clinical guidelines for patient management after percutaneous intervention.

In the near future additional potent glycoprotein IIa/IIIb inhibitors will be available; most of these compounds are peptides or small molecules with a short half-life and impressive selectivity for the receptor. The

Table 44-4. Events prevented per 1000 high-risk PTCA patients treated with c7E3 Fab

	Benefit for 1000 patients	
	30 day	6 month
Intention to treat analysis		
Death	0	3
Death + MI	35	39
Death + MI + urgent intervention	45	53
Death + MI + all intervention	—	81
Treated patients only		
Death	5	7
Death + MI	43	45
Death + MI + urgent intervention	54	62
Death + MI + all intervention	—	89

attributes of the IIa/IIIb blocker with the most favorable clinical profile will only be known once a series of large clinical trials has been completed comparing effects on both acute ischemic events and restenosis.

Thrombin inhibitors

Thrombin inhibitors have undergone a similar evolution to antiplatelet agents, although the strength of the evidence is less rigorous. The strongest case for the need for some thrombin inhibition in the setting of percutaneous intervention comes from a series of observational studies comparing the outcomes of patients with both stable and unstable angina treated with heparin vs. the outcomes of patients undergoing procedures without heparin.[22,23] These studies were extended specifically to patients with unstable angina when the investigators found a lower rate of abrupt closure when such patients were treated with a course of heparin for several days before undergoing a procedure.[24]

Over the past several years the critical importance of a high level of thrombin inhibition has been stressed in several observational studies that have shown that an activated clotting time in excess of 300 seconds leads to a lower rate of acute ischemic events.[23,25] Considerable data are now available concerning the use of heparin to provide the high ACT levels needed.[26,27] Increasing doses of heparin producing higher ACT levels are associated with fewer ischemic/thrombotic complications and more bleeding complications.[28,29] In a series of 438 patients treated at Duke, the mean ACT level during balloon inflation was 346 seconds in patients with abrupt closure, compared with 388 seconds ($P < 0.002$) in patients without abrupt closure.

The newer thrombin inhibitors currently in clinical trials have substantial theoretical advantages over heparin. These inhibitors are effective against clot-bound thrombin; are not neutralized by platelet factor IV, heparinase, and other platelet release compounds; and are not dependent on antithrombin III for their activity. Two of these direct thrombin inhibitors, hirudin and hirulog, are currently in clinical trials. Hirudin is the major anticoagulant of the medicinal leech, and is now available through recombinant DNA technology. Hirulog is a synthetic thrombin inhibitor designed as an analogue of hirudin. In a dose-ranging study in which 40% to 50% of patients had unstable angina, Topol et al. demonstrated that doses of hirulog achieving an ACT of over 300 seconds were associated with a lower risk of ischemic events than doses achieving an ACT of over 300 seconds.[30] These results do not compare hirulog with adequate doses of heparin and therefore should not be interpreted as evidence of an incremental benefit of hirulog; a large-scale randomized trial comparing the two has completed enrollment, but the results are not yet available. A randomized trial comparing hirudin with heparin has been reported recently; this 113-patient study was a pilot study for a larger randomized trial.[31] The use of hirudin was associated with a reduction in ischemic events in the first 30 days after the procedure and no increase in major bleeding events. Early reports from the larger randomized trial demonstrate a reduction in ischemic event rates in the first 30 days but no difference in 6-month event rates.

Thrombolytic agents

Systemic. At the time of diagnostic angiography in patients with unstable angina, the appearance of thrombus is common. Given the overwhelming evidence in favor of the use of thrombolysis in acute coronary occlusion and the angiographic evidence that systemic thrombolytic agent administration lyses thrombus,[32-35] the administration of a systemic thrombolytic agent is a rational approach to the problem. An overview of the available randomized trial information, however, shows a strong trend towards an *increase* in the rate of nonfatal infarction rather than a decrease (Fig. 44-2), probably as a result of the activity of clot-bound thrombin as the thrombus begins to resolve.[36,37] The largest randomized trial reported to date of systemic thrombolysis[38] as a prelude to balloon angioplasty demonstrated no clinical benefit and a significant increase in the rate of bleeding complications (Table 44-5). Accordingly, administration of systemic thrombolytic therapy cannot be recommended in the setting of unstable angina, regardless of the clot burden in the lesion.

Local. The reasons for the failure of systemic thrombolytic therapy to improve outcome in the setting of unstable angina remain unclear. One approach to reduce the thrombus burden while minimizing the

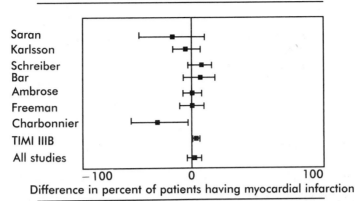

Source: Saran, Bhandari, Narain, et al., 1990; Karlsson Berglund, Bjorkholm, et al., 1992; Screiber, Rizik, White, et al., 1992; Bar, Verheught, Col, et al., 1992; Ambrose, Torre, Sharma, et al., 1992; Freeman, Langer, Wilson, et al., 1992; Charbonnier, Bernadet, Schiele, et al., 1992; TIMI-IIIB, in press.

Fig. 44-2. Influence of thrombolysis on MI in patients presenting with unstable angina. (From Braunwald E et al: Unstable angina: diagnosis and management, 1994, US Department of Health and Human Services.)

Table 44-5. Results of the TAUSA trial

Post-PTCA endpoint	Simple lesion		Complex lesion	
	UK ($N = 95$)	PL ($N = 111$)	UK ($N = 123$)	PL ($N = 117$)
Intracoronary thrombus	11.6%	12.6%	20.3%	26.5%
Acute closure	3.2%	0.9%	10.6%*	2.7%
Ischemia	4.2%	2.7%	9.8%*	2.7%

*$P < 0.05$, UK (urokinase) vs. PL (placebo).
(From Torre SR, Ambrose JA, Sharma SK, et al: *J Am Coll Cardiol* 105A, 1994.)

bleeding risk would be to administer thrombolytic therapy locally to the lesion. Several devices have been developed specifically for this purpose, and small observational series evaluating clot resolution using angiography have been promising. Recently, several randomized pilot studies have been mounted, but until these results are available, intracoronary thrombolytic administration cannot be recommended routinely.

Device selection

Standard balloon angioplasty. The vast majority of information concerning percutaneous intervention in the setting of unstable angina involves standard balloon angioplasty. No definitive information is available to lead to the selection of one type of balloon over another, although the results of the Perfusion Balloon Catheter Trial[39] indicated that in the setting of complex lesion morphology, including the angiographic appearance of thrombus, a gradual and prolonged dilation may be superior to routine balloon dilatation in preventing abrupt closure.

Directional atherectomy. Directional coronary atherectomy (DCA) has been studied in the setting of unstable angina in a large number of patients. The majority of available information indicates that the risk of acute complications with DCA increases as a function of the instability of the angina and the inverse of the duration of the instability. The CAVEAT data cited above indicate that the relative increase in acute complications with DCA was even greater in patients with unstable angina characterized by rest pain with documented ECG changes.[40] One of the most intriguing aspects of EPIC was the finding that the gradient of acute complications in the control group was almost identical to the gradient observed in CAVEAT; however, in the patients treated with c7E3 Fab, the complication rate was identical and low in both groups.

Transluminal extraction catheter. Little information is available specifically regarding the use of the TEC device in patients with unstable angina. The ability of the device to extract thrombus has been touted as a reason why it is preferably used in this setting, but empirical evidence to support this approach has not been published.

Rotational atherectomy. As with DCA, the complication rate after rotoblator is higher in patients with unstable angina. Unfortunately, no comparative data with other methods of intervention are available to determine whether this increased risk is proportionately greater or less with rotoblator compared with other methods of achieving revascularization in patients with unstable angina.

Coronary stenting. The major complication of coronary stenting is thrombosis; this complication has been reported to be higher in patients with unstable angina compared with patients with stable angina,[41] although the local thrombogenic environment produced by the struts of the stent itself is probably the most important risk. Currently, stenting is recommended only for "bail-out" of failed procedures, although recent evidence[42,43] points to advantages of primary stenting as a means of preventing the recurrence of stenosis.

THE FUTURE
Plaque stabilization

The goal of future therapies in patients with coronary heart disease will be the stabilization of the existing atherosclerotic plaques while attempting to prevent the development of new plaques. The approach will involve an effort to achieve a dynamic equilibrium involving the coagulation system, lipids, and the neurohormonal axis. Although progress will be substantial over the next decade, acute activation of this chronic disease will continue to be a major public health problem. From this perspective the goal of treating the acute event is to minimize the amount of myocardial damage with its associated complications while attempting to achieve stabilization of the acutely unstable plaque.

Conservative approach

The conservative approach to stabilizing the unstable plaque would relegate percutaneous intervention to a back-up method if pharmacologic efforts failed. Progressive improvement in antiplatelet and antithrombin therapy combined with new discoveries in the pharmacology of vessel wall physiology will increasingly enhance the ability of intensive medical therapy to prevent vessel closure and subsequent myocardial necrosis. In this scheme, patients with unstable ischemic syndromes would be treated aggressively and angiographic intervention would be contemplated only after there was convincing evidence of recurrent ischemia. The rationale for this approach is clear: angiographic intervention is a higher risk in patients with unstable lesions and use of angiographic facilities is expensive.

Aggressive approach

The alternate approach is to develop therapies that make early, aggressive intervention more effective and less risky. If patients could be admitted to the hospital, treated aggressively medically for a short period of time, and then subjected to angiography, it may be possible to reduce overall cost by treating the active lesion mechanically and discharging patients relatively early. This approach would avoid the cost of prolonged stay in a heavily monitored environment and the expensive non-invasive risk evaluations that frequently follow the stabilization of the patient. The best estimate from the TIMI IIIB trial already found a "toss-up" in the 1-year estimated cost between the aggressive and the conservative approach. Technologies with a higher initial success rate, a lower complication rate, and/or a lower rate of restenosis would allow the aggressive approach to have substantial clinical and financial advantages.

REFERENCES

1. Ambrose JA: Plaque disruption and the acute coronary syndromes of unstable angina and myocardial infarction: if the substrate is similar, why is the clinical presentation different? *J Am Coll Cardiol* 19:1653-1658, 1992.
2. Falk E: Plaque rupture with severe preexisting stenosis precipitating coronary thrombosis: characteristics of coronary atherosclerotic plaques underlying fatal occlusive thrombi, *Br Heart J* 50:127-134, 1983.
3. Falk E: Unstable angina with fatal outcome: dynamic coronary thrombosis leading to infarction or sudden death, *Circulation* 71:699-708, 1985.
4. Braunwald E, Mark DB, Jones RH, et al: Unstable angina: diagnosis and management, 1994, US Department of Health and Human Services.
5. Califf RM, Willerson JT: Percutaneous transluminal coronary angioplasty: prevention of occlusion and restenosis. In Fuster V, Verstraete M, (eds): *Thrombosis in cardiovascular disorder,* Philadelphia, 1992, WB Saunders.
6. de Feyter PJ, Serruys PW: Percutaneous transluminal coronary angioplasty for unstable angina. In Topol EJ, (ed): *Textbook of interventional cardiology,* Philadelphia, 1994, WB Saunders.
7. Myler RK, Shaw RE, Stertzer SH: Unstable angina and coronary angioplasty, *Circulation* 82(suppl II):II-88-II-95, 1990.
8. Parisi AF, Folland ED, Hartigan P: A comparison of angioplasty with medical therapy in the treatment of single-vessel coronary artery disease. Veterans Affairs ACME Investigators, *N Engl J Med* 326:10-16, 1992.
9. King SBI: Emory Angioplasty Surgery Trial (EAST). Presentation at 43rd Annual Scientific Session, American College of Cardiology, March 15, 1994.
10. Henderson RA: The Randomised Intervention Treatment of Angina (RITA) trial protocol: a long-term study of coronary angioplasty and coronary artery bypass surgery in patients with angina, *Br Heart J* 62:411-414, 1989.
11. Ischinger TA: German Angioplasty Bypass Investigation (GABI). Presentation at 43rd Annual Scientific Session, American College of Cardiology, March 15, 1994.
12. Mark DB, Nelson CL, Califf RM, et al: The continuing evolution of therapy for coronary artery disease: initial results from the era of coronary angioplasty, *Circulation* 89:2015-2025, 1994.
13. The TIMI IIIB Investigators: Effects of tissue plasminogen activator and a comparison of early invasive and conservative strategies in unstable angina and non-Q-wave myocardial infarction: results of the TIMI IIIB trial, *Circulation* 89:1545-1556, 1994.
14. Theroux P, Ouimet H, McCans J, et al: Aspirin, heparin, or both to treat acute unstable angina, *N Engl J Med* 319:1105-1111, 1988.
15. Miller JM, Granger CB, Bovill EG, et al: Rebound increase in thrombin activity after cessation of intravenous heparin, *Circulation* 88(Suppl I):I-202, 1993.
16. Curfman GD, Heinsimer JA, Lozner EC, et al: Intravenous nitroglycerin in the treatment of spontaneous angina pectoris: a prospective randomized trial, *Circulation* 67:276-282, 1982.
17. Lewis HD, Davis JW, Archibald DG: Protective effects of aspirin against acute myocardial infarction and death in men with unstable angina. Results of a Veterans Administration Cooperative Study, *N Engl J Med* 309:396-403, 1983.
18. Cairns JA, Gent M, Singer J: Aspirin, sulfinpyrazone, or both in unstable angina, *N Engl J Med* 313:1369-1375, 1985.
19. Wallentin LC, Research Group on Instability in Coronary Artery Disease in Southeast Sweden: Aspirin (75 mg/day) after an episode

of unstable coronary artery disease: long-term effects on the risk for myocardial infarction, occurrence of severe angina, and the need for revascularization, *J Am Coll Cardiol* 18:1617-1626, 1991.

20. ISIS-2: Randomised trial of intravenous streptokinase, oral aspirin, both, or neither among 17,187 cases of suspected acute myocardial infarction: ISIS-2, *Lancet* 2:349-360, 1988.

21. The EPIC Investigators: Use of a monoclonal antibody directed against the platelet glycoprotein IIb/IIIa receptor in high-risk coronary angioplasty, *N Engl J Med* 330:956-961, 1994.

22. Laskey MAL, Deutsch E, Barnathan E: Influence of heparin therapy on percutaneous transluminal coronary angioplasty outcome in unstable angina pectoris, *Am J Cardiol* 65:1425-1429, 1990.

23. Gabliani G, Deligonul U, Kern M, et al: Acute coronary occlusion occurring after successful transluminal coronary angioplasty: temporal relationship to discontinuation of anticoagulation, *Am Heart J* 116:696-700, 1988.

24. Hettleman BD, Aplin RL, Sullivan PR, et al: Three days of heparin pretreatment reduces major complications of coronary angioplasty in patients with unstable angina, *J Am Coll Cardiol* 15:154A, 1990.

25. Ogilby JD, Kopelman HA, Klein LW, et al: Adequate heparinization during PTCA: assessment using activated clotting times, *Cathet Cardiovasc Diagn* 18:206-209, 1989.

26. Narins CR, Hillegass WB, Jr, Nelson CL, et al: The relationship between activated clotting time during angioplasty and abrupt closure, *Circulation* (in press).

27. Fernandez-Ortiz A, Dougherty KG, Goas CM, et al: Relation between procedural activated coagulation time and outcome after percutaneous transluminal coronary angioplasty, *J Am Coll Cardiol* 23:1061-1065, 1994.

28. Narins CR, Hillegass WB, Nelson CL, et al: Activated clotting time predicts abrupt closure risk during angioplasty, *J Am Coll Cardiol* 23:470A, 1994.

29. Hillegass WB, Narins CR, Brott BC, et al: Activated clotting time predicts bleeding complications from angioplasty, *J Am Coll Cardiol* 23:184A, 1994.

30. Topol EJ, Bonan R, Jewitt D, et al: Use of a direct antithrombin, hirulog, in place of heparin during coronary angioplasty, *Circulation* 87:1622-1629, 1993.

31. van den Bos AA, Deckers JW, Heyndrickx GR, et al: Safety and efficacy of recombinant hirudin (CGP 39 393) versus heparin in patients with stable angina undergoing coronary angioplasty, *Circulation* 88(1):2058-2066, 1993.

32. The TIMI IIIA Investigators: Early effects of tissue-type plasminogen activator added to conventional therapy on the culprit lesion

in patients presenting with ischemic cardiac pain at rest: results of the Thrombolysis in Myocardial Ischemia (TIMI III) trial, *Circulation* 87:38-52, 1993.

33. Ambrose JA, Torre SR, Sharma SK, et al: Adjunctive thrombolytic therapy for angioplasty in ischemic rest angina: results of a double-blind randomized pilot study, *J Am Coll Cardiol* 20:1197-1204, 1992.

34. Bar FW, Verheugt FW, Col J, et al: Thrombolysis in patients with unstable angina improves the angiographic but not the clinical outcome: results of UNASEM, a multicenter, randomized, placebo-controlled, clinical trial with anistreplase, *Circulation* 86:131-137, 1992.

35. Nicklas JM, Topol EJ, Kander N, et al: Randomized, double-blind, placebo-controlled trial of tissue plasminogen activator in unstable angina, *Circulation* 13:434-441, 1989.

36. Eisenberg PR, Sobel BS, Jaffe AS: Activation of prothrombin accompanying thrombolysis with recombinant tissue type plasminogen activator, *J Am Coll Cardiol* 19:1065-1069, 1989.

37. Rapold HJ: Promotion of thrombin activity by thrombolytic therapy without simultaneous anticoagulation, *Lancet* 1:481-482, 1990.

38. Torre SR, Ambrose JA, Sharma SK, et al: Adjuvant intracoronary urokinase worsens the procedural outcome for PTCA of complex lesions in unstable angina: results of the thrombolysis and angioplasty in unstable angina (TAUSA) trial, *J Am Coll Cardiol* 105A, 1994.

39. Ohman EM, Marquis J, Ricci DR, et al, for the Perfusion Balloon Catheter Study Group: A randomized comparison of the effects of gradual prolonged versus standard primary balloon inflation on early and late outcome: results of a multicenter clinical trial, *Circulation* 89:1118-1125, 1994.

40. Harrington RA, Holmes DR, Berdan LG, et al, for the CAVEAT Investigators: Clinical characteristics and outcomes of patients with unstable angina undergoing percutaneous coronary intervention in CAVEAT, *J Am Coll Cardiol* 288A, 1994.

41. Nath FC, Muller DWM, Ellis SG, et al: Thrombosis of a flexible coil coronary stent: frequency, predictors and clinical outcome, *J Am Coll Cardiol* 21:622-627, 1993.

42. Fischman DL, Leon MB, Baim DS, et al: A randomized comparison of coronary-stent-placement and balloon angioplasty in the treatment of coronary artery disease, *N Engl J Med* 331:496-501, 1994.

43. Serruys PW, de Jaegere P, Kiemeneij F, et al: A comparison of balloon-expandable-stent implantation with balloon angioplasty in patients with coronary artery disease, *N Engl J Med* 331:489-495, 1994.

Chapter 45

CORONARY ARTERY BYPASS GRAFTING FOR UNSTABLE ANGINA OR NON–Q-WAVE MYOCARDIAL INFARCTION

Donald D. Glower
Joseph G. Reves

INDICATIONS AND PATIENT SELECTION FOR CORONARY BYPASS GRAFTING

Consideration of coronary bypass grafting in patients with unstable angina or non–Q-wave MI is primarily based on data that these two patient groups are at increased risk for refractory anginal symptoms, subsequent MI, and cardiac death. Unstable angina requiring hospital admission has been associated with an early mortality rate of 3% to 5%[1-4] and a 6% to 14% rate of early MI.[1,2,4] Within the first year after discharge, patients with unstable angina have had a 7% to 9% mortality rate, an 11% to 14% risk of MI, and a significant incidence of readmission for unstable angina.[3-5]

Non–Q-wave MI is classically defined by a small elevation of CPK-MB isoenzymes without development of electrocardiographic Q waves, and non–Q-wave infarctions generally involve smaller amounts of myocardium, often with little or no detectable wall motion abnormality. Like unstable angina, non–Q-wave MI places patients at increased risk for reinfarction, recurrent angina, and death as compared to patients with stable angina or even Q-wave MI. In a collected review, non–Q-wave infarction was associated with a 9% in-hospital and 28.5% long-term mortality rate vs. 17% and 21%, respectively, for Q-wave infarction. The risks of in-hospital reinfarction (11%), reinfarction after discharge (18%), and in-hospital postinfarction angina with ECG changes (38%) were all greater than after Q-wave infarction.[6] The risk of late death or reinfarction may be four times greater with anterior non–Q-wave infarction as compared with non–Q-wave infarction in other locations.[7]

Randomized studies have shown that several subsets of patients with unstable angina may benefit from coronary artery bypass grafting compared with medical therapy. In patients with severe rest angina associated with ST-T changes on electrocardiogram, the Veterans' Affairs Cooperative Study showed a significant survival benefit with coronary artery bypass grafting if three-vessel coronary disease (Fig. 45-1) or abnormal left ventricular dysfunction (Fig. 45-2) were present.[8,9] All patients with unstable angina, with or without ischemia at rest, were more likely to be free of angina (Fig. 45-3),

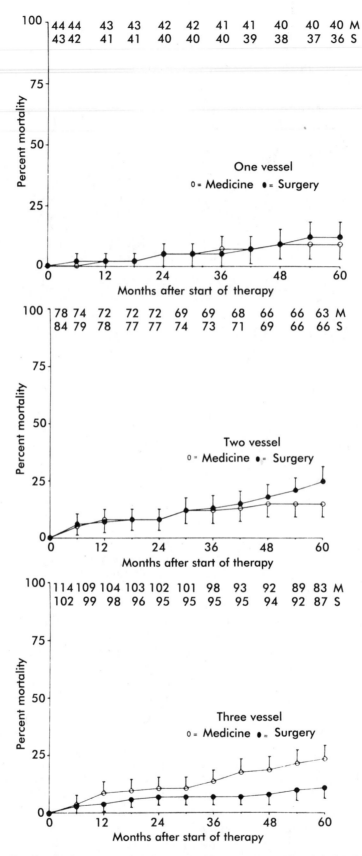

Fig. 45-1. Randomized comparison of medical therapy and coronary bypass grafting in patients with unstable angina and one-, two-, or three-vessel disease; $P < 0.02$ medicine vs. surgery for 3-vessel disease. (From Parisi AF, Khuri S, Deupree RH, et al: Medical compared with surgical management of unstable angina: 5-year mortality and morbidity in the Veterans' Administration Study, *Circulation* 80:1176-1189, 1989.)

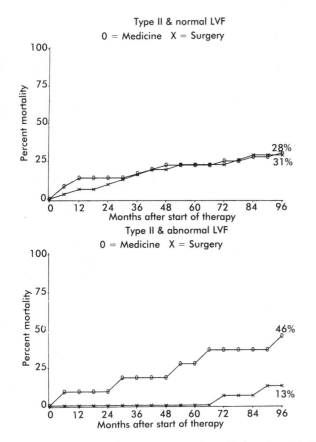

Fig. 45-2. Randomized comparison of medical and surgical therapy for Braunwald Type II unstable angina in patients with normal LV function (LVF) and with abnormal LVF; $P < 0.04$ medicine vs. surgery with abnormal LVF. (From Sharma GV, Deupree RH, Khuri SF, et al: Coronary bypass surgery improves survival in high-risk unstable angina. Results of a Veterans' Administration Cooperative study with an 8-year follow-up. Veterans' Administration Unstable Angina Cooperative Study Group, *Circulation* 84 (suppl III):260-267, 1991.)

had greater exercise tolerance (Fig. 45-4), required fewer antianginal medications, and were less likely to be readmitted for cardiac reasons (Fig. 45-5) after surgical than medical therapy.[10] The earlier randomized trial of the National Cooperative Study Group demonstrated that surgical treatment of unstable angina provided better relief of angina; however, no difference was observed in late infarction, employment, or survival after 2 years of follow-up, perhaps because of the short follow-up interval and limited statistical power of this study.[4]

Based on the results of these randomized studies, coronary artery bypass grafting is indicated in patients with unstable angina when angina is poorly controlled with medical therapy or when three-vessel coronary disease or left ventricular dysfunction are present. In addition, left main coronary disease or high-risk ischemia on exercise testing would indicate surgery in patients with angina initially stabilized on medical therapy, as suggested by nonrandomized studies finding decreased survival on medical therapy in these groups.[11-13] Although no randomized trials have compared medical and surgical therapy after non–Q-wave MI, the indications for coronary bypass grafting after non–Q-wave infarction are considered to be the same as those for unstable angina because the natural history of unstable angina and non–Q-wave infarction are similar.[6] In one series of 217 patients admitted with unstable angina, 50% had angina refractory to medical therapy, necessitating urgent revascularization by operation or angioplasty. Thus, 50% of patients were initially stabilized on medical therapy, but only 16% were ultimately managed with medical therapy alone[14] (Fig. 45-6).

Because percutaneous transluminal coronary angioplasty is a relatively recent phenomenon, little data exists

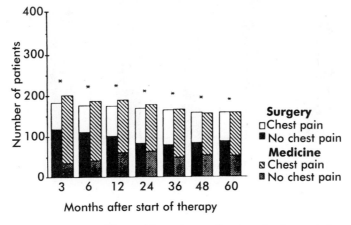

Fig. 45-3. Number of patients with or without chest pain at varying intervals in a randomized comparison of medical therapy and coronary bypass grafting for unstable angina; *$P < 0.05$ surgery vs. medicine. (From Booth DC, Deupree RH, Sharma GVRK, et al: Medical compared with surgical management of unstable angina; five-year mortality and morbidity in the Veterans' Administration study, *Circulation* 83:87-95, 1991.)

to define the relative roles of angioplasty versus coronary bypass grafting in patients with unstable angina or non–Q-wave MI. Nonetheless, several patient characteristics may be helpful in choosing operative revascularization vs. percutaneous angioplasty.[15] A failed coronary angioplasty resulting in myocardial ischemia generally indicates coronary bypass grafting. Significant aortoilio-femoral disease or coronary lesions anatomically unsuitable for coronary angioplasty would similarly favor surgical revascularization. Similarly, coronary bypass grafting may be preferable for coronary lesions with morphology less suitable for angioplasty (chronic total occlusion, tortuous vessels, bifurcated lesions, calcified vessels). Patients with significant concurrent valvular disease or ventricular septal defect likely to require surgical correction should undergo surgical revascularization to avoid multiple procedures. Finally, left main coronary disease (and, to a lesser extent, three-vessel coronary disease or impaired ejection fraction) would indicate coronary bypass grafting over angioplasty be-

cause of the decreased long-term success rate expected for left main or three-vessel angioplasty.

On the other hand, several factors may favor selection of percutaneous angioplasty over coronary bypass grafting in patients with unstable angina or non–Q-wave MI. In patients who have lesions that are anatomically suitable for angioplasty, one- or two-vessel disease may be relative indications for angioplasty. Because of increased operative risk, decreased likelihood of obtaining a complete revascularization, and increased likelihood of adverse outcome on medical therapy, prior coronary bypass grafting may be a relative indication for angioplasty in selected patients having anatomy that is suitable for angioplasty.[16] Severely depressed ejection fraction less than 25% may be a relative indication for angioplasty because of excessive surgical risk.[17] Other patients may have relative contraindications to surgical revascularization because of a limited life expectancy of less than 3 years, poor physical stamina to tolerate a surgical procedure, or a stroke in the previous 4 to 6 weeks.

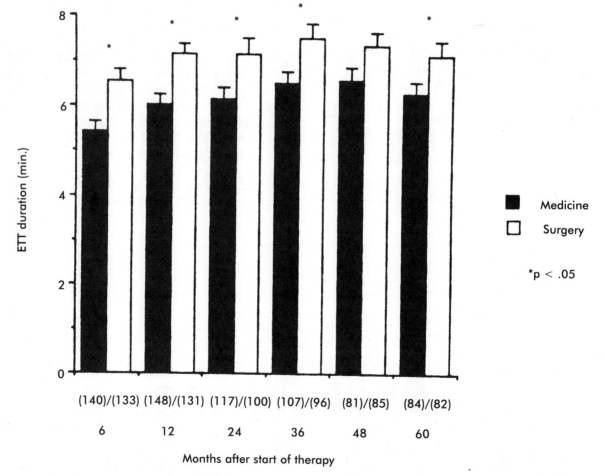

Fig. 45-4. Exercise treadmill test (ETT) duration at varying intervals in a randomized comparison of medical therapy and coronary bypass grafting for unstable angina; *$P < 0.05$ surgery vs. medicine. (From Booth DC, Deupree RH, Sharma GVRK, et al: Quality of life after bypass surgery for unstable angina. Five-year follow-up results of a Veterans' Affairs Cooperative Study, *Circulation* 83:87-95, 1991.)

TIMING OF CORONARY BYPASS GRAFTING

For those patients likely to benefit from coronary bypass grafting after a non–Q-wave MI or with postinfarction angina, considerable controversy surrounds the timing of surgery relative to the MI. Several investigators[17-20] have observed that patients undergoing coronary bypass grafting within 1 week of MI have an increased surgical mortality. In a large study of 993 patients undergoing coronary bypass grafting for unstable angina, in-hospital mortality increased from 7% to 22% if surgery was performed less than 24 hours after MI[18] (Fig. 45-7). Whether this increased risk was caused by unstable ischemia requiring urgent revascularization or by surgical intervention before adequate recovery from MI was unclear. On the other hand, many other investigators[21-23] have failed to find any increased surgical risk for coronary bypass grafting soon after MI. Although the data are not definitive, consideration should be given to delaying coronary bypass grafting after MI associated with significant reversible morbidity that might increase surgical risk, provided that the patient is sufficiently stable to make reinfarction during the recovery period unlikely. On the other hand, early revascularization *may* be considered for the remainder of patients to minimize the economic and physiologic costs of prolonged hospitalization.

Unlike the timing of coronary bypass grafting relative to MI, the timing of surgical revascularization relative to recent thrombolytic therapy is less controversial. Several studies[24,25] showed that operation within 12 hours of thrombolytic therapy significantly increased perioperative blood loss, transfusion requirements, and morbidity. Coronary bypass grafting should generally be delayed for 12 to 24 hours after acute thrombolytic therapy until coagulation status has normalized. Although these patients often continue to receive heparin therapy, measurement of the serum fibrinogen level and prothrombin time may be useful in determining when the thrombolytic effect has sufficiently cleared for safe surgery.

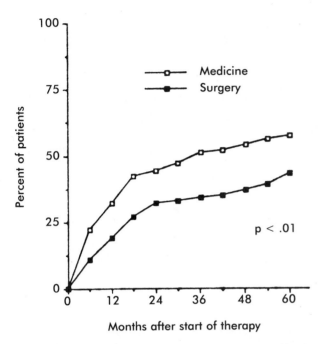

Fig. 45-5. Percentage of patients requiring rehospitalization for cardiac reasons in a randomized comparison of medical and surgical therapy for unstable angina; $P < 0.01$ medicine vs. surgery. (From Booth DC, Deupree RH, Sharma GVRK, et al: Medical compared with surgical management of unstable angina; five-year mortality and morbidity in the Veterans' Administration study, 83:87-95, 1991.)

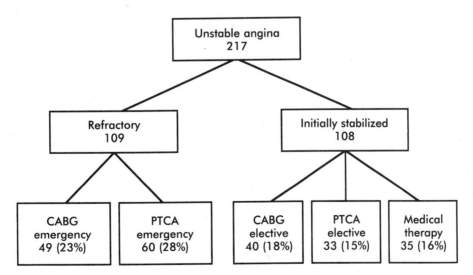

Fig. 45-6. Ultimate therapeutic distribution in one series of 217 patients with unstable angina. (From DeFeyter PJ, Serruys PW, VanDenBrand M, et al: Emergency coronary angioplasty in refractory unstable angina, *N Engl J Med* 313:342-346, 1985.)

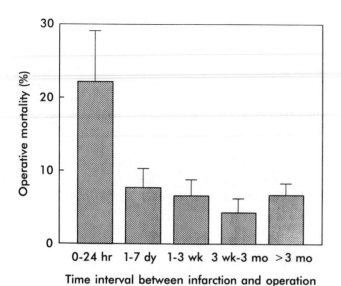

Fig. 45-7. Operative mortality from coronary bypass grafting as a function of time interval between infarction and operation in patients with unstable angina. (From Curtis JJ, Walls JT, Salam NH, et al: Impact of unstable angina on operative mortality with coronary revascularization at varying time intervals after myocardial infarction, *J Thorac Cardiovasc Surg* 102:867-873, 1991.)

In addition to MI and thrombolysis, several other acute events may increase surgical risk if immediately followed by surgical revascularization. A recent significant gastrointestinal bleed, a stroke within 4 to 6 weeks, acute reversible renal failure, or other recent major surgery that could produce bleeding during full heparinization are relative contraindications to early revascularization in the patient with unstable angina or non–Q-wave MI.

PATIENT PREPARATION

For those patients undergoing coronary bypass grafting for unstable angina or non–Q-wave MI, adequate patient preparation can minimize perioperative morbidity and risk. Surgery during ongoing ischemia has been reported to increase the rate of perioperative MI by up to 18%.[26] Therefore myocardial ischemia should be controlled before revascularization by maintaining these patients on intravenous heparin, beta blockers, and intravenous or topical nitroglycerin. Abrupt preoperative cessation of beta blockade has been associated with risk of ischemia and infarction.[27] In patients with unstable angina treated medically, immediate initiation of either aspirin or heparin therapy reduced the risk of

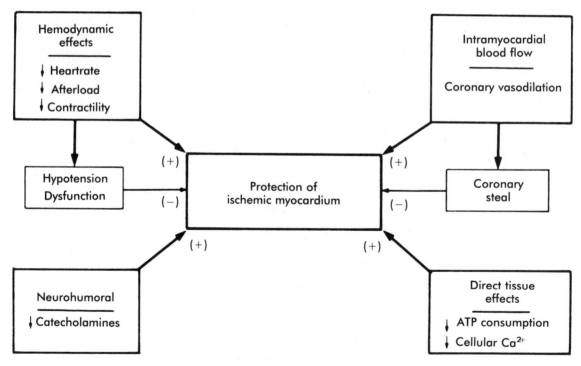

Fig. 45-8. Hemodynamic and oxygenation data throughout the procedure in the anesthetized and sedated patients. The vertical axis includes arterial Po_2, heart rate, mean blood pressure, and rate-pressure product. The horizontal axis indicates the time in minutes after baseline measurements. The times of intubation (8 minutes) and extubation (91 minutes) are indicated by arrows; *-$P < 0.05$; **$P < 0.005$ in intergroup comparisons. (From deBruijn NP, Hlatky MA, Jacobs JR, et al: General anesthesia during percutaneous transluminary coronary angioplasty for acute myocardial infarction: results of a randomized controlled clinical trial, *Anesth Analg* 68:201-207, 1989.)

MI or recurrent refractory angina in the randomized trial of Theroux et al.[28] Although this study lacked statistical power to detect an advantage of heparin and aspirin together, the randomized trial of Wallentin et al.[29] found that the combination of heparin and aspirin improved outcome relative to aspirin alone in men with unstable angina or non–Q-wave MI. For patients with AMI, immediate aspirin therapy reduced mortality in the randomized ISIS 2 trial.[30] Postoperative aspirin therapy begun within 1 hour of coronary bypass grafting improved long-term graft patency rates.[31] On the other hand, aspirin exposure within 7 days of surgery may increase perioperative bleeding.[31-33] At present the risks of increased perioperative bleeding appear to be outweighed by the benefits of preoperative aspirin therapy in most patients with unstable angina or non–Q-wave MI. For patients

with acute instability or ongoing ischemia poorly relieved with medical management, placement of an intraaortic balloon pump may improve survival[14] and allow patient stabilization to occur before coronary bypass grafting. With modern techniques of percutaneously inserting the intraaortic balloon pump, in this setting the incidence of significant complications has fallen to 6% or less.[34] The majority of these complications relate to false aneurysm or thrombosis of the femoral artery requiring repair; a minor degree of limb ischemia or blood loss caused by the balloon pump has been reported in up to 59% of patients, often after thrombolytic therapy.[34]

Preoperative hemodynamic optimization is a desirable goal in all patients because poorly controlled hypotension, hypertension, or congestive heart failure may add considerably to surgical risk. If significant hemodynamic instability is present, Swan-Ganz catheterization and intravenous drips may be necessary to control blood pressure and to optimize cardiac loading. Patients with cardiogenic shock requiring inotropic support do very poorly with surgery and frequently succumb perioperatively from heart failure. Therefore, we usually consider coronary bypass grafting only after the patient has been proven capable of generating a normal cardiac output without inotropic agents.

In addition to hemodynamics, other factors may be optimized to reduce perioperative risk. If possible, ongoing sepsis should be controlled before proceeding to surgery. To minimize the risk of anesthesia, serum glucose and electrolytes should be in the normal range before coronary bypass grafting is performed.

ANESTHETIC CONCERNS

We have postulated that anesthesia is an effective myocardial protective strategy;[35-37] this subject has been recently reviewed.[38] Patients with unstable angina or even ongoing MI can be safely anesthetized by experienced cardiac anesthesiologists. Support for this thesis comes from a study in which patients with AMI were randomized to receive either general anesthesia or sedation during diagnostic catheterization and PTCA.[39]

It is clear that stress is increased during induction of and emergence from anesthesia, but stress actually is reduced during the majority of anesthesia time[39] (Fig. 45-8). We have summarized the potential benefits of anesthesia on the ischemic heart in Figure 45-9.[40] As seen in Figure 45-8 and as widely believed, the benefits of general anesthesia largely are a result of decreased myocardial oxygen demand, as reflected by decreases in rate-pressure-product, and augmentation of oxygen delivery seen in higher oxygen-carrying capacity of the blood. It is not uncommon for the anesthesiologist to receive in the operating room a patient who has ongoing ischemia and to see the electrocardiographic evidence of ischemia disappear with the induction of general anes-

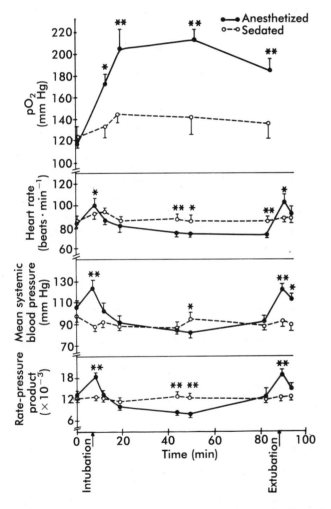

Fig. 45-9. A schematic diagram showing the overall affect of anesthetics during AMI. Note that salvage is achieved by enhancing oxygen delivery and reducing myocardial demand by direct and indirect actions. (From Kates RA, Hill RF, Reves JG: Reperfusion of the acute myocardial infarction: role of anesthesia. In Reves JG (ed): *Acute Revascularization of the Infarcted Heart,* Orlando, 1987, Grune and Stratton.)

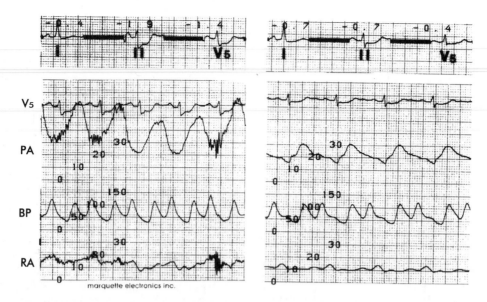

Fig. 45-10. Beneficial effects of anesthesia induction. Patient with ongoing ischemia despite intraaortic balloon pump (IABP) and intravenous nitroglycerin (IV NTG) therapy. *A,* Before induction, evidence of marked ischemia and elevated filling pressures; *B,* Ten minutes after induction, IABP and NTG unchanged. Note the dramatic improvement in ischemia and decreased filling pressures. (From Maccidi GM, Hill RF, McIntyre RW, et al.: Anesthesia—method of myocardial protection in patients with ischemic heart disease. In *Cardiac Surgery State of the Art Reviews,* Hanley and Belfus Series, 1988.)

thesia (Fig. 45-10). The anesthetic drugs may have inherent myocardial protective qualities such as calcium channel blocking properties, and certainly general anesthesia attenuates the catecholamine response that accompanies angina and infarction.

Anesthetic management of the ischemic patient is conducted promptly, and often the anesthesia induction is initiated before all hemodynamic monitoring is established to spare the patient the additional discomfort of placement of arterial and central venous cannulation. No one superior anesthetic technique is used; a host of drugs including benzodiazepines, opioids, and inhalation drugs are used for the induction and maintenance of general anesthesia.

The principles of anesthetic management are to: (1) minimize myocardial oxygen demand through reduction of preload, heart rate, and afterload; (2) optimize oxygen delivery by maintaining a normal or high Pao_2 and hemoglobin; and (3) treat ischemia aggressively with nitrates, beta-adrenergic antagonists, and, occasionally, calcium-channel blockers. With this form of management, anesthesia is a very effective myocardial protective strategy, and concerns about the risks of anesthesia should not be allowed to delay referral for needed bypass surgery in acute ischemic heart disease.

RESULTS OF CORONARY BYPASS GRAFTING

The results of coronary artery bypass grafting in patients with unstable angina or non–Q-wave MI are well documented and may be considered in terms of in-hospital morbidity, survival, ventricular function, and symptoms. No contemporary data are available to evaluate the cost effectiveness of coronary bypass grafting vs. medical therapy or percutaneous angioplasty for the patient with unstable angina or non–Q-wave MI.

In-hospital morbidity

Patients undergoing bypass grafting for unstable angina have slightly greater perioperative morbidity than patients undergoing elective bypass grafting for stable angina. Most frequent major complications include low cardiac output (5% to 21%), perioperative myocardial infarction MI (2% to 11%), reoperation for bleeding (1% to 3%), stroke (2% to 3%), and mediastinitis (1% to 2%).[21,41-43] In-hospital morbidity after coronary bypass grafting for non–Q-wave infarction has not differed significantly from that of unstable angina.[6,20]

Survival

In-hospital mortality after coronary bypass grafting for unstable angina has averaged from 4% to 6%,[42,44,45] significantly higher than the 1% to 2% mortality rate reported for stable angina. In-hospital mortality for coronary bypass in patients with non–Q-wave infarction and postinfarction angina has been even higher, averaging 8%.[17,23,46] Risk factors for perioperative death in unstable angina and postinfarction angina are similar to those for other coronary disease patients and include older age, left ventricular dysfunction, and prior bypass operation.[17,19,21,41,44]

Long-term survival in patients undergoing coronary bypass grafting for unstable angina or postinfarction angina has generally been good, ranging from 87% to 92% at 5 years and 75% to 83% at 10 years.[23,44,47,48] Of note, long-term survival was not affected by whether unstable angina occurred at rest, after MI, or was simply progressive or of recent onset.[48]

Ventricular function

The effects of coronary bypass grafting on left ventricular function in the patient with unstable angina have been poorly documented. However, several studies have suggested that patients receiving thrombolysis followed by coronary bypass grafting for AMI showed a greater degree of recovery in left ventricular ejection fraction and infarct zone regional function than in patients treated with thrombolysis alone.[49] Using repeat angiography after coronary bypass grafting, Rankin et al.[50] observed improvement in regional wall motion in 40% of patients with unstable angina.

Symptoms

One year after coronary bypass grafting for unstable angina, roughly 78% of the patients are pain free, and up to 73% of those who had worked before surgery have returned to work.[47,51] Booth et al.[10] reported that 55% of patients were painfree within 5 years of surgery, and only 12% developed angina on exercise testing.[10] In a series of older patients, the percentage of patients working 5 years after surgery has been as low as 28%.[10] The incidence of reoperation after 5 years or 10 years of follow-up was 6% and 17% respectively in a large series of patients operated on for unstable angina between 1970 and 1982.[48] The incidence of late reoperation would be expected to be lower in recent series with a greater utilization of internal mammary artery grafting.

REFERENCES

1. Heng MK, Norris RM, Singh BN, et al: Prognosis in unstable angina, *Br Heart J* 38:921-925, 1976.
2. Langer A, Freeman MR, Armstrong PW: ST segment shift in unstable angina:pathophysiology and association with coronary anatomy and hospital outcome, *J Am Coll Cardiol* 13:1495-1502, 1989.
3. Marmur JD, Freeman MR, Langer AL, et al: Prognosis in medically stabilized unstable angina: early Holter ST-segment monitoring compared with suspected unstable coronary artery disease, *Ann Int Med* 113:575-579, 1990.
4. National Cooperative Study Group: Unstable angina pectoris: national cooperative study group to compare surgical and medical therapy. II. In-hospital experience and initial follow-up results in patients with one-, two-, and three-vessel disease, *Am J Cardiol* 42:839-848, 1978.
5. Mulcahy R, Awadhi A, Buitleor M, et al: Natural history and prognosis of unstable angina, *Am Heart J* 109:753-758, 1985.
6. Gibson RS: Non-Q wave myocardial infarction: prognosis, chang-

ing incidence, and management. In Gersh BJ, Rahimtoola SH (eds): *Acute myocardial infarction,* New York, 1981, Elsevier.
7. Kao W, Khaja F, Goldstein S, et al: Cardiac event rate after non Q-wave acute myocardial infarction and the significance of its anterior location, *Am J Cardiol* 64:1236-1242, 1989.
8. Parisi AF, Khuri S, Deupree RH, et al: Medical compared with surgical management of unstable angina: 5-year mortality and morbidity in the Veterans' Administration Study, *Circulation* 80:1176-1189, 1989.
9. Sharma GV, Deupree RH, Khuri SF, et al: Coronary bypass surgery improves survival in high-risk unstable angina. Results of a Veterans' Administration Cooperative study with an 8-year follow-up. Veterans Administration Unstable Angina Cooperative Study Group, *Circulation* 84 (suppl III):260-267, 1991.
10. Booth DC, Deupree RH, Sharma GVRK, et al: Medical compared with surgical management of unstable angina: 5-year mortality and morbidity in the Veterans' Administration study, *Circulation* 83:87-95, 1991.
11. Califf RM, Harrell FE Jr, Lee KL, et al: The evolution of medical and surgical therapy for coronary artery disease. A 15-year perspective, *JAMA* 261:2077-2086, 1989.
12. Mark DB, Hlatky MA, Harrell FE Jr, et al: Exercise treadmill score for predicting prognosis in coronary artery disease, *Ann Intern Med* 106:793-800, 1987.
13. Takaro T, Hultgren HN, Lipton MJ, et al and participants in the Study Group: The VA cooperative randomized study of surgery for coronary arterial occlusive disease. II. Subgroup with significant left main lesions, *Circulation* 54 (suppl III):107-117, 1976.
14. DeFeyter PJ, Serruys PW, VanDenBrand M, et al: Emergency coronary angioplasty in refractory unstable angina, *N Engl J Med* 313:342-346, 1985.
15. DeFeyter PJ, Serruys PW, VanDenBrand M, et al: Percutaneous transluminal coronary angioplasty for unstable angina, *Am J Cardiol* 68:125B-135B, 1991.
16. Theroux P, Waters D: Unstable angina: special considerations in the postbypass patient, *Cardiovasc Clin* 21(2):169-191, 1991.
17. Hochberg MS, Parsonnet V, Hussain SM, et al: Timing of coronary revascularization after acute myocardial infarction, *J Thorac Cardiovasc Surg* 88:914-921, 1984.
18. Curtis JJ, Walls JT, Salam NH, et al: Impact of unstable angina on operative mortality with coronary revascularization at varying time intervals after myocardial infarction, *J Thorac Cardivasc Surg* 102:867-873, 1991.
19. Kennedy JW, Ivey TD, Misbach G, et al: Coronary artery bypass graft surgery early after acute myocardial infarction, *Circulation* 79(suppl I):73-78, 1989.
20. Kouchoukos NT, Murphy S, Philpott T, et al: Coronary artery bypass grafting for postinfarction angina pectoris, *Circulation* 79(suppl I):68-72, 1989.
21. Applebaum R, House R, Rademaker A, et al: Coronary artery bypass grafting within thirty days of acute myocardial infarction. Early and late results in 406 patients, *J Thorac Cardiovasc Surg* 102:745-752, 1991.
22. Connolly MW, Gelbfish JS, Rose DM, et al: Early coronary artery bypass grafting for complicated acute myocardial infarction, *J Cardiovasc Surg (Torino)* 29:375-382, 1988.
23. Gardner TJ, Stuart RS, Greene PS, et al: The risk of coronary artery bypass surgery for patients with postinfarction angina, *Circulation* 79(suppl I):79-80, 1989.
24. Lee KF, Mandell J, Rankin JS, et al: Immediate versus delayed coronary grafting after streptokinase treatment: postoperative blood loss and clinical results, *J Thorac Cardiovasc Surg* 95:216-221, 1988.
25. Skinner JR, Phillips SJ, Zeff RH, et al: Immediate coronary bypass following failed streptokinase infusion in evolving myocardial infarction, *J Thorac Cardiovasc Surg* 87:567-570, 1984.

26. Golding LAR, Loop FD, Sheldon WC, et al: Emergency revascularization for unstable angina, *Circulation* 58:1163-1166, 1978.

27. Miller RR, Alson HG, Amsterdam EA, et al: Propranolol withdrawal rebound phenomenon, *N Engl J Med* 293:416, 1975.

28. Theroux P, Ouimet H, McCans J, et al: Aspirin, heparin, or both to treat acute unstable angina, *N Engl J Med* 319:1105-1111, 1988.

29. Wallentin LC: Aspirin (75 mg/day) after an episode of unstable coronary artery disease: long-term effects on the risk for myocardial infarction, occurrence of severe angina and the need for revascularization. Research Group on Instability in Coronary Artery Disease in Southeast Sweden, *J Am Coll Cardiol* 18:1587-1593, 1991.

30. ISIS 2 (Second International Study of Infarct Survival) Collaborative Group: Randomized trial of intravenous streptokinase, oral aspirin, both, or neither among 17,187 cases of suspected acute myocardial infarction: ISIS-2, *Lancet* ii:349-360, 1988.

31. Gavaghan TP, Gebski V, Baron DW: Immediate postoperative aspirin improves vein graft patency early and late after coronary artery bypass graft surgery, *Circulation* 83:1526-1533, 1991.

32. Bashein G, Nessly ML, Rice AL, et al: Preoperative aspirin therapy and reoperation for bleeding after coronary artery bypass surgery, *Arch Intern Med* 151:89-93, 1991.

33. Sethi GK, Copeland JG, Goldman S, et al: Implications of preoperative administration of aspirin in patients undergoing coronary artery bypass grafting. Department of Veterans Affairs Cooperative Study on Antiplatelet Therapy, *J Am Coll Cardiol* 15:15-20, 1990.

34. Ohman EM, Califf RM, George BS, et al: The use of intraaortic balloon pumping as an adjunct to reperfusion therapy in acute myocardial infarction. The Thrombolysis and Angioplasty in Myocardial Infarction (TAMI) Study Group, *Am Heart J* 121:895-901, 1991.

35. Hill RF, Reves JG: Myocardial protection: role of anesthetic drugs. In Reves JG: *Anesthesiology clinics,* vol 6, Baltimore, 1988, WB Saunders.

36. Maccioli GM, Hill RF, McIntyre RW, et al: Reves JG: Anesthesia—method of myocardial protection in patients with ischemic heart disease. In *Cardiac Surgery State of the Art Reviews,* Hanley and Belfus Series, 1988.

37. McIntyre RW, Hlatky MA, Reves JG: General anesthesia in the patient with acute myocardial infarction. In Califf RM, Mark DB, Wagner GS (eds): *Acute coronary care in the thrombolytic era,* Chicago, 1988, Year Book Medical Publishers.

38. Mangano DT: Perioperative cardiac morbidity, *Anesthesiology* 72:153-184, 1990.

39. deBruijn NP, Hlatky MA, Jacobs JR, et al: General anesthesia during percutaneous transluminary coronary angioplasty for acute myocardial infarction: results of a randomized controlled clinical trial, *Anesth Analg* 68:201-207, 1989.

40. Kates RA, Hill RF, Reves JG: Reperfusion of the acute myocardial infarction: role of anesthesia. In Reves JG (ed): *Acute revascularization of the infarcted heart,* Orlando, 1987, Grune and Stratton.

41. Hammermeister KE, Morrison DA: Coronary bypass surgery for stable angina and unstable angina pectoris, *Cardiol Clin* 135-155, 1991.

42. Hannan EL, Kilburn H Jr, O'Donnell JF, et al: Adult open heart surgery in New York State. An analysis of risk factors and hospital mortality rates, *JAMA* 264:2768-2774, 1990.

43. Naunheim KS, Fiore AC, Arango DC, et al: Coronary artery bypass grafting for unstable angina pectoris: risk analysis, *Ann Thorac Surg* 47:569-574, 1989.

44. McCormick JR, Schick EC Jr, McCabe CH, et al: Determinants of operative mortality and long-term survival in patients with unstable angina. The CASS experience, *J Thorac Cardiovasc Surg* 89:683-688, 1985.

45. Rankin JS, Newton JR Jr, Califf RM, et al: Clinical characteristics and current management of medically refractory unstable angina, *Ann Surg* 200:457-465, 1984.

46. Breyer RH, Engelman RM, Rousou JA, et al: Postinfarction angina: an expanding subset of patients undergoing coronary artery bypass, *J Thorac Cardiovasc Surg* 90:532-540, 1985.

47. Kaiser GC, Schaff HV, Killip T: Myocardial revascularization for unstable angina pectoris, *Circulation* 79(suppl I):60-67, 1989.

48. Rahimtoola SH, Nunley D, Grunkemeier G, et al: Ten-year survival after coronary artery bypass surgery for unstable angina, *N Engl J Med* 308:676-681, 1983.

49. Kereiakes DJ, Califf RM, George BS, et al: Coronary bypass surgery improves global and regional left ventricular function following thrombolytic therapy for acute myocardial infarction—TAMI Study Group, *Am Heart J* 122:390-399, 1991.

50. Rankin JS, Newman GE, Muhlbaier LH, et al: The effects of coronary revascularization on left ventricular function in ischemic heart disease, *J Thorac Cardiovasc Surg* 90:818-832, 1985.

51. Huttunen K, Rehnberg S, Huttunen H, et al: Clinical characteristics and coronary anatomy in refractory unstable angina pectoris leading to coronary artery bypass grafting: the Kuopio experience, *Scand J Thorac Cardiovasc Surg* 23:19-23, 1989.

Chapter 46

CARDIOGENIC SHOCK

James R. Bengtson
Robert J. Goldberg
Andrew J. Kaplan

Shock is the manifestation of the rude unhinging of the machinery of life.

GROSS, 1972

Although advances in diagnosis, monitoring, and treatment of patients with myocardial infarction (MI) have contributed to an improved prognosis, survival rates in the subset of patients who develop cardiogenic shock continue to be very low. With improved understanding of the pathophysiology of shock and continued improvements in mechanical circulatory assistance and surgical revascularization, there is recent evidence that more patients whose MIs are complicated by shock may be able to survive their hospitalization.

In this chapter, we review current concepts regarding the epidemiology, pathophysiology, and management of cardiogenic shock.

DEFINITION

Circulatory shock is a pathophysiologic state in which the heart is unable to deliver enough tissue blood flow and oxygen to meet the metabolic demands of the body.[1] This state may result from derangements in any of the basic components of the circulation: the heart, blood volume, or the vascular system. Cardiogenic shock, a type of circulatory shock caused by severely impaired ventricular pump function, may be defined as all of the following:

1. Systolic blood pressure less than 80 to 90 mm Hg (or 30 mm Hg less than basal levels) for at least 30 minutes.
2. Persistence of shock after correction of extramyocardial factors contributing to hypotension and reduced cardiac output (hypovolemia, arrhythmias, hypoxemia, acidosis, etc.).

3. Evidence of tissue hypoperfusion, such as oliguria (< 20-30 ml/hr), cyanosis, or altered mental status.

It must be emphasized that hypotension is not synonymous with shock. The cardinal feature of shock is inadequate tissue perfusion. Patients with low blood pressure may have normal tissue perfusion if vascular resistance is also decreased or decreased perfusion despite "normal" blood pressure in the presence of severe reflex vasoconstriction.

ETIOLOGY

The syndrome of insufficient cardiac output leading to inadequate tissue perfusion may result from several causes (Table 46-1). Cardiogenic shock most commonly results from acute myocardial infarction (AMI) in which sufficient myocardium is lost to cause inadequate tissue perfusion. The most common type of infarction precipitating shock is anterior MI caused by occlusion of the left anterior descending artery.[2] However, occlusion of a dominant right coronary artery may cause a predominant right ventricular infarction with cardiogenic shock.[3] Because this type of infarction causes reduced diastolic compliance and systolic dysfunction of the right ventricle (see Chapter 60), it results in a volume-sensitive state, in contrast to the pressure-sensitive state after infarction of the left ventricle.

Cardiogenic shock may also result from mechanical complications after AMI. It is important to remember that in contrast to shock caused by large anterior infarcts, papillary muscle dysfunction or rupture (see Chapter 53) can cause shock without extensive infarction

Table 46-1. Etiologic classification of cardiogenic shock

Acute myocardial infarction
    Loss of critical left ventricular myocardium
    Right ventricular pump failure
    Mechanical complications
        Acute mitral regurgitation due to papillary muscle
            dysfunction or rupture
        Ventricular septal rupture
        Free wall rupture
        Left ventricular aneurysm
End-stage cardiomyopathy
Myocardial contusion
Myocarditis
Left ventricular outflow tract obstruction
    Aortic stenosis
    Hypertrophic obstructive cardiomyopathy
Left ventricular inflow tract obstruction
    Mitral stenosis
    Left atrial myxoma
Postcardiopulmonary bypass

---

or multivessel coronary artery disease.[4-6] Ventricular free-wall or septal rupture leads to cardiogenic shock in the majority of patients, particularly those suffering their first MI.[7-9]

INCIDENCE

Based on a number of studies of cardiogenic shock (Table 46-2), the incidence of cardiogenic shock complicating AMI ranges from 6% to approximately 20%.[10-18] Studies published between 1937 and 1952 that examined the incidence rates of cardiogenic shock exhibit similar variation in rates to those of more recent studies.[19] Variations in the incidence of cardiogenic shock after AMI may result from differences in the size and characteristics of the patient samples, the extent of patient delay in admission to the hospital after the onset of symptoms, criteria for the diagnosis of cardiogenic shock and MI, and variation in use of ancillary therapies. A recent population-based investigation of 4762 patients admitted to 16 hospitals in the Worcester, Massachusetts metropolitan area between 1975 and 1988 found an overall incidence of cardiogenic shock after MI of 7.5%.[8] In examining changes over time in the incidence of cardiogenic shock with AMI, the authors[8] did not find an appreciable change in rates between 1975 and 1988; the incidence rates ranged from 6.7% to 9.1% over the 13-year period under study. Using multivariable regression analysis to adjust for a variety of demographic and clinical characteristics, as well as therapeutic interventions that may have affected the incidence of cardiogenic shock and that may have changed over the periods under study, they observed a significant, albeit inconsistent, change over time in the adjusted risk estimates for cardiogenic shock. The highest adjusted risks for the

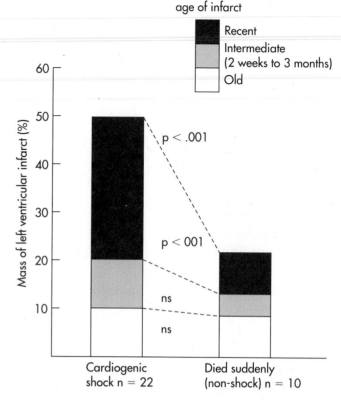

Fig. 46-1. Mass of left ventricular infarction in 22 patients who died of cardiogenic shock compared with 10 with sudden death. (From Alonso DR, Scheidt S, Post M, et al: *Circulation* 48:588, 1973. Used by permission.)

development of shock were found, however, in the most recent years under study (1986 and 1988).

PATHOLOGY

The mechanical failure associated with cardiogenic shock is thought to arise from a cumulative loss of at least 40% of left ventricular myocardium. Page et al.[20] compared autopsy specimens of 20 patients dying of AMI complicated by cardiogenic shock with those of AMI patients who had sudden arrhythmic deaths and those dying of shock of other etiologies. Almost all shock patients had lost 40% to 70% of left ventricular myocardium. Autopsy specimens demonstrated a ragged appearance at the border of the infarct with patches of dead or damaged myocytes interspersed in the border region (Fig. 46-1). A greater duration of cardiogenic shock before death correlated with an increased extent of damaged and dead cells at the border. Hearts from patients without shock showed a clear margination between dead myocardium, a zone of inflammation, and undamaged myocardium. Other autopsy studies have confirmed these findings, showing acute damage or recent damage combined with previous scarring.[21-25]

Table 46-2. Incidence of cardiogenic shock among patients with acute myocardial infarction*

Author	Study years	Study population	Population characteristics	Incidence of shock (%)
Malach and Rosenberg[10]	1954-1955	264 patients with AMI admitted to Kings County Hospital (NY)	Age 68 yr 61% male	9.5
Killip and Kimball[11]	1965-1967	250 patients with AMI admitted to NY hospital	Age 64 yr 72% male	18.8
Scheidt et al.[12]	1965-1969	547 patients with AMI admitted to NY hospital	Age 67 yr 75% male	13.3
Goldberg et al.[13]	1966-1971	1304 patients with AMI admitted to 20 metropolitan Baltimore hospitals	Age ≥60 yr: 43% 69% male	6.3 (1967) 7.2 (1971)
Kobayashi et al.[14]	1977-1982	264 patients with AMI admitted to Showa University School of Medicine	Age ≥70 yr: 36% 72% male	13.3
Takano et al.[15]	1977-1982	657 patients with AMI admitted to Nippon Medical School	–	11.4
Gheorghiade et al.[16]	1980-1984	2162 consecutive patients with suspected MI admitted to Henry Ford Hospital	Age 64 yr 59% male	6.0
Jugdutt and Warnica[17]	1981-1983	310 consecutive patients with AMI admitted to the University of Alberta hospital	Age 61 yr 76% male	10.0
Goldberg et al.[18]	1975-1988	4762 patients with AMI admitted to 16 metropolitan Worcester, Mass. hospitals	Age 61 yr 61% male	7.3 (1975) 7.1 (1978) 7.5 (1981) 6.7 (1984) 7.6 (1986) 9.1 (1988)

*AMI, Acute myocardial infarction; NY, New York.

Most patients have severe and extensive coronary artery disease, often involving all three major coronary arteries, with predominant involvement of the left anterior descending artery. In addition, patients frequently demonstrate extension of recent areas of necrosis and focal necrotic areas remote from the major location of recent infarction.[26] It should be noted, however, that loss of 40% to 60% of the myocardium may occur without necessarily causing cardiogenic shock.

PATHOPHYSIOLOGY

The primary defect in postinfarction shock is severely depressed ventricular function. The magnitude of this impairment is related to imbalances between myocardial oxygen supply and demand, which progress during the course of the infarction. Reduced cardiac output because of a drop in stroke volume causes systemic pressure to fall. Compensatory mechanisms, including increased heart rate, contractility, and wall tension, increase myocardial oxygen consumption. Fixed coronary stenoses limit flow despite maximal arteriolar vasodilation. Perfusion pressure then becomes the major determinant of coronary blood flow. Any slight decrease in systemic pressure can reduce coronary pressure and flow below critical levels.

The combination of severe diffuse coronary artery disease and prolonged hypotension are thus particularly detrimental to cardiac function in the shock patient. Severely impaired coronary perfusion results in further ischemia and necrosis of myocardium, both at the border zone of the infarct and in the distribution of other coronary arteries. This, in turn, further reduces cardiac output, systemic blood pressure, and coronary flow. A positive feedback cycle is established in which cardiac pump dysfunction leads to progressive myocardial ischemia and finally intractable circulatory failure (Fig. 46-2).

Feedback and compensatory mechanisms are enacted in the setting of shock. In the early stages, they operate to restore blood flow to vital organs, as follows:

1. Sympathetic nervous system. A rise in sympathetic tone is activated by baroreceptors and chemore-

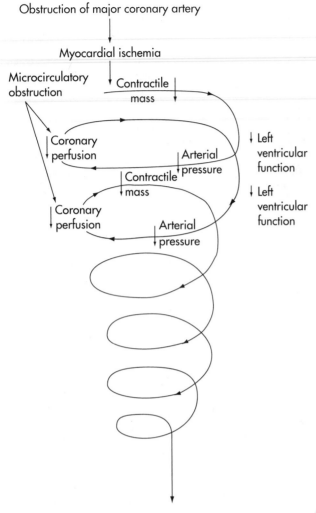

Obstruction of major coronary artery

Myocardial ischemia

Microcirculatory obstruction

Contractile mass

Coronary perfusion

Arterial pressure

↓ Left ventricular function

Contractile mass

↓ Left ventricular function

Coronary perfusion

Arterial pressure

Fig. 46-2. Sequence of events in the vicious cycle in which coronary artery obstruction leads to cardiogenic shock and progressive circulatory deterioration. (From Pasternak RC, Braunwald E: Acute myocardial infarction. In Wilson JD, Braunwald E, Isselbacher KJ, et al [eds]: *Harrison's principles of internal medicine,* New York, 1987, McGraw-Hill. Used by permission.)

ceptors. This triggers a rise in heart rate, myocardial contractility, venous tone, arterial vasoconstriction, catecholamine synthesis and release, and shift of fluid into the vascular compartment.

2. Endogenous vasoconstrictors and hormones. Decreased renal perfusion pressure and sympathetic stimulation of renal nerves activates the renin-angiotensin system. Angiotensin II levels rise, leading to peripheral vasoconstriction and synthesis of aldosterone. Aldosterone exerts a mineralocorticoid effect. Sodium and water resorption by the kidneys then is increased, raising blood volume. Hypotension also triggers baroreceptor reflexes, causing release of antidiuretic hormone (ADH). ADH acts on the kidneys to increase water resorption.

3. Local vasoregulatory mechanisms. Tissue ischemia leads to accumulation of vasoactive metabolites. These cause arteriolar and capillary vasodilation. Hypoxia also acts directly to dilate arteriolar beds. These effects increase regional blood flow and total capillary surface area, thereby improving blood-oxygen exchange. Local autoregulation in the coronary, cerebral, and renal circulations causes vasodilation to occur in response to a drop in perfusion pressure. Blood flow is redistributed away from the skin, intestines, and skeletal muscle to the vital organs.

As cardiogenic shock becomes more prolonged, tissue ischemia and organ dysfunction become more pronounced, causing deleterious positive feedback pathways to ensue:

1. Depressed cardiac function. Accumulated metabolic acids and toxic humoral factors reduce cardiac contractility.

2. Vasodilation. Prolonged hypoxia, acidosis, and an accumulation of vasodilatory metabolites counteract sympathetic vasoconstriction. Systemic hypotension then occurs, impairing blood flow to vital organs. Venous return is also decreased, impairing cardiac filling. Anatomic arteriovenous channels open, shunting blood from the tissue beds. Nutritive flow is thus further compromised.

3. Microvascular endothelial injury. The integrity of the endothelium is disrupted, leading to increased capillary permeability. Fluid and protein leave the intravascular space, reducing vascular volume, thereby lowering cardiac output and blood pressure. In the lungs, gas exchange is impaired by development of interstitial and alveolar edema. Mucosal damage in the intestines allows entry of bacteria and toxins into the bloodstream. Glomerular and tubular damage in the kidneys leads to fluid, electrolyte, and metabolic disturbances.

4. Intravascular clotting. Microthrombi and platelet aggregates form because of stasis secondary to decreased cardiac output, capillary endothelial damage resulting in fibrin deposition, and catecholamine-induced platelet aggregation.

The cumulative effect of these perturbations of homeostasis is multisystem organ failure and eventual death.

CLINICAL ASSESSMENT
History and physical examination

Patients who develop cardiogenic shock after MI tend to be older men.[12,77] A history of previous infarction is present in approximately one third of patients, as is a history of diabetes. The interval between the onset of infarct symptoms and shock is often prolonged[12,27]; in a recent series, this interval was 9 hours, with a quartile range of 4 to 31 hours.[2]

Patients in shock generally have an ashen or cyanotic appearance, with cold and clammy skin. Because of cerebral hypoperfusion, they may be disoriented or even unconscious.[12] Peripheral pulses are rapid and thready, with a narrow pulse pressure. Arrhythmias occur commonly. Respirations are shallow and rapid, and Cheyne-Stokes respirations may occur as a result of cerebral hypoperfusion, especially in the elderly and those treated with narcotics. Except in patients with predominant right ventricular infarction, pulmonary edema is present and associated with varying degrees of respiratory distress, hypoxemia, and carbon dioxide retention. Cardiac examination may reveal a prominent systolic impulse medial to the apex in the third to the fifth intercostal space, reflecting left ventricular dyskinesis. A systolic thrill along the left sternal border is consistent with ventricular septal rupture or severe mitral regurgitation. Heart sounds are decreased in intensity because of reduced cardiac contractility. Abnormal heart sounds, including S3, S4, and systolic murmurs caused by mitral regurgitation or septal rupture, are often present. As noted in Chapter 54, however, acute severe mitral regurgitation may manifest without an audible systolic murmur in up to 50% of patients, so the absence of a murmur should not be used to rule out this complication.

Laboratory values and electrocardiogram

In the majority of patients with cardiogenic shock after MI, the infarct location is anterior or anterolateral.[2,23,27] New Q waves are often present; however, as many as one third of patients may have non–Q-wave infarction without electrocardiographic (ECG) evidence.[2,28,29] Laboratory tests will generally show elevation of cardiac enzymes, lactic acidosis, hypoxemia, low mixed venous oxygen saturation, high arteriovenous oxygen difference, and low urinary sodium concentration.

Hemodynamic monitoring

For improvement in long-term outcome, institution of hemodynamic monitoring is not nearly as important as rapid revascularization. Nevertheless, insertion of a Swan-Ganz catheter is often useful for optimizing therapy in patients with cardiogenic shock, confirming the presence of mechanical complications such as ventricular septal rupture (by a step-up in oxygen saturation in the right ventricle) and acute mitral regurgitation (by v waves in the pulmonary capillary wedge tracing),[30] and for providing prognostic information.[31,32] Hemodynamic monitoring in cardiogenic shock generally will show a low cardiac index (< 2.2 L/min/m^2), arterial hypotension, elevated left ventricular filling pressure (mean pulmonary capillary wedge pres-

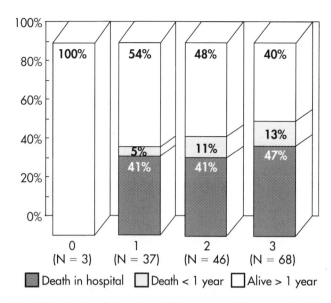

Fig. 46-3. In-hospital and postdischarge mortality rates for 154 patients with cardiogenic shock after acute myocardial infarction, categorized by the number (0-3) of significantly diseased vessels detected by cardiac catheterization. (From Bengtson JR, Kaplan AJ, Pieper KS, et al: *J Am Coll Cardiol* 20:1485, 1992. Used by permission.)

sure > 18 mm Hg), and elevated systemic vascular resistance (>30 Wood units).[32] The low output is usually associated with a low stroke volume index (<20 ml/m^2) and low stroke work index.

Echocardiography

Transthoracic echocardiography is often useful in determining the cause of cardiogenic shock. It can show the extent of myocardial damage, the contribution of right ventricular dysfunction, and mechanical complications (including valvular regurgitation, septal and free wall rupture, and compromise by pericardial fluid). Transesophageal echocardiography (TEE) can also be safely performed in patients with cardiogenic shock. In the only series published to date, none of 44 patients with cardiogenic shock who underwent TEE had clinically significant complications, and 13 (30%) underwent urgent cardiac surgery based on the results of the test.[33]

Cardiac catheterization and angiography

The feasibility of angiography after stabilization with intraaortic balloon counterpulsation and pharmacologic therapy was first demonstrated by Leinbach et al.[34] in 1972. Left ventriculography will generally show the ejection fraction to be decreased to less than 40%. In most patients with recent MI, the infarct-related coronary artery is the left anterior descending artery, the artery is occluded, and significant stenoses are present in all three major coronary arteries (Figs. 46-3 and 46-4).[2,12,24]

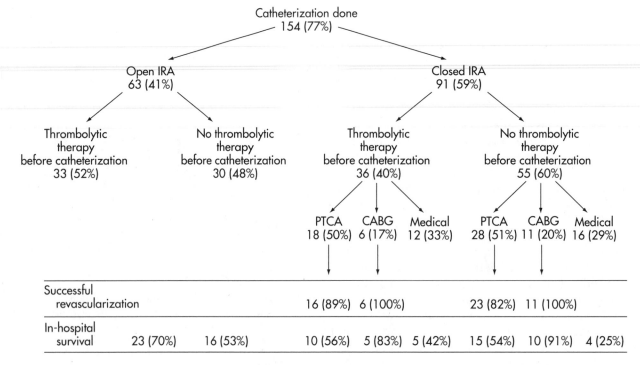

Fig. 46-4. Interventions in 200 patients with cardiogenic shock after acute myocardial infarction. Percentages add to 100% across rows except for bottom two rows, in which percentages are based on therapy received. *Cath,* Cardiac catheterization; *IRA,* infarct-related artery; *PTCA,* percutaneous transluminal coronary angioplasty; *CABG,* coronary artery bypass graft surgery. (From Bengtson JR, Kaplan AJ, Pieper KS, et al: *J Am Coll Cardiol* 20:1485, 1992. Used by permission.)

MANAGEMENT

The primary goal in treating cardiogenic shock from any cause is to maximize coronary blood flow, reduce myocardial work, and restore systemic blood flow. Because cardiogenic shock is often caused by progressive myocardial damage, rapid assessment and early institution of definitive therapy are essential. General resuscitative and supportive measures should be initiated immediately, including establishing and confirming adequate oxygenation and ventilation, correction of electrolyte and acid-base abnormalities, pain relief, and restoration of sinus rhythm.

Pharmacologic therapy

Although general guidelines for pharmacologic management of these critically ill patients can be offered, they should not be used dogmatically. If the patient does not respond adequately to therapy in an appropriate time frame or paradoxically seems to get worse, it is critical to reevaluate the strategies being used and to consider whether a change in strategy should be attempted.

Vasopressor and inotropic agents, including the sympathomimetic amines (dobutamine, dopamine, norepinephrine, isoproterenol) and phosphodiesterase in-

hibitors (amrinone, milrinone), are useful to help improve cardiac output, reduce left ventricular filling pressures, and maintain systemic pressures. However, these beneficial effects are generally achieved at the expense of increased myocardial oxygen consumption. Because we cannot directly measure myocardial oxygen demand, it is often difficult to recognize when increasing drug dosage may be counterproductive (i.e., because it results in more ischemia than increased cardiac output). *Dobutamine* is primarily a β_1-agonist, increasing myocardial contractility. It raises cardiac output and lowers left ventricular filling pressures while augmenting diastolic coronary blood flow and collateral blood flow to ischemic areas.[35,36] Relative to other sympathomimetic drugs, dobutamine is less arrhythmogenic. Dosing should be titrated to achieve a cardiac index above 2.2 L/min while observing for an improvement in peripheral perfusion. *Dopamine's* cardiovascular effects are dependent on dose. In usual therapeutic doses (2-15 μg/kg/min), it increases cardiac output and blood pressure. Urine output may increase as a result of enhanced renal perfusion, even at low infusion rates. Systemic hemodynamics may improve at the expense of increased myocardial oxygen consumption. Combined infusions of dobutamine and dopamine may have more benefit than infusions of either agent alone.[37] *Norepinephrine* is generally used as a last resort when systemic blood pressure remains too low for cerebral and coronary perfusion. *Isoproterenol* has both positive inotropic and chronotropic effects. However, it increases myocardial oxygen requirements, reduces coronary perfusion pressure, and frequently induces arrhythmias. In a study by Mueller et al.,[38] isoproterenol adversely affected myocardial cell metabolism despite an improvement in coronary arterial perfusion. Use of this drug in cardiogenic shock should be restricted to significant bradyarrhythmias, as a "bridge" to temporary transvenous pacemaker insertion. *Amrinone* and *milrinone,* phosphodiesterase inhibitors, increase myocardial contractility by increasing intracellular cyclic adenosine monophosphate (cAMP). In severe congestive heart failure, they increase cardiac output and stroke volume while reducing pulmonary capillary wedge pressure.

Digoxin is a weak inotropic agent that has not been shown to be of benefit in the setting of cardiogenic shock. Because this drug results in increased myocardial oxygen consumption, it may, in fact, be deleterious. Unless atrial arrhythmias develop, we do not use digoxin for acute phase management of cardiogenic shock.

Peripheral vasodilators reduce myocardial oxygen demands by decreasing both preload and afterload. Capillary flow is also improved and capillary hydrostatic pressure reduced. The potential risk is exacerbation of myocardial ischemia by either reduction in diastolic coronary perfusion pressure or "coronary steal," resulting in redistribution of collateral flow away from the ischemic region. *Nitroprusside* acts on both arterial and venous circulations. It improves hemodynamics in cases of shock where systemic vascular resistance and filling pressures are elevated but severe hypotension is not present. It is also temporarily useful in the setting of severe mitral regurgitation, where decreasing peripheral vascular resistance reduces regurgitation and enhances cardiac output. As with the inotropic agents, long-term prognosis is not favorably altered.

Diuretics should be used in the setting of elevated left ventricular pressures to relieve pulmonary edema and reduce heart size, thereby lowering wall tension and oxygen requirements. Intravenous (IV) *furosemide* or *bumetanide* should be administered to achieve a pulmonary capillary wedge pressure of 15 to 18 mm Hg.

Despite the beneficial hemodynamic effects of pharmacologic therapy in cardiogenic shock, it should be emphasized that these effects are only temporary. In fact, several studies have found pharmacologic therapy to have no effect on the high mortality of patients with cardiogenic shock who do not receive revascularization.[2,39-41]

Mechanical circulatory assistance

In addition to pharmacologic agents, mechanical circulatory assistance can be used to help stabilize patients with cardiogenic shock, especially in those for whom revascularization and repair of mechanical complications (mitral regurgitation, ventricular rupture) can be attempted within 2 to 4 days after balloon insertion. Of the several types of assist devices now available, intraaortic balloon counterpulsation (IABP), developed in 1962[42] and first used in cardiogenic shock in 1968,[43] has been most widely used. Counterpulsation simultaneously reduces afterload, resulting in decreased left ventricular work and myocardial oxygen demand, and increases diastolic aortic pressure, leading to improved coronary artery perfusion and subendocardial blood flow. The combined effect of decreased afterload and increased coronary blood flow is to reduce myocardial ischemia, left ventricular end diastolic pressure, mitral regurgitation, and left-to-right shunting across a ventricular septal rupture and to improve forward stroke volume and cardiac output. In contrast to therapy with sympathomimetic drugs, counterpulsation achieves improvements in coronary blood flow and cardiac output without increasing myocardial oxygen demand.

Although use of IABP generally results in temporary clinical and hemodynamic improvement,[28,44-47] counterpulsation without subsequent revascularization does not appear to appreciably affect survival in patients with shock (Table 46-3).* In one early study, 87 patients with cardiogenic shock were enrolled in a protocol of standardized IABP treatment. Despite favorable early hemodynamic responses, in-hospital survival was 17%, and 1-year survival was 9%.[45] DeWood et al.[54] found that in-hospital survival was 48% in patients with cardiogenic shock treated with IABP without subsequent coronary artery bypass grafting vs. 58% in patients who did go on to have surgical revascularization. The 1-year survival among patients discharged from the hospital was 60% vs. 91%, respectively. Patients who underwent surgical revascularization in this study had balloon counterpulsation instituted 3.1 hours earlier (6 vs. 9.1 hours mean) than those treated with IABP alone. The subgroup of patients treated with both IABP and surgical revascularization within 16 hours from the onset of infarction had a 75% 1-year survival rate.

Complications occur in approximately 5% to 36% of patients treated with IABP.[2,45,50,56-59] The most common complications include limb ischemia, femoral artery laceration, aortic dissection, infection, hemolysis, thrombocytopenia, thrombosis, and embolism. Absolute contraindications to use of IABP include aortic insufficiency

---

*References 2, 28, 34, 40, 44-46, 48-56.

Table 46-3. Intraaortic balloon counterpulsation in cardiogenic shock*

Authors	No. of patients	In-hospital survival (%)	Survival without revascularization (%)	Survival with revascularization (%)
Dunkman et al.[44]	40	10 (25)	4/25 (16)	6/15 (40)
Leinbach et al.[34]	11	3 (27)	0/4 (0)	2/7 (29)
Scheidt et al.[45]	87	15 (17)	NA	NA
O'Rourke et al.[48]	25	9 (36)	3/12 (25)	6/13 (46)
Willerson et al.[49]	23	2 (9)	1/19 (5)	1/4 (25)
Bardet et al.[28]	42	13 (31)	3/25 (12)	10/17 (59)
Beckman et al.[50]	40	8 (20)	7/29 (24)	1/11 (9)
Hagemeijer et al.[51]	17	9 (53)	9/17 (53)	NA
Jackson et al.[46]	23	5 (22)	5/21 (24)	0/2 (0)
Johnson et al.[52]	28	13 (46)	8/18 (44)	5/10 (50)
Forssell et al.[40]	15	1 (7)	1/15 (7)	NA
O'Rourke et al.[53]	74	25 (34)	7/18 (39)	18/56 (32)
DeWood et al.[54]	40	21 (53)	10/21 (48)	11/19 (58)
Pierri et al.[55]	47	18 (38)	1/13 (8)	12/34 (35)
Goldberger et al.[56]	20	4 (20)	3/19 (16)	0/1 (0)
Bengtson et al.[2]	99	51 (52)	16/43 (37)	35/56 (63)
TOTAL	631	207 (33)	78/299 (26)	107/245 (44)

*Odds ratio = 2.1 for IABP + revascularization vs. IABP alone. (95% confidence limits = 1.4 − 3.2.)

and aortic aneurysm. Severe peripheral vascular disease is a relative contraindication.

External counterpulsation is a noninvasive form of circulatory assistance, consisting of a water-filled bladder enclosed in a rigid plastic case. Diastolic pressure is augmented and afterload reduced by applying synchronous intermittent positive and negative pressure to the extremities. Although there are no data that conclusively demonstrate that external counterpulsation improves survival in cardiogenic shock, transient hemodynamic improvement comparable with that obtained with IAPB has been documented using this device.[60,61]

Percutaneous cardiopulmonary bypass using the femoral vessels has been used relatively recently to manage patients with cardiogenic shock. Shawl et al.[62] reported on eight patients with cardiogenic shock in whom bypass was initiated after a mean interval of 106 minutes, achieving flow rates of 3.2 to 5.2 L/min. Seven of the patients had successful angioplasty and were alive after a mean follow-up period of 8.2 months.[62] The major limitation to the use of percutaneous bypass is that blood cell destruction occurs progressively. In addition, perfusion is nonpulsatile, so that increases in coronary blood flow may be accompanied by increases in cardiac work.[1] Combined use of IABP and percutaneous bypass might be an optimal approach to improving hemodynamics. Phillips et al.[63] used this approach in 16 patients with shock persisting after IABP. Ten of the patients (63%) were successfully weaned from the combined therapy, and seven were alive 4 months to 5 years after discharge.[63]

Several types of ventricular assist devices using pulsatile flow or centrifugal flow have been described for management of patients with postcardiotomy cardiogenic shock, and uncontrolled series suggest that in-hospital survival may be improved in these patients.[29,64-69] The Hemopump, a transvalvular axial flow assist device inserted via femoral artery cut-down, has also had encouraging early clinical results.[70-72]

Thrombolytic therapy

The ability of thrombolytic therapy to restore arterial patency in a patient with cardiogenic shock after AMI was first demonstrated by Mathey et al.[73] in 1980. However, subsequent studies have shown that the arterial patency rate after such therapy for cardiogenic shock is poor. In the 1985 Society for Cardiac Angiography registry, reperfusion was documented in only 43% of 45 patients with shock treated with intracoronary streptokinase.[74] In a more recent study, patency of the infarct-related artery was documented in 48% of 69 patients with cardiogenic shock treated with thrombolytic therapy.[2] This disappointing patency rate is probably the result of reduced coronary perfusion pressure in cardiogenic shock.

In the Society for Cardiac Angiography registry, mortality was 42% among patients treated successfully with IV streptokinase and 84% in those without reperfusion. However, it is difficult to demonstrate from any of the large, randomized clinical trials that survival of patients with cardiogenic shock is improved by thrombolytic therapy. In the Gruppo Italiano Per Lo Studio Della Streptochinasi Nell'Infarto Miocardico-1 (GISSI-1) study, 280 patients with Killip class IV symptoms were enrolled.[75] The 146 patients treated with streptokinase had a 30-day mortality of 69.9% compared with 70.1% in

Table 46-4. Angioplasty in cardiogenic shock*

Authors	No. of patients	Reperfusion rate (%)	In-hospital survival (%)	Survival with reperfusion (%)	Survival without reperfusion (%)
O'Neill et al.[77]	27	89	20 (73)	19/24 (79)	1/3 (33)
Heuser et al.[78]	10	60	6 (60)	5/6 (83)	1/4 (25)
Shani et al.[79]	9	67	6 (67)	6/6 (100)	0/3 (0)
Disler et al.[80]	7	71	3 (43)	3/5 (60)	0/2 (0)
Landin et al.[81]	34	79	20 (59)	19/27 (70)	1/7 (14)
Laramee et al.[82]	39	85	23 (59)	NA	NA
Lee et al.[83]	24	54	12 (50)	10/13 (77)	2/11 (18)
Ellis et al.[84]	61	69	42 (69)	36/42 (86)	6/19 (32)
Gacioch and Topol[85]	25	72	14 (56)	14/18 (78)	0/7 (0)
Verna et al.[86]	6	100	1 (17)	1/6 (17)	0/0 (0)
Hibbard et al.[87]	45	62	25 (56)	20/28 (71)	5/17 (29)
Eltchaninoff et al.[88]	33	76	21 (64)	19/25 (76)	2/8 (25)
Lee et al.[89]	69	71	38 (55)	34/49 (69)	4/20 (20)
Bengtson et al.[2]	44	84	25 (57)	23/37 (62)	2/7 (29)
TOTAL	389	72	231 (59)	186/249 (75)	22/101 (22)

*Odds ratio = 9.8 for reperfusion vs. no reperfusion. (95% confidence limits = 5.7 − 17.0.)

134 patients treated with placebo. Importantly, the confidence limits for treatment effect in this group substantially overlap the 20% reduction in mortality observed in the total study population. The Second International Study of Infarct Survival (ISIS-2) showed a reduction in mortality in treated patients with a systolic blood pressure less than 100 mm Hg, but not all of these patients may have met criteria for shock.[76] In a recent pooled analysis by the Fibrinolytic Therapy Trialists of patients with a systolic blood pressure < 100 mm Hg, thrombolysis reduced 30-day mortality from 35% to 30% (P < .01). In the GISSI-2/International trial, 175 Killip class IV patients treated with streptokinase had a 30-day mortality of 65% compared with a 78% mortality in 148 patients treated with tissue-type plasminogen activator (t-PA) (P = 0.05). Similarly, in the recently completed GUSTO trial, the 30-day mortality rate with streptokinase (pooled) was 56%, whereas that with accelerated t-PA was 63%.

Overall, these data raise concern that thrombolytic therapy alone is not adequate to improve survival in patients with shock. However, in every other respect, more severely ill patients achieve a greater reduction in mortality with thrombolytic therapy. Therefore, use of small subset analyses to assess the benefit of thrombolytic therapy may be inappropriate, especially because the confidence limits for treatment effect overlap with the expected effect of this therapy in all treated patients. The apparent benefit of streptokinase over t-PA in these patients in two large international trials is intriguing but, as yet, unexplained. At present, we believe that the decision about which thrombolytic agent to use is substantially less important than the decision to move

the patient emergently to the cardiac catheterization laboratory.

Percutaneous transluminal coronary angioplasty

Although there are no randomized studies of percutaneous transluminal coronary angioplasty (PTCA) in cardiogenic shock, results from several uncontrolled studies (Table 46-4) suggest that PTCA can restore infarct artery patency and have beneficial effects on both in-hospital and long-term survival.[2,77-89] Interpretation of these uncontrolled studies requires caution. The selection of patients undergoing angiography is often biased by exclusion of the elderly and those with severe comorbid disease. Furthermore, in calculating survival, none of the published series has reported the number of patients who died after the decision was made to proceed with angiography or angioplasty but before these procedures could be done. Thus, these series may overstate the benefits of direct angioplasty in cardiogenic shock. Nevertheless, outcomes from these series appear substantially better than supportive measures or thrombolytic therapy alone, with reperfusion of the infarct-related artery achieved in approximately 72% of patients (95% confidence interval 68%-77%). In-hospital survival has averaged 75% (95% confidence interval 69%-80%) for patients with successful PTCA vs. 22% (95% confidence interval 14%-30%) in those with unsuccessful procedures. In one retrospective series of 83 patients with AMI complicated by cardiogenic shock, the 30-day survival among 24 patients who were treated with emergency PTCA was 50% vs. 17% in 59 patients treated medically.[83] Patients who had a successful PTCA had an even better 30-day survival rate of 77%. However, only

17% of patients with multivessel disease survived despite successful PTCA.

Coronary artery bypass surgery

The goal of surgery in the setting of postinfarction shock is to improve ventricular function and limit infarct size by restoring blood flow to ischemic but viable periinfarction tissue. The ideal patient should receive early revascularization to a region of large ongoing infarction and contracting noninfarcted segments supplied by stenotic vessels. Surprisingly, functional recovery has been found to be possible as long as 12 to 18 hours after infarction. Before 1980, nine studies reported an average in-hospital survival of 46% and a late survival (<2 years) of 41%. More current studies show marked improvement in early and late survival obtained by early surgical intervention. DeWood et al.[54] first reported the important reduction in mortality in patients receiving therapy with IABP plus surgery vs. those receiving IABP alone. Mortality was 25% if surgical revascularization was achieved within 16 hours. However, it remained close to that observed with IABP alone (71%) if delayed for more than 18 hours. Other investigators have confirmed that early intervention appears to be essential if substantial myocardial salvage is to be achieved. Laks et al.[90] found that in as many as 92% of patients, shock could be reversed through revascularization, allowing discontinuation of inotropes and IABP. The enthusiasm of the role of surgical revascularization in cardiogenic shock remains restrained, however, because of high operative mortality rates, inherent time delays, and the high degree of surgical expertise required.

Patients with surgically remediable mechanical lesions should also be considered for emergency intervention, even in the setting of cardiogenic shock. These include acute mitral regurgitation, especially secondary to papillary muscle rupture, acute ventricular septal rupture, and ventricular free wall rupture and tamponade. Approximately 50% of patients survive their hospital stay when repair of a ventricular septal defect or mitral valve replacement is done with or without coronary artery bypass surgery.[91] In patients with myocardial rupture that is detected early and where no delays occur between detection and arrival in the operating room, survival appears excellent, but the number of reported cases has been small.[92,93]

PROGNOSIS

The in-hospital survival among patients with AMI complicated by cardiogenic shock is poor (Table 46-5). The majority of patients with AMI developing cardiogenic shock die during the acute hospitalization. Using data from the population-based Worcester Heart Attack Study, the overall impact and time trends (1975-1988) of

Table 46-5. In-hospital case-facility rates in patients with acute myocardial infarction complicated by cardiogenic shock

Authors	Study years	No. with shock	Case fatality (%)
Binder et al.[19]	1950-1952	82	83
Malach and Rosenberg[10]	1954	25	100
Killip and Kimball[11]	1965-1967	47	81
Scheidt et al.[12]	1965-1969	73	86
Goldberg et al.[13]	1966-1967	32	81
	1971	58	52
Grande et al.[96]	1978-1979	31	72
Kobayashi et al.[14]	1977-1982	35	60
Goldberg et al.[18]	1975	57	74
	1978	60	77
	1981	75	76
	1984	48	79
	1986	58	79
	1988	60	82

the in-hospital case-fatality rate for cardiogenic shock complicating AMI were recently examined.[18] The adverse impact of cardiogenic shock on short-term survival after AMI was seen during each of the six periods examined in this community-wide study. The in-hospital survival of patients with cardiogenic shock failed to improve over time and actually worsened between 1975 and 1988. In 1975, 74% of patients developing cardiogenic shock during hospitalization for AMI died, whereas 82% of those developing cardiogenic shock in 1988 died during the acute hospitalization.[25,84]

CONCLUSIONS

Cardiogenic shock is the leading cause of death in patients hospitalized following AMI, and several lines of evidence exist to suggest that overall survival rates for these patients have not changed over the past several years. Our current approach to these patients is:

1. Rapid diagnosis of the underlying cause of shock, through careful physical examination, hemodynamic monitoring, emergency echocardiography, and cardiac catheterization. All patients with suspected cardiogenic shock should have an arterial line placed, because noninvasive blood pressure measurement correlates poorly with true blood pressure.[94] A Swan-Ganz catheter and Foley catheter should also be placed. The Swan-Ganz catheter is typically placed during or after cardiac catheterization.

2. Stabilization of the patient, through prompt correction of arrhythmias, abnormalities of electrolyte concentrations, acid-base status, and blood gas

values, and through the use of vasoactive drugs and mechanical circulatory assistance. Vasoactive drugs should be initiated at low doses (dopamine 2 µg/kg/min, dobutamine 2 µg/kg/min, amrinone 0.75 mg/kg bolus, followed by 5 µg/kg/min, Levophed 2 µg/min) and then titrated against the patient's hemodynamic response. The pulmonary capillary wedge pressure should be maintained at 15 to 18 mm Hg.

3. Early revascularization and correction of mechanical defects. Urgent surgical intervention is crucial for patients who survive the initial phase of ventricular free wall rupture. For patients with papillary muscle dysfunction or ventricular septal rupture, hemodynamic stabilization with afterload-reducing drugs, vasopressors, and IABP may be tried initially, proceeding to urgent surgery in patients who remain unstable. Patients with left ventricular power failure should undergo emergency catheterization to identify the perfusion status of the infarct-related artery.

It is our practice to attempt emergency revascularization in all of these patients when the infarct vessel is occluded (Thrombolysis in Myocardial Infarction [TIMI] grades 0-1) or has poor distal flow (TIMI grade 2). Patients with significant left main disease or a target lesion unsuitable for PTCA should be referred for immediate coronary artery bypass surgery. All others are managed initially with PTCA.

It cannot be overemphasized that all three of these steps must proceed simultaneously and with all possible speed. One of the most common management mistakes we see in this area is the adoption of a relatively leisurely pace in diagnosis and therapy, especially in a hypotensive patient who initially "looks good." If such patients do not have obviously reversible courses of hypotension or evidence of a right ventricular infarction and they do not correct with 1 L of normal saline solution infused rapidly, we initiate arrangements for emergency catheterization.

In spite of an aggressive therapeutic approach, many patients with cardiogenic shock will not be found to be candidates for definitive therapy because of extensive left ventricular damage. Therefore, the most promising approach to this syndrome ultimately is prevention of its development after AMI through aggressive reperfusion therapy applied as early as possible after symptom onset.

REFERENCES

1. Dole WP, O'Rourke RA: Pathophysiology and management of cardiogenic shock, *Curr Probl Cardiol* 8:1-72, 1983.
2. Bengtson JR, Kaplan AJ, Pieper KS, et al: Prognosis in cardiogenic shock after acute myocardial infarction in the interventional era, *J Am Coll Cardiol* 20:1482-1489, 1992.
3. Gewirtz H, Gold HK, Fallon JT, et al: Role of right ventricular infarction in cardiogenic shock associated with inferior myocardial infarction, *Br Heart J* 42:719-725, 1979.
4. Radford MJ, Johnson RA, Buckley MJ, et al: Survival following mitral valve replacement for mitral regurgitation due to coronary artery disease, *Circulation* 60(suppl I):39-47, 1979.
5. Wei JY, Hutchins GM, Bulkley BH: Papillary muscle rupture in fatal acute myocardial infarction: a potentially treatable form of cardiogenic shock, *Ann Intern Med* 90:149-152, 1979.
6. Nishimura RA, Schaff HV, Shub C, et al: Papillary muscle rupture complicating acute myocardial infarction: analysis of 17 patients, *Am J Cardiol* 51:373-377, 1983.
7. Friedman HS, Kihn LA, Katz AM: Clinical and electrocardiographic features of cardiac rupture following acute myocardial infarction, *Am J Med* 50:709-720, 1971.
8. Radford MJ, Johnson RA, Daggett WM, et al: Ventricular septal rupture: a review of clinical and physiologic features and an analysis of survival, *Circulation* 64:545-553, 1981.
9. Held AC, Cole PL, Lipton B, et al: Rupture of the interventricular septum complicating acute myocardial infarction: a multicenter analysis of clinical findings and outcome, *Am Heart J* 116:1330-1336, 1988.
10. Malach M, Rosenberg B: Acute myocardial infarction in a city hospital: III. Experience with shock, *Am J Cardiol* 5:487-492, 1960.
11. Killip T, Kimball JT: Treatment of myocardial infarction in a coronary care unit: a two year experience with 250 patients, *Am J Cardiol* 20:457-464, 1967.
12. Scheidt S, Ascheim R, Killip T: Shock after acute myocardial infarction: a clinical and hemodynamic profile, *Am J Cardiol* 26:556-564, 1970.
13. Goldberg R, Szklo M, Tonascia JA, et al: Time trends in prognosis of patients with myocardial infarction: a population-based study, *Johns Hopkins Med J* 144:73-80, 1979.
14. Kobayashi M, Nitani H, Hasegawa M, et al: Effect of medical treatment of acute myocardial infarction in coronary care unit—study on its effect mainly on the cases with complication, *Jpn Circ J* 48:650-658, 1984.
15. Takano T, Endo T, Saito H, et al: Clinical usefulness of intraaortic balloon pumping in acute myocardial infarction complicated with cardiogenic shock, ventricular septal perforation and mitral regurgitation, *Jpn Circ J* 48:678-689, 1984.
16. Gheorghiade M, Anderson J, Rosman H, et al: Risk identification at the time of admission to coronary care unit in patients with suspected myocardial infarction, *Am Heart J* 116:1212-1217, 1988.
17. Jugdutt BI, Warnica JW: Intravenous nitroglycerin therapy in limit myocardial infarct size, expansion and complications: effect of timing, dosage and infarct location, *Circulation* 78:906-919, 1988.
18. Goldberg RJ, Gore JM, Alpert JS, et al: Cardiogenic shock after acute myocardial infarction: incidence and mortality from a community-wide perspective, 1975 to 1988, *N Engl J Med* 325:1117-1122, 1991.
19. Binder MJ, Ryan JA, Marcus S, et al: Evaluation of therapy in shock following acute myocardial infarction, *Am J Med* 18:622-632, 1955.
20. Page DL, Caulfield JB, Kastor JA, et al: Myocardial changes associated with cardiogenic shock, *N Engl J Med* 285:133-137, 1971.
21. Harnarayan C, Bennett MA, Pentecost BL, et al: Quantitative study of infarcted myocardium in cardiogenic shock, *Br Heart J* 32:728-732, 1970.
22. Bolooki H: Emergency cardiac procedures in patients in cardiogenic shock due to complications of coronary artery disease, *Circulation* 79(suppl I):137-148, 1989.
23. Alonso DR, Scheidt S, Post M, et al: Pathophysiology of cardiogenic shock: quantification of myocardial necrosis, clinical, pathologic and electrocardiographic correlations, *Circulation* 48:588-596, 1973.
24. Wackers FJ, Lie KI, Becker AE, et al: Coronary artery disease in

patients dying from cardiogenic shock or congestive heart failure in the setting of acute myocardial infarction, *Br Heart J* 38:906-910, 1976.

25. Schreiber TL, Miller DH, Zola B: Management of myocardial infarction shock: current status, *Am Heart J* 117:435-443, 1989.

26. Gutovitz AL, Sobel BE, Roberts R: Progressive nature of myocardial injury in selected patients with cardiogenic shock, *Am J Cardiol* 41:469-475, 1978.

27. Hands ME, Rutherford JD, Muller JE, et al: The in-hospital development of cardiogenic shock after myocardial infarction: incidence, predictors of occurrence, outcome and prognostic factors, *J Am Coll Cardiol* 14:40-46, 1989.

28. Bardet J, Masquet C, Kahn JC, et al: Clinical and hemodynamic results of intraaortic balloon counterpulsation and surgery for cardiogenic shock, *Am Heart J* 93:280-288, 1977.

29. Joyce LD, Kiser JC, Eales F, et al: Experience with the Sarns centrifugal pump as a ventricular assist device, *ASAIO Trans* 36:M619-M623, 1990.

30. Daily EK: Use of hemodynamics to differentiate pathophysiologic causes of cardiogenic shock, *Crit Care Nurs Clin North Am* 1:589-602, 1989.

31. Ratshin RA, Rackley CE, Russell Jr. RO: Hemodynamic evaluation of left ventricular function in shock complicating myocardial infarction, *Circulation* 45:127-139, 1972.

32. Forrester JS, Diamond G, Chatterjee K, et al: Medical therapy of acute myocardial infarction by application of hemodynamic subsets, *N Engl J Med* 295:1356-1362, 1976.

33. Oh JK, Sinak LJ, Freeman WK, et al: Transesophageal echocardiography in patients with shock syndrome, *Circulation* 78(suppl II):127, 1991.

34. Leinbach RC, Dinsmore RE, Mundth ED, et al: Selective coronary and left ventricular cineangiography during intraaortic balloon pumping for cardiogenic shock, *Circulation* 45:845-852, 1972.

35. Gillespie T, Ambos HD, Sobel BE, et al: Effects of dobutamine in patients with acute myocardial infarction, *Am J Cardiol* 39:588-594, 1977.

36. Goldstein RA, Passamani ER, Roberts R: A comparison of digoxin and dobutamine in patients with acute infarction and cardiac failure, *N Engl J Med* 303:846-850, 1980.

37. Richard C, Ricome JL, Rimailho A, et al: Combined hemodynamic effects of dopamine and dobutamine in cardiogenic shock, *Circulation* 67:620-626, 1983.

38. Mueller H, Ayres SM, Gregory JJ, et al: Hemodynamics, coronary blood flow, and myocardial metabolism in cardiogenic shock: response to 1-norepinephrine and isoproterenol, *J Clin Invest* 49:1885-1902, 1970.

39. Gunnar RM, Loeb HS: Use of drugs in cardiogenic shock due to acute myocardial infarction, *Circulation* 45:1111-1124, 1972.

40. Forssell G, Nordlander R, Nyquist O, et al: Intraaortic balloon pumping in the treatment of cardiogenic shock complicating acute myocardial infarction, *Acta Med Scand* 206:189-192, 1979.

41. Resnekov L: Cardiogenic shock, *Chest* 83:893-898, 1983.

42. Moulopoulos SD, Topaz S, Kolff WJ: Diastolic balloon pumping (with carbon dioxide) in the aorta: a mechanical assistance to the failing circulation, *Am Heart J* 63:669-675, 1962.

43. Kantrowitz A, Tjonneland S, Freed PS, et al: Initial clinical experience with intraaortic balloon pumping in cardiogenic shock, *JAMA* 203:113-118, 1968.

44. Dunkman WB, Leinbach RC, Buckley MJ, et al: Clinical and hemodynamic results in intraaortic balloon pumping and surgery for cardiogenic shock, *Circulation* 46:465-477, 1972.

45. Scheidt S, Wilner G, Mueller H, et al: Intraaortic balloon pump counterpulsation in cardiogenic shock: report of a cooperative clinical trial, *N Engl J Med* 288:979-984, 1973.

46. Jackson G, Cullum P, Pastellopoulos A, et al: Intra-aortic balloon assistance in cardiogenic shock after myocardial infarction or cardiac surgery, *Br Heart J* 39:598-604, 1977.

47. Weiss AT, Engel S, Gotsman CJ, et al: Regional and global left ventricular function during intraaortic balloon counterpulsation in patients with acute myocardial infarction shock, *Am Heart J* 108:249-254, 1984.

48. O'Rourke MF, Chang VP, Windsor HM, et al: Acute severe cardiac failure complicating myocardial infarction: experience with 100 patients referred for consideration of mechanical left ventricular assistance, *Br Heart J* 37:169-181, 1975.

49. Willerson JT, Curry GC, Watson JT, et al: Intraaortic balloon counterpulsation in patients in cardiogenic shock, medically refractory left ventricular failure and/or recurrent ventricular tachycardia, *Am J Med* 58:183-191, 1975.

50. Beckman CB, Geha AS, Hammond GL, et al: Results and complications of intraaortic balloon counterpulsation, *Ann Thorac Surg* 24:550-557, 1977.

51. Hagemeijer F, Laird JD, Haalebos MP, et al: Effectiveness of intraaortic balloon pumping without cardiac surgery for patients with severe heart failure secondary to a recent myocardial infarction, *Am J Cardiol* 40:951-956, 1977.

52. Johnson SA, Scanlon PJ, Loeb HS, et al: Treatment of cardiogenic shock in myocardial infarction by intraaortic balloon counterpulsation and surgery, *Am J Med* 62:687-692, 1977.

53. O'Rourke MF, Sammuel N, Chang VP: Arterial counterpulsation in severe refractory heart failure complicating acute myocardial infarction, *Br Heart J* 41:308-316, 1979.

54. DeWood MA, Notske RN, Hensley GR, et al: Intraaortic balloon counterpulsation with and without reperfusion of myocardial infarction shock, *Circulation* 61:1105-1112, 1980.

55. Pierri MK, Zema M, Kligfield P, et al: Exercise tolerance in late survivors of balloon pumping and surgery for cardiogenic shock, *Circulation* 62(suppl I):138-141, 1980.

56. Goldberger M, Tabak SW, Shah PK: Clinical experience with intraaortic balloon counterpulsation in 112 consecutive patients, *Am Heart J* 111:497-502, 1986.

57. McCabe JC, Abel RM, Subramanian VA, et al: Complications of intra-aortic balloon insertion and counterpulsation, *Circulation* 57:769-773, 1978.

58. McEnany MT, Kay HR, Buckley MJ, et al: Clinical experience with intraaortic balloon pump support in 728 patients, *Circulation* 58(suppl 1):124-132, 1978.

59. Isner JM, Cohen SR, Virmani R, et al: Complications of intraaortic balloon counterpulsation device, clinical and morphological observations in 45 necropsy patients, *Am J Cardiol* 45:260-268, 1980.

60. Beckman CB, Romero LH, Shatney CH, et al: Clinical comparison of the intra-aortic balloon pump and external counterpulsation for cardiogenic shock, *Trans Am Soc Artif Intern Organs* 29:414-418, 1973.

61. Soroff HS, Hui J, Giron F: Current status of external counterpulsation, *Crit Care Clin* 2:277-295, 1986.

62. Shawl FA, Domanski MJ, Hernandez TJ, et al: Emergency percutaneous cardiopulmonary bypass support in cardiogenic shock from acute myocardial infarction, *Am J Cardiol* 64:967-970, 1989.

63. Phillips S, Zeff R, Spector M, et al: Combined benefit of intraaortic balloon pump and percutaneous bypass, *J Am Coll Cardiol* 17:358A, 1991.

64. Pae WE, Pierce WS, Pennock JL, et al: Long-term results of ventricular assist pumping in postcardiotomy cardiogenic shock, *J Thorac Cardiovasc Surg* 93:434-441, 1987.

65. Zumbro GL, Kitchens WR, Shearer G, et al: Mechanical assistance for cardiogenic shock following cardiac surgery, myocardial infarction, and cardiac transplantation, *Ann Thorac Surg* 44:11-13, 1987.

66. Parascandola SA, Pae WE, Davis PK, et al: Determinants of survival in patients with ventricular assist devices, *ASAIO Trans* 34:222-228, 1988.
67. Pennington DG, McBride LR, Swartz MT, et al: Use of the Pierce-Donachy ventricular assist device in patients with cardiogenic shock after cardiac operations, *Ann Thorac Surg* 47:130-135, 1989.
68. Deeb GM, Bolling SF, Nicklas J, et al: Clinical experience with the Nimbus pumb, *ASAIO Trans* 36:M632-M636, 1990.
69. Miller CA, Pae WE, Pierce WS: Combined registry for the clinical use of mechanical ventricular assist devices. Postcardiotomy cardiogenic shock, *ASAIO Trans* 36:43-46, 1990.
70. Frazier OH, Wampler RK, Duncan JM, et al: First human use of the Hemopump, a catheter-mounted ventricular assist device, *Ann Thorac Surg* 49:299-304, 1990.
71. Lincoff AM, Popma JJ, Bates ER, et al: Successful coronary angioplasty in two patients with cardiogenic shock using the Nimbus Hemopump support device, *Am Heart J* 120:970-972, 1990.
72. Phillips SJ, Barker L, Balentine B, et al: Hemopump support for the failing heart, *ASAIO Trans* 36:M629-M632, 1990.
73. Mathey D, Kuck K, Remmecke J, et al: Transluminal recanalization of coronary artery thrombosis: a preliminary report of its application in cardiogenic shock, *Eur Heart J* 1:207-212, 1980.
74. Kennedy JW, Gensini GG, Timmis GC, et al: Acute myocardial infarction treated with intracoronary streptokinase: a report of the Society for Cardiac Angioplasty, *Am J Cardiol* 55:871-877, 1985.
75. Gruppo Italiano Per Lo Studio Della Streptochinasi Nell'Infarto Miocardico (GISSI): Effectiveness of intravenous thrombolytic treatment in acute myocardial infarction, *Lancet* 1:397-401, 1986.
76. ISIS-2 (Second International Study of Infarct Survival) Collaborative Group: Randomized trial of intravenous streptokinase, oral aspirin, both, or neither among 17187 cases of suspected acute myocardial infarction: ISIS-2, *Lancet* 2:349-360, 1988.
77. O'Neill W, Erbel R, Laufer N, et al: Coronary angioplasty therapy of cardiogenic shock complicating acute myocardial infarction, *Circulation* 72(suppl III):III309, 1985.
78. Heuser RR, Maddoux GL, Goss JE, et al: Coronary angioplasty in the treatment of cardiogenic shock: the therapy of choice, *J Am Coll Cardiol* 7:219A, 1986.
79. Shani J, Rivera M, Greengart A, et al: Percutaneous transluminal coronary angioplasty in cardiogenic shock, *J Am Coll Cardiol* 7:149A, 1986.
80. Disler L, Haitas B, Benjamin J, et al: Cardiogenic shock in evolving myocardial infarction: treatment by angioplasty and streptokinase, *Heart Lung* 16:649-652, 1987.
81. Landin RJ, Rothbaum DA, Linnemeier TJ, et al: Hospital mortality of patients undergoing emergency angioplasty for acute myocardial infarction: relationship of mortality to cardiogenic shock and unsuccessful angioplasty, *Circulation* 78:11-16, 1988.
82. Laramee LA, Rutherford BD, Ligon RW, et al: Coronary angioplasty for cardiogenic shock following myocardial infarction, *Circulation* 78(suppl II):634, 1988.
83. Lee L, Bates ER, Pitt B, et al: Percutaneous transluminal coronary angioplasty improves survival in acute myocardial infarction complicated by cardiogenic shock, *Circulation* 78:1345-1351, 1988.
84. Ellis SG, O'Neill WW, Bates ER, et al: Implications for patient triage and survival and left ventricular functional recovery analyses in 500 patients treated with coronary angioplasty for acute myocardial infarction, *J Am Coll Cardiol* 13:1251-1259, 1989.
85. Gacioch GM, Topol EJ: Frontiers in cardiogenic shock management: integration of angioplasty and new support devices, *Circulation* 80(suppl II):624, 1989.
86. Verna E, Repetto S, Boscarini M, et al: Emergency coronary angioplasty in patients with severe left ventricular dysfunction or cardiogenic shock after acute myocardial infarction, *Eur Heart J* 10:958-966, 1989.
87. Hibbard MD, Holmes DR, Gersh BJ, et al: Coronary angioplasty for acute myocardial infarction complicated by cardiogenic shock, *Circulation* 82(suppl III):511, 1990.
88. Eltchaninoff H, Simpfendorfer C, Whitlow P: Coronary angioplasty improves both early and one year survival in acute myocardial infarction complicated by cardiogenic shock, *J Am Coll Cardiol* 17:167A, 1991.
89. Lee L, Erbel R, Brown TM, et al: Multicenter registry of angioplasty therapy of cardiogenic shock: initial and long-term survival, *J Am Coll Cardiol* 17:599-603, 1991.
90. Laks H, Rosenkranz E, Buckberg GD: Surgical treatment of cardiogenic shock after myocardial infarction, *Circulation* 74(suppl III):11-16, 1986.
91. Subramanian VA, Roberts AJ, Zema MJ, et al: Cardiogenic shock following acute myocardial infarction. Late functional results after emergency cardiac surgery, *NY State J Med* 80:947-952, 1980.
92. Hochreiter C, Goldstein J, Borer JS, et al: Myocardial free-wall rupture after acute infarction: survival aided by percutaneous intraaortic balloon counterpulsation, *Circulation* 65:1279-1282, 1982.
93. Pugliese P, Tommassini G, Macri R, et al: Successful repair of postinfarction heart rupture, *J Cardiovasc Surg* 27:332-335, 1986.
94. Cohn JN: Blood pressure measurement in shock. Mechanism of inaccuracy in auscultatory and palpatory methods, *JAMA* 199:972-976, 1967.
95. Takano H, Nakatani T, Noda H, et al: Clinical considerations of a left ventricular assist system for acute myocardial infarction with cardiogenic shock, *ASAIO Trans* 32:467-473, 1986.
96. Grande P, Christiansen C, Hansen BF: Myocardial infarct size and cardiogenic shock, *Eur Heart J* 4:289-294, 1983.

Chapter 47

RECURRENT ISCHEMIA AND REINFARCTION AFTER REPERFUSION

E. Magnus Ohman
Robert A. Harrington
Christopher B. Granger

The use of aggressive reperfusion strategies, including thrombolytic therapy and direct angioplasty in AMI has improved survival, decreased infarct expansion, and reduced morbidity. By restoring coronary perfusion early in AMI, an unstable plaque is exposed, and stabilization of this "culprit" lesion has become the focus of intense investigation to prevent its further reactivation, which can lead to reocclusion. Paradoxically, any therapy that substantially improves patency of the infarct-related artery may incur a higher risk of recurrent ischemic events, such as reocclusion or reinfarction. Thus, newer strategies aimed at improving patency and survival may also cause more ischemic events. In this chapter we will review the incidence, clinical characteristics, and consequences of recurrent ischemia, reocclusion of the infarct-related artery, and reinfarction. The aim is to provide a clinical perspective on prevention and management of this vexing problem.

Recurrent ischemia and reinfarction represent two extremes of a continuum of adverse events after successful thrombolysis. Although these events will be categorized in this chapter as separate entities, it must be borne in mind that for an individual patient, reocclusion of the infarct-related artery may be silent with relatively few clinical signs, modestly noticeable as recurrent ischemia with short-lived alterations in hemodynamics or the ECG, or clinically apparent as a reinfarction with persistent chest pain and ECG changes.[1,2] In addition, other factors such as vasospasm, inadequate collateral blood flow to viable areas of myocardium, or ischemia resulting from multivessel coronary artery disease may cause ischemia that is unrelated to the culprit lesion. Thus, recurrent ischemia represents a heterogeneous clinical picture after thrombolysis that is difficult to categorize given its underlying pathology. On the other hand, reocclusion of the infarct-related artery and reinfarction are outcomes that lack subjectivity, and therefore both represent a firm foundation from which predictions and accurate clinical observations can be made and for which prompt clinical action is warranted.

RECURRENT ISCHEMIA AND REINFARCTION IN THE PRETHROMBOLYTIC ERA

In-hospital recurrent ischemia was common in the era before the widespread use of thrombolytic therapy. Recurrent angina with or without ECG changes occurred in 19% to 37% of patients with MI[3-5] and was more common in patients with non–Q-wave infarction.[5] Reinfarction was also felt to be more commonly associated with non–Q-wave MI.[3,6] The incidence of reinfarction, as determined by serial CK-MB sampling in the MILIS study, was 8.4%, and the majority of reinfarctions occurred 7 to 14 days after the index infarction.[4] The factors that were independent predictors of reinfarction

Table 47-1. Rate of reinfarction

Study	N	Agent	Active	Control	P
0-24 hours					
ISAM[145]	1741	SK	2.3%	1.1%	0.06
GISSI-1[146]	11,806	SK	4.1%	2.1%	<0.05
ISIS-2[95]	16,981	SK	2.8%	2.4%	NS
ASSET[147]	13,318	t-PA	3.9%	4.5%	NS
ECSG[148]	721	t-PA	5.9%	6.2%	NS
AIMS[149]	1004	APSAC	6.1%	4.7%	<0.05
6-24 hours					
LATE[150]	5711	t-PA	2.9%	3.7%	NS
EMERAS[151]	4534	SK	1.8%	2.0%	NS

were recurrent chest pain, female gender, obesity, history of previous MI, ST segment depression on the admission ECG, and a non–Q-wave infarction.[3,4] However, in a larger population study of 2024 patients admitted to four hospitals between 1979 and 1984, there was no evidence of an increased risk of in-hospital reinfarction after non–Q-wave, compared with Q-wave infarction (7% vs. 6%).[5] The consequences of reinfarction in the prethrombolytic era were also serious. Patients enrolled in the MILIS study who suffered a reinfarction had an in-hospital mortality rate of 30%, and 24% developed cardiogenic shock.[4]

With the introduction of thrombolytic therapy it was speculated that the incidence of reinfarction might increase modestly.[7] In an overview by Yusuf et al. of the early randomized trials of thrombolytic therapy, the rate of reinfarction was similar in patients allocated to thrombolytic therapy vs. control (3.9% vs. 6.3%).[8] However, in subsequent large placebo-controlled thrombolytic trials the rate of reinfarction has tended to be higher in patients randomized to active therapy as shown in Table 47-1.

THE OPEN ARTERY HYPOTHESIS

With the introduction of early cardiac catheterization in AMI it became possible to study the changes in patency status of the infarct-related coronary artery during and after thrombolysis.[9,10] Several studies have examined the patency status of the infarct-related artery at hospital discharge in patients receiving reperfusion therapies.[11-17] In general these studies have documented an improved long-term survival in patients with antegrade flow established in the infarct-related artery at hospital discharge as shown in Table 47-2. The lack of sustained coronary artery patency is the main limitation of long-term benefit after reperfusion has been established,[18] and it has been found to be particularly important in patients with reduced left ventricular function.[19] Therefore reocclusion has been a major

therapeutic focus in the search to develop new thrombolytic and adjunctive strategies in AMI.

INCIDENCE AND TIMING OF REOCCLUSION OF THE INFARCT-RELATED ARTERY

Assessing the true incidence of reocclusion has been difficult because different studies have used different methodologies and definitions.[20] The rate of reocclusion has been between 4% and 45%, depending on agent studied, timing of repeat cardiac catheterization, and whether or not patients who had rescue PTCA were included.[21,22] A pooled analysis by Granger et al. of 1183 patients who had patency of the infarct-related artery documented during angiography twice during hospitalization found that the overall reocclusion rate was 10.8%.[20] The rate of reocclusion was higher in patients receiving t-PA (14%) compared with patients receiving non–fibrin-specific agents such as streptokinase, AP-SAC, or urokinase (8%, $P = 0.002$). The largest systematic evaluation of reperfusion and reocclusion rates was the angiographic substudy of the GUSTO trial.[23] In this study reocclusion was defined as TIMI grade flow 0 or 1 at follow-up angiography performed 5 to 7 days after the 90-minute acute cardiac catheterization. Only patients who did *not* have angioplasty during the follow-up period were included in the analysis, which artificially lowers the reocclusion rates compared with other studies. The reocclusion rate in the 586 patients with patent infarct-related artery was similar among the four treatment strategies. The reocclusion rate was 6.4% and 5.5% in patients receiving streptokinase with subcutaneous or intravenous heparin respectively, 5.9% with accelerated t-PA, and 4.9% in patients receiving a combination of t-PA and streptokinase. The rate of reocclusion in the GUSTO angiographic substudy is lower compared with other series, which may be because patients who had PTCA acutely were excluded from the analysis. In an overview of 1064 patients enrolled in five studies with acute and follow-up angiography performed by the

Table 47-2. Long-term mortality rates according to patency status of infarct-related arteries

Study	N	Intervention	Follow-up (mo)	Mortality by reperfusion status, n/n (%)		P value
				Open	Closed	
Kennedy et al.[11]	134	IC SK	12	5/93 (5)	6/41 (15)	0.008
Dalen et al.[152]	289	IV SK or IV t-PA	12	13/161 (8)	19/128 (15)	0.07
Mathey et al.[12]	227	IV SK or IV UK or PTCA	48	27/171 (16)	21/56 (37)	0.005
Simoons et al.[13]	234	IC SK or IV SK or PTCA	36	18/198 (9)	12/36 (33)	NA
Kander et al.[14]	293	IV SK or IV t-PA	21*	14/244 (5.8)	3/49 (6.1)	NA
Taylor et al.[16]	180	PTCA + IC SK or IV SK	74	8/137 (6)	8/43 (19)	0.024
Brodie et al.[15]	348	PTCA	40	15/317 (4.7)	2/31 (6.5)	0.67
Moliterno et al.[17]	200	PTCA or CABG	42	1/52 (2)	24/148 (16)	0.008
Total	1917			7.4% (6%-9%)†	17.9% (15%-21%)†	

*Mean.
†95% CI.
CABG, coronary artery bypass graft; IC, intracoronary; IV, intravenous; NA, not available; PTCA, percutaneous transluminal coronary angioplasty; SK, streptokinase; t-PA, tissue-type plasminogen activator; UK, urokinase.

TAMI study group, the overall rate of reocclusion was 8.4% in patients receiving thrombolytic therapy (t-PA, urokinase, or the combination of t-PA and urokinase) alone, compared with 14.8% in patients with angioplasty performed in combination with thrombolytic therapy.[24] It has been consistently documented that patients receiving accelerated t-PA and/or weight-adjusted doses of t-PA have had lower rates of reocclusion compared, with standard t-PA dosing over 3 hours.[24-26]

The timing of reocclusion of the infarct-related artery is difficult to ascertain. It is now well established that in the early phase of MI, coronary flow may be intermittent,[9] which makes the timing of angiography an important issue. The TAMI study group showed that symptoms that lead to early angiography occurred in approximately 58% of patients with reocclusions and occurred within 48 hours of the index infarction in over 80% of symptomatic reocclusions[1], as shown in Figure 47-1.

Reocclusion rates after hospital discharge in patients treated with thrombolytic therapy but without angioplasty has been shown to be approximately 30%.[27,28] The majority of late reocclusions appear to be "silent,"[27,28] but in some series patients have had some symptoms suggestive of a recurrent ischemic event.[29]

PATHOPHYSIOLOGY OF REOCCLUSION

Reocclusion after thrombolysis is a complex event that reflects a combination of mechanical factors related to the underlying lesion, along with the hematologic mileau of the clotting cascade and platelet activation.

Angiographic studies can help clarify the impact of lesion severity or morphology on the rate of reocclusion. However, the events leading to generation of fibrin or activation of platelets are more complex and difficult to examine because of the transient nature of these markers. For that reason the majority of studies of the hematologic aspects of reocclusion are based on animal experimentation or indirect observations in humans.

THE COAGULATION CASCADE AND REOCCLUSION

Administration of thrombolytic therapy with subsequent reperfusion is associated with a transient procoagulant state, which occurs despite fibrinolysis and intense concomitant anticoagulation. This phenomenon has been described after treatment with both t-PA and streptokinase.[30-32] Animal models of reperfusion have suggested that reocclusion following thrombolysis is partially mediated by an effect of persistent or recurrent thrombin activation and platelet activation.[33-38]

The conversion of fibrinogen to fibrin, the common pathway leading to clot formation, is stimulated by the presence of thrombin. During this conversion fibrinopeptide (FPA) is enzymatically cleaved from fibrinogen and can be measured in serum as shown in Figure 47-2. Thus, FPA has been used as an sensitive indirect marker of thrombin activity. A paradoxical increase in FPA levels after administration of streptokinase or t-PA has been documented by several investigators.[30-32] Eisenberg et al. have suggested that thrombin generation is occurring through the activation of prothrombin via

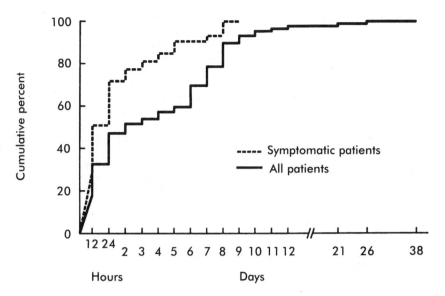

Fig. 47-1. Graph of time to angiographically documented reocclusion of infarct-related artery for patients with symptoms of reocclusion (broken line) and all patients (solid line). Cumulative percentage of patients with reocclusion is displayed on vertical axis and time to reocclusion is displayed on horizontal axis. Median time to symptomatic reocclusion ($N = 53$) was 0.91 days; in total cohort ($N = 91$), it was 2.2 days. (From Ohman EM, Califf RM, Topol EJ, et al: Consequences of reocclusion after successful reperfusion therapy in acute myocardial infarction. TAMI study group, *Circulation* 82:781-791, 1990. Used by permission.)

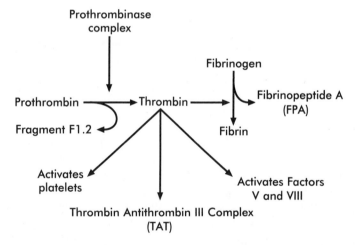

Fig. 47-2. Schematic representation of the link between the coagulation cascade and platelet activation. Thrombin is the central enzyme in the regulation of hemostasis. It is a potent activator of platelets and is responsible for the conversion of fibrinogen to fibrin. During this conversion, a small peptide is released *(FPA)* that may serve as a marker of thrombin activity. The thrombin-antithrombin III complex *(TAT)* is a marker of circulating thrombin while Fragment *(F)* 1.2 is a marker of thrombin generation.

activation of Factor V by plasmin with subsequent acceleration of generation of Factor Xa's action on prothrombin.[39] Once thrombin is absorbed into the fibrin clot during the conversion of fibrinogen to fibrin, a small amount of fibrin-bound thrombin remains enzymatically active.[40] The fibrin-bound thrombin only

slowly equilibrates within the circulation, and plasmin releases the active thrombin back into the circulation. Thus, the enzymatically active thrombin released by fibrinolysis (such as t-PA) may cause further platelet activation and thrombosis. In addition to the "new" thrombin being generated from clot dissolution, reexposure of collagen surfaces in the coronary plaque can cause further platelet activation and thrombin formation. It has not been possible to clarify which mechanism is the predominant force leading to reocclusion, but studies in man have observed that elevated levels of FPA have consistently been associated with reocclusion of the infarct-related artery,[41-43] although the findings have not been consistent.[44] It has been observed that FPA levels can be suppressed by the concomitant administration of intravenous heparin,[41] but its relationship to reocclusion remains controversial.[44]

Excess thrombin binds with anti-thrombin III in the circulation to form a thrombin-antithrombin III (TAT) complex, as shown in Figure 47-2. The TAT complex is no longer enzymatically active and can be measured in serum. In a study of 55 patients treated with t-PA or pro-urokinase, TAT levels were consistently elevated in patients who developed early reocclusion.[45] These data in aggregate suggest that thrombin generation plays a pivotal role in early reocclusion. Newer antithrombins have been developed to more fully suppress thrombin generation after thrombolysis as compared with intravenous heparin; these will be described later.

THE ROLE OF PLATELET ACTIVATION AND REOCCLUSION

The thrombus examined after the occurrence of reocclusion is typically rich in platelets (>90%) and resistant to further thrombolytic therapy.[46] The effect of thrombolytic agents on platelet function is complex, but both streptokinase and t-PA can activate platelets both in vitro and in vivo.[47,48] Studies have found increased excretion of thromboxane A2 metabolites, an indirect measure of platelet aggregability and activation, in patients receiving thrombolytic therapy.[47] Stimulation of platelets leading to aggregation and thrombus formation is a complex process involving several pathways. The platelet-activating substances include circulating catecholamines, local release of adenosine diphosphate (ADP) from activated platelets, circulating and fibrin-bound thrombin, and collagen in the coronary plaque, as shown in Figure 47-3. The activated platelets in turn supply further ADP and thrombin, causing a further escalation in thrombus formation.[49] In addition, platelets release Factor XIII, which helps to stabilize the clot further by cross-linking with fibrin.[50] Although the predominant force leading to platelet activation during thrombolysis has not been elucidated, therapies that have targeted any one or many pathways leading to platelet activation have been found to be able to reduce the rate of reocclusion or reinfarction. Aspirin, heparin, and beta blockers have all been found to reduce the rate of reocclusion or reinfarction.[22,51,52] In addition, potent inhibitors of the glycoprotein IIb/IIIa receptor, the final pathway for platelet activation, have been found to

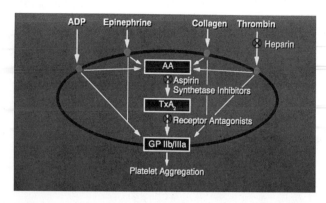

Fig. 47-3. Schematic representation of platelet activation and agents preventing platelet aggregation. Platelets are activated through multiple pathways either indirectly through the Arachadonic Acid (AA) pathway including Thromboxane A_2 (TxA$_2$) generation to the final pathway of the Glycoprotein (GP) IIb/IIIa receptor or directly to the GP IIb/IIIa receptor that allows platelets to aggregate. The effect of circulating thrombin on the platelet can be indirectly blocked (⊗) by heparin. The conversion of AA to TxA$_2$ can be blocked by aspirin or other TxA$_2$ synthetase inhibitors. In addition, specific TxA$_2$ receptor antagonists can prevent the direct action of Thromboxane on the GP IIb/IIIa receptor.

reduce the rate of abrupt closure after angioplasty[53] and perhaps to reduce ischemic events after thrombolysis.[54]

ANGIOGRAPHIC CHARACTERISTICS AND REOCCLUSION

Although the exact interplay between thrombin generation and platelet activation remains to be more fully explored, the direct pharmacologic attack on several pathways of the complex system has improved our understanding of the pathophysiology of reocclusion. In addition to the coagulation system, a mechanical factor that may play a role in the risk of reocclusion is the residual lesion. Early animal experimentation suggested that shear forces may directly stimulate platelets.[55] Elegant studies by Badimon et al. have shown that platelet deposition is proportional to the severity of the lesion in an in vitro model of flow in an injured vessel wall.[56] The lesions with the most severe stenosis and flow limitation had the most platelet deposition. However, the association between the rate of reocclusion after thrombolysis and the degree of residual stenosis in humans has been variable. Early angiographic studies with intracoronary streptokinase suggested that patients with more severe stenosis had a higher likelihood of reocclusion during follow-up.[57-61] Subsequent larger studies with a variety of intravenous thrombolytic therapies have failed to detect a relationship between residual lesion stenosis and reocclusion rates in the first week after infarction.[1,62,63] Importantly, late reocclusion of the infarct-related artery has been closely associated with lesion stenosis severity after thrombolysis during a

3-month follow-up period.[64] In this study the rate of reocclusion was 35% in patients with a residual stenosis ≥ 90%, as compared with 5% in patients with a stenosis < 90%. These data are especially noteworthy because no patients had angioplasty during the 3-month period after MI.

Selected studies have also explored the relationship between the residual lesion morphology and the risk of reocclusion. Ambrose et al. documented that ischemic events were more likely to occur in patients with unstable angina who had ulcerated lesion morphology.[65] After thrombolysis for AMI, patients with an ulcerated lesion or those with retained thrombus have also been shown by several small series to be more prone to reocclude.[57,66,67] However, these observations have not been confirmed in a larger series of patients receiving intravenous t-PA[62] or in the GUSTO trial.[63]

The most important angiographic variable predicting reocclusion is the degree of coronary perfusion. Several studies have noted a high rate of reocclusion in patients who have reduced TIMI grade flow (0-2) at acute cardiac catheterization,[1,68] although this may be partly explained by the fact that rescue angioplasty was performed on patients with TIMI grade flow 0 to 1.[69] Several series have noted a high rate of reocclusion in patients undergoing angioplasty in conjunction with thrombolytic therapy,[70] suggesting that the mechanical disruption of the plaque in the presence of thrombolytic therapy may further enhance a prothrombotic state or cause micro-embolization leading to flow impairment with subsequent reocclusion.[71] In addition, several investigations have shown that normal coronary perfusion (TIMI grade 3 flow) is optimal for enhanced myocardial salvage,[72,73] improved left ventricular function,[72,74,75] and improved morbidity and survival.[75-77] The reocclusion rate in patients with normal coronary flow has been low in the majority of studies with high rates of angiographic follow-up.[1,76]

CONSEQUENCES OF REOCCLUSION

The effect of reocclusion on myocardial function after reperfusion have been studied carefully both in animal models and in humans. In a canine model of reperfusion and reocclusion it was observed that animals suffering reocclusion had significant worsening of ischemic damage and dysfunction.[78] These findings were confirmed by the TAMI study group in patients treated with thrombolytic therapy.[1] In this study of 810 patients reocclusion occurred in 91 (12.4%) patients during hospitalization. Patients with reocclusion had significantly worse recovery of global and infarct zone function at the follow-up cardiac catheterization, as shown in Figure 47-4. In addition, patients with reocclusion had a significantly more complicated hospital course, with a higher incidence of pulmonary edema (19% vs. 14%), sustained

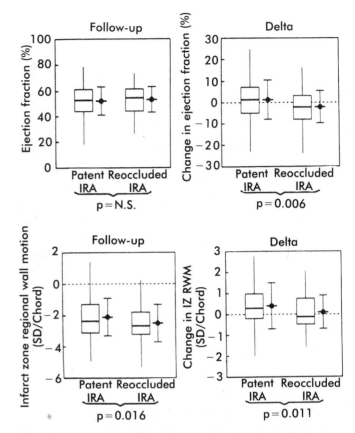

Fig. 47-4. Box (median and interquartile values) and whisker (mean ± 1 SD) plots of global left ventricular function in patients with patent (N = 479) and reoccluded (N = 72) infarct-related arteries at follow-up cardiac catheterization at a median of 7 days (left panel). Δ ejection fraction (acute minus follow-up) is given in right panel. There was a highly significant difference in change in ejection fraction between patients with patent (N = 444) and reoccluded infarct-related arteries (N = 65; P = 0.006). IRA, infarct-related artery; Delta, difference in ejection fraction between acute and follow-up left ventricular arteriography. Box (median and instraquartile values) and whisker (means ± 1 SD) plots of infarct-zone regional wall motion as determined by centerline method in patients with patent (N = 480) and reoccluded (N = 72) infarct-related arteries (left panel). Patients with reocclusion of infarct-related artery had a significantly worse infarct zone regional wall motion (P = 0.016). Δ (acute minus follow-up) infarct zone regional wall motion is shown in right panel. Patients with patent infarct-related artery (N = 443) had a highly significant improvement in infarct zone regional wall function, compared with patients with reocclusions (N = 65; P = 0.011). IRA, infarct-related artery; IZ RWM, infarct zone regional wall motion; SD/Chord, SDs per chord; Delta, difference in infarct zone regional wall motion between acute and follow-up left ventricular arteriography. (From Ohman EM, Califf RM, Topol EJ, et al: Consequences of reocclusion after successful reperfusion therapy in acute myocardial infarction. TAMI study group, *Circulation* 82:781-791, 1990. Used by permission.)

hypotension (25% vs. 17%), and second- or third-degree atrioventricular block (25% vs. 13%), compared with patients with sustained coronary artery patency. Most importantly, patients with reocclusion had a substantially higher in-hospital mortality (11% vs. 5%, $P = 0.01$). These findings suggest that reocclusion of the infarct-related artery is associated with a high morbidity and mortality and that prevention of this complication is important for further improvement in clinical outcomes in patients treated with thrombolytic therapy.

PREDICTION OF REOCCLUSION

The relationship between clinical and angiographic characteristics and the rate of reocclusion was explored using logistic regression analysis of 1331 patients enrolled in the TAMI studies.[24] Only four factors were found to be predictive of reocclusion of the infarct-related artery. The most important predictive variable was TIMI grade flow in the infarct-related artery at the 90-minute angiogram ($P < 0.0001$). Patients with TIMI grade flow between 0 and 1 had a reocclusion rate of 21%; patients with TIMI grade flow of 2 or 3 had reocclusion rates of 15% and 8%, respectively. Other variables predictive of reocclusion were the use of t-PA (14% vs. 8% for urokinase or combination therapy, $P = 0.0004$), occlusion of the right coronary artery (15% vs. 9% LAD and 6% CxA, $P = 0.004$), and slow heart rate on admission (<60 beats/min: 18% vs. >91 beats/min: 5%, $P = 0.0005$). Although these factors are helpful in understanding the incidence of reocclusion, only two of the variables (TIMI grade flow and the thrombolytic strategy) can be modified easily in the clinical setting. Coronary perfusion can be improved by a variety of adjunctive treatment strategies. In addition, lower reocclusion rates can be achieved when t-PA is front loaded.[25,76,79]

CONSEQUENCES OF RECURRENT ISCHEMIA AND REINFARCTION

The importance of recurrent ischemia after thrombolysis was clearly documented by Califf et al. in a review of the TAMI studies.[2] Among their 1221 patients 226 (19%) suffered from a recurrent ischemic event defined as recurrent chest pain associated with ECG changes in the absence of reinfarction. The in-hospital mortality was 11% in patients with recurrent ischemia, compared with 4% in those without any event ($P < 0.0001$). The morbidity in patients with recurrent ischemia was higher, with greater prevalence of congestive cardiac failure (31% vs. 17%). The average cost of the hospitalization was substantially higher in patients with recurrent ischemia ($23,609 vs. $19,712). The effect of recurrent ischemia after thrombolytic therapy on in-hospital morbidity and mortality has also been observed by the GISSI study group[80] and other investigators.[81] In addition,

early postinfarction angina has been found to be a strong predictor of cardiac death within 1 year of AMI.[82] In a study of 231 consecutive patients with a first MI the 1-year mortality rate was 15% in patients with early recurrent ischemia, as compared with 3% in those without ($P < 0.005$).

Observations from the TAMI studies have documented the in-hospital incidence of reinfarction to be low (3%) but with a high in-hospital mortality rate (23%).[2] In addition, patients with reinfarction had a high prevalence of heart failure during hospitalization (48%) and had a long CCU stay (6 days) and hospital stay (14 days). In the GUSTO trial the rate of in-hospital reinfarction was 4%, and the incidence was similar among commonly used thrombolytic therapies (streptokinase 4% and accelerated t-PA 4%).[83] The average time to reinfarction after index infarction was 4 days and this was also similar among the thrombolytic strategies. The 30-day mortality rate in patients with reinfarction ranged from 17% with accelerated t-PA to 20% with streptokinase with intravenous heparin. Reinfarction has also been shown to increase long-term mortality. In the TIMI 2 study reinfarction was found to be an independent predictor of death during a 3-year follow-up period.[84] In a study from Israel the 5-year mortality rate in patients with reinfarction was 40%, compared with 20% in patients without reinfarction.[85]

Recurrent ischemia and reinfarction are two of the most important complications occurring after thrombolysis. These events are at opposite ends of a spectrum of ischemic complications that occur after thrombolysis, and both contribute significantly to the in-hospital mortality of patients with AMI.[86] It is clear from these observations that recurrent ischemic events need to be reduced by prevention of reocclusion after thrombolysis. Ideally, treatment strategies aimed at preventing reocclusion should be applied to the groups of patients who are most likely to develop recurrent ischemia, reocclusion, or reinfarction.

PREDICTION OF RECURRENT ISCHEMIA AND REINFARCTION

Because of the serious nature of recurrent ischemia and reinfarction, much work has concentrated on attempting to predict recurrent ischemia or reinfarction.[87-89] In general it has not been possible to define clearly which patients will develop recurrent ischemia based on careful analyses of clinical and angiographic analysis,[87] although a higher incidence of postinfarction angina was observed in patients with multi-vessel coronary artery disease.[88] The incidence of recurrent ischemia occurring after angioplasty in combination with thrombolytic therapy has been varied, with some studies showing a higher incidence[90,91] and others a lower incidence.[92] This may be because of the different angioplasty strategies used in these studies. However, the incidence of recurrent ischemia has been particularly high in patients who developed a dissection of the infarct-related artery after angioplasty.[89]

It has also been difficult to identify patients who are susceptible to reinfarction after thrombolysis. In a substudy of the GISSI-2 study of 8907 patients, reinfarction occurring within the first 6 hours after index infarction could not be predicted by any clinical characteristics.[93] An evaluation of 456 patients treated with streptokinase or t-PA found only that continued smoking was a risk factor for reinfarction during the first year after thrombolysis.[94] Importantly, the risk of reinfarction could be reduced in smokers who stopped smoking after the index infarction.

PHARMACOLOGIC APPROACHES TO PREVENTION OF RECURRENT ISCHEMIC EVENTS

Aspirin has been used to prevent recurrent ischemic events in several clinical trials. In the ISIS-2 study patients assigned to aspirin had a 1.8% rate of reinfarction, compared with 3.3% of patients allocated to placebo ($P < 0.00001$).[95] In an overview of 32 studies reocclusion occurred in 11% of patients receiving aspirin as compared with 25% ($P < 0.001$) of those not[22]; the rate of recurrent ischemia was also significantly improved with aspirin therapy (25% vs. 41%, $P < 0.001$). Thus, antiplatelet therapy is essential for the early[96] and late[28] reduction of reocclusion, recurrent ischemia, and reinfarction after thrombolysis. Novel antiplatelet agents targeted towards the final pathway of platelet aggregation, the glycoprotein IIb/IIIa receptor, have also been studied in canine models of reperfusion and reocclusion.[97,98] Early clinical investigation of 7E3 (GP IIb/IIa receptor blocker) after t-PA has shown that this agent has the potential to reduce clinical events of recurrent ischemia.[54] Further investigation in this field is under way with other specific antiplatelet therapies.

Because of the large body of evidence that suggests that thrombin plays a pivotal role in mediating reocclusion, intravenous heparin has been advocated as an adjunctive therapy with thrombolysis. However, several large randomized trials have not documented a survival benefit of either subcutaneous heparin over placebo,[93,99] or intravenous over subcutaneous heparin.[23] In addition, intravenous heparin in conjunction with APSAC did not prevent recurrent ischemic events compared with APSAC alone,[100] and hemorrhagic complications were significantly more common in patients randomized to heparin. On the other hand, intravenous heparin has been advocated with t-PA in AMI.[96] The use of intravenous heparin has been advocated with a higher early patency rate,[101] but continuing the therapy failed to affect reocclusion rates.[51] In an overview by Granger et al. the patency rate was significantly higher in patients receiving intravenous heparin, but a clinical benefit could not be demonstrated[102] and these patients had significantly more bleeding complications (24% vs. 18%, $P < 0.01$). The duration of heparin administration after t-PA to reduce recurrent ischemic events has been studied in two randomized trials.[103,104] Although relatively small, both trials documented that intravenous heparin could be stopped after 24 hours of infusion without affecting the incidence of recurrent ischemia, reocclusion, or reinfarction during hospitalization. However, rebound ischemic events can occur after the cessation of intravenous heparin,[105] although some have suggested preventing such rebound with adequate aspirin therapy. Recent observation of hematologic markers of thrombosis have suggested a rebound of thrombin activity after cessation of heparin even in the presence of aspirin therapy. These findings suggest that intravenous heparin is not required with nonspecific thrombolytic therapies (streptokinase or APSAC), but that it is required for at least 24 hours after t-PA administration. The exact duration of intravenous heparin therapy remains controversial. It should be continued at least as long as patients remain clinically unstable. In low-risk patients it may be stopped early to facilitate early discharge.

One of the reasons for the relatively low efficacy of intravenous heparin in reducing ischemic complications after MI may be that clot-bound thrombin is not inactivated by heparin and that it is susceptible to inactivation by antithrombin-III-independent inhibitors.[106,107] As previously shown, numerous animal studies have delineated the clear importance of thrombin in the reocclusion process.[33-38] These studies have typically shown that reocclusion following experimentally induced thrombosis and thrombolysis can be prevented with a variety of direct thrombin inhibitors such as hirudin,[108-110] Hirulog,[111-114] Argatroban,[34,35,37,115,116] and D-phenylalanyl-L-prolyl-L-arginyl chloromethyl ketone (PPACK)[117,118] but not with heparin, as shown in a schematic representation in Figure 47-5. Intravenous recombinant hirudin has recently been studied in conjunction with t-PA and aspirin in a dose-escalation study[119] of 162 patients randomized to hirudin and 84 to heparin. Hirudin-treated patients were more likely to have patent infarct-related arteries (98% vs. 89%, $P = 0.01$) at 18- to 36-hour cardiac catheterization and had less reocclusion of the infarct-related artery (2% vs. 7%, $P = 0.07$). They also had less cardiac mortality and nonfatal reinfarction during hospitalization (7% vs. 17%, $P = 0.02$). The rebound phenomenon has also been observed with the specific antithrombins, suggesting that clinical recurrence may also be observed with these compounds.[120] Several large-scale clinical trials are currently being performed to explore the benefit of

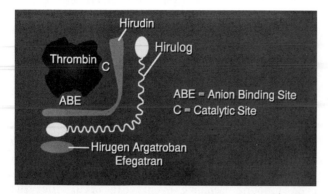

Fig. 47-5. Schematic representation of various direct thrombin inhibitors. First generation thrombin inhibitors (Hirudin and Hirulog) prevent thrombin to activate platelets or stimulate fibrinogen conversion to fibrin by binding to both the anion binding site and catalytic site. Newer agents (Hirugen, Argatroban, and Efegatran) bind directly to the anion binding site.

intravenous hirudin over heparin in the management of acute ischemic syndromes including AMI.

Beta blockers have been used to improve mortality in AMI, as is discussed in Chapter 30. Immediate intravenous beta blockade in conjunction with thrombolytic therapy has been shown to reduce the in-hospital rate of reinfarction (3% vs. 5%, $P = 0.02$) and recurrent angina (19% vs. 24%, $P < 0.02$), compared with deferred therapy.[52] Calcium antagonists, nitrates, ACE inhibitors, and warfarin have not been found to reduce recurrent ischemia or reinfarction in the early phase after thrombolysis.[96]

MECHANICAL APPROACHES TO PREVENT RECURRENT ISCHEMIC EVENTS

Early clinical trials of intracoronary thrombolytic therapy used adjunctive angioplasty to restore patency.[121,122] An early randomized clinical trial compared the efficacy of primary angioplasty (without prior thrombolytic therapy) with intracoronary streptokinase and found similar clinical outcomes in both groups but with an improved left ventricular function in patients assigned to angioplasty.[123] Subsequently, three clinical trials explored the role of adjunctive angioplasty after intravenous thrombolytic therapy.[70,91,92] All three trials documented that immediate coronary angiography coupled with angioplasty did not offer any clinical benefit over a deferred angioplasty strategy.[124] There was a trend towards a higher mortality rate in patients assigned to immediate angioplasty (6.1% vs. 3.2%), but the incidence of reocclusion was similar.[70] However, the three studies documented conflicting results on the incidence of recurrent ischemia and reinfarction, which may be explained partly by the different use of angioplasty strategies in these trials.[70] Recurrent ischemic events have been shown to be most pronounced in

patients who have rescue angioplasty after intravenous thrombolytic therapy has failed to restore patency.[69,81]

Primary angioplasty was initially compared with a strategy of combined intravenous streptokinase and angioplasty in a randomized trial of 122 patients.[125] The addition of streptokinase to angioplasty did not improve clinical outcomes but was associated with significantly higher vascular and bleeding complications. Four subsequent randomized clinical trials have compared intravenous streptokinase or t-PA with primary angioplasty.[126-129] In these trials primary angioplasty has consistently been shown to reduce the rates of recurrent ischemia and reinfarction, compared with thrombolytic therapy. These trials have in general been performed in high-volume centers known for their expertise with this procedure. Recent observations from the state of California have suggested that the outcome of patients undergoing angioplasty in AMI may be affected by the angioplasty volume at each hospital, with a less complicated course seen in hospitals that perform a higher volume of angioplasty.[130] For this reason the clinical expertise with this procedure in AMI needs to be considered. The relationship between operator expertise and clinical outcomes with primary angioplasty compared with front-loaded t-PA is currently being examined in the GUSTO-II study, which is also exploring the relative benefit of hirudin in conjunction with primary angioplasty.

Aortic counterpulsation has been found to reduce ischemia in patients with AMI.[131] More recently the TAMI study group in an observational study of 810 patients found that those treated with IABP had a lower rate of reocclusion.[132] To explore the risk-to-benefit ratio of IABP compared with standard therapy, a randomized trial of 182 patients was performed.[133] Patients assigned to IABP for 48 hours had less reocclusion (8% vs. 21%, $P < 0.03$), less need for emergency angioplasty (2% vs. 11%, $P < 0.02$), less recurrent ischemia (4% vs. 21%, $P < 0.001$), and less reinfarction (3% vs. 8%), compared with control therapy. The use of prophylactic IABP was not associated with a higher rate of hemorrhagic or vascular complications. Similar benefits of IABP therapy have also been observed in nonrandomized series of angioplasty in AMI.[134] The prophylactic use of IABP was also not associated with a longer duration of hospitalization or higher hospital costs. The use of IABP in conjunction with primary angioplasty is currently being examined in the PAMI-2 study.

SUMMARY OF STRATEGIES TO PREVENT RECURRENT ISCHEMIA, REOCCLUSION, AND REINFARCTION

Front-loaded weight-adjusted t-PA or primary angioplasty are the reperfusion strategies that have been associated with the lowest rate of recurrent ischemic events during the hospitalization. Adjunctive therapies found to be essential include aspirin and intravenous heparin. However, with nonspecific thrombolytic therapies (streptokinase or APSAC) there is no indication that heparin provides any clinical advantage. Beta blockers should also be used wherever possible. In patients undergoing angioplasty during AMI aortic counterpulsation has been found to reduce recurrent ischemia and reocclusion.

MONITORING TO DETECT RECURRENT ISCHEMIC EVENTS

Up to 40% of reocclusions that occur after thrombolysis are "silent," having no obvious clinical signs or ECG findings.[1] Careful surveillance in the first 48 hours after reperfusion is therefore particularly important. Reinfarction should be suspected when patients develop recurrent angina or alterations in hemodynamic findings, including congestive cardiac failure, sustained ventricular arrhythmias, or high-degree atrioventricular block. In addition, new ECG changes such as ST elevation or new ST-T wave changes are all indicative of threatened reinfarction. Continuous 12-lead ECG monitoring of ST segments has proven useful for detecting reocclusion during the first 48 hours after reperfusion. Typically patients with spontaneous or therapeutically induced reperfusion exhibit prompt resolution of ST segments on the ECG. On the other hand, patients with persistent occlusion of the infarct-related artery show no or minimal changes of the ST segments. Several studies have suggested that during the dynamic changes of the ST segments that occur during reperfusion further elevation of the ST segment after reperfusion is a sign of reocclusion.[135,136] However, the prognostic significance of reelevation of ST segments has been controversial: in one study it was associated with a favorable outcome,[137] whereas others have found a worse clinical outcome with the same abnormality.[138,139] In our experience, reelevation of the ST segment after thrombolysis is a serious event that should lead one to consider early angiography or other interventions.[140]

TREATMENT OF RECURRENT ISCHEMIA OR REINFARCTION

The goal of the management of patients with recurrent ischemia or threatening reinfarction is first to determine the perfusion status of the infarct-related artery. Management should then be directed towards restoring normal coronary blood flow as soon as possible. In a series of 303 patients, 74 of whom had early recurrent ischemia, the early and successful use of angioplasty to restore patency and normal perfusion was associated with improved survival and improved left ventricular function during follow-up.[81] Although a selection bias occurs when this type of observational

Table 47-3. Repeat thrombolytic therapy for reinfarction

Study	N	Time from index MI to reinfarction	Major bleeding	Patency	Mortality
White[144]	31	5 days	6%	73%	10%
Purvis[142]	30	5 days	10%	71%	17%
Simoons[153]	26	NA	12%	54%	NA
Barbash[154]	52	NA	4%	62%	6%

analysis is performed, the mortality was a striking 32% in patients with recurrent ischemia in whom patency could not be reestablished by angioplasty. These findings suggest that the combination of acute angiography and angioplasty where indicated may be the preferred strategy in patients with recurrent ischemia, reocclusion, or reinfarction.

Repeat administration of thrombolytic therapy is a common response to threatened reinfarction. It has been estimated that approximately 50% of patients with recurrent ischemia do not go on to reinfarction when given repeat thrombolysis.[141] In addition, as many as 83% of patients treated with rescue t-PA during reinfarction are alive 1 year after their hospitalization.[142] In the GUSTO trial thrombolysis was repeated in 46% of all suspected reinfarctions.[143] Repeat thrombolysis was more commonly used outside North America as a "rescue" therapy, whereas in the United States acute cardiac catheterization and angioplasty were most common. Patients treated with repeat thrombolytic therapy had a significantly lower mortality after adjusting for important baseline characteristics (11% vs. 24%, $P < 0.001$) compared with patients in whom this therapy was not used.

Several studies of repeat thrombolysis are shown in Table 47-3. In general, repeat thrombolysis has been found to be effective in improving clinical outcomes, while not significantly affecting the incidence of intracranial hemorrhage. To date, the rate of intracranial hemorrhage has been comparable in patients with suspected reinfarction treated with or without repeat thrombolysis, but the published series have been too small to assess this with confidence. Allergic reactions have occurred in patients who have been treated twice with streptokinase or APSAC during the hospitalization. In a study by White et al. readministration of streptokinase was associated with a 50% rate of allergic reactions, although most were benign.[144] Early and rapid identification of patients with reinfarction using prompt treatments with either t-PA or angioplasty is recommended for this high-risk population.

Recurrent ischemic events represent one of the major limitations of current reperfusion therapies. Although significant improvements have been made in the last decade in understanding the pathophysiology of this continuum of ischemia, it still causes considerable morbidity and mortality. Careful clinical vigilance in combination with repeated evaluations of the 12-lead ECG is the best method for early detection of recurrent ischemia. As the majority of reocclusions occur without symptoms or signs of recurrent ischemia, prevention represents the best strategy to reduce this event. Many new pharmacologic and mechanical therapies show promise in reducing recurrent ischemia, reocclusion, and reinfarction. Despite improvements in the management and prevention of reinfarction and recurrent ischemia these events will continue to require more rapid and effective therapies to restore sustained patency of the infarct-related artery with its associated important prognostic correlates.

REFERENCES

1. Ohman EM, Califf RM, Topol EJ, et al: Consequences of reocclusion after successful reperfusion therapy in acute myocardial infarction. TAMI study group, *Circulation* 82:781-791, 1990.
2. Califf RM, Topol EJ, Ohman EM, et al: Isolated recurrent ischemia after thrombolytic therapy is a frequent, important and expensive adverse clinical outcome (abstract), *J Am Coll Cardiol* 19:301A, 1992.
3. Marmor A, Geltman EM, Schechtman K, et al: Recurrent myocardial infarction: clinical predictors and prognostic implications, *Circ Res* 66:415-421, 1982.
4. Muller JE, Rude RE, Braunwald E, et al and The Mills Study Group: Myocardial infarct extension: occurrence, outcome, and risk factors in the multicenter investigation of limitation of infarct size, *Ann Intern Med* 108:1-6, 1988.
5. Nicod P, Gilpin E, Dittrich H, et al: Short- and long-term clinical outcome after Q wave and non-Q wave myocardial infarction in a large patient population, *Circulation* 79:528-536, 1989.
6. Hollander G, Ozick H, Greengart A, et al: High mortality early reinfarction with first nontransmural myocardial infarction, *Am Heart J* 108:1412, 1984.
7. Schaer DH, Leiboff RH, Katz RJ, et al: Recurrent early ischemic events after thrombolysis for acute myocardial infarction, *Am J Cardiol* 59:788-792, 1987.
8. Yusuf S, Collins R, Peto R, et al: Intravenous and intracoronary fibrinolytic therapy in acute myocardial infarction: overview of results on mortality, reinfarction and side effects from 33 randomized controlled trials, *Eur Heart J* 6:556-585, 1985.
9. Hackett D, Davies G, Chierchia S, et al: Intermittent coronary occlusion in acute myocardial infarction, *N Engl J Med* 317:1055-1059, 1987.
10. Rentrop P, Blanke H, Karsch KR, et al: Selective intracoronary thrombolysis in acute myocardial infarction and unstable angina pectoris, *Circulation* 63:307-317, 1981.
11. Kennedy JW, Ritchie JL, Davis KB, et al: The Western Washington randomized trial of intracoronary streptokinase in acute myocardial infarction, *N Engl J Med* 312:1073-1078, 1985.
12. Mathey DG, Schofer J, Sheehan FH, et al: Improved survival up to four years after early coronary thrombolysis, *Am J Cardiol* 61:524-529, 1988.
13. Simoons ML, Vos J, Tijssen JGP, et al: Long-term benefit of early thrombolytic therapy in patients with acute myocardial infarction: 5-year follow-up of a trial conducted by the Interuniversity Cardiology Institute of the Netherlands, *J Am Coll Cardiol* 14:1609-1615, 1989.
14. Kander NH, O'Neill W, Topol EJ, et al: Long-term follow-up of patients treated with coronary angioplasty for acute myocardial infarction, *Am Heart J* 118:228-233, 1989.
15. Brodie BR, Stuckey TD, Hansen CJ, et al: Importance of a patient infarct-related artery for hospital and late survival after direct coronary angioplasty for acute myocardial infarction, *Am J Cardiol* 69:1113-1119, 1992.
16. Taylor GJ, Moses HW, Katholi RE, et al: Six-year survival after coronary thrombolysis and early revascularization for acute myocardial infarction, *Am J Cardiol* 70:26-30, 1992.
17. Moliterno DJ, Lange RA, Willard JE, et al: Does restoration of antegrade flow in the infarct-related coronary artery days to weeks after myocardial infarction improve long-term survival? *Cor Art Dis* 3:299-304, 1992.
18. Fortin DF, Califf RM: Long-term survival from acute myocardial infarction: salutary effect of an open coronary vessel, *Am J Med* 88:9N-15N, 1990.
19. White HD, Cross DB, Elliott JM, et al: Long-term prognostic importance of patency of the infarct-related coronary artery after thrombolytic therapy for acute myocardial infarction, *Circulation* 89:61-67, 1994.
20. Granger CB, White H, Bates E, et al: Patency profiles and left ventricular function after intravenous thrombolysis: a pooled analysis, *Am J Cardiol* (in press) 1995.
21. Schaer DH, Ross AM, Wasserman AG: Reinfarction, recurrent angina, and reocclusion after thrombolytic therapy, *Circulation* 76(suppl II):II-57-II-62, 1987.
22. Roux S, Christeller S, Ludin E: Effects of aspirin on coronary reocclusion and recurrent ischemia after thrombolysis: a meta-analysis, *J Am Coll Cardiol* 19:671-677, 1992.
23. The GUSTO Investigators: An international randomized comparing of thrombolytic strategies for AMI, *N Engl J Med* 329(10):673-682, 1993.
24. Ohman EM, George BS, Kereiakes DJ, et al for the TAMI Study Group: Event-free hospitalization after early and sustained patency using combination thrombolytic therapy in acute myocardial infarction (abstract), *J Am Coll Cardiol* 17(suppl A):187A, 1991.
25. Wall TC, Califf RM, George BS, et al: Accelerated plasminogen activator dose regimens for coronary thrombolysis, *J Am Coll Cardiol* 19:482-489, 1992.
26. Neuhaus KL, Feuerer W, Jeep-Tebbe S, et al: Improved thrombolysis with a modified dose regimen of recombinant tissue-type plasminogen activator, *J Am Coll Cardiol* 14:1566-1569, 1989.
27. Takens BH, Brugemann J, van der Meer J, et al: Reocclusion three months after successful thrombolytic treatment of acute myocardial infarction with anisoylated plasminogen streptokinase activating complex, *Am J Cardiol* 65:1422-1424, 1990.
28. Meijer A, Verheugt FWA, Werter CJPJ, et al: Aspirin versus coumadin in the prevention of reocclusion and recurrent ischemia after successful thrombolysis: a prospective placebo-controlled angiographic study. Results of the APRICOT study, *Circulation* 87:1524-1530, 1993.
29. Uebis R, Dorr R, Reynen K, et al: Reocclusion following previously successful thrombolysis in acute myocardial infarction, *Klin Worchenschr* 66:115-118, 1988.
30. Eisenberg PR, Sherman L, Rich M, et al: Importance of continued activation of thrombin reflected by fibrinopeptide A to the efficacy of thrombolysis, *J Am Coll Cardiol* 7:1255-1262, 1986.
31. Owen J, Friedman KD, Grossman BA, et al: Thrombolytic therapy with tissue plasminogen activator or streptokinase induces transient thrombin activity, *Blood* 72:616-620, 1988.

32. Rapold HJ: Promotion of thrombin activity by thrombolytic therapy without simultaneous anticoagulation, *Lancet* 1:481-482, 1990.

33. Heras M, Chesebro JH, Webster MW, et al: Hirudin, heparin, and placebo during deep arterial injury in the pig. The in vivo role of thrombin in platelet-mediated thrombosis, *Circ Res* 82:1476-1484, 1990.

34. Fitzgerald DJ, FitzGerald GA: Role of thrombin and thromboxane A2 in reocclusion following coronary thrombolysis with tissue-type plasminogen activator, *Proc Nat Acad Sci USA* 86:7585-7589, 1989.

35. Jang I-K, Gold HK, Ziskind AA, et al: Prevention of platelet-rich arterial thrombosis by selective thrombin inhibition, *Circulation* 81:219-225, 1990.

36. Eidt JF, Allison P, Noble S, et al: Thrombin is an important mediator of platelet aggregation in stenosed canine coronary arteries with endothelial injury, *J Clin Invest* 84:18-27, 1989.

37. Mellott MJ, Connolly TM, York SJ, et al: Prevention of reocclusion by MCI-9038, a thrombin inhibitor, following t-PA-induced thrombolysis in a canine model of femoral arterial thrombosis, *Thromb Haemost* 66:526-534, 1990.

38. Chesebro JH, Fuster V: Dynamic thrombosis and thrombolysis. Role of antithrombins, *Circ Res* 83:1815-1817, 1991.

39. Eisenberg PR, Sobel BE, Jaffe AS: Activation of prothrombin accompanying thrombolysis with recombinant tissue-type plasminogen activator, *J Am Coll Cardiol* 19:1065-1069, 1992.

40. Francis CW, Markham, Jr, Barlow GH, et al: Thrombin activity of fibrin thrombi and soluble plasmic derivatives, *J Lab Clin Med* 102:220-230, 1983.

41. Eisenberg PR, Sherman LA, Jaffe AS: Paradoxic elevation of fibrinopeptide A after streptokinase: evidence for continued thrombosis despite intense fibrinolysis, *J Am Coll Cardiol* 10:527-529, 1987.

42. Rapold HJ, Kuemmerli H, Weiss M, et al: Monitoring of fibrin generation during thrombolytic therapy of acute myocardial infarction with recombinant tissue-type plasminogen activator, *Circ Res* 79:980-989, 1989.

43. Rapold HJ, Grimaudo V, Declerck PJ, et al: Plasma levels of plasminogen activator inhibitor type 1, beta-thromboglobulin, and fibrinopeptide A before, during, and after treatment of acute myocardial infarction with altephase, *Blood* 78:1490-1495, 1991.

44. Ring ME, Butman SM, Bruck DC, et al: Fibrin metabolism in patients with acute myocardial infarction during and after treatment with tissue-type plasminogen activator, *Thromb Haemost* 60:428-433, 1988.

45. Gulba DC, Barthels M, Westhoff-Bleck M, et al: Increased thrombin levels during thrombolytic therapy in acute myocardial infarction: relevance for the success of therapy, *Circulation* 83:937-944, 1991.

46. Jang IK, Gold HK, Ziskind AA, et al: Differential sensitivity of erythrocyte-rich and platelet-rich arterial thrombi to lysis with recombinant tissue-type plasminogen activator. A possible explanation for resistance to coronary thrombolysis, *Circ Res* 79:920-928, 1989.

47. Fitzgerald DJ, Catella F, Roy L, et al: Marked platelet activation in vivo after intravenous streptokinase in patients with acute myocardial infarction, *Circulation* 77:142-150, 1988.

48. Ohlstein EH, Storer B, Fujita T, et al: Tissue-type plasminogen activator and streptokinase induce platelet hyperaggregability in the rabbit, *Thromb Res* 46:575-585, 1987.

49. Coller BS: Platelets and thrombolytic therapy, *N Engl J Med* 322:33-42, 1990.

50. Greenberg JP, Packham MA, Guccione MA, et al: Survival of rabbit platelets treated in vitro with chymotrypsin, plasmin, trypsin or neuroaminidase, *Blood* 53:916-927, 1979.

51. Hsia J, Kleiman N, Aguirre F, et al for the HART investigators: Heparin-induced prolongation of partial thromboplastin time after thrombolysis: relation to coronary artery patency, *J Am Coll Cardiol* 20:31-35, 1992.

52. Roberts R, Rogers WJ, Mueller HS, et al for the TIMI investigators: Immediate versus deferred beta-blockade following thrombolytic therapy in patients with acute myocardial infarction. Results of the thrombolysis in myocardial infarction (TIMI) II-B study, *Circulation* 83:422-437, 1991.

53. The EPIC Investigators: Use of a monoclonal antibody directed against the platelet glycoprotein IIb/IIIa receptor in high-risk coronary angioplasty, *N Eng J Med* 330:956-961, 1994.

54. Kleiman NS, Ohman EM, Califf RM, et al: Profound inhibition of platelet aggregation with monoclonal antibody 7E3 fab after thrombolytic therapy: results of the thrombolysis and angioplasty in myocardial infarction (TAMI) 8 pilot study (abstract), *J Am Coll Cardiol* 22:381-389, 1993.

55. Wall TC, Phillips HR, Stack RS, et al: Results of high dose-intravenous urokinase for acute myocardial infarction, *Am J Cardiol* 65:124-131, 1990.

56. Badimon L, Badimon JJ: Mechanisms of arterial thrombosis in nonparallel streamlines: platelet thrombi grow on the apex of stenotic severely injured vessel wall: experimental study in the pig model, *J Clin Invest* 84:1134-1144, 1989.

57. Gash AK, Spann JF, Sherry S, et al: Factors influencing reocclusion after coronary thrombolysis for acute myocardial infarction, *Am J Cardiol* 57:175-177, 1986.

58. Koren G, Luria MH, Weiss AT, et al: Early treatment of acute myocardial infarction with intravenous streptokinase: a high-risk syndrome, *Arch Intern Med* 147:237-240, 1987.

59. Harrison DG, Ferguson DW, Collins SM, et al: Rethrombosis after repertusion with streptokinase: importance of geometry of residual lesions, *Circulation* 69:991-999, 1984.

60. Serruys PW, Wijns W, van den Brand M, et al: Is transluminal coronary angioplasty mandatory after successful thrombolysis? *Br Heart J* 50:257-265, 1983.

61. Badger RS, Brown BG, Kennedy JW, et al: Usefulness of recanalization to luminal diameter of 0.6 millimeter or more with intracoronary streptokinase during acute myocardial infarction in predicting "normal" perfusion status, continued arterial patency and survival at one year, *Am J Cardiol* 59:519-522, 1987.

62. Ellis SG, Topol EJ, George BS, et al: Recurrent ischemia without warning. Analysis of risk factors for in-hospital ischemic events following successful thrombolysis with intravenous tissue plasmin ogen activator, *Circulation* 80:1159-1165, 1989.

63. Reiner JS, Lundergan CF, van de Brand M, et al and for the GUSTO Angiographic Investigators: Early angiography cannot predict postthrombolytic coronary reocclusion: observations from the GUSTO angiographic study, *J Am Coll Cardiol* (in press).

64. Veen G, Meyer A, Verheugt FWA, et al: Culprit lesion morphology and stenosis severity in the prediction of reocclusion after coronary thrombolysis: angiographic results of the APRICOT study, *J Am Coll Cardiol* 22:1755-1762, 1993.

65. Ambrose JA, Winters SL, Arora RR, et al: Coronary angiographic morphology in myocardial infarction: a link between the pathogenesis of unstable angina and myocardial infarction, *J Am Coll Cardiol* 6:1233-1238, 1985.

66. Coste P, Durrieu C, Chevalier JM, et al: Rethrombosis after emergency angioplasty for acute myocardial infarction: importance of morphology of residual lesions, (abstract), *Eur Heart J* 11:23, 1990.

67. Hsia J, Kleiman NS, Aguirre F, et al: Angiographic predictors of reocclusion following initially successful thrombolysis (abstract), *Circulation* 82(suppl III):255, 1990.

68. Wall TC, Mark DB, Califf RM, et al: Prediction of early recurrent myocardial ischemia and coronary reocclusion after successful

thrombolysis: a qualitative and quantitative angiographic study, *Am J Cardiol* 63:423-428, 1989.

69. Abbottsmith CW, Topol EJ, George BS, et al: Fate of patients with acute myocardial infarction with patency of the infarct-related vessel achieved with successful thrombolysis versus rescue angioplasty, *J Am Coll Cardiol* 16:770-778, 1990.

70. Labinaz M, Ellis SG, Phillips HR, et al: The role of angioplasty after successful thrombolysis for acute myocardial infarction, *Cor Art Dis* 5:399-406, 1994.

71. Saber RS, Edwards WD, Bailey KR, et al: Coronary embolization after balloon angioplasty or thrombolytic therapy: an autopsy study of 32 cases, *J Am Coll Cardiol* 22:1283-1288, 1993.

72. Clemmensen P, Ohman EM, Sevilla DC, et al: Importance of early and complete reperfusion to achieve myocardial salvage after thrombolysis in acute myocardial infarction, *Am J Cardiol* 70:1391-1396, 1992.

73. Karagounis L, Sherman SG, Menlove RL, et al: Does thrombolysis in myocardial infarction (TIMI) perfusion grade 2 represent a mostly patent artery or a mostly occluded artery? Enzymatic and electrocardiographic evidence from the TEAM-2 study, *J Am Coll Cardiol* 19:1-10, 1992.

74. Lincoff AM, Topol EJ, Sigmon KN, et al: Is a coronary artery with TIMI grade 2 flow "patent"? Outcome in the thrombolysis and angioplasty in myocardial infarction trials, *Am J Cardiol* (in press) 1994.

75. Anderson JL, Karagounis LA, Becker LC, et al: TIMI perfusion grade 3 but not grade 2 results in improved outcome after thrombolysis for myocardial infarction: ventriculographic, enzymatic, and electrocardiographic evidence from the TEAM-3 study, *Circ Res* 87:1829-1839, 1993.

76. The GUSTO Angiographic Investigators: The effects of tissue plasminogen activator, streptokinase, or both on coronary artery patency, ventricular function, and survival after myocardial infarction, *N Engl J Med* 329:1615-1622, 1993.

77. Lincoff AM, Topol EJ: Illusion of reperfusion: does anyone achieve optimal reperfusion during acute myocardial infarction? *Circulation* 88:1361-1374, 1993.

78. Lim MJ, Gallagher MA, Ziadeh M, et al: Effect of coronary reocclusion after initial reperfusion on ventricular function and infarct size, *J Am Coll Cardiol* 18:879-885, 1991.

79. Topol EJ: Ultrathrombolysis, *J Am Coll Cardiol* 15:922-924, 1990.

80. Silva P, Galli M, Campolo L, and the IRES (Ischemia Residua) Study Group: Prognostic significance of early ischemia after acute myocardial infarction in low-risk patients, *Am J Cardiol* 71:1142-1147, 1993.

81. Ellis SG, Debowey D, Bates ER, et al: Treatment of recurrent ischemia after thrombolysis and successful reperfusion for acute myocardial infarction: effect on in-hospital mortality and left ventricular function, *J Am Coll Cardiol* 17:752-757, 1991.

82. Galjee MA, Visser FC, DeCock CC, et al: The prognostic value, clinical, and angiographic characteristics of patients with early postinfarction angina after a first myocardial infarction, *Am Heart J* 125:48-55, 1992.

83. Ohman EM, Armstrong PW, Guerci AD, et al and the GUSTO trial investigators: Reinfarction after thrombolytic therapy: experience from the GUSTO trial (abstract), *Circulation* 88(suppl I):I-490, 1993.

84. Mueller HS, Forman SA, Menegus MA, et al and TIMI II investigators: Prognostic significance of nonfatal reinfarction in TIMI II (abstract), *Circulation* 88(suppl I):I-490, 1993.

85. Kornowski R, Goldbourt U, Zion M, et al and the SPRINT study group: Predictors and long-term prognostic significance of recurrent infarction in the year after a first myocardial infarction, *Am J Cardiol* 72:883-888, 1993.

86. Ohman EM, Topol EJ, Califf RM, et al and the Thrombolysis Angioplasty in Myocardial Infarction Study Group: An analysis of the cause of early mortality after administration of thrombolytic therapy, *Cor Art Dis* 4:957-964, 1993.

87. Kahn JK, Rutherford BD, McConahay DR, et al: Outcome following emergency coronary artery bypass grafting for failed elective balloon coronary angioplasty in patients with prior coronary bypass, *Am J Cardiol* 66:285-288, 1990.

88. Bosch X, Theroux P, Waters DD, et al: Early postinfarction ischemia: clinical, angiographic, and prognostic significance, *Circulation* 75:988-995, 1987.

89. Ellis SG, Gallison L, Grines CL, et al: Incidence and predictors of early recurrent ischemia after successful percutaneous transluminal coronary angioplasty for acute myocardial infarction, *Am J Cardiol* 63:263-268, 1989.

90. The TIMI Research Group: Immediate versus delayed catheterization and angioplasty following thrombolytic therapy for acute myocardial infarction, *J Am Med Assoc* 260:2849-2858, 1988.

91. Simoons ML, Arnold AER, Betriu A, et al and the European Cooperative Study Group for Recombinant Tissue-Type Plasminogen Activator (rTPA): Thrombolysis with tissue plasminogen activator in acute myocardial infarction: no additional benefit from immediate percutaneous coronary angioplasty, *Lancet* 1:197-203, 1988.

92. Topol EJ, Califf RM, George BS, et al: A randomized trial of immediate versus delayed elective angioplasty after intravenous tissue plasminogen activator in acute myocardial infarction, *N Engl J Med* 317:581-588, 1987.

93. GISSI-2 Investigators, ANMCO and M. Negri Institute I: Predictors of nonfatal reinfarction in survivors of myocardial infarction after thrombolysis. Results from the GISSI-2 data-base (abstract), *Circulation* (suppl I):I-490, 1993.

94. Rivers JT, White HD, Cross DB, et al: Reinfarction after thrombolytic therapy for acute myocardial infarction followed by conservative management: incidence and effect of smoking, *J Am Coll Cardiol* 16:340-348, 1990.

95. ISIS-2 (Second International Study of Infarct Survival) Collaborative Group: Randomized trial of intravenous streptokinase, oral aspirin, both, or neither among 17,187 cases of suspected acute myocardial infarction, *Lancet* II:349-360, 1988.

96. Popma JJ, Topol EJ: Adjuncts to thrombolysis for myocardial reperfusion, *Ann Intern Med* 115:34-44, 1991.

97. Gold HK, Coller BS, Yasuda T, et al: Rapid and sustained coronary artery recanalization with combined bolus injection of recombinant tissue-type plasminogen activator and monoclonal antiplatelet GPIIb/IIIa antibody in a canine preparation, *Circulation* 3:670-677, 1988.

98. Yasuda T, Gold HK, Leinbach RC, et al: Lysis of plasminogen activator-resistant platelet-rich coronary artery thrombus with combined bolus injection of recombinant tissue-type plasminogen activator and antiplatelet GPIIb/IIIa antibody, *J Am Coll Cardiol* 16:1728-1735, 1990.

99. ISIS-3 (Third International Study of Infarct Survival) Collaborative Group. ISIS-3: A randomized comparison of streptokinase vs tissue plasminogen activator vs antistreplase and of aspirin plus heparin vs aspirin alone among 41,299 cases of suspected acute myocardial infarction, *Lancet* 339:753-770, 1992.

100. O'Connor CM, Meese R, Carney R, et al and the DUCCS group: A randomized trial of intravenous heparin in conjunction with anistreplase (anisoylated plasminogen streptokinase activator comples) in acute myocardial infarction: the Duke University clinical cardiology study (DUCCS) 1, *J Am Coll Cardiol* 23:11-18, 1994.

101. Hsia J, Hamilton WP, Kleiman N, et al: A comparison between heparin and low-dose aspirin as adjunctive therapy with tissue plasminogen activator for acute myocardial infarction Heparin-Aspirin Reperfusion Trial (HART) Investigators, *N Engl J Med* 323:1433-1437, 1990.

102. Granger CB, O'Connor CM, Bleich SD, et al: An overview of the effect of intravenous heparin on clinical endpoints following thrombolytic therapy for acute myocardial infarction (abstract), *Circulation* 86(suppl I):I-259, 1992.

103. Kander NH, Holland KJ, Pitt B, et al: A randomized pilot trial of brief versus prolonged heparin after successful reperfusion in acute myocardial infarction, *Am J Cardiol* 65:139-142, 1990.

104. Thompson PL, Aylward PE, Federman J, et al and the National Heart Foundation of Australia Coronary Thrombolysis Group: A randomized comparison of intravenous heparin with oral aspirin and dipyridamole 24 hours after recombinant tissue-type plasminogen activator for acute myocardial infarction, *Circ Res* 83:1534-1542, 1991.

105. Theroux P, Waters D, Lam J, et al: Reactivation of unstable angina after the discontinuation of heparin, *N Engl J Med* 327:141-145, 1992.

106. Hogg PJ, Jackson CM: Fibrin monomer protects thrombin from inactivation by heparin-antithrombin III: implications for heparin efficacy, *Proc Nat Acad Sci USA* 86:3619-3623, 1989.

107. Weitz JL, Hudoba M, Massel D, et al: Clot-bound thrombin is protected from inhibition by heparin-antithrombin III but is susceptible to inactivation by antithrombin III-independent inhibitors, *J Clin Invest* 86:385-391, 1990.

108. Mirshahi M, Soria J, Soria C, et al: Evaluation of the inhibition by heparin and hirudin of coagulation activation during r-tPA-induced thrombolysis, *Blood* 74:1025-1030, 1989.

109. Bleich SD, Nichols T, Schumacher R, et al: The role of heparin following coronary thrombolysis with tissue plasminogen activator (t-PA) (abstract), *Circulation* 80(suppl II):II-113, 1989.

110. Heras M, Chesebro JH, Penny WJ, et al: Effects of thrombin inhibition on the development of acute platelet-thrombus deposition during angioplasty in pigs. Heparin versus recombinant hirudin, a specific thrombin inhibitor, *Circ Res* 79:657-665, 1989.

111. Yao SK, Ober JC, Ferguson JJ, et al: Combination of inhibition of thrombin and blockade of thromboxane A2 synthetase and receptors enhance thrombolysis and delays reocclusion in canine coronary arteries, *Circ Res* 86:1993-1999, 1992.

112. Maraganore JM, Chao B, Joseph ML, et al: Anticoagulant activity of synthetic hirudin peptides, *J Biol Chem* 264:8692-8698, 1989.

113. Maraganore JM, Bourdon P, Jablonski J, et al: Design and characterization of hirulogs: a novel class of bivalent peptide inhibitors of thrombin, *Biochemistry* 29:7095-7101, 1990.

114. Topol EJ, Scarpace DG, Palabrica TM, et al: Hirulog: a direct thrombin inhibitor peptide, instead of heparin for routine coronary angioplasty: a pilot experience (abstract), *Circulation* 84 (suppl II):II-2354, 1993.

115. Yasuda T, Gold HK, Yaoita H, et al: Comparative effects of aspirin, a synthetic thrombin inhibitor and a monoclonal antiplatelet glycoprotein IIb/IIIa antibody on coronary artery reperfusion, reocclusion and bleeding with recombinant tissue-type plasminogen activator in a canine preparation, *J Am Coll Cardiol* 16:714-722, 1990.

116. Clarke RJ, Mayo G, FitzGerald GA, et al: Combined administration of aspirin and a specific thrombin inhibitor in man, *Circulation* 83:1510-1518, 1991.

117. Hanson SR, Harker LA: Interruption of acute platelet-dependent thrombosis by the synthetic antithrombin D-phenylalanyl-L-prolyl-L-arginyl chloromethyl ketone, *Proc National Academy of Sciences of the USA* 85:3184-3188, 1988.

118. Krupski WC, Bass A, Kelly AB, et al: Heparin-resistant thrombus formation by endovascular stents in baboons, *Circulation* 81:570-577, 1990.

119. Cannon CP, Henry TD, Schweiger MJ, et al and the TIMI 5 Investigators: A pilot trial of recombinant desulfatohirudin compared with heparin in conjunction with tissue-type plasminogen activator and aspirin for acute myocardial infarction: results of the thrombolysis in myocardial infarction (TIMI) 5 trial, *J Am Coll Cardiol* 23:993-1003, 1994.

120. Gold HK, Torres FW, Garabedian HD, et al: Evidence for a rebound coagulation phenomenon after cessation of a 4-hour infusion of a specific thrombin inhibitor in patients with unstable angina pectoris, *J Am Coll Cardiol* 21:1039-1047, 1993.

121. Stack RS, O'Connor CM, Mark DB, et al: Coronary perfusion during acute myocardial infarction with a combined therapy of coronary angioplasty and high-dose intravenous streptokinase, *Circulation* 1:151-161, 1988.

122. Hartzler GO, Rutherford BD, McConahay DR, et al: Percutaneous transluminal coronary angioplasty with and without thrombolytic therapy for treatment of acute myocardial infarction, *Am Heart J* 106:965-973, 1983.

123. O'Neill W, Timmis GC, Bourdillon PD, et al: A prospective randomized clinical trial of intracoronary streptokinase versus coronary angioplasty for acute myocardial infarction, *N Engl J Med* 314:812-818, 1986.

124. Holmes DR, Topol EJ: Reperfusion momentum: lessons from the randomized trials of immediate coronary angioplasty for myocardial infarction, *J Am Coll Cardiol* 14:1572-1578, 1989.

125. O'Neill WM, Weintraub R, Grines CL, et al: A prospective, placebo-controlled, randomized trial of intravenous streptokinase and angioplasty versus lone angioplasty therapy of acute myocardial infarction, *Circulation* 86:1710-1717, 1992.

126. Grines CL, Browne KF, Marco J, et al: A comparison of immediate angioplasty with thrombolytic therapy for acute myocardial infarction. The Primary Angioplasty in Myocardial Infarction Study Group, *N Engl J Med* 328:673-679, 1993.

127. Zijlstra F, De Boer MJ, Hoorntje JCA, et al: A comparison of immediate coronary angioplasty with intravenous streptokinase in acute myocardial infarction, *N Engl J Med* 328:680-684, 1993.

128. Gibbons RJ, Holmes DR, Reeder GS, et al and the Mayo Coronary Care Unit and Catheterization Laboratory Groups: Immediate angioplasty compared with the administration of a thrombolytic agent followed by conservative treatment for myocardial infarction, *N Engl J Med* 328:685-691, 1993.

129. Ribeiro EE, Silva LA, Carneiro R, et al: Randomized trial of direct coronary angioplasty versus intravenous streptokinase in acute myocardial infarction, *J Am Coll Cardiol* 22:376-380, 1993.

130. Ritchie JL, Phillips KA, Luft HS: Coronary angioplasty: statewide experience in California, *Circulation* 88:2735-2743, 1993.

131. Williams DL, Korr KS, Gerwirtz H, et al: The effect of intra-aortic balloon counterpulsation on regional myocardial blood flow and oxygen consumption in the presence of coronary artery stenosis in patients with unstable angina, *Circulation* 66:593-597, 1982.

132. Ohman EM, Califf RM, George BS, et al: The use of intraaortic balloon pumping as an adjunct to reperfusion therapy in acute myocardial infarction. The Thrombolysis and Angioplasty in Myocardial Infarction (TAMI) Study Group, *Am Heart J* 121:895-901, 1991.

133. Ohman EM, George BS, White CJ, et al and the Randomized IABP Study Group: The use of aortic counterpulsation to improve sustained coronary artery patency during acute myocardial infarction: results of a randomized trial, *Circulation* 90:792-799, 1994.

134. Ishihara M, Sato H, Tateishi H, et al: Effects of intraaortic balloon pumping on coronary hemodynamics after coronary angioplasty in patients with acute myocardial infarction, *Am Heart J* 124:1133-1138, 1992.

135. Krucoff MW, Wagner NB, Pope JE, et al: The portable programmable microprocessor-driven real-time 12-lead electrocardiographic monitor: a preliminary report of a new device for

the noninvasive detection of successful reperfusion or silent coronary reocclusion, *Am J Cardiol* 65:143-148, 1990.

136. Kwon K, Freedman B, Wilcox I, et al: The unstable ST segment early after thrombolysis for acute infarction and its usefulness as a marker of recurrent coronary occlusion, *Am J Cardiol* 67:109-115, 1991.

137. Shechter M, Rabinowitz B, Beker B, et al: Additional ST segment elevation during the first hour of thrombolytic therapy: an electrocardiographic sign predicting a favorable clinical outcome, *J Am Coll Cardiol* 20:1460-1464, 1992.

138. Kondo M, Tamura K, Tanio H, et al: Is ST segment re-elevation associated with reperfusion an indicator of marked myocardial damage after thrombolysis? *J Am Coll Cardiol* 21:62-67, 1993.

139. Dissmann R, Linderer T, Goerke M, et al: Sudden increase of the ST segment elevation at time of reperfusion predicts extensive infarcts in patients with intravenous thrombolysis, *Am Heart J* 126:832-839, 1993.

140. Krucoff MW, Croll MA, Pope JE, et al and the TAMI 7 Study Group: Continuous 12-lead ST-segment recovery analysis in the TAMI 7 study. Performance of a noninvasive method for real-time detection of failed myocardial reperfusion, *Circ Res* 88:437-446, 1993.

141. Becker RC: Repeat thrombolysis for early coronary arterial reocclusion, *Cor Art Dis* 3:499-512, 1992.

142. Purvis JA, McNeil AJ, Roberts MJD, et al: First-year follow-up after repeat thrombolytic therapy with recombinant-tissue plasminogen activator for myocardial reinfarction, *Cor Art Dis* 3:713-720, 1992.

143. Barbash GI, Ohman EM, White HD, et al and the GUSTO Investigators: Rescue thrombolysis for suspected reinfarction following thrombolytic therapy: experience from the GUSTO trial, *J Am Coll Cardiol* 29A, 1994.

144. White HD, Cross DB, Williams BF, et al: Safety and efficacy of repeat thrombolytic treatment after acute myocardial infarction, *Br Heart J* 64:177-181, 1990.

145. The ISAM Study Group: A prospective trial of intravenous streptokinase in acute myocardial infarction (ISAM). Mortality, morbidity, and infarct size at 21 days, *N Engl J Med* 314:1465-1471, 1986.

146. Gruppo Italiano per lo Studio della Streptochinasi nell'Infarto Miocardico (GISSI): Effectiveness of intravenous thrombolytic treatment in acute myocardial infarction, *Lancet* I:397-401, 1986.

147. Wilcox RG, Olsson CG, Skene AM, et al and the ASSET Study Group: Trial of tissue plasminogen activator for mortality reduction in acute myocardial infarction, *Lancet* II:525-530, 1988.

148. Van de Werf F, Arnold AER: Intravenous tissue plasminogen activator and size of infarct left ventricular function, and survival in acute myocardial infarction, *Br Med J* 297:1374-1379, 1988.

149. AIMS Trial Study Group: Long-term effects of intravenous anistreplase in acute myocardial infarction: final report of the AIMS study, *Lancet* 335:427-431, 1990.

150. LATE Study Group: Late assessment of thrombolytic efficacy (LATE) study with altephase 6-24 hours after onset of acute myocardial infarction, *Lancet* 342:759-766, 1993.

151. EMERAS (Estudio Multicentrico Estreptoquinasa Republicas de America del Sur) Collaborative Group: Randomised trial of late thrombolysis in patients with suspected acute myocardial infarction, *Lancet* 342:767-772, 1993.

152. Dalen JE, Gore JM, Braunwald E, et al: Six- and twelve-month follow-up of the phase 1 thrombolysis in myocardial infarction (TIMI) trial, *Am J Cardiol* 62:179-185, 1988.

153. Simoons ML, Arnout J, van den Brand M, et al for the European Cooperative Study Group: Retreatment with altephase for early signs of reocclusion after thrombolysis, *Am J Cardiol* 71:524-528, 1993.

154. Barbash GI, Hod H, Roth A, et al: Repeat infusions of recombinant tissue-type plasminogen activator in patients with acute myocardial infarction and early recurrent myocardial ischemia, *J Am Coll Cardiol* 16:779-783, 1990.

Chapter 48

PERICARDITIS AFTER MYOCARDIAL INFARCTION

Thomas C. Wall
Walter L. Floyd

Pericarditis after myocardial infarction (MI) may occur as either an early complication or remote from the acute event. Pericarditis associated with the acute phase of infarction is most accurately termed postmyocardial infarction pericarditis (PMIP). The syndrome of delayed pericarditis, as first described by Dressler[1,2] and others,[3] can be considered reactive inflammation to a variety of myocardial injuries. This clinical entity is best referred to as postcardiac injury syndrome (PCIS). Such a clinical distinction between these two types of pericardial disease is important from a diagnostic, therapeutic, and prognostic perspective.

PMIP

PMIP usually occurs 2 to 6 days after the onset of an acute myocardial infarction (AMI). It characteristically resolves to become clinically inapparent within several days. The diagnosis is exclusively dependent on the observation of a pericardial friction rub. Because of the evanescent nature of this auscultatory finding, the clinical incidence has been reported to vary from 7% to 20%.[4-9] However, with the advent of thrombolytic therapy, the reported frequency of a pericardial friction rub has been only around 5%.[10-13] Theoretically, by achieving earlier reperfusion of the infarct-related artery, the use of thrombolytic therapy may prevent progression to transmural myocardial necrosis, thereby reducing the risk of developing pericarditis.[13-15]

The pericardial rub of PMIP is not only transient but usually well localized to the left sternal border. Commonly the extracardiac sound does not have the typical "three-component" character but may have only one or two components during each cardiac cycle. Although the pericardial rub is often an incidental finding with no associated symptoms, the patient may complain of a pleuritic discomfort substernally that can radiate to the left trapezial ridge or left upper extremity. As with other forms of pericarditis, the pain is often exacerbated by a change in position, coughing, or deep breathing.

Fever, as well as an elevated sedimentation rate and white blood cell count, may be present; however, these findings may also occur as a natural sequela to the initial myocardial injury. The electrocardiogram (ECG) is usually not helpful in making a diagnosis of PMIP.[9,16,17] Because of the evolving ST-segment changes with the index infarction, additional findings may be observed. Occasionally, PR depression is noted along with further J-point elevation in other ECG leads distant from the site of infarction. The chest x-ray film is most commonly nonspecific but may demonstrate pleural effusion. Concomitant pericardial effusion can occur and has a reported incidence of approximately 25% between day 3 and 6 postinfarction.[18-22] There is poor correlation, however, between a pericardial friction rub and the presence of an effusion. Pericardial effusions, like pericarditis, are more commonly associated with anterior as opposed to inferior or posterior infarctions.

Despite the frequent occurrence of pericardial effusions with PMIP, adverse consequences, including hemorrhagic tamponade, are quite rare.[23-29] Before the advent of thrombolytic therapy, several cases were reported with the use of anticoagulation with and without cardiac rupture. However, most of these patients were overanticoagulated by current standards. Even with aggressive anticoagulation with concomitant thrombolytic therapy, the occurrence of hemodynamically significant pericardial effusions with tamponade is surprisingly uncommon.[13,30-32] At present, pericarditis should not be considered a contraindication to anticoagulant therapy.[13,29,33] However, late treatment (> 11 hours) with thrombolytic therapy can increase cardiac rupture and associated hemorrhagic tamponade.[5] Finally, constrictive pericarditis after anticoagulant therapy has been reported but is extremely rare.[34]

The incidence of pericarditis in patients dying of transmural infarction at autopsy is high.[35] Historically a pericardial friction rub has been a harbinger of more extensive myocardial injury. Clinically the duration of the rub appears to correlate with a worse outcome.[36] Patients with a pericardial rub have a higher frequency of anterior MI with ventricular aneurysmal formation, elevated pulmonary capillary wedge pressures, and higher alveolar arterial oxygen differences.[37] Likewise, in the era of thrombolytic therapy, a pericardial friction rub has been shown to be useful in predicting the amount and extent of myocardial damage. In one large prospective study, patients with PMIP had a lower baseline and follow-up ejection fraction, worse regional left ventricular function, and a higher frequency of left ventricular failure.[13] In fact, the presence of a pericardial friction rub predicted left ventricular damage, as measured by global ejection fraction independent of infarct location. Finally, the in-hospital mortality was 15% vs. 6%, respectively, in those with as opposed to those without a pericardial rub.

In general, the therapy of PMIP should be dependent on the severity of pain. Because the pain is usually of short duration, the use of aspirin in doses up to 650 mg orally every 4 to 6 hours may be used as necessary. In one prospective study, the majority of patients obtained relief from their chest discomfort within 48 hours of initiating therapy.[16] Nonsteroidal anti-inflammatory agents such as indomethacin or ibuprofen can be used in refractory or aspirin allergic patients. Unfortunately, their use has been associated with impaired myocardial healing and early infarct expansion. Concomitant afterload therapy with nitrates, nifedipine, or angiotensin-converting enzyme inhibitors may attenuate this potential adverse effect.[38] In recalcitrant cases, oral or intravenous (IV) corticosteroids can provide prompt and dramatic relief of pain. Because of the impairment with infarct healing, their use should be brief, with aspirin being substituted once pain relief is achieved.[39]

POSTCARDIAC INJURY SYNDROME

PCIS can occur after MI, cardiac surgery, or trauma.[40] The delayed form of postmyocardial infarction syndrome was first described by Dressler[1] in 1956. From a subsequent series, Dressler[3] estimated that this complication occurred in 3% to 4% of all MIs. However, more recent reports have reported a much lower incidence, with the most recent account finding no cases in 229 patients.[5,41]

PCIS is characterized by the onset of pleuritic or pericarditic pain, a pericardial friction rub, and fever. Typically these features are noted 1 week or more after an AMI. In one study, 65% of patients who developed the syndrome did so within 3 months, and all of them developed it by 12 months.[42] Rarely the onset can occur less than 1 week from the signal infarction. Physical signs include fever, sinus tachycardia, a pericardial friction rub, and often a pleuritic rub. Signs related to the previous MI such as left ventricular enlargement, gallop rhythm, or murmurs may also be present. Cardiac tamponade is rare but has been reported with or without concomitant anticoagulant therapy.

Leukocytosis with white blood cell counts up to 21,000/mm^3 are common. Likewise, the erythrocyte sedimentation rate is nearly always increased. The ECG may show diffuse ST-segment or T-wave changes; however, residual abnormalities from the previous infarction are likely to obscure such observations. Often these changes are difficult to distinguish from those occurring with recurrent ischemia. The chest x-ray film generally shows cardiomegaly, pleural effusion (usually on the left), and acute pulmonary infiltrates.[17] Echocardiography frequently demonstrates a pericardial effusion, which is generally small.

The exact cause of the syndrome remains elusive, although an immunopathic one appears to be most likely. Antibodies to cardiac tissue have been detected in this syndrome.[43] Theoretically myocardial injury facilitates release of cardiac antigens into the circulation, promoting the formation of circulating immune complexes. These complexes, when deposited in the pleura, lungs, pericardium, and joints, initiate an inflammatory reaction. Eventually, the immune complexes are cleared by the reticuloendothelial system, with ultimate regression of the syndrome.[44] Unfortunately, recurrences are common and they can occur over a period as long as 28 months.

Therapy of PCIS is dependent on the severity of symptoms or the unusual evidence of hemodynamic compromise. Analgesics frequently relieve the pain but do not suppress the inflammatory response. Nonsteroidal inflammatory drugs such as aspirin or indomethacin should be used initially. Therapy should be continued for 10 to 14 days. The patient should be advised of the high probability of recurrence even for extended periods. If possible, oral or parenteral corticosteroid compounds should be reserved for patients having severe or refractory pain or showing evidence of cardiac tamponade. Because relapses occur regardless of the type of therapy, multiple recurrences should not lead one to consider the treatment with nonsteroidal drugs to have failed. Additional simple measures during recurrence such as bedrest or activity modification should not be overlooked. However, the emotional support provided to the patient discouraged by a relapsing and prolonged illness is likely to be the most important therapy the clinician can provide.[45]

REFERENCES

1. Dressler W: Post-myocardial infarction syndrome: Preliminary report of a complications resembling idiopathic, recurrent, benign pericarditis, *JAMA* 160:1379-1384, 1956.
2. Dressler W: The post-myocardial infarction syndrome, *Arch Intern Med* 103:28-42, 1959.
3. Dressler W, Yurkofsky J, Starr MC: Hemorrhagic pericarditis, pleurisy, and pneumonia complicating recent myocardial infarction, *Am Heart J* 54:42-49, 1957.
4. Parkinson J, Bedford DR: Cardiac infarction and coronary thrombosis, *Lancet* 2:4-11, 1928.
5. Thadani U, Chopra MP, Aber COP, et al: Pericarditis after acute myocardial infarction, *Br Med J (Clin Res)* 2:135-137, 1971.
6. Lichstein E, Liu H-M, Gupta P: Pericarditis complicating acute myocardial infarction: incidence of complications and significance of electrocardiogram on admission, *Am Heart J* 87:246-252, 1974.
7. Toole J, Silverman ME: Pericarditis of acute myocardial infarction, *Chest* 67:647-653, 1975.
8. Tofler GH, Muller JE, Stone PH, et al: Pericarditis in acute myocardial infarction: characterization and clinical significance, *Am Heart J* 117:86-90, 1989.
9. Kranin FM, Flessas AP, Spodick DH: Infarction-associated pericarditis, *N Engl J Med* 311:1211-1214, 1984.
10. Franzosi MG, Mauri F, Pampallona S, et al: The GISSI study further analysis, *Circulation* 76(suppl II):II53-II56, 1987.
11. Van de Werf F, European Cooperative Study Group: Lessons from the European cooperative recombinant tissue-type plasminogen activator (rt-PA) versus placebo trial, *J Am Coll Cardiol* 12:14A-19A, 1988.
12. Simoons ML, Brand M, DeZwaan C, et al: Improved survival after early thrombolysis in acute myocardial infarction, *Lancet* 2:578-581, 1985.
13. Wall TC, Califf RM, Harrelson-Woodlief L, et al: Usefulness of a pericardial friction rub after thrombolytic therapy during acute myocardial infarction in predicting amount of myocardial damage, *Am J Cardiol* 66:1418-1421, 1990.
14. Reimer KA, Lowe JE, Rasmussen MM, et al: The wave front phenomenon of ischemic cell death. Myocardial infarct size vs duration of coronary occlusion in dogs, *Circulation* 56:786-794, 1977.
15. Honan MB, Harrell FE, Reimer KA, et al: Cardiac rupture, mortality, and the timing of the thrombolytic therapy: a meta-analysis, *J Am Coll Cardiol* 16:359-367, 1990.
16. Berman J, Haffajee CI, Alpert JS: Therapy of symptomatic pericarditis after myocardial infarction: Retrospective and prospective studies of aspirin, indomethacin, prednisone, and spontaneous resolution, *Am Heart J* 101:750-753, 1981.
17. Spodick DH: Electrocardiographic changes in acute pericarditis. In Fowler NO (ed): *The pericardium in health and disease,* Mount Kisco, NY, 1985, Futura, pp 79-98.
18. Wunderink RG: Incidence of pericardial effusions in acute myocardial infarctions, *Chest* 85:494-496, 1984.
19. Kaplan K, Davison R, Parker M, et al: Frequency of pericardial effusion as determined by M-mode echocardiography in acute myocardial infarction, *Am J Cardiol* 55:335-337, 1985.
20. Pierard LA, Albert A, Henrard L, et al: Incidence and significance of pericardial effusion in acute myocardial infarction as determined by two-dimensional echocardiography, *J Am Coll Cardiol* 8:517-520, 1986.
21. Galve E, Garcia-Del-Castillo H, Evangelista A, et al: Pericardial effusion in the course of myocardial infarction: incidence, natural history, and clinical relevance, *Circulation* 73:294-299, 1986.
22. Belkin RN, Mark DB, Aronson L, et al: Pericardial effusion after intravenous recombinant tissue-type plasminogen activator for acute myocardial infarction, *Am J Cardiol* 67:496-500, 1991.
23. Goldstein R, Wolff L: Hemorrhagic pericarditis in acute myocardial infarction treated with bishydroxycoumarin, *JAMA* 146:616-621, 1951.
24. Anderson M, Christensen NA, Edwards JE: Hemopericardium complicating myocardial infarction in the absence of cardiac rupture, *Arch Intern Med* 90:634-645, 1952.
25. Rose OA, Ott Jr RH, Maier HC: Hemopericardium with tamponade during anticoagulant therapy of myocardial infarct, *JAMA* 152:1221-1223, 1953.
26. Lange HF, Aarseth S: The influence of anticoagulant therapy on the occurrence of cardiac rupture and hemopericardium following heart infarction: II. A controlled study of a selected treated group based on 1,044 autopsies, *Am Heart J* 56:257-263, 1958.
27. Guberman BA, Fowler NO, Engel PJ, et al: Cardiac tamponade in medical patients, *Circulation* 64:633-640, 1981.
28. Miller RL: Hemopericardium with use of oral anticoagulant therapy, *JAMA* 209:1362-1363, 1969.
29. Chalmers TC, Matta RJ, Smith Jr H, et al: Evidence favoring the use of anticoagulants in the hospital phase of acute myocardial infarction, *N Engl J Med* 297:1091-1096, 1977.
30. Barrington WW, Smith JE, Himmelstein SI: Cardiac tamponade following treatment with tissue plasminogen activator: an atypical hemodynamic response to pericardiocentesis, *Am Heart J* 121:1227-1229, 1991.
31. Walker WD, Furntes F, Adams PR, et al: Hemopericardium and tamponade following intracoronary thrombolysis with streptokinase, *Tex Heart Inst J* 12:203-206, 1985.
32. Valeix B, Labrunie P, Jahjah F, et al: Hemopericardium after coronary recanalization by streptokinase during acute myocardial infarction, *Arch Mal Coeur* 76:1081-1084, 1983.
33. Khandheria BK, Shub C, Nishimura RA, et al: To anticoagulate or not: implications for the management of patients with acute myocardial infarction complicated by both left ventricular thrombus and pericardial effusion, *Can J Cardiol* 3:173-176, 1987.
34. Karim AH, Salomon J: Constrictive pericarditis after myocardial infarction: sequela of anticoagulant-induced hemopericardium, *Am J Med* 79:389-390, 1985.
35. Roberts WC, Spray TL: Pericardial heart disease: a study of its causes, consequences and morphologic features, *Cardiovasc Clin* 7:11-65, 1976.
36. Niarchos AP, McKendrick CS: Prognosis of pericarditis after acute myocardial infarction, *Br Heart J* 35:49-54, 1973.
37. Sugiura T, Kwasaka T, Takayama Y, et al: Factors associated with pericardial effusion in acute Q wave myocardial infarction, *Circulation* 81:477-481, 1990.
38. Jugdutt BI, Basualdo CA: Myocardial infarct expansion during indomethacin obuprofen therapy for symptomatic post infarction pericarditis. Influence of other pharmacologic agents during early remodeling, *Can J Cardiol* 5:211-221, 1989.
39. Roberts R, de Mello V, Sobel BE: Deleterious effect of methyl-

prednisolone in patients with myocardial infarction, *Circulation* 53:(suppl I):204-206, 1976.

40. Khan AH: The postcardiac injury syndromes, *Clin Cardiol* 15:67-72, 1992.

41. Lichstein E, Arsura E, Hollander G, et al: Current incidence of postmyocardial infarction (Dressler's) syndrome), *Am J Cardiol* 50:1269-1271, 1982.

42. Welin L, Vedin A, Wilhelmsson C: Characteristics, prevalence, and prognosis of postmyocardial infarction syndrome, *Br Heart J* 50:140-145, 1983.

43. Uuskiula MM, Lamp KM, Martin SI: Relationship between the clinical course of acute myocardial infarction and specific sensitization of lymphocytes and lymphotoxin production, *Kardiologia* 26:57-62, 1987.

44. Lessof MH: Postpericardiotomy syndrome: pathogenesis and management, *Hosp Pract* II:81-86, 1976.

45. Floyd WL: Pericarditis following myocardial infarction. In Califf RM, Wagner GS (eds): *Acute coronary care: principles and practice,* Hingham, Mass, 1985, Martinus Nijhoff, pp 459-461.

Chapter 49

SUPRAVENTRICULAR ARRHYTHMIAS AND HEART BLOCK IN ACUTE MYOCARDIAL INFARCTION

Damian A. Brezinski

Supraventricular arrhythmias and heart block are common in patients with AMI.[1-3] The clinical presentation can range from a benign, asymptomatic ECG finding to catastrophic hemodynamic collapse. Some of these arrhythmias have long-term adverse prognostic significance, whereas others do not. The diagnosis and treatment of these dysrhythmias have advanced in the thrombolytic era,[2,3] mostly as a result of improved understanding of the arrhythmia mechanisms and the ability to tailor specific therapies.

Virtually every known rhythm disturbance has been described in the setting of AMI.[2-5] A 10% to 30% incidence of arrhythmia has been confirmed by a number of studies[1-6]; this incidence, however, appears to be reduced in patients who are treated with reperfusion therapy.[7] Supraventricular arrhythmias are associated with a variety of predictors of poor outcome in AMI,[1-10] but it is unclear whether these rhythm disturbances alone are independent risk factors or whether they simply reflect the severity of underlying disease. Studies on whether supraventricular tachycardia in the setting of MI is an independent predictor of death, however, are contradictory[11,12] and limited by small sample size. Despite this controversy, physicians generally treat supraventricular arrhythmia in patients with AMI because these patients are often symptomatic and have a worse outcome regardless of the independence of the

prognostic significance. This chapter reviews the diagnosis of supraventricular arrhythmia and heart block and discusses therapies used in the treatment of these disorders.

APPROACH TO THE PATIENT

A patient with acute ischemic heart disease and a supraventricular arrhythmia may manifest (1) an asymptomatic rhythm disturbance noted on the ECG, (2) a symptomatic but stable dysrhythmia, or (3) a hemodynamically unstable rhythm or conduction disturbance. In each case the clinician must select appropriate diagnostic and therapeutic maneuvers. In overtly unstable patients, diagnosis and management must proceed rapidly and simultaneously; in clinically stable patients, a more orderly sequential assessment is possible.

Initial assessment begins with a brief history to elicit symptoms of ischemia or hemodynamic compromise, a directed physical examination, and a 12-lead ECG or rhythm strip to assess the cardiac rhythm adequately. From this initial assessment the physician determines the degree of hemodynamic stability of the patient (usually through the history and physical examination), the cardiac rhythm of the patient (using the ECG), and the need for diagnostic or therapeutic maneuvers such as carotid sinus massage, adenosine challenge, or esophageal electrode tracings. From this brief assessment a diagnosis and management plan can usually be made.

Initial history and physical examination — is the patient stable?

Every patient with AMI should receive a thorough, complete history and physical examination. However, in the setting of a supraventricular arrhythmia the threat of rapid hemodynamic collapse may necessitate a limited, directed history and physical examination to determine if immediate intervention (e.g., electrocardioversion or pharmacologic intervention) is indicated. In the absence of symptoms, hemodynamic instability, or electrocardiographic evidence of ongoing ischemia, the physician may expand upon the initial examination and carefully assess the 12-lead ECG.

The 12-lead electrocardiogram and single-lead rhythm monitor

One of the first questions that must be addressed in the AMI patient with a new rhythm disturbance is whether there is evidence of recurrent ischemia. In making this determination a complete 12-lead ECG is essential; ST changes should not be read off the standard cardiac monitor strip. The 12-lead ECG is often crucial in diagnosing certain types of arrhythmia, such as wide complex tachycardia. A long continuous tracing of one or two selected leads (a rhythm strip) is a very helpful supplement for assessing many types of supraventricular arrhythmias and heart blocks. A number of excellent textbooks have been written describing the assessment of ischemia and dysrhythmia,[13-15] and a number of classification schemes have been described.

The first goal of analysis of the rhythm strip or ECG is to look for evidence of dissociation between the atrial and ventricular complexes. When AV dissociation is observed, for practical purposes the rhythm can be assumed to be ventricular, although rare atrial arrhythmias can occur with AV dissociation. Fusion or capture beats are evidence of AV dissociation.

Because a QRS complex < 0.12 seconds in duration is almost always supraventricular, a QRS complex greater than 0.12 seconds requires differentiation of supraventricular and ventricular tachyarrhythmias. A rhythm strip alone should not be used to determine QRS duration because a simple lead can be misleading.

The rhythm is defined as a supraventricular tachycardia if the QRS width is less than 0.12 seconds in multiple leads and the ventricular rate exceeds 100/min. These supraventricular tachycardias are further classified and discussed later in this chapter. If the ventricular rate is less than 60/min the rhythm is defined as a bradycardia. Bradycardias are further described later in this chapter.

Carotid sinus massage and adenosine challenge

The patient's response to carotid sinus massage provides important diagnostic information. This maneuver increases vagal tone, slows the rate of sinus nodal discharge, and prolongs atrioventricular nodal conduction time and refractoriness. It is especially useful in differentiating supraventricular tachycardias either by abruptly terminating the tachycardia or by slowing ventricular response and allowing better assessment of P-wave morphology and the relationship of the P wave to the QRS complex.

During carotid sinus massage the patient should be monitored by 12-lead ECG or single-lead monitor; be sure the tracing is relatively free of artifact. Before this maneuver is performed, the carotids should be auscultated carefully; massage should be avoided in a patient with carotid bruits. The patient is placed in a supine position, the neck is hyperextended with the head turned away from the side being massaged, the sternocleidomastoid muscle is relaxed or gently pushed out of the way, and the carotid impulse is located at the angle of the jaw. The carotid bifurcation is touched gently initially with the palmar portion of the fingertips to detect hypersensitive responses. If no change in cardiac rhythm occurs, pressure is applied more firmly for approximately 5 seconds, first on one side and then on the other (never on both sides simultaneously) with a gentle rotating massaging motion. External pressure stimulates baroceptors in the carotid sinus to trigger a reflex increase in vagal activity and sympathetic withdrawal.

Adenosine is an endogenous nucleoside present throughout the body, and rapid intravenous injection of adenosine is steadily becoming the method of choice for initial assessment of supraventricular tachycardias.[16,17] Its extremely short half-life (1-6 seconds) makes it a very safe assessment method. A number of studies[17,18] have demonstrated that adenosine is more effective than and at least as safe as carotid sinus massage. As for carotid sinus massage, the patient is supine and an adequate continuous rhythm strip should be established. Rapid injection of an intravenous bolus of 6 mg (consider 3 mg in very small or elderly patients) is followed by careful monitoring of the cardiac rhythm. If no effect is seen at 1 minute, an intravenous bolus of 12 mg should be injected.[18] Approximately 92% of specific supraventricular tachycardias that use the atrioventricular node as a part of their reentrant circuit respond to a 12-mg adenosine dose.[17] The patient may experience transient side effects, such as flushing, dyspnea, or chest pressure, which usually resolve in less than 1 minute. Transient heart block often occurs but resolves spontaneously; atropine is rarely necessary. Cases of rapid acceleration of atrial flutter and precipitation of ventricular fibrillation have been reported, so pacing support and defibrillators should be available.

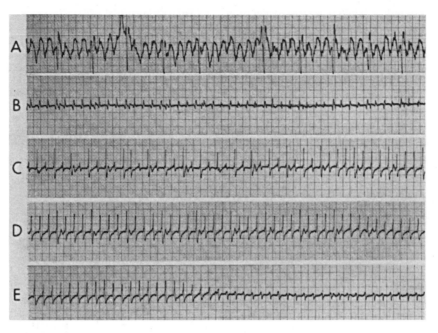

Fig. 49-1. Esophageal tracing. Panel *A* is a tracing of the surface lead of a patient with clear flutter waves. An esophageal lead is first placed all the way into the stomach (just as the nasogastric tube is positioned) and then slowly pulled up the esophagus. The panels show the lead *(B)*, in the stomach, *(C)*, behind the left ventricle, *(D)*, behind the atrium and *(E)*, passing the atrium and going to the upper esophagus.

Bronchospasm may also occur and should be treated promptly. Dipyridamole may potentiate the effects of adenosine.

Esophageal tracings

Esophageal electrode tracings may provide useful diagnostic information, especially when the 12-lead ECG and adenosine challenge are insufficient to establish the diagnosis of supraventricular arrhythmia.[6] The esophageal lead can provide detailed atrial activity tracings, particularly when the P waves are not demonstrable on rhythm strips or the 12-lead ECG. As is shown in Figure 49-1, the esophageal lead should be manipulated until the P waves are as large as possible. Should the esophageal lead show 1:1 atrioventricular conduction, vagal maneuvers or adenosine can be used to increase AV nodal refractoriness to further define the relationship of the P wave to the QRS complex. Atrial pacing through the esophageal lead can also be used to entrain the atrial activity.

SPECTRUM OF ARRHYTHMIAS

The frequency of supraventricular arrhythmias observed in patients with AMI is dependent upon the intensity with which the patient is monitored.[6] A 10% to 30% incidence of these conduction disturbances is generally noted,[1-6] and they are associated with poor outcome.[12] In the following sections we present the most commonly observed supraventricular arrhythmias in the early phases of AMI and the current treatment recommendations we routinely make.

The supraventricular tachycardias

Table 49-1 lists the commonly encountered supraventricular tachycardias in AMI. Atrial fibrillation and flutter are included, although they do not always present with a ventricular rate greater than 100/min. However, in the setting of AMI the response rate of atrial fibrillation and atrial flutter is frequently rapid.

Sinus tachycardia. Approximately 30% of patients with AMI develop sinus tachycardia[6] (Table 49-1, Fig. 49-2). Sinus tachycardia is important because it is usually a marker of abnormal physiologic stresses such as ischemia, pain, anxiety, hypovolemia, hypotension, heart failure, hypoxemia, anemia, pericarditis, or fever (Fig. 49-2). Consequently its appearance should prompt a clinical examination and laboratory testing to identify the underlying cause. Sinus tachycardia may also be seen with the use of drugs commonly administered in AMI (e.g., atropine, dopamine, dobutamine). The prognostic importance of this rhythm depends upon the underlying cause, but sinus tachycardia in the setting of MI is generally associated with worse outcome.[1,3,5] It is undesirable in AMI because it increases myocardial work and decreases disastolic coronary perfusion time and may thereby provoke or worsen ischemia. In the prethrombolytic era we observed isolated sinus tachycardia in the absence of other obvious causes such as

Table 49-1. Common supraventricular tachycardias in acute myocardial infarction

Arrhythmia	12-lead	P-wave	QRS complex	Esophag	CSM	Physical exam
Sinus tachycardia	P wave same as NSR	R = 100-180; Rhy = reg; C = peaked	R = 100-180; Rhy = reg; C = normal	1 P wave for QRS	Rate slowed	a-wave = nl; S1 = nl; S2 = nl
NSR with PACs	P wave same as NSR	R = 60-100; Rhy = irreg; C = variable	R = 60-100; Rhy = irreg; C = variable	1 P wave for QRS	Rate slowed	a-wave = irreg; S1 = variable; S2 = nl
Atrial flutter	Saw-tooth pattern	R = 250-350; Rhy = reg; C = saw-tooth	R = 75-125; Rhy = reg; C = nl	Many saw-tooth waves	Vent rate slowed, flutter	a-wave = flutter; S1 = nl; S2 = nl
Atrial fibrillation	Irreg QRS complex seen	R = 400-600; Rhy = irreg; C = no P-wave	R = 100-160; R = irreg; C = nl	Irreg P-wave >350/min	Slowed, fib remains	a-wave = absent; S1 = variable; S2 = nl
Multifocal atrial tachycardia	Irreg P + QRS complex	R = 100-160; Rhy = irreg; C = multiform	R = 100-160; R = irreg; C = nl	One P wave for 1 QRS	Slowed, MAT remains	a-wave = irreg; S1 = variable; S2 = nl

Abbreviations: R = rate, Rhy = rhythm, C = wave contour, reg = regular, irreg = irregular, nl = normal, abnl = abnormal, fib = fibrillation, 12-lead = 12-lead ECG, Esophag = esophageal lead, CSM = carotid sinus massage or adenosine, Abs = absent, NSR = normal sinus rhythm, PACs = premature atrial complexes.

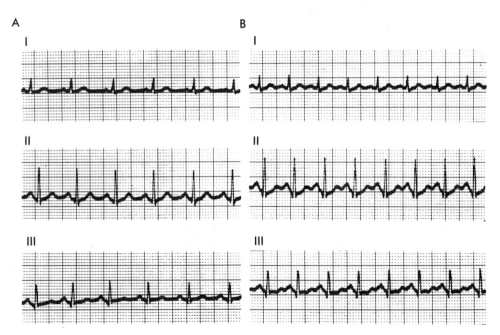

Fig. 49-2. Sinus tachycardia electrocardiogram. Both tracings **A** and **B** were recorded within a period of a few minutes from a 19-year-old man with considerable anxiety but no evidence of organic heart disease. **A,** The rate is 108 beats/min; **B,** the rate is 148 beats/min. There is a slight increase in the amplitude of the P waves when the heart rate is more rapid. There is also junctional ST-segment depression in tracing **B.** The T waves in lead III are biphasic during the more rapid rate.

clinically evident heart failure in 16% of 610 consecutive MI admissions.[19] These patients had both a higher in-hospital and long-term mortality rate than patients without this finding.

The treatment of sinus tachycardia should focus upon identifying its cause and administering the appropriate therapy (e.g., fever treated with antipyretics, hypovolemia treated with volume). Beta-adrenergic blockade can slow sinus tachycardia, but this should be considered only after the underlying disorders have been identified and left ventricular decompensation has been ruled out as a cause. Usually a carefully focused examination,

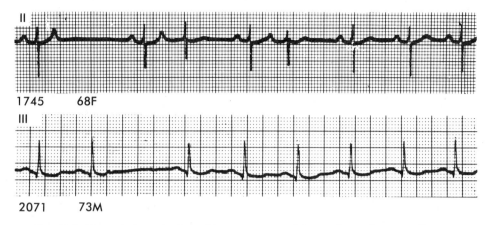

Fig. 49-3. Normal sinus rhythm with premature atrial complexes electrocardiogram.

including blood pressure measurement, auscultation of the lungs for rales, and palpation of the extremities for coolness, can provide direction for choice of therapy. In difficult cases we have used a pulmonary artery catheter to rule out occult heart failure as a cause.

Normal sinus rhythm with premature atrial complexes. Atrial premature complexes occur in at least 50% of all patients with AMI[1] (Table 49-1, Fig. 49-3). They may be particularly frequent in patients with heart failure, atrial ischemia/infarction, and pericarditis. They are not specifically associated with increased mortality in patients with AMI and, as such, require no specific therapy.

Atrial flutter. Atrial flutter (Table 49-1, Fig. 49-4) occurs in at least 1% of patients with AMI.[4] The ECG shows identically recurring sawtooth flutter waves at a rate of 250 to 300 per minute, often best visualized in the inferior leads (II, III, or AVF) or in lead VI. The ventricular response rate can vary from 75 to 175 per minute, depending upon the atrial rate and the degree of atrioventricular block (typically 2:1; other blocks include 3:1, 4:1, and variable block). Atrial flutter may revert spontaneously to normal sinus rhythm or degenerate into atrial fibrillation. During an episode the physical examination may reveal rapid flutter waves in the jugular venous pulse. If the relationship of the flutter waves to the conducted QRS complexes remains constant, the first heart sound will often have a constant intensity. Atrial flutter with variable conduction will often vary in the intensity of the first heart sound.

Rapid atrial flutter may precipitate hemodynamic instability or exacerbate ischemia (especially if 1:1 AV conduction occurs), necessitating cardioversion. Synchronous direct current cardioversion with 50 to 100 J is the treatment of choice for patients with hemodynamic instability or ongoing ischemia. If the patient is clinically stable in atrial flutter, management usually has two principal objectives: to control the ventricular rate by blocking the AV node and to convert the rhythm to

normal sinus rhythm. Rate control of this arrhythmia is often difficult to achieve and may require more than one agent. The main drugs used for rate control are beta blockers, calcium channel blockers, or digoxin. After the ventricular response has been controlled, pharmacologic cardioversion, either with Class IA or Class III antiarrhythmic drugs, or direct current electrocardioversion can be attempted if the atrial flutter has not resolved spontaneously. The use of Class IA or III antiarrhythmic drugs is somewhat controversial and will be discussed further in subsequent sections.

Atrial fibrillation. Atrial fibrillation (Table 49-1, Fig. 49-5) is one of the most common supraventricular arrhythmias in the setting of AMI, occurring in approximately 10% to 15% of all patients.[20-24] Often patients will alternate between atrial fibrillation and flutter before ultimately settling into atrial fibrillation as the sustained rhythm. Atrial fibrillation is abrupt in onset and can cause rapid hemodynamic instability, usually by one of three mechanisms: (1) the loss of the atrial component of the cardiac output, (2) increased ventricular response rate with decreased diastolic filling time, or (3) irregular ventricular filling.[21]

The ECG in atrial fibrillation demonstrates an irregular atrial baseline of variable morphology at a rate of 350 to 600 per minute (Fig. 49-5). The ventricular response is irregularly irregular; in the setting of AMI it is usually at a rate of 100 to 160 per minute. The physical findings include variation in the intensity of the first heart sound, absence of a-waves in the jugular venous pulse, and an irregularly irregular pulse. Typically the rate of the auscultated precordial pulse is faster than the rate palpated at the wrist because each contraction is not sufficiently strong to transmit pressure waves to the peripheral arterial system (this phenomenon is known as *pulse deficit*).

The treatment of new-onset atrial fibrillation in AMI, like atrial flutter, has two principal objectives: rate control and rhythm conversion. As in atrial flutter, the

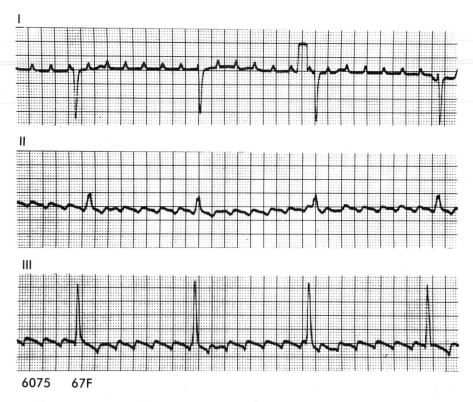

6075   67F

Fig. 49-4. Atrial flutter electrocardiogram. Atrial flutter with complete AV block. Variation of the PR interval and a constant RR interval are seen. The patient was receiving digitalis. The escape rhythm probably is idioventricular in origin.

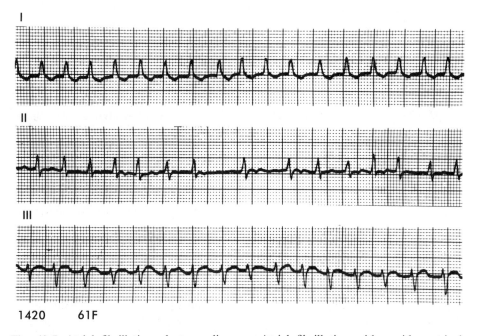

1420   61F

Fig. 49-5. Atrial fibrillation electrocardiogram. Atrial fibrillation with rapid ventricular response. The ventricular rate is about 180 beats/min in leads I and III; the ventricular rhythm appears regular but is not.

Lead II

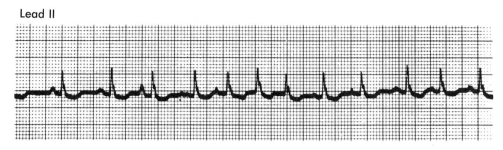

Fig. 49-6. Multifocal atrial tachycardia electrocardiogram.

most commonly used rate control agents are beta blockers, calcium channel blockers, and digoxin. Beta-adrenergic blockade should be used whenever possible. Direct current cardioversion and a variety of antiarrhythmic drugs have been demonstrated to be effective for rhythm conversion.[20] As with atrial flutter, clinically unstable patients should undergo synchronized electrocardioversion, with a starting energy of 100 J.

Recent data has suggested that thrombolytic therapy alone reduces the occurrence of atrial fibrillation in AMI. Nielsen et al.[7] retrospectively analyzed patients with AMI and new-onset atrial fibrillation. In patients who received thrombolytic therapy there was a dramatic decrease in the occurrence of atrial fibrillation (16% vs. 3%; $P = 0.009$), although the lack of randomization led to differences in baseline characteristics that were not controlled for in the analysis. Confirmatory information for the effect of reperfusion in preventing atrial fibrillation has come from the GUSTO I trial.[25] In this study, which included only thrombolytic therapy candidates, among patients randomized to t-PA 8.7% had atrial fibrillation or flutter, compared with 9.9% among patients randomized to streptokinase.

Atrial fibrillation in the setting of MI is associated with an increased mortality, predominately because of its association with worse left ventricular function. In GUSTO I, the mortality was 14.3% in the 3819 patients with atrial fibrillation/flutter, compared with 6.2% in 36,891 patients without atrial fibrillation/flutter. However, atrial fibrillation is also associated with an increased risk of stroke in the acute phase of the infarction, independently of other risk factors. In the Duke experience before thrombolytic therapy[26] atrial fibrillation occurred in 33% of patients with stroke compared with 14% of patients without stroke. In the TAMI experience atrial fibrillation was not independently associated with stroke, although the sample size was small, whereas in GUSTO I atrial fibrillation was associated with a three-fold increase in the risk of stroke in a case-control study within the trial comparing 592 patients with stroke and 548 age-matched controls without stroke in the trial.

Multifocal atrial tachycardia. Multifocal atrial

tachycardia (MAT; Table 49-1, Fig. 49-6) occurs in 5% to 7% of patients with AMI.[27] It is an irregular supraventricular arrhythmia with multiform (at least three different P-wave morphologies) and irregularly spaced P waves at rates of 100 per minute or more. The ventricular rhythm is irregular and rapid, secondary to the atrial mechanism. Atrial activity of MAT, unlike that of atrial fibrillation, is well organized, and the baseline is isoelectric between P waves. Multifocal atrial tachycardia is often a secondary rhythm associated with AMI, especially common in patients with lung disease and ventilatory failure.[28] The physical examination includes variation in the intensity of the first heart sound, but jugular a-waves are present and irregular; an irregularly irregular pulse is present. Significant disease is often evident on the lung examination.

The treatment of MAT is difficult and should include therapy directed at the underlying causes. Improvement in oxygenation is key to the correction of the arrhythmia in those with decompensated lung disease. Sympathomimetic agents are often used to treat the lung disease, but may exacerbate MAT; aminophylline should be avoided. If MAT is rapid and unstable, the rate can often be controlled with intravenous calcium-channel blockade. Beta blockers should be used with great caution, as they may worsen the chronic lung disease. Conversion usually occurs without pharmacologic agents, after correction of the underlying cause of the arrhythmia.

Uncommon supraventricular tachycardias in AMI. Table 49-2 identifies and lists the treatment of a variety of less common supraventricular tachycardias in AMI. The less common rhythms, when they occur, are generally stable and can be assessed carefully by the noted methods. Recommended treatments should only be administered when the diagnosis is certain. Adenosine or carotid sinus massage is frequently helpful in identifying the location and morphology of P waves; esophageal lead tracings are also very useful.

Bradycardia and heart block

Sinus bradycardia. Sinus bradycardia (Fig. 49-7, Table 49-3A) is an extremely common rhythm in the early hours of MI, occurring in up to 40% of patients in

Table 49-2. Uncommon supraventricular tachycardias in acute myocardial infarction

Arrhythmia	12-lead	P-wave	QRS complex	Esophag	CSM	Treatment
Atrial tachycardia	P waves = diff contour	R = 100-160; Rhy = reg/irr; C = (−) in II, III, AVF	R = 100-160; Rhy = reg/irr; C = nl	1 P for 1 QRS	Some slow	Adenosine, IV diltiazem or type IA
SA nodal reentrant tachycardia	Looks like sinus tachycardia	R = 100-160; Rhy = reg; C = long RP, short PR	R = 100-160; Rhy = reg; C = nl	1 + P wave for QRS	Abrupt break of rhythm	IV beta, type IA or III, adenosine
AV nodal reentrant tachycardia	Narrow complex tachycardia	R = 150-200; Rhy = reg; C = retrograde	R = 150-200; Rhy = reg; C = nl	P at same time as QRS	Abrupt break of rhythm	IV diltiazem, esmolol, digoxin, adenosine
Orthodromic reciprocating tachycardia	Preexcited tachycardia	R = 100-160; Rhy = reg; C = P halfway between QRS	R = 100-160; Rhy = reg; C = may be preexcited	P halfway between QRS	Abrupt break of rhythm	Seen in WPW; type IA type III

R = rate, Rhy = rhythm, C = wave contour, reg = regular, irreg = irregular, nl = normal, 12-lead = 12-lead ECG, Esophag = esophageal lead, CSM = carotid sinus massage or adenosine, SA = sinoatrial, AV = atrioventricular.

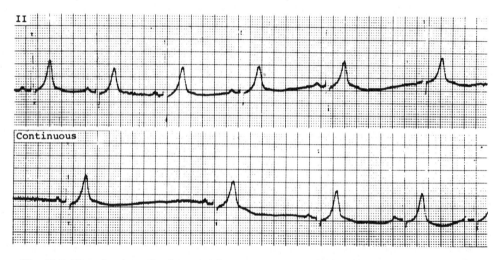

Fig. 49-7. Sinus bradycardia electrocardiogram. Symptomatic sinus bradycardia. The patient is a 75-year-old man with dizziness. The tracing was recorded during a dizzy spell. Considerable variation in heart rate is seen. The last complex in the upper strip is probably an ectopic atrial escape beat. Although sinus arrest or SA block cannot be excluded during the long pause in the bottom strip, sinus bradycardia is more likely because of the gradual change. The cause of the sinus bradycardia was unknown.

the first hour of symptoms.[29] It is particularly common in inferior wall infarctions and typically reflects enhanced vagal tone. In the TAMI 1 study sustained sinus bradycardia was seen in 21% of patients overall but was more than twice as common in RCA or LCX infarcts as compared to LAD infarcts.[30] The atria and the SA and AV nodes are richly innervated by the vagus nerve, and stimulation (e.g., upon reperfusion) may produce both bradycardia and hypotension (the Bezold-Jarisch reflex). In an early European Cooperative Study Group

trial, sinus bradycardia was twice as common in t-PA–treated patients as in the placebo group (14% vs. 6%).[31]

Other causes of enhanced vagal tone in AMI include severe pain and the use of morphine sulfate for its treatment. Management of symptomatic bradycardia (usually less than 40 beats per minute) includes the administration of atropine (0.3 to 0.5 mg every 3 to 5 minutes for a total dose of 2 mg), with isoproterenol or pacing reserved for patients in whom atropine fails. Atropine and isoproterenol should be dosed carefully, as

Table 49-3A. Bradycardia and heart block in acute myocardial infarction

Arrhythmia	12-lead	P-wave	QRS complex	Esophag	CSM	Physical exam
Sinus brady-cardia	P wave same as NSR	R = <60; Rhy = reg; C= nl	R = <60; Rhy = reg; C= nl	1 P wave for QRS	Avoid CSM	a-wave = nl; S1 = nl; S2 = nl
First-degree AV block	Long PR	R = 60-100; Rhy = reg; C = nl	R = 60-100; Rhy = reg; C = nl	Long PR	Avoid CSM	a-wave = nl; S1 = nl; S2 = nl
Type I second-degree AV block	Long PR skipped QRS	R = 60-100; Rhy = reg; C = nl	R = 30-100; Rhy = irreg; C = nl	QRS lost	Increased AV block	a-wave = abnl; S1 = cyclic; S2 = cyclic
Type II second-degree AV block	Constant PR; QRS skipped	R = 60-100; Rhy = reg; C = nl	R = 30-100; Rhy = irreg; C = nl	QRS lost	Sinus slowed only	a-wave = abnl; S1 = cyclic; S2 = cyclic
Complete heart block	P-QRS not as-sociated	R = 60-100; Rhy = reg; C = nl	R = <40; Rhy = reg; C = nl	P-QRS not as-sociated	Avoid CSM	a-wave = cannon; S1/S2 = abnl

R = rate, Rhy = rhythm, C = wave contour, reg = regular, irreg = irregular, nl = normal, abnl = abnormal, fib = fibrillation, 12-lead = 12-lead ECG, Esophag = esophageal lead, CSM = carotid sinus massage or adenosine, Abs = absent.

Table 49-3B. Indications for pacemaker placement

Arrhythmia	Temporary pacer	Permanent pacer
Sinus bradycardia	When symptoms occur	Symptoms severe and prolonged
First-degree AV block	When symptomatic or requiring repeated or constant treatment	Symptoms severe and prolonged
Type I second-degree AV block	When symptomatic or requiring repeated or constant treatment	Symptoms severe and prolonged
Type II second-degree AV block	All AMIs	All post-MI patients
Complete heart block	All anterior infarctions; all that progress via type II mechanisms	All post-MI patients

these drugs may lead to "overshoot" tachycardia and subsequent ischemia or hemodynamic instability. Sinus bradycardia has no adverse prognostic significance. Persistent sinus bradycardia or advanced sinus node dysfunction in this setting suggests sinus node or atrial ischemia/infarction.

Heart block (Fig. 49-8, Table 49-3A). The most common types of conduction blocks and suggested treatments are noted in Tables 3A and 3B. The incidence, significance, and treatment of heart block depend upon the clinical setting and the type(s) of conduction block present.[6] Heart block in an inferior MI is frequently a result of increased vagal tone or ischemia, with consequent block within the atrioventricular node. This usually results in first-degree AV block or Mobitz type I second-degree AV block and requires only simple observation unless there is associated hemodynamic instability. When significant hemodynamic compromise is observed, atrioventricular sequential pacing leads to the best improvement in hemodynamics in these patients. Higher-order atrioventricular block, when ob-

served in the setting of inferior MI, often is asymptomatic and well tolerated.

Substantial information has become available recently concerning the development of complete heart block after inferior infarction. In both the TAMI[32] and the TIMI trials the occurrence of complete heart block was associated with a two- to three-fold increase in mortality, after adjusting for differences in baseline characteristics between patients with and without complete heart block. In the TAMI studies 13% of inferior MI patients had complete heart block, and this conduction disturbance occurred within 6 hours of symptom onset in over half the patients and within 72 hours of symptom onset in 96% of patients. Complete heart block patients not only had a higher mortality, but they also had a decrease in global and regional left ventricular function, a higher rate of reocclusion, and more ventricular fibrillation, pulmonary edema, and sustained hypotension. The mortality could not be attributed to the heart block per se, as almost all patients had temporary pacing instituted as needed. Indeed, posthospital mortality was

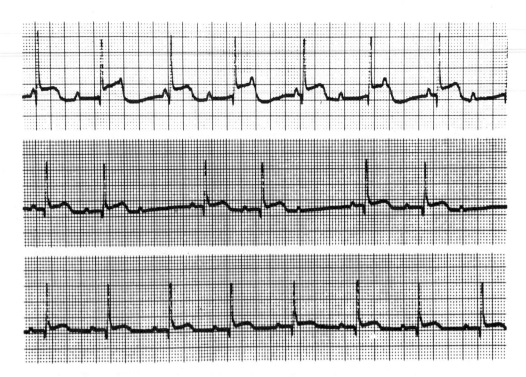

Fig. 49-8. Cardiac conduction block. AV block resulting from acute inferior MI. The upper strip shows complete AV block with junctional escape rhythm. The middle and lower strips show type I second-degree and first-degree AV block, respectively. All the rhythm strips were recorded on the same day.

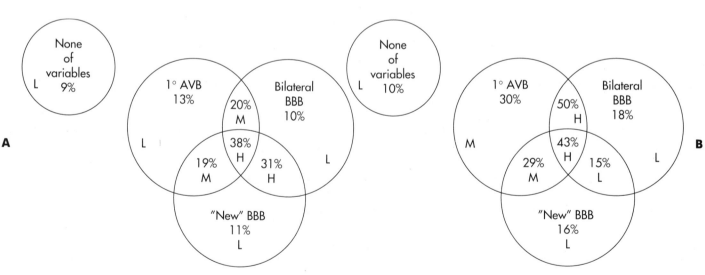

Fig. 49-9. A, Risk of progression to high-grade AV block—multicenter data. Venn diagram of the results of a multicenter study illustrating the risk of progression to high-grade AV block during AMI using three variables to stratify risk: first-degree AV block (AVB), new bundle branch block (BBB), and bifascicular (bilateral) block. L = low risk; M = moderate risk; H = high risk. **B,** Risk of progression to high-grade AV block—LA County Hospital data. Venn diagram of the results from the Los Angeles County Hospital study illustrating the risk of progression to high-grade AV block using same "risk" factors as the multicenter study in Fig. 49-9, **A.**

	None	AV Block	Mobitz I	Mobitz II	Hemiblock	RBBB	LBBB
A None	6/495	4/42	2/17	0/8	1/20	1/18	2/12
1° AVB	—	—	9/21	0/3	0/3	1/3	0/6
Mobitz I	—	—	—	2/6	0/0	0/0	0/2
Mobitz II	—	—	—	—	0/1	0/0	1/1
Hemiblock	—	—	—	—	—	6/26	0/3
RBBB	—	—	—	—	—	—	0/1

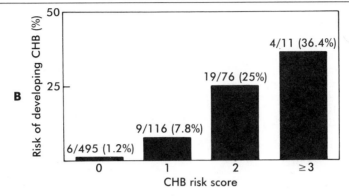

Fig. 49-10. A, The occurrence of complete heart block in patients with AMI and various combinations of risk factors. *Complete heart block risk scores of 0, 1, and 2 expressed as the number of patients developing complete heart block/the number of patients having that combination of risk factors. **B,** The risk of developing complete heart block in patients with increasing risk scores. The risk of developing complete heart block in patients with increasing risk scores increases progressively. Numerators are number of patients developing complete heart block; denominators are number of patients having that risk score. CHB = complete heart block.

not affected by the occurrence of heart block, which is strong evidence that permanent pacing is unnecessary.

Higher-degree atrioventricular block in the setting of anterior MI or MI of indeterminate location, especially Mobitz Type II AV block and complete heart block, is a much more ominous sign and should be treated aggressively. A number of studies have demonstrated a very high mortality rate for these patients, although as with inferior MI the deaths are often the result of ventricular fibrillation and not heart block per se.

The factors determining progression to high-grade AV block in a population of patients with AMI were described by Hindman et al.[29] and later by DeGuzman and Rahimtoola.[33] In both studies (Fig. 49-9A and 49-9B), the high-risk patients were those with new bundle branch block and bilateral bundle branch block (e.g., right bundle branch block and either left anterior hemiblock, left posterior hemiblock, or left bundle branch block). In addition DeGuzman and Rahimtoola also showed high risk in those patients with first-degree AV block and bilateral bundle branch block, as is shown in Figure 49-9B. Prophylactic temporary pacing is recommended for these high-risk patient populations.

Lamas et al.[34] noted that a variety of conduction abnormalities are at risk for complete heart block, as is seen in Figure 49-10A, and they developed a complete heart block risk score, as shown in Figure 49-10B. Patients had one point added to their risk score for each of the following abnormalities: first-degree atrioventricular block, Mobitz I block, Mobitz II block, left anterior hemiblock, left posterior hemiblock, right bundle branch block, or left bundle branch block. An increasing score was associated with increasing incidence of progression to complete heart block (Fig. 49-10A). Whereas patients with a 0 score had a risk of 1.2%, those with a score of 2 had a risk of 25%, and those with a score of 3 or more had a risk of 36%. Prophylactic temporary pacing is recommended for patients with a score of 3 or more.

Thus, temporary prophylactic pacemaker placement should be considered in a variety of clinical settings: (1) in patients with high-degree AV block or severe symptoms (Table 49-3A), (2) in new bundle branch block and bilateral bundle branch block, or first-degree AV block and bundle branch block (Fig. 49-9A and 49-9B), or (3) with risk scores of 3 or greater, as is shown in Figures 49-10A and 49-10B. In each case temporary transvenous or transcutaneous pacing should be considered. Now that transcutaneous pacers are available in most areas, these devices may be used to replace prophylactic transvenous pacers, especially in patients who receive thrombolytic therapy. Because of the risk of inability of a transcutaneous pacer to capture the ventricle of

Table 49-4. Pharmacologic agents used in supraventricular arrhythmias

Agents	Maintenance dosage range	Efficacy	Comments
Rate-controlling agents			
Diltiazem	17-25 mg	>85%	Less likely to induce hypotension
Verapamil	5-15 mg	>85%	Hypotension, CHF
Esmolol	0.1-0.2 mg/kg/min	50%	Less efficacy, short half-life
Digoxin	0.25-1 mg	50%	Generally safe, less effective in high adrenergic states
Rhythm-terminating agents			
Adenosine	6-18 mg	>90%	Ultrashort half-life, rapid onset
Quinidine sulfate	600 mg q6h	60	Controversial, risk of torsades
Procainamide	3 mg/kg/hr	60%	Proarrhythmic risk
Flecanide/encainide	Not recommended		
Propafenone	100-200 mg	>80%	Proarrhythmic risk
Amiodarone	200 mg	80%	Acute effects mediated by Class III and beta-blocking actions; long-term toxicity limits use; proarrhythmic risk
Sotalol	80 mg BID	80%	Proarrhythmic risk

patients with large anterior MIs, it should be tested before use in all patients, and, if at all possible, transvenous pacing should be considered in patients with large anterior infarction.

Indications for permanent pacemaker placement are shown in Table 49-3B. In general, permanent pacing should be considered in all patients in whom symptoms from their conduction disturbance are prolonged and severe. Additionally, all patients with type II second-degree atrioventricular block and/or complete heart block in a setting other than inferior MI (regardless of symptoms) should be considered for permanent pacemaker. In alternating bundle branch block with a persistent conduction block, the possible benefits of permanent pacemaker placement are not known, although some authors recommend permanent pacing in this setting.

One uncommon but interesting problem occurs when a patient with inferior MI has hemodynamically stable complete heart block that persists for days. Although the natural history of this problem is to gradually disappear, the economic advantage may accrue to permanent pacing in this situation.

CAVEATS OF THERAPY

The first line of therapy for a supraventricular arrhythmia in patients with MI has not changed from the recommendations of the American Heart Association in the Advanced Cardiac Life Support guidelines.[35] Adenosine can be considered first-line therapy for most regular supraventricular tachyarrhythmias[16,17,35] because of its ability to terminate a wide variety of rhythms. If the rhythm is not terminated, adenosine will transiently increase atrioventricular nodal refractoriness, thus allowing better differentiation of P waves. Carotid

sinus massage may also be considered, but is generally less helpful than adenosine. If these maneuvers fail, a variety of pharmacologic agents can be used, as outlined in Table 49-4.

In general we recommend rate control (initially with intravenous diltiazem, beta blocker, or digoxin), especially with very rapid supraventricular rhythms that threaten to produce hemodynamic instability. We prefer to use beta-blocking agents as the first line of treatment because they also have the beneficial effects of reducing mortality, reinfarction, and recurrent ischemia. Although esmolol has theoretical advantages because of its short half-life, we use either metoprolol or atenolol except in patients with a relative contraindication to beta blockers (severe left ventricular dysfunction, broncho spastic lung disease, pulmonary rales, or mild conduction disorder) because of the cost implications. Digoxin, although used for many years in this setting, is generally not preferred acutely because of its rather long onset of action. Calcium channel blockers are generally avoided in AMI because of evidence of increased mortality when used in the setting of left ventricular dysfunction. One of the most difficult quandaries in the Cardiac Care Unit arises when a patient develops atrial fibrillation/flutter with a rapid ventricular response that is hemodynamically stable in the setting of substantial left ventricular dysfunction with manifest heart failure. We generally use intravenous esmolol or diltiazem in this setting, again with careful monitoring because of the risk of precipitating deterioration. After the rate has been controlled, conversion to normal sinus rhythm can be attempted with Class IA or Class III antiarrhythmic therapy, or with synchronized direct current cardioversion. In unstable patients immediate electrocardioversion should be performed, starting at 100 J.

Because arrhythmias occurring in the first 48 hours of AMI may simply reflect transient electrical instability, we often discontinue antiarrhythmic therapy if it has been started after 48 to 72 hours (or when the patient is clinically stable) to reassess the need for therapy. In patients who continue to have symptomatic arrhythmias, long-term therapy should be considered with caution.[6] In most arrhythmias, especially atrial fibrillation and atrial flutter, the combination of a rate-controlling agent (such as beta-adrenergic blockade) and a Class IA (e.g., procainamide) or Class III (e.g., sotalol) antiarrhythmic drug often is required. Whenever possible we choose sotalol for long-term therapy because of accruing evidence that it has less arrhythmogenic potential than other available agents. Recent evidence has demonstrated that intravenous sotalol is a very effective agent to terminate arrhythmias, but this form of sotalol is not currently available in the United States.

The long-term use of antiarrhythmic therapy has come under intense scrutiny. Coplen et al.[36] and the Stroke Prevention in Atrial Fibrillation (SPAF) investigators[37] have demonstrated increased mortality in selected patient populations who received Class IA or Class III antiarrhythmic medications. The Class IC antiarrhythmic drugs (e.g., flecainide and encainide, the latter of which is no longer available), are contraindicated following AMI because of their increased mortality risk, as demonstrated by the Cardiac Arrhythmia Suppression Trial (CAST) investigators.[38] Together these studies have raised concerns about the safety of antiarrhythmic drugs in the setting of AMI. Although further study is needed, current data suggest that treatment with any antiarrhythmic may increase the risk of morbidity and mortality in selected patients with structural heart disease following MI. Until the degree of this risk and the patient population involved are better defined, we use antiarrhythmic therapy with caution, almost always in patients in whom symptoms from the arrhythmia are severe and prolonged. In general, we subject patients to this unknown risk of antiarrhythmic drugs only when the arrhythmia is very poorly tolerated (because of exacerbation of ischemia, hemodynamic instability, or severe symptoms from the dysrhythmia) following AMI; otherwise, we simply control the ventricular response.

In patients with persistent or chronic atrial fibrillation after MI, anticoagulation should be used unless an absolute contraindication is present. In the elderly or those in whom chronic anticoagulation is contraindicated, aspirin is an alternative that reduces the risk of thromboembolic stroke. Recently evidence has been accumulating that the combination of aspirin and warfarin in lower doses of each (81 mg of aspirin and 1 to 3 mg of coumadin) may be beneficial.

Although not included in the Vaughn-Williams clas-

sification of antiarrhythmic therapy, magnesium has been intensely studied as therapy following AMI. In a metaanalysis by Horner[39] and prospective data by the Leicester Intravenous Magnesium Intervention Trial II (LIMIT II),[40] use of magnesium has been shown to decrease mortality following AMI. More recent prospective work in 50,000 patients with AMI in the International Study of Infarct Survival (ISIS-4)[41] has shown no demonstrable benefit of magnesium therapy in early AMI. Further analysis is needed, but we do not recommend aggressive magnesium in AMI at this time.

The use of radiofrequency catheter ablation to eliminate accessory pathways, AV nodal reentrant tachycardia, atrial flutter, and ectopic arrhythmic foci has gained widespread recognition recently.[42] The mapping and ablation techniques require specialized electrophysiology laboratories and experienced electrophysiologists.

The treatment of supraventricular arrhythmias and heart block in the setting of AMI remains dynamic. To maximize effects of reperfusion and patient survival, efficient treatment of cardiac rhythm and conduction disturbances is mandatory. Fortunately, advances in pharmacology and electrophysiology have improved the ability of the physician in the treatment of these rhythm disturbances.

ACKNOWLEDGMENTS

I wish to thank Dr. Marcus Wharton, Dr. Carlton Nibley, and Dr. Mark Hamer for their comments and suggestions during the preparation of this chapter.

REFERENCES

1. Pasternak RC, Braunwald E, Sobel BE: Acute myocardial infarction. In Braunwald E, (ed): *Heart disease: a textbook of cardiovascular medicine,* Philadelphia, 1992, WB Saunders.
2. Metzler LE, Cohen HE: The incidence of arrhythmias associated with acute myocardial infarction. In Metzler LE, Dunning LE, (eds): *Textbook of coronary care,* Bowie, Md, 1972, Charles Press.
3. DeSanctis RW, Block P, Hutter AM: Tachyarrhythmias in myocardial infarction, *Circulation* 65:681, 1972.
4. Imperial ES, Carballo R, Zimmerman HA: Disturbances of rate, rhythm and conduction in acute myocardial infarction: a statistical study of 153 cases, *Am J Cardiol* 6:24, 1960.
5. Metzler LE, Kitchell JB: The incidence of arrhythmias associated with acute myocardial infarction, *Prog Cardiovas Dis* 9:50, 1966.
6. Irwin JM: In-hospital monitoring and management of arrhythmias following thrombolytic therapy. In Califf RM, Mark DB, Wagner GS (eds): *Acute coronary care in the thrombolytic era,* Chicago, 1988, Year Book Medical.
7. Nielsen FE, Sorensen HT, Christensen JH, et al: Reduced occurrence of atrial fibrillation in acute myocardial infarction treated with streptokinase, *Eur Heart J* 12:1081, 1991.
8. Rechavia E, Strasberg B, Mager A, et al: The incidence of atrial arrhythmias during inferior wall myocardial infarction with and without right ventricular involvement, *Am Heart J* 124:387, 1992.
9. Zoni Berisso M, Ferroni A, DeCaro E, et al: Clinical significance of supraventricular tachyarrhythmias after acute myocardial infarction, *Eur Heart J* 7:743, 1986.
10. Zoni Berisso M, Carratino L, Ferroni A, et al: Frequency,

characteristics and significance of supraventricular tachyarrhythmias detected by 24-hour electrocardiographic recording in the late hospital phase of acute myocardial infarction, *Am J Cardiol* 65:1064, 1990.

11. Zoni Berisso M, Ferroni A, Molini D, et al: Supraventricular tachyarrhythmias during acute myocardial infarction, *G Ital Cardiol* 21:49, 1991.

12. Kobayashi Y, Katoh T, Takano T, et al: Paroxysmal atrial fibrillation and flutter associated with acute myocardial infarction: hemodynamic evaluation in relation to the development of arrhythmias and prognosis, *Jap Circ J* 56:1, 1992.

13. Goldberger AL, Goldberger E: *Clinical electrocardiography: a simplified approach,* Baltimore, 1990, Mosby.

14. Grauer K, Curry RW: *Clinical electrocardiography: a primary care approach,* Boston, 1992, Blackwell Scientific.

15. Zipes DP: Specific arrhythmias: diagnosis and treatment. In: Braunwald E (ed): *Heart disease: a textbook of cardiovascular medicine,* Philadelphia, 1992, WB Saunders.

16. Belardinelli L, Linden J, Berne RM: The cardiac effects of adenosine, *Prog Cardiovasc Dis* 32:73, 1989.

17. Dimarco JP, Miles W, Akhtar M, et al: Adenosine for paroxysmal supraventricular tachycardia: dose ranging and comparison with verapamil: assessment in placebo-controlled, multicenter trials, *Ann Intern Med* 113:104, 1990.

18. Dunham G, Allen-LaPointe N, Bellinger R: *The Heart Center at Duke University Hospital dosing guide,* Durham, 1990, Duke University.

19. Crimm A, Severance HW Jr, Coffey K, et al: Prognostic significance of isolated sinus tachycardia during first three days of acute myocardial infarction, *Am J Med* 76:983-988, 1984.

20. Pritchett ELC: Management of atrial fibrillation, *N Engl J Med* 326:1264, 1992.

21. Kyriakidis M, Barbetseas J, Antonopoulos A, et al: Early atrial arrhythmias in acute myocardial infarction: role of the sinus node artery, *Chest* 101:944, 1992.

22. Hod H, Lew AS, Keltai M, et al: Early atrial fibrillation during evolving myocardial infarction: a consequence of impaired left atrial perfusion, *Circulation* 75:146-150, 1987.

23. Sugiura T, Iwasaka T, Takahashi N, et al: Factors associated with atrial fibrillation in Q wave anterior myocardial infarction, *Am Heart J* 21:1409, 1991.

24. Flugelman MY, Hasin Y, Shefer A, et al: Atrial fibrillation in acute myocardial infarction, *Isr J Med* 22:355, 1986.

25. The GUSTO Investigators: An international randomized trial comparing four thrombolytic strategies for acute myocardial infarction, *N Engl J Med* 329:673-682, 1993.

26. Komrad MS, Coffey CE, Coffey KS, et al: Myocardial infarction and stroke, *Neurology* 34:1403-1409, 1984.

27. Scher DL, Arsura EL: Multifocal atrial tachycardia: mechanisms, clincal correlates and treatment, *Am Heart J* 118:574, 1989.

28. Yurchak P, McGovern BA: Supraventricular arrhythmias. In Eagle KA, Haber E, DeSanctis RW, et al (eds): *The practice of cardiology,* Boston, 1980, Little, Brown.

29. Hindman MC, Wagner GS, JaRo M, et al: The clinical significance of bundle branch block complicating acute myocardial infarction, *Circulation* 58:689, 1978.

30. Bates ER, Califf RM, Stack RS, et al: Thrombolysis and angioplasty in Myocardial Infarction (TAMI-1) Trial: influence of infarct location on arterial patency, left ventricular function and mortality, *J Am Coll Cardiol* 13:12-18, 1989.

31. Verstraete M, Bernard R, Bory M, et al: Randomised trial of intravenous recombinant tissue-type plasminogen activator versus intravenous streptokinase in acute myocardial infarction. Report from the European Cooperative Study Group for Recombinant Tissue-type Plasmninogen Activator, *Lancet* 1:842-847, 1985.

32. Clemmenson P, Bates ER, Califf RM, et al: Complete atrioventricular block complicating inferior wall acute myocardial infarction treated with reperfusion therapy—TAMI study group, *Am J Cardiol* 67:225-230, 1991.

33. DeGuzman M, Rahimtoola SH: What is the role of pacemakers in patients with coronary artery disease and conduction abnormalities? In Rahimtoola SH (ed): *Current controversies in coronary heart disease,* Philadelphia, 1983, FA Davis.

34. Lamas GA, Muller JE, Turi ZG, et al: A simplified method to predict occurrence of complete heart block during acute myocardial infarction, *Am J Cardiol* 57:1213, 1986.

35. Proceedings of the National Conference on Cardiopulmonary Resuscitation and Emergency Cardiac Care, Dallas, Texas, Feb 22-25, 1992, *Ann Emerg Med* 22:275, 1993.

36. Coplen SE, Antman EM, Berlin JA, et al: Efficacy and safety of quinidine therapy for maintenance of sinus rhythm after cardioversion: a meta-analysis of randomized control trials, *Circulation* 82:1106, 1990.

37. Flaker GC, Blackshear JL, McBride R, et al: Antiarrhythmic drug therapy and cardiac mortality in atrial fibrillation, *J Am Coll Cardiol* 20:527, 1992.

38. Echt DS, Lisbow PR, Mitchell B, et al: Mortality and morbidity in patients receiving encainide, flecainide or placebo: The Cardiac Arrhythmia Suppression Trial, *N Engl J Med* 324:781, 1991.

39. Horner SM: Efficacy of intravenous magnesium in acute myocardial infarction in reducing arrhythmias and mortality: meta-analysis of magnesium in acute myocardial infarction, *Circulation* 86:774, 1992.

40. Woods KL, Fletcher S, Roffe C, et al: Intravenous magnesium sulphate in suspected acute myocardial infarction: results of the second Leicester Intravenous Magnesium Intervention Trial (LIMIT-2), *Lancet* 339:1553, 1992.

41. ISIS Collaborative Group: Randomized study of intravenous magnesium in over 50,000 patients with suspected acute myocardial infarction, *Circulation* 88:I-292, 1993.

42. Haines DE, DiMarco JP: Current therapy for supraventricular tachycardia, *Curr Prob Cardiol* 17:8, 1992.

Chapter 50

VENTRICULAR ARRHYTHMIAS AFTER ACUTE MYOCARDIAL INFARCTION

Jodie L. Hurwitz
Eric N. Prystowsky

Ventricular arrhythmias commonly complicate acute myocardial infarction (AMI). The mechanisms, prognosis, and treatment options differ, depending on the clinical circumstances and the time of occurrence of the ventricular arrhythmias after the acute infarct event. The evaluation of post-MI ventricular arrhythmias can be separated conceptually and practically into three phases: *early in-hospital phase* (first 48 to 72 hours), the *late in-hospital phase* (72 hours to discharge), and the *out-of-hospital phase* (after hospital discharge). It should be noted that the prognostic demarcation time of early postinfarction ventricular arrhythmias at 48 to 72 hours is arbitrary, and the last 24 hours of this period is truly a gray zone.

EARLY IN-HOSPITAL PHASE (FIRST 48 TO 72 HOURS)

Ventricular arrhythmias that occur in the first 48 to 72 hours after AMI are usually considered to be a consequence of the pathophysiologic milieu of the AMI itself. They are frequently secondary to reversible causes such as ischemia, for example, during the acute phase of the MI or from reperfusion, or because of electrolyte abnormalities such as low potassium or magnesium.[1] These arrhythmias do not have the same adverse

long-term prognostic implications as similar arrhythmias that occur several days after an MI.

Ventricular fibrillation

Ventricular fibrillation (VF) and sustained rapid polymorphic ventricular tachycardia (PMVT-S) require immediate defibrillation. When these arrhythmias occur early after an MI, evaluation for recurrent ischemia should be performed. Prophylactic lidocaine therapy to prevent VF or PMVT-S within the first few days after infarction is controversial[2-4] (see Chapter 31). Its use has not been shown to decrease mortality and may cause substantial side effects if serum lidocaine levels are too high, or in certain patients, even with usual lidocaine levels. However, the psychologic trauma of undergoing defibrillation and "being brought back from the dead" can be substantial and can instill long-lasting fear in some patients. In our opinion prophylactic lidocaine use is optional, depending on physician preference. In patients who are hospitalized in acute care settings where physicians are not easily accessible (i.e., no on-call staff in the hospital) the prophylactic use of lidocaine is very reasonable. In patients who have an episode of VF or PMVT-S we recommend lidocaine for at least 24 hours, although no specific information is available concerning these patients. Importantly, prophylactic lidocaine therapy should be discontinued after 48 to 72 hours to allow telemetry monitoring of the patient's rhythm in the drug-free state for several days before hospital discharge.

Sustained monomorphic ventricular tachycardia

Few data are available about sustained monomorphic ventricular tachycardia (MVT-S) when it occurs within the first 2 to 3 days after AMI. Some consider it related to the acute ischemic event and recommend no long-term therapy.[5] We think that the occurrence of MVT-S even within the first 3 days after MI usually warrants further evaluation with electrophysiology testing before hospital discharge.[6-8] If MVT-S is inducible we recommend antiarrhythmic treatment guided by electrophysiology study. If sustained VT is not induced, no therapy is recommended.

Ventricular tachycardia is a wide QRS complex tachycardia that is by definition greater than 100 beats per minute. A sustained episode of ventricular tachycardia lasts 30 seconds or longer, or causes hemodynamic compromise in less than 30 seconds. There are several features that help differentiate ventricular from supraventricular tachycardia with aberrancy.[9] The diagnosis of ventricular tachycardia can be made relatively reliably when at least one of the following is present: AV dissociation, fusion beats, QRS duration > 140 ms (RBBB) or > 160 ms (LBBB), far right axis, and positive or negative QRS concordance across the precordial leads.

The initial treatment of MVT-S depends on the symptoms it causes. If the patient has substantial hemodynamic compromise or clear evidence of ongoing ischemia, emergency electrical cardioversion is recommended. Successful termination of ventricular tachycardia can usually be accomplished with direct current shocks of 20 to 50 watts per second. If the sustained ventricular tachycardia does not cause significant hemodynamic effects, or ischemia, we suggest administration of intravenous procainamide to terminate ventricular tachycardia. In our experience lidocaine is not as effective as procainamide for this purpose. Procainamide is given at 50mg/min to a dose of 10 to 14 mg/kg, with blood pressure monitoring (see Chapter 39). Electrical cardioversion will be needed if drugs fail to convert ventricular tachycardia.

All antiarrhythmic medications should be discontinued several days before electrophysiology study. If ventricular tachycardia recurs in the absence of medication but before the electrophysiology study, then initiation of a treatment protocol becomes necessary (see below). The electrophysiology study is performed to determine if the patient has inducible sustained ventricular tachycardia. We prefer to study patients at least

7 days post MI. In some patients it may not be possible to perform an electrophysiology study in the drug-free state because of frequent recurrent ventricular tachycardia; suppressive therapy is obviously needed in this situation.

Whenever possible a 12-lead electrocardiogram of the patient's spontaneous ventricular tachycardia should be obtained. This can usually be performed, even if a patient's hemodynamic status is marginal. Evaluation of the 12-lead electrocardiogram at the bedside is invaluable in making the diagnosis of ventricular tachycardia vis-a-vis the criteria listed above. The 12-lead electrocardiogram allows confirmation that the ventricular tachycardia induced during the electrophysiology study represents the clinical arrhythmia.

Nonsustained ventricular tachycardia

Nonsustained ventricular tachycardia is not necessarily a harbinger of more serious ventricular arrhythmias. When the patient is mildly symptomatic, which usually means the patient has palpitations, reassurance rather than antiarrhythmic medication is recommended. In those patients with frequent episodes of nonsustained ventricular tachycardia or in whom reassurance is not adequate treatment for symptoms, short-term treatment (24 to 48 hours) with intravenous procainamide or lidocaine can be given. Postinfarction patients with nonsustained ventricular tachycardia occurring only in the first 72 hours do not need further evaluation with electrophysiology study or Holter monitoring. It is very important that antiarrhythmic medication be discontinued several days before hospital discharge in order to assess adequately the patient's rhythm in the absence of drugs.

Asymptomatic ventricular arrhythmias

Previously it was thought that many types of nonsustained ventricular arrhythmias (VA) in the early postinfarction period were markers for high risk of future sustained ventricular arrhythmias, and that suppressing them would lower the future risk. Thus, frequent premature ventricular complexes (PVCs), pairs, and R on T PVCs were considered warning arrhythmias, and some recommended the use of antiarrhythmic medication in order to suppress them.[10] We recommend no treatment for these arrhythmias. The Cardiac Arrhythmia Suppression Trial (CAST) investigated whether suppression of asymptomatic or mildly symptomatic VAs with IC antiarrhythmic agents would decrease mortality.[11,12] In this study 1498 postinfarction patients in whom ventricular ectopy could be suppressed with encainide, flecainide, or moricizine were prospectively randomized to receive drug or placebo. Seven hundred and fifty-five patients were randomized to receive drug, and 743 patients were randomized to receive placebo.

Part of the study was stopped early, after about 2 years, when it became apparent after a mean follow-up of 10 months that there was a higher mortality in the group receiving encainide or flecainide (43 deaths), compared with the placebo group (16 deaths, $P = 0.0004$). This significant difference in mortality held true regardless of the demographics of the patients. There were no differences between the two groups in the incidence of nonlethal disqualifying ventricular tachycardia, recognized proarrhythmia requiring discontinuation of the drug, syncope, need for pacemaker placement, congestive heart failure, recurrent MI or angina, or coronary artery bypass grafting or angioplasty.

CAST II continued for about 2 more years using moricizine vs. placebo, but this was also stopped early.[13] Of note, the patients treated with moricizine had a higher mortality rate than the placebo group in the first 14 days of therapy, and overall there was no significant difference in mortality. Thus it was discovered that suppression of asymptomatic ventricular arrhythmias after MI with encainide, flecainide, or moricizine increased rather than decreased mortality. In our opinion the results of CAST and CAST II are applicable to patients in the in-hospital and out-of-hospital phases after MI.[14,15] Thus, regardless of the postMI phase a patient is in, we recommend no treatment for asymptomatic PVCs.

Accelerated idioventricular rhythm (AIVR) is a slow ventricular tachycardia that can occur post MI. It is a wide complex arrhythmia that is by definition less than 100 beats per minute. It is ventricular in origin and therefore satisfies many of the criteria for ventricular tachycardia; it often looks identical to the previously discussed VT except that the rate is slower. This is often an escape arrhythmia during a period of time when the SA node and AV node are ischemic and not functioning appropriately. AIVR is usually asymptomatic and rarely needs treatment; it rarely occurs after the first 48 hours of the AMI.

LATE IN-HOSPITAL PHASE (72 HOURS TO HOSPITAL DISCHARGE)
Ventricular fibrillation

When ventricular fibrillation occurs in a postMI hospitalized patient more than 3 days after the infarction, recurrent ischemia should be considered. Reinfarction with extension or expansion needs to be ruled out with serial cardiac enzymes and electrocardiograms. Consideration for urgent cardiac catheterization should be given to patients with late ventricular fibrillation in whom recurrent ischemia can be documented. Electrolyte abnormalities (such as low potassium or magnesium) or proarrhythmia caused by drugs (such as antiarrhythmic drugs or adrenergic agonists) may also play a significant but usually very small role in initiating the arrhythmia. Unless acute ischemia is documented or significant electrolyte imbalances or other reversible problems are obvious, these patients should be considered at risk for recurrent ventricular fibrillation and an electrophysiology study recommended. Long-term treatment may include drugs or nonpharmacologic approaches, (e.g. implantable defibrillators). In general we prefer an implantable cardioverter defibrillator if the patient has a left ventricular ejection fraction of $<30\%$.[16]

Prophylactic intravenous lidocaine or procainamide may be used until the electrophysiology study is performed after direct current cardioversion is used to treat the immediate arrhythmia. These antiarrhythmic medications should be discontinued at least 5 half-lives before the electrophysiology study.

Sustained ventricular tachycardia

When sustained monomorphic ventricular tachycardia occurs several days postinfarction, it is an indication for further electrophysiologic evaluation. If the sustained ventricular tachycardia causes hemodynamic collapse, then immediate electrical cardioversion is necessary. If the patient is hemodynamically stable, treatment with intravenous procainamide as an initial choice, or lidocaine as a second choice can be used. Electrolyte status should be checked, although hypokalemia or hypomagnesemia are almost never the cause of recurrent monomorphic ventricular tachycardia. Five to seven days postinfarction is an appropriate time to consider electrophysiology study, which should be performed before hospital discharge. When sustained monomorphic ventricular tachycardia has been reproducibly initiated and terminated in the electrophysiology laboratory, several treatment options are available, such as surgery, antiarrhythmic drugs, or implantable cardioverter-defibrillator.[17,18]

Surgery. There are several indications for coronary artery bypass surgery in a postinfarction patient. When bypass surgery is being contemplated in a patient with sustained ventricular tachycardia, the prospects of performing electrophysiology-guided resection should also be considered.[19] Those patients who may be ideal candidates for resection have a left ventricular aneurysm and a single morphology of sustained ventricular tachycardia.[20] At baseline, electrophysiology study localization of the site of origin of the ventricular tachycardia can be accomplished using various mapping techniques. In the operating room the site of origin of the ventricular tachycardia is again determined and the subendocardial area(s) are resected. Repeat electrophysiology testing postsurgery should always be performed. If sustained ventricular tachycardia is still inducible after surgery, antiarrhythmic drugs or implantation of cardioverter-defibrillator can be chosen.

Antiarrhythmic drugs. If a patient does not require bypass surgery, initial treatment in most patients for inducible sustained monomorphic ventricular tachycardia should be with antiarrhythmic medication and repeat electrophysiology studies.[21] The initial drug choice depends on several factors (e.g., history of congestive heart failure) and should be individualized. The goal is to provide effective therapy with the fewest side effects to the patient.[22] As such, procainamide is often unsuitable orally because of its frequent long-term side effects, including systemic lupus erythematosus. Quinidine is often our initial drug, although sotalol and, in selected patients, disopyramide can be given.[23] If sustained hemodynamically unstable ventricular tachycardia is initiated at repeat electrophysiology study during drug therapy, treatment with a different antiarrhythmic agent is warranted. Other agents include propafenone or combination treatment with quinidine or disopyramide plus mexiletine. Propafenone has a variable half-life, depending on its degree of metabolism, but should reach steady state after about 3 days on a specific dose. We use a slightly more aggressive dosing schedule than is recommended in the package insert. We begin with a dose of 150 mg TID and increase this to 225 mg TID after 1 to 2 days. The patients can either undergo electrophysiology study after 2 to 3 days of 225 mg TID, or they can have the medication increased to 300 mg TID and be studied 3 days after this dose is initiated.

Sotalol is now approved and fared well in the recently published ESVEM trial.[24] Although the data showed that sotalol can prevent induction of VT in up to 40% of patients, the patient population studied was very specific and small. Entry criteria into ESVEM included documentation of substantial amounts of spontaneous ventricular arrhythmias as well as inducible VT-S with electrophysiology study. Importantly and inexplicably there was nearly a 33% 1-year arrhythmia recurrence rate in patients who were considered to have been controlled. We initiate treatment with 80 mg of sotalol twice a day, increasing the dosage relatively quickly in patients who can tolerate it. We usually give a patient one to two doses of 80 mg in the first 12 to 24 hours of treatment. If there is no symptomatic bradycardia or prolongation of the QT interval to ≥ 520 ms, we increase the dose to 120 mg twice a day and then to 160 mg BID. Electrophysiology testing should be performed when the patient is at a steady-state dose of approximately 320 to 480 mg a day.

Should inducible hemodynamically unstable ventricular tachycardia still be present after two or more drug trials, amiodarone, primary VT surgery, or implantation of a cardioverter-defibrillator should be considered. The latter option is becoming more desirable with the newer nonthoracotomy lead defibrillator systems. Amiodarone is recommended for those patients with sustained ventricular tachycardia who are not candidates for EPS or ICD.

Implantable cardioverter-defibrillator. Patients with spontaneous sustained ventricular tachycardia without sustained ventricular tachycardia induced at electrophysiology study, or patients with ventricular fibrillation and no sustained ventricular arrhythmias at electrophysiology study are candidates for implantation of a cardioverter-defibrillator as initial treatment.[25,26]

Newer models of implantable defibrillators (third-generation devices) available now have several therapy options, including antitachycardia pacing capability, which is often successful in terminating sustained ventricular tachycardia. Antitachycardia pacing algorithms are evaluated in the electrophysiology laboratory before the device is implanted and before the patient is discharged from hospital in order to enhance the chances for successful termination of a spontaneous recurrence of the arrhythmia. Even when termination of the ventricular tachycardia by pacing is reproducible, it is possible to accelerate the ventricular tachycardia with pacing to a hemodynamically unstable rhythm; therefore back-up defibrillator therapy is always programmed.

It is important to remember that ICDs will not prevent arrhythmias, only treat them when they occur. Therefore it is necessary at times to continue an antiarrhythmic medication after device implantation for several reasons. These may be to decrease the frequency of either nonsustained or sustained supraventricular and ventricular arrhythmias, to slow the rate of ventricular tachycardia to prevent syncope before therapy is given, or to enhance the chance for antitachycardia pacing success.

Nonsustained ventricular tachycardia

If nonsustained ventricular tachycardia occurs after the first 72 hours, patients should be separated into relatively low-risk and high-risk groups. The relative risk of sudden cardiac death is high in a patient with nonsustained ventricular tachycardia and a left ventricular ejection fraction of $\leq 40\%$. A positive signal averaged ECG (SAECG) may also be predictive of subsequent ventricular tachyarrhythmias, and is thought to represent an area of slow conduction in the ventricle, one of the prerequisites for reentrant ventricular tachycardia.[27-29] In a study by Kuchar et al.[30] patients with a left ventricular ejection fraction of $<40\%$ and a positive SAECG were at high risk for sudden cardiac death.

The proper treatment for post-MI patients who have nonsustained ventricular tachycardia and a decreased left ventricular ejection fraction is presently unknown. Several clinical trials are currently examining the major therapeutic options for these patients. The Multicenter Unsustained Tachycardia Trial (MUSTT)[31] is enrolling patients with documented coronary artery disease, left ventricular ejection fraction of 40% or less, and nonsustained ventricular tachycardia documented 5 days or more postinfarction. The patients undergo electrophysiology study, and if sustained VT is initiated, they are randomized into a drug treatment group or to a "no therapy" group. The drug treatment group includes initial treatment with an IA agent, sotalol, or propafenone. Further treatment can include other drugs, including amiodarone, or cardioverter-defibrillator implantation. All patients, including those who are noninducible (and therefore not treated) are followed prospectively. Signal-averaged electrocardiograms are also being obtained in these patients to help determine the sensitivity, specificity, and predictive accuracy of positive SAECG for the occurrence of future sustained ventricular arrhythmias.

The Multicenter Automatic Defibrillator Implantation Trial (MADIT)[32] includes patients with documented coronary artery disease, at least 1 month post MI, left ventricular ejection fraction less than or equal to 35%, and nonsustained ventricular tachycardia. Those patients who have inducible ventricular tachyarrhythmias that are not suppressible with IV procainamide are randomized to receive conventional pharmacologic therapy or an implantable cardioverter-defibrillator.

These large-scale clinical trials should improve our understanding of which patients, if any, with nonsustained ventricular tachycardia require treatment to prevent sudden cardiac death or decrease mortality.

There are several large studies evaluating the use of prophylactic amiodarone post MI.[33-35] One recent double-blind placebo-controlled study compared amiodarone with placebo therapy in patients after recent MI who could not receive beta blockers.[33] Three hundred and five patients received amiodarone, and 308 received placebo. There were 33 deaths in the placebo group and 21 deaths in the patients receiving amiodarone. All 33 deaths in the placebo group occurred secondary to cardiac causes, whereas 19 of the 21 deaths in the patients receiving amiodarone occurred secondary to cardiac causes. There was a significant decrease in Lown grade 4 (couplets or salvos) ventricular arrhythmias in the amiodarone group. Side effects, however, were significantly more frequent in the amiodarone group (30% vs. 10%).

The Basel Antiarrhythmic Study of Infarct Survival (BASIS) randomized post-MI patients who had asymptomatic complex ventricular ectopic activity on 24-hour electrocardiographic recording before hospital discharge into groups treated with antiarrhythmic therapy ($N = 100$), low-dose amiodarone therapy ($N = 98$), or no antiarrhythmic therapy ($N = 114$).[34] There were 27 cardiac deaths and 3 noncardiac deaths during the 1-year followup. The cumulative mortality rates at 12 months

were 13% in the control group, 10% in the individualized therapy group, and 5% in the amiodarone treatment group. The problems with this study were the use of only short-term electrocardiographic monitoring periods, the concomitant uses of beta blockers in some of the patients, and the nonblinded format. Of interest is the results of a continuation of this trial with longer-term followup of the amiodarone-treated group and the control group.[35] For the total followup period (55 to 125 months) both total mortality as well as cardiac death remained significantly lower in the group that received amiodarone as compared with the control group.

There are several ongoing multicenter trials evaluating the use of amiodarone in the post-MI population, including the Canadian Amiodarone Myocardial Infarction Arrhythmias Trial (CAMIAT) and the European Myocardial Infarction Amiodarone Trial (EMIAT). We reserve judgment concerning prophylactic amiodarone use in this patient population until the outcome of these studies is known.

OUT-OF-HOSPITAL PHASE (AFTER DISCHARGE)
Ventricular fibrillation and sustained ventricular tachycardia

If ventricular fibrillation or sustained polymorphic ventricular tachycardia occur after hospital discharge, the evaluation and treatment are the same as if these arrhythmias occurred during the late MI in-hospital phase. Recurrent infarction or ischemia should be considered first. If a diagnosis of recurrent ischemia cannot be made, subsequent evaluation should include electrophysiology study. Treatment would include pharmacologic agents or nonpharmacologic approaches such as the implantable cardioverter-defibrillator, depending on the outcome of electrophysiology testing and the degree of left ventricular (LV) dysfunction. Intravenous antiarrhythmic drug prophylaxis once the patient is hospitalized is usually not necessary.

If sustained monomorphic ventricular tachycardia occurs during the late post-MI period, it is recommended that the patient undergo electrophysiology testing and treatment as previously recommended. The three treatment options of surgery, pharmacology, and device implantation all still apply. Tests should be performed to evaluate the patient for ischemia, and its presence may suggest one method of treatment over another, such as surgery and subendocardial resection.

Premature ventricular complexes and nonsustained ventricular tachycardia

Symptomatic nonsustained ventricular tachycardia in the late post-MI period can be classified according to the degree of accompanying symptoms: minor symptoms, (e.g., palpitations) and potentially serious symptoms, (e.g., presyncope). For minor symptoms we rely on reassurance and try to avoid specific antiarrhythmic therapy unless they are very bothersome; an increase in the dose of beta-blocker therapy would be our first-line treatment. If more severe symptoms such as presyncope are present, we recommend electrophysiology evaluation to determine whether a more serious arrhythmia, (e.g., sustained ventricular tachycardia), is inducible; if so, the patient should receive treatment for the sustained ventricular tachycardia.

There is a group of patients with asymptomatic nonsustained ventricular tachycardia who appear to be at low risk for serious future arrhythmic events. These are patients with coronary artery disease with a left ventricular ejection fraction of > 40%. We recommend no treatment for these patients. There is also little clinical evidence that currently supports treating patients with nonsustained ventricular tachycardia and left ventricular ejection fraction of < 40%. Our own approach to these patients is to enter them, when possible, into one of the prospective ongoing trials in this area as previously discussed.

Although we have divided the post-MI period into three arbitrary time phases according to the timing of the ventricular arrhythmias after the AMI, there are some general guidelines that apply to all three.

Hemodynamically significant arrhythmias should be treated with electrical cardioversion, whereas sustained hemodynamically tolerated arrhythmias can be treated with IV medication, such as procainamide. Whenever ventricular fibrillation occurs, ischemia should be at the top of the differential diagnosis list. The occurrence of sustained monomorphic ventricular tachycardia mandates further testing, preferably with electrophysiology studies. Only about 30% to 40% of these patients will be successfully treated with medication, and the rest will require nonpharmacologic treatment, such as an implantable cardioverter-defibrillator. If nonsustained ventricular tachycardia occurs less than 5 days post MI, we recommend repeat Holter evaluation 5 days after the MI. If nonsustained ventricular tachycardia occurs 5 days or more post MI in a patient with a depressed (≤40%) left ventricular ejection fraction, individual clinical judgment must suffice until the results of the major multicenter nonsustained ventricular tachycardia trials are available. Enrollment of these patients into these trials should be considered whenever possible. Whenever possible, specific therapy to suppress PVCs should be avoided.

REFERENCES

1. Kloner RA: Does reperfusion injury exist in humans? *J Am Coll Cardiol* 21:537-545, 1993.
2. Hine IK, Laird N, Hewitt P, et al: Meta-analytic evidence against prophylactic use of lidocaine in acute myocardial infarction, *Arch Intern Med* 149 (12):2694-2698, 1989.
3. Nattel S, Arenal A: Antiarrhythmic prophylaxis after acute myocardial infarction. Is lidocaine still useful? *Drugs* 45(1):9-14, 1993.
4. MacMahon S, Collins R, Peto R, et al: Effects of prophylactic lidocaine in suspected acute myocardial infarction. *JAMA* 260: 1910-1916, 1988.
5. Eldar M, Sievner Z, Goldbourt U, et al: Primary ventricular tachycardia in acute myocardial infarction: clinical characteristics and mortality, *Ann Intern Med* 117:31-36, 1992.
6. Welch WJ, Blackwell WH, Whitlock RA, et al: Sustained monomorphic ventricular tachycardia with acute myocardial infarction, *Circulation* 78:4; II-236, 1988.
7. Pogwizd SM, Corr PB: Mechanisms underlying the development of ventricular fibrillation during early myocardial ischemia, *Circ Res* 66:672-695, 1990.
8. Waldo AL, Henthorn RW, Carlson MD: A perspective on ventricular arrhythmias: patient assessment for therapy and outcome, *Am J Cardiol* 65:30B-35B, 1990.
9. Ahktar M, Shenasa M, Jasayeri M: Wide QRS complex tachycardia: reappraisal of a common clinical problem, *Ann Intern Med* 109:905-912, 1988.
10. Lown B, Wolf M: Approaches to sudden death from coronary artery disease, *Circulation* 44:330-342, 1971.
11. The Cardiac Arrhythmia Suppression Trial Investigators: Preliminary report: effect of encainide and flecainide on mortality in a randomized trial of arrhythmia suppression after myocardial infarction, *N Engl J Med* 321:406-412, 1989.
12. Echt DS, Liebson PR, Mitchell LB, et al and the CAST Investigators: Mortality and morbidity in patients receiving encainide, flecainide or placebo, *N Eng J Med* 324:782-788, 1991.
13. The Cardiac Arrhythmia Suppression Trial II Investigators: Effect of the antiarrhythmic agent moricizine on survival after myocardial infarction, *N Engl J Med* 327(4):227-233, 1992.
14. Hine LK, Laird NM, Pegttewilit MS, et al: Meta-analysis of empirical long-term antiarrhythmic trials after myocardial infarction, *JAMA* 262:3037-3040, 1989.
15. Teo KK, Yusuf S, Furberg CD: Effects of prophylactic antiarrhythmic drug therapy in acute myocardial infarction, *JAMA* 270:1589-1595, 1993.
16. Knilans TK, Prystowsky EN: Antiarrhythmic drug therapy in management of cardiac arrest survivors, *Circulation* 85(suppl I): I-118-I-124, 1992.
17. DiMarco JP, Lerman BB, Kron IL, et al: Sustained ventricular tachyarrhythmias within 2 months of acute myocardial infarction: results of medical and surgical therapy in patients resuscitated from the initial episode, *J Am Coll Cardiol* 6:759-768, 1985.
18. Brugada P, Andries EW: Early postmyocardial infarction ventricular arrhythmias. In Albert Brest (ed): *Cardiovascular Clinics*, Philadelphia, 1992, FA Davis.
19. Hargrove WC, Miller JM: Risk stratification and management of patients with recurrent ventricular tachycardia and other malignant ventricular arrhythmias, *Circulation* 79(suppl I): I-178-I-181, 1989.
20. Miller JM, Kienzle MG, Harken AH, et al: Subendocardial resection for ventricular tachycardia: predictors of surgical success, *Circulation* 70:624-631, 1984.
21. Wyse DG: Pharmacologic therapy in patients with ventricular tachyarrhythmias, *Cardiol Clin* 11(1):65-83, 1993.
22. Vaughan-Williams EM: Classification of antiarrhythmic drugs. In Sandoe E, Flensted-Jensen E, Olsen KH, (eds): *Symposium on cardiac arrhythmias,* Södertälje, Sweden, 1970, AB Astra.
23. Mason JW: Comparison of electrophysiologic testing with Holter monitoring to predict antiarrhythmic-drug efficacy for ventricular tacharrhythmias, *N Engl J Med* 329(7):445-451, 1993.
24. Mason JW Comparison of seven antiarrhythmic drugs in patients with ventricular tachyarrhythmias, *N Eng J Med* 329:452-458, 1993.

25. Kutalek SP, Dreifus LS: Implantable cardioverter-defibrillators, *Adv Intern Med* 38:421-438, 1993.
26. Capucci A, Boriani G: Drugs, surgery, cardioverter defibrillator: a decision based on the clinical problem, *PACE* 16(II):519-526, 1993.
27. Simson MB: Use of signals in the terminal QRS complex to identify patients with ventricular tachycardia after myocardial infarction, *Circulation* 64(2):235-242, 1981.
28. Vatterott PJ, Hammill SC, Bailey KR, et al: Signal-averaged electrocardiography: a new noninvasive test to identify patients at risk for ventricular arrhythmias, *Mayo Clin Proc* 63:931-942, 1988.
29. Cain ME: Predicting sustained VT by ECG signal averaging, *Cardiology* 54-58, 1986.
30. Kuchar DL, Thorburn CW, Sammel NL: Signal-averaged electrocardiogram for evaluation of recurrent syncope, *Am J Cardiol* 58:949-953, 1986.
31. Buxton AE, Fisher JD, Josephson ME, et al: Prevention of sudden death in patients with coronary artery disease: the multicenter unsustained tachycardia trial (MUSTT), *Prog Cardiovascular Dis* XXXVI(3):215-226, 1993.
32. Multicenter Automatic Defibrillator Implantation Trial (MADIT): Design and clinical protocol, *PACE* 14:633-635, 1991.
33. Ceremuzynski L, Kleczar E, Krzeminska-Pakula M, et al: Effect of amiodarone on mortality after myocardial infarction: a double-blind, placebo-controlled, pilot study, *J Am Coll Cardiol* 20:1056-1062, 1992.
34. Burkart F, Pfisterer M, Kiowski W, et al: Effect of antiarrhythmic therapy on mortality in survivors of myocardial infarction with asymptomatic complex ventricular arrhythmias: Basel antiarrhythmic study of infarct survival, *J Am Coll Cardiol* 16:1711-1718, 1990.
35. Pfisterer M, Kiowski W, Brunner H, et al: Long-term benefit of 1-year amiodarone treatment for persistent complex ventricular arrhythmias after myocardial infarction, *Circulation* 87:309-311, 1993.

Chapter 51

EXTRACRANIAL HEMORRHAGIC COMPLICATIONS OF THROMBOLYTIC THERAPY

David C. Sane

One of the many important lessons learned from the trials of thrombolytic therapy for acute myocardial infarction (AMI) is that the hemostatic system is quite resilient and usually effective despite the use of numerous drugs and interventions that interfere with its function. Combinations of plasminogen activators, aspirin, and heparin are routinely administered to critically ill patients with usually mild and acceptable hemorrhagic complications. Even more aggressive regimens of antiplatelet agents such as glycoprotein IIb/IIIa antagonists and potent antithrombins such as hirudin are currently being investigated as adjunctive therapy during thrombolysis. These strategies will challenge the hemostatic system even more and will undoubtedly lead to a further appreciation of the fact that hemostasis can be both friend and foe. Greater success at reducing thrombotic complications such as reocclusion will likely be accompanied by higher bleeding rates.

Despite the usual resilience of the hemostatic system, occasional dramatic failures such as intracranial hemorrhage or massive gastrointestinal bleeding occur, reminding the physician that hemorrhage is the principal complication of thrombolytic therapy. This chapter reviews the patient characteristics and hematologic factors that contribute to increased systemic bleeding risk and makes recommendations for the management of hemorrhagic events. Because the management, outcome, and etiologic factors of intracranial hemorrhage differ from systemic bleeding, this topic is covered in a separate chapter. For a thorough discussion of hemorrhage during thrombolytic therapy, the reader is referred to several recent reviews.[1-5]

ASSESSING THE PATIENT BEFORE THROMBOLYTIC THERAPY

It is of primary importance to ascertain that the patient is experiencing an AMI before administering a plasminogen activator. Several case reports have detailed adverse outcomes when patients with pericarditis or aortic dissection were treated for mistaken diagnosis of AMI.[6-8] In the Anglo-Scandinavian Study of Early Thrombolysis (ASSET) study, in which ST-segment elevation was not required as an entry criterion, 13 out of 5005 (0.26%) patients had a final diagnosis of acute aortic dissection.[9] In the Thrombolysis and Angioplasty in Myocardial Infarction (TAMI) studies, 20 out of 1387 (1.4%) patients did not have a final diagnosis of AMI.[10] The requirement for ST-segment elevation in at least two contiguous leads on the electrocardiogram (ECG) will reduce the risk of adverse outcome because of inappropriate treatment of acute aortic dissection.

RELATIVE CONTRAINDICATIONS

Several placebo-controlled studies have demonstrated that thrombolytic therapy reduces 30-day mortality by approximately 25%, whereas less than 0.1% of patients will experience fatal extracranial hemorrhage. Despite this perspective, it is often difficult for the physician to decide whether to exclude a patient with one or more relative contraindications from the benefits of thrombolytic therapy. A majority of patients admitted to the community hospital with an AMI will have one or more relative contraindications or other exclusion criteria.[11] The mortality rate among these ineligible patients has been reported to be fivefold higher than patients treated with thrombolytic therapy.[11] Therefore, for the majority of patients with relative contraindications, withholding therapy carries a higher mortality. On the other hand, greater morbidity and mortality are suspected but not proved to be associated with treatment of subsets of patients with one or more relative contraindications. The physician's task is to discriminate the small number of patients for whom treatment represents an excessive risk. Unfortunately, this decision must be made within minutes without the aid of a substantial clinical database on this subject.

Cardiopulmonary resuscitation (CPR) has traditionally been listed as a relative contraindication to thrombolytic therapy, but patients requiring less that 10 minutes of compressions do not have significantly increased risk of hemorrhage.[12] A case of fatal intrathoracic hemorrhage was reported in a patient with CPR complicated by rib fractures,[13] however, so strict vigilance is warranted in these patients. Current warfarin sodium (Coumadin) administration is a relative contraindication and was noted to increase intracranial hemorrhage in one study.[14] In the TAMI studies, thrombolytic therapy was administered to seven patients under current warfarin treatment. The prothrombin time (PT) was mildly prolonged (13.0–15.7 seconds; ratio 1.1-1.4) at the time of therapy. One patient experienced an extensive hematoma resulting from placement of an internal jugular catheter. This access site was necessary because the patient had an inferior vena cava filter for history of deep venous thrombosis and pulmonary embolism. No other unusual bleeding complications were noted in these patients. At present, we believe that mild prolongation (≤3 seconds) of the PT by warfarin is an acceptable risk for patients with a strong indication for thrombolytic therapy, if primary angioplasty is not readily available. There is virtually no information on hemorrhage in diabetics with retinal disease, and we currently do not exclude these patients from thrombolysis. Recent cataract surgery predisposes to hyphema, but this is usually well tolerated.[15,16]

PATIENT CHARACTERISTICS CONTRIBUTING TO HEMORRHAGE

Low body weight (<70 kg), female gender, older age, history of hypertension, and physical signs of cardiac decompensation have been associated with increased bleeding risk.[17,18] The use of weight-adjusted dosing regimens for tissue-type plasminogen activator (t-PA) in patients less than 70 kg may reduce bleeding.[19] The association of high t-PA antigen levels with hemorrhage[18,20] may result in part from weight-independent dosing. Elderly patients appear to have a higher bleeding complication rate than younger patients.[17,21] Because most studies also demonstrate a greater reduction in absolute mortality rate in elderly than younger patients,[22] age itself should not be a contraindication to thrombolysis.[23]

The presence of comorbid medical conditions and a poor performance status increases the risk of hemorrhage during anticoagulation with heparin and warfarin.[24] Although patients with multiple medical problems have not been studied in depth, it is likely that they also have increased bleeding risks during thrombolytic therapy.

INCIDENCE OF SYSTEMIC HEMORRHAGE

The reported rates of systemic hemorrhage vary dramatically in the literature. In general, rates are lower in large trials in which mortality is the primary endpoint and secondary endpoints are not examined as closely. The criteria for major and minor bleeds vary considerably between studies. Also, not all studies have classified a drop in hematocrit without transfusion or a detectable bleeding site as a hemorrhagic outcome.

In a 1989 review of the literature, Fennerty et al.[3] reported that the incidence of major hemorrhage with streptokinase was 15% in invasive studies vs. only 0.8% in noninvasive studies. For trials with t-PA, the average rate of major bleeding was 12.7% (invasive) vs. 4% (one noninvasive study). The rates of fatal hemorrhage were 0.04% vs. 0.1% for streptokinase and recombinant t-PA (rt-PA), respectively.

SITES OF HEMORRHAGE

The major sites of extracranial hemorrhage are listed in Table 51-1. When thrombolysis is followed by invasive procedures, up to 45% of patients will develop significant groin hematomas at the access site. In the TAMI-I study, 4% of patients needed repair of the femoral arterial access site to control bleeding.[17] Recent studies using color-flow Doppler have demonstrated a significant prevalence of pseudoaneurysms among patients with large periaccess hematomas. Careful placement of arterial clamps using color-flow Doppler as a guide can result in successful closure of these pseudoaneurysms. A recent study comparing the Sones vs. Judkins ap-

Table 51-1. Frequency of extracranial hemorrhage by site

	%
Catheterization site hematoma	25-45
Other puncture sites	1-5
Gastrointestinal	4-10
Genitourinary	1-5
Retroperitoneal	≤1
Epistaxis	≤1
Unknown site	≤5

proaches for emergency cardiac catheterization during thrombolytic therapy has demonstrated a reduction in the need for vascular repair with the brachial approach (1% vs. 3%).[25] If intervention is delayed, the most common site of detectable bleeding is from the gastrointestinal tract, the majority of which is occult blood loss.

Retroperitoneal hemorrhage occurs in up to 1% of patients. Patients with femoral arterial or venous punctures above the inguinal ligament are at increased risk for retroperitoneal hemorrhage,[26] but this complication may rarely occur spontaneously during thrombolysis without invasive procedures or in patients with cardiac catheterizations performed by the brachial approach.[25] The first sign is usually hypotension with variable abdominal tenderness. Computed tomography is usually necessary for diagnosis.

Epistaxis may occur spontaneously in 1% of patients or may be precipitated by nasal intubations. If intubation is necessary, the oral route with direct visualization is strongly preferred in the patient who has recently received thrombolytic therapy.

OTHER BLEEDING SITES

Rarely hemorrhage occurs at other sites. Several cases of spontaneous hemorrhagic pericardial effusion have been reported.[27-30] These appear to occur in patients with extensive MI complicated by postinfarction pericarditis. In one retrospective study, 1% of patients treated with thrombolytic therapy for AMI developed hemorrhagic pericardial effusions, causing tamponade physiology.[27] In a small prospective study, echocardiograms performed in 52 patients enrolled in TAMI-1 documented a 24% (10/42) incidence of pericardial effusions at day 6 after t-PA.[31] Only one of these (10%) was classified as a large effusion, and no patients developed echocardiographic or hemodynamic signs of tamponade.[31] Myocardial hemorrhage is exacerbated by thrombolytic therapy and may increase the risk of myocardial rupture if extensive bland necrosis is already present.[32] Localized hemorrhage has been reported in the iliopsoas muscle,[33] spleen,[34] breast,[35] and joints.[36,37] A case of hemospermia[38] has also been reported.

BLOOD LOSS WITHOUT IDENTIFIED SITE

In the TIMI-II study, 7.8% of the invasive strategy group and 6.2% of the conservative group had declines in hemoglobin between 40 and 50 g/L without identified bleeding site.[18] This blood loss is accounted for in studies using a bleeding index (units transfused + Δ hematocrit/ 3); bleeding at cryptic sites such as the retroperitoneum and thoracic cavity should be excluded by computed tomography in these cases.

IATROGENIC LOSS

Patients in intensive care units may have more than 40 ml of blood drawn daily for diagnostic tests. Patients with arterial lines have more blood drawn than those without arterial lines. This iatrogenic blood loss contributes to transfusion requirements.[39]

INVASIVE PROCEDURES AND HEMORRHAGE

Most postthrombolysis bleeding (70%) occurs at the catheterization site. "Conservative" or "delayed" angiography strategies have been reported to reduce hemorrhagic complications.[18] As expected, the early use of cardiopulmonary bypass after failed thrombolysis and PCTA increase bleeding.[40-42] If delayed until 3 to 5 days after thrombolytic therapy, coronary artery bypass grafting (CABG) can be performed with no excess hemorrhage compared with elective cases.[43,44]

The use of intraaortic balloon counterpulsation (IABP) requires heparin anticoagulation, as well as insertion of a large-bore arterial catheter. In a recent series of patients requiring IABP, a mean decrease in hematocrit of 17% ± 7% was reported vs. 12% ± 5% when IABP was not used.[45]

COAGULATION PARAMETERS AND HEMORRHAGE

Several studies have shown weak but significant correlation between levels of coagulation parameters and hemorrhagic risk,[17,18,20,46] especially for therapy with rt-PA (Table 51-2). Low nadir fibrinogen (<1 g/L) at 5 hours after therapy has been associated with increased bleeding risk. This association is understandable given the crucial role that fibrinogen serves as the precursor of fibrin and as the "bridge" between activated platelets. Elevated fibrinogen degradation product levels (FDP) at 5 hours have also been linked to increased hemorrhage. The rise in FDP levels is significant not only because it reflects fibrinogen depletion but also because of the unique anticoagulant and antiplatelet effects of these compounds. FDPs interfere with fibrin polymerization, block fibrinogen binding to platelets, and serve as a site for systemic generation of plasmin.[47] Thus, the generation of FDPs contributes to the lack of fibrin specificity of t-PA and enhances fibrinogenolysis. Elevated t-PA antigen levels have been associated with increased bleeding. It is important to note that the mean peak t-PA level at a 100-mg dose is about half that at a 150-mg dose.[18] This finding is consistent with a saturable clearance mechanism and supports weight-adjusted dosing in lighter patients. Prolongation of the activated thromboplastin time (aPTT) greater than 90 seconds has recently been reported as a risk for hemorrhage, pointing to the need for close scrutiny of adjuvant heparin anticoagulant therapy.[18] Platelet function[48] and number have also been established as important factors in the bleeding risk profile. The same coagulation profile that is associated with excess hemorrhage may also contribute to improved clinical outcome, however. Optimal anticoagulation with heparin appears to reduce the incidence of coronary rethrombosis,[49] again pointing to

Table 51-2. Patient characteristics, procedures, and laboratory findings associated with increased risk of hemorrhage*

Patient characteristics
  Low body weight (< 70 kg)
  Female gender
  Older age
  History of hypertension
  Physical signs of cardiac decompensation

Procedures
  Coronary artery bypass grafting
  Early angioplasty
  Intra aortic balloon pump insertion

Laboratory findings
  Low fibrinogen level (< 1 g/L at 5 hr)
  High FDP levels (≥ 300 mg/L at 5 hr)
  High t-PA level (≥ 1500 mg/L at 50 min)
  aPTT prolonged > 90 sec
  Thrombocytopenia (≤ 100 × 10^9/L)
  Bleeding time prolonged > 9 min

*FDP, Fibrinogen degradation product; t-PA, tissue-type plasminogen activator; aPTT, activated thromboplastin time.

the tightrope that must be walked when administering thrombolytic therapy.

THROMBOCYTOPENIA

Thrombocytopenia has recently been recognized as an important independent risk factor for hemorrhage during thrombolytic therapy (Table 51-3).[18,50] Thrombocytopenia was noted in six patients (3%) treated with rt-PA, heparin, and invasive procedures during the TIMI-I trial.[46] The streptokinase-treated group had a 2.0% incidence of thrombocytopenia. No assessment of excess hemorrhage attributable to thrombocytopenia was made in this trial. In the TIMI-II trial, 1.5% of patients treated with 100 mg of rt-PA in the conservative arm had thrombocytopenia. In this study, the occurrence of thrombocytopenia correlated very significantly with both major and minor hemorrhagic events.[18] In the composite analysis of TAMI trials II, III, and V (which included patients treated with rt-PA, urokinase, or combination therapy), a much higher incidence of 16.4% of thrombocytopenia was noted. As expected, thrombocytopenia was much more common in patients undergoing CABG and IABP. When a linear regression analysis was used with age, IABP, and CABG as variables, thrombocytopenia was a significant independent predictor of increased hemorrhagic risk. In the nonsurgical population, the occurrence of thrombocytopenia was by far the variable with the most predictive power for hemorrhage.[50]

As yet, none of these studies has determined the cause of thrombocytopenia during thrombolytic therapy. If patients undergoing early catheterization, CABG, and IABP are excluded, a significant incidence of 1.5% is still observed.[18] Because the nadir platelet count occurs at 3 to 5 days, a direct effect of the plasminogen activator seems unlikely. The nearly uniform incidence of thrombocytopenia in TAMI trials II, III, and V using different plasminogen activators (rt-PA, urokinase, or combination) also argues against a direct effect.[50] The universal use of heparin in all studies describing thrombocytope-

Table 51-3. Incidence of thrombocytopenia

Study	Definition of T	Treatment	Incidence of T	Hemorrhagic risk
TIMI-I	< 150,000/μl	rt-PA, 80 mg IS	6.3%	NR
		SK, 1.5 mu IS	2.0%	NR
TIMI-II	< 100,000/μl	rt-PA, 100 mg CS	1.5%	ODDs Ratio 7.5 for major hemorrhage, 3.3 for minor hemorrhage
TAMI-II, III, V	< 100,000/μl or < 50% baseline	rt-PA, rt-PA + UK, UK (variable doses)	16.4%	P < 0.0001 for increased blood loss with T vs. no T

T, Thrombocytopenia; IS, Invasive Strategy; NR, Not Reported; SK, Streptokinase; mu, million units; CS, Conservative Strategy; UK, Urokinase. Excludes patients with thrombocytopenia prior to treatment.

nia drug thrombolysis makes heparin-induced thrombocytopenia (HIT) a plausible cause. The timing of thrombocytopenia and its overall incidence are consistent with HIT.

Other potential mechanisms for thrombocytopenia include increased clearance of platelets because of an alteration of surface glycoproteins (e.g., cleavage of glycoproteins Ib and IIb/IIIa by plasmin) or adherence of FDPs to the platelet surface. These mechanisms are unlikely to be major etiologies because of the lack of correlation of thrombocytopenia with the extent of plasmin generation and fibrinogenolysis. Another potential mechanism for increased clearance would be the formation of antistreptokinase/streptokinase-plasminogen complexes on the platelet surface. This mechanism also appears to be an unlikely cause because excess thrombocytopenia was not observed in the TIMI-I study with streptokinase therapy.

PLATELET FUNCTION INHIBITION

Platelets play a pivotal role in achieving primary hemostasis. One study has found a weak ($P = 0.04$)

association between hemorrhage and prolonged bleeding time.[48] A variety of mechanisms for platelet inhibition occur in patients treated with thrombolytic agents. Almost all patients receive aspirin for primary prevention, unstable angina, or mortality reduction during thrombolytic therapy for MI. The use of more potent platelet inhibitors, such as monoclonal antibodies to glycoprotein IIb/IIIa, is likely to expand in the future. Thus, the minimal platelet function necessary to prevent excess hemorrhage during thrombolysis will undergo closer scrutiny in the near future.

Other causes of platelet inhibition include direct and indirect effects of plasminogen activators (Fig. 51-1). There is some evidence that plasmin degrades surface receptor glycoproteins Ib and IIb/IIIa that mediate von Willebrand's factor and fibrinogen binding, respectively.[51,52] FDPs also have antiplatelet effects, in part by binding to the platelet surface and occupying the fibrinogen receptor.[52] This prevents the formation of the fibrinogen bridge between platelets that is necessary for aggregation. There is also evidence that preformed

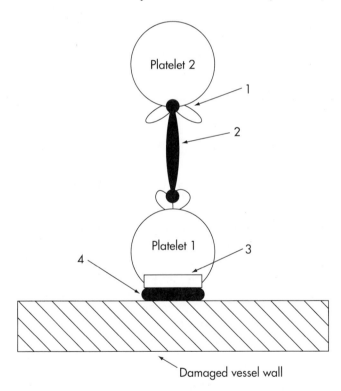

Fig. 51-1. Plasmin-mediated disruption of primary hemostasis. Two platelets participating in the early events of primary hemostasis are diagrammed. Platelet 1 is bound to von Willebrand's factor (which is attached to the damaged vessel wall) via the receptor glycoprotein Ib. Platelets 1 and 2 are connected through a fibrinogen "bridge." Fibrinogen is bound to activated platelets by the receptor glycoprotein IIb/IIIa. Plasmin can disrupt this early event in hemostasis by (1) degrading glycoprotein IIb/IIIa, (2) proteolyzing the connecting fibrinogen molecule, (3) degrading glycoprotein Ib, and (4) cleaving von Willebrand's factor.

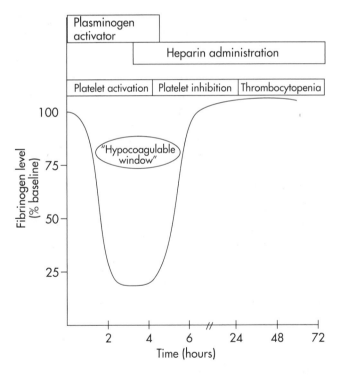

Fig. 51-2. Time-dependent changes in parameters influencing hemorrhage. The decline in fibrinogen from baseline is shown after administration of thrombolytic therapy. The nadir fibrinogen level occurs at 3 to 6 hours. High levels of fibrinogen degradation products (FDPs) also occur at 3 to 6 hours (not shown) and exert independent anticoagulant and antiplatelet effects. The time interval of 3 to 6 hours may be considered a "hypocoagulable window" because (1) the fibrinogen level is at its nadir, (2) the FDP level is at its peak, (3) early platelet activation is followed by inhibition, (4) heparin administration is usually started at this time, and (5) residual levels of plasminogen activator may persist at this time.

platelet aggregates may be disrupted by plasmin-mediated degradation of fibrinogen.[53]

In addition to degrading glycoprotein Ib (the VWF receptor), plasmin may directly degrade VWF itself.[54] The adjuvant administration of high-dose heparin may further disrupt platelet adhesion by inhibiting the binding of VWF to glycoprotein Ib.[55] Together, in the extreme case, these effects could produce a bleeding diathesis similar to mild von Willebrand's disease.

A variety of other causes of platelet inhibition occur in this setting. Contrast media (especially ionic varieties), β-blockade, and calcium channel blockade all have mild antiplatelet effects.

TIME DEPENDENCE OF HEMOSTATIC CHANGES

The hemostatic state of the patient undergoes a predictable sequence of changes after the administration of plasminogen activator (Fig. 51-2). With the generation of systemic plasmin, plasminogen is depleted, and the principal plasmin inhibitor (α_2-antiplasmin) is consumed. Soon thereafter, fibrinogen is degraded by plasmin, releasing FDPs. The nadir fibrinogen level (maximum FDP level) occurs 3 to 6 hours after initiation of thrombolytic therapy.[46] Although the extent of fibrinogen depletion varies from patient to patient and is greater with fibrin-nonspecific than fibrin-specific agents, the nadir typically occurs at 3 to 6 hours. During this time interval, plasminogen activator is cleared from the circulation, although it may still be active at sites of fibrin deposits, especially with fibrin-specific agents. After the infusion of plasminogen activator is completed, heparin is often started. In addition, preliminary experiments indicate that platelet activation by thrombolytic agents occurs early (< 1 hour), whereas inhibition occurs later (after 1 hour).[56,57] Thus, the time interval between 3 and 6 hours may represent a particularly hypocoagulable "window" during which hemorrhage is likely. By 24 hours, the plasma fibrinogen level is approximately two thirds of baseline, and between 48 hours and hospital discharge, the fibrinogen level returns to pretreatment levels. Some studies have demonstrated an overshoot of the fibrinogen level, with discharge levels being almost 150% of pretreatment levels.[46]

THERAPEUTIC IMPLICATIONS

The time at which hemorrhage occurs may influence the treatment approach if initial conservative management fails. Bleeding at up to 3 hours is less likely to result from platelet dysfunction, fibrinogen depletion, cofactor degradation, or α_2-antiplasmin consumption. Therefore, transfusion products such as cryoprecipitate, platelets, and fresh frozen plasma (FFP) are less likely to be beneficial. Because high plasminogen activator and plasmin levels occur early, ε-aminocaproic acid (Amicar) is more likely to be useful, although its use is strictly reserved because of potential thrombogenicity. In the 3 to 6-hour window, cryoprecipitate and FFP are more likely to be useful. Heparin is usually started at this time, and reversal with protamine should be considered. Platelets are likely to be useful only after platelet dysfunction emerges, 3 to 4 hours into therapy. ε-Aminocaproic acid is less likely to be useful at later times, especially for fibrin-nonspecific agents. There is evidence that t-PA and other fibrin-specific agents may remain bound and active at fibrin deposits for hours after the agents are cleared from the systemic circulation. Because of the fear of precipitating rethrombosis, however, antifibrinolytic agents are usually reserved for life-threatening hemorrhage, as last resort therapy. At 6 to 24 hours, variable degrees of hypofibrinogenemia persist. After 24 hours, the fibrinogen level should be adequate for primary hemostasis. It is not known how well fibrin that is formed during thrombolytic therapy is stabilized by factor XIIIa. Incorporation of certain FDPs (e.g., Fragment X) into a hemostatic plug may produce fragile clots not fully cross-linked between fibrinogen chains or to α_2-antiplasmin. Thus, hemorrhage occurring after 24 hours may represent fibrinolysis by physiologic t-PA levels of poorly stabilized hemostatic plugs. Bleeding after 24 hours is more likely caused by breakdown of these plugs or the anticoagulant effects of heparin administration, thrombocytopenia, or a combination of these factors.

TRANSFUSION THERAPY

A few patients will fail conservative management and require transfusion therapy. We have previously outlined an approach to the sequence of transfusion products to be used (Fig. 51-3).[1] Cryoprecipitate is rich in fibrinogen and factor VIII and should be considered first, especially 4 to 6 hours after initiation of treatment when fibrinogen levels are lowest. FFP may be useful to replenish α_2-antiplasmin and factor V, but only partial repletion can be achieved because this blood product is not concentrated for any coagulation factor. If the patient continues to bleed, platelets should be considered, especially if antiplatelet agents have been administered, if the platelet count is less than 100,000/μl, or if a bleeding time is prolonged more than 9 minutes.

The decision to transfuse should be weighed against the potential risks of this therapy: up to 1:40,000 chance of human immunodeficiency virus infection from screened blood products[58]; 0.5% risk of hepatitis[59]; and allergic reactions, volume overload, and theoretical risks such as precipitating a coronary rethrombosis. Stricter criteria for transfusion have recently been tested in the setting of thrombolysis. In the TAMI-V study, transfusion was limited to patients with a hematocrit of 22% or

General principles of transfusion therapy

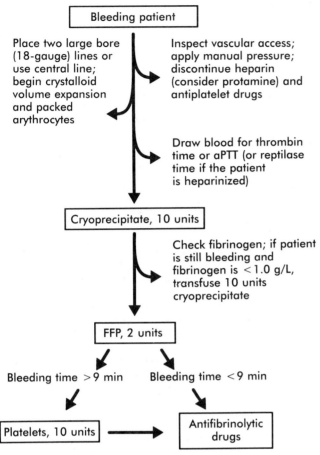

Fig. 51-3. Severe extracranial hemorrhage causing hemodynamic compromise, unresponsive to manual compression, fluids, protamine, and other conservative measures. Cryoprecipitate 10 units intravenously once or twice is recommended as initial therapy. If hemorrhage persists, give platelets (especially if platelet count is < 100,000 μl or bleeding time is > 9 minutes). If hemorrhage persists, give 5 g of ε-aminocaproic acid intravenously 30 to 60 minutes, then a 0.5 to 1.0 g/hr continuous infusion until hemorrhage is controlled. Consider ε-aminocaproic acid (Amicar) earlier for massive life-threatening bleeding or if reperfusion attempts are known to have failed.

less unless they were unstable. Only 10% of nonsurgical patients required transfusion with 2 or more units of packed red blood cells.[60]

ANTIFIBRINOLYTIC THERAPY

We consider antifibrinolytic agents (e.g., Amicar) as last resort therapy because of the fear that these drugs could precipitate rethromboses. Antifibrinolytic agents should be used immediately, however, in intracranial hemorrhage where the mortality rate (> 50%) is significantly greater than that of a coronary rethrombosis. Early administration should also be encouraged in massive, poorly controlled hemorrhage or in patients

with serious bleeding and known failure at attempts to achieve reperfusion.

FUTURE DIRECTIONS

Additional studies defining the appropriate use of invasive procedures such as angioplasty and IABP will likely make the greatest impact on hemorrhage during thrombolytic therapy. Several new pharmacologic agents may have some potential in this setting. Plasminogen activator inhibitor-1 (PAI-1) has been produced by recombinant DNA technology[61] and has been shown to reduce bleeding in rabbits administered rt-PA and aspirin.[62] Aprotinin, an inhibitor of plasmin and streptokinase-plasmin, also decreases bleeding in the rabbit model.[63] Desmopressin (DDAVP) decreases the bleeding time prolongation in rabbits administered streptokinase and aspirin.[64] If these findings are confirmed in clinical trials, these agents could be useful in patients with severe hemorrhagic episodes, such as central nervous system bleeding, or in patients who refuse blood product transfusions.[65]

Large-scale clinical trials with direct, antithrombin III–independent thrombin inhibitors such as hirudin and hirulog have recently been initiated (Global Utilization of Streptokinase and Tissue Plasminogen Activator for Occluded Coronary Arteries-II and TIMI-IX). These agents should not cause thrombocytopenia or accelerate plasminogen activation as heparin does, thus potentially lowering bleeding risks. Their more potent antithrombin effects may outweigh these marginal benefits, however.

Closer monitoring of the anticoagulant effects of heparin and other adjuvant therapy could reduce bleeding risks. Several devices that can measure prothrombin time, aPTT, or global fibrinolytic parameters have undergone initial testing.[66,67] Bedside monitoring, with rapid assay turnaround, could help avoid wide swings in levels of anticoagulation.

REFERENCES

1. Sane DC, Califf RM, Topol EJ, et al: Bleeding during thrombolytic therapy for acute myocardial infarction: mechanisms and management, *Ann Intern Med* 111:1010-1022, 1989.
2. Sherry S: Bleeding complications in thrombolytic therapy, *Hosp Pract* 25(suppl 5):1-21, 1990.
3. Fennerty AG, Levine MN, Hirsh J: Hemorrhagic complications of thrombolytic therapy in the treatment of myocardial infarction and venous thromboembolism, *Chest* 95:88S-97S, 1989.
4. Marder VJ: Bleeding complications of thrombolytic therapy, *Am J Hosp Pharmacol* 47(suppl 2):S15-S19, 1990.
5. Samama M: Haemorrhagic aspects of thrombolytic therapy, *Eur Heart J* 11(suppl F):15-18, 1990.
6. Blankenship JC, Almquist AK: Cardiovascular complications of thrombolytic therapy in patients with a mistaken diagnosis of acute myocardial infarction, *J Am Coll Cardiol* 14:1579-1582, 1989.
7. Tilly WS, Harston WE: Inadvertent administration of streptokinase to patients with pericarditis, *Am J Med* 81:541-544, 1986.
8. Satler LF, Levine S, Kent KM, et al: Aortic dissection masquerading as acute myocardial infarction: implications for thrombolytic

therapy without cardiac catheterization, *Am J Cardiol* 54:1134-1135, 1984.

9. Wilcox RG, Olsson CG, Skene AM, et al: Trial of tissue plasminogen activator for mortality reduction in acute myocardial infarction: Anglo-Scandinavian Study of Early Thrombolysis (ASSET), *Lancet* 2:525-530, 1988.

10. Chapman GD, Ohman EM, Topol EJ, et al: Minimizing the risks of inappropriately administering thrombolytic therapy, *Am J Cardiol* 71:783-787, 1993.

11. Cragg DR, Friedman HZ, Bonema JD, et al: Outcome of patients with acute myocardial infarction who are ineligible for thrombolytic therapy, *Ann Intern Med* 115:173-177, 1991.

12. Tenaglia AN, Califf RM, Candela RJ, et al: Thrombolytic therapy in patients requiring cardiopulmonary resuscitation, *Am J Cardiol* 68:1015-1019, 1991.

13. Oakley CM: Fatal intrathoracic haemorrhage after cardiopulmonary resuscitation and treatment with streptokinase and heparin, *Br Heart J* 63:69, 1990.

14. De Jaegere PP, Arnold AA, Balk AH, et al: Intracranial hemorrhage in association with thrombolytic therapy: incidence and clinical predictive factors, *J Am Coll Cardiol* 19:295-296, 1992.

15. Cahane M, Ashkenazi I, Avni I, et al: Total hyphema following streptokinase eight days after cataract extraction, *Br J Ophthalmol* 74:447, 1990.

16. Glikson M, Feinberg M, Hod H, et al: Thrombolytic therapy for acute myocardial infarction following recent cataract surgery, *Am Heart J* 121:1542-1543, 1991.

17. Califf RM, Topol EJ, George BS, et al: Hemorrhagic complications associated with the use of intravenous tissue plasminogen activator in the treatment of acute myocardial infarction, *Am J Med* 85:353-359, 1988.

18. Bovill EG, Terrin ML, Stump DC, et al: Hemorrhagic events during therapy with recombinant tissue-type plasminogen activator, heparin, and aspirin for acute myocardial infarction. Results of the thrombolysis in myocardial infarction (TIMI), phase II trial, *Ann Intern Med* 115:256-265, 1991.

19. Topol EJ, George BS, Kereiakes DJ, et al: Comparison of two dose regimens of intravenous tissue plasminogen activator for acute myocardial infarction, *Am J Cardiol* 61:723-728, 1988.

20. Stump DC, Califf RM, Topol EJ, et al: Pharmacodynamics of thrombolysis with recombinant tissue-type plasminogen activator. Correlation with characteristics of and clinical outcomes in patients with acute myocardial infarction, *Circulation* 80:1222-1230, 1989.

21. Lew AS, Hod H, Cercek B, et al: Mortality and morbidity rates of patients older and younger than 75 years with acute myocardial infarction treated with intravenous streptokinase, *Am J Cardiol* 59:1-5, 1978.

22. ISIS-2 (Second International Study of Infarct Survival) Collaborative Group: Randomized trial of intravenous streptokinase, and aspirin, both, or neither among 17,187 cases of suspected acute myocardial infarction: ISIS-2, *Lancet* 2:349-360, 1988.

23. Wittry MD, Thornton TA, Chaitman BR: Safe use of thrombolysis in the elderly, *Geriatrics* 44:28-30, 1989.

24. Nieuwenhuis HK, Albada J, Banga JD, et al: Identification of risk factors for bleeding during treatment of acute venous thromboembolism with heparin or low molecular weight heparin, *Blood* 78:2337-2343, 1991.

25. George BS, Candela RJ, Topol EJ, et al: Brachial approach to emergency cardiac catheterization during thrombolytic therapy for acute myocardial infarction, *Cathet Cardiovasc Diagn* 20:221-226, 1990.

26. Donovan BC: How to give thrombolytic therapy safely, *Chest* 95:290S-292S, 1989.

27. Renkin J, de Bruyne B, Benit E, et al: Cardiac tamponade early after thrombolysis for acute myocardial infarction: a rare but not reported hemorrhagic complication, *J Am Coll Cardiol* 17:280-285, 1991.

28. Barrington WW, Smith JE, Hammelstein SI: Cardiac tamponade following treatment with tissue plasminogen activator: an atypical hemodynamic response to pericardiocentesis, *Am Heart J* 121:1227-1229, 1991.

29. Walker WE, Fuentes F, Adams PR, et al: Hemopericardium and tamponade following intracoronary thrombolysis with streptokinase, *Tex Heart Inst J* 12:203-206, 1985.

30. Valeix B, Labrunie P, Jahjah F, et al: Hemopericardium after coronary recanalization by streptokinase during acute myocardial infarction, *Arch Mal Coeur* 76:1081-1084, 1983.

31. Belkin RN, Mark DB, Aronson L, et al: Pericardial effusion after intravenous recombinant tissue-type plasminogen activator for acute myocardial infarction, *Am J Cardiol* 67:496-500, 1991.

32. Honan MB, Harrell Jr FE, Reimer KA, et al: Cardiac rupture, mortality and the timing of thrombolytic therapy: a meta analysis, *J Am Coll Cardiol* 16:359-367, 1990.

33. Gillanders IA, Nakielny R, Channer KS: Spontaneous iliopsoas haemorrhage — an unusual complication of streptokinase therapy, *Postgrad Med J* 66:862-863, 1990.

34. Blanklenship J, Indeck M: Splenic hemorrhage after tissue plasminogen activator for acute myocardial infarction, *N Engl J Med* 3225:969, 1991.

35. Leor J, Livschitz S, Vered Z: Giant breast hematoma requiring blood transfusion: an unusual complication after an echocardiographic study during thrombolytic therapy, *J Am Soc Echocardiogr* 3:502-504, 1990.

36. Sanders PA: Haemarthrosis associated with thrombolytic therapy, *Br J Rheumatol* 30:236-237, 1991.

37. Oldroyd KG, Hornung RS, Jones AM, et al: Spontaneous haemarthrosis following thrombolytic therapy for myocardial infarction, *Postgrad Med J* 66:387-388, 1990.

38. Keeling PJ, Lawson CS: Haemospermia: a complication of thrombolytic therapy, *Br J Hosp Med* 44:244, 1990.

39. Smoller BR, Kruskall MS: Phlebotomy for diagnostic laboratory tests in adults. Pattern of use and effect in transfusion requirements, *N Engl J Med* 314:1233-1235, 1986.

40. Skinner JR, Phillips SJ, Zeff RH, et al: Immediate coronary bypass following failed streptokinase infusion in evolving myocardial infarction, *J Thorac Cardiovasc Surg* 87:567-570, 1984.

41. Ferguson Jr TB, Muhlbaier LH, Salai DL, et al: Coronary bypass grafting after failed elective and failed emergent percutaneous angioplasty, *J Thorac Cardiovasc Surg* 95:761-772, 1988.

42. Kereiakes DJ, Topol EJ, George BS, et al: Emergency coronary artery bypass surgery preserves global and regional left ventricular function after intravenous tissue plasminogen activator therapy for acute myocardial infarction, *J Am Coll Cardiol* 11:899-907, 1988.

43. Wellens Jr HA, Scheider JA, Mikell FL, et al: Early operative intervention after thrombolytic therapy for acute myocardial infarction, *J Vasc Surg* 2:186-191, 1985.

44. Anderson JL, Battistessa SA, Clayton PD, et al: Coronary bypass surgery early after thrombolytic therapy for acute myocardial infarction, *Ann Thorac Surg* 41:176-183, 1986.

45. Ohman EM, Califf RM, George BS, et al: The use of intra-aortic balloon pumping as an adjunct to reperfusion therapy in acute myocardial infarction, *Am Heart J* 121:895-901, 1991.

46. Rao AK, Pratt C, Berke A, et al: Thrombolysis in Myocardial Infarction (TIMI) Trial–Phase I: hemorrhagic manifestations and changes in plasma fibrinogen and the fibrinolytic system in patients treated with recombinant tissue plasminogen activator and streptokinase, *J Am Coll Cardiol* 11:1-11, 1988.

47. Weitz JI, Leslie B, Ginsberg J: Soluble fibrin degradation products potentiate tissue plasminogen activator–induced fibrinogen proteolysis, *J Clin Invest* 87:1082-1090, 1991.

48. Gimple LW, Gold HK, Leinbach RC, et al: Correlation between

template bleeding times and spontaneous bleeding during treatment of acute myocardial infarction with recombinant tissue-type plasminogen activator, *Circulation* 80:581-588, 1989.

49. Arnout J, Simoons M, de Bono D, et al: Correlation between level of heparinization and patency of the infarct-related coronary artery often treatment of acute myocardial infarction with alteplase (rt-PA), *J Am Coll Cardial* 20:513-519, 1992.

50. Harrington RA, Sane DC, Califf RM, et al: Clinical importance of thrombocytopenia occurring in the hospital phase after administration of thrombolytic therapy for acute myocardial infarction. The Thrombolysis and Angioplasty in Myocardial Infarction Study Group, *J Am Coll Cardiol* 23:891-898, 1994.

51. Adelman B, Michelson AD, Loscalzo J, et al: Plasmin effect on platelet glycoprotein Ib–von Willebrand factor interactions, *Blood* 65:32-40, 1985.

52. Pasche B, Collins L, Ouimet H, et al: Modulation of platelet function by plasmin and fibrinogen degradation products during thrombolysis [abstract], *Blood* 78:558, 1991.

53. Loscalzo J, Vaughan DE: Tissue plasminogen activator promotes platelet disaggregation in plasma, *J Clin Invest* 79:1749-1755, 1987.

54. Federici AB, Berkowitz SD, Zimmerman TS, et al: Proteolysis of von Willebrand factor after thrombolytic therapy in patients with acute myocardial infarction, *Blood* 79:38-44, 1992.

55. Sobel M, McNeill PM, Carlson PL, et al: Heparin inhibition of von Willebrand factor dependent platelet function in vitro and in vivo, *J Clin Invest* 87:1787-1793, 1991.

56. Coller BS: Platelets and thrombolytic therapy, *N Engl J Med* 322:33-42, 1990.

57. Rudd MA, George D, Amarante P, et al: Temporal effects of thrombolytic agents on platelet function in vivo and their modulation by prostaglandins, *Circ Res* 67:1175-1181, 1990.

58. Ward JW, Holmberg SD, Allen JR, et al: Transmission of human immunodeficiency virus (HIV) by blood screened as negative for HIV antibody, *N Engl J Med* 318:473-478, 1988.

59. Walker RH: Special report: transfusion risk, *Am J Clin Pathol* 88:374-378, 1987.

60. Wall TC, Califf RM, Ellis SG, et al: Lack of impact of early catheterization and fibrin specially on bleeding complications after thrombolytic therapy, *J Am Coll Cardiol* 21:597-603, 1993.

61. Reilly TM, Seetharam R, Duke JL, et al: Purification and characterization of recombinant plasminogen activator inhibitor-1 from *Eschericia coli, J Biol Chem* 265:9570-9574, 1990.

62. Vaughan DE, Declerck PJ, DeMol M, et al: Recombinant plasminogen activator inhibitor-1 reverses the bleeding tendency associated with the combined administration of tissue-type plasminogen activator and aspirin in rabbits, *J Clin Invest* 84:586-591, 1989.

63. Clozel JP, Banken L, Roux S: Aprotinin: an antidote for recombinant tissue-type plasminogen activator active in vivo, *J Am Coll Cardiol* 16:507-510, 1990.

64. Johnstone MT, Andrews T, Ware JA, et al: Bleeding time prolongation with streptokinase and its reduction with 1-desamino-8-D-arginine vasopressin, *Circulation* 82:2142-2151, 1990.

65. Sugarman J, Churchill LR, Moore JK, et al: Medical, ethical and legal issues regarding thrombolytic therapy in the Jehovah's witness, *Am J Cardiol* 68:1525-1529, 1991.

66. Sane DC, Gresalfi NJ, O'Mara N, et al: Exploration of rapid bedside monitoring of coagulation and fibrinolytic parameters during thrombolytic therapy, *Blood Coag Fibrinol* 3:47-54, 1991.

67. Lucas FV, Duncan A, Jay R, et al: A novel whole blood capillary technique for measuring the prothrombin time, *Am J Clin Pathol* 88:442-446, 1987.

Chapter 52

STROKE DURING ACUTE MYOCARDIAL INFARCTION

Christopher M. O'Connor

Stroke following AMI is a devastating complication afflicting up to 30,000 patients per year, often within the first few days after their heart attack.[1-7] This catastrophic complication is associated with a mortality rate of at least 40%, and among survivors over half have significant disability. Acute myocardial infarction patients who suffer stroke have longer and costlier hospital stays.[6,8-15] In the prethrombolytic era, stroke was reported in up to 3% of patients suffering an AMI, usually 2 to 3 days after the index MI. Two thirds of these patients died in hospital. Most of these strokes were caused by cerebral embolism, although there were other types of cerebral infarcts, including simultaneous strokes caused by atherosclerosis and ischemic injury secondary to the hemodynamic consequences of the infarct.[3-6,15] The thrombolytic era has brought about a change in the spectrum of cerebral events,[8,16-19] and this chapter will examine this change in detail.

DEFINITION

The World Health Organization defines stroke as a rapidly developing clinical condition with signs of focal or global disturbance of cerebral function lasting 24 hours or longer or leading to death with no apparent cause other than that of vascular origin.[20] As defined in the TAMI trials, stroke is a new focal neurologic deficit lasting longer than 24 hours, confirmed by a neurologist's examination and by computed tomography or magnetic resonance imaging of the head.[8,21-24] Most studies of patients experiencing stroke during AMI that were conducted before and in the early years

of the thrombolytic era used different definitions of stroke, which in part accounts for the differences in reported rates.[3-5,9-12,15,21-29] Some clinical trials did not require brain imaging or neurologist confirmation. Furthermore, strokes were not well distinguished from transient ischemic attacks and reversible ischemic neurologic deficits in some of these reports. In addition, differences in inclusion criteria, particularly with respect to a history of cerebrovascular disease, admission blood pressure, cardiogenic shock, and age, directly affect the rates and types of strokes seen in various clinical reports.*

Stroke represents a heterogeneous group of disorders that may present as intracranial masses, vascular abnormalities, systemic conditions, drug sensitivities, and, in particular in the AMI setting, may result from hemodynamic or electrical disturbances in addition to traditional causes. Despite this heterogeneity most stroke subtypes can be broadly categorized as embolic or vascular in the setting of AMI.[1-5,8,18,29]

PATHOGENESIS OF STROKE AND STROKE SUBTYPES

In order to better understand the underlying basis of brain injury from stroke, the pathogenesis of this type of cerebrovascular disease can be separated into two distinct processes: (1) vascular events that result in a reduction in or cessation of cerebral blood flow and (2)

---

*References 3, 5, 9, 11-13, 15, 21-28.

the subsequent abnormalities, caused by oxygen and nutrient (glucose) deprivation, which produce death of the neuron.[29-33] The damage inflicted by a stroke depends on the degree and duration of impaired cerebral blood flow as well as the extent of collateral support. After only 1 hour of interrupted blood flow, cerebral infarction occurs, resulting in the death of the neuron and supportive cells. Because vascular collaterals maintain partial blood flow to this territory, occlusion of cerebral blood vessels reduces but seldom abolishes the delivery of oxygen and nutrients to the brain in the affected territory.

When the occluded thrombus undergoes spontaneous lysis and initiates reperfusion to the ischemic area, reversible cellular dysfunction can occur in some cells and trigger lethal processes. This is known as *reperfusion injury of the brain* and is similar to the process that occurs following thrombolysis in the myocardium.[34-36] The progressive death of cardiac cells after vascular occlusion, known as the *wavefront phenomenon of myocardial necrosis,* has been extensively described by Reimer and Jennings in the cardiovascular literature[37]; these same general principles may apply to the brain. Ischemia lasting 5 minutes but less than 1 hour kills vulnerable neurons selectively within the affected vascular bed. When ischemia lasts for more than 1 hour in the brain, infarction begins in the central zone and progressively enlarges in a circumferential fashion over at least 6 to 8 hours, which is quite similar to the model described by Reimer and Jennings.[37] Time delays in the recognition and treatment of stroke may thus result in further damage and a less favorable outcome, especially if blood flow can be restored or the metabolic demands on brain tissue can be reduced.[29-34,37,38]

Several different types of stroke can occur in the setting of AMI and are distinguished from each other because of their different pathogenesis, clinical characteristics at onset, and outcome. The two main types of stroke are parenchymal intracranial hemorrhages and strokes secondary to cardiogenic embolism, which is the predominant type of nonhemorrhagic stroke; an important clinical feature of the embolic stroke is the conversion to hemorrhagic stroke.* It is important for the clinician to know the type of stroke the patient suffers because it dictates major differences in management strategies, ranging from the discontinuation or reversal of anticoagulation (which increases the risk of reinfarction and extension of MI) to the safe continuation of anticoagulation (which reduces not only cardiovascular complications but also the risk of recurrent embolic stroke and stroke-related complications).[39-41]

---

*References 3, 5, 8, 18, 25, 39-41.

Cardiogenic embolization

Most strokes in the prethrombolytic era were cardioembolic, were associated with anterior wall MIs, and were presumably caused by left ventricular thrombi.[3-5,19] These usually occurred during the first week of AMI, sometimes within 4 hours of onset. They occurred more commonly in patients with wall motion abnormalities in the anteroapical region, clinical congestive heart failure, and atrial fibrillation. An increased risk of embolization has been demonstrated in AMI patients with left ventricular thrombi seen on echocardiography. Specific characteristics of the left ventricular thrombi (mobile and protruding) may increase the risk of cerebral embolization.[3-5,39,41-48]

The clinical diagnosis of cardiogenic brain embolism as a cause of stroke is challenging. Clinical evidence such as site of ischemia, abruptness of onset, and diminished consciousness provide clues concerning the cause of the stroke but are insufficiently predictive for an exact diagnosis. The old diagnostic standard of early arteriography demonstrating embolic arterial occlusions without atherosclerosis is not practical in the setting of AMI. Even when arteriography is performed, the source may not be easily definable because severe cervical carotid stenosis or diffuse ascending aortic atherosclerosis coexists in 10% to 15% of patients with suspected cardioembolic stroke and cannot be ignored as a potential cause.[25,49-52] In the absence of cerebrovascular disease the presence of a cardioembolic source is adequate for deeming a stroke cardioembolic in origin.[29,53,54] Because cardioembolic strokes can undergo secondary hemorrhagic transformation, continued or early anticoagulation has been recommended only in limited circumstances.[25,39-41] Previous studies using multiple computed tomographic scan images have found spontaneous hemorrhagic transformation in 25% to 40% of patients with cardioembolic stroke. However, in the GUSTO analysis of 589 strokes, only 10% demonstrated hemorrhagic conversions. Large embolic infarctions (> 20 cm^2), which are visible on early computed tomographic imaging (<6 hours) and which display mass effect (displacement of intracranial structures by blood or edema), may be especially prone to secondary hemorrhage.[25,40,41,51,55]

Spontaneous hemorrhagic transformation occurs usually within the first 4 days of cardioembolic stroke.[25,40,56] In patients who develop an early hemorrhagic component, there is often an initial delay of at least 6 hours from stroke onset as detected by imaging techniques (computed tomography or magnetic resonance imaging). Spontaneous hemorrhagic transformation is not usually associated with clinical deterioration, but anticoagulants could cause further neurologic impairment.[29,39,41,51,57] Computed tomographic imaging of hemorrhagic transformations of embolic strokes usually shows mixed areas of attenuation with no significant mass effect on early imaging, and the hemorrhage appears to be related to a specific vascular territory.[18,39,41,57] Parenchymal intracranial hemorrhage, in contrast, is often homogeneous in appearance and extends into multiple vascular territories.[25,39-41,51,55-56,58] Although the issue of hemorrhagic transformation has been broadly studied, adequate information about observer variability of brain imaging readings to make the diagnosis, and the clinical consequences of the entity itself or its treatment have not yet been published.

Parenchymous intracerebral hemorrhage

Intracerebral hemorrhage is defined as bleeding into the brain parenchyma with formation of a focal hematoma. Approximately 10% of all strokes are intracerebral hemorrhages, which are more common among African-Americans and those of Asian descent.[59-61] In the population not exposed to thrombolytic therapy, most intracerebral hemorrhages are associated with chronic or acute arterial hypertension, and the bleeding may be caused by rupture of arteries damaged by chronic hypertension.[62] Long-term changes in blood pressure may also lead to infiltration of the walls of penetrating arteries by lipid and hyaline material (lipohyalinosis), resulting in microaneurysmal outpouchings (Charcot-Bouchard aneurysms).[16,31-32,56,62-68] Often, however, autopsy examination of patients with acute intracranial hemorrhage shows breakage of penetrating arteries without aneurysmal changes.

Most patients who are subsequently found to have an intracranial hemorrhage have an elevated systolic blood pressure on arrival to the hospital. Some of them have no history of hypertension and no cardiac, renal, or retinal evidence of hypertensive changes on clinical examination. Factors related to transient acute rises in blood pressure that can result in intracerebral hemorrhage include use of drugs such as cocaine and amphetamines, environmental stressors such as exposure to extreme cold or trigeminal nerve stimulation, and postsurgical states including carotid endarectomy, heart transplantation, and correction of congenital heart lesions. The less common causes of intracranial hemorrhage include vascular malformations, traumatic hematomas, and aneurysmal ruptures.[29,42,59-60,62-63,69-71]

Since the advent of thrombolytic therapy for AMI, parenchymal intracranial hemorrhage has become an important and more frequent complication facing the clinician. This type of stroke constitutes one half of all strokes seen in the setting of MI following thrombolytic therapy.[8,15,17-19] In the GUSTO trial 47% of the strokes were intracranial hemorrhages in the setting of an overall stroke rate of 1.45%.[14] These hemorrhages have unique clinical characteristics. They are not confined to any particular vascular territory and are most often seen as a confluent blood collection with homogeneous density and sharp edges, often with surrounding mass effect.[16,18,55,72] It is believed that the breakage of capillaries, arterioles, or small arteries leads to extravasation of blood into the brain parenchyma and results in the hematoma that causes an increase in pressure locally, which disrupts the surrounding brain parenchyma and vascular structures. The hematoma enlarges on the outer surface in direct response to increased systemic blood pressure and decreased clotting ability. These hematomas can expand along fiber track pathways and may decompress by dissecting into a ventricle, resulting in significant morbidity.[18,29,55,59,73]

Most patients with intracranial hemorrhage demonstrate neurologic symptoms within the first 24 hours of thrombolytic therapy, which should prompt early computed tomographic scanning of the brain.[8,16,18,55,74-75] Computed tomographic scanning is invaluable in delineating the types and extent of intracranial hemorrhage and is helpful in defining the characteristics that are predictive of clinical outcome.[18,55,76] Although the computed tomographic patterns of intracranial hemorrhage are varied, 84% of all nonventricular hemorrhages were supratentorial in location in the Duke Myocardial Infarction Databank analysis. The most common sites of intracranial hemorrhage were supratentorial and intraparenchymal. Computed tomographic findings of multiple intracranial bleeding sites, significant mass effect with midline shift, enlarged volume, or parenchymal hematomas were associated with increased mortality.[8,55]

Other strokes

Subarachnoid hemorrhage is a cause of 6% to 13% of all strokes. In the setting of AMI, subarachnoid hemorrhage is far less common, occurring in less than one patient in one thousand. Subarachnoid hemorrhages are secondary to aneurysms that take years to develop; most are not congenital. Weight lifting and sexual intercourse have been described as risk factors by some investigators. Importantly, premonitory headaches occur in the preceding weeks in up to 50% of patients; these tend to be diffuse, severe, and of sudden onset. The pattern of bleeding seen on computed tomography can be used to infer the site of the ruptured aneurysm.*

A subdural hematoma is a collection of blood between the outer layers of the brain surface. It may be remote from a point of traumatic impact. It is usually caused by tearing of the vein that bridges the cortical surface to an intracranial venous sinus. A small percentage of acute subdural hematomas are secondary to arterial bleeding from a damaged cortical artery. Computed tomographic scanning shows a crescent-shaped,

---

*References 10, 14, 18, 55, 69, 77, 78.

high-density area conforming to the cortical surface and frequently covering much of the surface of the frontal and parietal occipital lobes.[14,18,55,79]

An acute epidural hematoma is a focal collection of blood, usually arterial, between the dura and the inner part of the skull. Most commonly, it is located beneath the point of traumatic impact, usually in the region of the middle meningeal artery. In the typical presentation, acute epidural hematomas are associated with a period of normal consciousness preceded by transient unconsciousness at initial injury and followed by a rapid decline in level of consciousness. Computed tomographic scanning in acute epidural hematoma reveals a high-density lenticular-shaped lesion.[55,59-61,79]

Each of these stroke types may be encountered by the clinician during the course of caring for an AMI patient. Although a variety of immediate actions are mandated when a focal neurologic change occurs, distinguishing the type of stroke is an important step in developing a management strategy for these patients.

STROKE IN THE THROMBOLYTIC ERA
Incidence and prevalence

With the advent of thrombolytic therapy for AMI, the overall stroke rate has appeared to increase slightly, but the spectrum has changed dramatically to include more strokes complicated by intracranial bleeding and characterized by different risk factors.[15,17,19] The overall stroke rate is higher in patients undergoing thrombolytic therapy than in those given placebo in randomized clinical trials (1.2% vs. 0.8%).[15] This difference results in a small (3.9%) but significant excess of strokes per 1000 patients treated with thrombolytic therapy.[15] Most of the excess appears to occur in the first day, probably related to an increase in intracranial hemorrhages.[12,15] In the ISIS-2 study there was an early peak in strokes within 24 hours in patients treated with thrombolytic therapy but fewer strokes in the post 24-hour period[12]; the GISSI I study showed a similar trend.[9] In the Fibrinolytic Therapy Trialists' (FTT) analysis, the total stroke rate was lower on days 2 to 35 (0.4 per 1000) in the thrombolysis group. This may reflect a lower nonhemorrhagic stroke rate caused by smaller infarct size and less risk of left ventricular thrombi.[15,42-47,80] Despite the slightly higher stroke rate in thrombolytic-treated patients compared with control patients, the trend over the past 20 years (compared to historical controls) has been toward fewer strokes in the overall MI population.[3,5,15]

Several factors play a role in the lower-than-expected absolute stroke rate in the thrombolytic trials. The inclusion criteria for thrombolytic trials are much more selective with respect to previous cerebrovascular disease, older age, and cardiogenic shock, all of which are risk factors for stroke.[81-83] Widescale use of antithrombotic therapy with aspirin and heparin reduces strokes by

reducing MI size and the occurrence of left ventricular thrombus.[48] Furthermore, early studies were unable to classify accurately the types of strokes after AMI[9,10,12,13]; in the ISIS 2 and 3 and GISSI 1 and 2 trials, up to one third of strokes were classified as uncertain or were not specified. The diagnosis was based on the treating physician's impression without detailed analysis of information by neurologists or radiologists. In addition, many patients did not undergo routine computed tomography scanning.[9,10,12,13]

Risk factors for ischemic cerebral infarction

Because of the catastrophic consequences of a stroke following AMI, many investigators have sought to delineate risk factors for stroke. However, most studies to date have had limited ability to detect true differences among possible risk factors because of the small number of strokes available for analysis. Although many reports have demonstrated a weak association with one to three risk factors, many other variables have been deemed not important when in fact the studies were underpowered. Other studies have described weak associations without correcting for multiple comparisons.

The risk factors for ischemic cerebral infarction in both the pre- and postthrombolytic eras are related to MIs prone to the development of left ventricular thrombi: increased age, anterior apical infarcts, poor Killip Class, nonwhite race, and atrial fibrillation during the hospital course.* The TAMI trials evaluated previous atrial fibrillation, previous cerebrovascular disease, and anterior wall MI with ejection fraction < 45%, predictors that had been identified in earlier studies. Only anterior wall MI with an ejection fraction < 45% was significantly associated with stroke, occurring in 75% of the nonhemorrhagic stroke group and 18% of the no-stroke group ($P = 0.0015$), but the study was underpowered.[8]

In the GUSTO trial nonhemorrhagic stroke was more common in patients with hypertension (54% vs. 38%), diabetes mellitus (23.5% vs. 15%), previous MI (27% vs. 16%), anterior wall MI (45% vs. 39%), female gender (32% vs. 25%), and increased age (69 vs. 61 yrs.).[14] When adjusted for the presence of other risk factors, increased age, descriptors of hemodyamic compromise (higher Killip Class, higher heart rate, elevated systolic blood pressure), lower body weight, and history of hypertension or cerebrovascular disease appeared to be important.[72] Patients with atrial fibrillation also had a markedly increased risk of stroke.

Risk factors for intracranial hemorrhage

Because of the potential catastrophic outcome of patients suffering intracranial hemorrhage following

---

*References 3-6, 8-9, 12, 14-15, 17-19, 84.

Table 52-1. Risk factors for stroke following thrombolytic therapy in acute myocardial infarction

Risk factor	Cerebral infarction	Intracranial hemorrhage
Age	X	X
Female gender		X
History of hypertension	X	X
Hemodynamic compromise	X	
Anterior MI	X	
Higher Killip class	X	
History of cerebral vascular disease	X	X
Diabetes mellitus		X
History of anticoagulation		X
Lower body weight		X
Elevated blood pressure		X
Elevated pulse pressure		X
Heparin		X
Thrombolytic therapy type		X
Thrombolytic therapy dose		X
Calcium blocker		X

thrombolytic therapy for AMI, several investigators have attempted to distinguish risk factors for intracranial hemorrhage from risk factors for ischemic cerebral infarct. Although most studies to date have had limited power, several risk factors have emerged as important in multiple studies (Table 52-1).

Age. The mortality rate is known to be higher in elderly patients undergoing treatment for AMI. It is also known that thrombolytic therapy benefits this age group to a greater extent in terms of mortality reduction,[9,12-15,82,83] although at the expense of increased bleeding complications.[14,82,83] Large randomized clinical trials of AMI and thrombolysis have shown an increasing risk of stroke in patients with increasing age.

The risk of stroke in patients over the age of 70 is felt to be the result of a reduction in the integrity of the cerebrovascular system. Some patients have had previous silent cerebral ischemic events that may increase their risk for subsequent events after receiving thrombolytic therapy. In addition, cerebral amyloid angiopathy may occur to a much greater extent in the elderly, and this angiopathy may play a pathogenic role in some intracerebral hemorrhages associated with thrombolytic therapy.[64-66,85-88] The frequency of cerebral hemorrhage in the GISSI-2 and the ISIS-3 trials suggested that the increased risk of cerebral hemorrhage in the elderly was predominantly seen in patients treated with t-PA and not in patients treated with streptokinase. In the case control study by Simoons, using the databases of six thrombolytic therapy trials, age over 65 years proved to be an important independent risk factor for intracranial hemorrhage (odds

ratio = 2.2).[89] This effect was magnified in elderly patients treated with t-PA (odds ratio = 3.2) as compared to streptokinase (odds ratio = 1.3). This trend was also seen in the GUSTO trial, where the hemorrhagic stroke rate in patients over 75 years was 2.1% with t-PA and 1.2% with streptokinase. In patients < 75 years treated with t-PA, the hemorrhagic stroke rate was 0.5% compared with 0.4% in the streptokinase group. However, when the combined endpoint of death or nonfatal disabling stroke was compared between the two treatment regimens, t-PA was still favored because for both thrombolytic agents the substantial mortality benefit outweighed the strokes that occurred (Fig. 52-1).

Sex. In nearly all thrombolytic trials women have demonstrated an increased risk of serious bleeding complications.[36,48] Until recently, however, analyses have not taken into account the lighter body weight of women. Although some investigators in small studies did not find gender to be an independent predictor of stroke,* large trials such as the GISSI study found female gender significantly related to a higher incidence of hemorrhagic stroke but not ischemic stroke. In DeJaegere's analysis, female gender was not a significant predictor for intracranial hemorrhage, but low body weight (< 70 kg) was associated with a threefold increase in risk of intracranial hemorrhage.[90] Simoons also confirmed that female gender was an univariate predictor of intracranial hemorrhage but not significant when age, weight, and blood pressure were accounted for. However, White found that even after accounting for weight and thrombolytic agent, women had an increased risk of intracranial hemorrhage (odds ratio = 2.9).[48] In the FTT overview the stroke rate for women was 1.4% vs. 0.9% for men, resulting in an excess of 2 strokes per 1000 patients.[15] Importantly, after adjusting for age and weight, female gender was not associated with any increased risk of stroke in the GUSTO trial.[14] It appears that if gender is an important risk factor at all, its independent contribution is modest and may be explained by other risk factors.

Race. Very few studies have investigated the impact of race on stroke during AMI. In the TIMI analysis, cerebral infarction occurred at a higher rate in the nonwhite population than in the white population (1.6% vs. 0.6%; P = .03). The univariate association of race, however, was not statistically significant when other important variables were accounted for.[18] In the GUSTO trial, African-Americans had a substantially higher risk of nonhemorrhagic stroke than whites (2.2% vs. 1.4%; P = .03).

Hypertension. Randomized clinical trials to date have reached varying conclusions about the relationship

---

*References 8, 9, 12, 18, 89, 90.

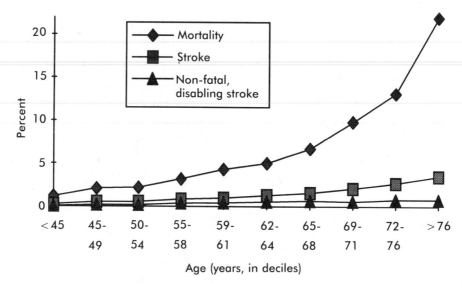

Fig. 52-1. Older patients in the GUSTO trial were at increased risk of both stroke in general and nonfatal, disabling stroke over their younger counterparts. The eldest decile has a 3.3% higher stroke rate than the youngest decile and a .8% higher nonfatal, disabling stroke rate.

between a history of hypertension and the risk of intracranial hemorrhage in AMI. This problem appears to have arisen because of inadequate power and the intercorrelation between history of hypertension and the presenting blood pressure. In GUSTO, patients with a hemorrhagic stroke were much likelier to have a history of hypertension (51%), even after adjusting for other factors. Most studies suggest that the presenting blood pressure is more important than the history of hypertension, perhaps reflecting the importance of adequate chronic blood pressure control.

Previous cerebrovascular disease. A history of neurologic disease within the previous 2 to 3 months has generally been an exclusion criterion from administration of thrombolytic therapy. In an analysis by the TIMI investigators, Gore found that patients who had a history of stroke, intermittent cerebral ischemic attack, or other neurologic disease 6 months and beyond had an intracranial hemorrhage risk of 10% vs. 1.2% in those without such a history ($P < .0001$).[18] This finding was the basis of a change in the TIMI protocol to exclude all patients with a history of stroke; a similar policy was incorporated into the GUSTO trial. However, it is important to remember that although patients with a history of cerebral vascular disease are at an increased risk, this risk may be less than the risk of death or severe disability from a large complicated MI that goes untreated with thrombolytic therapy (Fig. 52-2).

Previous anticoagulation. Anticoagulation use has been shown to be a risk factor for intracranial hemorrhage in patients treated chronically post-MI and in patients treated for atrial fibrillation.[91,92] In the case

control study by DeJaegere this was an important risk factor for intracranial hemorrhage. In their analysis, anticoagulation therapy before admission carried the highest risk with an odds ratio of 5.7 (95% confidence intervals 1.1 to 29.4). With inclusion of additional datasets in an expanded analysis by Simoons, this trend was no longer present. Anticoagulants are known to be associated with spontaneous intracerebral hemorrhage, and this risk appears to be enhanced when thrombolytic therapy is superimposed. The underlying mechanism of this interaction is not well understood.[64] In GUSTO a case control study found that patients with a history of warfarin use had odds ratios of 2.7 for any stroke and 1.8 for hemorrhagic stroke.

Diabetes mellitus. Diabetes mellitus has been inconsistently associated with an increased risk of stroke. In several studies, diabetes mellitus did not confer increased risk.[8,18,89,90] In the FTT overview the stroke rate following thrombolysis was 1.9% in patients with diabetes and 1% in patients without diabetes. Diabetes was not associated with increased risk in the case control study of six thrombolytic datasets. This excess was seen entirely in the first 24 hours following treatment, suggesting that the strokes were hemorrhagic in origin.[15] In the GUSTO trial diabetes was associated with nonhemorrhagic stroke, but not with hemorrhagic stroke.

Body weight. One of the more important physical characteristics associated with increased risk of hemorrhagic stroke following thrombolytic therapy appears to be body weight; however, studies conducted in the TIMI, TAMI, and GISSI datasets did not find such an

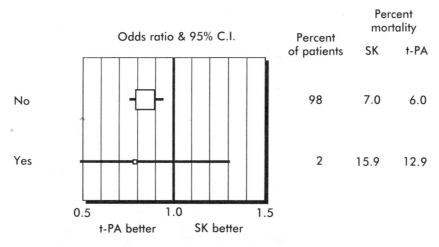

Fig. 52-2. A history of cerebrovascular disease imparted an increased risk of mortality in the GUSTO trial, both for patients given streptokinase (SK) and those randomized to t-PA.

association, although the GISSI analysis used body mass index as an indicator of obesity. The analysis by DeJaegere's group found that body weight < 70 kg was associated with an risk of intracranial hemorrhage increased 3.7 times. Among patients treated with streptokinase, the dose index (dose divided by body weight) was higher in patients with intracranial hemorrhage (20,000 ± 1000 units/kg) than in control patients (18,000 ± 1000 units/kg; $P < 0.05$). A difference in the dose index of t-PA was not found in this study. In their expanded case control analysis, lighter body weight (< 70 kg) still confirmed independent risk of intracranial hemorrhage (odds ratio = 2) In the GUSTO trial, patients who suffered hemorrhagic stroke had a lower median weight (70 kg) than those without hemorrhagic stroke (78 kg) (Fig. 52-3). Based on these observations, future studies may lead to better weight-adjusted regimens, as has occurred with t-PA and heparin, and lower stroke rates.[24]

Presenting blood pressure. Both systolic and diastolic blood pressure have been found to be consistent risk factors for intracranial hemorrhage.[8,15,87,89] In the Western Washington database, transient elevations in blood pressure were a risk factor for intracranial hemorrhage independent of whether the patient had a baseline history of hypertension.[93] Simoons found that hypertension on admission (systolic BP ≥ 65 mm Hg, diastolic BP ≥ 95 mm Hg or both) was independently associated with an increase risk of intracranial hemorrhage (odds ratio = 2). Although the GISSI investigators found no correlation between blood pressure and risk of stroke, the ISIS investigators found that a higher systolic blood pressure was associated with an increased risk of stroke, particularly in patients treated with t-PA. They proposed that the lower risk of intracranial hemorrhage with streptokinase compared with t-PA in patients with

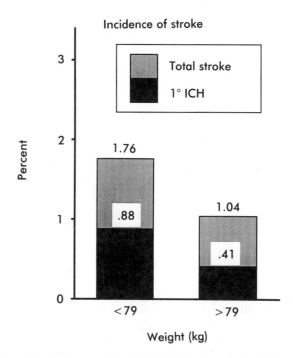

Fig. 52-3. Lighter patients in GUSTO were much likelier to have a stroke and to be in the subclass of patients who had intracerebral hemorrhages.

elevated systolic blood pressure may in part result from its hypotensive effects. In the GUSTO trial systolic and diastolic blood pressures were higher in patients who suffered both nonhemorrhagic and hemorrhagic strokes (Fig. 52-4).[14,94] It had been hoped that in patients with an elevated blood pressure on admission, antihypertensive therapy could lower the risk of hemorrhagic stroke. Unfortunately the GUSTO trial demonstrated that medical therapy for acute hypertension did not lower the risk of hemorrhagic stroke.[94]

Incidence of stroke

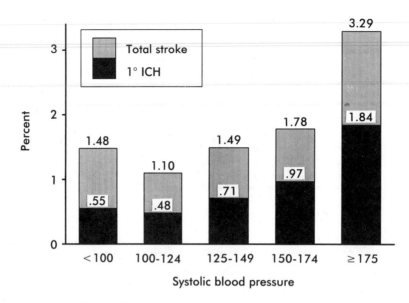

Fig. 52-4. Patients with very high systolic blood pressure were at much higher risk of suffering either any stroke or an intracerebral hemorrhage. Note that patients with very low systolic blood pressure had a somewhat increased risk of stroke as well.

Pulse pressure. Until recently, pulse pressure had not been recognized as a risk factor for stroke.[95] Pulse pressure is a reflection of reduced arterial wall compliance and the subsequent "pressure hammer" on cerebral vessels. In an evaluation of the Thrombolytic Predictive Instrument database made up of 12 clinical trials and registries, 19 intracranial hemorrhages were confirmed by computed tomography and compared with 175 matched controls. The mean pulse pressure in patients developing intracranial hemorrhage was 34% higher than the mean pulse pressure among those who did not develop hemorrhage.[95] On the contrary, pulse pressure conferred no independent risk once both systolic and diastolic blood pressure were considered in an analysis of the GUSTO data.[18,72] This aggregated information demonstrates that both the systolic and diastolic blood pressure are important risk factors.

Type and dose of thrombolytic agent. There has been considerable debate over the differences in hemorrhagic complications between the nonspecific fibrinolytic agents such as streptokinase and the specific fibrinolytic agents such as t-PA. In the GISSI studies, patients older than 70 years randomized to streptokinase had a 0.3% risk of intracranial hemorrhage and those randomized to t-PA had a 0.7% risk, an excess of 4 per 1000. In the ISIS 3 study there was a 0.3% risk of intracranial hemorrhage with streptokinase and 1.2% risk with t-PA, an excess of 9 per 1000 with t-PA.[10,13] In the Simoons analysis, standard dose t-PA was associated with a higher risk of intracranial hemorrhage (odds ratio = 1.6). This risk

was compounded in elderly patients who were lighter and presented with hypertension.

In the GUSTO trial, combination therapy with t-PA plus streptokinase had the highest primary intracranial hemorrhage rate. In the accelerated t-PA arm, which was frontloaded and weight adjusted, there was a 0.7% risk of primary intracranial hemorrhage vs. a 0.5% risk in the streptokinase arms. Despite the higher stroke rate with t-PA, the death or nonfatal disabling stroke combined endpoint was lower for t-PA than streptokinase.[14,96] This combined endpoint is probably the most important from the patient's point of view, and it avoids the pitfalls of counting deaths and strokes twice, and thus may be more appropriate for comparing thrombolytic regimens.[14,97]

The dose of thrombolytic therapy is a well-known risk factor for intracranial hemorrhage. The TIMI-2 study using high-dose alteplase (150 mg) was associated with an unusually high intracranial hemorrhage rate of 1.5%. After a reduction in dose to 100 mg, the hemorrhagic stroke rate declined to 0.5%.[18] The differences in the reported stroke rates from the GUSTO, ISIS, and GISSI trials may reflect the weight-adjusted dosing of t-PA.[10,12,14]

Adjunctive therapy. Adjunctive therapies have been associated with an increased risk of intracranial hemorrhage. Subcutaneous heparin therapy in the ISIS-3 study produced a 2 per 1000 increase in the risk of intracranial hemorrhage over patients randomized to no heparin. In the streptokinase arms of the GUSTO trial, intravenous heparin was associated with a 1 per 1000 increased risk of primary intracranial hemorrhage over the subcutaneous heparin treatment arm. Interestingly, the nonhemorrhagic infarct rate was also slightly higher in the intravenous heparin arm (.64% vs. .56%).

The intensity of the physiologic effect of heparin has also been associated with an increased risk of intracranial hemorrhage. In six patients who had intracranial hemorrhages, Kase et al. demonstrated that the partial thromboplastin time was greater than 80 seconds and less than 150 seconds in four of these patients.[16] In an analysis of the Duke Cardiac Care Unit intracranial hemorrhage registry, 10 of 13 patients had partial thromboplastin times of less than 100 seconds at the time of their intracranial hemorrhages.[74,75] Most recently the GUSTO II trial was discontinued early because of an excess intracranial hemorrhage rate, which was associated with aPTT values above 100 seconds in both the hirudin and heparin groups.[98]

Aspirin therapy has been shown to reduce the overall risk of stroke following AMI,[12,99] and there is no clear evidence that aspirin therapy increases the risk of acute stroke during AMI following thrombolytic therapy. A slight trend towards increased risk of hemorrhagic stroke was present in ISIS-2 with aspirin, but this was more than offset by the reduction in risk of nonhemorrhagic stroke. Simoons found that in-hospital aspirin use was associated with no increased risk of intracranial hemorrhage. Unless there is a significant contraindication, all patients should receive aspirin therapy during the early stages of AMI.[12]

Other types of adjunctive therapy have been associated with an increased risk of intracranial hemorrhage. Among the medications patients take before and during AMI, calcium channel blockers were associated with an increased frequency of intracranial hemorrhage in the TIMI-2 trial; this effect did not appear to depend on the type of calcium channel blocker. On the other hand, beta-blocker therapy administered immediately appeared to be associated with a lower risk of intracranial hemorrhage. There was a 0.3% intracranial hemorrhage rate in the group randomized to immediate intravenous beta-blocker therapy and a 1% intracranial hemorrhage rate in the group randomized to beta-blocker therapy at hospital discharge in the TIMI 2 study.[18,100] These associations with calcium channel blockers and beta blockers were not seen in the GUSTO study, and further work is necessary to see if these associations remain firm.[14,18]

Other risk factors. Other factors that have been less clearly associated with an increased risk of intracranial hemorrhage include smoking history[18] and heavy alcohol ingestion.[8,101] Head trauma has not been formally evaluated as an independent risk factor, and most patients with a history of such trauma have been excluded from admission. We have seen an intracranial hemorrhage occur in a patient with no neurologic abnormalities on initial physical examination and who had suffered a remote closed head injury.[74,75] A preliminary analysis of the GUSTO case control study identified head trauma as a major risk factor and dementia as a modest risk factor.[102]

DIAGNOSIS OF STROKE

The initial diagnosis of acute stroke in a patient with MI can be complicated. Patients presenting with an AMI, particularly elderly patients, often may have altered sensorium from concomitant medications, hypoperfusion, or deterioration in their clinical status.[8,74,75] In the Duke Cardiac Care Unit experience, the initial presenting neurologic symptom was profound nausea and vomiting in 46% of patients with intracranial hemorrhage. Agitation and confusion were found in 15% and severe headache was found in 15% of patients. The initial symptom or sign of focal weakness or abrupt onset of coma occurred in a small minority (1%) of patients. Given the often subtle and nonspecific symptoms, the diagnosis of stroke can be delayed up to 6 hours in the setting of AMI,[8,74,75] and thus result in further extension and delayed treatment.

Head computed tomographic imaging is the initial diagnostic test of choice, given its accuracy in acute cerebral syndromes and the relative ease of performing it in critically ill patients. A wide variety of patterns of intracranial hemorrhage can be found on computed tomography. Although the majority of intraparenchymal hemorrhages are supratentorial, subdural hematomas and subarachnoid hemorrhages are not uncommon. Multiple sites of hemorrhage are more characteristic of these strokes than primary hypertensive bleeds.[18,55] Patients with multiple areas of hemorrhage are at increased risk of dying, as are patients who demonstrate severe mass effect with midline shift resulting in uncal or transtentorial herniation, demonstrated by computed tomography. Intraparenchymal hemorrhages were also associated with slightly increased risk of dying. Other modalities such as magnetic resonance imaging can be useful, particularly if nonhemorrhagic stroke is the only consideration in a patient who has fewer complications.[55]

Patients being treated at a hospital without computed tomography will need to be transferred to a facility with 24-hour computed tomographic capability.[6] Until the transfer can be accomplished, the patient's anticoagulation should be discontinued and close neurologic observation should be maintained. The hemodynamic status of the patient should be optimized, and the patient should be accompanied by a physician or a highly skilled nurse during transport to a tertiary care hospital in case the patient becomes unstable. Cryoprecipitate should be on hand during transport and should be administered

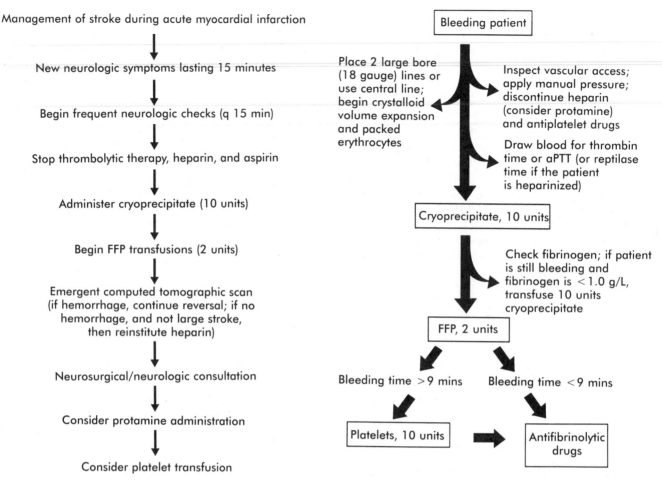

Management of stroke during acute myocardial infarction

New neurologic symptoms lasting 15 minutes

Begin frequent neurologic checks (q 15 min)

Stop thrombolytic therapy, heparin, and aspirin

Administer cryoprecipitate (10 units)

Begin FFP transfusions (2 units)

Emergent computed tomographic scan (if hemorrhage, continue reversal; if no hemorrhage, and not large stroke, then reinstitute heparin)

Neurosurgical/neurologic consultation

Consider protamine administration

Consider platelet transfusion

Fig. 52-5. Patients who appear to have developed a stroke following AMI require close and frequent attention in the acute period. Note especially the different care prescribed following computed tomographic determination of the type of stroke.

Bleeding patient

Place 2 large bore (18 gauge) lines or use central line; begin crystalloid volume expansion and packed erythrocytes

Inspect vascular access; apply manual pressure; discontinue heparin (consider protamine) and antiplatelet drugs

Draw blood for thrombin time or aPTT (or reptilase time if the patient is heparinized)

Cryoprecipitate, 10 units

Check fibrinogen; if patient is still bleeding and fibrinogen is <1.0 g/L, transfuse 10 units cryoprecipitate

FFP, 2 units

Bleeding time >9 mins   Bleeding time <9 mins

Platelets, 10 units   Antifibrinolytic drugs

Fig. 52-6. A typical strategy for the management of major bleeding causing hemodynamic compromise that is not immediately life-threatening. aPTT = activated partial thromboplastin time; FFP = fresh frozen plasma. (Reprinted with permission from Sane DC, Califf RM, Topol EJ, et al: Bleeding during thrombolytic therapy for acute myocardial infarction: mechanisms and management, *Ann Intern Med* 111:1010-1022, 1989.)

empirically. If the patient cannot be transferred and his or her neurologic status continues to deteriorate, the physician should assume the stroke is hemorrhagic and act accordingly.[6,103] These high-risk patients are best managed in a center that has had experience in managing severe bleeding complications following thrombolytic therapy and has readily available 24-hour emergency consultative neurologic and neurosurgical capabilities.[5,6,36]

Treatment

Management of stroke during AMI. The management of acute hemorrhagic stroke following thrombolytic therapy for AMI is enhanced when adequate preparations have been made and high-risk patients have been identified (Fig. 52-5). Patients with important risk factors for stroke (particularly a history of severe hypertension, elevated presenting systolic blood pressure, or older age; see Table 52-1) should receive intensive nursing and physician observation for the first

24 hours because 70% of hemorrhagic strokes occur in this time period. Neurologic assessments should be performed frequently. In the event of a new neurologic change (coma or a focal deficit) from baseline that persists for greater than 15 minutes and is unexplained by medications or hemodynamic, metabolic, or arrhythmic disturbances, thrombolytic therapy, heparin, and aspirin therapy should be discontinued. The presence of disorientation or confusion should prompt a detailed physical examination to look for a focal deficit. Appropriate blood work should be sent, including a coagulation assessment consisting of a fibrinogen level and a partial thromboplastin time as well as a hemogram and platelet count[5,103] (Fig. 52-6).

If coma or a focal deficit occurs within the first 48 hours, intracranial hemorrhage should be suspected and anticoagulation should be discontinued before conduct-

GUSTO severity of strokes

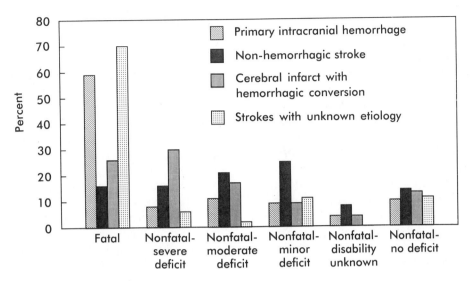

Fig. 52-7. Among 41,021 patients randomized in the GUSTO trial, 592 had strokes. This figure shows how the strokes were distributed according to resultant disability and by type of stroke.

ing imaging studies. If there is evidence of a persistent lytic state as manifested by a serum fibrinogen < 100 mg/L, 10 units of cryoprecipitate should be administered, followed by 2 units of fresh frozen plasma. Heparin therapy should be discontinued, and protamine should be administered. Platelets should be transfused if aspirin therapy was recent and the bleeding time is greater than 9 minutes. As the coagulation state is being normalized (fibrinogen > 100, PTT < 40 seconds, PT < 1.2 seconds), plans for emergency computed tomographic scanning should be under way. It is important not to wait until computed tomography confirmation to begin reversal of the anticoagulated state when a severe or progressive focal neurologic deficit is present because time delays in some cases of up to 3 hours may result in further irreversible brain damage. Once the diagnosis of intracranial hemorrhage is established, efforts to reverse the coagulation defect completely should be continued. Neurologic and neurosurgical consultation should be obtained immediately.[5,36,64,103,104]

During this period every effort should be made to stabilize the patient hemodynamically. If there is no evidence of an intracranial hemorrhage and an ischemic infarct is suspected, anticoagulation should be maintained unless the ischemic infarct is large (infarct territory > 20 cm^3 on computed tomography imaging) or displaces intracranial structures.[5,55]

Surgical management of acute intracranial hemorrhage. Rapid neurosurgical evaluation and intervention may be the most promising form of treatment in some cases. It is not necessary to delay performing craniotomy in order to reverse the anticoagulant state. During a rapid craniotomy on an anticoagulated patient, an anesthesiologist may transfuse blood products temporarily at a rate sufficient for blood volume and oxygenation while continuing to reverse the anticoagulant state. In select cases, rapid evacuation of hematoma and relief of intracranial pressure in the setting of deteriorating neurologic status is mandatory. If the intracranial hemorrhage involves a ventricular bleed, ventriculostomy may be indicated.[64,104] In our experience emergency neurosurgical intervention may be indicated in up to 15% of patients experiencing intracranial hemorrhage. The overall high mortality of these patients should not preclude surgical intervention. In the GUSTO trial, approximately 5% (50) of patients with intracranial hemorrhage underwent acute neurosurgical intervention. Although not corrected for baseline differences, patients who underwent emergent craniotomies tended to have a more favorable outcome than patients treated conservatively (neurosurgical events).[18,72]

Complications of stroke

Overall, stroke-related mortality approximates 40%, ranging from 15% for supratentorial and brainstem ischemic infarcts to 60% for intracranial hemorrhage.[8,18,55] The mortality rate for infratentorial hemorrhages is 30%. In the GUSTO trial the mortality rate for all strokes was 41% (Fig. 52-7). Intracranial hemorrhages had the highest death rate at 59% and the lowest moderate or severely disabled rate at 19%. In cerebral infarction with hemorrhagic conversion, which represented only 10% of the ischemic infarctions, the moderate-severe disability rate was higher at 47%. The nonhemorrhagic stroke mortality was 16%, with a moderate-severe disability of 37%. The GUSTO stroke analysis supports work by others that hemorrhagic strokes confer a higher mortality and consequent lower disability.

Neurologic complications. One of the most important complications of acute stroke is transtentorial herniation from cerebral edema. This remains the most common cause of death during the first week, peaking at 24 hours for hemorrhagic strokes and at 2 to 5 days for nonhemorrhagic strokes.[8,105-107]

Brainstem compression with subsequent hemorrhage and infarction accounts for the serious morbidity and mortality associated with herniation. Herniation is a result of raised intracranial pressures caused by cerebral edema seen with large strokes. Treatment of this life-threatening condition remains challenging. Steroid treatment for cerebral edema has been disappointing. Other means of fluid reduction have been used, but these interventions have not been demonstrated to improve long-term outcome using rigorous clinical trial methodology. Mannitol therapy may be effective by decreasing total cerebral volume; its benefits, however, are only temporary. In addition, hyperventilation via mechanical ventilation may help decompression, especially in patients with cerebellar stroke and signs of brainstem compression.[5,106-108]

Hemorrhagic transformation of cardioembolic strokes usually occurs within 4 days. It occurs in 5% to 20% of all ischemic strokes following thrombolytic therapy and may lead to clinical deterioration and, at times, death. Hemorrhagic transformation may more commonly lead to herniation than bland infarcts because of a greater frequency of concomitant cerebral edema. Neurologic deterioration during hemorrhagic transformation seldom occurs without mass effect and can usually be explained by stroke size and the presence of cerebral edema. Risk factors for hemorrhagic conversion in addition to cardioembolic source include large infarct volume, midline shift, and increased age. Interestingly, hypertension and anticoagulation therapy have not been identified as independent risk factors for hemorrhagic transformation of ischemic infarcts, but the available studies are small and underpowered.[29,39,41,55,106-109]

Acute hydrocephalus caused by compression of the aqueduct by blood or edema may complicate cerebral hemorrhage and lead to rapid deterioration or death. Management in this setting includes emergent neurosurgical ventricular shunting and hematoma evacuation, preceded by reduction of cerebral edema with mannitol hyperventilation.[59,110] Other neurologic complications include seizure activity, which can occur in over 10% of stroke patients. Depression is quite common and results in significant functional impairment.

Medical complications. Independent of the neurologic complications, stroke following thrombolytic therapy can result in a number of medical sequelae that lead to significant morbidity and mortality. Acute stroke can result in deranged glucose metabolism, which in turn can increase the risk of stroke extension, enhance morbidity, and reduce long-term survival. Importantly, an elevated blood sugar, which can be seen in 20% to 30% of acute stroke patients with a history of diabetes, has been associated with higher fatality rates. Hyperglycemia is associated with reduced cerebral blood flow, increased cerebral edema, and larger infarcts, although the degree to which hyperglycemia is a cause of bad outcomes or simply a consequence of bad outcomes remains unclear. Patients with blood glucose levels in the diabetic range should be treated with insulin by infusion in the acute phase and subsequently investigated for the presence of diabetes.[108,109] The use of intravenous glucose solution should be discouraged during volume infusions.

Inappropriate antidiuretic hormone secretion occurs in 10% of cerebral infarctions or cerebral hemorrhages and may exacerbate cerebral edema. Complications may include clinical deterioration, hyponatremia, and seizure activity.

An elevation in blood pressure can occur in up to 80% of acute stroke patients with a previous history of hypertension, and its treatment is controversial. Recent data from the GUSTO trial suggest that attempts to control elevated blood pressure do not reduce the risk of stroke. Whether this finding can be applied to the risk of recurrent stroke or stroke extension is unclear. Severe hypertension (systolic > 200 mm Hg, diastolic > 120 mm Hg) probably should be treated with short-acting agents such as nitroglycerin and intravenous beta blockers.[96]

Other medical complications that are associated with a worse outcome include fever, which is a common complication in over 40% of patients and correlates with stroke severity,[111] thromboembolic complications (deep venous thrombosis or pulmonary embolus), aspiration and urinary tract infections.[112,113]

Rehabilitation

Approximately one third of patients who sustain a stroke will survive the acute event and will be left with considerable residual disability. In the GUSTO trial, 41% of stroke patients died, 12% suffered a severe deficit, 14% a moderate deficit, 16% a mild deficit, 5% no deficit, and 12% were unclassified. The highest rate of residual severe deficit occurred in patients with nonhemorrhagic infarcts. Patients with hemorrhagic strokes were more likely to die and therefore less likely to be alive and to have a severe deficit.[14]

Forty percent of patients who survive a stroke for 6 months will require help with one or more routine activities of living such as bathing, dressing, feeding, and mobility. Ten percent of stroke survivors live in the open community whereas the majority need long-term nursing care. Efforts to improve the outcome of patients suffering stroke after an AMI through aggressive rehabilitation are continuing.[114]

Secondary prevention of stroke

Nonhemorrhagic stroke. The risk of recurrent stroke outside the setting of AMI after the first stroke is approximately 10% in the first year and 5% to 7% per year subsequently, which is seven times the risk of stroke in a normal population of the same age. It is not clear whether this trend will also be seen in stroke patients post-MI. There are no carefully controlled randomized clinical trials of risk-factor modification in stroke patients. The primary prevention studies suggest that blood pressure control and smoking cessation are imperative. Antiplatelet therapy with aspirin reduces the risk of stroke by 25% following MI with as little as 162 mg of aspirin a day.[12] Ticlopidine can be prescribed for patients who cannot tolerate aspirin, and may have an advantage in women.[115] Oral anticoagulation has also been shown to be effective in reducing ischemic stroke rates post-MI, but this therapy has not been shown to provide significant benefit over antiplatelet therapy.[91] In patients with strokes that are not cardioembolic in origin, an investigation of the carotid vasculature is imperative. For patients with recent mild carotid distribution of ischemic event and severe (70% to 99%) luminal diameter stenosis of the origin of the symptomatic and internal carotid artery, carotid endarterectomy is beneficial in centers that have a low risk of strokes that result from surgery.[112,116-118]

Hemorrhagic stroke. The secondary prevention of hemorrhagic strokes includes modifying risk factors for primary intracranial hemorrhage, such as controlling arterial hypertension with appropriate antihypertensive medical therapy. Chronic anticoagulation with warfarin is contraindicated, and even the use of antiplatelet therapy with aspirin should be examined carefully. There is a small increased risk of first hemorrhagic stroke in patients taking low-dose prophylactic aspirin.[119]

Hemorrhagic conversion of an embolic stroke may require low-dose anticoagulation after a week or more of convalescence and observation. The risk of recurrent embolic stroke is highest during the first week following the initial embolic stroke; thus attempts to reduce this risk by controlling heart failure, controlling and maintaining sinus rhythm, and providing some degree of anticoagulation if indicated remain the cornerstone of management.[39,41]

Stroke following AMI continues to be an important complication of thrombolytic therapy for AMI. The combined incidence of death and severe neurologic deficit appears to be lower in the thrombolytic than in the prethrombolytic era. Prevention is best achieved by knowing who is at increased risk and by carefully weighing the risk vs. the total clinical benefit of therapy. High-risk patients should be considered for alternative reperfusion strategies such as direct angioplasty. If thrombolytic therapy is administered, a heightened awareness can result in prompt recognition of an evolving neurologic deficit and subsequent swift management. As more is known about the net clinical benefit of therapeutic strategies, we will increasingly be able to select the optimal strategy for each patient. The information presented in this chapter provides some guidance into the decision-making process that can maximize outcomes. Currently, front-loaded, weight-adjusted t-PA appears to be the favored thrombolytic strategy when the combined endpoint of death and nonfatal disabling stroke is taken into account,[14] but the routine use of t-PA will lead to a modest excess of strokes, further emphasizing the importance of rapid diagnosis.

Once the stroke has occurred after the AMI, prompt diagnosis and early intervention are essential to improve outcome. The focus in patients with intracranial hemorrhage should be an immediate reversal of the fibrinolytic state; early surgical intervention is sometimes necessary. The medical management of the complications of stroke throughout the hospitalization is imperative to improve neurologic outcome in this illness that carries up to a 40% mortality. Secondary prevention and stroke rehabilitation are important to improve the long-term outcome of these patients. Further research is being conducted to determine the instantaneous risk of stroke with AMI and allow that risk to be detected before thrombolytic therapy is administered.[99]

REFERENCES

1. American Heart Association: *Heart and stroke facts,* Dallas, 1994, the Association.
2. American Heart Association: *Heart and stroke facts:* 1994 statistical supplement, Dallas, 1994, the Association.
3. Komrad MS, Coffey CE, Coffey KS, et al: Myocardial infarction and stroke, *Neurology* 34:1403-1409, 1984.
4. Thompson PL, Robinson JS: Stroke after acute myocardial infarction: relation to infarct size, *Br Med J* 2:457-459, 1978.
5. Califf RM, Massey EW: Myocardial infarction and stroke in the thrombolytic era. In: Califf RM, Mark DB, Wagner GS, (eds): *Acute coronary care in the thrombolytic era,* Chicago, 1988, Year Book Medical Publishers.
6. Mark DB, Hlatky MA, O'Connor CM, et al: Administration of thrombolytic therapy in the community hospital: established principles and unresolved issues, *J Am Coll Cardiol* 12(suppl): 32A-43A, 1988.
7. Bonita R: Epidemiology of stroke, *Lancet* 339:342-344, 1992.
8. O'Connor CM, Califf RM, Massey EW, et al: Stroke and acute myocardial infarction in the thrombolytic era: clinical correlates and long-term prognosis, *J Am Coll Cardiol* 16:533-540, 1990.
9. Gruppo Italiano per lo Studio della Streptochinasi nell'Infarto Miocardico (GISSI): Effectiveness of intravenous thrombolytic treatment in acute myocardial infarction, *Lancet* 1:397-402, 1986.

10. Gruppo Italiano per lo Studio della Sopravvivenzae Nell'Infarto Miocardico: GISSI-2: a factorial randomised trial of alteplase versus streptokinase and heparin versus no heparin among 12,490 patients with acute myocardial infarction, *Lancet* 336:65-71, 1990.

11. ISAM Study Group: A prospective trial of intravenous streptokinase in acute myocardial infarction (ISAM): mortality, morbidity and infarct size at 21 days, *N Engl J Med* 314:1465-1471, 1986.

12. ISIS-2 (Second International Study of Infarct Survival) Collaborative Group: Randomised trial of intravenous streptokinase, oral aspirin, both or neither among 17,187 cases of suspected acute myocardial infarction: ISIS-2, *Lancet* 2:349-360.

13. ISIS-3 (Third International Study of Infarct Survival) Collaborative Group: ISIS-3: a randomised comparison of streptokinase vs. tissue plasminogen activator vs. anistreplace and of aspirin plus heparin vs. aspirin alone among 41,299 cases of suspected acute myocardial infarction, *Lancet* 339:753-770, 1992.

14. The GUSTO Investigators: An international randomized trial comparing four thrombolytic strategies for acute myocardial infarction, *N Engl J Med* 329:673-682, 1993.

15. Fibrinolytic Therapy Trialists' (FTT) Collaborative Group: Indications for fibrinolytic therapy in suspected acute myocardial infarction: collaborative overview of early mortality and major morbidity results from all randomised trials of more than 1000 patients, *Lancet* 343:311-322, 1994.

16. Kase CS, O'Neal AM, Fisher M, et al: Intracranial hemorrhage after use of tissue plasminogen activator for coronary thrombolysis, *Ann Intern Med* 112:17-21, 1990.

17. Maggioni AP, Fronzosi MG, Farina ML, et al: Cerebrovascular events after myocardial infarction: analysis of the GISSI Trial, *Br Med J* 302:1428-1431, 1991.

18. Gore JM, Sloan M, Price TR, et al, and the TIMI Investigators: Intracerebral hemorrhage, cerebral infarction, and subdural hematoma after acute myocardial infarction and thrombolytic therapy in the Thrombolysis in Myocardial Infarction Study. Thrombolysis in Myocardial Infarction, Phase II, Pilot and Clinical Trial, *Circulation* 83:448-459, 1991.

19. Longstreth WT Jr, Litwin PE, Weaver WD, et al and the MITI Project Group: Myocardial infarction, thrombolytic therapy, and stroke. A community-based study, *Stroke* 24:587-590, 1993.

20. WHO MONICA Project, principal investigators: The World Health Organization MONICA Project (monitoring trends and determinants in cardiovascular disease): a major international collaboration, *J Clin Epidemiol* 41:105-114, 1988.

21. Topol EJ, Califf RM, George BS, et al: A randomized trial of immediate versus delayed elective angioplasty after intravenous tissue plasminogen activator in acute myocardial infarction, *N Engl J Med* 317:581-588, 1987.

22. Topol EJ, Califf RM, George GS, et al: Coronary arterial thrombolysis with combined infusion of recombinant tissue-type plasminogen activator and urokinase in patients with acute myocardial infarction, *Circulation* 77:1100-1107, 1988.

23. Topol EJ, George BS, Kereiakes DJ, et al: A randomized controlled trial of intravenous tissue plasminogen activator and early intravenous heparin in acute myocardial infarction, *Circulation* 79:281-286, 1989.

24. Topol EJ, Califf RM: The risk of stroke after thrombolytic therapy, *N Engl J Med* 327:1531-1532, 1992.

25. Cerebral Embolism Study Group: Immediate anticoagulation of embolic stroke: brain hemorrhage and management options, *Stroke* 15:779-789, 1984.

26. Van de Werf F, Arnold FER, for the European Study Group for Recombinant Tissue-Type Plasminogen Activator: Intravenous tissue plasminogen activator and size of infarct, left ventricular function, and survival in acute myocardial infarction, *Br Med J* 297:1374-1379, 1988.

27. Wilcox RG, von der Lippe G, Olsson CG, et al: Trial of tissue plasminogen activator for mortality reduction in acute myocardial infarction: Anglo-Scandinavian Study of Early Thrombolysis (ASSET), *Lancet* 2:525-530, 1988.

28. TIMI Study Group: Comparison of invasive and conservative strategies after treatment with intravenous tissue plasminogen activator in acute myocardial infarction: results of Thrombolysis in Myocardial Infarction (TIMI) Phase II trial, *N Engl J Med* 320:618-627, 1989.

29. Barnett HJM, Mohr JP, Stein BM, et al (eds): *Stroke: pathophysiology, diagnosis, and management,* New York, 1986, Churchill Livingstone.

30. Fischer CM: Pathological observations in hypertensive cerebral hemorrhages, *J Neuropathol Exp Neurol* 30:536-550, 1971.

31. Fisher CM, Adams RD: Observation of brain embolism with special reference to the mechanisms of hemorrhagic infarction, *J Neuropathol Exp Neurol* 10:92-93, 1951.

32. Farris AS, Harden CA, Poser CM: Pathogenesis of hemorrhage infarction of the brain, *Arch Neurol* 9:468-476, 1963.

33. Pulsinelli W: Pathophysiology of acute ischemic stroke, *Lancet* 339:533-536, 1992.

34. Califf RM, Herzog WR: Efforts to prevent reperfusion injury. In Califf RM, Mark DB, Wagner GS, (eds): *Acute coronary care in the thrombolytic era,* ed 2, Chicago, 1994, Year Book.

35. Zivin JA, Lyden PD, Degirolami U, et al: Tissue plasminogen activator: reduction of neurologic damage after experimental embolic stroke, *Arch Neurol* 45:387-391, 1988.

36. Califf RM, Topol EJ, George BS, et al: Hemorrhagic complications associated with the use of intravenous tissue plasminogen activator in treatment of acute myocardial infarction, *Am J Med* 85:353-359, 1988.

37. Reimer KA, Lowe JE, Rasmussen MM, et al: The wavefront phenomenon of ischemic cell death: 1. myocardial infarct size versus duration of coronary occlusion in dogs, *Circulation* 56:786-794, 1977.

38. Gillman S: Neurological complications of open heart surgery, *Am Neurol Assoc* 475-476, 1990.

39. Hart RG, Easton JD: Hemorrhagic infarcts, *Stroke* 17:586-589, 1986.

40. Ramirez-Lassepas M, Quinones MR: Heparin therapy for stroke: hemorrhagic complications and risk factors for intracerebral hemorrhage, *Neurology* 34:114-117, 1984.

41. Sherman DG, Hart RG: Stroke and transient ischemic attack: thromboembolism and antithrombotic therapy. In Fuster V, Verstraete M (eds): *Thrombosis in cardiovascular disorders,* Philadelphia, 1992, WB Saunders Co.

42. Eigler N, Maurer G, Shah PK: Effect of early systemic thrombolytic therapy on left ventricular mural thrombus formation in acute anterior myocardial infarction, *Am J Cardiol* 54:261-263, 1984.

43. Lavie CJ, O'Keefe JH, Chesebro JH, et al: Prevention of left ventricular dilatation by successful thrombolytic reperfusion, *Am J Cardiol* 66:31-36, 1990.

44. Sharma B, Carvalho A, Wyeth R, et al: Left ventricular thrombi diagnosed by echocardiography in patients with acute myocardial infarction treated with intracoronary streptokinase followed by intravenous heparin, *Am J Cardiol* 56:422-425, 1985.

45. Stratton JR, Speck SM, Caldwell JH, et al: Late effects of intracoronary streptokinase on regional wall motion, ventricular aneurysm and left ventricular thrombus in myocardial infarction: results from the Western Washington Ramdomized Trial, *J Am Coll Cardiol* 5:1023-1028, 1985.

46. Kouvaras G, Chronopoulos G, Soufras G, et al: The effects of long-term antithrombotic treatment of left ventricular thrombi in patients after an acute myocardial infarction, *Am Heart J* 199:73-78, 1990.

47. Turpie AGG, Robinson JG, Doyle DJ, et al: Comparison of high-dose with low-dose subcutaneous heparin to prevent left ventricular mural thrombus in patients with acute transmural anterior myocardial infarction, *N Engl J Med* 320:352-357, 1989.

48. White H, Barbash GI, Modan M, et al for the Investigators of the International Tissue Plasminogen Activator/Streptokinase Mortality Study: After correcting for worse baseline characteristics, women treated with thrombolytic therapy for acute myocardial infarction have the same mortality and morbidity as men except for a higher incidence of hemorrhagic stroke, *Circulation* 88(1): 2097-2103, 1993.

49. Zanette EM, Fieschi C, Bozzao L, et al: Comparison of cerebral angiography and transcranial Doppler sonography in acute stroke, *Stroke* 20:899-903, 1989.

50. Zeumer H: Vascular recanalizing techniques in interventional neuroradiology, *J Neurol* 231:287-294, 1985.

51. Lodder J: Hemorrhagic transformation in cardioembolic stroke, *Stroke* 19:1482-1484, 1988.

52. Bogousslavsky J, Cachin C, Regli F, et al: Cardiac sources of embolism and cerebral infarction: clinical consequences and vascular concomitants, *Neurology* 41:855-859, 1991.

53. Bamford J: Clinical examination in diagnosis and subclassification of stroke, *Lancet* 339:400-402, 1992.

54. Landi G: Clinical diagnosis of transient ischaemic attacks, *Lancet* 339:402-405, 1992.

55. Uglietta JP, O'Connor CM, Boyko OB, et al: CT patterns of intracranial hemorrhage complicating thrombolytic therapy for acute myocardial infarction, *Radiology* 181:555-559, 1991.

56. Horning CR, Dorndorf W, Agnoli AL: Hemorrhagic cerebral infarction: a prospective study, *Stroke* 17:179-185, 1986.

57. Babikian VL, Kase CS, Pessin MS, et al: Intracerebral hemorrhage in stroke patients anticoagulated with heparin, *Stroke* 20:1500-1503, 1989.

58. Sloan M, Gore JM: Ischemic stroke and intracranial hemorrhage following thrombolytic therapy for acute myocardial infarction: a risk-benefit analysis, *Am J Cardiol* 69:21A-38A, 1992.

59. Caplan LR: Intracerebral hemorrhage revisited, *Neurology* 38: 624-627, 1988.

60. Caplan LR: Intracerebral haemorrhage, *Lancet* 339:656-658, 1992.

61. Feldman E: Intracerebral hemorrhage, *Stroke* 22:684-691, 1991.

62. Brott T, Thalinger K, Hertzbefy V: Hypertension as a risk factor for spontaneous intracerebral hemorrhage, *Stroke* 17:1078-1083, 1986.

63. Brott T: Thrombolytic therapy for stroke. In *Cardiovascular and Brain Metabolism Reviews,* New York, 1991, Raven Press.

64. DaSilva VF, Bormanis J: Intracerebral hemorrhage after combined anticoagulant-thrombolytic therapy for myocardial infarction: two case reports and a short review, *Neurosurgery* 30:943-945, 1992.

65. del Zoppo GJ, Mori E: Hematologic causes of intracerebral hemorrhage and their treatment, *Neurosurg Clin North Am* 3:637-658, 1992.

66. Ramsay DA, Penswick JL, Robertson DM: Fatal streptokinase-induced intracerebral hemorrhage in cerebral amyloid angiopathy, *Can J Neurol* 17:336-341, 1990.

67. Kalyan-Raman UP, Kalyan-Raman K: Cerebral amyloid angiopathy causing intracranial hemorrhage, *Ann Neurol* 16:321-329, 1984.

68. The International Study Group: In-hospital mortality and clinical course of 20,891 patients with suspected acute myocardial infarction randomised between alteplase and streptokinase with or without heparin, *Lancet* 336:71-75, 1990.

69. Hijdra A, Braakman R, van Gijn J, et al: Aneurysmal subarachnoid hemorrhage: complications and outcome in a hospital population, *Stroke* 18:1061-1067, 1987.

70. Okazaki H, Reagen TJ, Campbell RJ: Clinicopathologic studies of primary cerebral amyloid angiopathy, *Mayo Clin Proc* 54:22-31, 1979.

71. Proner J, Rosenblum BR, Rothman A: Ruptured arteriovenous malformation complicating thrombolytic therapy with tissue plasminogen activator, *Arch Neurol* 47:105-106, 1990.

72. Gore JM, Barbash GI, White HD, et al for the GUSTO Trial: Functional status following stroke after thrombolytic therapy — results from the GUSTO Trial, *J Am Coll Cardiol* 28A, 1994.

73. Samama M: Hemorrhagic aspects of thrombolytic therapy, *Eur Heart J* 11:15-18, 1990.

74. O'Connor CM, Aldrich H, Massey EW, et al: Intracranial hemorrhage after thrombolytic therapy for acute myocardial infarction: clinical characteristics and in-hospital outcome, *J Am Coll Cardiol* 15:213A, 1990.

75. O'Connor CM, Aldrich H, Uglietta J, et al: Risk factor profile of patients with intracranial hemorrhage after thrombolytic therapy for acute myocardial infarction, *Neurology* (suppl.): April 1990.

76. Stroke. Towards better management. Summary and recommendations of a report of the Royal College of Physicians, *J R Coll Physicians Lond* 24:15-17, 1990.

77. Gijn JV: Subarachnoid haemorrhage, *Lancet* 339:653-655, 1992.

78. Verwey RD, Wijdicks EFM, van Gijn J: Warning headache in aneurysmal subarachnoid hemorrhage, *Arch Neurol* 45:1019-1020, 1988.

79. Mattle H, Kohler S, Huber P, et al: Anticoagulation-related intracranial extracerebral hemorrhage, *J Neurol Neursurg Psych* 52:829-837, 1989.

80. Held AC, Gore JM, Paraskos J, et al: Impact of thrombolytic therapy on left ventricular mural thrombi in acute myocardial infarction, *Am J Cardiol* 62:310-311, 1988.

81. Grines CL, DeMaria AN: Optimal utilization of thrombolytic therapy for acute myocardial infarction: concepts and controversies, *J Am Coll Cardiol* 16:223-231, 1990.

82. O'Connor CM, Califf RM: Aggressive therapy of acute MI in the elderly, *Hosp Prac* 27:59-76, 1992.

83. Lew AS, Hod H, Cercek B, et al: Mortality and morbidity rates of patients older and younger than 75 years with acute myocardial infarction treated with intravenous streptokinase, *Am J Cardiol* 59:1-5, 1987.

84. Behar S, Tanne D, Abinader E, et al for the SPRINT Study Group: Cerebrovascular accident complicating acute myocardial infarction:incidence, clinical significance, and short- and long-term mortality rates, *Am J Med* 91:45-50, 1991.

85. Wittry MD, Thornton TA, Chaitman BR: Safe use of thrombolysis in the elderly, *Geriatrics* 44:28-36, 1989.

86. More RS, Vincent R: Intracerebral hemorrhage after thrombolytic therapy for acute myocardial infarction, *Postgrad Med J* 68:800-803, 1992.

87. Anderson JL, Karagounis L, Allen A, et al: Older age and elevated blood pressure are risk factors for intracerebral hemorrhage after thrombolysis, *Am J Cardiol* 68:166-170, 1991.

88. Pendlebury WW, Iole ED, Tracy RP, et al: Dill BA. Intracerebral hemorrhage related to cerebral amyloid angiopathy and t-PA treatment, *Ann Neurol* 29:210-213, 1991.

89. Simoons ML, Maggioni AP, Knatterud G, et al: Individual risk assessment for intracranial haemorrhage during thrombolytic therapy, *Lancet* 342:1523-1528, 1993.

90. De Jaegere PP, Arnold AA, Balk AH, et al: Intracranial hemorrhage in association with thrombolytic therapy: incidence and clinical predictive factors, *J Am Coll Cardiol* 19:289-294, 1992.

91. Smith P, Arnesen H, Holme I: The effect of warfarin on mortality and reinfarction after myocardial infarction, *N Engl J Med* 323:147-152, 1990.

92. Stroke Prevention in Atrial Fibrillation Investigators: Stroke

Prevention in Atrial Fibrillation Study: final results, *Circulation* 84:527-539, 1991.

93. Althouse R, Maynard C, Olsufka M, et al: Risk factor for hemorrhagic and ischemic stroke in myocardial infarct patients treated with tissue plasminogen activator, *J Am Coll Cardiol* 13 (suppl A):153A, 1989.

94. Aylward P, Wilcox R, Granger C, et al for the GUSTO Investigators: Higher arterial blood pressure is associated with lower mortality but higher risk of stroke: results from the GUSTO Trial, *J Am Coll Cardiol* 28A, 1994.

95. Selker HP, Schmid CH, Beshansky JR, et al and the TPI Investigators: Pulse pressure predicts thrombolysis-related hemorrhagic stroke, *Circulation* 86(suppl I):I-67, 1992.

96. Barbash GI, White HD, Gore JM, et al for the GUSTO Trial: More aggressive thrombolytic treatment increases stroke risk: results from the GUSTO trial, *J Am Coll Cardiol* 28A, 1994.

97. Hillegass WB, Jollis JG, Granger CB, et al: Intracranial hemorrhage risk and new thrombolytic therapies in acute myocardial infarction, *Am J Cardiol* 73:444-449, 1994.

98. The GUSTO IIa Investigators: Increase in intracerebral hemorrhage with more aggressive antithrombin therapy for acute coronary syndromes: the GUSTO IIa preliminary results, *Circulation* 1994; in press.

99. Antiplatelet Trialists' Collaboration: Secondary prevention of vascular disease by prolonged antiplatelet treatment, *Br Med J* 296:320-331, 1988.

100. Roberts R, Rogers WJ, Mueller HS, et al for the TIMI investigators: Immediate versus deferred B-blockade following thrombolytic therapy in patients with acute myocardial infarction. Results of the Thrombolysis In Myocardial Infarction (TIMI) II-B study, *Circulation* 83:422-437, 1991.

101. Gill JS, Shipley MJ, Tsementzis SA, et al: Alcohol consumption—a risk factor for hemorrhagic and nonhemorrhagic stroke, *Am J Med* 90:489-497, 1991.

102. Granger C, White H, Aylward P, et al for the GUSTO Investigators: Risk factors for stroke following thrombolytic therapy: case-control study from the GUSTO trial, *Circulation* 1994; in press.

103. Sane DC, Califf RM, Topol EJ, et al: Bleeding during thrombolytic therapy for acute myocardial infarction: mechanisms and management, *Ann Intern Med* 111:1010-1022, 1989.

104. Eleff SM, Borel C, Bell WR, et al: Acute management of intracranial hemorrhage in patients receiving thrombolytic therapy: case reports, *Neurosurgery* 26:876-869, 1990.

105. Reith KG, Fujiwara K, DiChiro G, et al: Serial measurements of CT attentuation and specific gravity in experimental cerebral edema, *Radiology* 135:343-348, 1980.

106. Oppenheimer S, Hachinski V: Complications of acute stroke, *Lancet* 339:721-724, 1992.

107. Sandercock P, Willems H: Medical treatment of acute ischaemic stroke, *Lancet* 339:537-539, 1992.

108. Oppenheimer SM, Cechetto DF, Hachinski VC: Cerebrogenic cardiac arrhythmias, *Arch Neurol* 47:513-519, 1990.

109. Oppenheimer SM, Hoffbrand BI, Oswald GA, et al: Diabetes mellitus and early mortality from stroke, *Br Med J* 291:1015-1016, 1985.

110. Gupta SR, Naheedy MH, Elias D, et al: Post-infarction seizures: a clinical study, *Stroke* 19:1477-1481, 1988.

111. Busto R, Dietrich WD, Globus M, et al: The importance of brain temperature in cerebral ischemic injury, *Stroke* 20:1113-1114, 1989.

112. Warlow C: Secondary prevention of stroke, *Lancet* 339:724-727, 1992.

113. Horner J, Massey EW, Rishi JE, et al: Aspiration following stroke: clinical correlates and outcome, *Neurology* 38:1359-1362, 1988.

114. Wade DT: Stroke: rehabilitation and long-term care, *Lancet* 339:791-793, 1992.

115. Gent M, Blakely JA, Easton JD, et al: The Canadian American Ticlopidine Study (CATS) in thromboembolic stroke, *Lancet* 1:1215-1220, 1989.

116. North American Symptomatic Carotid Endarterectomy Trial Collaborators: Beneficial effect of carotid endarterectomy in symptomatic patients with high-grade carotid stenosis, *N Engl J Med* 325:445-453, 1991.

117. Krul JMJ, van Gijn J, Ackerstaff RGA, et al: Site and pathogenesis of infarcts associated with carotid endarterectomy, *Stroke* 20:324-328, 1989.

118. EC-IC Bypass Study Group: Failure of extracranial-intracranial arterial bypass to reduce the risk of ischemic stroke: results of an international randomized trial, *N Engl J Med* 313:1191-1200, 1985.

119. The Steering Committee of the Physicians' Health Study Research Group: Preliminary report: findings from the aspirin component of the ongoing Physicians' Health Study, *N Engl J Med* 318:262-264, 1988.

Chapter 53

ISCHEMIC MITRAL REGURGITATION AND OTHER MECHANICAL COMPLICATIONS

James E. Tcheng
James M. Douglas, Jr.

The therapeutics of the modern thrombolytic era, including intensive cardiac care, administration of thrombolytic therapy, use of anticoagulation and antiplatelet therapeutics, and percutaneous interventional and surgical revascularization, have succeeded in dramatically reducing the mortality of acute myocardial infarction (MI). Even with the success of these strategies, significant morbidity and mortality occur as a result of untoward mechanical and electrical complications of myocardial cellular ischemia and necrosis. This chapter reviews a number of these mechanical complications, specifically those that result in loss of mechanical functional or structural integrity involving the left ventricle. Also included are general guidelines for the recognition, diagnosis, management, and treatment of these syndromes.

These disorders present the clinician with some of the most difficult diagnostic and management challenges and comprise a significant portion of the differential diagnosis of hypotension and cardiogenic shock complicating MI (Table 53-1). All share in common the principle of myocardial ischemia leading to alteration of the normal mechanical function and geometric structure of the left ventricle. Although this review concentrates on mechanical etiologies of hypotension and cardiogenic shock, other reversible etiologies as listed in the table must be considered and corrected when present.

MITRAL REGURGITATION COMPLICATING AMI
Anatomy and pathogenesis

Acute mitral regurgitation caused by MI, defined as mitral valvular incompetence after acute MI without preceding mitral valvular pathologic conditions, is one of the most common of the mechanical complications of acute MI. Some degree of mitral regurgitation has been documented angiographically in 18% to 19% of patients hospitalized for MI.[1,2]

The anatomy of the mitral apparatus includes the mitral papillary muscles, chordae tendinae, mitral leaflets, and mitral annulus (Fig. 53-1). The papillary muscles are actually groups of muscles that consist of two or three well-defined, closely associated heads. These groups of muscles exist anatomically as anterolateral and posteromedial papillary muscle groups. Attached to the heads of the papillary muscles are the chordae tendinae, fibrous, trabeculated structures that serve as guy wires for the mitral leaflets. Chordae from each muscle group attach to both mitral leaflets; thus compromise of one papillary muscle will affect the systolic coaptation of both leaflets.

The vascular supply of the muscles is via penetrating arteries arising from the epicardial coronary vessels. Because of their relatively large size and their distance from the epicardial vessels, the papillary muscles are

Table 53-1. Differential diagnosis of hypotension and cardiogenic shock complicating myocardial infarction

Primary left ventricular failure
Primary right ventricular failure
Cardiac tamponade
Hypovolemia, bleeding
Mechanical complications
   Mitral regurgitation
      Papillary muscle dysfunction
      Mitral annular dilation
      Global left ventricular dysfunction
      Papillary muscle rupture
   Rupture of the interventricular septum
   Rupture of the ventricular free wall
      True rupture
      Left ventricular pseudoaneurysm
Dysrhythmias
Vasovagal reactions
Septicemia
Pulmonary embolism
Pneumothorax
Drugs
Iatrogenic causes

particularly sensitive to ischemia.[3] The anterolateral papillary muscles are supplied predominantly via obtuse marginal branches of the circumflex but also typically receive a second collateral blood supply from diagonal branches of the left anterior descending artery. The posteromedial muscles usually have a single blood supply arising from the posterior descending artery. As a consequence, the posteromedial papillary muscles tend to be more susceptible to ischemia and infarction than the anterolateral group.

The etiologies of mitral regurgitation secondary to ischemia have been classified into three distinct entities: papillary muscle dysfunction, generalized left ventricular or mitral annular dilation (or both), and papillary muscle or chordal rupture.[4] Any one or combination of these factors may contribute to the development of acute mitral regurgitation.

The most common cause of acute ischemic mitral regurgitation is the syndrome classically referred to as papillary muscle dysfunction. In this syndrome, ischemia of the papillary muscle alters the functional integrity of the mitral apparatus primarily by compromising systolic mitral leaflet coaptation, resulting in valvular regurgitation.[5,6] Papillary muscle necrosis without rupture is common in this setting.[7] Of note, in animal models it is unusual to have mitral regurgitation with primary, isolated ischemia of the papillary muscle unless there is also ischemia or infarction of the adjacent left ventricular myocardium.[8,9] More recent experimental evidence further suggests that global left ventricular dysfunction must be present before incomplete mitral leaflet coaptation can occur. In an animal model, Kaul et al.[10] noted

that mitral insufficiency was not observed even when one or both papillary muscles and the adjacent regions of myocardium were made ischemic and dysfunctional; regurgitation occurred only when there was significant global left ventricular impairment as well.

When there is generalized left ventricular or mitral annular dilation, valvular coaptation is compromised because of the unfavorable alterations in the geometry and spatial relationships of the papillary muscles, chordae tendinae, and mitral valvular leaflets.[11,12] This syndrome typically results from extensive myocardial injury, diffuse or recurrent infarction, or ventricular aneurysm formation. Poor overall left ventricular function typical of this class of patients serves only to compound the management of mitral regurgitation.

The least frequent cause is papillary muscle rupture. Rupture can occur in the body of the papillary muscle proper or at the point of attachment of the papillary muscle to the chordae tendinae. Even though this syndrome occurs in less than 1% of all patients hospitalized for MI, this form of ischemic mitral regurgitation is typically the most dramatic, because patients may suddenly develop pulmonary edema and cardiogenic shock 2 to 7 days after an otherwise uncomplicated infarction.[13-15] Similar to rupture of the ventricular septum or ventricular free wall, this syndrome should be managed as a true surgical emergency, because the complications of shock and pulmonary edema are consequences not of primary ventricular dysfunction but of a mechanical defect.[14,16] The diagnosis should be suspected especially in patients with a first infarction involving the posterior or inferior walls and can be confirmed by echocardiography or angiography.[17] Emergency surgical reattachment or mitral valve replacement remains the mainstay of treatment.

Diagnosis

The auscultatory findings of ischemic mitral regurgitation are quite different than the holosystolic murmur of rheumatic mitral disease. A crescendo-decrescendo murmur delayed in onset well after the first heart sound and heard best at the apex is typical.[18,19] The most specific characteristic of the murmur is that it has a delayed onset into middle or late systole; the murmur may be evanescent after infarction.[19,20] Unfortunately, the murmur of ischemic mitral regurgitation is a relatively insensitive finding and may not be appreciated in a considerable number of patients, including half of those with the most severe grades of regurgitation.[2,21,22] Thus, a high index of suspicion should be maintained for the presence of mitral regurgitation in all patients with acute MI, especially in the presence of hypotension, pulmonary edema, or cardiogenic shock (see Table 54-1). Echocardiography should be performed to evaluate right and left ventricular function, differentiate among

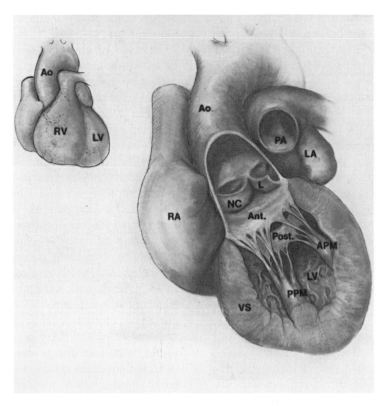

Fig. 53-1. Normal anatomy of the mitral valvular apparatus. The right ventricle *(RV, upper left)* has been removed in the principal illustration. The anterior mitral leaflet *(Ant.)* and the posterior mitral leaflet *(Post.)* receive insertions from both the anterolateral papillary muscle *(APM)* group and the posteromedial papillary muscle *(PPM)* group. Although not depicted, the anterolateral papillary muscle group receives a dual blood supply from obtuse marginal branches of the left circumflex and diagonal branches of the left anterior descending, whereas the posteromedial papillary muscle group receives only a single blood supply from the posterior descending. *Ao,* Aorta; *LV,* left ventricle; *RA,* right atrium; *PA,* pulmonary artery; *LA,* left atrium; *NC,* noncoronary aortic cusp; *L,* left coronary aortic cusp; *VS,* interventricular septum.

etiologies of mitral regurgitation, and exclude other etiologies of hemodynamic compromise; color-flow Doppler echocardiography permits quantitation of the severity of the incompetence.[23,24] Transesophageal Doppler echocardiography may have special utility in this setting as the most sensitive and specific indicator of regurgitation and should be performed when transthoracic echocardiography is equivocal or nondiagnostic.[25] Cardiac catheterization can confirm the diagnosis but is more useful in defining coronary anatomy in preparation for surgical revascularization; of note, cardiac catheterization is relatively insensitive in differentiating etiologies of mitral regurgitation, particularly papillary muscle rupture.

The clinical manifestations of acute mitral regurgitation are highly variable and are related to the degree of mitral incompetence, as well as overall left ventricular performance. Manifestations may range from a transient murmur to florid pulmonary edema, shock, rapid clinical deterioration, and death. Risk factors for the development of ischemic mitral regurgitation include advanced age, depressed left ventricular ejection fraction, congestive heart failure, severity of coronary artery disease, history of prior infarction, and associated medical illnesses.[1,2,26-28] With significant grades of mitral regurgitation, Swan-Ganz catheterization may demonstrate elevated mean pulmonary capillary wedge pressures and large V waves; these findings, however, are neither sensitive nor specific for this disorder and may be found in association with acute ventricular septal defect and left-sided heart failure.[29-31]

Treatment

Because of the high mortality rates associated with advanced degrees of mitral regurgitation, treatment of this disorder should be both interventional and symptomatic. Every attempt should be made to open the infarct-related artery of the patient with mitral regurgitation; small case series have documented reversal of mitral insufficiency and restoration of valvular competence with direct angioplasty during the acute phase of an MI, as well as with angioplasty in the elective setting.[32-34] Similar results have been noted in patients with mild to moderately severe regurgitation after surgical revascularization, even without valvular repair or replacement.[1] Unfortunately, patients with moderately severe to severe mitral regurgitation remain at substantial risk of death even with successful thrombolysis or direct angioplasty; despite the therapies of the modern thrombolytic era, 3+ or 4+ regurgitation has been identified as an independent predictor of mortality in multivariable analysis and is associated with a 1-year survival of only 48%.[2] Because of this high mortality, patients with 3+ or 4+ regurgitation should be managed most aggressively, with early consideration for surgical revascularization and repair or replacement of the mitral valve, especially when serial assessment indicates continued mitral valvular insufficiency despite coronary reperfusion.

Symptomatic treatment should be tailored to the degree of hemodynamic compromise induced by valvular compromise. In the patient with severe pulmonary edema, diuresis and afterload reduction may reverse pulmonary edema; nitroprusside has been shown to be of benefit in the stable patient.[35] Intraaortic balloon counterpulsation should also be considered, particularly in the patient with hypotension or refractory pulmonary edema.[36] For the rapidly deteriorating patient, percutaneous extracorporeal support may be implemented as a temporary bridge to the operating room. In any event, stabilization of the critically ill patient should be viewed as only temporary; definitive therapy should be considered at the earliest possible moment, because deterioration is unpredictable and may be rapid.

The timing and implementation of definitive therapy remain complex and controversial; no prospective randomized clinical trials comparing the various treatment options have been published to date. Nonetheless, a reasonable therapeutic approach can be derived from a survey of the published retrospective examinations in combination with clinical experience. The therapeutic options for patients with ischemic mitral regurgitation include thrombolytic therapy alone or combined with coronary angioplasty, coronary angioplasty alone, coronary artery bypass grafting, combined coronary artery bypass grafting with mitral valve replacement or repair, and isolated mitral valve replacement. This broad range of therapeutic options is a direct result of the diversity of the etiologies and clinical spectrum of this disorder. Patients may have reversible or irreversible acutely ischemic myocardium; they may have global left ventricular dilation, restricted mitral leaflet motion, leaflet prolapse, or acute papillary muscle rupture. Furthermore, the congestive heart failure frequently observed in this setting may be caused by global left ventricular pump

dysfunction, pump inefficiency secondary to severe regurgitation, or both.

Because of the variety of clinical manifestations, definitive therapy must be individualized. Serial echocardiography is an extremely useful tool in diagnosing, assessing, and guiding treatment in the patient with ischemic mitral regurgitation. Emergency echocardiography performed in patients suspected of having mitral valvular insufficiency will confirm the diagnosis and help define the mechanism of regurgitation. This is of particular importance in the patient with papillary muscle rupture, because early surgical intervention is desirable. In some patients, successful reperfusion with thrombolytic therapy or direct angioplasty may result in restoration of valvular competence. In this setting, echocardiography will document recovery of valvular competence. Serial echocardiography will also identify those patients with varying degrees of mitral insufficiency in whom regurgitation becomes significant only during myocardial ischemia. In these patients, coronary angioplasty or coronary artery bypass grafting alone would be indicated to reverse mitral insufficiency.

In patients with stable moderate to severe mitral regurgitation in whom spontaneous reversibility has not been demonstrated by serial echocardiography, surgical revascularization with valve repair or replacement confers a significant long-term benefit in contrast to medical therapy alone.[1,4,37-48] Furthermore, repair of the valvular apparatus rather than replacement offers additional benefits by reducing both short- and long-term morbidity and mortality.[37-39,41-43,45,46,48] Though surgical mortality in patients with ischemic mitral regurgitation remains higher than that seen in the general population undergoing coronary artery bypass graft surgery, medical management carries with it an even higher mortality.[2,49,50]

Occasionally the clinical significance of mitral regurgitation is unclear at the time of proposed surgical revascularization. In these instances, we have found it helpful to observe the hemodynamic changes and the degree of mitral regurgitation occurring in response to volume challenge and increased afterload induced intraoperatively. During these tests, filling pressures are monitored continuously and valvular function assessed using transesophageal echocardiography. Development of severe mitral regurgitation in response to volume or afterload challenge mandates valve repair or replacement. In patients with mild to moderate regurgitation, the ultimate decision to address the valve is additionally influenced by the patient's general clinical condition and the surgical accessibility of the mitral valve. Patients without hemodynamic compromise from mitral regurgitation will probably benefit from restoration of valvular competence only in terms of late mortality.

Rarely, isolated mitral valve repair or replacement will be performed in patients with ischemic mitral regurgitation. For the most part, this approach is reserved for the patient with severe hemodynamic compromise secondary to valvular dysfunction in association with nongraftable coronary artery disease.

When is surgery unlikely to be of benefit? Although no studies have systematically defined this group of patients, it is evident that certain patients have an extremely high risk of perioperative morbidity and mortality. These patients require a greater degree of surgical judgment in determining the advisability and timing of surgical intervention. For example, patients with oliguric renal failure who can be medically stabilized (with or without the use of intraaortic balloon pump counterpulsation) should have surgery delayed until renal function plateaus or improves. In these patients, if sufficient hemodynamic improvement cannot be quickly accomplished and ventricular function is well preserved (e.g., ejection fraction $\geq 50\%$), urgent operation with dialysis access should be considered. Another group of patients with a high perioperative risk profile are patients with significant impairment of left ventricular function. In this group of patients, it may be more appropriate to stabilize the patient with medical therapy and intraaortic balloon pump counterpulsation for several days before surgical treatment. Surgical risk increases as ejection fraction decreases; patients with a left ventricular ejection fraction of less than 35% and severe mitral regurgitation can be expected to have a very high risk of perioperative morbidity and mortality, and those with ejection fractions of less than 25% are unlikely to benefit from surgical intervention at all. In the latter situation, symptomatic (comfort) support is perhaps the most appropriate approach.

In conclusion, ischemic mitral regurgitation is an important clinical entity with multiple functional etiologies and protean manifestations. Only through an aggressive combined interventional and surgical approach coupled with astute clinical management can further reductions in mortality be made in this setting.

VENTRICULAR SEPTAL RUPTURE
Anatomy and pathogenesis

Ventricular septal rupture is one of two syndromes of rupture of the myocardial wall that may occur after MI (the second being rupture of the lateral free wall). Septal rupture creates a ventricular septal defect between the left and right ventricles; communication to the coronary sinus is also anatomically possible but extremely rare. The actual rupture is frequently a catastrophic event manifesting as acute hypotension, biventricular failure, and a new pansystolic murmur; a thrill is present in 50% of patients.[51] Although the size of the defect largely determines the relative volume of the resultant shunt, the extent of hemodynamic compromise induced by the combination of the shunt and the infarction is more

closely correlated with mortality.[52] Ventricular septal rupture should always be considered in the presence of refractory cardiogenic hypotension, even in the absence of a typical murmur. Paradoxically, defects with impressive palpable and audible examination findings may actually represent the smallest of defects and occur in patients whose hemodynamic perturbations are most easily managed.

Acquired ventricular septal defect is a relatively uncommon complication of MI, occurring in less than 1% to 2% of patients; this represents only about 10% of all patients sustaining any form of myocardial rupture.[53,54] Early reperfusion, especially with thrombolytic therapy, may further reduce the propensity for this complication by augmenting recovery of ischemic myocardium adjacent to necrotic tissue and promoting scar formation and healing. Acquired ventricular septal defects may be classified into one of two anatomic locations: anterior, typically high septal defects, occurring in the membranous, trabeculated septum of the anterior portion of the septum (Fig. 53-2); and inferior, typically located along the posteroinferior portion of the muscular septum and occasionally extending out to the apex. Infarcts of the membranous septum generally result from infarction of the left anterior descending, whereas posterior defects are the consequence of infarction of the posterior descending artery. Ruptures may be simple, limited to a direct through-and-through defect, or complex, including multiple holes, multiple fenestrations within a single communication, linear tears, and serpiginous dissection tracts.[55] Anterior defects tend to be limited in size and dimension compared with posterior defects; right ventricular infarction frequently complicates posterior defects. Risk factors are similar to those of ventricular free wall rupture and include poor collateral flow to the septum; septal rupture is more common during a first infarction and posterior infarction and is commonly associated with right ventricular infarction.[51,55-59] The distribution of diseased coronary arteries is skewed toward one-vessel disease.[51,57,59]

Diagnosis

The diagnosis of acute ventricular septal defect should be entertained in the patient with cardiogenic hypotension, biventricular failure (with right-sided failure frequently masking left-sided failure), and a new murmur or thrill after MI. Echocardiography is of particular utility in this setting, with two-dimensional imaging providing information about regional and global biventricular performance and color-flow Doppler imaging demonstrating location and type of septal rupture, as well as qualitative estimation of the severity of the shunt.[60-62] Similarly, transesophageal echocardiography can be performed, particularly in the patient with an

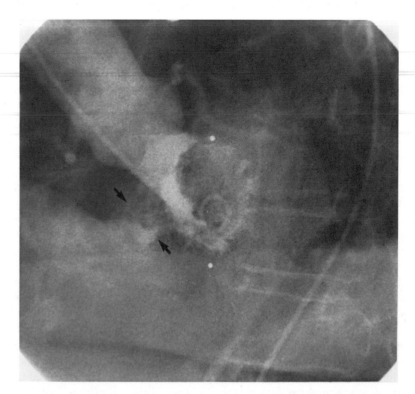

Fig. 53-2. Left anterior oblique cineangiographic view of an acute ventricular septal defect. Arrows indicate the margins of the communication between the left and right ventricular chambers. This acute septal rupture was an anterior septal defect, suggested by the well-defined margins and the proximity of the defect to the atrioventricular septum.

intubated airway, when transthoracic imaging proves inconclusive.[63] Giant left atrial V waves mimicking severe mitral regurgitation may be observed during Swan-Ganz catheterization.[29-31] Diagnostic left-sided heart catheterization should be performed primarily to document coronary anatomy before surgical repair and revascularization; left ventriculography may not be required, especially after high-quality echocardiographic studies, provided left ventricular function is well maintained and the defect well defined. If desired, right-sided heart catheterization with oximetry can provide quantitative assessment of the severity of the shunt; however, this is useful primarily to justify delay of definitive surgical repair by documentation of a small, hemodynamically insignificant shunt.

Therapy

Definitive therapy of ventricular septal rupture remains surgical repair. In patients fortunate enough to survive 6 or more weeks after the initial infarct, favorable operative and long-term mortality rates have been documented in early retrospective studies.[64,65] These patients, however, were composed of the minority of patients with the smallest of defects; indeed, their outcomes would be expected to be favorable in view of the minimal hemodynamic perturbation associated with a small defect. Unfortunately, the majority of patients

with acute ventricular rupture develop severe hemodynamic compromise that, if left unrepaired, quickly evolves into refractory forward output failure and death.[66,67] Management of these patients is at best difficult; medical management should be directed at restoration of metabolic abnormalities, primarily by augmentation of forward cardiac output with intraaortic balloon counterpulsation and vasodilators. Diuretics should be used judiciously to manage volume overload, as should pressors; the use of pressor agents may paradoxically increase shunt flow by increasing systemic resistance out of proportion to salutary inotropic effects. Where available, percutaneous cardiopulmonary support may be placed to provide extracorporeal support of vital organs as a bridge to the operating theater; this will improve peripheral perfusion, reduce myocardial ischemia, unload the heart, and reduce the shunt fraction. However, this can be implemented only on agreement in advance for emergency surgical operative repair, because the support is limited to a duration of up to only 6 to 8 hours. The best indication for application of this technology is in the patient with limited infarction and well-preserved overall left ventricular function, a large shunt fraction, and a relatively brief period ($<$ 12-24 hours) of relative hypoperfusion without true organ failure, because this type of patient would be expected to have a better surgical outcome than the patient with severely compromised ventricular performance. Indeed, overall left ventricular function is preserved in most cases of septal rupture.[51]

Surgical intervention should be performed at the earliest possible time, especially in the hypotensive patient in cardiogenic shock, because delay may contribute to organ failure and poorer surgical outcome. Although delay of definitive repair may seem judicious, especially in the stable patient, clinical deterioration is unpredictable and may be rapid; early surgical intervention may preempt clinical deterioration.[68] Operative mortality, especially in the acute setting, has been approximately 45% overall in reported series of operative repair. Mortality is higher in the setting of inferior MI compared with anterior infarction, being approximately 70% vs. 25% respectively. Furthermore, initial surgical outcome is clearly influenced by preoperative right ventricular dysfunction; poor right ventricular function is an important risk factor for postoperative mortality. Although most series demonstrate a survival advantage for patients operated on subacutely, these patients represent primarily those with the least hemodynamic compromise. Finally, as with patients with acute ischemic mitral regurgitation, there may be a subset in whom the surgical approach is unjustified because of an excessive perioperative mortality; although this group has not been systematically defined, such patients might include those with irreversible end-organ damage, severe impairment of overall left ventricular function, or large, multiple defects of the inferior wall combined with a large biventricular infarct. In conclusion, despite the high operative mortality, early surgical intervention remains the therapy of choice, especially in the hemodynamically compromised patient,[49,50,69,70] because medical mortality can be expected to be as high as 80% in the first week.[66,67]

VENTRICULAR WALL RUPTURE

Rupture of the left ventricular myocardial wall results in creation of a communication between the ventricular chamber and the pericardial space and is typically a sudden, unexpected, and catastrophic event. Anatomically, ventricular rupture differs from ventricular septal defect only by location of the disruption, with the rupture involving the lateral wall of the heart instead of the ventricular septum. If left untreated, this complication can result in the rapid accumulation of blood in the pericardial space (hemopericardium), pericardial tamponade, and death.

Ventricular rupture may be manifest in two forms, free rupture and pseudoaneurysm. The rupture event represents the creation of a hole or rent in the lateral myocardial wall, formed in an area of necrosis because of the pressure differential between the intraventricular cavity and the pericardial space. Free cardiac rupture is characterized by the unimpeded distribution of blood within the entire pericardial space after the rupture event. The same pathophysiology leading to free rupture results in pseudoaneurysm (false aneurysm) formation; in this situation, however, blood does not become freely distributed but instead becomes trapped within a limited portion of the pericardial space by pericardial adhesions, fibrin, or organized thrombus. Angiographically, pseudoaneurysm superficially resembles true left ventricular aneurysm formation by the appearance of a narrow neck communicating from the ventricular cavity to another saccular cavity; clues to differentiating the two include location and appearance. The true left ventricular aneurysm is typically apical and is thus best visualized angiographically in the right anterior oblique view; the pseudoaneurysm, on the other hand, involves the lateral free wall and thus is more easily appreciated angiographically in the left anterior oblique view. Margins of the true ventricular aneurysm are defined by the left ventricular free wall and are thus smooth and rounded (except when intraventricular thrombus or incomplete opacification obscures the margins), whereas pseudoaneurysm may be shaped more like a saucer or bowl (Fig. 53-3).

Ventricular free wall rupture accounts for approximately 10% to 20% of all deaths after MI or 2% to 4% of all patients admitted with MI.[71-74] One third of rupture events occur within 24 hours of manifestation; the remaining are distributed over several weeks, with 10% occurring more than 2 weeks from the time of infarction.[71,72] Risk factors for cardiac rupture include advanced age, female gender, hypertension, first infarction, and transmural infarction in the absence of collateral flow.[75-79] Persistent postinfarction hypertension, especially in the presence of a small initial infarct, infarct expansion, or wall thinning may create additional mechanical stresses contributing to cardiac rupture.

Most cases of free cardiac rupture are catastrophic. Some patients may develop sudden onset of chest pain with a "tearing" sensation. The clinical picture is one of rapidly progressive severe hypotension resistant to volume expansion and pressors, followed by electromechanical dissociation and death. Cardiac rupture should thus be suspected in the stable patient with sudden deterioration, as well as in any patient with unexplained severe hypotension after infarction. Definitive therapy remains immediate surgical repair; emergency pericardiocentesis, with repetitive aspiration of the pericardial space, should be performed as a bridge to the operating theater. Even with aggressive management, however, this manifestation is associated with an exceedingly high mortality, largely because of the rapidly progressive demise typical of this complication.

Subacute rupture, defined solely by a more indolent time course compared with acute rupture, should always

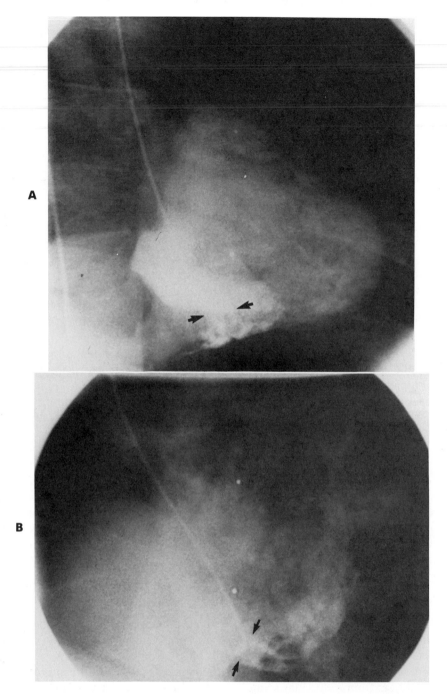

Fig. 53-3. Right anterior oblique (**A**) and left anterior oblique (**B**) cineangiographic views of a pseudoaneurysm originating along the inferior wall. Arrows indicate the margins of the communication between the pseudoaneurysm and the left ventricular cavity. Note the saucerlike shape of the pseudoaneurysm.

be considered in the differential diagnosis of the patient with refractory cardiogenic shock.[53] The primary presentation is that of pericardial tamponade physiology, typically with right-sided heart failure out of proportion to left-sided failure 3 or more days after infarction.[80-82] Swan-Ganz catheterization findings are consistent with pericardial tamponade, and echocardiography confirms the presence of fluid throughout the pericardial space. Even though not necessarily catastrophic, this complication should be treated as a true emergency, because clinical deterioration is unpredictable. Again, emergency pericardiocentesis may result in temporary stabilization of the patient while arrangements are being made for definitive surgical repair. Angiography is generally confirmatory of the diagnosis; time permitting, angiography should be performed primarily to assess the significance of coronary arterial disease in other coronary distributions in preparation for thoracotomy.

Pseudoaneurysm is more difficult to diagnose, primarily because it may remain clinically silent until catastrophic rupture of the pseudoaneurysm into the remaining free pericardial space. In fact, this diagnosis is made primarily at postmortem examination.[83] Nonspecific findings that may be present include a persistent pericardial friction rub, apical pansystolic murmur, mitral regurgitation, persistent ST-segment elevation, and an abnormal protrusion of the left ventricular lateral wall shadow on chest x-ray film.[53] Diagnosis is often an ancillary finding on performance of left ventriculography and can also be made by echocardiography. Once diagnosed, however, definitive surgical resection and repair should be performed as soon as feasible to preclude the possibility of catastrophic rupture, hemopericardium, and death.[84]

Management of the patient with cardiac rupture should be directed at expedient surgical repair. Stabilization with repetitive pericardiocentesis, intraaortic balloon counterpulsation, and correction of electrolyte abnormalities, electrical disturbances, and hemodynamic perturbations should be performed as part of the preoperative preparation of the patient. Sterile placement of a pigtail catheter within the pericardial space by exchange over a guidewire may augment the process of repetitive pericardiocentesis. When available, percutaneous cardiopulmonary support should be implemented, especially in the patient with free wall acute or subacute rupture, or rupture of a pseudoaneurysm; this will provide a window of approximately 6 to 8 hours during which the patient can be referred to the operating suite. In this setting, percutaneous support will not only maintain noncardiac organ viability but also unload and relax the heart, reducing the potential for further myocardial ischemia, infarction, or necrosis. Prognosis of these patients is dependent on definitive repair; long-term outcome after surgical treatment is excellent.[83,84]

CONCLUSION

Mechanical complications of acute MI occur infrequently but are typically dramatic and life threatening. These complications present the practicing clinician the most difficult diagnostic challenges and management quandaries. In general, prevention is the best intervention; specifically, early reperfusion, either with thrombolytic therapy, rescue angioplasty, or direct angioplasty, may reduce the propensity for these complications.[85-87] Once the patient has sustained an infarction, the clinician should maintain a high index of suspicion for the appearance of mechanical complications, especially evaluating the patient with hemodynamic compromise;

emergency echocardiography may prove enlightening in securing an accurate diagnosis. Once a mechanical complication becomes manifest, the risk to the patient is generally exceedingly high, justifying aggressive intervention and management. All of these complications are amenable to surgical repair, which remains the therapy of choice; the use of percutaneous cardiopulmonary support may provide a critical window of time during which extracorporeal support permits the mobilization of the surgical team for definitive repair.

REFERENCES

1. Hickey MS, Smith LR, Muhlbaier LH, et al: Current prognosis of ischemic mitral regurgitation, *Circulation* 78(suppl):I51, 1988.
2. Tcheng JE, Jackman Jr JD, Nelson CL, et al: Outcome of patients sustaining acute ischemic mitral regurgitation during myocardial infarction, *Ann Intern Med* 117:18, 1992.
3. Estes Jr EH, Dalton FM, Entman ML, et al: The anatomy and blood supply of the papillary muscle of the left ventricle, *Am Heart J* 71:356, 1966.
4. Rankin JS, Hickey MS, Smith LR, et al: Ischemic mitral regurgitation, *Circulation* 79(suppl):I116, 1989.
5. Burch GE, DePasquale NP, Phillips JH: The syndrome of papillary muscle dysfunction, *Am Heart J* 75:399, 1968.
6. Godley RW, Wann LS, Rogers EW, et al: Incomplete mitral leaflet closure in patients with papillary muscle dysfunction, *Circulation* 63:565, 1981.
7. Lie, JT, Wright Jr KE, Titus JL: Sudden appearance of a systolic murmur after acute myocardial infarction, *Am Heart J* 90:507, 1975.
8. Mittall AK, Langston Jr M, Cohn KE, et al: Combined papillary muscle and left ventricular wall dysfunction as a cause of mitral regurgitation, *Circulation* 44:174, 1971.
9. Underwood FO, Sybers RG, Ferrier FL, et al: Cineangiographic studies of the pathophysiology of experimental papillary muscle damage in dogs, *AJR* 108:702, 1970.
10. Kaul S, Spotnitz WD, Glasheen WP, et al: Mechanism of ischemic mitral regurgitation: an experimental evaluation, *Circulation* 84:2167, 1991.
11. Balu V, Hershowitz S, Zaki Masud AR, et al: Mitral regurgitation in coronary artery disease, *Chest* 81:550, 1982.
12. Bulkley BH, Roberts WC: Dilatation of the mitral annulus, *Am J Med* 59:457, 1975.
13. Cederquist L, Soderstrom J: Papillary muscle rupture in myocardial infarction, *Acta Med Scand* 176:287, 1964.
14. Nishimura RA, Schaff HV, Shub C, et al: Papillary muscle rupture complicating acute myocardial infarction: analysis of 17 patients, *Am J Cardiol* 51:373, 1983.
15. Wei JT, Hutchins GM, Bulkley BH: Papillary muscle rupture in fatal acute myocardial infarction: a potentially treatable cause of cardiogenic shock, *Ann Intern Med* 90:149, 1979.
16. Clements Jr SD, Story WE, Hurst JW, et al: Ruptured papillary muscle, a complication of myocardial infarction: clinical presentation, diagnosis, and treatment, *Clin Cardiol* 8:93, 1985.
17. Barbour DJ, Roberts WC: Rupture of a left ventricular papillary muscle during acute myocardial infarction: analysis of 22 necropsy patients, *J Am Coll Cardiol* 8:558, 1986.
18. Burch GE, DePasquale NP, Phillips JH: Clinical manifestations of papillary muscle dysfunction, *Arch Intern Med* 112:112, 1963.
19. Phillips JH, Burch GE, DePasquale NP: Syndrome of papillary muscle dysfunction, *Ann Intern Med* 59:508, 1963.
20. Maisel AS, Gilpin EA, Klein L, et al: The murmur of papillary muscle dysfunction in acute myocardial infarction: clinical features and prognostic implication, *Am Heart J* 112:705, 1986.

21. Forrester JS, Diamond G, Freedman S, et al: Silent mitral insufficiency in acute myocardial infarction, *Circulation* 44:877, 1982.

22. Roberts WC, Perloff JK: Mitral valvular disease: a clinicopathologic survey of the conditions causing the mitral valve to function abnormally, *Ann Intern Med* 77:939, 1972.

23. Izumi S, Miyatake K, Beppu S, et al: Mechanism of mitral regurgitation in patients with myocardial infarction: a study using real-time two-dimensional Doppler flow imaging and echocardiography, *Circulation* 76:777, 1987.

24. Nishimura RA, Shub C, Tajik AJ: Two dimensional echocardiographic diagnosis of partial papillary muscle rupture, *Br Heart J* 48:598, 1982.

25. Sheikh KH, Bengtson JR, Rankin JS, et al: Intraoperative transesophageal Doppler color flow imaging used to guide patient selection and operative treatment of ischemic mitral regurgitation, *Circulation* 84:594, 1991.

26. Barzilai B, Gessler Jr C, Perez JE, et al: Significance of Doppler-detected mitral regurgitation in acute myocardial infarction, *Am J Cardiol Cardiol* 61:220, 1988.

27. De Servi S, Vaccari L, Assandri J, et al: Clinical significance of mitral regurgitation in patients with recent myocardial infarction, *Eur Heart J* 9(suppl):F5, 1988.

28. Loperfido F, Biasucci LM, Pennestri F, et al: Pulsed Doppler echocardiographic analysis of mitral regurgitation after myocardial infarction, *Am J Cardiol* 58:692, 1986.

29. Bethea CF, Peter RH, Behar VS, et al: The hemodynamic simulation of mitral regurgitation in ventricular septal defect after myocardial infarction, *Cathet Cardiovasc Diagn* 2:97, 1976.

30. Drobach M, Schwartz L, Scully HE, et al: Giant left atrial V-waves in post-myocardial infarction ventricular septal defect, *Ann Thorac Surg* 27:347, 1979.

31. Fuchs RM, Heuser RR, Yin FC, et al: Limitations of pulmonary wedge v-waves in diagnosing mitral regurgitation, *Am J Cardiol* 49:849, 1982.

32. Heuser RR, Maddoux GL, Goss JE, et al: Coronary angioplasty for acute mitral regurgitation due to myocardial infarction, *Ann Intern Med* 107:852, 1987.

33. Reinfeld HB, Samet P, Hildner FJ: Resolution of congestive failure, mitral regurgitation, and angina after percutaneous transluminal coronary angioplasty of triple vessel disease, *Cathet Cardiovasc Diagn* 11:273, 1985.

34. Shawl FA, Forman MB, Punja S, et al: Emergent coronary angioplasty in the treatment of acute ischemic mitral regurgitation: long-term results in five cases, *J Am Coll Cardiol* 14:986, 1989.

35. Goodman DJ, Rossen RM, Holloway EL, et al: Effect of nitroprusside on left ventricular dynamics in mitral regurgitation, *Circulation* 50:1025, 1974.

36. Gold HK, Leinbach RC, Sanders CA, et al: Intraaortic balloon pumping for ventricular septal defect or mitral regurgitation complicating acute myocardial infarction, *Circulation* 47:1191, 1973.

37. Angell WW, Oury JH, Shah P: A comparison of replacement and reconstruction in patients with mitral regurgitation, *J Thorac Cardiovasc Surg* 93:45, 1987.

38. Bonchek LI, Olinger GN, Siegel R, et al: Left ventricular performance after mitral reconstruction for mitral regurgitation, *J Thorac Cardiovasc Surg* 88:122, 1984.

39. Cohn LH, Kowalker W, Bhatia S, et al: Comparative morbidity of mitral valve repair versus replacement for mitral regurgitation with and without coronary artery disease, *Ann Thorac Surg* 45:284, 1988.

40. Connolly MW, Gelbfish JS, Jacobowitz IJ, et al: Surgical results for mitral regurgitation from coronary artery disease, *J Thorac Cardiovasc Surg* 91:379, 1986.

41. David TE, Ho WC: The effect of preservation of chordae tendineae on mitral valve replacement for postinfarction mitral regurgitation, *Circulation* 74(suppl):I116, 1986.

42. Kay GL, Kay JK, Zubiate P, et al: Mitral valve repair for mitral regurgitation secondary to coronary artery disease, *Circulation* 74:I88, 1986.

43. Kay GL, Kay JH, Mendez MA, et al: Long-term results of operations for mitral regurgitation secondary to coronary artery disease, *Cardiovasc Clin* 17:41, 1987.

44. Magovern JA, Pennock JL, Campbell DB, et al: Risks of mitral valve replacement and mitral valve replacement with coronary artery bypass, *Ann Thorac Surg* 39:346, 1985.

45. Rankin JS, Feneley MP, Hickey MS, et al: A clinical comparison of mitral valve repair versus valve replacement in ischemic mitral regurgitation, *J Thorac Cardiovasc Surg* 95:165, 1988.

46. Rankin JS, Livesey SA, Smith LR, et al: Trends in the surgical treatment of ischemic mitral regurgitation: effects of mitral valve repair on hospital mortality, *Thorac Cardiovasc Surg* 1:149, 1989.

47. Replogle RL, Campbell CD: Surgery for mitral regurgitation associated with ischemic heart disease, *Circulation* 79(suppl):I122, 1989.

48. Sand ME, Naftel DC, Blackstone EH, et al: A comparison of repair and replacement for mitral valve incompetence, *J Thorac Cardiovasc Surg* 94:208, 1987.

49. Nishimura RA, Schaff HV, Gersh BJ, et al: Early repair of mechanical complications after acute myocardial infarction, *JAMA* 256:47, 1986.

50. Scanlon PJ, Montoya A, Johnson SA, et al: Urgent surgery for ventricular septal rupture complicating acute myocardial infarction, *Circulation* 72(suppl):II185, 1985.

51. Radford MJ, Johnson RA, Daggett Jr WM, et al: Ventricular septal rupture: A review of clinical and physiologic features and an analysis of survival, *Circulation* 64:545, 1981.

52. Feneley MP, Chang VP, O'Rourke MF: Myocardial rupture after acute myocardial infarction. Ten year review, *Br Heart J* 49:550, 1983.

53. Lavie CJ, Gersh BJ: Mechanical and electrical complications of acute myocardial infarction, *Mayo Clin Proc* 65:709, 1990.

54. Vlodaver Z, Edwards JE: Rupture of ventricular septum or papillary muscle complicating myocardial infarction, *Circulation* 55:815, 1977.

55. Edwards BS, Edwards WD, Edwards JE: Ventricular septal rupture complicating acute myocardial infarction: identification of simple and complex types in 53 autopsied hearts, *Am J Cardiol* 54:1201, 1984.

56. Cummings RG, Reimer KA, Califf R, et al: Quantitative analysis of right and left ventricular infarction in the presence of postinfarction ventricular septal defect, *Circulation* 77:33, 1988.

57. Mann JM, Roberts WC: Acquired ventricular septal defect during acute myocardial infarction: analysis of 38 unoperated necropsy patients and comparison with 50 unoperated necropsy patients without rupture, *Am J Cardiol* 62:8, 1988.

58. Moore CA, Nygaard TW, Kaiser DL, et al: Postinfarction ventricular septal rupture: the importance of location of infarction and right ventricular function in determining survival, *Circulation* 74:45, 1986.

59. Reddy SG, Roberts WC: Frequency of rupture of the left ventricular free wall or ventricular septum among necropsy cases of fatal acute myocardial infarction since introduction of coronary care units, *Am J Cardiol* 63:906, 1989.

60. Smyllie JH, Dawkins K, Conway N, et al: Diagnosis of ventricular septal rupture after myocardial infarction: value of colour flow mapping, *Br Heart J* 62:260, 1989.

61. Smyllie JH, Sutherland GR, Geuskens R, et al: Doppler color flow mapping in the diagnosis of ventricular septal rupture and acute

mitral regurgitation after myocardial infarction, *J Am Coll Cardiol* 15:1449, 1990.

62. Zachariah ZP, Hsiung MC, Nanda NC, et al: Diagnosis of rupture of the ventricular septum during acute myocardial infarction by Doppler color flow mapping, *Am J Cardiol* 59:162, 1987.

63. Oh JK, Seward JB, Khandheria BK, et al: Transesophageal echocardiography in the intensive care unit [abstract], *Circulation* 78(suppl):II-298, 1988.

64. Daggett WM, Guyton RA, Mundth ED, et al: Surgery for post-myocardial infarct ventricular septal defect, *Ann Surg* 186: 260, 1977.

65. Giuliani ER, Danielson GK, Pluth JR, et al: Postinfarction ventricular septal rupture: surgical considerations and results, *Circulation* 49:455, 1974.

66. Sanders R, Kern W, Blount S: Perforation of the interventricular septum complicating myocardial infarction, *Am Heart J* 51:736, 1956.

67. Sanders RJ, Neubuerger KT, Ravin A: Rupture of papillary muscles: occurrence of rupture of the posterior muscle in posterior myocardial infarction, *Dis Chest* 31:316, 1957.

68. Montoya A, McKeever L, Scanlon P, et al: Early repair of ventricular septal rupture after infarction, *Am J Cardiol* 45:345, 1980.

69. Cohn LH: Surgical treatment of acute myocardial infarction, *Cardiology* 76:167, 1989.

70. Thomas Jr CS, Alford Jr WC, Burrus GR, et al: Urgent operation for acquired ventricular septal defect, *Ann Surg* 195:706, 1982.

71. Dellborg M, Held P, Swedberg K, et al: Rupture of the myocardium. Occurrence and risk factors, *Br Heart J* 54:11, 1985.

72. Rasmussen S, Leth A, Kjoller E, et al: Cardiac rupture in acute myocardial infarction: a review of 72 consecutive cases, *Acta Med Scand* 205:11, 1979.

73. Sievers J: Cardiac rupture in acute myocardial infarction, *Geriatrics* 21:125, 1966.

74. Solberg S, Nordrum I, Fausa D, et al: Cardiac ruptures in northern Norway. A retrospective study of 104 cases, *Acta Med Scand* 224:303, 1988.

75. Bates RJ, Buetler S, Resnekov L, et al: Cardiac rupture—challenge in diagnosis and management, *Am J Cardiol* 40:429, 1977.

76. Christensen DJ, Ford M, Reading J, et al: Effect of hypertension in myocardial rupture after acute myocardial infarction, *Chest* 72:618, 1977.

77. Mann JM, Roberts WC: Rupture of the left ventricular free wall during acute myocardial infarction: analysis of 138 necropsy patients and comparison with 50 necropsy patients with acute myocardial infarction without rupture, *Am J Cardiol* 62:847, 1988.

78. Nakano T, Konishi T, Takezawa H: Potential prevention of myocardial rupture resulting from acute myocardial infarction, *Clin Cardiol* 8:199, 1985.

79. Oblath RW, Levinson DC, Griffith GC: Factors influencing rupture of the heart after myocardial infarction, *JAMA* 149:1276, 1952.

80. Coma-Canella I, Lopez-Sendon J, Nu-nez GL, et al: Subacute left ventricular free wall rupture following acute myocardial infarction: bedside hemodynamics, differential diagnosis, and treatment, *Am Heart J* 106:278, 1983.

81. O'Rourke MF: Subacute heart rupture following myocardial infarction: clinical features of a correctable condition, *Lancet* 2:124, 1973.

82. O'Rourke MF, Sammel N, Chang VP: Arterial counterpulsation in severe refractory heart failure complicating acute myocardial infarction, *Br Heart J* 41:308, 1979.

83. Gueron M, Wanderman KL, Hirch M, et al: Pseudoaneurysm of the left ventricle after myocardial infarction: a curable form of myocardial rupture, *J Thorac Cardiovasc Surg* 69:736, 1975.

84. Rittenhouse EA, Sauvage LR, Mansfield PB, et al: False aneurysm of the left ventricle: report of four cases and review of surgical management, *Ann Surg* 189:409, 1979.

85. Gertz SD, Kragel AH, Kalan JM, et al: Comparison of coronary and myocardial morphologic findings in patients with and without thrombolytic therapy during fatal first acute myocardial infarction. The TIMI Investigators, *Am J Cardiol* 66:904, 1990.

86. Honan MB, Harrell Jr FE, Reimer KA, et al: Cardiac rupture, mortality and the timing of thrombolytic therapy: a meta-analysis, *J Am Coll Cardiol* 16:359, 1990.

87. Kahn JK, O'Keefe Jr HJ, Rutherford BD, et al: Timing and mechanism of in-hospital and late death after primary coronary angioplasty during acute myocardial infarction, *Am J Cardiol* 66:1045, 1990.

Chapter 54

ACUTE CARE OF THE PATIENT WITH PREVIOUS CORONARY BYPASS SURGERY

Michael H. Sketch, Jr.
Marino Labinaz
Paul E. Nathan
Joseph A. Puma
Robert M. Califf

Coronary artery bypass grafting is an effective method of revascularization in the patient with obstructive coronary artery disease.[1,2] Although several studies have demonstrated its benefit in improving long-term survival in specific patient populations, bypass surgery is performed in the majority of cases for symptom relief. For both indications, bypass surgery is a palliative rather than a curative form of therapy, with the long-term results dependent on the attrition rate of the bypass conduits as well as the progression of atherosclerosis in the native coronary circulation.[3]

Over the last several years the marked increase in the use of this procedure has resulted in an ever-increasing population of patients with unstable angina and AMI who have had previous bypass grafting. In some series, up to 20% of the patients who present with unstable angina have had previous bypass surgery.[4] Over a decade ago only 2% of all patients presenting with an AMI had previous bypass surgery; the current incidence is 10% to 15%.[5] Despite this large patient population there is a paucity of data regarding their management in the setting of unstable angina and AMI. While awaiting the results of randomized clinical trials, an appropriate

understanding of the pathoanatomy, pathophysiology, and observational treatment evaluations of this clinical problem may aid the clinician in making rational decisions about therapy.

PATHOANATOMY
Native coronary arteries

Progression of native coronary artery disease (worsening of a preexisting lesion or appearance of a new diameter narrowing greater than 49%) in patients with previous bypass surgery occurs at an approximate annual rate of 5%.[6-9] In 1971, Aldridge and Trimble were the first to suggest that the atherosclerotic process displayed an accelerated course in the recipient native artery after bypass surgery.[10] This phenomenon occurred in 5 of 8 recipient arteries and was always observed proximal to the anastomosis. Bousvaros et al. corroborated these observations and emphasized that this process may play a role in the development of unstable angina and AMI. These findings were subsequently contradicted by Gensini et al. who demonstrated in a retrospective analysis of 220 patients with serial angiograms that the progression of coronary artery disease was greater in the nonoperated group.[12] The results of this study should be interpreted with caution, however, because the follow-up period was significantly longer in the nonoperated group. Subsequently, the majority of studies have supported the original observations of Aldridge and Trimble.[6-9,13,14]

The incidence of new native coronary occlusions ranges from 40% to 60% in grafted arteries vs. 2% to 6% in nongrafted arteries.[13] Various theories have been proposed to explain these observations and include (1) surgical manipulation of an already diseased coronary artery; (2) reduction in the pressure gradient across a severely stenotic proximal segment, producing turbulence and stasis at that point, which may lead to thrombus formation and occlusion; and (3) reversal of flow.[13] The reversal of flow may have two effects. First, because the blood in the grafted vessel will move from a narrow segment to one of wider caliber and because flow velocity is inversely related to the cross-sectional area of the vessel, the flow will be less in the proximal segment. Second, the reversal of flow may result in retrograde perfusion of the branches proximal to the graft insertion. The branching pattern of the coronary tree will demand that the current of blood flow negotiate acute angles to perfuse the proximal branches and will thus create increased turbulence at branch points.

These results are disturbing insofar as they suggest that saphenous vein (and probably internal mammary artery) bypass grafting is associated with native coronary artery deterioration. It is equally clear from the study by Maurer et al. that arteries with significant but less critical (50% to 75%) stenoses are almost as likely to close following bypass grafting as are those arteries with major stenoses.[13] This finding questions the wisdom of operating on vessels with borderline stenoses.

Saphenous vein grafts

The rate of vein graft closure in the perioperative and early postoperative period (up to 1 month) ranges from 5% to 20%.[15] Thrombosis is the usual cause of graft closure during this period. Damage to the venous endothelium may lead to platelet deposition and stimulation of the coagulation cascade. This damage may be produced by the sudden exposure to the high-pressure arterial system, impaired nutrition of the venous wall, and injury secondary to the venotomy and arteriotomy. Technical factors that may stimulate thrombus formation include twisting of the graft and implantation of the graft under tension. Low vein-graft blood flow and a small luminal size of the grafted artery may predispose to an increase in the early occlusion rate of bypass grafts.[16]

All patent vein grafts develop intimal hyperplasia between the first and twelfth postoperative month.[17] The intimal hyperplasia is inversely related to flow.[18] All layers of the graft are involved in this unique process, and the result is a homogeneous and diffuse reduction in graft vessel caliber approaching that of the recipient artery by 1 year following surgery. By the twelfth postoperative month, approximately 10% of patent vein grafts have $\geq$ 50% segmental luminal diameter narrowing.[15,19] This narrowing is most common at the distal anastomosis. The most frequent mechanism of graft closure during this time period is the development of occlusive thrombi superimposed upon intimal hyperplasia.[20]

Atherosclerotic lesions in vein grafts are usually not apparent until 3 years following graft insertion. These lesions resemble native coronary lesions in that they contain foam cells, blood product debris, cholesterol clefts, fibrocollagenous tissue, and calcific deposits. However, in contrast to native coronary lesions, the predominant cell type in vein graft lesions is the foam cell, resulting in less fibrocollagenous tissue and calcific deposits. These foam cells appear to erode the intima and predispose to plaque fissure or rupture. These characteristics account for the fragility of vein graft lesions and the frequent presence of blood in the atheroma.[18,21]

In summary, occlusion occurs in 10% to 25% of grafts during the first postoperative year. Graft occlusion between years 1 and 7 is less common, with a yearly graft occlusion rate of 0.5% to 3%. After the seventh year the closure rate may increase two- to threefold. With this occlusion rate only 30% to 40% of vein grafts are without significant (>50% luminal reduction) atherosclerotic narrowing 12 years after the surgery.[22] This attrition rate, combined with the apparent accelerated progression of disease in native vessels, presumably explains the reduction in the survival benefit of surgery that is observed beyond the first 5 to 10 years after the operation.

Internal mammary artery grafts

In sharp contrast to the saphenous vein graft, the internal mammary artery graft is much less prone to intimal thickening. In order to understand this observation, Svendsen et al. examined the morphologic differences between the left anterior descending coronary artery and the internal mammary artery in 62 autopsies from individuals of various age groups.[23] The amount of intimal thickening was assessed for each vessel in all patients. They found that intimal thickening was more marked and occurred earlier in life in the left anterior descending coronary artery than in the internal mammary artery. When fibrointimal proliferation does occur, it is most common at the distal anastomosis and occurs predominately within the first year following bypass surgery. The 10-year attrition rate of this graft has been reported to be 10% to 15% at the Cleveland Clinic;

however, little multicenter long-term data has been published.[22] The use of this conduit has shown a substantial beneficial effect on long-term patient survival.[24]

CORONARY RISK FACTORS

Because saphenous vein and internal mammary artery grafts appear to be susceptible to atherosclerosis, modification of cardiovascular risk factors may alter their long-term outcome. The modifiable risk factors for coronary artery disease that may influence the results of coronary artery bypass surgery are hypertension, tobacco abuse, hypercholesterolemia, and diabetes mellitus.

Saphenous vein grafts

Several pathologic and angiographic studies have documented an association between atherosclerosis and hypercholesterolemia in saphenous vein grafts. In a postmortem study of 56 patients, the mean serum cholesterol level of patients whose grafts had atherosclerosis was over 300 mg/dl, whereas the mean serum cholesterol level of patients whose grafts had only intimal hyperplasia was 170 mg/dl.[25] A follow-up pathologic study supported the association between serum cholesterol and atherosclerosis by univariate analysis.[26] Both these pathologic studies found no association between serum triglyceride levels and graft atherosclerosis. Similar findings were documented in angiographic studies. In a retrospective study of 501 patients with serial arteriograms following bypass surgery, a multivariate analysis revealed a significant association between progression of vein graft disease and hypercholesterolemia.[22] The Cholesterol-Lowering Atherosclerosis Study demonstrated that lipid modification with colestipol and niacin resulted in a lower incidence of graft attrition and less progression of disease in native vessels.[27] In a clinical study by Lytle et al., event-free survival was decreased in patients with an elevated cholesterol following bypass surgery.[28]

Several clinical studies have documented an association between the progression of saphenous vein graft atherosclerosis and diabetes, smoking, and hypertension, in addition to hypercholesterolemia.[28-32] In a study involving 2004 patients after bypass surgery, diabetes mellitus was found to be significantly associated with postoperative mortality.[31] Another study found smoking and diabetes to correlate with a decreased event-free survival in 107 patients following bypass surgery.[28]

Epidemiologic studies have found an association between high levels of factor VII a, fibrinogen, and Lp[a] and native coronary atherosclerosis.[33,34] Similar thrombotic risk factors have not been defined for bypass graft atherosclerosis.

The combination of several risk factors may have a cumulative effect on the long-term postoperative outcome. Tschan et al. found a significant reduction in favorable outcome in postoperative patients having two or more coronary risk factors vs. patients with less than two risk factors.[35] In a similar study of patients following bypass surgery, there was a significantly higher incidence of MI in patients who had four to five coronary risk factors.[36]

Internal mammary artery grafts

In contrast to data on saphenous vein grafts, little data is available on the influence of coronary risk factors on the outcome of internal mammary artery grafts. As discussed earlier the internal mammary artery graft attrition rate is reported to be only 10% to 15% at 10 years after surgery. With this low attrition rate it seems unlikely that traditional coronary risk factors impact significantly on these conduits.

MANAGEMENT OF UNSTABLE ANGINA IN THE POSTBYPASS PATIENT

Annually approximately 5% to 10% of postbypass patients experience a worsening or recurrence of their ischemic symptoms.[3,37] As the interval following surgery increases beyond the first 5 to 10 years, there is an increase in the frequency of recurrent anginal symptoms and a decrease in the survival benefit.[3,24] The clinical characteristics of patients with unstable angina postbypass appears to be similar to patients without previous bypass surgery.[4]

An understanding of the mechanism of graft closure is important in the management of patients following coronary artery bypass grafting. As discussed earlier, early graft closure (up to 1 month postoperative) is related to thrombosis, in which platelet deposition and activation of the coagulation system play an important role. Between the first and twelfth month the most frequent mechanism of graft closure is the development of occlusive thrombi superimposed on intimal hyperplasia, whereas atherosclerotic lesions begin to appear following the first year. Based on these pathophysiologic observations, possible management options in the setting of unstable angina will be discussed.

Antiplatelet and antithrombotic agents

Antiplatelet and antithrombotic agents play a crucial role in the control of platelet aggregation and thrombus formation in unstable angina. Aspirin is the prototype antiplatelet agent, whereas heparin is the prototype antithrombotic agent.

In several prospective randomized clinical trials the use of aspirin compared to placebo for the treatment of unstable angina has been found to be associated with a significant reduction in the subsequent incidence of fatal and nonfatal MI.[38,39] Although studies have not specifically examined the impact of aspirin on the management of unstable angina in postbypass patients, numerous studies have examined the impact of aspirin on the early and late postoperative patency of saphenous vein grafts.[40-48] Some early studies evaluated the utility of aspirin initiated during the preoperative period. Although the patency rates compared favorably to trials in which aspirin was started after surgery, these patients experienced more postoperative bleeding, increased transfusion requirements, and an increased frequency of reoperation.[49] In a study by Chesebro et al., a regimen of preoperative dipyridamole and postoperative dipyridamole and aspirin resulted in a reduction in the rate of graft occlusion at both 1 and 12 months postsurgery.[42] At a median of 12 months there was a reduction in the occlusion rate from 25% to 11% with aspirin.

In contrast to saphenous vein grafts, thrombosis and intimal hyperplasia are rare in internal mammary artery grafts. However, antiplatelet therapy is recommended to further decrease the low incidence of thrombosis in these conduits.

The optimal combination, dose, and duration of antiplatelet therapy has not been clarified. Despite the inclusion of dipyridamole in the postoperative regimen of many studies, no clear benefit of aspirin and dipyridamole over aspirin alone has been shown. Within 24 hours following surgery a loading dose of 325 mg of aspirin should be administered and followed by a maintenance dose of 80 to 325 mg daily. Therapy should be continued for a minimum of 1 year following surgery but probably should be continued indefinitely.

Heparin is the most effective anticoagulant currently available for the treatment of unstable angina. Although its anticoagulant property primarily involves the activation and modulation of antithrombin III, several additional properties of heparin may increase its beneficial role in the management of unstable angina. Binding to endothelial cells, heparin helps to restore electronegativity to the injured endothelial surface. It also prevents thrombin-induced platelet aggregation, inhibits leukocyte lysosomal enzyme release and free radical generation, and inhibits smooth muscle cell proliferation.[50]

The combination of heparin and aspirin should theoretically have a favorable impact on the management of postbypass patients with unstable angina. However, in a subset of 88 patients with unstable angina and previous bypass surgery, Théroux et al. retrospectively analyzed the effect of aspirin, heparin, or both on the clinical endpoints of death, MI, and severe refractory angina.[51] Surprisingly, no effect of aspirin could be detected in these patients for any of the three endpoints, whereas heparin did decrease the incidence of these events. Although these results should be interpreted with caution as with any retrospective analysis, especially with such a small sample size, the superiority of heparin in this study suggests that thrombin activation may be more important than platelet aggregation in the genesis of graft closure and untoward events in patients with previous bypass surgery. In a subsequent randomized trial comparing aspirin and heparin for the prevention of MI during the acute hospitalization phase of unstable angina, the superiority of heparin over aspirin was demonstrated again.[52]

Calcium antagonists, beta blockers, and nitrates

The efficacy of calcium antagonists, beta-adrenergic blockers, and nitrates in relieving angina is well established. Although these agents differ in their mechanisms of action, they all reduce myocardial oxygen demand and therefore should be beneficial in unstable angina. The specific impact of these agents on patients with unstable angina and previous bypass surgery has not been documented.

Intravenous nitroglycerin is the mainstay of antiischemic therapy in the management of unstable angina. In addition to the reduction in preload and afterload, nitroglycerin's inhibitory effect on platelet aggregation may be important in its overall mechanism of action. Platelets taken from patients treated with intravenous nitroglycerin exhibit attenuated aggregation responses ex vivo and may exhibit similar responses in vivo.[53] This finding may further support the use of nitrates in the postbypass patient with unstable angina.

Although several randomized trials have examined the role of beta blockers and calcium antagonists in the management of unstable angina, none were specifically designed to address patients with previous bypass surgery. In patients presenting with unstable angina and not receiving beta-blocker therapy, the addition of a beta blocker appears to reduce the symptoms of recurrent ischemia and the incidence of MI.[54,55] With respect to the calcium channel blockers, nifedipine and other similar agents that do not decrease heart rate are associated with an increased risk of MI or recurrent ischemia.[54,56] Diltiazem, which does decrease heart rate, has been shown to be neither beneficial nor detrimental.[57] Furthermore, in the post-MI patient with depressed left ventricular function, diltiazem has been shown to have a detrimental effect. Therefore calcium channel blockers should only be used for treating refractory symptoms in the unstable angina patient after other agents have failed.

Thrombolytic therapy

In 1980 Rentrop et al. described the successful application of selective thrombolysis in a patient with unstable angina and previous bypass surgery.[58] Restoration of graft patency was obtained with 140,000 units of intragraft streptokinase. Since this initial report, documentation of the safety and efficacy of thrombolytic therapy in the management of unstable angina has been limited to isolated case reports and small series of patients.[58-62]

In the largest series of patients receiving intragraft thrombolytic therapy, Hartman et al. describe a method of administering a prolonged, low-dose infusion of urokinase directly into the proximal portion of the graft.[61,62] Via this method 46 consecutive patients with 47 occluded grafts were treated with a urokinase infusion at a dose of 100,000 to 250,000 u/l over 7.5 to 77 hours. Successful recanalization was achieved in 79% of the grafts. Procedure-related complications occurred in 32% of the patients, including 6 patients with chest pain and ST-segment elevation suggestive of infarction and 10 patients with a significant hematoma. Of the successfully treated patients, 61% remained free of symptoms during a mean follow-up interval of 27 months. However, in a study by Levine et al. on the late follow-up of 10 patients who received a prolonged urokinase infusion for occluded vein grafts, all patients either reoccluded, suffered an MI, or died.[63] Although early patency of occluded vein grafts can be achieved in the majority of patients with prolonged thrombolytic therapy with or without adjunctive balloon angioplasty, the overall value of this strategy is uncertain.

Reoperation and coronary angioplasty

Before the introduction of percutaneous transluminal coronary angioplasty (PTCA) by Gruentzig in 1979,[64] reoperation was the only available option for the treatment of recurrent anginal symptoms refractory to medical therapy. Reoperations account for 5% to 10% of all coronary artery bypass graft procedures.[65,66] Despite improvements in myocardial protection and increased surgical experience, the risks of reoperation still exceed those for the initial revascularization. The perioperative mortality rate for the first reoperation varies from 2% to 7.5%, whereas the perioperative mortality rate for the second reoperation has been reported to be as high as 9%.[67-74] Perioperative MI occurred in 2% to 9.2% of patients, and postoperative bleeding requiring reexploration occurred in 1.3% to 6.8% of patients undergoing a reoperation. In addition to the higher operative mortality rate associated with reoperation, there is less relief of angina in the first year after the reoperation than after the initial operation.

PTCA is a potential alternative to reoperation for select saphenous vein and internal mammary artery grafts. In an initial series of 25 patients, balloon angioplasty resulted in a 56% angiographic success rate.[75] Subsequent studies have reported higher success rates ranging from 78% to 94%.[76-81] MI, emergency CABG, and death were reported in up to 8%, 3.5%, and 2% of patients, respectively. The reported restenosis rates vary from 33% to 73% of patients undergoing angiographic follow-up.[76-81] The age of a vein graft at the

time of angioplasty may influence the incidence of restenosis. In the series of 672 saphenous vein graft lesions reported by Douglas et al., restenosis occurred in 32% of lesions dilated within 6 months of surgery, 43% from 6 months to 1 year, 61% from 1 to 5 years, and 64% over 5 years.[81] Even though these studies do not specifically address the unstable angina patient, one would expect a lower acute procedural success rate and a higher restenosis rate.

The results of coronary artery bypass surgery in patients who fail PTCA of coronary bypass conduits is associated with significant morbidity and mortality. Weintraub et al. reviewed the outcomes of 46 patients who underwent reoperation for failed angioplasty during the same hospital stay.[82] Thirty-three of the 46 patients had acute ischemia. In this group with ischemia, three patients (9.1%) died and eleven (33.3%) had a nonfatal Q-wave MI.

MANAGEMENT OF AMI IN THE POSTBYPASS PATIENT

During the last decade there has been a significant increase in the number of patients with previous coronary bypass surgery who present with an AMI. Treatment strategies in the management of an AMI have not been adequately validated in this cohort of patients.

Because of differences in pathophysiology, the clinical features and prognosis following an AMI in postbypass patients are different from patients without surgery.[83,84] The Coronary Artery Surgery Study (CASS) Registry was used by Davis et al. to evaluate the 30-day mortality of AMI in patients with and without prior bypass surgery.[85] The mortality rate in the group with previous bypass surgery was 21%, which was significantly lower than the 36% mortality rate seen in patients treated medically. Although the surgical group had more two-vessel disease and less ventricular dysfunction at baseline, the difference in mortality remained significant despite adjusting for age, extent of disease, left ventricular dysfunction, angina, prior MI, and sex. Left ventricular dysfunction was an important predictor of mortality in both groups, whereas the number of diseased vessels appeared to be an important risk factor only in the nonbypass group.

To define the long-term prognosis of patients who suffered an MI late after bypass surgery, Wiseman et al. compared a cohort of patients who had an MI >60 days after bypass surgery to a similar cohort of patients without previous bypass surgery.[83] The cumulative 5-year cardiac mortality was similar in both patient groups. However, there was a significantly higher incidence of reinfarctions, admissions for unstable angina, and revascularization procedures in the postbypass group.

In a retrospective analysis of prospectively collected

data in the Duke University Databank for Cardiovascular Diseases, all patients who underwent immediate angiography for a suspected AMI between March 1986 and July 1990 were examined.[86] Patients were subdivided into those with and without a history of previous coronary bypass surgery. The group of patients with an AMI and a history of previous bypass surgery had more extensive coronary artery disease, a higher incidence of congestive heart failure, an infarct-related artery that was more difficult to identify, and a reperfusion rate that was lower compared to patients without a previous history of bypass surgery. Although the early survival was equivalent, the unadjusted late mortality was higher in the patients with previous bypass surgery.

The recently completed GUSTO trial has also provided some important insights in the management of AMI in patients with previous bypass surgery.[87] In this trial, which compared different thrombolytic strategies in 41,021 patients who presented with an AMI, 4% of patients had previous bypass surgery. This group of patients was significantly older, had a higher incidence of prior MIs, and significantly more risk factors for coronary artery disease in comparison to the group without previous CABG. These significant clinical differences probably account for the higher 30-day mortality rate (10.6% vs. 6.7%) and higher reinfarction rate (5.4% vs. 3.7%) seen in the patients with a previous bypass operation.

In summary, most studies demonstrate a worse prognosis in patients presenting with an AMI who have had prior bypass surgery compared to those without prior surgery. This difference in outcome has been attributed to the advanced age, more extensive coronary artery disease, and greater left ventricular dysfunction of the postbypass patient. Further studies to analyze new therapeutic strategies are needed in this ever-increasing cohort of patients.

Antiplatelet and antithrombotic agents

Aspirin has been found to decrease vascular mortality significantly in patients with AMI and to decrease mortality and recurrent cardiovascular events in the chronic phase after MI.[88] Although these beneficial effects have not been specifically examined in postbypass patients, similar benefits would be expected.

The use of heparin in the setting of an AMI has been very controversial over the years. In the prethrombolytic era several small studies failed to show any beneficial effect of heparin. However, in a metaanalysis of these trials, heparin therapy was associated with a significant decrease in mortality and reinfarction.[89] More recently, GISSI-II and ISIS-III evaluated the use of adjunctive heparin therapy following thrombolytic therapy.[90,91] In these studies no beneficial effect was found, but in both studies heparin was administered subcutaneously. Nei-

ther study specifically addressed patients with prior bypass surgery. In the GUSTO trial no significant difference was noted in patients receiving either subcutaneous or intravenous heparin therapy following streptokinase.[92] However, patients with or without previous bypass surgery who received an accelerated dose of t-PA with intravenous heparin demonstrated an increased survival rate compared with other groups.

Calcium antagonists, beta blockers, and nitrates

Diltiazem has been shown to be effective in reducing the incidence of reinfarction following a non–Q-wave MI.[93,94] With the increased prevalence of non–Q-wave MIs in the postbypass patient, it is tempting to postulate that a similar beneficial impact of diltiazem should be present, though this has not yet been examined. However, several factors may limit the use of diltiazem in the postbypass patient with a non–Q-wave MI. The diagnosis of a non–Q-wave infarct may be difficult secondary to the distorted QRS complexes often seen in the postbypass patient. In addition, because many postbypass patients have impaired ventricular function, diltiazem may be associated with a higher mortality, as seen in the MDPIT study.[95] Numerous trials have examined the other calcium channel blockers in patients who present with an AMI. Agents such as nifedipine, which do not decrease heart rate but may cause reflex tachycardia, have been associated with an increased mortality. In contrast, verapamil may have a beneficial effect by decreasing the heart rate; however, further study is warranted.[96] In general, the routine use of calcium channel blockers to reduce the incidence of reinfarction in the postbypass patient cannot be recommended.

β-adrenergic blockers have been demonstrated in several clinical trials to reduce mortality and the rate of reinfarction in patients surviving an AMI.[97-99] Although no study has specifically addressed their use in the postbypass patient, their use in this subgroup is strongly recommended.

The ability of nitrates to improve myocardial oxygen consumption by reducing both preload and afterload make these agents useful in the management of AMI. These agents may also help to reduce coronary vasospasm and inhibit platelet aggregation, adding to their beneficial effect. Several small trials have examined both oral and intravenous nitrates (nitroglycerin and nitroprusside). In a metaanalysis by Yusuf et al., the use of nitrates resulted in a 35% reduction in mortality, whereas oral nitrates produced a 21% reduction in mortality.[100,101] The recent ISIS-IV trial demonstrated no adjunctive benefit of nitrates in the treatment of AMI.[102] No study has specifically addressed patients with previous bypass surgery.

The use of ACE-inhibitors following an AMI has

been shown to be beneficial in patients with depressed left ventricular function regardless of symptoms.[103,104] The intravenous use of these agents in the acute phase of an MI does not appear to have a beneficial effect on mortality.[105] However, the recently completed ISIS-4 and GISSI-3 trials demonstrated a survival advantage when oral captopril or lisinopril was started in the acute phase of an AMI and continued for 4 to 6 weeks.[106,107] Although not specifically addressed in the postbypass patient, similar recommendations regarding the use of ACE inhibitors can be made, as in patients who have not had prior bypass surgery.[103,104]

Thrombolytic therapy

Despite the growing number of patients with previous bypass surgery presenting with an AMI, data regarding the most appropriate reperfusion strategy is limited. These patients have been excluded from most reperfusion trials because of the difficulty encountered in identifying the infarct-related artery.[108]

The initial reported data on the efficacy of intravenous thrombolytic therapy in patients with prior bypass surgery presenting with an AMI included five patients treated with intravenous tissue plasminogen activator.[108] Clinical evidence of reperfusion was present in four patients (80%); all five patients had a patent bypass graft in the distribution of the infarct at the time of angiography. This study is limited by the small number of patients and the relatively long time interval (up to 9 days) between the infarct and subsequent coronary angiography.

In another study, Grines et al. retrospectively reviewed 50 patients who presented with an infarct at least 1 year after undergoing bypass surgery.[109] The infarct-related vessel was a native coronary artery in 16%, a saphenous vein graft in 76%, and unidentifiable in 8% of the patients. Of the 11 patients who received intravenous thrombolytic therapy, successful reperfusion occurred in three of three (100%) native coronary arteries and two of eight (25%) saphenous vein grafts. In four of the occluded grafts, "salvage angioplasty" or intragraft thrombolytic therapy resulted in successful reperfusion. The authors suggest that the potential superiority of salvage angioplasty and/or intragraft thrombolytic therapy may be the result of the large thrombus burden in vein grafts and the inability of delivering intravenously administered thrombolytics to these conduits.

The effect of various thrombolytic strategies in the GUSTO trial was examined in the patients with previous bypass surgery. In those patients treated with accelerated t-PA, the 30-day mortality rate was 9.4%, whereas in patients treated with streptokinase, the mortality rate was 11.4%. In contrast, the patients with no previous bypass surgery had a mortality rate of 6.1% with accelerated t-PA and 7.1% with streptokinase. Prior

bypass surgery was an independent risk factor for mortality regardless of the thrombolytic strategy. This observation emphasizes the importance of determining the optimum treatment for these patients in future clinical trials.

Coronary angioplasty

Recent clinical trials have demonstrated the utility of direct angioplasty for the treatment of AMI in native coronary arteries (see Chapter 26). Although not specifically examined, the patient with previous bypass surgery may also benefit from this form of therapy. However, in view of the large thrombus burden and diffuse disease within vein grafts, direct angioplasty may be associated with a lower acute success rate and a higher incidence of complications. Kahn et al. retrospectively analyzed 72 patients with prior coronary artery bypass surgery who underwent direct balloon angioplasty without antecedent thrombolytic therapy.[110] Angioplasty was successful in 41 of 48 (85%) vein grafts and 24 of 24 (100%) native arteries. There were five in-hospital deaths (10%) in the vein graft cohort and two in-hospital deaths (8%) in the native artery cohort. There were no strokes, urgent bypass operations, transfusions, or clinical evidence of distal embolization. Again, prospective randomized clinical trials comparing direct angioplasty to thrombolytic therapy (intravenous or intragraft) are warranted.

The role of new interventional devices in the management of AMI in the postbypass patient has not been defined. The transluminal extraction catheter, a wire-based, motor-driven, rotating flexible torque tube with two stainless steel blades at the conical head of the catheter that can excise and extract atherosclerotic plaque, may have a niche in this cohort of patients (see Chapter 36). In a preliminary series of nine patients with an AMI and an occluded vein graft, the procedural success rate with the transluminal extraction catheter was 93%.[111] One patient died. There were no postprocedural infarcts or emergency bypass surgeries. Although these results are encouraging, randomized clinical trials are needed.

SUMMARY

The management of patients with prior coronary bypass surgery who present with unstable angina or an AMI is one of the most complex and challenging areas of cardiology. Developing a management strategy for these patients requires an understanding of the natural history of bypass conduits, the importance of risk factor modification, and the risks and benefits of various management options.

A key component to understanding the natural history of saphenous vein and internal mammary artery grafts is the time-dependent changes in these vessels. Thrombosis is the primary cause of graft failure in the early postoperative period up to 1 month, whereas occlusive thrombi superimposed upon intimal hyperplasia is the primary cause of graft failure between the first and twelfth postoperative months. Antiplatelet agents are effective in reducing the incidence of early graft thrombosis.

The development of a management strategy in these patients is limited by the small number of reported studies examining the efficacy of various antianginals and thrombolytic agents. Because patients with prior coronary bypass surgery have largely been excluded from major thrombolytic trials, the relative risks and benefits of these agents in this patient population is unknown. Furthermore, to provide optimal care for these patients, better methods of ischemia detection are needed. The 12-lead ECG and coronary angiography often fail to localize the affected myocardial region and the infarct-related vessel.

By increasing the use of the internal mammary artery as a bypass conduit, aggressive risk-factor modification, and the use of antiplatelet agents, the incidence of unstable angina and AMI may be minimized in these patients.

REFERENCES

1. Kirklin JW, Akins CW, Blackstone EH, et al: Guidelines and indications for coronary artery bypass graft surgery: a report of the American College of Cardiology/American Heart Association Task Force on Assessment of Diagnostic and Therapeutic Cardiovascular Procedures (Subcommittee on Coronary Artery Bypass Graft Surgery), J Am Coll Cardiol 17:543-589, 1991.
2. Gersh BJ, Califf RM, Loop FD, et al: Coronary bypass surgery in chronic stable angina, Circulation 79:I46-I59, 1989.
3. Campeau L, Lesperance J, Hermann J, et al: Loss of improvement of angina between 1 and 7 years after aortocoronary bypass surgery: correlations with changes in vein grafts and in coronary arteries, Circulation 60:1-5, 1979.
4. Waters DD, Walling A, Roy D, et al: Previous coronary artery bypass grafting as an adverse prognostic factor in unstable angina pectoris, Am J Cardiol 58:465-469, 1986.
5. Campeau L: Late changes in saphenous vein coronary artery bypass grafts and their implications in clinical practice, Can J Cardiol 3:23A, 1987.
6. Guthaner DF, Robert EW, Alderman EL, et al: Long-term serial angiographic studies after coronary artery bypass surgery, Circulation 60:250-259, 1979.
7. Nitter-Hauge S, Levorstad K: Does aortocoronary saphenous vein bypass surgery change the native coronary arteries? Acta Med Scand 207:189-193, 1980.
8. Bourassa MG, Enjalbert M, Campeau L, et al: Progression of atherosclerosis in coronary arteries and bypass grafts: ten years later, Am J Cardiol 53:102C-107C, 1984.
9. Bourassa MG, Lesperance J, Corbara F, et al: Progression of obstructive coronary artery disease 5 to 7 years after aortocoronary bypass surgery, Cleve Clin Q 45:175-176, 1978.
10. Aldridge HE, Trimble AS: Progression of proximal coronary artery lesions to total occlusion after aortocoronary saphenous vein bypass grafting, J Thorac Cardiovasc Surg 62:7-11, 1971.
11. Bousvaros G, Piracha AR, Chaudhry MA: Increase in severity of proximal coronary disease after successful distal aortocoronary grafts: its nature and effect, Circulation 46:870-879, 1972.
12. Gensini GG, Esente P, Kelly A: Natural history of coronary disease in patients with and without coronary bypass graft surgery, Circulation 50:II-98-II-102, 1974.
13. Maurer BJ, Oberman A, Holt JH, et al: Changes in grafted and nongrafted coronary arteries following saphenous vein bypass grafting, Circulation 50:293-300, 1974.
14. Bulkley BH, Hutchins GM: Accelerated "atherosclerosis": a morphologic study of 97 saphenous vein coronary artery bypass grafts, Circulation 55:163-169, 1977.
15. Lawrie GM, Lie JT, Morris GC Jr, et al: Vein graft patency and intimal proliferation after aortocoronary bypass: early and long-term angiopathologic correlations, Am J Cardiol 38:856-862, 1976.
16. Brody WR, Angell WW, Kosec JC: Histologic fate of venous coronary artery bypass in dogs, Am J Pathol 66:111-130, 1972.
17. Campeau L, Enjalbert M, Lesperance J, et al: The relation of risk factors to the development of atherosclerosis in saphenous vein bypass grafts and the progression of disease in the native circulation: a study 10 years after aortocoronary bypass surgery, N Engl J Med 311:1329-1332, 1984.
18. Smith SH, Greer JC: Morphology of saphenous vein coronary artery bypass grafts 7 to 116 months postoperative, Arch Pathol Lab Med 107:13-18, 1983.
19. Fuster V, Chesebro JH: Role of platelet and platelet inhibitors in aortocoronary artery vein-graft disease, Circulation 73:227-232, 1986.
20. Israel DH, Adam PC, Stein B, et al: Antithrombotic therapy in the coronary vein graft patient, Clin Cardiol 14:283-295, 1991.
21. Waller BF, Rothbaum DA, Gorfinkel HJ, et al: Morphologic observations after percutaneous transluminal balloon angioplasty of early and late aortocoronary saphenous vein bypass grafts, J Am Coll Cardiol 4:784-792, 1984.
22. Lytle BW, Loop FD, Cosgrove DM, et al: Long-term (5 to 12 years) serial studies of internal mammary artery and saphenous vein coronary bypass grafts, J Thorac Cardiovasc Surg 89:248-258, 1985.
23. Svendson E, Dregelid E, Eide GE: Internal elastic membrane in the internal mammary and left anterior descending coronary arteries and its relationship to intimal thickening, Atherosclerosis 83:239-248, 1990.
24. Loop FD, Lytle BW, Cosgrove DM, et al: Influence of the internal mammary artery graft on 10-year survival and other cardiac events, N Engl J Med 314:1-6, 1986.
25. Atkinson JB, Foman MB, Vaughan WK, et al: Morphologic changes in long-term saphenous vein bypass grafts, Chest 88:341-348, 1985.
26. Solymoss BC, Nadeau P, Campeau L: Factors related to atherosclerosis of saphenous vein coronary bypass grafts, J Am Coll Cardiol 9:85A, 1987.
27. Blankenhorn DH, Nessim SA, Johnson RL, et al: Beneficial effects of combined colestipol-niacin therapy on coronary atherosclerosis and coronary venous bypass grafts, JAMA 257:3233-3240, 1987.
28. Lytle BW, Kramer JR, Golding LAR, et al: Young adults with coronary atherosclerosis: influence of risk factors on the ten-year results of myocardial revascularization, J Am Coll Cardiol 3:504A, 1984.
29. Cosgrove DM, Loop FD, Lytle BW, et al: Predictors of reoperation after myocardial revascularization, J Thorac Cardiovasc Surg 92:811-821, 1986.
30. Fox MH, Gruchow HW, Barboriak JJ, et al: Risk factors among patients undergoing repeat aortocoronary bypass procedures, J Thorac Cardiovasc Surg 93:56-61, 1987.
31. Adler DS, Goldman L, O'Neill A, et al: Long-term survival of more than 2000 patients after coronary bypass grafting, Am J Cardiol 58:195-202, 1986.

32. Lawrie GM, Morris GC Jr, Glasser DH: Influence of diabetes mellitus on the results of coronary bypass surgery: follow-up of 212 diabetic patients 10 to 15 years after surgery, *JAMA* 256:2967-2971, 1986.

33. Meade TW, Mellows S, Brozovic M, et al: Haemostatic function and ischaemic heart disease: principal results of the Northwick Park Heart Study, *Lancet* 2:533-537, 1986.

34. Dahlen GH, Guyton JR, Attar M, et al: Association of levels of lipoprotein Lp(a), plasma lipids, and other lipoproteins with coronary artery disease documented by angiography, *Circulation* 74:758-765, 1986.

35. Tschan W, Hoffman A, Brukart F, et al: Coronary artery bypass grafts: influence of preoperative risk factors on the late postoperative course, *Chest* 88:185-189, 1985.

36. Lambert M, Kouz S, Campeau L: Preoperative and operative predictive variables of late clinical events following saphenous vein coronary artery bypass surgery, *Can J Cardiol* 5:87-92, 1989.

37. Seides SF, Borer JS, Kent KM, et al: Long-term anatomic fate of coronary artery bypass grafts and functional status of patients five years after operation, *N Engl J Med* 298:1213-1217, 1978.

38. Lewis HD, David JW, Archibald DG, et al: Protective efffects of aspirin against acute myocardial infarction and death in men with unstable angina, *N Engl J Med* 309:396-403, 1983.

39. Cairns JA, Gent M, Singer J, et al: Aspirin, sulfinpyrazone, or both in unstable angina: results of a Canadian Multicenter Trial, *N Engl J Med* 313:1369-1375, 1985.

40. Hennenkens CH, Buring JE, Sandercock P, et al: Aspirin and other antiplatelet agents in the secondary and primary prevention of cardiovascular disease, *Circulation* 80:749-756, 1989.

41. Goldman S, Copeland J, Moritz T, et al: Saphenous vein graft patency one year after coronary artery bypass surgery and effect of antiplatelet therapy: results of a Veterans Administration Cooperative Study, *Circulation* 80:1190-1197, 1989.

42. Chesebro JH, Fuster V, Elveback LR, et al: Effect of dipyridamole and aspirin on late vein graft patency after coronary bypass operation, *N Engl J Med* 310:209-214, 1984.

43. Verstraete M, Brown BG, Chesebro JH, et al: Evaluation of antiplatelet agents in the prevention of aortocoronary bypass occlusion, *Eur Heart J* 7:4-13, 1986.

44. Goldman S, Copeland J, Moritz T, et al: Internal mammary artery and saphenous vein graft patency: effects of aspirin, *Circulation* 82:IV-237-242, 1990.

45. Sanz G, Pajaron A, Alegria E, et al: Prevention of early aortocoronary bypass occlusion by low-dose aspirin and dipyridamole, *Circulation* 82:765-773, 1990.

46. Garaghan TP, Gebski V, Baron DW: Immediate postoperative aspirin improves vein graft patency early and late after coronary artery bypass graft surgery: a placebo-controlled, randomized trial, *Circulation* 85:1526-1533, 1991.

47. Goldman S, Copeland J, Moritz T, et al: Starting aspirin after operation: effects on early graft patency — Department of Veteran's Affairs Cooperative Study Group, *Circulation* 84:520-526, 1991.

48. Chesebro JH: Effect of dipyridamole and aspirin on vein graft patency after coronary bypass operations, *Thromb Res* 12:5-10, 1990.

49. Goldman S, Copeland J, Mortiz T, et al: Improvement in early saphenous vein graft patency after bypass surgery with antiplatelet therapy: results of a Veterans Administration Cooperative Study, *Circulation* 77:1324-1332, 1988.

50. Théroux P, Latour JG: Anticoagulants and their use in acute ischemic syndrome. In Topol EJ (ed): *Interventional cardiology,* Philadelphia, 1989, WB Saunders.

51. Théroux P, Quimet H, McCans J, et al: Aspirin, heparin, or both to treat acute unstable angina, *N Engl J Med* 319:1105-1111, 1988.

52. Théroux P, Waters D, Qiu S, et al: Aspirin versus heparin to

prevent myocardial infarction during the acute phase of unstable angina, *Circulation* 88:2045-2048, 1993.

53. Stamler J, Cunningham M, Loscalzo J: Reduced thiols and the effect of intravenous nitroglycerin on platelet aggregation, *Am J Cardiol* 62:377-380, 1988.

54. HINT Research Group: Early treatment of unstable angina in the coronary care unit: a randomized, double-blind, placebo-controlled comparison of recurrent ischemia in patients treated with nifedipine and metoprolol or both, *Br Heart J* 56:400-413, 1986.

55. Tijssen JG, Lubsen J: Early treatment of unstable angina with nifedipine and metoprolol — the HINT trial, *J Cardiovasc Pharmacol* 12:S71-S77, 1988.

56. Held PH, Yosuf S, Furberg C: Calcium channel blockers in acute myocardial infarction and unstable angina: an overview, *Br Med J* 2:1187-1192, 1989.

57. Theroux PO, Taeymans Y, Morissette D, et al: A randomized study comparing propranolol and diltiazem in the treatment of unstable angina, *J Am Coll Cardiol* 5:717-722, 1985.

58. Rentrop P, Blanke H, Karsch KR, et al: Recanalization of an acutely occluded aortocoronary bypass by intragraft fibrinolysis, *Circulation* 62:1123-1126, 1980.

59. Slysh S, Goldberg S, Dervan JP, et al: Unstable angina and evolving myocardial infarction following coronary bypass surgery: pathogenesis and treatment with interventional catheterization, *Am Heart J* 109:744-752, 1985.

60. Vetrovec GW, Leinbach RC, Gold HK, et al: Intracoronary thrombolysis in syndromes of unstable ischemia: angiographic and clinical results, *Am Heart J* 104:946-952, 1982.

61. Hartmann J, McKeever L, Teran J, et al: Prolonged infusion of urokinase for recanalization of chronically occluded aortocoronary bypass grafts, *Am J Cardiol* 61:189-191, 1988.

62. Hartmann J, McKeever LS, Stamato NJ, et al: Recanalization of chronically occluded aortocoronary saphenous vein bypass grafts by extended infusion of urokinase: initial results and short-term clinical follow-up, *J Am Coll Cardiol* 18:1517-1523, 1991.

63. Levine DJ, Sharaf BL, Williams DO: Late follow-up of patients with totally occluded saphenous vein grafts treated by prolonged selective urokinase infusion, *J Am Coll Cardiol* 19:292A, 1992.

64. Gruentzig AR, Senning A, Siegenthaler WE: Nonoperative dilatation of coronary artery stenosis: percutaneous transluminal coronary angioplasty, *N Engl J Med* 301:61-68, 1979.

65. Foster ED, Fisher LD, Kaiser GC, et al: Comparison of operative mortality for initial and repeat coronary artery bypass grafting: the Coronary Artery Surgery Study (CASS) registry experience, *Ann Thorac Surg* 38:563-570, 1984.

66. Cameron A, Kemp HG, Green GE: Reoperation for coronary artery disease: 10 years of clinical follow-up, *Circulation* 78:I-158-I-162, 1988.

67. Osaka S, Barratt-Boyes BG, Brandt PW, et al: Early and late results of reoperation for coronary artery disease: a 13-year experience, *Aust N Z J Surg* 58:537-541, 1988.

68. Reul GJ, Cooley DA, Ott DA, et al: Reoperation for recurrent coronary artery disease: causes, indications and results in 168 patients, *Arch Surg* 114:1269-1275, 1979.

69. Schaff HV, Orszulah TA, Gersh BJ, et al: The morbidity or mortality of reoperation for coronary artery disease and analysis of late results with use of actuarial estimate of event-free interval, *J Thorac Cardiovasc Surg* 85:508-515, 1983.

70. Pidgeon J, Brooks N, Magee P, et al: Reoperation for angina after previous aortocoronary bypass surgery, *Br Heart J* 53:269-275, 1985.

71. Laird-Meeter K, Vandomburg R, Van Den Brand MJBM, et al: Incidence, risk, and outcome of reintervention after aortocoronary bypass surgery, *Br Heart J* 57:427-435, 1987.

72. Lytle BW, Loop FD, Cosgrove DM, et al: Fifteen hundred

coronary reoperations: results and determinants of early and late survival, *J Thorac Cardiovasc Surg* 93:847-859, 1987.

73. Verhaul HA, Moulijn AC, Hondema S, et al: Late results of 200 repeat coronary artery bypass operations, *Am J Cardiol* 67:24-30, 1991.

74. Lytle BW, Cosgrove DM, Taylor PC, et al: Multiple coronary reoperations: early and late results, *Circulation* 80:II-626, 1989.

75. Kent KM, Bentivogio LG, Block PC: Percutaneous transluminal coronary angioplasty: report from the registry of the National Heart, Lung, and Blood Institute, *Am J Cardiol* 49:2011-2020, 1982.

76. Block PC, Cowley MJ, Kaltenbach M, et al: Percutaneous angioplasty of stenoses of bypass grafts or of bypass graft anastomotic sites, *Am J Cardiol* 53:666-668, 1984.

77. Corbelli J, Franco I, Hollman J, et al: Percutaneous transluminal coronary angioplasty after previous coronary artery bypass surgery, *Am J Cardiol* 56:398-403, 1985.

78. Pinkerton CA, Slack JD, Orr CM, et al: Percutaneous transluminal angioplasty in patients with prior myocardial revascularization surgery, *Am J Cardiol* 61:15G-22G, 1988.

79. Platko WP, Hollman J, Whitlow PL, et al: Percutaneous transluminal angioplasty at saphenous vein graft: long-term follow-up, *J Am Coll Cardiol* 14:1645-1650, 1989.

80. Meester BJ, Samson M, Suryapranata H, et al: Long-term follow-up after attempted angioplasty of saphenous vein grafts: the Thoraxcenter experience 1981-1988, *Eur Heart J* 12:648-653, 1991.

81. Douglas JS, Weintraub WS, Liberman HA, et al: Update of saphenous graft angioplasty: restenosis and long-term outcome, *Circulation* 84:II-249A, 1991.

82. Weintraub WS, Cohen CL, Curling PE, et al: Results of coronary surgery after failed elective coronary angioplasty in patients with prior coronary surgery, *J Am Coll Cardiol* 16:1341-1347, 1990.

83. Wiseman A, Waters DD, Walling A, et al: Long-term prognosis after myocardial infarction in patients with previous coronary artery surgery, *J Am Coll Cardiol* 12:873-880, 1988.

84. Crean PA, Waters DD, Bosch X, et al: Angiographic findings after myocardial infarction in patients with previous bypass surgery: explanations for smaller infarcts in this group compared with control patients, *Circulation* 71:693-698, 1985.

85. Davis KB, Alderman EL, Koanski AS, et al: Early mortality of acute myocardial infarction in patients with and without prior coronary revascularization surgery: a Coronary Artery Surgery Study Registry Study, *Circulation* 85:2100-2109, 1992.

86. Nathan PE, Sketch MH Jr, Fortin DF, et al: Acute myocardial infarction in patients with previous coronary bypass surgery: association of complex anatomy and lower reperfusion rates with poor long-term survival, *J Am Coll Cardiol* 21:349A, 1993.

87. The GUSTO Investigators: An international randomized trial comparing four thrombolytic strategies for acute myocardial infarction, *N Engl J Med* 329:673-682, 1993.

88. Stein B, Fuster V, Israel DH, et al: Platelet inhibitor agents in cardiovascular disease: an update, *J Am Coll Cardiol* 14:813-836, 1989.

89. MacMahon S, Collins R, Knight C, et al: Reduction in major morbidity and mortality by heparin in acute myocardial infarction, *Circulation* 78:II-98, 1988.

90. Third International Study of Infarct Survival (ISIS 3) Collaborative Group: ISIS 3: a randomized trial of streptokinase vs. tissue plasminogen activator vs. anistreplase and of aspirin plus heparin vs. aspirin alone among 41,299 cases of suspected acute myocardial infarction, *Lancet* 339:753-770, 1992.

91. Groupo Italiano per lo Studio della Sopravvivenza nell'Infarcto Miocardico: GISSI-2: a factorial randomized trial of alteplase versus streptokinase and heparin versus no heparin among 12,490 patients with acute myocardial infarction, *Lancet* 336:65-71, 1990.

92. The GUSTO Investigators: An international randomized trial comparing four thrombolytic strategies for acute myocardial infarction, *N Engl J Med* 329:673-682, 1993.

93. Gibson RS, Boden WE, Théroux P, et al and the Diltiazem Reinfarction Study Group: Diltiazem and reinfarction in patients with non-Q-wave myocardial infarction, *N Engl J Med* 315:423-429, 1986.

94. Gibson RS, Young PM, Boden WH, et al: Prognostic significance and beneficial effect of diltiazem on the incidence of early recurrent ischemia after non-Q-wave myocardial infarction: results from the Multicenter Diltiazem Reinfarction Study, *Am J Cardiol* 60:203-209, 1987.

95. The effect of diltiazem on mortality and reinfarction after myocardial infarction: the Multicenter Diltiazem Postinfarction Trial Research Group, *N Engl J Med* 319:385-392, 1988.

96. Held PH, Teo KK, Yusuf S: Effects of beta-blockers, calcium channel blockers, nitrates, and magnesium in acute myocardial infarction and unstable angina pectoris. In Topol EJ (ed): *Textbook of interventional cardiology,* Philadelphia, 1993, WB Saunders.

97. Gundersen T, Abrahamsen AM, Kjekshos J, et al for the Norwegian Multicenter Study Group: Timolol-related reduction in mortality and reinfarction in patients ages 65-75 years surviving acute myocardial infarction, *Circulation* 66:1179-1184, 1982.

98. Chadda K, Goldstein S, Byington R, et al: Effect of propranolol after acute myocardial infarction in patients with congestive heart failure, *Circulation* 73:503-510, 1986.

99. Furberg CD, Hawkins CM, Lichstein E, for the Beta Blocker Heart Attack Trial Study Group: Effect of propranolol in postinfarction patients with mechanical or electrical complications, *Circulation* 69:761-765, 1984.

100. Yusuf S, Collins R, MacMahon S, et al: Effect of intravenous nitrates on mortality in acute myocardial infarction: an overview of the randomized trials, *Lancet* 1:1088-1092, 1988.

101. Held PH, Teo KK, Yusuf S: Effects of beta blockers, calcium channel blockers, and nitrates in acute myocardial infarction and unstable angina pectoris. In Topol EJ, (ed): *Textbook of interventional cardiology,* Philadelphia, 1990, WB Saunders.

102. ISIS-4 Collaborative Group: ISIS-4: randomized study of oral isosorbide mononitrate in over 50,000 patients with suspected acute myocardial infarction, *Circulation* 88:I-394, 1993.

103. Pfeffer MA, Braunwald E, Moye LA, et al: Effect of captopril on mortality and morbidity in patients with left ventricular dysfunction after myocardial infarction. Results of the survival and ventricular enlargement trial. The SAVE Investigators, *N Engl J Med* 327:669-677, 1992.

104. The SOLVD Investigators: Effect of enalapril on survival in patients with reduced left ventricular ejection fractions and congestive heart failure. The SOLVD Investigators, *N Engl J Med* 325:293-302, 1991.

105. Swedberg K, Held P, Kjekshus J, et al: Effects of the early administration of enalapril on mortality in patients with acute myocardial infarction. Results of the Cooperative New Scandinavian Enalapril Survival Study II (CONSENSUS II), *N Engl J Med* 327:678-684, 1992.

106. GISSI-3 Investigators: The third Gruppo Italiano per lo Studio della Sopravvivenza nell'Infarcto Miocardico (GISSI-3) trial—Thrombolysis and International Infarction (Ninth International Workshop), Milan, November 1993.

107. ISIS-4 Collaborative Group: ISIS-4: randomized study of oral captopril in over 50,000 patients with suspected acute myocardial infarction, *Circulation* 88:I-394, 1993.

108. Kleiman NS, Berman DA, Gaston WR, et al: Early intravenous thrombolytic therapy for acute myocardial infarction in patients with prior coronary bypass grafts, *Am J Cardiol* 63:102-104, 1989.

109. Grines CL, Booth DC, Nissen SE, et al: Mechanism of acute myocardial infarction in patients with prior coronary artery bypass grafting and therapeutic implications, *Am J Cardiol* 65:1292-1296, 1990.

110. Kahn JK, Rutherford BD, McLonahay DR, et al: Usefulness of angioplasty during acute myocardial infarction in patients with prior coronary artery bypass grafting, *Am J Cardiol* 65:698-702, 1990.

111. Labinaz M, Sketch MH Jr, O'Neill WW, et al: Transluminal extraction-endarterectomy catheter. In Roubin GS, Califf RM, O'Neill WW, et al (eds): *Interventional cardiovascular medicine: principles and practice,* New York, 1993, Churchill Livingstone.

Chapter 55

ACUTE RENAL FAILURE IN THE CORONARY CARE UNIT

Eugene Kovalik
Steven J. Schwab

In the mid-1960s coronary care units (CCUs) were developed to provide specialized intensive care for patients with acute coronary artery disease. Initially these units focused on the early recognition and treatment of cardiac arrhythmias. Recently there has been rapid expansion in technologic, pharmacologic, and mechanical interventions for coronary disease that have taken acute coronary care far beyond arrhythmia recognition and treatment. These interventions are responsible, at least in part, for the 21% decrease in mortality from coronary disease observed since 1968.[1] As the population receiving aggressive intervention has shifted to include more older and less stable patients, many with hypotension, the risk of developing acute renal insufficiency has increased. Overall, approximately 5% of hospitalized patients develop some degree of renal impairment, 55% of the time from iatrogenic causes. If the serum creatinine rises less than 3 mg/dl, hospital mortality is less than 15%, whereas in more severe cases there is a hospital mortality rate exceeding 50%.[2] Many patients admitted to the CCU already have some degree of chronic renal insufficiency, placing them at risk for further loss. In this chapter we discuss the diagnosis of acute renal failure (ARF) and the therapeutic options available to the cardiologist caring for these complex patients and review several areas of particular concern to the CCU physician.

ARF is defined as an abrupt decline in renal function sufficient to cause retention of nitrogenous and other metabolic byproducts. ARF is traditionally divided into three categories based on urine output: nonoliguric ARF

(>400 ml/day of urine output), oliguric ARF (between 100 and 400 ml/day), and anuric ARF (<100 ml/day). These divisions have important prognostic and patient management implications.

The relative frequency of these three forms depends on how ARF is defined. If all patients with an acute rise of 0.5 to 1.0 mg/dl in their serum creatinine are included, nonoliguric renal failure predominates, accounting for 50% to 90% of ARF. If only patients requiring some form of dialytic therapy are taken into consideration, the percentage of nonoliguric ARF falls to 5% to 20%.[3] The number of nephrons damaged and the severity of the injury determine into which group patients fall. The causes of ARF are numerous but can generally be divided into three groups for evaluation: prerenal, intrarenal, and postrenal causes (Table 55-1).[3] The clinical evaluation of the patient with ARF starts by placing the patient into one of these categories to direct further diagnosis and therapy.

EVALUATION
History and physical examination

Points in the history of a patient with ARF that are particularly important involve any previous history of renal insufficiency, diabetes, or peripheral vascular disease. A recent history of hypotensive episodes, exposure to intravenous (IV) or intraarterial contrast administration should also be sought. Previous vascular manipulation (e.g., aortography, cardiac catheterization, or intraaortic balloon counterpulsation) may be a clue to a cholesterol emboli syndrome. The use of prescription

Table 55-1. Causes of acute renal failure

Prerenal failure
  Decreased cardiac output
    Myocardial infarction
    Cardiac arrhythmia
    Decompensated congestive heart failure
    Cardiac tamponade
    Pulmonary embolism
    Positive-pressure mechanical ventilation
  Hypovolemia with or without hypotension
    Decreased intake
    External losses of extracellular fluid
      Renal losses
      Gastrointestinal losses
      Dermal losses
    Internal losses, redistribution, or third spacing
      Hypoalbuminemia
      Cirrhosis of the liver
      Nephrotic syndrome
      Pancreatitis
      Traumatized tissues
      Peritonitis
      Intestinal obstruction
      Burns
  Peripheral vasodilation
    Sepsis
    Shock
    Liver failure
    Antihypertensive agents
    Drug overdose
  Renal vascular occlusion
    Atherosclerosis
    Embolism
    Thrombosis
    Vasculitis
    Renal pedicle compression
  Disruption in renal autoregulation
    Prostaglandin inhibitors
    Angiotensin-covering enzyme inhibitors

Postrenal failure (obstruction)
  Intraureteral obstruction
    Blood clots
    Stones
    Papillary necrosis
    Fungus balls
  Extraureteral obstruction
    Ligation
    Malignancy
    Endometriosis
    Retroperitoneal fibrosis, tumors
  Lower urinary tract obstruction

Urethral stricture
Prostatic hypertrophy or cancer
Bladder cancer
Cervical cancer
Neurogenic bladder

Intrinsic renal failure
  Vascular diseases
    Malignant hypertension
    Vasculitis
    Hemolytic-uremic syndrome
    Thrombotic thrombocytopenic purpura
    Toxemia of pregnancy
    Postpartum nephrosclerosis
    Cholesterol emboli
  Glomerular diseases
    Acute postinfectious glomerulonephritis
    Goodpasture's syndrome
    Rapidly progressive glomerulonephritis
    Lupus nephritis
    IgA nephropathy
  Interstitial nephritis
    Infectious causes
      Staphylococcus, gram-negative bacteria, leptospirosis, brucellosis, viruses, fungi, acid-fast bacilli
    Infiltrative causes
      Leukemia, lymphoma, sarcoidosis, other granulomas
    Related to drugs
      Penicillins, cephalosporins, nonsteroidal antiinflammatory drugs, allopurinol, thiazide diuretics, cimetidine, phenytoin, furosemide, analgesics
    Idiopathic causes
  Tubular diseases—"acute tubular necrosis"
    Ischemic injury
      Prolonged prerenal azotemia
      Shock, postoperative
      Crush syndrome, major trauma
    Nephrotoxic injury
      Antibiotics, radiographic contrast media, anesthetic agents, chemotherapeutic agents, immunosuppressive agents, organic solvents, pesticides, heavy metals
    Pigment injury
      Myoglobinuria
      Hemoglobinuria
    Crystal-induced injury
      Uric acid nephropathy
      Oxalate nephropathy
    Metabolic causes
      Hypercalcemia
      Myeloma proteins
      Light-chain nephropathy

From Jacobson HR, Stricker GE, Klahr S (eds): *The principles and practice of nephrology*, Philadelphia, 1991, BC Decker, p 632. Used by permission.

and nonprescription medications (e.g., nonsteroidal agents, angiotensin-converting enzyme (ACE) inhibitors, antihypertensives, diuretics) are common precipitants of ARF in the susceptible patient. Symptoms of bladder outlet obstruction suggest a possible postrenal cause.

The volume status of the patient should be deter-

mined, and if hypovolemia is present, it should be rapidly corrected. If the assessment proves difficult because of anasarca, hypotension, or cor pulmonale, central monitoring with a Swan-Ganz catheter becomes important to direct fluid management. Hypotension deserves rapid attention because prolonged low blood pressure can convert reversible prerenal conditions to established ARF.

Table 55-2. Characteristics of the urinalysis in various forms of renal failure*

Disorders	Findings
Prerenal failure	Specific gravity: >1.015 pH: <6 Protein: trace-1+ Sediment: sparse hyaline and fine granular casts or bland
Postrenal failure	Specific gravity: 1.010 pH: >6 Protein: trace-1+ Hemoglobin + Sediment: RBCs, WBCs
Glomerular diseases	Specific gravity: >1.020 pH: <6 Protein: 1-+ Sediment: RBCs, RBC casts, WBCs, oval fat bodies, free fat droplets, fatty casts
Vascular diseases	Specific gravity: >1.020 if preglomerular pH: <6 Protein: trace-2+ Sediment: RBCs and RBC casts with glomerular involvement
Interstitial diseases	Specific gravity: 1.010 pH: 6-7 Protein: trace-1+ Sediment: WBCs, WBC casts, eosinophils, RBCs, RTE cells
Acute tubular necrosis	Muddy brown urine Specific gravity: 1.010 pH: 6-7 Protein: trace-1+ Blood: + Sediment: RBCs, WBCs, RTE cells, RTE casts, pigmented casts
Ethylene glycol intoxication	Same as ATN except for the presence of calcium oxalate monohydrate and dihydrate crystals; intracellular crystals may be seen
Acute uric acid nephropathy	Same as ATN except for the presence of uric acid crystals

From Jacobson HR, Stricker GE, Klahr S (eds): *The principles and practice of nephrology*, Philadelphia, 1991, BC Decker, p 635. Used by permission.
RTE, Renal tubular epithelial; *RBC*, red blood cells; *WBC*, white blood cells; *ATN*, acute tubular necrosis.

Table 55-3. Urinary indices in various forms of acute renal failure*†‡

	Prerenal	ATN
Specific gravity	>1.020	<1.010
Urinary osmolality (mOsm/kg H_2O)	>500	<350
Uosm/Posm	>1.3	<1.1
Urinary sodium (mEq/L)	<20	>40
U/P Urea nitrogen	>8	<3
U/P Creatinine	>40	<20
RFI	<1	>1
FE Na (%)	<1	>1

From Jacobson HR, Stricker GE, Klahr S (eds): *The principles and practice of nephrology*, Philadelphia, 1991, BC Decker, p 637. Used by permission.
ATN, Acute tubular necrosis; *U*, urine; *P*, plasma; *RFI*, renal failure index.
†FE Na (fractional excretion of sodium)(%) $= \dfrac{U/P\ Na}{U/P\ Cr} \times 100$
‡RFI $= \dfrac{U\ Na}{U/P\ Cr}$

pression in these patients and to clarify the diagnosis in the remaining 10%.

Laboratory evaluation

The initial manifestation of ARF is usually either a fall in urine output or a rise in the serum creatinine (Cr) and blood urea nitrogen (BUN) levels. The urinalysis is essential in the differential diagnosis of ARF. The key findings are summarized in Table 55-2.[3] Urine electrolyte indices supplement the physical examination in differentiating between prerenal conditions and established ARF (Table 55-3).[3] A low urinary sodium level suggests a prerenal condition that may be readily reversible by improvement in renal perfusion by either volume replacement or improvement in cardiac output. These urinary studies are not applicable to someone who has received diuretics within 12 hours of the test, however, because those agents cause obligatory salt wasting and loss of urine concentrating ability.

Radiologic procedures

The renal ultrasound is the best single radiologic procedure in the evaluation of ARF. It can evaluate the upper tract for obstruction and delineate the number and size of kidneys present (bilateral small kidneys suggesting chronic renal disease and asymmetric size suggesting possible renal artery disease). The radionuclide renal scan is of limited value unless obstruction of the renal arteries is considered likely, as can occur in the setting of a dissecting aortic aneurysm. Renal artery duplex scanning is of limited use in the evaluation of the renal vasculature because it is highly operator depen-

The patient should be examined for mottling of the skin, especially on the distal extremities, as evidence of cholesterol emboli. Abdominal and peripheral bruits indicative of vascular disease should be sought. Catheterization of the bladder for measurement of a postvoid residual evaluates the lower urinary tract for obstruction. These basic bedside steps usually allow the clinician to classify the patient as prerenal, intrarenal, or postrenal ARF in 90% of cases.[3] Further laboratory and radiologic evaluations serve to confirm the initial im-

dent with poor reproducibility and is not considered to be a reliable test.

Renal biopsy

Renal biopsy is considered in the rare coronary care patient in whom a clear reason for a severe and persistent decline in renal function cannot be found. In critically ill patients in the CCU it is usually contraindicated secondary to the active coronary problem and the frequent use of systemic anticoagulation. Even when indicated in these patients, biopsy can usually be deferred for several weeks until the patient has passed safely through the acute illness.

Additional interventions

In most instances of CCU-related ARF the diagnostic approach detailed earlier will rapidly allow classification into one of the three broad pathophysiologic categories. Prerenal conditions require correction of renal perfusion by either repleting circulatory volume or increasing blood pressure or cardiac output. In some instances in unstable patients, central hemodynamic monitoring is required to direct or withhold volume replacement. Once adequate volume and blood pressure are established, diuretics should be used to encourage urine output. Initial doses of furosemide at 40 to 80 mg intravenously are appropriate. A maximum IV dose of 200 mg of furosemide or equivalent should be the follow-up dose if the initial dose does not prompt a response. Combination therapy with a distal tubule diuretic (e.g., metolazone) can occasionally be helpful in patients resistant to a loop diuretic alone. Repetitive large doses in a nonresponding patient should not be employed because they can lead to significant ototoxicity. Patients with established oliguric ARF require conservative management and consideration for dialysis as described later in the chapter.

Postrenal conditions such as bladder neck obstruction caused by prostate disease or hydronephrosis secondary to stones should prompt a urologic consultation and corrective management.

Intrarenal conditions require further evaluation. Toxins such as aminoglycosides, ACE inhibitors, radiographic contrast media, and cholesterol emboli occur frequently in the CCU, as discussed later on. In contrast, primary renal diseases such as the glomerulonephritides, characterized by proteinuria and hematuria, usually do not manifest de novo in a CCU patient.

COMMON CAUSES
Ischemic ARF

Ischemia is the most common cause of an acute reduction in renal function, accounting for almost 50% of ARF in intensive care unit (ICU) patients.[4] The hallmark of ischemia at the pathologic level is acute tubular necrosis (ATN). Ischemic ARF can occur for many reasons, but hypotension associated with acute coronary ischemia, cardiac arrest, or cardiogenic shock is most common. Renal ischemia occurs on a continuum ranging from reversible prerenal azotemia to established oliguric ARF. The rapid resolution of renal hypoperfusion by restoration of blood volume or blood pressure ameliorates the injury. Serial assessment of urinary electrolytes is frequently helpful in determining if a reversible prerenal condition still exists (see Table 55-3).

In addition, many patients seen in the CCU have unsuspected compromise of renal blood flow. In a study from this institution, out of 1235 abdominal aortograms performed as part of routine cardiac catheterization, 30% had some degree of renal artery disease, and 15% had significant (> 50%) stenosis (11% unilateral and 4% bilateral).[5] Thus, coronary artery disease (CAD) patients are particularly at risk for reduced renal perfusion during episodes of pump failure, hypovolemia, or hypotension.[6]

Despite the kidneys receiving 25% of the cardiac output, their oxygen extraction is only 20%. When perfusion pressure falls, regulatory mechanisms come into play to constrict the efferent arteriole preferentially and thereby preserve filtration pressure. Unfortunately, this compromises the low-pressure capillary bed supplying the renal parenchyma with oxygen.[3] The primary injury occurs in the medullary thick ascending limb of the loop of Henle, which is an area of relative hypoxia where cells are very metabolically active in pumping ions. Any decrease in blood flow can result in renal "angina" with oxygen demand exceeding the supply.[7] Blocking these pumps with furosemide[8] or ouabain[9] has been shown to decrease the damage in ischemic animal models of ATN but has not been proved to be of clinical benefit in human trials.[7]

The manifestation and evaluation of patients with ischemic ATN are similar to those of any other patient with ARF, as described earlier. Prognosis depends on the underlying medical problems, age of the patient, preexisting renal disease, and duration of the oliguric phase if present. Return of renal function, when it occurs, typically appears between 1 and 2 weeks,[7] with 30% to 70% of patients having some permanent loss of glomerular filtration rate (GFR).[10] In general, despite the period of oliguria, patients with good premorbid renal function will regain their kidney function.[11]

Contrast nephropathy

Radiographic contrast agents are useful in radiology because of their triiodinated benzene ring structure, which allows them to absorb x-rays more completely, thereby enhancing visualization of contrast-containing structures. Both ionic and nonionic agents are available with osmolalities ranging from 300 to 2400 mOsm/kg of water. The incidence of contrast nephrotoxicity related to these agents varies from 1% to 12%, depending on the patients undergoing the procedure and the definition of toxicity.[12] Contrast agents have also been implicated as a cause of ARF in 12% of episodes occurring in the hospital setting.[13]

Pathophysiologically multiple theories exist to explain what happens at the level of the kidney during contrast nephrotoxicity. Unlike other arterial beds, which on exposure to contrast agents vasoconstrict and then subsequently vasodilate, the renal vasculature vasodilates initially, followed by progressive vasoconstriction with increased vascular resistance and concomitant decrease in both renal plasma flow and GFR.[13] This effect usually resolves within 1 to 2 hours after the procedure and cannot account for the delayed loss of renal function. There are striking similarities between experimental contrast nephropathy and the proposed mechanisms of nonsteroidal antiinflamatory–mediated renal injury as reviewed by Porter[14] and Levenson et al.[15] At the present time, the best data support an alteration of intrarenal hemodynamics as the pathophysiologic event leading to the decline in renal function.[12] Other theories include the direct toxicity of contrast agents, changes in red blood cell morphology, intratubular obstruction by urinary protein and uric acid crystals (because of the uricosuric effect of contrast agents), and immunologic reactions as summarized by Byrd and Sherman.[16]

Contrast nephrotoxicity, when defined as an increase in serum creatinine level of more than 0.5 mg/dl, occurs in 2% to 6% of an unselected population undergoing cardiac catheterization.[17] Stricter requirements to establish a diagnosis of contrast nephrotoxicity will yield a lower incidence. Diminished renal function or elevated serum creatinine level is the single largest risk factor for both clinical and subclinical contrast nephropathy.[17-19] This risk increases in a linear fashion above serum creatinine measurements of 1.2 mg/dl (Fig. 55-1).[17] Diabetes is an additional significant risk factor when combined with a baseline abnormality of renal function.[19,20] Diabetes alone, however, does not appear to predispose to contrast toxicity.[17,18] When the serum creatinine level is less than 2.5 mg/dl, there does not appear to be an advantage in using nonionic agents vs. ionic agents to reduce the risk of renal toxicity, although other systemic side effects are decreased.[18,21] However, small decreases in the incidence of contrast nephrotoxicity may occur at levels of serum creatinine greater than 2.5 mg/dl when nonionic contrast agents are used in preference to ionic agents.[22] Patients greater than age 70 years are at higher risk only if their baseline renal function is abnormal.[23]

Animal studies suggest volume depletion and prostaglandin inhibition contribute to the risk of developing

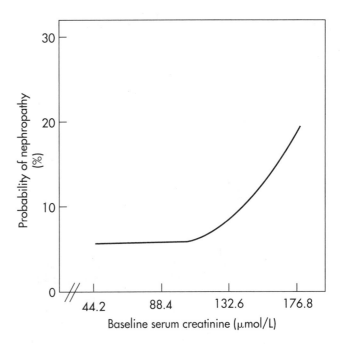

Fig. 55-1. Model for predicting risk for contrast-induced nephrotoxicity. (From Davidson CJ, Hlatky M, Morris KG, et al: *Ann Intern Med* 110:119, 1989. Used by permission.)

nephrotoxicity.[3] There is a general consensus based on animal studies that volume depletion predisposes to contrast nephrotoxicity.[12] Because of these observations, hydration before contrast exposure is warranted in most patients. Treatment with diuretics, mannitol, and other agents has not been shown to be of any clinical value. The volume of contrast used is also probably a risk factor, although most clinical trials have been unable to find a difference in contrast nephrotoxicity at the doses commonly used for cardiac catheterization.[18] In contrast, when less than 30 ml of dye was used in high-risk patients, the risk of nephrotoxicity was significantly decreased.[20]

Patients who develop contrast nephrotoxicity may have either oliguric or nonoliguric ARF, with the latter predominating.[14] The serum creatinine level begins to rise within 24 hours, peaking on average in 4.2 days.[3,24] Recovery to baseline is usually the rule by day 10, with less than 10% of affected individuals requiring dialytic support.[14] Of note, the fractional excretion of sodium tends to be less than 1 in patients after contrast exposure. Persistent nephrograms can be seen 24 to 48 hours after the procedure in patients with significant impairment. At the present time, maintaining euvolemia before dye use appears to be the only intervention that has been shown to have clinical utility.[3]

A difficult question that frequently is raised in patients in the CCU is the risk of contrast exposure in patients with ARF. There is no definitive answer. We believe that once ARF occurs, the kidney is relatively protected from further damage by its poor perfusion and decreased oxygen consumption. Dye can be used if urgently needed. A kidney recovering from ARF is at extreme risk from radiographic agents because of its increased metabolic requirements associated with recovery. However, patients who urgently need a contrast study because of an ongoing cardiac condition should not have it withheld if it is believed to be essential for survival. Contrast toxicity only rarely results in permanent loss of renal function, whereas acute cardiac syndromes remain the leading cause of death in the United States.

Cholesterol emboli

With the extensive use of invasive procedures to diagnose and treat patients with CAD, the problem of cholesterol embolization is gaining in importance as a cause of ARF in the CCU. The first reports on cholesterol embolization date to 1862 when Panum[25] described his findings in the German literature. The topic was forgotten for the most part until 1945 when Flory[26] reviewed his autopsy findings in patients with atheromatous disease of the aorta. He found 1.3% of those with mild to moderate atheromatous disease had evidence of cholesterol emboli as opposed to 12% of those with severe disease.[26] The pathologic lesions seen consist of acicular or needle-shaped spaces surrounded by amorphous debris, later giant cells, and finally concentric fibrosis.[27,28] In paraffin sections the cholesterol itself is dissolved, leaving only empty clefts. When frozen specimens and appropriate stains are used, the cholesterol appears as birefringent crystals under polarized light. The crystals have continued to be present up to 4 months after embolization in experimental animal models.[27]

Thurlbeck and Castleman[29] noted that 77% of patients dying after the newly introduced procedure of abdominal aortic aneurysm repair were shown to have cholesterol emboli to their kidneys. In reviewing the literature between 1965 and 1985, Fine et al.[30] found that the kidney was the most frequent organ involved (Table 55-4). In patients undergoing invasive vascular procedures, Ramirez et al.[31] found the incidence of cholesterol emboli during aortography to be 30% (25% of these events occurring in the kidney) and coronary angiography 25.5% (2% of these events occurring in the kidney) vs 4.3% in controls.

The typical patient is male with previous medical problems as outlined in Table 55-5,[13] having had a recent vascular procedure.[30] Of special note is the frequency of anticoagulant use, a common therapeutic measure used in the CCU. Cholesterol embolization occurring after thrombolytic use is becoming more widely reported.[32,33] The mechanism of embolization in these various causes involves either the physical disruption of an atheroma

Table 55-4. Location of premortem histologic diagnosis of cholesterol emboli

Histologic site	No.*
Muscle	19
Skin	19
Kidney	17
Amputated toe	6
Gastrointestinal mucosa	5
Prostate†	4
Lymph node	1
Amputation stump	1
Ureters‡	1
Spleen§	1
Bone marrow	1
TOTAL	75

From Fine MJ, Kapoor W, Falanga V: *Angiology* 38:769, 1987. Used by permission.
*Frequency of site.
†The prostatic tissue was obtained from a transurethral resection of the prostate in all 4 cases.
‡The ureter was resected because of structure, and cholesterol crystals were found in the periurethral arterioles.
§The spleen was resected because of hemolytic anemia, and cholesterol crystals were discovered within the organ.

Table 55-5. Profiles of patients suffering from cholesterol emboli

60-year-old man
Extensive atherosclerosis, especially aorta
Large-vessel bruits
Amaurosis fugax (transient monocular blindness)
Transient ischemic episodes
Cerebrovascular accident
Intermittent claudication
Coronary artery disease
Longstanding hypertension
Renovascular hypertension
Retinal artery cholesterol emboli

From Cronin RE: *Am J Med Sci* 298:342, 1989. Used by permission.

and cholesterol release or an inhibition or dissolution of a clot over an exposed plaque, thereby preventing endothelialization.

Patients usually have either an acute syndrome or a more chronic course as outlined in Tables 55-6 and 55-7.[13] Of particular note is the difficult to control hypertension and livedo reticularis. The development of renal failure is often insidious in the nonacute form, occurring 1 to 2 weeks after an angiographic procedure[34] (in contrast to dye nephrotoxicity, which occurs within 24 to 48 hours). An increased sedimentation rate, peripheral eosinophilia (up to 80% in other reports[35]) and elevation of Cr and BUN are the major laboratory findings.[30] The best histologic sites for diagnosis are skin, muscle, and kidney.[30]

Table 55-6. Characteristics of the acute cholesterol emboli syndrome

Agitation, sweating
Pain in legs or feet
Abdominal and back pain
Numbness or paralysis of extremities
Skin discoloration (livedo reticularis and purple toes)
Acute hypertension
Acute renal failure
Hypotension
Death

From Cronin RE: *Am J Med Sci* 298:342, 1989. Used by permission.

Table 55-7. Characteristics of the nonacute cholesterol emboli syndrome

Malignant or episodic hypertension
Post angiography or postoperative chronic renal failure
Acute pancreatitis
Myopathy
Peritonitis, bowel ischemia (melena, hematochezia)
Livedo reticularis
Gangrene of extremity

From Cronin RE: *Am J Med Sci* 298:342, 1989. Used by permission.

There are no good therapies to treat cholesterol emboli. Anticoagulation in itself may worsen the problem[36] and, if possible, should probably be discontinued. Corticosteroids, low-molecular-weight dextran, intraarterial vasodilators, and sympathetic blockade have not been shown to be effective.[28,34,37] Mortality has been reported anywhere from 73% to 81% and is usually cardiac or multifactorial in nature.[30] Less severe cases have been reported with a return of renal function although the usual course is slow progression of the renal failure.[34] If a catheterization is contemplated in someone who is at high risk for cholesterol emboli, the brachial route may be preferable, if possible, to avoid passing catheters through severely diseased abdominal aortas.[37]

Nephrotoxins

ACE inhibitors. ACE inhibitors have been in clinical use since the 1980s and have become one of the mainstays of therapies in congestive heart failure and hypertension. Unfortunately, they are not without risk. In patients with compromised renal blood flow, as in bilateral renal artery stenosis and severe congestive heart failure, the kidneys are dependent on angiotensin to constrict the efferent arteriole to maintain GFR. Inhibition of this pathway clinically leads to a fall in GFR and consequently a fall in urine output and rise in serum creatinine. The effects are reversible if the agent is withdrawn, but prolonged exposure can lead to ATN.

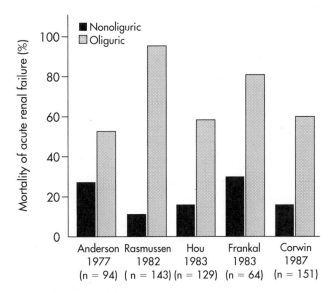

Fig. 55-2. Mortality rates of oliguric and nonoliguric forms of acute renal failure. (From Jacobson HR, Stricker GE, Klahr S [eds]: *The principles and practice of nephrology,* Philadelphia, 1991, BC Decker, p 665. Used by permission.)

Longer-acting ACE inhibitors are probably worse than shorter-acting ones such as captopril because they do not allow for any recovery of glomerular perfusion between doses.[38-42] Concomitant use of a diuretic predisposes the patient to renal injury by causing volume contraction and further decreasing renal perfusion. Diuretic dosage should be reduced when an ACE inhibitor is started.

Patients with hyporeninemic hypoaldosteronism, such as diabetics, are also at risk of developing complications with ACE inhibitors. They depend on what little circulating aldosterone exists to help in potassium secretion in the distal tubule. Inhibition of angiotensin stimulation of aldosterone secretion can clinically manifest itself as the sudden onset of hyperkalemia.[3,43,44] Frequent monitoring of serum potassium is essential in any of these patient groups on initiating ACE inhibitor therapy.

Nonsteroidal antiinflammatory agents. These agents are used for pain relief and, more important, to inhibit platelet aggregation and clot formation. Unfortunately, they too can interfere with renal function. Patients with compromised renal perfusion depend on intrarenally produced vasodilatory prostaglandins to oppose vasoconstrictor forces in the kidney. Inhibition of their production can lead to a fall in GFR, decrease in urine output, and rise in serum Cr level. Because these prostaglandins also stimulate renin release and the activation of the angiotensin-aldosterone axis, their inhibitory loss may also manifest itself as hyperkalemia.[3,45,46] Acute and chronic interstitial nephritis are other potential complications of nonsteroidal therapy.[3]

Aminoglycosides. These antibiotics are the leading

Table 55-8. Protocols to improve bleeding time in uremia

Agent*	Usual dose	Onset of action	Peak action	Duration of effect	Comments (ref.)
Cryoprecipitate (IV)	10 units over 30 min	<4 hr	4-12 hr	12-18 hr	Effective on repeat dosing; hepatitis or AIDS risk equivalent to transfusion of 10 units of blood (Janson et al.)
IV DDAVP	0.3 µg/kg in 50 ml saline	<1 hr	1-4 hr	4-8 hr	May not be effective on repeated dosing (Mannucci et al.)
Intranasal DDAVP	3.0 µg/kg	Same?	Same?	Same?	Convenient, but only limited clinical experience (Shapiro et al.)
IV estrogen	0.6 mg/kg/day for 5 days (days 1-5)	6 hr (day 1)	Day 5-7	14 days	No reported adverse effects (Livio et al.) For oral regimens see Liu et al: *Lancet* 2:887, 1984, or Bronner et al: *Ann Intern Med* 105:371, 1986.

From Daugirdas J, Ing T (eds): *Handbook of dialysis*, Boston, 1988, Little, Brown p 351. Used by permission.
*Desmopressin (DDAVP) is available from Armour Pharmaceutical Co., Kankakee, Ill. Conjugated estrogen (Emopremarin) is available from Ayerst Pharmaceutical Co., New York, N.Y.

Table 55-9. Indications for dialysis in acute renal failure

Blood urea nitrogen level >100 mg/dl, or Cr >8 mq/dL
Acidemia, serum HCO_3 <15 mEq/L
Hyperkalemia, serum K >6.0 mEq/L
Hyponatremia, serum Na <120 mEq/L
Pulmonary edema
Seizures or coma
Uremic bleeding
Protracted vomiting

Cr, Serum creatinine
From Jacobson HR, Stricker GE, Klahr S (eds): *The principles and practice of nephrology*, Philadelphia, 1991, BC Decker, p 673. Used by permission.

cause of antibiotic-induced renal damage. Patients present with gradual onset of nonoliguric renal failure. The serum creatinine level may be a poor reflection of the degree of renal damage, and recovery may take months.[3] Toxicity can occur even with therapeutic predose and postdose levels. Given the multitude of antibiotics available, the use of these agents should be reserved to appropriate situations.

MANAGEMENT

The conservative management of ARF is well established. Prerenal causes should be reversed. Possible nephrotoxins as outlined earlier in the chapter should be avoided. Daily weights and strict intake and output measurement should be followed to maintain the patient euvolemic. This should include the insensible volume losses of roughly 500 to 700 ml/day. Because survival is

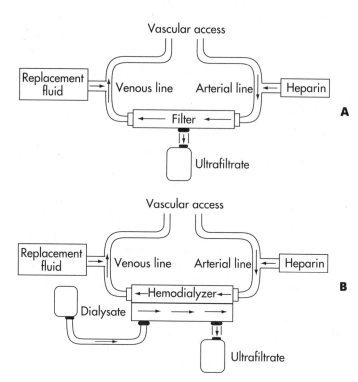

Fig. 55-3. Schematic representation of **(A)** continuous arteriovenous hemofiltration and **(B)** continuous arteriovenous hemodialysis. (From Nahman NS, Middendorf DF: *Med Clin North Am* 74:975, 1990. Used by permission.)

improved in the nonoliguric form of ARF (Fig. 55-2),[3] attempts should be made initially to convert oliguric to nonoliguric ARF with the use of diuretics. We favor using increasing doses of furosemide, up to 200 mg intravenously, with a distal tubule diuretic (e.g., meto-

Table 55-10. Factors favoring various dialysis modalities

Peritoneal dialysis	Hemodialysis	Arteriovenous hemofiltration
Minimal increase in catabolic rate	High catabolic rate	Moderately high catabolic rate
Slow fluid-electrolyte correction required	Rapid fluid-electrolyte correction required	Rapid fluid correction required
Intact peritoneum without infection or adhesions	Hemodynamically stable patient	Moderately fast electrolyte correction required
Hemodynamically unstable patient	Hemodynamically stable patient	Hemodynamically unstable patient
Untrained or minimally trained staff	Trained staff; equipment	Intermediate level of staff training and equipment relative to peritoneal dialysis and hemodialysis

From Jacobson HR, Stricker GE, Klahr S (eds): *The principles and practice of nephrology*, Philadelphia, 1991, BC Decker, p 673. Used by permission.

Table 55-11. Risks and complications of various dialysis modalities

Peritoneal dialysis	Hemodialysis	Arteriovenous hemofiltration
Slow fluid and solute removal	Hemodynamic instability	Volume depletion
Drainage failure	Hypoxemia	Hemorrhage
Unpredictable fluid removal	Hemorrhage	Electrolyte disturbances
Peritonitis	Osmolar dysequilibrium	Filter clotting
Puncture of abdominal viscus	Dialyzer clotting	Vascular thrombosis
Respiratory compromise	Access thrombosis	Infection
Hyperglycemia	Infection	Arrhythmias
	Arrhythmias	

From Jacobson HR, Stricker GE, Klahr S (eds): *The principles and practice of nephrology*, Philadelphia, 1991, BC Decker, p 674. Used by permission.

lazone) if a loop diuretic alone fails. If the attempt to convert the type of ARF fails, diuretics should be discontinued as ototoxicity can develop. Although low-dose dopamine (1-4 μ/kg/min) has been used in experimental models of ARF to maintain renal vasodilation, no controlled studies have been performed to evaluate its use in human ischemic renal failure.[3]

Electrolyte abnormalities can be handled conservatively by limiting the intake of phosphate (<800 mg/day) and potassium (<60 mEq/day), using oral phosphate binders with meals (500-1000 mg of calcium carbonate, 250-500 mg of calcium acetate, or 30-60 ml of aluminum hydroxide) and exchange resins to control potassium (sodium polystyrene sulfonate [Kayexylate] orally or as a retention enema). Mild acidosis can be treated with bicarbonate. Because acute illness and renal failure cause insulin resistance, hyperglycemia should be treated with insulin as needed. Drug dosages must be reduced and dosing schedules changed as required. Bleeding problems can be treated initially as outlined in Table 55-8.[47] Ultimately, when conservative measures fail, some form of dialytic therapy becomes necessary.

Renal replacement therapies

Once conservative management fails, renal replacement therapy is needed. The usual indications are listed in Table 55-9.[3] Dialysis, however, is usually begun electively to improve patient management and allow improved nutrition. This early initiation of renal replacement therapy allows parenteral nutrition, as well an easing of volume and transfusion restrictions.

Currently three methods of renal replacement therapy are available: hemodialysis, peritoneal dialysis, and continuous arteriovenous hemofiltration/dialysis (CAVH/CAVHD) (Fig. 55-3).[48] Factors favoring one mode of therapy over the other are listed in Table 55-10[3] and their complications in Table 55-11.[3] Access is obtained by a doubled lumen venous catheter in the femoral, subclavian, or internal jugular veins in the case of hemodialysis, Tenckhoff catheter into the peritoneal cavity for peritoneal dialysis, and a combination of large venous and arterial catheters or Scribner shunt in the case of CAVH/CAVHD.

The major drawbacks to hemodialysis are the large changes in blood pressure that can occur and the risk of bleeding from heparin use. This latter problem has been resolved with the development of a no-heparin technique[49] and with citrate regional anticoagulation.[50] Unfortunately, both CAVH and CAVHD require the need for anticoagulation and arterial access. Regional anticoagulation with CAVH is possible, but its high complication rate has prevented its widespread acceptance. We favor peritoneal dialysis if technically feasible in CCU patients because it has limited hemodynamic consequences, avoids the need for anticoagulation, and allows continual ultrafiltration. This therapy can be

Table 55-12. Nutritional requirements in acute renal failure*†

Calories

Maintain body weight in normal range, 2000 kcal/day (29 kcal/kg)
ARF, uncomplicated, increase by 10%
ARF, complicated by trauma, surgery, or sepsis, increase by 50%
ARF, complicated by severe trauma or burn injury (>50% body surface area), increase by 100%
Give as dextrose, fat emulsion, or both

Protein

Oral feeding, 0.5-1.0 g/kg/day
Parenteral feeding, essential amino acids 10-20 g/day; with dialysis, increase essential amino acids or add 10-20 g/day nonessential amino acids

Water-electrolytes

Sufficient to replace previous days losses plus determined deficits

Assessment

Daily body weights, levels of BUN, glucose, Na^+, K^+, Cl^-, HCO_3^-, Ca^{2+}, and phosphorus; twice weekly levels of Mg^{2+}, AST, ammonia, triglycerides, arterial blood gases

Goals

Minimize negative nitrogen balance; avoid volume overload and other complications of nutritional therapy

---

From Jacobson HR, Stricker GE, Klahr S (eds): *The principles and practice of nephrology*, Philadelphia, 1991, BC Decker, p 671. Used by permission.
*Based on an average-sized 70-kg adult.
†*ARF*, Acute renal failure; *BUN*, blood urea nitrogen; *AST*, aspartate aminotransferase.

continued outside the ICU setting, whereas CAVH and CAVHD require ICU monitoring.

NUTRITION

Patients in the CCU are usually catabolic and require nutritional support to recover, particularly those who develop ARF of whatever etiology. Early consultation with the nutrition service and implementation of feeding strategies will play an important role in supporting the patient to recovery. In general adequate calories (25-50 kcal/kg/day) are required. Protein is restricted to 0.5 g/kg/day during conservative management. When renal replacement therapy is instituted, protein intake is increased to 1 to 1.5 g/kg/day. All magnesium-containing compounds should be discontinued. In patients unable or unwilling to eat, either enteral or parenteral hyperalimentation is indicated. There are many formulas available, and discussion of the various categories is beyond the scope of this chapter. A rough guide of basic requirements is given in Table 55-12.[3]

CONCLUSION

ARF is a serious problem in patients with cardiovascular disease. Given the interventional nature of modern cardiology, progressively less stable patients will undergo diagnostic and therapeutic procedures. This will result in a more frequent exposure of cardiologists to ARF, especially in the CCU. Certain renal insults associated with cardiac catheterization and coronary angioplasty will occur frequently. These injuries were discussed in depth in this chapter and include ischemic ARF, cholesterol emboli, and contrast nephrotoxicity. An understanding of these conditions and a thorough approach to these problems will improve care for CCU patients.

REFERENCES

1. Satler LW, Rackley CE: Changing outcome in acute myocardial infarction, *Cardiol Clin* 20:19-26, 1989.
2. Hou SH, Bushinsky DA, Wish JB, et al: Hospital-acquired renal insufficiency: a prospective study, *Am J Med* 74:243-248, 1983.
3. Jacobson HR, Stricker GE, Klahr S ed: *The Principles and practice of nephrology*, Philadelphia, 1991, BC Decker.
4. Corwin HL, Bonventre JV: Acute renal failure in the intensive care unit: I and II, *Intensive Care Med* 14:10-16, 86-96, 1988.
5. Harding MB, Smith LB, Himmelstein SI, et al: Renal artery stenosis: prevalence and associated risk factors in patients undergoing routine cardiac catheterization, *J Am Soc Nephrol* 2:1-9, 1992.
6. Jacobson HR: Ischemic renal disease: an overlooked clinical entity? *Kidney Int* 34:729-743, 1988.
7. Brezis M, Rosen S, Silva P, et al: Renal ischemia: a new perspective, *Kidney Int* 26:375-383, 1984.
8. Kramer HJ, Schuurmann J, Wassermann C, et al: Prostaglandin-independent protection by furosemide from oliguric ischemic renal failure in conscious rats, *Kidney Int* 17:455-464, 1980.
9. Siegel M, Rice J, Barnes J, et al: Protective effect of mini-dose ouabain in ischemic renal failure in the dog [abstract], *Clin Res* 3:518A, 1983.
10. Finn WF: Diagnosis and management of acute tubular necrosis, *Med Clin North Am* 74:873-917, 1990.
11. Spurney R, Fulkerson W, Schwab S: Acute renal failure in critically ill patients: prognosis for recovery of kidney function following prolonged dialysis support, *Crit Care Med* 19:8-11, 1991.
12. Vari RC, Natarajan LA, Whitescarver SA, et al: Induction, prevention and mechanisms of contrast media–induced acute renal failure, *Kidney Int* 33:699-707, 1988.
13. Cronin RE: Southwestern Internal Medicine Conference: renal failure following radiologic procedures, *Am J Med Sci* 298:342-356, 1989.
14. Porter GA: Experimental contrast-associated nephrophathy and its clinical implications, *Am J Cardiol* 66:18F-22F, 1990.
15. Levenson DJ, Simmons CE Jr, Brenner BM: Arachidonic acid metabolism, prostaglandins, and the kidney, *Am J Med* 72:354-374, 1982.
16. Byrd L, Sherman RL: Radiocontrast-induced acute renal failure: a clinical and pathophysiologic review, *Medicine (Baltimore)* 58:270-279, 1979.
17. Davidson CJ, Hlatky M, Morris KG, et al: Cardiovascular and renal toxicity of a nonionic radiographic contrast agent after cardiac catheterization: a prospective trial, *Ann Intern Med* 110:119-124, 1989.
18. Schwab SJ, Hlatky MA, Pieper KS, et al: Contrast nephrotoxicity: a randomized controlled trial of a nonionic and an ionic radiographic contrast agent, *N Engl J Med* 320:149-153, 1989.

19. Pafrey PS, Griffiths SM, Barrett BJ, et al: Contrast material–induced renal failure in patients with diabetes mellitus, renal insufficiency, or both: a prospective controlled study, *N Engl J Med* 320:143-149, 1989.

20. Manske CL, Sprafka JM, Strony JT, et al: Contrast nephropathy in azotemic diabetic patients undergoing coronary angiography, *Am J Med* 89:615-620, 1990.

21. Harding MB, Davidson CJ, Pieper KS, et al: Comparison of cardiovascular and renal toxicity after cardiac catheterization using a nonionic versus ionic radiographic contrast agent, *Am J Cardiol* 68:1117-1119, 1991.

22. Barrett BJ, Parfrey PS, Vavasour HM, et al: Contrast nephropathy in patients with impaired renal function: high versus low osmolar media, *Kidney Int* 41:1274-1279, 1992.

23. Rich MW, Crecelius CA: Incidence, risk factors, and clinical course of acute renal insufficiency after cardiac catheterization in patients 70 years of age or older, *Arch Intern Med* 150:1237-1242, 1990.

24. Porter GA: Contrast associated nephropathy, *Am J Cardiol* 64:22E-26E, 1989.

25. Panum, PL: Experimentelle Beitrage Zur Lehre Von Der Embolie, *Virchow Arch (A)* 25:308, 1862.

26. Flory CM: Arterial occlusions produced by emboli from eroded aortic atheromatous plaques, *Am J Pathol* 21:549-565, 1945.

27. Gore I, McCombs HL, Lindquist RL: Observation on the fate of cholesterol emboli, *J Atheroscler Res* 4:526-535, 1964.

28. Kassirer JP: Atheroembolic renal disease, *N Engl J Med* 280:812-818, 1969.

29. Thurlbeck WM, Castleman B: Atheromatous emboli to the kidneys after aortic surgery, *N Engl J Med* 257:442-447, 1957.

30. Fine MJ, Kapoor W, Falanga V: Cholesterol crystal embolization: a review of 221 cases in the English literature, *Angiology* 38:769-784, 1987.

31. Ramirez G, O'Neill WM, Lambert R, Bloomer HA: Cholesterol emboli, *Arch Intern Med* 138:1430-1432, 1978.

32. Glassock RJ (ed): Acute renal failure, hypertension and skin necrosis in a patient with streptokinase therapy, *Am J Nephrol* 4:193-200, 1984.

33. Queen M, Biem HJ, Moe GW, et al: Development of cholesterol embolization syndrome after intravenous streptokinase for acute myocardial infarction, *Am J Cardiol* 65:1042-1043, 1990.

34. Smith MC, Ghose MK, Henry AR: The clinical spectrum of renal cholesterol embolization, *Am J Med* 71:174-180, 1981.

35. Kasinath BS, Corwin HL, Bidani AK, et al: Eosinophilia in the diagnosis of atheroembolic renal disease, *Am J Nephrol* 7:173-177, 1987.

36. Darsee JR: Cholesterol emboli: the great masquerader, *South Med J* 72:174-180, 1979.

37. Colt HG, Begg RJ, Saporito JJ, et al: Cholesterol emboli after cardiac catheterization: eight cases and a review of the literature, *Medicine (Baltimore)* 67:389-400, 1988.

38. Keane WF, Anderson S, Aurell M, et al: Angiotensin converting enzyme inhibitors and progressive renal insufficiency: current experiences and future directions, *Ann Intern Med* 111:503-516, 1989.

39. Packer M, Lee WH, Medina N, et al: Functional renal insufficiency during long-term therapy with captopril and enalapril in severe chronic heart failure, *Ann Intern Med* 106:346-354, 1987.

40. Suki WN: Renal hemodynamic consequences of angiotensin-converting enzyme inhibition in congestive heart failure, *Arch Intern Med* 149:669-673, 1989.

41. Badr KF, Ichikawa I: Prerenal failure: a deleterious shift from renal compensation to decompensation, *N Engl J Med* 319:623-629, 1988.

42. Packer M, Lee WH, Yushak M, et al: Comparison of captopril and enalapril in patients with severe chronic heart failure, *N Engl J Med* 315:847-853, 1986.

43. DeFronzo RA: Hyperkalemic and hyporeninemic hypoaldosteronism, *Kidney Int* 17:118-134, 1980.

44. Abraham PA, Opsahl JA, Halstenson CE, et al: Efficacy and renal effects of enalapril therapy for hypertensive patients with chronic renal insufficiency, *Arch Intern Med* 148:2358-2343, 1988.

45. Whelton A, Stout RL, Spilman PS, et al: Renal effects of ibuprofen, piroxicam, and sulindac in patients with asymptomatic renal failure, *Ann Intern Med* 112:568-576, 1990.

46. Murray MD, Brater DC: Adverse effects of nonsteroidal anti-inflammatory drugs on renal function, *Ann Intern Med* 112:559-560, 1990.

47. Daugirdas J, Ing T, (ed): *Handbook of dialysis,* Boston, 1988, Little, Brown, p. 351.

48. Nahman NS, Middendorf DF: Continuous arteriovenous hemofiltration, *Med Clin North Am* 74:975-984, 1990.

49. Schwab S, Onorato J, Sharar L, et al: Hemodialysis without anticoagulation: results of a one year prospective trial in hospitalized patients at risk for bleeding, *Am J Med* 83:405-410, 1987.

50. Pinnick RV: Regional citrate anticoagulation in the patient at high risk for bleeding, *N Engl J Med* 308:258-263, 1983.

Chapter 56

VASCULAR COMPLICATIONS OF CARDIAC CATHETERIZATION

Lewis B. Schwartz
Richard L. McCann

Since the advent of coronary angiography, complications occurring at the vascular access site have remained a persistent problem. Both the original brachial arteriotomy approach[1,2] and the femoral percutaneous approach[3,4] can cause significant vascular injury, resulting in a threat to limb or even life. This chapter describes the incidence, risk factors, diagnosis, and therapeutic options for complications of cardiac catheterization occurring specifically at the access artery. Other complications of catheterization, including coronary artery dissection, cerebrovascular accident, and cardiac dysrhythmias, are discussed elsewhere.

COMPLICATIONS OF CATHETERIZATION VIA THE FEMORAL ARTERY
Incidence and risk factors

Cardiac catheterization via the femoral percutaneous route is now considered the method of choice at many institutions because vascular complications are less frequent compared with brachial artery access (see later discussion). Large clinical series have shown that vascular complications occur in less than 1% of catheterizations (Table 56-1). The reported complication rate varies from 0% to 5.8% according to institution, size of the series, and definition of complication. At our own institution, a rate of 0.59% has been observed in more than 24,000 examinations over a 5-year period.[5]

Much has been written regarding risk factors for femoral vascular complications in hopes of identifying subpopulations in which alternate approaches could be used. Some studies have shown that females tend to have a higher risk than males,[5,6,20,26] although the data are not uniform.[23,27] Advanced age has been implicated as a risk factor by some groups[5,6] but not others.[23,27] Preexisting lower extremity peripheral vascular disease is generally accepted as a risk factor,[5,11,28] and its presence should be considered in the decision to use femoral access. Absent or diminished femoral pulses or known severe atherosclerotic disease should be considered relative contraindications to femoral access unless such an approach is clearly justified by the clinical circumstances. Similarly, puncture of a previously placed Dacron aortobifemoral bypass graft is more difficult than the native femoral artery, although the increased risks of thrombosis and hemorrhage may be acceptable if the clinical setting is compelling.

In adults, both obesity[11,29] and extremely low body weight[5] have been associated with an increased complication rate. Other reported risk factors include large catheter size,[11] the use of multiple catheters,[30] or multiple punctures,[10,23] prolonged procedure time,[19,23,31] operator experience,[19,22,31] and the presence of congestive heart failure[5] or hypertension.[21,28,30]

It is generally accepted that the use of heparin during catheterization decreases thrombotic complications, and this practice should be routine.[19,32-35] The relationship between complications and continuing anticoagulation after the procedure is less well established, however.

Table 56-1. Vascular complications of cardiac catheterization via the femoral artery

Authors	Year	Catheter- izations	Complications		Hemorrhage/ hematoma	Pseudo- aneurysm	Thrombo- embolism	Arteriovenous fistula	Other*
			No.	%					
McCann et al.[5]	1991	24820	146	0.59	NR†	64	7	8	0
Oweida et al.[6]	1990	4988	55	1.10	6	35	5	8	1
Kaufman et al.[7]	1989	3548	35	0.99	20	4	5	0	6
Richardson et al.[8]	1989	295	6	2.03	2	1	2	0	1
Babu et al.[9]	1989	10500	14	0.13	8	4	1	1	0
Sheikh et al.[10]	1989	5526	22	0.39	0	14	0	8	0
Skillman et al.[11]	1988	7124	55	0.77	8	31	6	10	0
Chiverton and Murie[12]	1986	2603	3	0.12	0	0	2	0	0
Bredlau et al.[13]	1985	3500	31	0.89	9	22	NR	NR	NR
McMillan and Murie[14]	1984	3413	11	0.32	0	7	3	0	1
Dorros et al.[15]	1983	1500	22	1.47	6	2	12	1	1
Dodek et al.[16]	1983	713	7	0.98	6	0	1	0	0
Kennedy[17]	1982	28933	44	0.15	17	0	27	0	NR
Davis et al.[18]	1979	6328	15	0.24	NR	NR	15	NR	NR
Adams and Adams[19]	1979	45999	192	0.42	64	21	107	NR	NR
Bourassa and Noble[20]	1976	5250	45	0.86	0	9	36	0	0
Schoonmaker and King[21]	1974	6800	38	0.56	16	0	22	0	NR
Adams et al.[22]	1973	22780	322	1.41	37	14	271	NR	NR
Brener and Couch[23]	1973	223	13	5.83	0	4	9	0	0
Green et al.[24]	1972	445	16	3.6	9	0	7	0	0
Aguilar et al.[25]	1966	253	0	0.0	0	0	0	0	0
TOTAL		185626	1092	0.59	208 (19%)	232 (21%)	605 (55%)	36 (3%)	10 (1%)

*Other, Aortic/femoral dissection, catheter embolization, aortic thrombosis, venous thrombosis, puncture site infection, mesenteric ischemia, and femoral artery aneurysm.
†NR, Not reported.

Some authors[6,11,30] have reported that continuation of heparin after catheterization leads to a higher incidence of vascular complications, whereas others[18,27] maintain that no such association exists. Postprocedure heparinization probably decreases thrombotic complications but increases bleeding complications; the predominant factor has not yet been established. It is clear, however, that the use of thrombolytic therapy at the time of catheterization does increase the risk of femoral artery bleeding complications.[5,6,10,36]

Whether cardiac catheterization accompanied by therapeutic maneuvers such as percutaneous transluminal coronary angioplasty (PTCA) or balloon valvuloplasty increases vascular complications remains controversial. In one study by Lilly et al.[27] the risk of complications in 1758 patients undergoing either PTCA or valvuloplasty was no different than the risk in 5890 patients undergoing diagnostic catheterization alone (0.63% vs. 0.53%, respectively). Other investigators[7,37] have confirmed this finding. On the other hand, a similar retrospective study of 16,350 patients showed that patients with complications were more likely to have undergone PTCA (34%) compared with patients without complications (24%).[5] In addition, a recent study of 6912 catheterizations showed that the risk of vascular complications was five times greater when an interventional procedure such as PTCA, valvuloplasty, or intraaortic balloon pump insertion was performed.[28] Although the relationship between femoral complications and PTCA remains unclear, there is general agreement that balloon valvuloplasty does result in increased complications because of the larger-bore catheters required for the procedure.[5,11,37-39]

One particularly interesting and well-studied risk factor for catheterization-induced femoral complications is the anatomic location of the arterial puncture site. It has been proposed that puncture of the common femoral artery (CFA) is optimal because the femoral sheath is circumferentially intact, and it enables compression over the hard bony surface of the femoral head

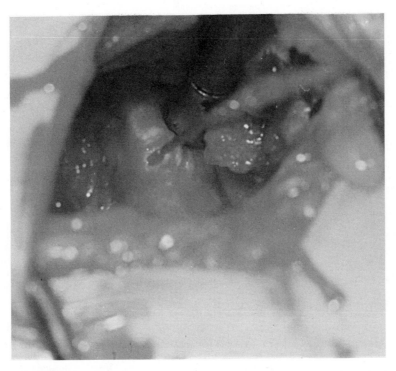

Fig. 56-1. Repair of femoral artery pseudoaneurysm 3 years after cardiac catheterization. Note the defect in the artery near the tip of the suction catheter.

for hemostasis.* The CFA bifurcation is located approximately 6 cm below the inguinal crease or, fluoroscopically, at the level of the inferior cortical margin of the femoral head.[41] Neither the external iliac, superficial femoral, or profunda femoris arteries are as easily compressed as the CFA and should be avoided. Catheterization via the CFA does not preclude the development of vascular complications, of course,[30,42] but their incidence can be minimized.

Hematoma, hemorrhage, and pseudoaneurysm

Hematoma, hemorrhage, and pseudoaneurysm are the most frequent vascular complications of cardiac catheterization. They represent a continuum of the same basic defect—inadequate hemostasis. The most benign form is hematoma, or extravasated blood into the perivascular tissues of the thigh. Because this complication is so frequent and benign, it is rarely reported. The incidence of uncomplicated hematomas that resorb spontaneously is probably about 5% to 10%,[43,44] although the incidence is clearly increasing with the growing use of thrombolytic therapy for AMI.[28,36,45] Surgical intervention is required for complications of hematomas, including acute expansion, frank hemorrhage, and skin necrosis. The incidence of femoral hematomas or persistent hemorrhage requiring surgery

is estimated at 0.08% to 0.68%, depending on the series.[5-9,11,15,19] Vascular surgical consultation and intervention should be instituted early because blood loss is poorly tolerated in these patients and early hematoma evacuation may avoid skin necrosis and arterial compression and thrombosis. Surgical evacuation and repair can usually be performed expeditiously under regional anesthesia with little morbidity. Local anesthesia is usually inadequate except for the smallest hematomas.

A more complicated problem arises when the arterial entry site is just above the inguinal ligament in the distal external iliac artery and compression on the femoral head is less effective. Extravasation then occurs into the retroperitoneal space, where large quantities of blood may accumulate. Exploration is generally indicated for either mass effect in the retroperitoneum or if the hemorrhage is uncontrolled or persistent.

When blood loss is controlled but the femoral artery puncture site fails to heal, a perivascular hematoma forms that may contain a central area that remains fluid. This has been traditionally referred to as a pseudoaneurysm (false aneurysm) because there is no aneurysm wall per se, only a rim of thrombus. It is the persistence of liquid blood in the center of the lesion that distinguishes a pseudoaneurysm from an uncomplicated hematoma. Most pseudoaneurysms are asymptomatic; occasionally patients will complain of pain or neuropathy. Most are diagnosed shortly after catheterization, although the interval between injury and diagnosis may be years (Fig.

---

*References 8, 11, 12, 14, 27, 40, 41.

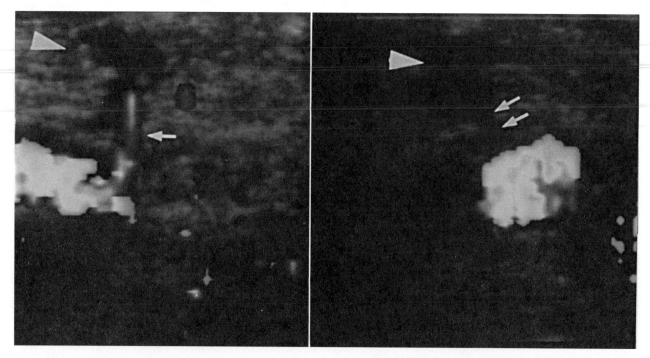

Fig. 56-2. A, Groin duplex ultrasonography with color flow Doppler imaging 2 days after cardiac catheterization. There is a relatively long passage (*single arrow*) leading from the femoral artery to the cavity (*arrowhead*). **B,** Follow-up 2 days later after treatment with only reduced activity shows no flow within the passage (*double arrow*) and complete thrombosis of the mass.

56-1). The classic physical finding is a pulsatile groin mass. Although an uncomplicated hematoma may transmit a pulse, a pseudoaneurysm is pulsatile in a radial direction on palpation of the lateral edges of the mass. The clinical impression can be easily and accurately confirmed by duplex ultrasound examination[5,10,30,46-49] (Fig. 56-2), and angiography is rarely required.

The treatment of pseudoaneurysms should be individualized according to the morphology of the lesion and the overall status of the patient. Many pseudoaneurysms will seal spontaneously shortly after catheterization. Sonographic characteristics that suggest imminent closure include a small cavity size and a long neck between the native vessel and pseudoaneurysm,[5] but these criteria are not strictly reliable.[50] If the lesion does not close within 3 to 4 days, continued observation may be complicated by frank rupture or pressure necrosis of the skin, and an attempt at closure is indicated.

Compression therapy has recently been introduced for false aneurysms occurring after catheterization.[50-52] Under sonographic guidance, the liquid center is compressed externally to the point of obliteration while still allowing flow in the native vessel. Compression is maintained for 30 to 60 minutes as tolerated, and in many cases thrombosis is induced, obviating the need for surgical intervention. Initial reports indicate that compression therapy may be successful in greater than 80% of cases.[52]

When nonoperative therapy fails, surgical repair is usually straightforward and can be performed under local or regional anesthesia. It is wise to obtain proximal control via the iliac artery through the use of a separate suprainguinal incision. Once proximal control has been secured, the pseudoaneurysm can be entered with digital control of backbleeding and the defect closed directly (see Figure 56-1). Arterial reconstruction is rarely required.

The results of more than 200 pseudoaneurysm repairs after cardiac catheterization are published in various small series (see Table 56-1).* Mortality from the operation is infrequent and usually occurs as a result of the underlying cardiac condition for which the catheterization was performed.[5,27] Morbidity is also limited, although troublesome wound infections have been reported.[8]

Thromboembolism

One of the most dreaded vascular complications of cardiac catheterization is femoral artery thromboembolism, which occurs between 0.01% and 1.1% of cases in more recent series (see Table 56-1).† Thromboembolism may occur as a result of local thrombosis at the puncture site or from distal embolization from the puncture site or

*References 5-11, 13-15, 19, 20, 23, 27-30, 37, 39, 41, 42, 47, 53-55.
†References 5-9, 11, 14-20, 23, 27-29, 37, 39, 56.

indwelling catheter. The signs and symptoms classically include pain, pallor, pulselessness, paresthesias, and paralysis. If the iliac artery becomes occluded, the foot typically becomes pale and pulseless, but rest pain only rarely results. Occlusion of the common or superficial femoral artery causes more pronounced symptoms, including rest pain. The most severe symptoms occur in patients with preexisting superficial femoral disease in whom the deep femoral system is acutely thrombosed. These patients have severe, unremitting extremity pain and constitute a surgical emergency. Because the condition of the femoral and distal pulses is critical, precatheterization evaluation should include a thorough investigation for peripheral vascular disease, including solicitation of a history of claudication or rest pain and evaluation and accurate documentation of the peripheral pulses by an experienced examiner.

Vascular surgical consultation should be sought when peripheral pulses are diminished, the limb is pale, or the patient complains of extremity pain. Paresthesias and paralysis are late signs and suggest irreversible tissue loss. When acute ischemia is manifested by neurologic changes or a clear deterioration from the precatheterization examination, immediate groin exploration and revascularization offer the best chance for limb salvage. Arteriography is generally not indicated because it only delays therapy, and intraoperative studies may be performed if needed. Groin exploration with the patient under local anesthesia is performed promptly and the puncture site exposed. The puncture site defect may be used for access for thromboembolectomy catheters and inspection of the lumen for intimal damage or the presence of an intimal flap. Fogarty thromboembolectomy, followed by repair, is all that is required in most cases. More extensive vascular reconstruction, including local endarterectomy, patch angioplasty, short segment resection, and formal bypass, is required in 10% to 40% of operations.[5,6,24,27]

The morbidity and mortality from peripheral ischemia after catheterization are significant. Surgical morbidity may occur in 20% to 80% of cases and includes hematoma, wound infection, deep venous thrombosis, myocardial infarction, sepsis, and multiple system organ failure.[8,9,15,28,29] In some series, amputation has been required in up to 5% of cases, primarily because of either extensive thrombosis or delay in therapy.[5,28,29,57] Mortality is also significant, occurring in 6% to 17% of cases, but almost always results from the underlying cardiac disease process and reflects the severity of illness of the patient population.* Long-term functional results are rarely reported. One study has suggested, however, that up to one third of patients will have persistent

procedure-related complaints, including leg pain, thigh anesthesia, or chronic incisional pain.[29]

Arteriovenous fistula

Arteriovenous fistula (AVF) creation is an unusual consequence of cardiac catheterization and is surprisingly rarely reported.* Like femoral pseudoaneurysms, it has been suggested that AVFs are more likely to occur after high or low arterial punctures[40,61] and after simultaneous artery and vein cannulation.[40,58,61] AVFs may manifest in a variety of ways, including as an asymptomatic thrill or bruit in the early postcatheterization period[5] or later with congestive heart failure, increasing angina, claudication, or leg swelling.[11,54] The diagnosis may be confirmed by duplex Doppler ultrasonography (Fig. 56-3)[5,62]; arteriography is not necessary for diagnostic purposes but may be helpful in planning the operative approach.

Many AVFs will close spontaneously; therefore, AVFs diagnosed in the early postcatheterization period without arterial, venous, or cardiac insufficiency may be observed. If the fistula has not resolved after about 6 weeks, spontaneous resolution is unlikely, and repair may be considered to obviate hemodynamic and infectious sequelae.[5,50] AVFs do not respond to compression therapy as do pseudoaneurysms, and most should be approached surgically. At the time of exploration, the arterial defect usually can be repaired primarily. Proximal and distal control of all four vessels before fistulotomy is critical to minimize blood loss.[63] Whether the involved vein should be repaired or simply ligated is a matter of some controversy. Some authors advocate venorrhaphy[60]; however, long-term patency is rare, and the risk of deep venous thrombosis probably outweighs the risk of venous stasis. Results of hemodynamically significant AVF repair are excellent, with prompt resolution of congestive failure[54] and rare recurrence.

COMPLICATIONS OF CATHETERIZATION VIA THE BRACHIAL ARTERY
Incidence and risk factors

Several studies have conclusively shown that access for catheterization via the brachial artery is accompanied by more vascular complications than the femoral route.† Although early reports estimated the risk of brachial artery thrombosis to be as high as 20% to 30%,[23,65-68] larger, more recent series quote more reasonable rates of 0.87% to 5.63% (Table 56-2).[9,18,22,61,69-71] The brachial approach is used primarily in some institutions or is indicated when femoral puncture is hazardous because of significant aortoiliac or

*References 5, 8, 14, 24, 27, 28.

*References 5, 6, 9-11, 15, 27, 50, 54, 55, 58, 59.
†References 9, 12, 17-19, 22, 23, 26, 64.

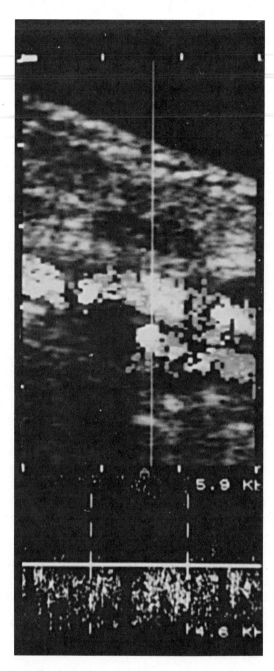

Fig. 56-3. Duplex ultrasound and color flow Doppler imaging of an arteriovenous fistula. Note continuous flow in the artery (*top*), as well as flow in the vein (*bottom*) from the site of the fistula toward the heart. The Doppler signal demonstrates diastolic augmentation of the flow waveform.

femoropopliteal atherosclerotic disease. Risk factors for the development of vascular complications using brachial access include female gender,[26,62] prior PTCA,[62] inadequate operator experience,[22,62] faulty arteriotomy closure,[62] brachial artery atherosclerosis,[62] lengthy procedure duration,[23,62,65,67,70] and failure to use heparin.[62] Although most authors recommend cut-down and brachial arteriotomy, acceptable preliminary results have

also been reported using percutaneous access.[73-78] The axillary approach is mentioned for completeness, although this method is technically more difficult and fraught with complications.* Even small axillary hematomas are poorly tolerated and may result in significant brachial plexus injury with permanent neurologic deficit.[53,81-86]

Thrombosis

The most common complication of brachial artery access is brachial artery thrombosis, which accounts for the majority of vascular complications using this approach (see Table 56-2). It is believed that the small size of the brachial artery is responsible for its poor tolerance of indwelling catheters and arteriorrhaphy.[26,62] Because of the abundant collateral circulation about the elbow, brachial artery thrombosis seldom produces severe or limb-threatening symptoms. Complaints of hand coolness, paresthesias, and ischemic pain are likely to lead to recognition of brachial artery thrombosis.[62,70] The most common mode of manifestation is the finding of absent brachial or radial pulses after catheterization.[70] Loss of pulses should never be attributed to arterial spasm; the deficit is caused by thrombosis until proved otherwise. The diagnosis can be confirmed by Doppler waveform and pressure studies, and angiography is usually not required.

When the diagnosis of brachial artery thrombosis has been made, prompt vascular surgical consultation and exploration are indicated. Thrombosis managed expectantly leads to the development of late claudication in 30% to 40% of cases.[67,69,87] Significant delay in surgery results in poor operative outcome, with increased likelihood of rethrombosis and persistent neurologic deficit.[9,70-72] Repair can often be performed by Fogarty thrombectomy alone or thrombectomy followed by resection of the affected arterial segment and primary reanastomosis. Formal vascular reconstruction with a vein patch or interposition vein graft is required in 1% to 20% of cases.[9,62,70,72,88] Results of surgery are generally excellent, with long-term secondary patency and good clinical outcome exceeding 90%.[9,62,70,72] The single most important factor affecting patency and the need for subsequent reexploration is the expediency of diagnosis and repair.† Because this procedure is easily performed with the patient under local anesthesia, delay is justified in only the most unstable patients. In one study by Babu et al.,[9] none of 48 patients who underwent early exploration suffered untoward sequelae, whereas 3 of 12 patients in whom the diagnosis and repair were delayed suffered significant permanent neurologic dis-

*References 57, 60, 63, 77, 79, 80.
†References 9, 23, 62, 65, 67, 70, 72, 88, 89.

Table 56-2. Vascular complications of cardiac catheterization via the brachial artery

Authors	Year	Catheterizations	Complications No.	Complications %	Hemorrhage/ hematoma	Pseudoaneurysm	Thromboembolism	Arteriovenous fistula
Kline et al.[72]	1990	34291	532	1.55	0	0	532	0
Babu et al.[9]	1989	5850	60	1.03	6	4	50	0
McCollum and Mavor[62]	1986	12158	106	0.87	12	2	92	0
Kitzmiller et al.[70]	1982	6518	100	1.53	0	0	100	0
Kennedy[17]	1982	23039	134	0.58	36	0	92	0
Davis et al.[18]	1979	1187	22	1.85	NR*	NR	22	NR
Adams and Adams[19]	1979	43080	523	1.21	21	16	486	NR
Karmody et al.[69]	1976	1084	61	5.63	0	0	61	0
Nicholas and DeMuth[71]	1976	553	21	3.80	0	0	21	0
Adams et al.[22]	1973	24124	435	1.80	17	14	404	NR
TOTAL		151884	1994	1.31	92 (5%)	36 (2%)	1866 (93%)	0 (0%)

*NR, Not reported.

ability. Balloon angioplasty and thrombolytic therapy for brachial artery occlusion have been reported and may be useful in selected patients.[90]

Other complications

Complications of bleeding occur much less frequently than thromboses when the brachial approach is used, probably because of the relative ease of compressibility of the brachial artery in the antecubital fossa. Less than 100 cases of hemorrhage requiring surgical exploration have been reported (see Table 56-2). Simple repair of the laceration is usually all that is required. Pseudoaneurysm and arteriovenous fistula formation are also rare but have been reported.[9,62,69,74]

MINIMIZING VASCULAR COMPLICATIONS

Effective limitation of vascular complications of cardiac catheterization revolves around three main issues: choice of access site, adequate mechanical hemostasis, and early vascular surgical referral.

As previously stated, the preferred access site for diagnostic and therapeutic cardiac catheterization is the common femoral artery. Both the brachial and axillary approaches carry higher incidences of complications, as does puncture of the common iliac, superficial femoral, or profunda femoris arteries. It should also be noted, however, that femoral complications, although infrequent, are generally more serious, with a small but real risk of limb loss.

Adequate mechanical hemostasis after catheterization cannot be overemphasized. Mechanical compression can be performed by the operator or by specially designed compression clamps, so-called C clamps.[44] The method of compression is not as important as the technique. Both methods require steady, evenly applied pressure so that the local tissues occlude the entry site but flow through the arterial lumen is maintained. Any lapse in pressure application leads to primary clot disruption and hemostatic failure.

When complications do occur, the key to successful management is early recognition and repair. There is virtual universal agreement that outcome for vascular complications is directly related to the expediency of the diagnosis and treatment.* It should be borne in mind that ischemia leads to immediate tissue damage, which may become irreversible after only 4 to 6 hours. The ability to reopen thrombosed vessels and reestablish blood flow far exceeds the ability to salvage ischemic tissue. Interventional cardiologists, radiologists, and vascular surgeons should maintain a team approach that rapidly identifies and treats complications to avoid their possible devastating consequences.

REFERENCES

1. Sones FM, Shirey EK: Cine coronary arteriography, *Mod Con Cardiovasc Dis* 31:735-738, 1962.
2. Zimmerman JA, Scott RW, Brecker ON: Catheterization of the left side of the heart in man, *Circulation* 1:357-359, 1950.
3. Judkins MP: Selective coronary arteriography: I. percutaneous transfemoral technic, *Radiology* 89:815-824, 1967.
4. Seldinger SI: Catheter replacement of the needle in percutaneous angiography: a new technique, *Acta Radiol* 39:368-376, 1953.
5. McCann RL, Schwartz LB, Pieper KS: Vascular complications of cardiac catheterization, *J Vasc Surg* 14:375-381, 1991.
6. Oweida SW, Roubin GS, Smith RB, et al: Postcatheterization vascular complications associated with percutaneous transluminal angioplasty, *J Vasc Surg* 12:310-315, 1990.

*References 9-11, 19, 23, 28, 29, 37, 57, 62, 65, 67, 70, 72, 79, 88, 89, 91.

7. Kaufman J, Moglia R, Lacy C, et al: Peripheral vascular complications from percutaneous transluminal coronary angioplasty: a comparison with transfemoral cardiac catheterization; *Am J Med Sci* 297:22-25, 1989.

8. Richardson JD, Shina MA, Miller FB, et al: Peripheral vascular complications of coronary angioplasty, *Am Surg* 55:675-680, 1989.

9. Babu SC, Piccorelli GO, Shah PM, et al: Incidence and results of arterial complications among 16,350 patients undergoing cardiac catheterization, *J Vasc Surg* 10:113-116, 1989.

10. Sheikh KH, Adams DB, McCann RL, et al: Utility of Doppler color flow imaging for identification of femoral arterial complications of cardiac catheterization, *Am Heart J* 117:623-628, 1989.

11. Skillman JJ, Ducksoo K, Baim DS: Vascular complications of percutaneous femoral cardiac interventions: incidence and operative repair, *Arch Surg* 123:1207-1212, 1988.

12. Chiverton SG, Murie JA: Incidence and management of arterial injuries from left heart catheterization, *J R Coll Physicians Lond* 20:126-128, 1986.

13. Bredlau CE, Roubin GS, Leimgruber PP, et al: In-hospital morbidity and mortality in patients undergoing elective coronary angioplasty, *Circulation* 72:1044-1052, 1985.

14. McMillan I, Murie JA: Vascular injury following cardiac catheterization, *Br J Surg* 71:832-835, 1984.

15. Dorros G, Cowley MJ, Simpson J, et al: Percutaneous transluminal coronary angioplasty: Report of complications from the National Heart, Lung, and Blood Institute PTCA Registry, *Circulation* 67:723-730, 1983.

16. Dodek A, Boone JA, Hooper RO, et al: Complications of coronary arteriography, *Can Med Assoc J* 128:934-936, 1983.

17. Kennedy JW: Complications associated with cardiac catheterization and angiography, *Cathet Cardiol Diagn* 8:5-11, 1982.

18. Davis K, Kennedy JW, Kemp HG, et al: Complications of coronary arteriography from the Collaborative Study of Coronary Artery surgery (CASS), *Circulation* 56:1105-1112, 1979.

19. Adams HL, Adams HL: Complications of coronary arteriography: a follow-up report, *Cardiovasc Radiol* 2:89-96, 1979.

20. Bourassa MG, Noble J: Complication rate of coronary arteriography: a review of 5250 cases studied by a percutaneous femoral technique, *Circulation* 53:106-114, 1976.

21. Schoonmaker FW, King SB: Coronary arteriography by the single catheter percutaneous femoral technique, *Circulation* 50:735-740, 1974.

22. Adams DF, Fraser DB, Abrams HL: The complications of coronary arteriography, *Circulation* 48:609-618, 1973.

23. Brener BJ, Couch NP: Peripheral arterial complications of left heart catheterization and their management, *Am J Surg* 125:521-526, 1973.

24. Green GS, McKinnon CM, Rösch J, et al: Complications of selective percutaneous transfemoral coronary arteriography and their prevention: a review of 445 consecutive examinations, *Circulation* 45:552-557, 1972.

25. Aguilar S, Kaulbach MG, Hugenholtz PG: Retrograde arterial catheterization of the left ventricle in 388 patients with special reference to aortic-valve disease and coarctation of the aorta, *N Engl J Med* 274:312-316, 1966.

26. Harris JM: Coronary angiography and its complications: the search for risk factors, *Arch Intern Med* 144:337-341, 1984.

27. Lilly MP, Reichman W, Sarazen AA, et al: Anatomic and clinical factors associated with complications of transfemoral arteriography, *Ann Vasc Surg* 4:264-269, 1990.

28. Messina LM, Brothers TE, Wakefield TW, et al: Clinical characteristics and surgical management of vascular complications in patients undergoing cardiac catheterization: Interventional versus diagnostic procedures, *J Vasc Surg* 13:593-600, 1991.

29. Cohen JR, Sardari F, Glener L, et al: Complications of diagnostic cardiac catheterization requiring surgical intervention, *Am J Cardiol* 67:787-788, 1991.

30. Fitzgerald EJ, Bowsher WG, Ruttley MST: False aneurysm of the femoral artery: computed tomographic and ultrasound appearances, *Clin Radiol* 37:585-588, 1986.

31. Lang EK: A survey of the complications of percutaneous retrograde arteriography, *Radiology* 81:257-263, 1963.

32. Eyer KM: Complications of transfemoral coronary arteriography and their prevention using heparin, *Am Heart J* 86:428, 1973.

33. Judkins MP, Gander MP: Prevention of complications of coronary arteriography, *Circulation* 44:599-602, 1974.

34. Walker WJ, Mundall SL, Broderick HG, et al: Systemic heparinization for femoral percutaneous coronary arteriography, *N Engl J Med* 288:826-828, 1973.

35. Weaver WF, Wilson CS, Forker AD, et al: Selective coronary arteriography: risk in a community hospital, *JAMA* 235:819-822, 1976.

36. Topol EJ, O'Neill WW, Langburd AB, et al: A randomized, placebo-controlled trial of intravenous recombinant tissue-type plasminogen activator and emergency coronary angioplasty in patients with acute myocardial infarction, *Circulation* 45:420-428, 1987.

37. Wyman RM, Safian RD, Portway V, et al: Current complications of diagnostic and therapeutic cardiac catheterization, *J Am Coll Cardiol* 12:1400-1406, 1988.

38. Burrows PE, Benson LN, Williams WG, et al: Iliofemoral arterial complications of balloon angioplasty for systemic obstructions in infants and children, *Circulation* 82:1697-1704, 1990.

39. Criber A, Savin T, Berland J, et al: Percutaneous transluminal balloon valvuloplasty of adult aortic stenosis: report of 92 cases, *J Am Coll Cardiol* 9:381-386, 1987.

40. Altin RS, Flicker S, Naidech HJ: Pseudoaneurysm and arteriovenous fistula after femoral artery catheterization: association with low femoral punctures, *AJR* 152:629-631, 1989.

41. Rapoport S, Sniderman KW, Morse SS, et al: Pseudoaneurysm: A complication of faulty technique in femoral arterial puncture, *Radiology* 154:529-530, 1985.

42. Roberts SR, Main D, Pinkerton J: Surgical therapy of femoral artery pseudoaneurysm after angiography, *Am J Surg* 154:676-680, 1987.

43. Block PC, Ockene I, Goldberg RJ, et al: A prospective randomized trial of outpatient versus inpatient cardiac catheterization, *N Engl J Med* 319:1251-1255, 1988.

44. Semler HJ: Transfemoral catheterization: mechanical versus manual control of bleeding, *Radiology* 154:234-235, 1985.

45. Taylor GJ, Song A, Moses HW, et al: The primary care physician and thrombolytic therapy for acute myocardial infarction: comparison of intravenous streptokinase in community hospitals and the tertiary referral center, *J Am Board Fam Pract* 3:1-6, 1990.

46. Abu-Yousef MM, Wiese JA, Shamma AR: The 'to-and-fro' sign: duplex Doppler evidence of femoral artery pseudoaneurysm, *AJR* 150:632-634, 1988.

47. Cohen GI, Chan KL: Physical examination and echo Doppler study in the assessment of femoral arterial complications following cardiac catheterization, *Cathet Cardiol Diagn* 21:137-143, 1990.

48. Helvie MA, Rubin JM, Silver TM, et al: The distinction between femoral artery pseudoaneurysms and other causes of groin masses: value of duplex Doppler sonography, *AJR* 150:1177-1180, 1988.

49. Mitchell DG, Needleman L, Bezzi M, et al: Femoral artery pseudoaneurysm: Diagnosis with conventional duplex and color Doppler ultrasound, *Radiology* 165:687-690, 1987.

50. Kent KC, McArdle CR, Kennedy B, et al: A prospective study of the clinical outcome of femoral pseudoaneurysms and arteriovenous fistulas induced by arterial puncture, *J Vasc Surg* 17:125-133, 1993.

51. Cox GS, Young JR, Gray BH, et al: Ultrasound-guided compression of traumatic pseudoaneurysms [abstract], *J Vasc Surg* 16:471, 1992.

52. Fellmeth BD, Roberts AC, Bookstein JJ, et al: Postangiographic femoral artery injuries: nonsurgical repair with US-guided compression, *Radiology* 178:671-675, 1991.

53. Eriksson I, Jorulf H: Surgical complications associated with arterial catheterization, *Scand J Thor Cardiovasc Surg* 4:69-75, 1970.

54. Glaser RL, McKellar D, Scher KS: Arteriovenous fistulas after cardiac catheterization, *Arch Surg* 124:1313-1315, 1989.

55. Ross RS: Arterial complications, *Circulation* 37(suppl III):III39-III41, 1968.

56. Gwost J, Stoebe T, Chesler E, et al: Analysis of the complications of cardiac catheterization over nine years, *Cathet Cardiol Diagn* 8:13-21, 1982.

57. Youkey JR, Clagett GP, Rich NM, et al: Vascular trauma secondary to diagnostic and therapeutic procedures; 1974 through 1982, *Am J Surg* 146:788-791, 1983.

58. Heystraten FMJ, Fast JH: Arteriovenous fistula as a complication of the Seldinger procedure of the femoral artery and vein: report of two cases, *Diagn Imag Clin Med* 52:197-201, 1983.

59. Kron J, Sutherland D, Rosch J, et al: Arteriovenous fistula: a rare complication of arterial puncture for cardiac catheterization, *Am J Cardiol* 55:1445-1446, 1985.

60. Hansen KJ, Link KM, Dean RH: Iatrogenic vascular injuries. In Bongard FS, Wilson SE, Perry MO (eds): *Vascular injuries in surgical practice,* Norwalk, Mass, 1991, Appleton & Lange, pp 289-305.

61. Picus D, Totty WG: Iatrogenic femoral arteriovenous fistulae: evaluation by digital vascular imaging, *AJR* 142:567-570, 1984.

62. McCollum CH, Mavor E: Brachial artery injury after cardiac catheterization, *J Vasc Surg* 4:355-359, 1986.

63. Rutherford RB, Pearce WH: Acute problems following diagnostic and interventional radiologic procedures. In Bergan JJ, Yao JST (eds): *Vascular surgical emergencies,* Orlando, Fla, 1987, Grune & Statton, pp 417-430.

64. Chahine RA, Herman MV, Gorlin R: Complications of coronary arteriography: comparison of the brachial to the femoral approach, *Ann Intern Med* 5:862, 1976.

65. Barnes RW, Petersen JL, Krugmire RB, et al: Complications of brachial artery catheterization: prospective evaluation with the Doppler ultrasonic velocity detector, *Chest* 66:363-367, 1974.

66. Jeresaty RM, Liss JP: Effects of brachial artery catheterization on arterial pulse and blood pressure in 203 patients, *Am Heart J* 4:481-485, 1968.

67. Machleder HI, Sweeney JP, Barker WF: Pulseless arm after brachial-artery catheterization, *Lancet* 1:407-409, 1972.

68. Voci G, Hamer NA: Retrograde arterial catheterization of the left ventricle, *Am J Cardiol* 5:493-497, 1960.

69. Karmody AM, Lempert N, Jarmolych J: The pathology of post-catheterization brachial artery occlusion, *J Surg Res* 20:601-606, 1976.

70. Kitzmiller JW, Hertzer NR, Beven EG: Routine surgical management of brachial artery occlusion after cardiac catheterization, *Arch Surg* 117:1066-1071, 1982.

71. Nicholas GG, DeMuth WE: Long-term results of brachial thrombectomy following cardiac catheterization, *Ann Surg* 183:436-438, 1976.

72. Kline RM, Hertzer NM, Beven EG, et al: Surgical treatment of brachial injuries after cardiac catheterization, *J Vasc Surg* 12:20-24, 1990.

73. Fergusson DJG, Kamada RO: Percutaneous entry of the brachial artery for left heart catheterization using a sheath, *Cathet Cardiovasc Diagn* 7:111-114, 1981.

74. Fergusson DJG, Kamada RO: Percutaneous entry of the brachial artery for left heart catheterization using a sheath: further experience, *Cathet Cardiovasc Diagn* 12:209-211, 1986.

75. Kamada RO, Fergusson DJG, Itagaki RKS: Percutaneous entry of the brachial artery for transluminal coronary angioplasty, *Cathet Cardiovasc Diagn* 15:132-133, 1988.

76. Korr KS, Januski V: Percutaneous brachial coronary angioplasty utilizing a standard side arm introducer system, *Cathet Cardiovasc Diagn* 18:121-124, 1989.

77. Maouad J, Hebert JL, Fernandez F, et al: Percutaneous brachial approach using the femoral artery sheath for left heart catheterization and selective coronary angiography, *Cathet Cardiovasc Diagn* 11:539-546, 1985.

78. Pepine CJ, VonGunten C, Hill JA, et al: Percutaneous brachial catheterization using a modified sheath and new catheter system, *Cathet Cardiovasc Diagn* 10:637-642, 1984.

79. Mills JL, Wiedeman JE, Robison JG, et al: Minimizing mortality and morbidity from iatrogenic arterial injuries: the need for early recognition and prompt repair, *J Vasc Surg* 4:22-27, 1986.

80. Molnar W, Paul DJ: Complications of axillary arteriotomies, *Radiology* 104:269-279, 1972.

81. Antonovic R, Rosch J, Dotter CT: Complications of percutaneous transaxillary catheterization for arteriography and selective chemotherapy, *Radiology* 126:386-393, 1976.

82. Carroll SE, Wilkins WW: Two cases of brachial plexus injury following percutaneous arteriograms, *Can Med Assoc J* 102:861-862, 1970.

83. Dudrick S, Masland W, Mishkin M: Brachial plexus injury following axillary artery puncture, *Radiology* 88:271-273, 1967.

84. Hessel SJ, Adams DF, Abrams HL: Complications of angiography, *Radiology* 138:273-281, 1981.

85. Roy P: Percutaneous catheterization via the axillary artery: a new approach to some technical roadblocks in selective arteriography, *AJR* 94:1-18, 1965.

86. Staal A, van Voorthuisen AE, van Dijk LM: Neurological complications following arterial catheterization by the axillary approach, *Br J Radiol* 39:115-116, 1966.

87. Menozian JO, Corson JD, Bush HL, et al: Management of the upper extremity with absent pulses after cardiac catheterization, *Am J Surg* 135:484-487, 1978.

88. Page CP, Hagood CO, Kemmerer WT: Management of postcatheterization: brachial artery thrombosis, *Surgery* 72:619-623, 1972.

89. Orcutt MB, Levinbe BA, Gaskill HV, et al: Iatrogenic vascular injury: a reducible problem, *Arch Surg* 120:384-385, 1985.

90. Angelini P, Bush HS: Brachial artery injury as a complication of cardiac catheterization: percutaneous transluminal angioplasty and streptokinase as a treatment alternative, *Cathet Cardiol Diagn* 15:243-246, 1988.

91. Booth P, Redington AN, Shinebourne EA, et al: Early complications of interventional balloon catheterization in infants and children, *Br Heart J* 65:109-112, 1991.

Chapter 57

MANAGEMENT OF THE ELDERLY PATIENT WITH ACUTE MYOCARDIAL INFARCTION

Frederick Feit
Bernard R. Chaitman

In excess of 500,000 patients are hospitalized annually in the United States with a confirmed diagnosis of acute myocardial infarction (AMI), a condition that accounts for approximately one fourth of all deaths in this country.[1,2] The recognition and management of AMI in the elderly have become increasingly important, given the relatively poor prognosis in this group and their increasing actual and proportional representation in our population.[3] Although people more than age 65 years currently constitute only 12% of our population, it is remarkable that approximately 80% of all deaths from MI occur in this age group, with the majority of those occurring in patients older than 75 years of age.[4] Furthermore, if current trends continue, the proportion of the American population over the age of 65 years will nearly double over the next 40 years, with the greatest increase being seen in those more than 80 years of age.[3]

It is not wise to impose a strict numerical limit to define the elderly, because chronologic age alone may not be the predominant predictor of clinical outcome or response to therapy. Although it has been established that there are significant changes in the cardiovascular system with aging, it is equally clear that the observed higher frequency of comorbidity and prior cardiac events contribute significantly to the poor prognosis in the elderly.[5] Therefore, when the independent effect of advanced age on the clinical outcome of new therapies is evaluated, it is important that multivariate analyses be performed. The fact that age alone should not exclude a patient from new therapies has become increasingly recognized over the past 30 years by investigators in the design of major clinical trials. For example, the Coronary Artery Surgery Study (CASS) performed in the 1970s excluded patients more than age 65 years; the Thrombolysis in Myocardial Infarction (TIMI) trial performed in the 1980s excluded patients more than age 75 years, whereas the recently completed Global Utilization of Streptokinase and Tissue Plasminogen Activator for Occluded Coronary Arteries (GUSTO) trial had no upper age limit.[6-8]

AGING AND THE CARDIOVASCULAR SYSTEM

To more completely understand the consequences of MI in the elderly, one must review the changes in the cardiovascular system that occur with aging.[5,9-13] On a cellular basis, there is an increase in myocyte size and degenerative changes, including "dropout" of myocytes, tubular dilation, lipid deposition, and the appearance of lipofuscin granules, which probably represent peroxidized mitochondrial membranes. The peroxidation of mitochondria results in the production of a monaldehyde that irreversibly denatures DNA, decreasing the production of ribosomal RNA and therefore protein synthesis. This series of events may in part account for the important clinical observation that the aged heart is less able to respond to acute hemodynamic challenges. Other anatomic changes observed include some degree of left ventricular hypertrophy, an increase in the myocardial content of fat, collagen, fibrous tissue, and calcium, and a marked decrease in the cellularity of the sinus node.

On a functional basis, there is a prolongation of myocardial relaxation time and a decrease in left ventricular compliance. These changes contribute to a decreased rate of left ventricular filling and an increase in end-diastolic pressure, both at rest and with exercise. A loss of compliance in the peripheral vasculature may further exacerbate this phenomenon. The aging heart also becomes progressively less responsive to the inotropic and chronotropic effects of β-adrenergic stimuli.

These changes in cardiac structure and function are often exacerbated by the effects of other conditions, including diabetes and hypertension, or by the presence of intrinsic cardiac disease.[14] Although the precise role that these changes play in the unfavorable prognosis of elderly patients with AMI remains undefined, there is little doubt that they do contribute to it.

DATA FROM THE PRETHROMBOLYTIC ERA
Incidence and presentation

A vast amount of information has been collected on the incidence, clinical course, and early and late mortality rate of AMI in the elderly. These data come from single center reports, longitudinal studies, registries, and controlled clinical trials.[15-23]

The Worcester Heart Attack Study was a community-based study that analyzed the population of patients with a primary or secondary discharge diagnosis of an initial AMI at 16 general acute care hospitals.[23] Four different calendar years (1975, 1978, 1981, and 1984) were analyzed. The incidence of hospitalization for initial AMI in patients greater than 75 years of age varied between 526 and 954 per 100,000 population (0.5%-1.0%) in the 4 years sampled. This was approximately ten times the incidence seen in the 25- to 54-year age group and twice that in patients 55 to 64 years of age. These figures significantly understate the actual incidence of MI, because patients with prior MI, those who died before reaching the hospital, and those who did not seek hospitalization were excluded. In a multicenter trial from England, more than 40% of patients greater than 75 years of age with AMI were dead on arrival at the hospital in contrast to less than 15% of those less than 45 years of age.[17] Presumably even more patients died at home. Furthermore, because symptoms in the elderly may be quite atypical, a significant number of these individuals may not even seek hospitalization. In a

retrospective multicenter review of 100 patients greater than 85 years of age hospitalized for AMI, only 41% complained of chest pain, whereas 22% had acute confusion. Vomiting and diaphoresis occurred with approximately half the frequency of that observed in younger patients.

Given these realities, the actual incidence of AMI in the elderly can best be estimated by longitudinal population studies that feature regular periodic cardiac evaluation. Such was the case in the Bronx Aging Study, in which 390 community-based subjects, 75 to 85 years of age, underwent annual cardiac examinations, including electrocardiograms, and in the Framingham Study in which such examinations were conducted biennially.[18,19] In the former study 115 new Q-wave infarctions occurred over an average follow-up of 76 months.[18] Fifty of these were unrecognized. Thus, the annual incidence of AMI was 5.6%, with 43% of these being unrecognized. Similarly, in the Framingham Study, more than one third of MIs in men more than 75 years of age were "silent."[19] This was more than twice the frequency of silent infarctions observed in younger men. From these population studies it is concluded that the incidence of AMI is dramatically increased in the elderly even though it is frequently unrecognized as a result of an atypical presentation.

Clinical features, hospital course, and long-term outcome

Data are also available on clinical features, hospital course, and long-term outcome in the elderly in contrast to the younger patients with an AMI.[21-26] Information collected from 2115 patients in the Worcester Heart Attack Study, 848 patients from the Multicenter Investigation on the Limitation of Infarct Size (MILIS), and 2026 patients from a prospective multicenter series are presented in Table 57-1.[21,23,25] It should be noted that in contrast to the latter two reports, the Worcester series included only patients with an initial MI, resulting in differing baseline characteristics and outcome. The most striking feature in these reports is the dramatic increase in the representation of female patients with increasing age, particularly in advance of 75 years. There is a higher prevalence of a history of angina pectoris or of congestive heart failure in patients greater than 75 years of age. Similarly, the prevalence of hypertension and diabetes increases with age, although there was no further incremental increase in patients more than age 75 years compared with those 65 to 74 years of age.

In terms of clinical course, the elderly patients were significantly more likely to develop congestive heart failure or cardiogenic shock. In fact, more than half of the patients older than 75 years developed congestive heart failure. This is particularly interesting because the elderly were more likely to have non–Q-wave MI and

Table 57-1. Acute myocardial infarction—baseline features and clinical course*

Baseline features	Worcester[23]				Smith et al.[25]		MILIS[21]	
Age groups (yr)	<55	55-64	65-74	≥75	65-75	>75	<65	65-75
No. of patients	465	533	548	570	702	1321	631	217
Female sex (%)	21	28	41	61	29	44	24	37
Medical history								
Angina pectoris (%)	14	15	20	24	44	50	34	42
Hypertension (%)	38	42	50	47	48	47	17	24
Diabetes (%)	12	17	23	22	20	17	17	24
Prior MI (%)	NA				33	33	22	28
Congestive heart failure					14	23	7	14
Outcome								
Congestive heart failure	21	29	42	55	28	44	53	65
Shock	2	6	7	8	7	15		
Atrial fibrillation					8	14	19	29
Non–Q-wave MI	24	28	26	41	34	38	24	28
Use of β-blocker	51	43	33	27			27	27
Mortality								
In-hospital	5	8	16	32	7	14	12	20

*MILIS, Multicenter Investigation on the Limitation of Infarct Size; MI, myocardial infarction; NA = not applicable—by definition patients in the Worcester Study could not have had a prior MI.

had significantly less creatine phosphokinase (CPK) release, although the method of reporting varied (Worcester: peak CPK ≥5 times normal occurred in 56% of patients 65-74 years vs. 45% of those >75 years; MILIS: peak CK-MB (IU/L), 153 in patients <65 years vs. 128 in those 65-74 years of age; Smith et al.[25]: peak CK (IU/L) 1.16×10^3 in patients 65 to 74 vs. 1.01×10^3 in patients ≥75 years of age). Thus, despite a lower incidence of Q-wave infarction and significantly less CPK release, the elderly patient with AMI was more likely to develop congestive heart failure or cardiogenic shock. This paradox may be explained in part by a higher incidence of prior known or undiagnosed MI and the cardiovascular changes associated with aging.

The mortality rates during hospitalization, which increase dramatically with age, are also shown in Table 57-1. Age remains an important *independent* predictor of in-hospital death when a multiple regression analysis adjusting for sex, history of angina, Q-wave vs. non–Q-wave MI, peak CPK level, occurrence of shock or congestive heart failure, and use of medications is carried out.[23] The multivariate adjusted odds ratio and 95% confidence limits for in-hospital mortality are 7.51 (4.43, 12.73) times as great for patients greater than 75 years old as for those less than 55 years old. Of interest is a decline over time in the in-hospital mortality rates in patients greater than 75 years old during the four time periods studied (1975, 40%; 1978, 36%; 1981, 31%; 1984, 23%). Approximately one in five patients in this age group surviving the initial hospitalization will die within 1 year of discharge, almost all because of a cardiovascular cause.[23-25]

INSIGHTS FROM CLINICAL TRIALS IN THE PRETHROMBOLYTIC ERA

Clinical trials performed during the prethrombolytic era assessing the effects of β-adrenergic blocking agents and anticoagulants offer insights into events that would unfold during the thrombolytic era. Forman et al.[27] analyzed the relationship between mortality reduction and patient age in studies involving the acute intravenous (IV) administration of β-blockers and the oral administration of these agents several days after the infarction is complete.[28-33] Data from these trials were presented in a variable fashion, with the elderly most often defined as either greater than 60 years of age or greater than 65 years of age. The pooled data indicate that with the acute administration of β-blockers intravenously (n = 23,200) mortality was reduced by 5% in the younger patients and 23% in the elderly, whereas with their late administration by the oral route (n = 7116), mortality was reduced by 28% in the younger patients and 40% in the elderly. Clearly, in either case the benefit of β-adrenergic blocking agents was greatest in the elderly. Unfortunately, it remains evident that many physicians resist prescribing β-blockers to elderly patients, even in the absence of contraindications.[34]

One controlled trial of oral anticoagulant therapy after MI involving 878 patients greater than 60 years of age revealed that this treatment significantly reduced mortality from 13% to 8% and recurrent MI from 16% to 6% over a 2-year period.[35] There were trends toward fewer total strokes (3.1% vs. 5.6%; p = ns) but more intracranial hemorrhages (1.6% vs. 0.2%) in the anticoagulated patients.

Table 57-2. Major trials of intravenous thrombolytic therapy: mortality by age*

Age groups (yr)	No. of patients	Control (%)	rt-PA (%)	Reduction (%)	Lives saved (No.)
ASSET					
<55	1493	4.4	3.8	13.6	6
55-65	1859	7.9	6.5	17.7	14
66-75	1679	16.4	10.8	34.1	56
GISSI					
≤65	7608	7.7	5.7	26.0	20
65-75	2886	8.1	16.6	8.3	15
>75	1215	33.1	28.9	12.7	42
ISIS-II					
<60	7720	5.8	4.2	27.6	16
60-69	6056	14.3	10.6	26.4	37
≥70	3411	21.6	18.2	15.8	34

*ASSET, Anglo-Scandinavian Study of Early Thrombolysis; GISSI, Grupo Italian per lo Studio della Streptochinasi nell' Infarto Miocardico; ISIS-II, International Study of Infart Survival; rt-PA, recombinant tissue-type plasminogen activator; lives saved, the theoretical number of lives saved for every 1000 patients receiving thrombolytic vs. conventional therapy.

A large number of trials evaluating antiplatelet therapy after MI have shown that these agents reduce morbidity and mortality.[36-40] The Antiplatelet Trialist Collaboration performed an overview of 31 randomized trials including about 29,000 patients with a history of transient ischemic attack, occlusive stroke, unstable angina, or MI.[41] Overall, allocation to antiplatelet therapy resulted in a reduction in vascular mortality by about 15% and nonfatal vascular events (stroke and MI) by approximately 30%. Although many of the postinfarction trials had an upper age limit of 65 years, others included patients up to 70 years of age (GAMIS, ARIS, and AMIS),* and the PARIS† I and II trials included those up to 75 years of age.[36-40] These individual trials, as well as the pooled data from the Antiplatelet Trialist Collaboration, clearly demonstrate that the benefit of aspirin and other antiplatelet therapies is relevant in the elderly patient.

Thus, randomized controlled trials assessing β-blockers, antiplatelet agents, and oral anticoagulants showed very favorable outcomes in elderly patients with AMI. Nonetheless, these findings did not translate into widespread use of these therapies.[34,42]

THROMBOLYTIC ERA

Although as early as 1912, Herrick[43] had suggested that acute coronary thrombosis resulted in MI, necroscopy studies from the 1970s led some[44] to the erroneous conclusion that coronary thrombosis was a result rather than the immediate cause of AMI. Although streptokinase was discovered in 1933 and administered in 1958,

the thrombolytic era was ushered in 20 years later with the pioneering studies of Rentrop and DeWood.[45-50] The former demonstrated through the findings at very early coronary angiography and those at early bypass surgery that coronary thrombosis was present in the majority of patients with AMI. The latter found that these thrombi could be lysed by the administration of intracoronary streptokinase, proving its efficacy in recanalizing occluded arteries and suggesting benefits on left ventricular function and survival. Subsequently, several large controlled trials assessed the effects of thrombolytic therapy administered intravenously both on left ventricular function and mortality.[51-64] It is not the goal of this chapter to rehash these trials in detail but to contrast the effects of therapy on these endpoints and complications in the elderly compared with those observed in younger patients with AMI.

MORTALITY

During the second half of the 1980s, six large trials comparing IV thrombolytic therapy with conventional treatment in patients with suspected AMI specifying mortality as the primary endpoint were performed.[60-65] The three largest trials were the Anglo-Scandinavian Study of Early Thrombolysis (ASSET), which tested recombinant tissue-type plasminogen activator (rt-PA) in patients up to 75 years of age, and the Second International Study of Infarct Survival (ISIS-II) and Gruppo Italiano per lo Studio della Streptochinasi nell'Infarto Miocardico (GISSI), both of which evaluated streptokinase and had no upper age limit.[60,63,64] Mortality rates were assessed at 21 days in the GISSI trial, 30 days in ASSET, and 35 days in ISIS-II. The effect of thrombolytic therapy on mortality with respect to age group is depicted in Table 57-2. Several important observations are readily apparent from these data. First, just as in the prethrombolytic era, there is a dramatic

*GAMIS, German Austrian Myocardial Infarction Study; ARIS, Anturane Reinfarction Italian Study; AMIS, Aspirin Myocardial Infarction Study.
†PARIS, Persantine Aspirin Reinfarction Study.

increase in mortality rate in the elderly patients treated conventionally, with approximately a fourfold greater rate in the "oldest" compared with the "youngest" subgroup in each of these trials. Second, although there is no clear trend in percent reduction in mortality by thrombolytic therapy according to age group, there is a clear trend as to which group receives the greatest *absolute* benefit. As shown in the last column of Table 57-2, given the high absolute mortality rate in the elderly, a similar percent reduction in the rate of mortality produces a greater absolute reduction. Thus, for any number of patients treated, several times as many lives will be saved in the subgroup of the oldest in contrast to that of the youngest patients. Furthermore, in a separate analysis of the extreme elderly (> 80 years of age) from the ISIS-II trial, combined therapy with streptokinase and aspirin resulted in a 46% reduction in mortality rate from 37% to 20%, potentially resulting in 170 lives saved for every 1000 patients treated.[66] It must be remembered that the patients in these trials were without such evident contraindications to the administration of a thrombolytic agent as uncontrolled hypertension, recent cerebrovascular accident, known bleeding disorder, recent surgery, or advanced or terminal illness. Although employing such exclusion criteria may select a subset of patients at lower risk than the overall population of elderly patients with infarction, the observed mortality rates in the control groups were still high, and the survival benefit conferred by the intravenously administered thrombolytic therapy was dramatic.

LEFT VENTRICULAR FUNCTION

Several well-designed prospective controlled trials have assessed the effect of the IV administration of a thrombolytic agent on left ventricular ejection fraction.[67-69] Unfortunately, the only report that specifically compared these results in older vs. younger patients excluded patients greater than 70 years of age, resulting in an "elderly" group defined as patients 60 to 70 years of age. In this elderly group, mean contrast left ventricular ejection fraction 3 weeks after infarction was 57% in patients treated with thrombolytic therapy compared with 50% in those treated conventionally, whereas in the younger patients these values were 59% and 54%, respectively. These findings indicate that patients in their sixties had an equivalent degree of preservation of left ventricular function as younger patients. Only one study, the Thrombolytic Therapy in an Older Patient Population (TTOPP) trial, specifically limited enrollment to patients greater than age 75 years.[70] Patients were randomly assigned to receive a "weight-adjusted" dose of rt-PA, followed by heparin and aspirin or heparin and aspirin alone. Although only 69 patients (mean age 81 years) were enrolled, mean left ventricular ejection fraction obtained before hospital

discharge was 52% in the group who received rt-PA compared with 41.5% in the control group (p< 0.05). These data further enforce the notion that the observed benefit on left ventricular function conferred by thrombolytic therapy is not age dependent and extends into the extreme elderly.

NONCEREBROVASCULAR HEMORRHAGIC COMPLICATIONS

Two reports involving the early experience with rt-PA[71,72] and one small uncontrolled series in which streptokinase was used have been widely cited as providing evidence that hemorrhagic complications are more likely to occur in elderly patients.[71-73] The latter study included only 24 patients greater than 75 years of age, and its findings were not confirmed by the larger GISSI and ISIS-II trials in which increasing age was not independently associated with a greater likelihood of hemorrhage with streptokinase therapy.[63,64] The two reports in which IV rt-PA was utilized involved the early experience of the TIMI and Thrombolysis and Angioplasty in Myocardial Infarction (TAMI) study groups.[71,72] In the former, the incidence of major hemorrhagic events was 8.7%, 14.5%, and 24.7% in patients less than 65, 65 to 69, and 70 or more years of age, respectively (p< 0.001). Similarly, the TAMI group noted that advanced age was an independent risk factor for the development of hemorrhage. The relevance of these studies to clinical practice has diminished, because most patients in both received 150 mg of rt-PA (a dose no longer utilized), and the majority of hemorrhagic events occurred as a result of local bleeding at the vascular access site for coronary angiography, performed acutely to assess coronary artery patency. Furthermore, a detailed analysis of patients assigned to the conservative strategy in the larger phase II of the TIMI trial, in which patients received 100 mg of rt-PA intravenously, in addition to oral aspirin and intravenous heparin, indicated that increasing age was not an independent risk factor for the development of hemorrhage.[74] Thus, the weight of the evidence from these larger trials did not suggest that increasing age was a significant independent risk factor for noncerebrovascular hemorrhagic events with therapy with either rt-PA or streptokinase as long as early cardiac catheterization is not routinely employed.[63,64,74] However, this conclusion may have been prematurely drawn, because a small gradient of risk with age could have been missed, given the low rate of hemorrhagic complications. In fact, initial data from the large GUSTO trial demonstrates a small but significant age-associated increase in the risk of noncerebrovascular hemorrhage.[8]

CEREBROVASCULAR COMPLICATIONS

No other complication of AMI in patients receiving thrombolytic therapy has received more attention than

Table 57-3. GUSTO—cerebrovascular accident by treatment group and age*

	Streptokinase groups	Accelerated t-PA	Odds ratio (95% CI)
Age ≤75 yr	n = 17,804	n = 9039	
Any stroke	1.08%	1.20%	1.21 (0.88-1.42)
Hemorrhagic stroke	0.42%	0.52%	1.24 (0.86-1.78)
Age >75 yr	n = 2358	n = 1297	
Any stroke	3.05%	3.93%	1.30 (0.90-1.87)
Hemorrhagic stroke	1.23%	2.08%	1.71 (1.01-2.88)

*t-PA, Tissue-type plasminogen activator; CI, confidence interval; odds ratio for t-PA vs. streptokinase.

the occurrence of a stroke. Detailed analyses of this complication have been provided from a number of large studies.[69-73]

An analysis of all cerebrovascular accidents in the GISSI trial showed that the incidence of 0.92% in streptokinase-treated patients did not differ significantly from that of 0.77% observed in conventionally treated patients.[75] Although most of the events were "undefined," treatment with streptokinase did result in a higher incidence of hemorrhagic cerebrovascular accidents, which generally occurred within 24 hours of admission. Older patients had an increased likelihood of developing a cerebrovascular accident in both treatment and control groups. The in-hospital mortality rate in patients with a cerebrovascular accident was 47%.

In a detailed analysis of the 3016 patients who received 100 mg of rt-PA in phase II of the TIMI trial, the incidence of cerebral infarction was 0.7%, of intracerebral hemorrhage 0.4%, and of subdural hematoma 0.1%.[76] The overall mortality rate within 6 weeks of manifestation was 48% in patients having such events. Older patients had a significantly increased frequency of both intracerebral hemorrhage and of cerebral infarction when age was treated as a continuous variable. A recent report from a registry in the Netherlands in which streptokinase was used in the majority of 2469 cases also identified increased age as an independent predictor of intracranial hemorrhage.[77]

The ISIS-III and International Study groups also assessed the rate of cerebrovascular events in elderly patients receiving thrombolytic therapy.[78,79] In the former trial patients received one of three thrombolytic agents: streptokinase, duteplase (a preparation of rt-PA no longer being evaluated), or anisoylated plasminogen streptokinase activator complex (APSAC). In the latter trial streptokinase and rt-PA were the agents tested. In both trials all patients received aspirin and were randomly assigned to receive heparin subcutaneously starting several hours after the completion of thrombolytic therapy or to receive no anticoagulant therapy. It must be pointed out that the administration of bolus doses of heparin subcutaneously every 12 hours does not result in consistent and reliable anticoagulation.[80] In

both studies the overall incidence of stroke increased dramatically in patients more than 70 years of age compared with those less than 70 years of age (2.3% vs. 0.6% in ISIS-III and 2.1% vs. 0.9% in the International Study). Further analysis of the latter data indicates that patients more than 70 years of age were 3.99 times as likely to have a stroke than those less than 60 years of age.[73] Even when covariates were considered, the adjusted relative risk for stroke in the older population was 2.72 times that of the younger group. Advanced age was independently predictive of both hemorrhagic and ischemic strokes. In the ISIS-III report there was a striking effect of increasing age on the occurrence of cerebral hemorrhage in patients treated with rt-PA: 1.6% in patients more than 70 years vs. 0.48% in patients less than 70 years but not those treated with streptokinase, where this occurred in 0.25% of patients more than 70 years vs. 0.23% of patients less than 70 years.

Data from the recently presented GUSTO trial again demonstrated that the risk of both any cerebrovascular accident and intracranial hemorrhage is significantly higher in the elderly (Table 57-3). As shown in the table, a front-loaded weight-adjusted regimen of rt-PA combined with aspirin and IV heparin resulted in an increased incidence of hemorrhagic stroke in the elderly compared with a regimen of streptokinase, aspirin, and IV or subcutaneous heparin. Furthermore, the mortality rate in patients with stroke was nearly 80% in octagenarians compared with 40% in the younger subgroup. As a result, the number of nonfatal disabling strokes was similar in the elderly and the younger patients (0.5%-0.6%).[8]

In summary, advanced age is an independent risk factor for the development of strokes in patients with AMI receiving thrombolytic therapy and in those treated conventionally. The administration of thrombolytic therapy results in an increased likelihood of intracerebral hemorrhage but may not increase the overall occurrence rate of stroke compared with patients treated conventionally.[75] Treatment with rt-PA rather than streptokinase may further increase the likelihood of intracranial hemorrhage in the elderly.[8,78] Finally, intracranial hemorrhage is much more likely to result in death in the elderly.[8]

DIRECT CORONARY ANGIOPLASTY

An intriguing alternative therapy in the elderly patient with AMI is emergency coronary angioplasty without the prior administration of a thrombolytic agent (direct PTCA). One large single center series of 105 consecutive patients greater than 70 years of age receiving this therapy revealed an angiographic success rate of 91% and an in-hospital mortality rate of 18%.[81] Although direct comparisons are not possible, this outcome compares favorably with that observed in patients in this age group treated with thrombolytic therapy, particularly when we consider that 11% of the patients in this series were in cardiogenic shock when first seen. There were no strokes, and only two patients had complications involving the site of vascular access. More recently a prospective, randomized multicenter trial involving 395 patients comparing direct PTCA with thrombolytic therapy utilizing rt-PA was reported.[82] The incidence of death plus reinfarction (the prespecified primary end point) occurred significantly less often in the direct PTCA than in the thrombolytic arm. Of particular interest was the observation of trends favoring direct PTCA specifically in the elderly population.[83] Treatment with direct PTCA in contrast to that with rt-PA resulted in rates of mortality of 6% vs. 15% and of stroke of 0% vs. 6% in the 150 patients greater than 65 years of age. Although these subgroup differences did not quite achieve statistical significance, the trends are of interest. These findings indicate that when experienced personnel and facilities are available, direct PTCA is a viable therapeutic option in the elderly patient with AMI. It is the treatment of choice when thrombolytic therapy is contraindicated.

CURRENT PRACTICE IN THE ELDERLY PATIENT

Despite the significant volume of data demonstrating the favorable risk/benefit ratio of thrombolytic therapy in the elderly patient with AMI, this therapy has not been universally embraced. In a recent report from the Myocardial Infarction Triage Investigation (MITI) study group, demographic, clinical, and treatment data on 3256 patients with AMI admitted to 19 coronary care units in the Greater Seattle area were reported.[42] As in the reports from the prethrombolytic era, a high percentage (56%) of patients over the age of 75 years were women. Furthermore, a history of angina pectoris 50% vs. 37%, of prior MI 35% vs. 23%, of hypertension 52% vs. 40%, and of congestive heart failure 24% vs. 3% were all more common in patients greater than 75 compared to those less than 55 years old. Of great interest was the decreased number of interventions and medications employed in the elderly compared with the younger patients. Coronary angiography was performed in 22% vs. 76%; coronary angioplasty in 7% vs. 29%; thrombolytic therapy in 5% vs. 39%; aspirin in 57% vs. 82% and heparin in 35% vs. 78% of patients greater than 75 years compared with those less than 55 years of age. Although more than 25% of patients in the elderly group were "good candidates" for thrombolytic therapy (i.e., seen within 6 hours of onset of pain, absence of severe hypertension, stroke, recent surgery, trauma, or confounding illness), only 5% received such therapy. Therefore, it appears that even at centers with extensive experience with thrombolytic therapy, there may be an inherent bias against its administration in the elderly. This may be due to a higher incidence of multiple relative contraindications in these patients or to the supposition on the part of some clinicians that because advanced age was an exclusion criterion for participation in many trials of thrombolytic therapy, it is a contraindication for the general use of such therapy. Perhaps some of the reluctance is related to the package inserts of both rt-PA and streptokinase, each of which contains a warning regarding the administration of these agents in patients older than 75 years of age. Whatever the reason, these practices continue despite a chorus of voices, with which we agree, calling for the use of thrombolytic therapy regardless of a patient's chronologic age if no other specific contraindications to its use are present.[66,84,85]

SUMMARY AND CONCLUSION

One of the great remaining challenges is our approach to AMI in the treatment of elderly patients, given their poor prognosis and increasing representation in our population. The characteristics of this group, which include a higher percentage of women and an increased likelihood of a prior history of angina pectoris, hypertension, diabetes, congestive heart failure, and prior MI, have been well defined. The clinical manifestation is often atypical.

Chronologic age alone is not a contraindication to the administration of thrombolytic therapy, to the performance of direct PTCA or, for that matter, to pharmacologic therapy with β-blockers, aspirin, or oral anticoagulants. In fact, the absolute benefit of many of these therapies appears to be greatest in the elderly. Paradoxically, among patients without specific contraindications to these therapies, they are applied with the lowest frequency in the elderly.

In conclusion, there is no chronologic age limit for the administration of thrombolytic therapy in patients with AMI. The detailed results of the GUSTO trial will further define the optimal thrombolytic and anticoagulant regimen in the elderly. Future trials and registry data will define the merit of direct percutaneous transluminal coronary angioplasty as a therapeutic alternative to thrombolytic therapy in these patients.

REFERENCES

1. Hillis LD: Myocardial ischemia, *N Engl J Med* 296:1034-1093, 1977.
2. National Center for Health Statistics: Utilization of short stay hospitals, United States, 1987, *Health Stat* 31:197, 1987.
3. Wei JY, Gersh BJ: Heart disease in the elderly. In O'Rourke RA, Crawford MH (eds): *Current problems in cardiology,* Chicago, 1987, Mosby, pp 7-65.
4. Gurwitz JH, Osganian V, Goldberg RJ, et al: Diagnostic testing in acute myocardial infarction: Does patient age influence utilization patterns? *Am J Epidemiol* 134:948-957, 1991.
5. Wei JY: Age and the cardiovascular system, *N Engl J Med* 327:1735-1739, 1992.
6. Principle Investigators of CASS et al: The National Heart, Lung, and Blood Institute Coronary Artery Surgery Study, *Circulation* 68(suppl I):I1-I81, 1983.
7. TIMI Study Group: Comparison of invasive and conservative strategies after treatment with intravenous tissue plasminogen activator in acute myocardial infarction. Results of the Thrombolysis in Myocardial Infarction (TIMI) Phase II Trial, *N Engl J Med* 320:618-627, 1989.
8. GUSTO Investigators: Thrombolysis for myocardial infarction: the Global Utilization of Streptokinase and Tissue Plasminogen Activator for Ocluded Coronary Arteries Trial, *N Engl J Med* 329:673-682, 1993.
9. Marcus FL, Friday K, McCans J, et al: Age-related prognosis after acute myocardial infarction (the Multicenter Diltiazem Postinfarction Trial), *Am J Cardiol* 65:559-566, 1990.
10. Goldberg RJ, Gore JM, Gurwitz JH, et al: The impact of age on the incidence and prognosis of initial acute myocardial infarction: the Worcester Heart Attack Study, *Am Heart J* 117:543-549, 1989.
11. Weisfeldt ML, Wright JR, Shreiner DP, et al.: Coronary flow and oxygen extraction in perfused hearts of senescent male rats, *J Appl Physiol* 30:44, 1971.
12. Pearson AC, Gudipati CV, Kabovitz, AJ: Effects of aging on left ventricular structure and function, *Am Heart J* 121:871, 1991.
13. Zerman, FD, Rodstein M: Cardiac rupture complicating myocardial infarction in the aged, *Arch Intern Med* 105:431, 1960.
14. Connolly DC, Elveback LR, Oxman HA: Coronary heart disease in residents of Rochester, Minnesota 1950-75. Effect of hypertension and its treatment in survival of patients with coronary artery disease, *Mayo Clin Proc* 58:249-254, 1983.
15. Olmsted WL, Groden DL, Silverman ME, et al: Prognosis in survivors of acute myocardial infarction occurring at age 70 years or older, *Am J Cardiol* 60:971-975, 1987.
16. Day JJ, Bayer AJ, Pathy MS, et al: Acute myocardial infarction: Diagnostic difficulties and outcome in advanced old age, *Age Aging* 16:239-243, 1987.
17. Wilcox RG, Hampton JR: Importance of age in prehospital and hospital mortality of heart attacks, *Br Heart J* 44:503-507, 1980.
18. Nadelmann J, Frishman WH, Ooi WL, et al: Prevalence, incidence and prognosis of recognized and unrecognized myocardial infarction in persons aged 75 years or older: The Bronx Aging Study, *Am J Cardiol* 66:533-537, 1990.
19. Kannel WB, Abbott RD: Incidence and prognosis of unrecognized myocardial infarction. An update on the Framingham Study, *N Engl J Med* 311:1144-1152, 1984.
20. Williams BO, Begg TB, Semple T, et al: The elderly in a coronary care unit, *Br Med J (Clin Res)* 2:451-453, 1976.
21. Tofler GH, Muller JE, Stone PH, et al: Factors leading to shorter survival after acute myocardial infarction in patients ages 65 to 75 years compared with younger patients, *Am J Cardiol* 62:860-867, 1988.
22. Marcus FI, Friday K, McCans J, et al: Age-related prognosis after acute myocardial infarction (The Multicenter Diltiazem Postinfarction Trial), *Am J Cardiol* 65:559-566, 1990.
23. Goldberg RJ, Gore JM, Gurwitz JH, et al: The impact of age on the incidence and prognosis of initial acute myocardial infarction: The Worcester Heart Attack Study, *Am Heart J* 117:543-549, 1989.
24. Merrilees MA, Scott JR, Norris RM: Prognosis after myocardial infarction: results of 15 year follow up, *Br Med J (Clin Res)* 288:3569, 1984.
25. Smith SC, Gilpin E, Ahnve S, et al: Outlook after acute myocardial infarction in the very elderly compared with that in patients aged 65 to 75 years, *J Am Coll Cardiol* 16:784-792, 1990.
26. Hands ME, Rutherford JD, Muller JE, et al: The in-hospital development of cardiogenic shock after myocardial infarction: incidence, predictors of occurrence, outcome and prognostic factors, *J Am Coll Cardiol* 14:40-46, 1989.
27. Forman DE, Gutierrez Bernal JL, Wei JY: Management of acute myocardial infarction in the very elderly, *Am J Med* 93:315-326, 1992.
28. ISIS-I (First International Study of Infarct Survival) Collaborative Group: Randomized trial of intravenous atenolol among 16,027 cases of suspected acute myocardial infarction, *Lancet* 2:57-66, 1986.
29. Herlitz J, Elmfeldt D, Holmberg S, et al: Goteborg Metoprolol Trial: Mortality and causes of death, *Am J Cardiol* 53:9D-14D, 1984.
30. MIAMI Trial Research Group: Metoprolol in acute myocardial infarction (MIAMI). A randomized placebo-controlled international trial, *Eur Heart J* XX:19, 1985.
31. Beta-Blocker Heart Attack Study Group: The beta-blocker heart attack trial, *JAMA* 246:2073-2074, 1981.
32. Beta-Blocker Heart Attack Trial Research Group: A randomized trial of propanolol in patients with myocardial infarction, *JAMA* 247:1701-1714, 1982.
33. Norwegian Multicenter Study Group: Timolol-induced reduction in mortality and reinfarction in patients surviving acute myocardial infarction, *N Engl J Med* 304:801-807, 1981.
34. Forman DE, Wei JY: Beta-blockers in older patients with myocardial infarction [letter], *JAMA* 226:2222, 1991.
35. Sixty Plus Reinfarction Study Group, de Vries WA, Loeliger EA, et al: A double-blind trial to assess longterm oral anticoagulant therapy in elderly patients after myocardial infarction, *Lancet* 2:989-994, 1980.
36. Breddin K, Loew D, Lechner K, et al: Secondary prevention of myocardial reinfarction a comparison of acetylsalicylic acid, placebo and phenprocoumon, *Haemostasis* 313:1369-375, 1980.
37. Anturan Reinfarction Italian Study; Sulphinpyrazone in post-myocardial infarction, *Lancet* 1:237-242, 1982.
38. Aspirin Myocardial Reinfarction Study Research Group: A randomized, controlled trial of aspirin in persons recovered from myocardial infarction, *JAMA* 243:661-669, 1980.
39. Persantine-Aspirin Reinfarction Study Research Group: Persantine and aspirin in coronary heart disease, *Circulation* 62(suppl II):1-22, 1980.
40. Klimt CR, Knatterud GL, Stamler J, et al: Persantine-aspirin reinfarction study, II: Secondary prevention with persantine and aspirin, *J Am Coll Cardiol* 7:251-69, 1986.
41. Antiplatelet Trialist Collaboration: Secondary prevention of vascular disease by prolonged antiplatelet treatment, *Br Med J (Clin Res)* 296:320-331, 1988.
42. Weaver WD, Litwin PE, Martin JS, et al: Effect of age on use of thrombolytic therapy and mortality in acute myocardial infarction, *J Am Coll Cardiol* 18:657-662, 1991.
43. Herrick JB: Clinical features of sudden obstruction of the coronary arteries, *JAMA* 59:2015, 1912.
44. Roberts WC, Buja LM: The frequency and significance of coronary artery thrombi in fatal acute myocardial infarction, *Am J Med* 52:425, 1972.
45. Tillet WS, Garner RL: The fibrinolytic activity of hemolytic streptococci, *J Exp Med* 58:485, 1933.

46. Schroeder R, Blamino G, vonLietner ER: Intravenous short-term thrombosis in acute myocardial infarction [abstract]. *Circulation* 64(suppl IV):10, 1981.

47. Blanke H, Karsch KR, Kreuzer H, et al: Changes in coronary anatomy and left ventricular function from the acute to chronic stage of myocardial infarction, *Clin Cardiol* 3:61, 1980.

48. De Wood MA, Spores JN, Notski R: Prevalence of total coronary occlusion during the early hours of transmural myocardial infarction. *N Engl J Med* 303:897, 1980.

49. Rentrop P, Blanke H, Karsch KR, et al: Initial experience with transmural recanalization or the recently occluded infarct-related coronary artery in acute myocardial infarction. Comparison with conventionally treated patients, *Clin Cardiol* 2:92, 1979.

50. Ganz W, Buckbinder N, Marcus H, et al: Intracoronary thrombolysis in evolving myocardial infarction, *Am Heart J* 101:4, 1981.

51. Khaja F, Walton JA Jr, Bryme JF, et al: Intracoronary fibrinolytic therapy in acute myocardial infarction, *N Engl J Med* 308:1305, 1983.

52. Anderson JL, Marshall HW, Bray BE, et al: A randomized trial of intracoronary streptokinase in the treatment of acute myocardial infarction, *N Engl J Med* 308:1312, 1983.

53. Kennedy J, Ritchie JL, Davis KB, et al: Western Washington randomized trial of intracoronary streptokinase in acute myocardial infarction, *N Engl J Med* 309:1477, 1983.

54. Rentrop KP, Feit F, Blanke H, et al: Effects of intracoronary streptokinase and intracoronary nitroglycerin infusion in coronary angiographic patterns and mortality in patients with acute myocardial infarction, *N Engl J Med* 311:1457-1463, 1984.

55. Rentrop KP, Feit F, Sherman W, et al: Major complications and interventions in the Mount Sinai–NYU Reperfusion Trial [abstract]. *Circulation* 76(suppl II):002, 1987.

56. Rao AK, Pratt C, Berke A, et al: Thrombolysis in Myocardial Infarction (TIMI) Trial—Phase I: Hemorrhagic manifestations and changes in plasma fibrinogen and the fibrinolytic system in patients treated with recombinant tissue plasminogen activator and streptokinase, *J Am Coll Cardiol* 11:1-11, 1988.

57. Sane DC, Califf RM, Topol EJ, et al: Bleeding during thrombolytic therapy for acute myocardial infarction: mechanisms and management, *Ann Intern Med* 111:1010-1022, 1989.

58. O'Rourke M, Baron D, Keogh, A et al: Limitation of myocardial infarction by early infusion of recombinant tissue-type plasminogen activator, *Circulation* 776:1311-1315, 1988.

59. White HD, Norris RM, Brown MA, et al: Effect of intravenous streptokinase on left ventricular function and early survival after acute myocardial infarction, *N Engl J Med* 317:850-855, 1987.

60. Wilcox RG, Olsson CG, Skene AM, et al: Trial of tissue plasminogen activator for mortality reduction in acute myocardial infarction. Anglo-Scandinavian Study of Early Thrombolysis (ASSET), *Lancet* 1:525-530, 1988.

61. AIMS Trial Study Group: Effect of intravenous APSAC on mortality after myocardial infarction: preliminary report of a placebo-controlled clinical trial, *Lancet* 8585:545-549, 1988.

62. Kennedy JW, Martin GV, Davis KB, et al: The Western Washington intravenous streptokinase in acute myocardial infarction randomized trial, *Circulation* 77:345-352, 1988.

63. Gruppo Italiano per lo Studio della streptochinasi nell'Infarto Miocardico (GISSI): Effectiveness of intravenous thrombolytic treatment in acute myocardial infarction, *Lancet* 2:397-402, 1986.

64. ISIS-II (Second International Study of Infarct Survival) Collaborative Group: Randomized trial of intravenous streptokinase, oral aspirin, both, or neither among 17,187 cases of suspected acute myocardial infarction: ISIS-2, *Lancet* 349-359, 1987.

65. I.S.A.M. Study Group: A prospective trial of intravenous streptokinase in acute myocardial infarction (I.S.A.M.). Mortality, morbidity and infarct size at 21 days, *N Engl J Med* 314:1465-1471, 1986.

66. Muller DW, Topol EJ: Selection of patients with acute myocardial infarction for thrombolytic therapy, *Ann Intern Med* 113:949-960, 1990.

67. National Heart Foundation of Australia Coronary Thrombolysis Group: Coronary thrombolysis and myocardial salvage by tissue plasminogen activator given up to 4 hours after onset of myocardial infarction, *Lancet* 1:203-208, 1988.

68. Guerci AD, Gerstenblith G, Brinker JA, et al: A randomized trial of intravenous tissue plasminogen activator for acute myocardial infarction with subsequent randomization to elective coronary angioplasty, *N Engl J Med* 317:1613-1618, 1987.

69. White HJ, Cross D, Scott M, et al: Comparison of effects of thrombolytic therapy on left ventricular function in patients over with those under 60 years of age, *Am J Cardiol* 67:913-918, 1991.

70. Feit F, Breed J, Anderson JL, et al: A randomized, placebo-controlled trial of tissue plasminogen activator in elderly patients with acute myocardial infarction, *Circulation* 82(III suppl):666, 1990.

71. Chaitman BR, Thompson B, Wittry MD, et al: The use of tissue-type plasminogen activator for acute myocardial infarction in the elderly: results from Thrombolysis In Myocardial Infarction in the elderly: results from Thrombolysis In Myocardial Infarction Phase I, open label studies and the Thrombolysis In Myocardial Infarction Phase II pilot study, *J Am Coll Cardiol* 14:1159-1165, 1989.

72. Califf, RM, Topol EJ, George BS, et al: Hemorrhagic complications associated with the use of intravenous tissue plasminogen activator in treatment of acute myocardial infarction, *Am J Med* 85:353-359, 1988.

73. Lew AS, Hod H, Cercek B, Shah P, et al: Mortality and morbidity rates of patients older and younger than 75 years with acute myocardial infarction treated with intravenous streptokinase, *Am J Cardiol* 59:1-5, 1987.

74. Bovill EG, Terrin ML, Stump DC, et al: Hemorrhagic events during therapy with recombinant tissue-type plasminogen activator, heparin, and aspirin for acute myocardial infarction. Results of the Thrombolysis in Myocardial Infarction (TIMI), Phase II Trial, *Ann Intern Med* 115:256-265, 1991.

75. Maggioni AP, Franzosi MG, Farina ML, et al: Cerebrovascular events after myocardial infarction: analysis of the GISSI trial, *Br Med J (Clin Res)* 302:1428-1421, 1991.

76. Gore, JM, Sloan M, Price TR, et al: Intracerebral hemorrhage, cerebral infarction, and subdural hematoma after acute myocardial infarction and thrombolytic therapy in the Thrombolysis in Myocardial Infarction Study, *Circulation* 83:448-459, 1991.

77. De Jaegere PP, Arnold AA, Balk AH, et al: Intracranial Hemorrhage in association with thrombolytic therapy: Incidence and clinical predictive factors, *Am Coll Cardiol* 19:289-294, 1992.

78. Third International Study of Infarct Survival Collaborative Group: ISIS-3: A randomized comparison of streptokinase vs. tissue plasminogen activator vs. anistreplase and of aspirin plus heparin vs aspirin alone among 41,299 cases of suspected acute myocardial infarction, *Lancet* 1:753-770, 1992.

79. International Study Group: In-hospital mortality and clinical course of 20,891 patients with suspected acute myocardial infarction randomized between alteplase and streptokinase with or without heparin, *Lancet* 1:71-75, 1990.

80. Sobel BE, Hirsh J: Principles and practice of coronary thrombolysis and conjunctive treatment, *Am J Cardiol* 68:382-388, 1991.

81. Lee TC, Laramee LA, Rutherford BD, et al: Emergency percutaneous transluminal coronary angioplasty for acute myocardial infarction in patients 70 years of age and older, *Am J Cardiol* 66:663-667, 1990.

82. Grines CL, Browne KF, Marco J, et al: A comparison of immediate angioplasty with thrombolytic therapy for acute myocardial infarction, *N Engl J Med* 328:673-679, 1993.

83. Stone GW, Grines CL, Vlietstra R, et al: Primary angioplasty is the preferred therapy for women and the elderly with acute myocardial infarction—results of the Primary Angioplasty in Myocardial Infarction (PAMI) Trial, *J Am Coll Cardiol* 21:330A, 1993.

84. Grines, CL, De Maria AN: Optimal utilization of thrombolytic therapy for acute myocardial infarction: concepts and controversies, *J Am Coll Cardiol* 16:223-231, 1990.

85. Sherry S, Marder VJ: Mistaken guidelines for thrombolytic therapy of acute myocardial infarction in the elderly, *J Am Coll Cardiol* 17:1237-1238, 1991.

Chapter 58

EVALUATION OF VALVULAR HEART DISEASE IN THE CCU
Anatomic and physiologic considerations

J. Kevin Harrison
Thomas M. Bashore

Cardiac care units (CCUs) have evolved in the last 20 years based on the premise that intensive hemodynamic and arrhythmia monitoring allow for rapid intervention and prevention of serious complications in critically ill patients with heart disease. The focus of these specialized intensive care units has been on patients with acute ischemic syndromes. This seems appropriate because about 6 million Americans have known coronary disease, and 1.5 million acute myocardial infarctions (AMIs) occur each year. It is important to appreciate, however, that rheumatic heart disease also affects 3 million individuals, another 300,000 patients have congenital heart disorders, and about 20,000 hospital admissions occur each year for endocarditis.[1]

It stands to reason that there will be patients with valvular or congenital heart disease who also suffer from acute ischemic syndromes (primarily because of coexistent atherosclerotic coronary artery disease). These patients present a particular challenge to busy clinicians, housestaff, and nurses on the CCU. Many of the routine hemodynamics that provide clinical estimates of disease severity and therapeutic success in acute ischemia are perturbed when there is associated valvular disease. In addition, therapies meant to improve hemodynamics in patients with acute ischemia may actually worsen the clinical picture when valvular or other structural heart

disease is superimposed. Although specific valvular diseases are discussed in Chapter 59, this chapter is designed to provide an overview of the anatomy and physiology that are relevant to understanding and caring for the CCU patient with valvular heart disease.

MONITORING THE PATIENT WITH COMPLEX CARDIOVASCULAR DISEASE IN THE CCU
Basic anatomic considerations

It is important to review some basic cardiovascular anatomic, hemodynamic, and physiologic principles to appreciate better the clinical complexity that occurs when ischemia is superimposed on hemodynamic derangements as a result of structural heart disease.

Certain anatomic relationships can be better appreciated by studying Figs. 58-1 to 58-3. A schematic of the normal structures one might observe in the anteroposterior view using chest x-ray film or bedside fluoroscopy is shown in Fig. 58-1. Fig. 58-2 represents a similar lateral schematic, and Fig. 58-3 shows a cross section. The traditional view of the heart as a right-sided and a left-sided structure is more accurately represented anatomically by considering it an anteroposterior organ.

The right atrium (RA) is divided into two parts: the large RA appendage (trabeculated with pectinate muscles and forming the right lateral border of the heart

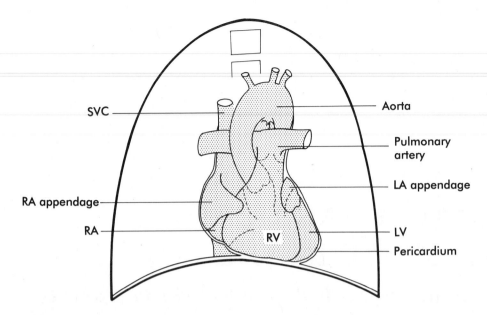

Fig. 58-1. Anteroposterior schematic of the heart as might be seen on fluoroscopy of the bedside. *SVC,* Superior vena cava; *RA,* right atrium; *LA,* left atrium; *RV,* right ventricle; *LV,* left ventricle. (From Bashore TM [ed]: *Invasive cardiology: principles and techniques,* Philadelphia, 1990, BC Decker, p 80. Used by permission.)

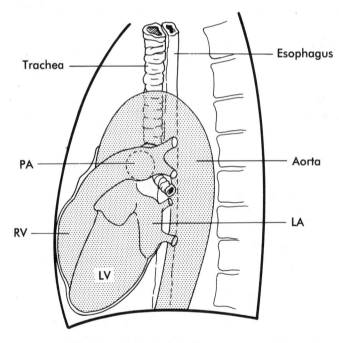

Fig. 58-2. Lateral schematic of the heart. *PA,* Pulmonary artery. (From Bashore TM [ed]: *Invasive cardiology: principles and techniques,* Philadelphia, 1990, BC Decker, p 81. Used by permission.)

silhouette) and the smoother RA body. The RA is thin walled (about 2 mm) and holds about 50 ml of blood. It receives blood from three sources: the superior vena cava (SVC), the inferior vena cava (IVC), and the coronary sinus (CS). The SVC, IVC, and CS all contribute variable amounts of blood to the RA, and each contribution has a different oxygen saturation. Blood from the IVC contains renal vein blood that is highly saturated, because the kidneys receive disproportionately high flow (about 25% of the cardiac output) compared with their oxygen requirements. The CS contributes only a small volume of blood to the RA, but

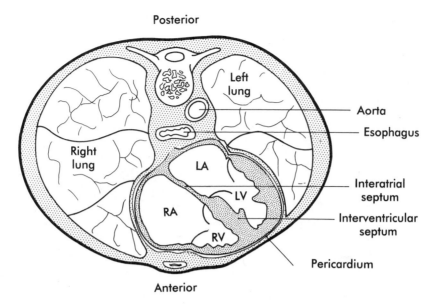

Fig. 58-3. Cross-sectional schematic of the heart. (From Bashore TM [ed]: *Invasive cardiology: principles and techniques,* Philadelphia, 1990, BC Decker, p 81. Used by permission.)

this efflux consists of drainage from the coronary bed, where very high oxygen extraction occurs. In point of fact, one of the problems with the coronary system from a teleologic standpoint is that myocardial oxygen extraction is almost always at a maximum. The only way to increase oxygen delivery to the heart, therefore, is to increase coronary flow, which becomes a problem when atherosclerotic disease intervenes and impairs the coronary flow reserve normally present. The SVC saturation reflects the venous saturation from the periphery. The SVC receives blood from both the upper extremities and the lower extremities through the azygous venous system that drains into it just above the RA-SVC junction. The important point is that oxygen saturations in the RA are mixed.

This variability becomes important when one is attempting to define "step-ups" in oxygen saturation because of a left-to-right shunt. Because of this, a step-up in oxygen saturation from the SVC to the RA must be of at least 11% (1.9 vol%) to ensure that it is greater than what one would expect solely because of the high saturation of blood from the IVC entering the RA. The oxygen saturations are more homogeneous in the RV and even more so in the pulmonary artery (PA). Table 58-1 reflects the minimum step-ups in oxygen saturation generally believed necessary to detect a left-to-right shunt at the atrial and ventricular levels. Because of this natural variability in saturations, the use of oxygen step-ups to detect a shunt is not very sensitive (at least a 1.3:1 shunt must be present). Although there are several mixed venous (MV) saturation formulas to help normalize for this heterogeneity, the most popular is:

Table 58-1. Minimum oxygen saturation step-ups required to detect an intracardiac shunt*

Shunt	Step-up sites	Minimal change in oxygen saturation (%)
Ventricular septal defect	RA to RV	7
Atrial septal defect	Mixed venous to RA	11

*RA, Right atrium; RV, right ventricle.

$$\frac{3\,(SVC) + 1\,(IVC)}{4} = MV$$

This MV saturation should be assumed to be the saturation of blood entering the RA and used in determining the magnitude of a shunt using oximetry.

In the fetus most of the blood from the SVC flows through the RA, to the right ventricle (RV), to the PA, and then skips the lungs by flowing through the open ductus arteriosus into the descending aorta. Blood from the IVC also skips the lungs by being deflected across a patent foramen ovale to the LA via a ridge of tissue (the eustachian valve). At birth the ductus closes, and the increased LA pressure closes the embryologic septum primum flap over the foramen ovale. In about 25% of adults the foramen remains "probe patent," and this can become an issue in certain disease states where the atria become stretched (opening the foramen) or when the RA pressure exceeds the LA pressure (e.g., with RV

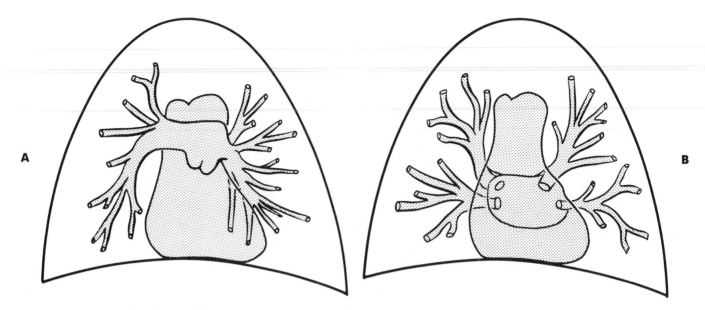

Fig. 58-4. A, Pulmonary arteries. Note how they spread from the hilum to the periphery. **B,** Pulmonary veins. The pulmonary veins can usually be distinguished from the pulmonary arteries on fluoroscopy and chest x-ray film by noting their vertical and horizontal shadows. (From Bashore TM [ed]: *Invasive cardiology: principles and techniques,* Philadelphia, 1990, BC Decker, p 88. Used by permission.)

infarction and pulmonary hypertension), resulting in a right-to-left shunt with arterial desaturation.

The RV is a crescent-shaped, thin-walled cardiac chamber that is designed for volume but not pressure work. The action of the RV has been likened to a bellows with the free wall pushing against the interventricular septum. The RV volume is greater than the LV; therefore, assuming both chambers produce a similar stroke volume, the RV ejection fraction is normally less than the LV (normal right ventricular ejection fraction >40%-45%; normal left ventricular ejection fraction >55%-60%). Flow of blood from the RA into the RV must take a 90-degree turn to proceed to the PA. A moderator band usually crosses the RV and contains Purkinje fibers of the right bundle branch (resulting in occasional right bundle branch block when banged with catheters). The RV outflow has few Purkinje fibers and contracts last. The RV, therefore, virtually squeezes blood toward the PA. The tricuspid annulus and valve separate the RA and RV. The tricuspid valve has three leaflets (anterior, posterior, and septal), and although certain discrete papillary muscles are present, unlike the mitral valve, many chordae attach haphazardly directly to the ventricular wall. This helps explain why tricuspid regurgitation (TR) is so common when the RV dilates and enlarges and why "TR begets TR." TR is common in CCU patients and is often clinically overlooked.

Blood flows through the main PA to both left and right lungs via the left and right PAs. The PAs radiate out from the hilum (Fig. 58-4, *A*), whereas the pulmonary veins drain vertically from the upper lobes and horizon-

tally from the lower lobes to the left atrium (LA) (Fig. 58-4, *B*). These relationships are worth recalling when one is examining the routine chest x-ray film for evidence of pulmonary arterial or venous hypertension.

The LA is anchored posteriorly by the pulmonary veins. The LA walls are thicker than the RA because it must generate pressures greater than the RA as it pushes blood toward the left ventricle (LV). The combination of these conditions results in the LA compliance being less than the RA, which affects the LA pressure waveform as described later on.

The LV is an ellipsoid, thick-walled chamber with spiral fibers theoretically traversing along the endocardial surface, then reversing and traveling up the epicardial surface to the base of the heart. Concentric, transverse fibers are sandwiched between the spiral muscle fibers everywhere except at the LV apex. The apex is therefore much thinner than the lateral walls. This contributes to the wall stress being greatest at the LV apex in accordance with the law of Laplace:

$$\text{Wall stress} \propto \frac{\text{Chamber radius} \times \text{Pressure}}{\text{Wall thickness}}$$

This heterogeneity in wall stress affects the visual interpretation of ventriculography and is consistent with the observation that up to 85% of the LV stroke volume results from short-axis shortening, whereas only 15% results from long-axis shortening.[2]

Blood enters the LV through the mitral valve and then must take almost a 180-degree turn to proceed out the LV outflow through the aortic valve. The mitral valve

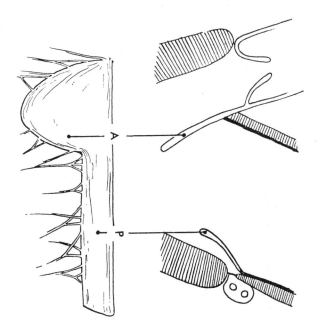

Fig. 58-5. Mitral valve and its attachments. The anterior mitral leaflet forms the left side of the aortic outflow tract. The mitral valve shares a portion of the aortic annulus with the aortic valve. These relationships are particularly important to understand when the hemodynamics of diseases such as idiopathic hypertrophic subaortic stenosis are considered. The shared annulus results in the calcified mitral annulus appearing as C rather than O shaped. It also explains contiguous disease processes that often affect both valves (e.g., rheumatic fever, endocarditis).

has two major leaflets: a triangular anterior and a rectangular posterior leaflet. The anterior mitral leaflet shares the posterior portion of the aortic valve anulus (Fig. 58-5). A totally calcified mitral annulus, for example, is C shaped and not O shaped for this reason. The attachment of the anterior mitral leaflet to the aortic anulus means the LV outflow tract is formed by the interventricular septum on one side and the anterior leaflet of the mitral valve on the other. This latter relationship is particularly important in certain disease states, as in hypertrophic obstructive cardiomyopathy where the dynamic outflow obstruction is contributed to by the anterior mitral valve leaflet, as well as the interventricular septum. This relationship is also important in bacterial endocarditis where infection of the anterior mitral leaflet and aortic valve often coexist because of their anatomic continuity.

In contrast to the tricuspid valve leaflets and their attachments, there are two discrete papillary muscles (posteromedial and anterolateral) that attach via chordae to the mitral valve. Chordae from each papillary muscle attach to both mitral leaflets. Chordae attach not only along the leaflet edges but also underneath on the body of the leaflets. Both papillary muscles, although supplied by end arteries, often have dual blood supplies.

The anterolateral papillary muscle tends to have one major head and receive its blood supply from diagonal branches of the left anterior descending, marginal branches of the circumflex coronary artery, or both. The posteromedial papillary muscle usually receives blood from distal branches of the circumflex and right coronary arteries and usually has multiple heads. The anatomy of the mitral apparatus has clinical relevance with respect to the normal function of the valve and the pathologic derangements which affect it.

Blood is ejected from the LV through the trileaflet aortic valve. The aortic valve is located deep inside the heart behind the RV outflow tract adjacent to the interatrial septum. It is composed of right coronary, left coronary, and noncoronary cusps. Under normal circumstances, the aortic valve, similar to all the heart valves, presents little or no obstruction to outflow.

Basic hemodynamic considerations

Contraction and relaxation of the myocardium. In the very simplest terms, excitation of the myocardial membrane results in the efflux of calcium into the cellular cytosol. This cytosolic calcium triggers release of calcium from the sarcoplasmic reticulum (SR) to the actin-myosin apparatus and contraction ensues. When calcium is subsequently removed from actin-myosin apparatus and returned to the SR, the process reverses and active relaxation occurs. The process of moving calcium in and out of the cell and the SR is an active one requiring cyclic adenosine monophosphate (cAMP) for energy.

This broad concept of how contraction and relaxation ensues has ready clinical relevance in many situations. For instance, both contraction and relaxation of the heart is improved by use of therapeutic agents that increase cAMP (i.e., catecholamines, phosphodiesterase inhibitors). When a drug such as digitalis is used, contraction may be improved by increasing cytosol calcium levels, but this increased cytosol calcium level may inhibit later removal of calcium from the actin-myosin apparatus to the cytosol during the active relaxation process. Digitalis thus improves contraction and may not help or may actually worsen myocardial relaxation. Conversely, drugs that deplete calcium in the cytosol, such as calcium channel blockers, may reduce contractility but can improve active relaxation. Ischemia results in a profound depletion of cAMP and thus adversely affects both myocardial contraction and relaxation.

Normal pressures and waveforms. Whenever a cardiac chamber contracts or blood flows into a closed chamber, the pressure in the chamber rises. Conversely, when the blood flows out of a cardiac chamber or active relaxation of that chamber occurs, the pressure falls. These simple concepts help explain the various pressure

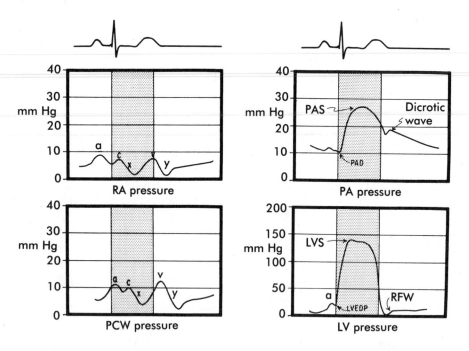

Fig. 58-6. Normal pressure waveforms. The normal right atrial *(RA)*, pulmonary capillary wedge *(PCW)*, pulmonary artery *(PA)*, and left ventricular *(LV)* waveforms are shown. Note the a wave is greater than the v wave in the RA, whereas the reverse is true in the PCW. Also note delayed PA closure at the dicrotic notch because of "hangout" phenomenon. See text for details.

waveforms observed in the heart. Fig. 58-6 schematically summarizes normal pressure waveforms.

The atrial pressure waveforms are the most complex to understand. There are five separate components. Three are positive waves: the *A wave* occurs during atrial contraction, the *C wave* occurs when the atrioventricular (AV) valve bulges into the atrium during initial ventricular contraction, and the *V wave* occurs during passive filling of the atrium. The V wave ceases when the AV valve opens. Two of the atrial waves are negative waves: the *X descent* caused by atrial diastolic relaxation and the "pulling" of the AV valve annulus into the ventricle during ventricular systole and the *Y descent* that begins at the peak of the V wave and represents the early decline in atrial pressure as blood flows into the ventricle from the atria.

The jugular venous pulsation (JVP) is a reflection of right atrial pressure waveform. Clinically, only the A and V waves are detectable at bedside. From a practical standpoint one should simultaneously palpate the opposite carotid while observing the JVP waveform with the patient reclining at about 60 degrees. The peak of ventricular systole (when the carotid pulse taps your finger) should time precisely with the X descent in the JVP. The wave observed immediately before the carotid upstroke is the A wave, and the wave after the carotid upstroke is the V wave. With practice this can be readily perceived. Diseases that affect RV compliance raise the

JVP and result in a very large A wave. Tricuspid regurgitation obliterates the normal X descent and results in a gradual filling in of the X descent (a C-V wave) that can be seen as systolic expansion of the JVP at the same time the carotid pulsation is felt.

Although the waveforms of the RA and LA are similar in their generation, the A wave is normally greater than the V in the RA, whereas the opposite occurs in the LA. This is because of the lower LA compliance. Recall the LA is thicker and literally trapped posteriorly, so that passive filling would be expected to result in a greater increase in pressure during late atrial diastole, whereas the RA is relatively open to the SVC and IVC. The pulmonary wedge pressures (PCWs) generally reflect the LA pressure because no valves are present between the PCW and the LA.

The RV and LV pressure waveforms are similar except for their magnitude. An initial pressure increase occurs when the atrium "kicks" blood toward the ventricles at end-diastole. The abrupt pressure rise during ventricular contraction then slams the AV valves shut. The AV valves remain closed until diastole has reduced the ventricular pressure to a level lower than that in the atria. Early filling of the ventricles is best appreciated as an active process related to myocardial relaxation, whereas the later stages of ventricular filling generally are considered a more passive phenomenon.

Ventricular ejection opens the semilunar valves, and

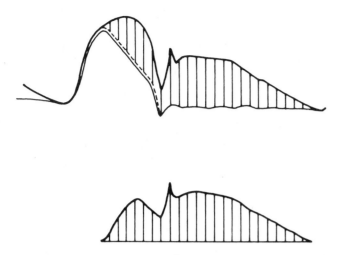

Fig. 58-7. Components of the aortic waveform. The top panel displays the outline of the aortic pressure waveform with the aortic flow waveform superimposed. The difference between aortic flow and pressure is shown in the hatched area and redisplayed below. The initial pressure wave is caused by aortic flow (percussion wave). A second pressure wave (tidal wave) represents a reflected wave primarily from the upper extremity, and the third wave (dicrotic wave) represents reflection from the lower extremity. (From O'Rourke MF: *Arterial function in health and disease,* New York, 1982, Churchill Livingstone, p 77. Used by permission.)

blood is ejected into the PA and aorta, respectively. The compliance of the pulmonary and aortic vasculature are vastly different though, resulting in differing pressure waveforms. Systemic vascular resistance is normally about ten times greater than pulmonary. The pulmonary resistance is so low that there is little discernable pressure rise even with large left to right shunts (e.g., in atrial septal defects). In addition, one lung can often be surgically removed without a substantial increase in pulmonary pressure. Pulmonary resistance is so low that the inertia of the blood propelled forward in systole tends to continue even after RV diastole begins. This latter phenomenon (known as hangout) is primarily responsible for delayed closure of the pulmonary valve (P_2) after the aortic valve (A_2).

The aortic pressure waveform is made up of three components that have clinical relevance: a percussion wave that correlates with flow into the aorta, a tidal wave that represents a reflected wave probably from the upper extremity, and a dicrotic wave that represents a reflected wave probably from the lower extremity.[3] Fig. 58-7 reviews those waveforms. In aortic stenosis, for instance, the percussion wave is lost and a "delay" in the carotid pulsation is perceived. A similar delay is felt at the femoral artery in patients with coarctation of the aorta. In hypertrophic cardiomyopathy the opposite occurs because rapid ejection of blood from the LV into the aorta occurs. This results in a separation between the percussion and the tidal waves (creating a bisferiens

pulse). When stroke volume is reduced and peripheral resistance high (a common scenario in the CCU), the pulse pressure is often quite low and the dicrotic wave may be markedly accentuated, again creating a bisferiens-type pulsation.

The normal arterial pressure waveforms vary throughout the body because of variation in the contributions of these three components. For instance, as noted in Fig. 58-8, as one approaches the periphery, the reflected waves begin to summate and the pulse pressure rises. In contrast, the highly elastic central aorta absorbs the impact of ejection. The central aortic pressure is therefore often lower than peripheral pulse pressure. This can be an issue when peripheral resistance is high, because myocardial ischemia and hypoperfusion may exist in the face of what appears to be adequate systemic pressure measured from a femoral or radial arterial line.

Basic physiologic principles with clinical relevance in the CCU

The fundamental relationship between myocardial chamber filling pressure and contractility and the resultant cardiac output was formulated years ago by Sarnoff and Berglund[4] and has been termed the ventricular function curve (Fig. 58-9). This relationship defines the cardiac output (or stroke work) as a function of the end-diastolic filling pressure. Its curvilinear nature is a consequence of the exponential relationship between the LV volume and the diastolic filling *pressure* (Fig. 58-10). The relationship between LV end-diastolic *volume* and cardiac output is actually quite linear and has been termed the preload recruitable stroke work.[5] As is evident from the ventricular function curve, under normal conditions an adequate cardiac output can be generated at a filling pressure that does not result in pulmonary congestion. When myocardial failure ensues, the curve flattens, and to generate an acceptable cardiac output, the LV filling pressure increases. There is thus a tradeoff between having a low output or pulmonary congestion when the curve flattens in CHF.

Therapeutic agents affect this curve in a variety of important ways (Fig. 58-11). For instance, diuretics and nitrates reduce filling pressure at the price of reducing cardiac output. Inotropic agents increase cardiac output but have only a minor effect on filling pressures. Afterload reducing agents improve both cardiac output and filling pressures. Because angiotensin II has been found to be present in myocardial cells and peripheral endothelial cells alike, resulting in an increase in intracellular calcium, the use of angiotensin-converting enzyme inhibitors reduces vascular tone and may also improve diastolic relaxation.

The same concepts can be alternatively represented by examining the pressure-volume relationship throughout the cardiac cycle. A pressure-volume loop represents isovolumic contraction, ventricular ejection, isovolumic relaxation, and, finally diastolic filling. This loop can be dramatically affected by changes in afterload without implying a change in myocardial contractility (Fig. 58-12). An increase in afterload increases peak ventricular pressure and increases the LV end-systolic volume (LVESV). Assuming LV end-diastolic volume (LVEDV) does not change, when the LV end-systolic volume increases, the calculated ejection fraction (EF) then necessarily falls:

$$EF = \frac{LVEDV - LVESV}{LVEDV}$$

Similarly, if afterload is reduced, as in mitral regurgitation, the LV end-diastolic volume increases disproportionately to the LV end-systolic volume, and the calculated ejection fraction is greater than normal (see Fig. 58-12). Afterload changes can therefore profoundly effect ejection phase indices such as the ejection fraction independent of changes in myocardial contractility.

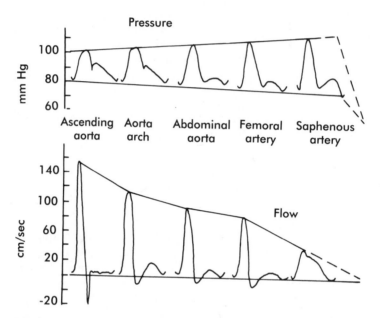

Fig. 58-8. Relationship of aortic pressure and flow as the periphery is approached. Approaching the origin of reflected waves causes them to summate with forward flow waveforms. Thus, as one approaches the periphery, the pulse pressure rises despite an actual decrease in forward flow. (From McDonald DA: *Blood flow in arteries,* Baltimore, 1974, Williams & Wilkins, p 358. Used by permission.)

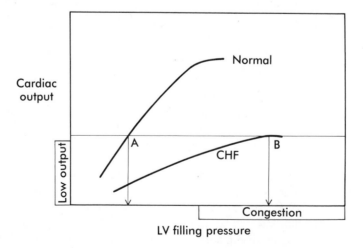

Fig. 58-9. Sarnoff's ventricular function curve. The classic ventricular function curve relates output to filling pressure in a curvilinear manner. In patients with congestive heart failure *(CHF)* the curve is depressed, and often cardiac output can be maintained only at a high filling pressure that results in pulmonary congestion.

Thus, LV ejection fraction may not accurately reflect LV systolic function when valvular heart disease coexists.

Changes in contractility also affects the systolic portion of the pressure-volume relationship. In a classic series of studies, Sagawa et al.[6] noted that when afterload was increased in a stepwise fashion in isolated heart preparations, a series of pressure-volume loops could be obtained. They noted that a linear relationship appeared to exist between these loops at similar time increments. For instance, at 10 msec, 20 msec, 30 msec, and so forth, a straight line could be drawn connecting each of these loops. The slope of this isochronic relationship was termed elastance. Eventually a maxi-

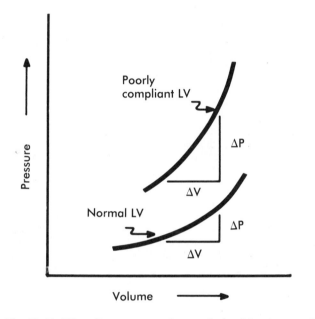

Fig. 58-10. Diastolic pressure-volume relationship. A normal left ventricular tracing is shown compared with a poorly compliant left ventricle. See text for discussion.

mum slope was reached (termed E_{max}) that appeared to represent the contractile state of the LV, independent of preload and afterload conditions. A change in this slope thus reflected a change in contractility independent of loading conditions. Although these relationships may not be truly linear under all conditions,[7] the concepts are useful in understanding clinical phenomena. If the slope of the E_{max} relationship flattens, the LV end-systolic volume rises and the ejection fraction falls. Thus, when myocardial failure occurs, the LV end-systolic volume rises and the ejection fraction falls. Both of these criteria have been used to help assess systolic function clinically.

The important message in all this is that the use of any ejection phase index, such as the ejection fraction, must be interpreted in light of not only the contractile state of the myocardium, but also the loading conditions placed on the ventricle. Abnormal loading conditions created by valvular disease or shunts may greatly effect these traditional indices and the hemodynamic monitoring being used in the CCU. Such effects need to be appreciated to avoid therapeutic misadventures.

Measurement of cardiac output and vascular resistance. Cardiac output in the CCU is generally measured with thermodilution methods. Thermodilution techniques use the indicator-dilution approach with temperature as the indicator to determine cardiac output. A Swan-Ganz or equivalent catheter is used to inject iced saline solution through a proximal port into the right atrium, and the change in temperature at the distal thermistor (located in the PA) is plotted versus time. The output is calculated by a rather complex equation that takes into account the temperature of the injectant, the temperature of the blood, the injectant volume, and specific gravity. The important concept is that the cardiac output is inversely related to the area under the

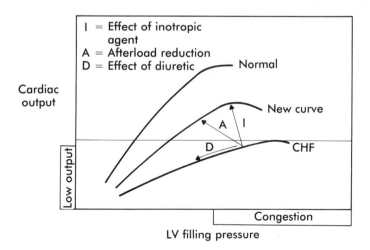

Fig. 58-11. Effect of various pharmacologic agents on the ventricular function curve. See text for discussion.

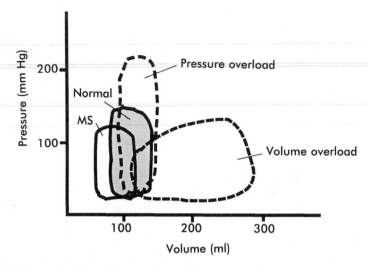

Fig. 58-12. Effect of various disease states on the pressure-volume (PV) relationship. The width of the PV loop represents stroke volume (left ventricular end-diastolic volume–left ventricular end-systolic volume [LVEDV-LVESV]). A normal loop is schematically represented in gray. The ejection fraction (EF) represents the stroke volume/LVEDV. In mitral stenosis, the EF is usually normal or even increased slightly compared with normal. With pressure overload, the work on the heart increases (area of the loop) and the width decreases (reduces EF). With volume overload (mitral regurgitation [MR] or aortic insufficiency [AI]), the LVEDV increases and the stroke volume (SV) increases; the result is an increase in EF. The EF alone, therefore, may reflect variable loading conditions (assuming similar contractile function in each of the situations shown above).

Table 58-2. Normal values for vascular resistance*

Measurement	Sites	Absolute units (dyn · sec · cm^{-5})	Wood units (mm Hg · min · L^{-1})
Pulmonary vascular resistance	Mean PA to mean PCW	67 ± 30	1 ± 0.5
Systemic vascular resistance	Mean peripheral to mean RA	1170 ± 270	15 ± 3.5

*PA, Pulmonary artery; PCW, pulmonary capillary wedge; RA, right atrium.

curve. At high outputs the curve rises rapidly and dissipates rapidly. At low outputs, the curve rises slowly and is relatively flat. The smaller the area under the curve, the higher the cardiac output. It is also important to appreciate that this method has a variability of between 10% and 15%, so that minor fluctuations should not be overinterpreted.

Cardiac output by thermodilution represents right-sided heart output only. Tricuspid regurgitation can be a particular problem for this technique, because the refluxing blood dissipates up the iced saline bolus. Similarly, in low output states, there is excessive loss of the cold temperature to surrounding blood and cardiac structures and therefore decreased accuracy. The measured cardiac output may be falsely high or low, depending on the thermodilution equipment and equation used.[8]

Cardiac output measurements can be used to calculate peripheral resistance using the analogy to Ohm's law (pressure = flow × resistance). The method assumes flow occurs only in systole and is uniform without fluctuations. This is obviously not true or systolic pressure would be very high and diastolic pressure would equal RA. To determine resistance (R) across any vascular bed, one uses the mean pressure (without fluctuations) entering the bed (P_1), the mean pressure distal to the bed (P_2), and cardiac output (CO). Flow increases proportionally to the pressure difference across the bed and inversely proportionally to the resistance:

$$\text{Flow} \propto \frac{P_1 - P_2}{R} \quad R = \frac{\overline{mP_1} - \overline{mP_2}}{CO}$$

Rearranging the equation allows determination of the resistance across any vascular bed. The normal resistance values are shown in Table 58-2. Wood units are used when pressure is recorded in millimeters of mercury and cardiac output in liters per minute.

Absolute units can be derived by simply multiplying
Wood units × 80.

An understanding of these pressure waveforms,
cardiac output, and resistance measurements are critical
in providing effective care for the patient with valvular
heart disease in the CCU. How these measurements are
perturbed and appropriate management of the individual valvular diseases are discussed in Chapter 59.

REFERENCES

1. Dustin HP, Chaplan LR, Curry CL, et al: Report of the task force
   in the availability of cardiovascular drugs to the medically indigent,
   Circulation 85:849-860, 1991.
2. Rankin JS, McHale PA, Arentzen CE, et al: The three-
   dimensional dynamic geometry of the left ventricle in the
   conscious dog, *Circ Res* 39:304-311, 1976.
3. O'Rourke MF: Contour of the arterial pulse and its interpretation.
   In O'Rourke MF (ed): *Arterial function in health and disease,* New
   York, 1982, Churchill Livingstone, pp 133-152.
4. Sarnoff SJ, Berglund E: Starling's law of the heart studied by
   means of simultaneous right and left ventricular function curves in
   the dog, *Circulation* 9:706-718; 1954.
5. Glower DD, Spratt JA, Snow NK, et al: Linearity of the
   Frank-Starling relationship in the intact heart; the concept of
   preload recruitable stroke work, *Circulation* 71:944-1009; 1985.
6. Sagawa K, Suga H, Shoukas AA, et al: End-systolic pressure/
   volume ratio: a new index of ventricular contractility, *Am J Cardiol*
   40:748-753, 1977.
7. Kass DA, Bexas R, Lankfor E, et al: Influence of contractile state
   on curvilinearity of in situ end-systolic pressure-volume relations,
   Circulation 79:167-178, 1989.
8. Cigarroa RG, Lange RA, Williams RH, et al: Underestimation of
   cardiac output by thermodilution in patients with tricuspid
   regurgitation, *Am J Med* 86:417-420, 1989.

Chapter 59

ASSESSMENT AND MANAGEMENT OF THE CRITICALLY ILL PATIENT WITH VALVULAR HEART DISEASE

J. Kevin Harrison
Thomas M. Bashore

Valvular heart disease may result in symptoms identical to those of isolated coronary artery disease, and it may also coexist with coronary disease. Management routinely beneficial to patients with isolated coronary disease, however, may be detrimental in certain valvular diseases. This chapter discusses the etiology, evaluation, and therapeutic options of the more common valvular disorders encountered in the cardiac care unit (CCU).

AORTIC STENOSIS
Etiology and diagnosis

The etiology of the overwhelming majority of cases of aortic stenosis (AS) in adults is degenerative calcific disease of the valve. This is a disease of the elderly, with the majority of patients in their seventies and eighties. With the population age increasing, the prevalence of AS continues to increase. About 50% of patients with AS have coexisting coronary disease.[1] These valves are heavily calcified, with nodular calcified plaques, impeding movement of the valve leaflets (Fig. 59-1, *A*). This degenerative calcific process may involve the conduction system of the heart as well, leading to atrioventricular block, and may also involve the adjacent mitral valve

apparatus, causing mitral regurgitation (MR). The latter problem of coexisting severe AS and MR is extremely difficult to manage and carries a particularly poor prognosis.

Aortic stenosis may also result from a congenitally bicuspid valve. Bicuspid AS is the most common congenital cardiac anomaly, occurring in about 1% of the population.[2] Symptoms related to severe bicuspid AS usually do not become manifest until the fifth and sixth decades of life, when fibrosis and calcification of the valve further impede its function (Fig. 59-1, *B*).

Rheumatic AS is less frequently encountered. It rarely exists alone; rather, it is most often associated with coexisting rheumatic involvement of the mitral valve. This inflammatory process causes scarring of the aortic valve cusps and fusion of individual leaflets (Fig. 59-1, *C*). The valvular deformity may lead to subsequent calcification, further impeding valve mobility. Rheumatic involvement of the aortic valve may also result in poor leaflet coaptation and is often associated with significant aortic insufficiency.

Regardless of the cause, AS is usually a progressive disease manifesting with symptoms of congestive heart failure, angina, or both. Sudden death caused by AS,

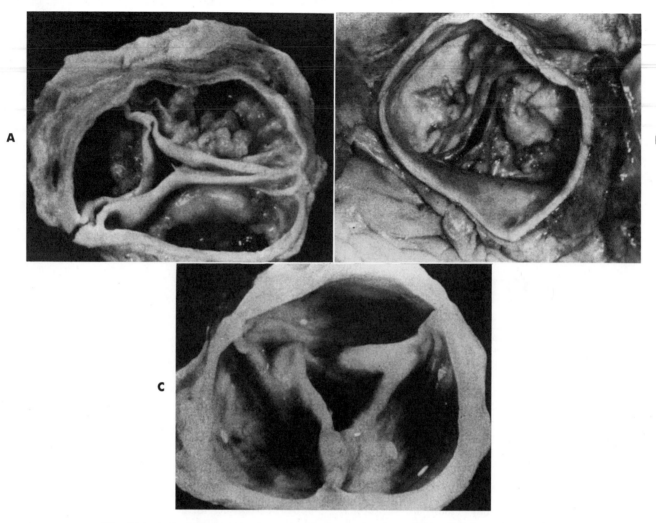

Fig. 59-1. A, Postmortem specimen showing degenerative calcific aortic stenosis. Note the nodular calcified plaque in the aortic valve sinuses. **B,** Postmortem specimen showing congenital bicuspid aortic stenosis. Note also the calcified plaque in both valve cusps. **C,** Postmortem specimen showing rheumatic aortic stenosis. Note the thickening and fusion of the commissures. (From Sutton GC, Anderson RH [eds]: *Slide atlas of cardiology,* London, 1978, Medi-Cine Productions.)

although often talked about, is unusual in the absence of preceding angina or heart failure symptoms.

The increased afterload created by aortic outflow obstruction stimulates compensatory left ventricular (LV) hypertrophy by mechanisms still unclear. This hypertrophy not only can lead to subendocardial ischemia and angina but also can impair LV diastolic function and filling and produce symptoms of pulmonary congestion.[3] Hypertrophy involves both individual myocytes and interstitial myocardial collagen. When compensatory hypertrophy is inadequate to reduce LV wall stress or when other diseases of the myocardium coexist (e.g., ischemic coronary artery disease), the systolic function of the ventricle deteriorates. Inappropriate LV dilation ensues. When this occurs, fatigue because of low output may be the major presenting complaint. Although

diastolic dysfunction of the left ventricle regardless of systolic function leads to congestive symptoms, LV systolic function (i.e., ejection fraction) has been shown to be the single most powerful predictor of survival in this disease[4] despite its afterload dependence.

Patients with severe AS commonly develop progressive symptoms of heart failure and angina, culminating in pulmonary edema and respiratory failure. The development of atrial fibrillation with loss of the atrial "kick" and shortening of the diastolic filling period may be hemodynamically catastrophic and cause abrupt pulmonary edema. In addition, myocardial infarction caused by coexisting coronary disease precipitates pulmonary edema not infrequently in these patients.

Syncope in patients with AS is usually multifactorial. It may be caused by profound peripheral vasodilation as a result of stimulation of LV baroreceptors, because the LV pressure rises during exercise or periods of stress. Syncope may also result from atrial or ventricular tachyarrhythmias or may be caused by AV block from associated degenerative, calcific disease of the conduction system. Treatment of the latter condition with transvenous pacing may be lifesaving, because patients with critical AS tolerate bradycardia and hypotension poorly.

In the acute care setting, prompt recognition of AS by physical examination is critical, although the classic findings may be lacking in some patients, particularly the elderly. Patients with AS usually have normal or low systolic blood pressure; conversely, it is unusual (but possible) for a patient with a systolic blood pressure of 170 mm Hg or more to have severe AS. The normal LV is capable of generating up to 340 to 350 mm Hg peak pressure. The characteristic high-pitched crescendo-decrescendo systolic murmur is usually best appreciated at the right upper sternal border and radiates to the base of the neck and carotid arteries. As the lesion severity worsens, the murmur peaks progressively later in systole and may also produce a systolic thrill. The delayed, plateaued carotid pulse (pulsus parvus et tardus) is helpful when present but may be masked by "stiff" peripheral vessels in the elderly. If the aortic valve is mobile, an aortic ejection click may be appreciated in early systole. With severe AS this ejection sound is lost, and the aortic closure sound is also characteristically diminished or absent because of the decreased mobility of the valve. The pulmonary closure sound may be accentuated in patients who have developed pulmonary hypertension. An audible and often palpable atrial filling wave (S4) is frequently present, and the apical impulse is characteristically sustained. When systolic LV failure ensues, the apical impulse becomes enlarged and a third heart sound may be present. The systolic murmur of AS is often appreciated at the apex, as well as the base, of the heart. The apical murmur may have a higher frequency and be more blowing in quality (the Gallaverdin phenomenon), making the distinction with coexisting MR more difficult. A key distinction is that the aortic murmur begins after closure of the mitral valve (S1) and ends before aortic closure (S2). In contrast, the murmur of MR blurs S1 and usually continues through S2 until mitral valve opening occurs.

Noninvasive evaluation of valvular heart disease with two-dimensional and Doppler echocardiography has revolutionized the evaluation of AS. Echocardiography typically demonstrates thickened aortic valve leaflets with reduced mobility. Short-axis views of the aortic valve usually can differentiate bicuspid from tricuspid valves. Estimation of the LV systolic function is also available. The presence of mitral annular calcification and the severity of any coexisting MR can also be estimated from the color-flow Doppler images. Heavily calcified mitral valves, however, may cause "shadowing" of the Doppler signal and thereby reduce the accuracy of estimates of MR severity.

The severity of AS can be semiquantitatively assessed using continuous-wave Doppler. The peak velocity (V) of the Doppler signal in m/sec can be converted to the peak *instantaneous* pressure gradient in mm Hg (P) across the valve by the equation: $P = 4V^2$. The valve area can also be estimated from the Doppler gradient using the continuity equation that assumes the area under the valve times the peak velocity of blood flow is equal to the area times peak velocity in the valvular orifice:

$$A_1V_1 = A_2V_2 \text{ or } AVA = \frac{A_1 \cdot V_1}{V_2}$$

where A_1 is the area of aortic annulus measured just beneath the aortic valve, V_1 is the mean Doppler velocity measured at site of A_1, and V_2 is the mean Doppler velocity in the maximum aortic Doppler profile just downstream from the aortic valve. This technique is quite reliable and correlates reasonably well with hemodynamically derived gradients and valve areas, but a few points of caution need be made in interpreting these data. In the presence of significantly reduced LV function, a moderate gradient (i.e., peak Doppler velocity of 3.5-4.0 m/sec) may be associated with severe AS; the absence of a high gradient is caused by decreased flow across the valve. This is at least partially compensated for in the continuity equation, as this equation takes into account a reduced LV outflow tract velocity in this situation. More important, errors in the acquisition and interpretation of the raw Doppler signal can lead to gross errors in the interpretation of the severity of the gradient. Whenever it is difficult to collect the Doppler sample from the maximum jet of blood, the severity of the aortic Doppler gradient may be lower than the true gradient (Fig. 59-2, *A*). This can be identified by noting an erratic continuous-wave Doppler envelope. The Doppler signal from coexistent MR may also be mistakenly interpreted as that from AS (Fig. 59-2, *B*). This is especially true when the MR jet is directed anteriorly and medially toward the interatrial septum and the ascending aorta (Fig. 59-3). This problem should be suspected when the aortic valve appears fairly mobile by two-dimensional imaging, yet the Doppler velocity profile suggests critical AS.

Symptomatic adults with AS by clinical and echocardiographic evaluation should undergo cardiac catheterization, including coronary angiography. By fluoroscopy the aortic valve is almost invariably calcified. Decreased cusp mobility can be visualized during ventriculography and ascending aortography. Ventriculography defines the presence and severity of associated MR, as well as

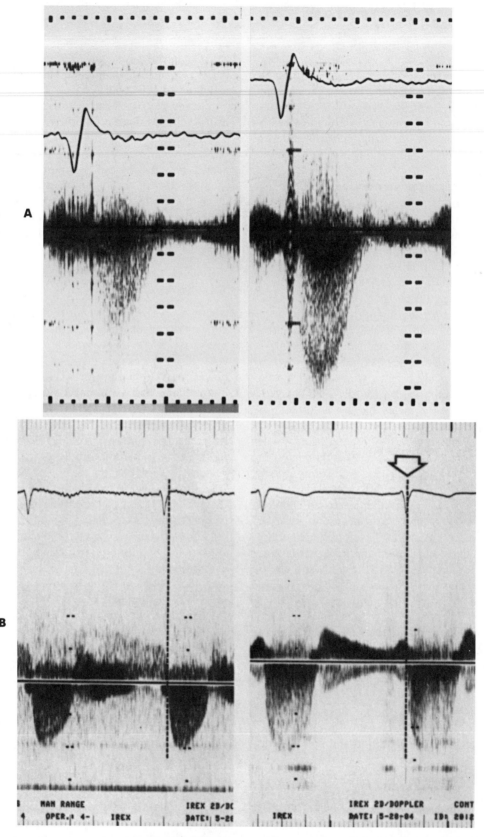

Fig. 59-2. A, Continuous-wave Doppler evaluation of aortic stenosis. *Panel A,* Note the erratic quality of the Doppler contour. The Doppler signal is not being sampled from the maximum velocity jet and thus underestimates the severity of the aortic stenosis. *Panel B,* The maximum Doppler signal is recorded, thus estimating the true severity of the aortic stenosis. **B,** Continuous-wave Doppler signals of aortic stenosis *(panel A)* and mitral regurgitation, *(panel B).* Note their similarity and ease with which they may be confused. In *panel A,* the Doppler signal of aortic stenosis begins slightly later following the QRS complex and has a more rounded contour.

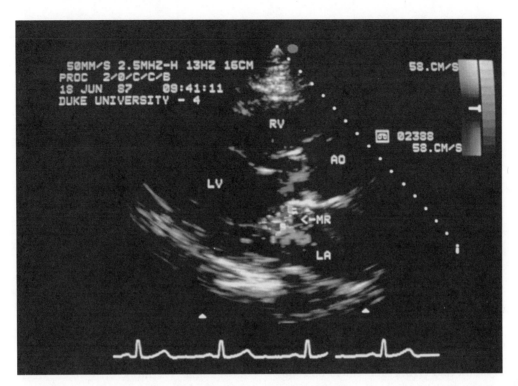

Fig. 59-3. Two-dimensional, Doppler echocardiogram demonstrating mitral regurgitation, which is directed anteriorly just beneath the LV outflow tract. This results from improper leaflet coaptation with relative posterior leaflet "prolapse." *MR,* Doppler color-flow mitral regurgitation; *LA,* left atrium; *LV,* left ventricle; *AO,* aorta; *RV,* right ventricle.

LV systolic function. Aortography defines the severity of aortic insufficiency. Dilation of the ascending aorta is not uncommon in patients with bicuspid aortic valves. Calcification of the ascending aorta itself may also be apparent. Occasionally "egg shell" calcification is seen extensively throughout the aorta and is associated with a brittle "porcelain" aorta. This type of aorta presents poor tissue for the surgeon to sew into and increases the risk of fragmentation and embolization during aortic cross-clamping.

The aortic valve gradient is most accurately determined by simultaneous measurement of LV and aortic pressures. This can be accomplished using a catheter with 2 micromanometer pressure transducers (Millar), using a double-lumen, fluid-filled catheter by "pullback" from the left ventricle to the aorta with superimposition of the pressure tracings or by simultaneous LV and peripheral artery pressures being recorded. When the latter technique is used, any difference between the peripheral artery and central aortic pressure must be adjusted for.

Once the pressure gradient is recorded, the peak-to-peak gradient, the mean gradient, and the peak instantaneous gradient can be determined (Fig. 59-4); the peak *instantaneous* gradient is similar to the peak Doppler velocity. The aortic valve area may determined by use of the Gorlin formula.[5] The Gorlin formula assumes

laminar flow (obviously not truly present) and is derived from the mean pressure gradient, the flow across the valve (the cardiac output), and the length of time the valve is open per minute (the systolic ejection period):

$$\text{Aortic valve area} = \frac{\text{CO}/(\text{HR SEP})}{44.3 \sqrt{\text{mean gradient}}}$$

where CO is cardiac output, HR is heart rate, SEP is systolic ejection period, and 44.3 is an empiric constant. A rough estimate of the aortic valve area can be made by simply dividing the cardiac output by the square root of the mean gradient.

The cardiac output is the most difficult part of this equation to determine accurately and is thus the weakest link in all hemodynamic valve area calculations. The Fick is the most accurate method of determining output, especially at low outputs, but this requires measurement of the arterovenous oxygen difference and *measurement* of oxygen consumption using a metabolic cart or similar instrument. Thermodilution techniques are inherently less accurate, especially in low-output states and in the presence of associated tricuspid regurgitation (TR; see previous chapter). To complicate matters further, in the presence of moderate or more severe aortic regurgitation (AR), the angiographic cardiac output must be used to define the aortic valve flow (i.e., forward plus regurgitant flow). Angiographic output is determined

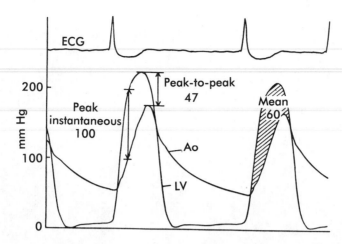

Fig. 59-4. Simultaneously left ventricular *(LV)* and aortic pressures *(Ao)* are shown in a patient with aortic stenosis. Various types of pressure gradient measurements, including the peak instantaneous, peak to peak, and mean gradient *(shaded area)*, are illustrated. The peak Doppler echocardiographic measurement correlates with the peak instantaneous hemodynamic measurement, whereas the mean gradient is used in the Gorlin equation for hemodynamically calculating the aortic valve area. (From Bashore, TM [ed]: *Invasive cardiology: principles and techniques,* Philadelphia, 1990, BC Decker, p 258. Used by permission.)

from ventriculography, and errors inherent in absolute volume measurements make it the least accurate of the three. Thus, when discrepancies arise between Doppler and hemodynamic indices of valvular stenosis severity, the strengths and the potential sources of error inherent in each technique need to be considered.

Acute management of AS in the CCU

The management of the critically ill patient with AS is treacherous. Patients with pulmonary edema and respiratory failure often require airway intubation and mechanical ventilation. In addition to improving pulmonary gas exchange and acid-base disturbances, this allows blood flow going to the respiratory muscles (which may be up to 30% of the cardiac output in this situation) to be redirected to the kidneys, which may result in profound diuresis and hemodynamic stabilization.

New-onset atrial fibrillation in patients with AS should be promptly terminated using electrical cardioversion, especially when associated with pulmonary edema, angina, or hypotension. Intravenous (IV) procainamide may be useful in less emergent instances or to maintain sinus rhythm after cardioversion. Ventricular arrhythmias require prompt treatment as well. Nonsustained ventricular tachycardia usually responds to treatment with IV lidocaine in concert with continued efforts directed toward improving hemodynamic, acid-base, and electrolyte derangements.

IV diuretics are the mainstay of treatment for pulmonary congestion, but like most other medical treatments for AS, even diuretics are potentially hazardous. Patients with AS and LV hypertrophy, with or without decreased systolic function, may require elevated LV diastolic pressures to maintain ventricular filling, stroke volume,

and cardiac output. Overly rapid, aggressive diureses may precipitate life-threatening hypotension. Invasive hemodynamic monitoring is helpful in critically ill patients with AS, especially when there is congestive heart failure (CHF) with associated borderline or low systolic pressures. Although there is no "magic" number, pulmonary capillary wedge (PCW) pressures of 15 to 20 mm Hg are generally associated with clinical and radiographic improvement. Because some patients have very stiff ventricles and clinically may be used to filling pressures in the 20 to 25 mm Hg range, the lowest PCW pressure at which adequate cardiac output and peripheral organ perfusion are maintained should be the goal. The level is frequently higher than that one would strive to achieve in patients with coronary disease alone. With a pulmonary artery catheter, one can frequently ensure that additional diureses is not associated with significant decrease in thermodilution cardiac output or widening of the arteriovenous oxygen difference. Systemic hypotension in AS patients needs to be avoided at all cost. Even prompt, aggressive cardiopulmonary resuscitation is usually unsuccessful in these patients with their increased myocardial blood flow requirements and LV outflow obstruction.

In patients with angina or congestive failure associated with hypotension, intraaortic balloon pump counterpulsation (IABP) can improve coronary flow. These devices, however, have less effect on afterload reduction because of the fixed outflow obstruction created by the AS and carry significant risk, especially in the elderly, in whom aortic atherosclerosis and peripheral vascular disease are common. In addition, IABP may worsen aortic insufficiency, and these devices are contraindicated in patients with more than mild AR. The potential risks and benefits of IABP therapy need to be considered in each case.

Coronary disease coexists in 50% of adult patients with AS. Aspirin and IV heparin are beneficial in those suspected of coexistent coronary disease, especially patients with angina, electrocardiographic (ECG) changes suggesting ischemia, or with serum evidence of myocardial damage. IV nitroglycerin may also be beneficial in the treatment of angina or pulmonary congestion in patients with AS. Like diuretics, IV nitrates must be used cautiously, often in conjunction with invasive monitoring to ensure that LV preload (PCW pressure) does not drop too rapidly and decrease cardiac output. In addition, IV nitrates decrease afterload and can cause hypotension. Mild afterload reduction associated with IV nitrates may improve cardiac output in the subgroup of patients with systolic pressures 130 mm Hg or more. This, however, is not predictable and needs to be documented by invasive monitoring.

More powerful afterload reducing agents such as IV nitroprusside should be avoided. Nitroprusside does not cause significant increase in cardiac output because of the fixed aortic valve obstruction and profound peripheral vasodilation from the drug can result in life-threatening hypotension.

Digoxin, given intravenously or orally, is important in controlling the ventricular response rate of those patients in atrial fibrillation. As pointed out earlier, rapid atrial fibrillation associated with hypotension, pulmonary edema, or angina should be corrected immediately with electrical cardioversion. Digoxin may be beneficial as an inotropic agent, at least in the short term, in patients with AS and depressed LV systolic function, but it is not of benefit and may further impair diastolic function in patients with LV hypertrophy and preserved systolic function.

β-Blockers and calcium channel blockers generally should be avoided in critically ill patients with severe AS. In the subgroup with impaired LV systolic function, they can cause worsening heart failure and can precipitate hypotension. However, in patients with LV hypertrophy and preserved systolic function, these agents may prove to be of benefit for congestive failure or angina refractory to other treatments. They may improve the intrinsic diastolic function of the myocardium. Their major effect, however, is slowing of the sinus rate, thereby decreasing myocardial oxygen requirements and increasing the diastolic filling period. β-Blockers are more effective in this respect than calcium channel blockers and IV esmolol is an optimal initial choice because of its short half-life. This drug can be instituted cautiously in low doses with invasive monitoring of the hemodynamic response. In contrast to the beneficial effects and routine use of β-blockers in patients with isolated coronary artery disease, the use of β-blockers in severe AS is potentially quite

Table 59-1. Acute treatment of CHF in patients with severe aortic stenosis*

Monitoring
Keep PCW in 15-20 mm Hg range depending on CO
Pharmacologic therapy
Effective
Diuretics (intravenous)
Arrhythmia control
Selectively useful
Nitrates
Digoxin
Low-dose inotropic agents
Aortic balloon counterpulsation
Calcium channel blockers
β-Blockers
Avoid
Most inotropic agents
Afterload reduction (nitroprusside, ACE inhibitors)
High-dose calcium blockers

*CHF, Congestive heart failure; PCW, pulmonary capillary wedge; CO, cardiac output; ACE, angiotensin-converting enzyme.

hazardous, and their use should be the exception rather than the rule.

In patients with profound hypertrophy or associated hypertrophic cardiomyopathy and AS, use of calcium channel blockers and β-blockers may reduce the heart rate and improve diastolic filling time. In addition, these agents may improve diastolic relaxation. These benefits may improve diastolic filling and reduce pulmonary congestion.

Although IV inotropic agents may be beneficial in selected patients with AS associated with reduced LV systolic function, they can also be hazardous and their effects may be paradoxic. As is the case with other cardiac disease states, IV dopamine and dobutamine can precipitate ischemia and tachyarrhythmias. More importantly, inotropic agents in patients with AS can precipitate paradoxical, profound hypotension. Recall that normotensive patients with AS may have LV systolic pressures in excess of 200 to 300 mm Hg. Inotropic agents, such as dobutamine, may further increase LV systolic pressure and stimulate LV baroreceptors, leading to profound reflex peripheral vasodilation. This vasodilation, with the relatively fixed cardiac output reserve because of the AS, can result in life-threatening hypotension. In addition, in patients with combined AS and MR, IV inotropes may increase the severity of the MR and worsen pulmonary congestion. This can be recognized by an increasing PCW pressure with an increasing V wave. Thus, in patients with depressed LV systolic function refractory to other measures, inotropic agents may be tried with careful invasive monitoring. We recommend beginning with very low doses (e.g., 2.5 μg/kg/min) of dobutamine and slowly increasing the dose with frequent hemodynamic measurements, realizing that paradoxical effects of

Table 59-2. Estimates of operative risk*

Operation†	Operative mortality (%)
CABG	1-2
AVR ± CABG	2-5
MVR	5-10
MVR + CABG	10-15

*Advanced age, advanced functional class, reduced left ventricular ejection fraction, cardiogenic shock, need for emergency surgery negatively influence the operative risk.
†CABG, Coronary artery bypass grafting; AVR, aortic valve replacement; MVR, mitral valve replacement.

these drugs may be encountered, requiring prompt discontinuation of the drug.

Vasoconstricting agents that further increase afterload, such as norepinephrine, should be avoided. In cases of cardiogenic shock, this drug must occasionally be used to restore blood pressure until other supportive measures such as insertion of an IABP can be accomplished. The prognosis of such patients is obviously extremely poor.

Thus, critically ill patients with AS are a tremendous challenge in even the most sophisticated and well equipped cardiac care units (CCUs). Table 59-1 summarizes the approach on the CCU when these patients have CHF.

Aortic valvular procedures

Aortic valve replacement remains the best therapeutic choice for patients with severe AS. Aortic valve replacement, with or without coronary bypass grafting, carries an operative mortality of about 5% (Table 59-2).[6-8] The strongest predictors of operative mortality have been poor preoperative functional class and advanced age.[8] Double-valve surgery requiring aortic and mitral valve replacement increases the operative mortality to about 10% to 15%.[7,9] Thus, for patients with severe AS and mild to moderate MR, aortic valve replacement alone may be prudent. The subsequent decrease in LV systolic pressure and decrease in LV chamber size may serve to eventually reduce the severity of the MR.[10]

Efforts toward aortic valve repair, with preservation of the native valve, have generally been unsatisfactory. Recently aortic valve decalcification with an ultrasonic calcium-debriding device showed improvement in the severity of stenosis, but the majority developed significant aortic regurgitation (AR) and we have abandoned this technique.[11]

Balloon aortic valvuloplasty has been increasingly employed over the past decade. Although the immediate hemodynamic results of this procedure were encouraging, the 6-month valvular restenosis rate is about 75%.[1] One-year survival after balloon aortic valvuloplasty is poor (65% in our experience[4]), and thus we consider balloon aortic valvuloplasty for palliative use only. It may be of symptomatic benefit in patients with symptoms of

heart failure or angina who are not surgical candidates because of coexisting illness. It may also be of benefit in patients with refractory congestive failure caused by AS and severely depressed LV systolic function in whom surgery is not possible because of continued pulmonary edema. In this circumstance balloon aortic valvuloplasty may be useful as a bridge to improve ventricular function and CHF before valve replacement. If ventricular function improves, this occurs within the first month after balloon valvuloplasty, and surgery needs to be performed in this time frame before restenosis occurs and LV function again deteriorates. With these rare exceptions, balloon aortic valvuloplasty should not be advised, and surgical aortic valve replacement remains the procedure of choice for the overwhelming majority of these patients.

HYPERTROPHIC CARDIOMYOPATHY

Hypertrophic cardiomyopathy or idiopathic hypertrophic subaortic stenosis (IHSS) is similar to AS in several respects. Both diseases have in common LV outflow obstruction and marked LV hypertrophy, resulting in impaired diastolic function and filling of the left ventricle. Although many of the hallmark physical findings in patients with IHSS are caused by the dynamic LV outflow obstruction, the major pathophysiology in this disease is related to LV diastolic dysfunction.

As with AS, these patients typically manifest clinically with symptoms of heart failure, angina, or syncope. Anginal symptoms are related to the extreme ventricular hypertrophy and subendocardial ischemia. Epicardial coronary obstructive disease is much less common than in AS. The preserved systolic ventricular function in these patients with severe CHF initially appears paradoxical, and the mainstay of treatment (β-blockers and calcium channel blockers) are in contrast to that employed for the more common patient with CHF caused by impaired systolic function.

Diagnosis

Physical examination and echocardiography are critical in making the proper diagnosis. A bisferiens character to the carotid and peripheral pulses may be appreciated. This is caused by the initial rapid ejection, attenuated late systolic aortic flow resulting from the LV outflow obstruction, followed by the augmented reflected pressure waves caused by the rapid early ejection. The apical impulse is sustained, and a palpable atrial filling wave is often present. The systolic murmur has a crescendo-decrescendo quality, is loudest along the upper sternal border, and may produce a palpable thrill. Unlike severe AS, the aortic closure sound in IHSS is preserved. In addition, diagnostic maneuvers that decrease preload, such as standing or Valsalva, increase the systolic murmur of IHSS, whereas these maneuvers have the opposite effect in AS. In addition, AR or MR may also be present in

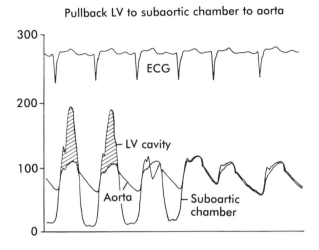

Pullback LV to subaortic chamber to aorta

Fig. 59-5. The intraventricular systolic gradient *(shaded area)* in idiopathic hypertrophic subaortic stenosis *(IHSS)* is demonstrated by simultaneous measurement of the left ventricular and aortic pressures as the catheter is withdrawn from deep in the left ventricular chamber *(left),* into the outflow area (subaortic chamber center), and then into the ascending aorta *(right).* No aortic valve gradient is demonstrated. (From Bashore TM [ed]: *Invasive cardiology: principles and techniques,* Philadelphia, 1990, BC Decker, p 271. Used by permission.)

patients with IHSS, and these murmurs may be appreciated on examination as well.

Echocardiography demonstrates severe LV hypertrophy. The ventricular cavity is usually small, and there may be near obliteration of the LV chamber at end-systole. Asymmetric hypertrophy of the septum is apparent. A Doppler gradient in the LV outflow may be evident at rest or can be precipitated by afterload reduction with amyl nitrate. Recall that the anterior leaflet of the mitral valve makes up part of the LV outflow tract. With the increased blood flow velocity through the LV outflow, the pressure around the accelerated blood flow drops (the Venturi effect), and the mitral leaflet is pulled into the LV outflow. This is referred to as systolic anterior motion (SAM) in echocardiography and may contribute to the dynamic left ventricular outflow tract obstruction observed. Doppler color-flow imaging will also demonstrate associated mitral or aortic insufficiency.

Noninvasive diagnosis of this disease can be made in almost all cases using two-dimensional Doppler echocardiography. Cardiac catheterization is confirmatory in this disease and is used to exclude associated coronary disease. Systolic contraction ("bridging") of the coronary vessels is often observed. A systolic pressure gradient can be demonstrated in the LV outflow tract beneath the aortic valve (Fig. 59-5). The decrease in the aortic pulse pressure after a premature ventricular contraction (Brockenbrough's phenomenon) is characteristic of IHSS (Fig. 59-6).

Acute therapy in the CCU

IV inotropes and digoxin, drugs routinely used to treat CHF because of systolic dysfunction, may worsen

CHF caused by hypertrophic cardiomyopathy. Afterload reduction also adversely affects patients with IHSS by further decreasing LV cavity size. Because symptoms are primarily a function of diastolic dysfunction, β-blockers and calcium channel blockers are the drugs of choice in hypertrophic cardiomyopathies. These drugs improve the intrinsic diastolic performance of the myocardium and, importantly, slow the sinus rate and lengthen the diastolic filling period. High doses of these drugs may be required, but the majority of patients can be effectively treated medically. Digoxin increases contractility by increasing calcium movement into the cytosol. The increased calcium cytosol may reduce cellular relaxation because the cell may be less able to remove calcium from a contractile apparatus. Digoxin thus may worsen the hemodynamics in IHSS by reducing diastolic relaxation. Calcium channel blockers reduce intracellular calcium and thus improve early relaxation.

As in AS, it is important to try to maintain sinus rhythm. Atrial contribution to forward output may be critical in patients with IHSS, and atrial fibrillation must be rapidly controlled and converted to prevent significant deterioration. Mitral annular calcium is common. MR may be present because of the systolic anterior motion of the mitral leaflet or annular calcium. MR is poorly tolerated in these patients and may predispose to atrial fibrillation.

Surgery with septal myomectomy is only occasionally required for IHSS patients with refractory symptoms or those unable to tolerate medical therapy. The pathophysiology of the clinical improvement after myomectomy is not completely clear, because it is the diastolic abnormalities rather than the outflow gradient that primarily determine the symptoms of this disease. Because the mitral valve is inherently involved in the pathophysiology of the disorder, mitral valve replacement has been advocated by some. Table 59-3 summarizes the management strategy.

Aortic regurgitation

The management of aortic regurgitation (AR) critically depends on the acuity of the valvular dysfunction. Patients with new-onset, acute AR need to be distinguished from patients with symptoms caused by chronic aortic valve leakage. The former disease process is hemodynamically distinct, because LV dilation and hypertrophy have not had time to develop (Fig. 59-7). Severe acute AR can progress rapidly from an asymptomatic state to severe CHF and death, and prompt surgical intervention is mandatory.

Acute AR

Acute AR is most often associated with endocarditis. Other etiologies include aortic dissection, trauma or connective tissue disorders, and rupture of a sinus of Valsalva's aneurysm (Table 59-4).

Patients with acute AR may abruptly develop pul-

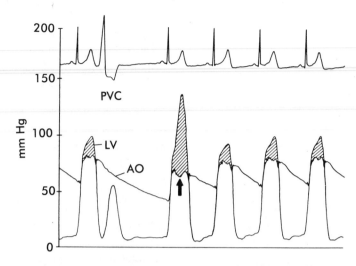

Fig. 59-6. Simultaneous measurement of the left ventricular and aortic pressure in idiopathic hypertrophic subaortic stenosis demonstrating the Brockenbrough phenomenon. The electrocardiogram is shown at the top of the panel. After a premature ventricular contraction *(PVC)*, the aortic systolic pressure is lower *(arrow)* than the baseline aortic systolic pressure. After the PVC, the compensatory pause results in a fall in aortic pressure (reduced afterload), and the contractility of the ventricle is increased in the post-PVC beat. The combination of reduced afterload and increased contractility results in greater left ventricular outflow obstruction. This causes the reduction in aortic systolic pressure and increase in the systolic interventricular gradient *(shaded)*. (From Bashore TM [ed]: *Invasive cardiology: principles and techniques,* Philadelphia, 1990, BC Decker, p 272. Used by permission.)

Table 59-3. Acute treatment of CHF in patients with hypertrophic cardiomyopathy*

Monitoring
  Keep PCW in 15-20 mm Hg range depending on CO
Pharmacologic therapy
  Effective
    Diuretics
    Arrhythmia control
    Calcium channel blockers
    β-Blockers
  Selectively useful
    Nitrates
  Avoid
    Inotropic agents
    Digoxin
    Afterload reduction (ACE inhibitors, nitroprusside)

*CHF, Congestive heart failure; *PCW*, pulmonary capillary wedge; *ACE*, angiotensin-converting enzyme.

Table 59-4. Causes of aortic insufficiency

A. Bacterial endocarditis
B. Rheumatic disease
C. Degenerative calcific disease
D. Traumatic valve rupture
E. Bicuspid aortic valve
F. Aneurysm of sinus of Valsalva
G. Congenital cusp fenestration
H. Associated subvalvular aortic stenosis
I. Aortic dissection
J. Ankylosing spondylitis
K. Reiter's disease
L. Rheumatoid arthritis
M. Associated with aortic root dilation
  1. Chronic hypertension
  2. Cystic medial necrosis/annuloaortic ectasia
    a. Marfan syndrome
    b. Idiopathic
  3. Syphilis
  4. Ehlers-Danlos syndrome

monary edema. Angina may occur in the absence of coronary disease because of reduced coronary perfusion pressure from the low aortic diastolic pressure and high LV diastolic pressure. On examination, a resting tachycardia is invariably present, but the wide pulse pressure characteristic of chronic AR is often lacking. The aortic closure sound is diminished or absent. The decrescendo diastolic blowing murmur is usually loudest at the left sternal border. The murmur may diminish or abate in late diastole. As the severity of the aortic insufficiency worsens, the murmur may become almost inaudible as pressures equalize in early diastole between the aorta and left ventricle. This disappearance of the diastolic murmur in association with worsening pulmonary edema is an ominous physical finding. The first heart sound is often diminished in intensity because of partial opposition of the mitral valve leaflets

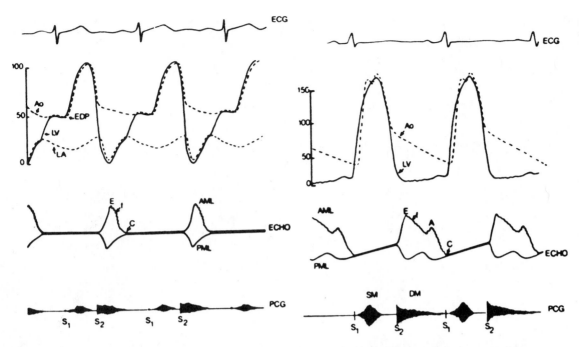

Fig. 59-7. Hemodynamic, echocardiographic *(ECHO)*, and phonocardiographic *(PCG)* manifestations of acute severe *(panel A)* and chronic aortic insufficiency *(panel B)*. Acute aortic regurgitation *(panel A)* results in a marked, steep increase in left ventricular diastolic pressure *(EDP)*. Note also that the aortic pulse pressure *(Ao)* is normal and the left atrial pressure *(LA)* is elevated. The M-mode echocardiogram *(ECHO)* demonstrates premature closure of the mitral valve *(C)* and the phonocardiogram *(PCG)* demonstrates the abbreviated duration of the diastolic murmur after S_2. In chronic severe aortic regurgitation *(panel B)*, the left ventricular end-diastolic pressures may be normal, and the characteristic widened aortic pressure *(Ao)* is demonstrated. The mitral valve closes normally at the onset of left ventricular systole, and the diastolic murmur is apparent throughout diastole. (From Morganroth JL: *Ann Intern Med* 87:225, 1977. Used by permission.)

before ventricular systole (mitral preclosure). An S_3 gallop is often audible because of the rapid diastolic reflux of blood.

Echocardiography may help define the cause of AR (e.g., vegetations in endocarditis, aortic tear in dissection). The left ventricle is usually hypercontractile and not significantly dilated. Color-flow Doppler imaging can help assess the severity of the AR (Fig. 59-8). Occasionally, however, if the AR is extremely severe, little turbulence exists because of rapid equalization of aortic and LV diastolic pressures, and thus no diastolic Doppler flow pattern is identifiable. Fluttering of the anterior mitral valve leaflet is seen on M-mode and two-dimensional imaging. In addition, mitral valve "preclosure" (Fig. 59-9) before ventricular systole can be identified, indicating severe aortic insufficiency. This sign warrants preparation for surgical intervention. The echocardiogram should also be used to evaluate other structural abnormalities that may need to be corrected during surgery (e.g., multiple valve endocarditis, aortic root disease). In patients with angina or adults at risk for coronary disease, coronary angiography should be emergently performed before

surgery. It must be emphasized, however, that there should be minimal delay in getting these patients to surgery. One must especially resist the temptation to get a few doses of antibiotics into patients with aortic endocarditis and severe acute AR, because surgical delay may be life-threatening in this condition. Many patients can proceed to surgery based only on the echocardiographic findings.

Medical treatment is aimed at temporary stabilization in preparation for valve replacement. Invasive hemodynamic monitoring is useful. Mechanical ventilation may be required and may also help provide hemodynamic stability. IV diuretics are required to reduce preload and improve pulmonary congestion. In those with normal or elevated systolic pressures, afterload reduction with IV nitroprusside may improve cardiac output and reduce pulmonary venous pressures. IV nitroglycerin is probably less effective than nitroprusside in this respect but may be the preferred drug in those with suspected coexistent coronary disease.

The majority of these patients are hyperadrenergic with hypercontractile left ventricles. Hypotension is an ominous sign. IV digoxin, dobutamine, or dopamine can

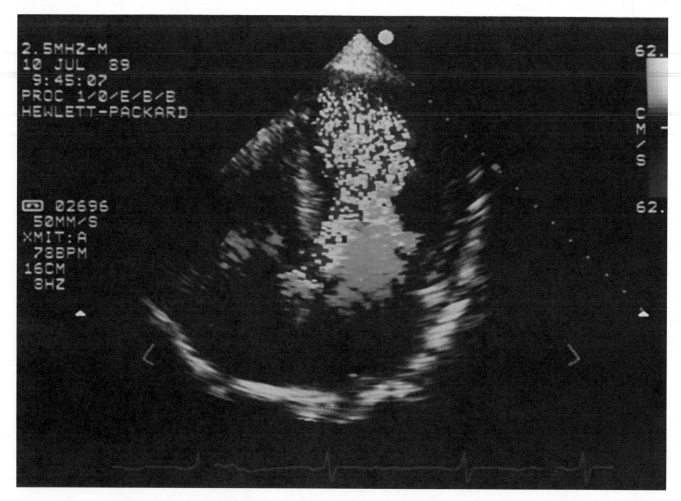

Fig. 59-8. Color-flow Doppler echocardiographic evaluation of severe aortic insufficiency. The diastolic color-flow Doppler mosaic fills the left ventricular chamber.

be employed for inotropic support for hypotensive patients with reduced LV systolic function. Arterial constricting drugs, β-blockers, and calcium channel blockers should be avoided. The slower the heart rate, the larger the diastolic time; brady arrhythmias should therefore be avoided. (In some patients, this may require pacemaker therapy.) IABP is contraindicated. It deserves emphasis that medical treatment in acute aortic insufficiency is useful only as a brief, temporizing measure in preparation for aortic valve replacement.

The operative mortality for valve replacement in acute aortic insufficiency is about 5%, whereas medically treated the condition is almost universally fatal.[12]

Chronic AR

Chronic aortic insufficiency may be tolerated for years but may eventually lead to symptoms of CHF. The left ventricle in this condition dilates and hypertrophies to compensate for the regurgitant volume, culminating in some of the largest ventricles encountered, so-called cor bovinum.

On physical examination, the pulse pressure is characteristically widened and may exceed 100 mm Hg. The diastolic pressure is usually less than 60 mm Hg with moderate or severe chronic AR. The carotid and peripheral pulses are hyperdynamic, with a rapid upstroke and fall in the arterial pressure. This basic hemodynamic phenomenon leads to the numerous peripheral stigmata, which carry various eponyms (Quincke's sign, Duroziez's sign, etc.). In addition, the increased stroke volume (forward plus regurgitant volume) leads to increased reflected pressure waves from the peripheral circulation. This is responsible for the increased systolic arterial pressure as one goes more peripherally, resulting in another physical finding in severe AR, Hill's sign (systolic pressure in the lower extremities exceeding that in the upper extremities by more than 40 mm Hg). In combined aortic stenosis and insufficiency, the increased reflected waves produce a bifid, bisferiens pulse that is often best detected in the brachial artery.

The apical impulse is often markedly enlarged and

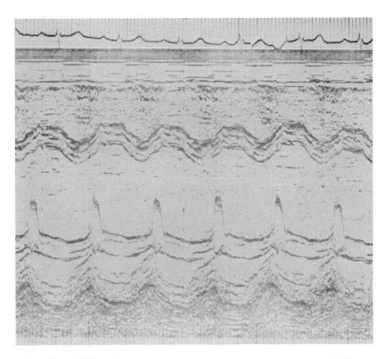

Fig. 59-9. M-mode echocardiogram in a patient with severe acute aortic regurgitation demonstrating mitral valve preclosure. The bottom part of the panel demonstrates the M-mode echocardiogram of the mitral valve showing closure of the valve before ventricular systole (onset of QRS complex). The ECG is shown at the top of the panel.

displaced laterally. There may be a palpable gallop associated with a loud S_3. The diastolic murmur is of blowing quality and is usually loudest at the left sternal border. It may, however, be most prominent at the right lower sternal border in those with associated dilation of the ascending aorta. The murmur is best heard with the patient sitting forward at end-expiration. The murmur may have a low-pitched rumbling quality at the apex (Austin-Flint murmur) simulating mitral stenosis. The aortic closure sound is often diminished or absent. The first heart sound may be diminished as well.

Echocardiography demonstrates a dilated left ventricle and fluttering of the anterior mitral valve leaflet caused by the regurgitant aortic jet. Doppler color-flow imaging can be used to estimate the severity of the aortic insufficiency (see Fig. 59-8). MR may be present in those with severe LV and mitral annular dilation or in patients with coexistent disease of the mitral valve. The diameter of the aortic root can be assessed by echocardiography as well.

Coronary angiography should be performed before surgery in adults. Catheterization is also of use in further defining the severity of AR and MR and in assessing the LV systolic function. One should realize that Doppler echocardiographic measurements are based on blood *velocity* profiles rather than *volume*. As such, Doppler echocardiography is very sensitive to picking up even small-volume, high-velocity turbulent flow. Thus, Dop-

pler echocardiography may *overestimate* the severity of valvular regurgitation and should be interpreted in conjunction with the physical examination and angiographic data. Angiography assesses the volume of regurgitant blood (contrast) and thus is affected by the volume of the blood without contrast in the chamber into which the contrast moves. Thus, when the regurgitant contrast leaks back into a large chamber, the contrast is "diluted" and the technique may thereby underestimate the severity of regurgitation. Thus, the severity of valvular regurgitation by any method can be only semiquantitated. In making therapeutic decisions, the clinician must integrate the physical examination, hemodynamic, echocardiographic, and angiographic data, realizing the strengths and weaknesses of each.

CHF caused by worsening chronic aortic insufficiency can be managed with a combination of preload reduction, afterload reduction, and inotropic agents. Diuretics, digoxin, nitrates, nitroprusside, angiotensin-converting enzyme (ACE) inhibitors, dopamine, and dobutamine in some combination may improve pulmonary congestion caused by AR. β-Blockers and calcium channel blockers should be avoided, especially in those with compromised LV systolic function. Unlike the emergent situation with acute aortic insufficiency, these patients are best treated medically toward resolution of their CHF. Once this is accomplished, cardiac catheterization can be performed and management decisions

Table 59-5. Acute treatment of CHF in patients with aortic regurgitation*

Monitoring
  Keep PCW in 15-20 mm Hg range depending on CO
Pharmacologic therapy
  Effective
    Diuretics
    Afterload reduction (nitroprusside, ACE inhibitors)
    Nitrates
    Inotropic agents
  Avoid
    β-Blockers
    Calcium channel blockers
    Intraaortic balloon pump counterpulsation

*CHF, Congestive heart failure; PCW, pulmonary capillary wedge; CO, cardiac output; ACE, angiotensin-converting enzyme.

Table 59-6. Causes of mitral regurgitation

A. Myxomatous degeneration
B. Rheumatic disease
C. Mitral valve prolapse
D. Annular stretching due to ventricular enlargement
E. Papillary muscle ischemia/infarction
F. Bacterial endocarditis
G. Associated with idiopathic hypertrophic stenosis
H. Connective tissue disorders
  1. Marfan syndrome
  2. Elhers-Danlos syndrome
I. Parachute mitral valve complex
J. Ruptured chordae
K. Degenerative mitral annular calcification
L. Libman-Sacks endocarditis (systemic lupus erythematosus)

made. Table 59-5 summarizes the medical approach to these patients.

The timing of surgical intervention for chronic aortic insufficiency is difficult. In the asymptomatic individual, if the aortic insufficiency is mild with preserved LV systolic function, patients may be managed medically for years with diuretics and afterload reduction. Systolic dysfunction may be masked, however, because of the effect of the altered loading conditions on measure of LV function such as the ejection fraction. Such patients should be followed for the development of symptoms and should have baseline and yearly evaluations of LV function using echocardiography, radionuclide angiography, or both. If the left ventricle begins to dilate or evidence exists that systolic function has begun to deteriorate, valve replacement should be strongly considered, even in the absence of symptoms.[13]

The prognosis of medically treated patients with symptoms caused by aortic insufficiency is poor. The median survival rate of patients with angina is 5 years, whereas it is 2 years for those with CHF symptoms.[14] In addition, if the AR is severe or the left ventricle is dilated or hypocontractile, valve replacement rather than medical therapy should initially be recommended even in the absence of symptoms. A severely dilated, hypocontractile left ventricle, however, increases the operative risk.[15] Although recovery of LV systolic function is the rule, it may be incomplete, even after successful aortic valve replacement.[16] The operative mortality from elective aortic valve replacement for aortic insufficiency is 5% to 10%.[6,8]

Mitral regurgitation

Mitral regurgitation (MR) in the CCU setting is frequently caused by ischemia but may also be caused by primary diseases of the mitral valve. A list of the more common etiologies of MR is shown in Table 59-6. MR secondary to ischemic myocardial disease is most com-

monly secondary to LV and mitral annular dilation. Papillary muscle ischemia or infarction may also cause MR. Although both papillary muscles potentially have dual blood supply, ischemia of the posteromedial papillary muscle causing MR is clinically more common, resulting from disease in the right coronary or circumflex coronary artery. Uncommonly, infarction may result in rupture of chordae and a flail mitral leaflet.

Primary disease of the mitral valve such as myxomatous degeneration or mitral annular calcification usually results in progressive symptoms of CHF. Abrupt pulmonary edema secondary to MR may result from rupture of a chordae associated with mitral valve prolapse or destruction of a leaflet in acute bacterial endocarditis.

In cases of acute, severe MR, the systolic blood pressure is usually low (<100 mm Hg), and there is a resting tachycardia. Patients may develop atrial fibrillation because of left atrial volume and pressure overload. The carotid pulse is often of decreased volume. The apical impulse is often enlarged and laterally displaced in those with chronic MR, whereas it may be unremarkable in those with acute MR. A gallop may be palpable as well and may be associated with a third or fourth heart sound. The characteristic holosystolic blowing murmur of MR is associated with a diminished or absent S_1 and most frequently radiates laterally from the apex toward the axilla. The direction of the regurgitant jet may lead to atypical radiation of the murmur, however, depending on the coaptation abnormality of the valve. This may result in radiation toward the aortic outflow region when the regurgitation is caused by posterior leaflet prolapse or radiation to the spine or occiput with a flail anterior leaflet. An early systolic click preceding the MR murmur suggests mitral valve prolapse as the cause of the disorder. The pulmonary closure sound may be accentuated in those who have developed pulmonary hypertension.

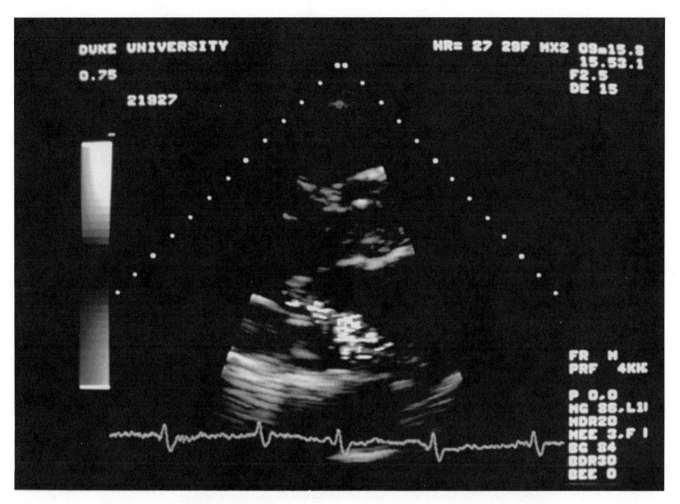

Fig. 59-10. Color-flow Doppler evaluation of mitral regurgitation caused by mitral valve anterior leaflet prolapse. Prolapse of the anterior mitral valve leaflet results in a regurgitant jet, demonstrated by color-flow Doppler, which is directed posteriorly and laterally toward the left atrial free wall.

Mitral valve morphology, determined by echocardiography, can often define the cause of the valvular regurgitation. The directional morphology of the color-flow Doppler regurgitant jet can also help define the cause of the regurgitation. Prolapse of one leaflet causes the jet to be directed in the opposite direction (Fig. 59-10). Posterior leaflet prolapse yields a regurgitant jet that is directed anteriorly and medially toward the atrial septum and ascending aorta (see Fig. 59-3). This type of regurgitation results in a murmur that radiates out the aortic outflow tract and can be confused with AS. In distinction to the murmur of aortic stenosis, however, this murmur has a blowing, holosystolic quality. It is not associated with a diminished A_2, and S_1 is diminished or absent. Occasionally in obese patients or when the MR is so severe that little turbulence results, the characteristic holosystolic murmur may be subtle or absent on physical examination. In addition, when the severity of MR is temporally dynamic, most commonly seen with ischemic MR, the murmur may vary greatly in intensity and, at times, be absent.

Invasive monitoring in the CCU can be useful in monitoring the results of pharmacologic interventions and may also be helpful diagnostically, demonstrating a large "C-V wave" when the diagnosis of MR is in doubt (Fig. 59-11). It must be realized, however, that the magnitude of the C-V wave does not depend solely on the severity of MR. For a given amount of MR, the C-V wave will be larger when the left atrial pressure is elevated and the atrium is noncompliant and already distended.

Diuresis and afterload reduction are the mainstays of medical treatment for MR. When the cause of the MR is ischemia, treatment is aimed toward resolution and prevention of further ischemia. Although β-blockers are generally avoided in patients with MR, they may be beneficial in patients with transient MR precipitated by coronary insufficiency. Inotropic agents (e.g., dob-

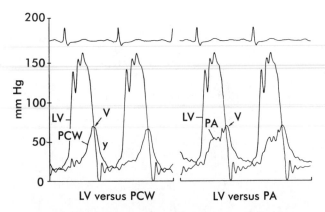

Fig. 59-11. Simultaneous recordings of left ventricular *(LV)* and pulmonary capillary wedge *(PCW)* pressure in a patient with severe mitral regurgitation is shown in the left panel. Note the large regurgitant V wave *(v)* in the PCW pressure tracing. The V wave is closely related temporally to the T wave of the electrocardiogram. In the right panel the V wave is evident even in the pulmonary artery *(PA)* pressure tracing. (From Bashore TM [ed]: *Invasive cardiology: principles and techniques,* Philadelphia, 1990, BC Decker, p 267. Used by permission.)

Table 59-7. Acute treatment of CHF in patients with mitral regurgitation*

Monitoring
  PCW pressures do not reflect LVEDP
Pharmacologic therapy
  Effective
    Diuretics
    Afterload reduction (nitroprusside, ACE inhibitors)
    Nitrates
    Inotropic agents
    Arrhythmia control
    Digoxin
    Intraaortic balloon counterpulsation
  Selectively effective (in ischemic MR)
    β-Blockers
    Calcium channel blockers

*CHF, Congestive heart failure; *PCW*, pulmonary capillary wedge; *LVEDP*, left ventricular end-diastolic pressure; *ACE*, angiotensin-converting enzyme; *MR*, mitral regurgitation.

utamine) in combination with afterload reduction (e.g., nitroprusside) are often effective in clearing pulmonary edema. Afterload reduction is usually the initial treatment of choice. If necessary, inotropic agents may then be added, assessing their success by repeated hemodynamic measurements. Digoxin is often required to control the ventricular response rate in patients with atrial fibrillation. Digoxin may also be of some acute benefit as an inotropic agent. Once the acute CHF has cleared, oral afterload reduction with ACE inhibitors may be substituted. In the hypotensive patient with severe MR, IABP is extremely effective. This is especially true of the patient with severe acute MR caused by acute myocardial ischemia or infarction, where the use of the device may be lifesaving. In addition to improving coronary perfusion pressure, the device improves forward output and decreases pulmonary congestion through its mechanical effects on afterload reduction, thereby reducing the severity of MR. Table 59-7 summarizes the medical strategy for treating MR.

Cardiac catheterization should be performed once the patient is stabilized, evaluating coronary anatomy, the severity of mitral regurgitation, and LV systolic function. Like aortic insufficiency, the timing of mitral valve surgery for chronic MR is difficult. Mild to moderate MR associated with normal LV function can be successfully managed medically for years with afterload reduction and diuretics. LV function and the severity of MR can be noninvasively followed with chest radiographs, echocardiography, and radionuclide angiography. With deterioration of LV ejection fraction or with LV dilation, mitral valve surgery should be recom-

mended even in the absence of symptoms. It should be recalled that MR may "falsely" elevate LV ejection fraction because of the decrease in end-systolic volume resulting from the MR. Ejection fractions of 40% or less associated with MR represent considerable myocardial dysfunction. Valve replacement in these patients entails increased operative risk, and many that survive surgery have severe residual LV dysfunction (ejection fractions of 20%-30%). The goal in asymptomatic patients with MR is to perform mitral valve repair or replacement before significant LV dysfunction ensues. Early signs of ventricular dysfunction are decreases in baseline or exercise radionuclide ejection fraction or increase in LV cavity size determined by echocardiography.

The use of mitral valve repair to preserve the native valve has been expanded over the last decade,[17,18] although mitral valve replacement continues to be the mainstay of mitral surgery to correct regurgitation. Mitral valve repair involves combinations of ring annuloplasty, leaflet resection, and chordal shortening. This is most often possible in those with myxomatous disease of the valve or stretching of the annulus because of LV dilation. This is not feasible with severe fibrosis and calcification of the mitral valve, as may occur with rheumatic disease and the long-term results when repair is applied to rheumatic disease are less favorable.[18]

The St. Jude's and Starr-Edwards mechanical valves have produced the most durable surgical results.[9,19] These valves, however, are associated with increased thromboembolic and bleeding complications compared with porcine valves. The rate of thromboembolic complications with mechanical valves is 2% to 3%/patient-year, as is the rate of warfarin-associated bleeding complications.[9,19] Although the risk of thromboembolism because of porcine valves is about half this, late

2

valvular degeneration beyond 5 years is a major limitation.[19-21] Because of the development of prosthetic insufficiency, especially in the mitral position, porcine valves should be reserved for those patients unable to tolerate long-term anticoagulation.[18]

Mitral valve replacement alone carries an operative risk of about 10% to 15%.[18,21] Surgical treatment of ischemic MR requiring combined bypass grafting and valve replacement markedly increases the operative risk. Operative mortality rates approaching 30% to 50% have been reported.[22-24] Thus, unless the MR is severe, it may be prudent to perform bypass grafting alone.[23] This may indirectly improve the MR, with resolution of ischemia and LV dilation.

Mitral stenosis

Mitral stenosis complicated by CHF and frank pulmonary edema requiring CCU care may be precipitated by the development of rapid atrial fibrillation, concurrent infections, anemia, hyperthyroidism, or pregnancy. Although the majority of patients develop symptoms of pulmonary congestion, some patients follow an insidious course with the gradual development of pulmonary hypertension, low cardiac output, and even cardiogenic shock.[25] Atypical chest pain is frequent in patients with mitral stenosis, but coexistent coronary disease is uncommon.

Rheumatic disease is almost always the cause of mitral stenosis, although rarely congenital abnormalities or degenerative calcific disease of the valve results in stenosis.

The diastolic rumbling murmur of mitral stenosis may be subtle and may be especially difficult to appreciate in patients with depressed cardiac output. The murmur is made more prominent at the bedside by measures aimed at increasing cardiac output, such as having the patient do a few sit-ups. The first heart sound is prominent and may be palpable, caused by the mitral valve thickening, and wide displacement of the leaflets in late diastole (the latter caused by the elevated left atrial driving pressure in late diastole). The pulmonary closure sound may be accentuated, and a right ventricular lift is appreciable in patients who have developed pulmonary hypertension and RV dilation. After S_2, an opening snap, characteristic of rheumatic mitral stenosis, is present. The opening snap is caused by the springing open of the thickened valve apparatus driven by the increased left atrial pressure. The interval between S_2 and the opening snap correlates with the severity of the mitral stenosis; the shorter the S_2-OS interval, the more severe the stenosis (Fig. 59-12).

Echocardiography has become the main stay for assessing the severity of mitral stenosis (Fig. 59-13). The severity of MS can be estimated using the half-time of the Doppler mitral valve inflow pattern or by two-

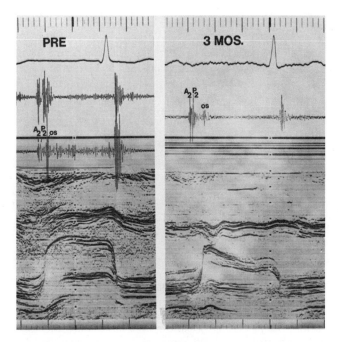

Fig. 59-12. Phonocardiographic and M-mode evaluation of a patient with mitral stenosis before *(PRE)* and 3 months after *(3 MOS)* balloon mitral commissurotomy. The electrocardiogram is shown at the top of the panel, the phonocardiogram in the center, and the M-mode echocardiogram through the mitral valve apparatus at the bottom of the figure. Note the improvement in the E-F slope of the anterior mitral valve leaflet after balloon commissurotomy and the increase in the A_2-OS interval on the phonocardiogram reflecting the reduced severity of mitral stenosis after balloon commissurotomy. *Pre*, Mitral valve area = 1.0 cm²; *3 MOS*, mitral valve area = 1.9 cm²; A_2, aortic valve closure; P_2, pulmonic valve closure; *os*, opening snap of the mitral valve.

dimensional planimetry of the mitral valve opening during diastole. When present, the Doppler velocity of TR can be used to estimate the pulmonary artery systolic pressure:

$$PA \text{ systolic pressure [mm Hg]} \simeq 4V^2 + RA \simeq 4V^2 + 5$$
where V = maximal TR Doppler velocity in m/sec.

Invasive hemodynamic monitoring of the patient with CHF due to MS is not particularly helpful. The PCW pressure does not reflect true LV filling pressure. Table 59-8 summarizes the key therapeutic strategy. Supplying IV diuretics and controlling the heart rate between 60 to 80 beats/min are most important. Atrial fibrillation is often associated with this disease. When it is of new onset and associated with severe pulmonary edema, electrical cardioversion is warranted. The ventricular response rate of atrial fibrillation should be controlled with digoxin or IV diltiazem. Inotropic agents that increase heart rate may worsen the hemodynamics by shortening diastolic filling. These are best avoided. β-Blockers may be useful in slowing the rate of patients in sinus rhythm. Verapamil may also be used but has less

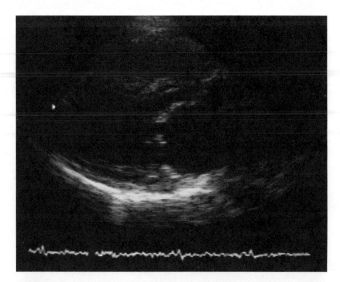

Fig. 59-13. Two-dimensional echocardiogram (long-axis, longitudinal view) of a patient with rheumatic mitral stenosis. Note the characteristic bowing of the mitral valve leaflets *(arrow)* during diastole because of tethering of the leaflet tips. *LA,* Left atrium; *LV,* left ventricle; *RV,* right ventricle; *Ao,* ascending aorta.

Table 59-8. Acute treatment of CHF in patients with mitral stenosis*

Monitoring
  PCW does not reflect LVEDP
Pharmacologic therapy
  Effective
    Diuretics
    Rate control
      Digoxin
      Calcium channel blockers
      β-Blockers
    Nitrates
  Selectively effective
    Aldactone (if right-sided heart failure present)
  Avoid
    Inotropic agents

---

*CHF, Congestive heart failure; *PCW,* pulmonary capillary wedge; *LVEDP,* left ventricular end-diastolic pressure; *ACE,* angiotensin-converting enzyme.

effect on the heart rate in sinus rhythm. In those with severe right-sided heart failure in addition to pulmonary congestion, the combination of aldactone with IV furosemide may be effective when furosemide alone is not. IV nitrates may also be acutely effective in further reducing preload.

Patients with appropriate mitral valve morphology can now be effectively treated with percutaneous balloon mitral commissurotomy at the time of cardiac catheterization (Fig. 59-14). This procedure carries an operative mortality of less than 1%.[26] Transesophageal echocardiography is a preoperative requirement to eliminate

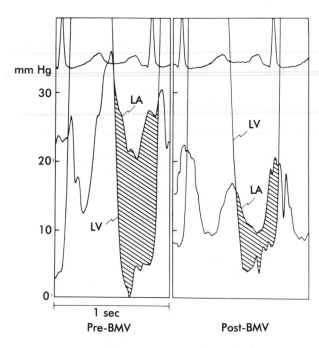

Fig. 59-14. Simultaneous measurement of left atrial *(LA)* and left ventricular pressures *(LV)* before *(left panel)* and immediately after *(right panel)* balloon mitral commissurotomy. The electrocardiogram is shown at the top. Note the marked reduction in the mitral valve diastolic gradient (mean gradient is shaded).

patients with left atrial thrombus. Balloon commissurotomy can also be safely and successfully performed in pregnant women who have CHF because of mitral stenosis.[27]

Surgical commissurotomy can be performed with low operative risk as well, but the percutaneous balloon technique has been shown to produce equivalent results and has less morbidity with an average hospital stay of only 2 days.[28] Patients not appropriate for balloon commissurotomy require mitral valve replacement, preferably with a mechanical prosthesis. Porcine valves are preferable in those unable to tolerate long-term anticoagulation or in women of childbearing age who are considering future pregnancies. The operative risk of surgical commissurotomy is about 1% and that of mitral valve replacement for mitral stenosis is about 5% to 10%.[21,29,30]

Tricuspid stenosis

Tricuspid stenosis is rarely encountered in the acute CCU setting and therefore will only be briefly mentioned. Rheumatic disease is the most frequent cause of tricuspid stenosis and it may be encountered in combination with rheumatic disease of the mitral or aortic valve. Tricuspid stenosis results in elevated right-sided filling pressures, and on examination there is evidence of elevated jugular venous pressure with a

Table 59-9. Causes of tricuspid regurgitation

A. Right ventricular dilation
B. Pulmonary hypertension
C. Rheumatic disease
D. Myxomatous disease
E. Bacterial endocarditis
F. Carcinoid heart disease
G. Congenital heart disease
  1. Ebstein's anomaly
  2. Atrioventricular canal defect
H. Right atrial myxoma

Table 59-10. Acute treatment of CHF in patients with tricuspid regurgitation*

Monitoring
  Thermodilution cardiac output becomes inaccurate in the face of TR
Pharmacologic therapy
  Effective
    Diuretics
      Add aldactone if hepatomegaly or ascites
      Use IV diuretics initially
    Nitrates
    Reduce pulmonary pressures
      Oxygen
      Reduce PCW if elevated
    Digoxin

*CHF, Congestive heart failure; TR, tricuspid regurgitation; CO, cardiac output; IV, intravenous; PCW, pulmonary capillary wedge.

prominent "a wave" in patients in sinus rhythm. The diastolic rumbling murmur of tricuspid stenosis is similar in quality to that of mitral stenosis but is usually located at the left sternal border and increases in intensity with inspiration.

Echocardiography is the most useful technique for evaluating the tricuspid valve. The normally "lacy" leaflets of the tricuspid valve are thickened, and there is restricted diastolic mobility in tricuspid stenosis. Doppler examination of the tricuspid inflow demonstrates turbulence and a velocity gradient across the valve. A mean gradient of only 4 or 5 mm Hg may be sufficient to cause peripheral congestion and limitation of exercise cardiac output. If tricuspid stenosis is not suspected, it can be overlooked during catheterization. Accurate measurement requires simultaneous measurement of the right atrial and RV pressures. Although rarely clinically significant, rheumatic tricuspid stenosis can also be effectively treated with percutaneous balloon valvotomy if significant TR does not coexist.[31]

Tricuspid regurgitation

Tricuspid regurgitation (TR) is frequently present in patients with severe CHF of any cause in the CCU. It is most commonly caused by volume overload and pulmonary hypertension with RV and tricuspid annular dilation. TR is most frequently encountered as a result of disease of other valves or the myocardium. Occasionally diseases affect the tricuspid valve primarily (Table 59-9).

The characteristic finding on physical examination is elevated venous pressures with a prominent "CV wave" in the jugular venous pulsations (Fig. 59-15). The CV wave occurs during or just after the carotid upstroke. The murmur of TR is a blowing, holosystolic murmur heard at the lower sternal border often radiating rightward. It characteristically increases in intensity with inspiration (Carvallo's sign). There is often a palpable right ventricular lift. A right-sided S_3, heard at the right upper sternal border, may be audible. If associated with elevated pulmonary pressures, P_2 may be increased in intensity or palpable.

Color-flow Doppler echocardiography can be used to judge the severity of the TR and the morphology of the valve itself to help to decipher the cause. In addition, the size and systolic function of the right ventricle can be estimated and the pulmonary artery pressures estimated from the peak TR Doppler velocity. Right-sided heart catheterization can be performed, but the majority of the data can be gathered noninvasively from echocardiographic and physical examination. When catheterization is performed, right ventriculography is useful in assessing the RV function and severity of TR. Some TR, however, may be created by the catheter lying across the tricuspid valve. As has been pointed out, thermodilution cardiac output measurement becomes quite unreliable in the presence of significant TR because of the thermal "diluting" effects of the valvular regurgitation.

In the majority of cases, TR is secondary to volume overload and elevated pulmonary pressures, and treatment is directed toward reduction of the pulmonary pressures and preload reduction with diuretics (Table 59-10). Digoxin may also be helpful in cases of severe right-sided heart failure with right ventricular dilation and reduced systolic function. IV inotropic drugs such as dobutamine may be temporarily helpful but are not of long-term benefit. Oral diuretics are frequently not successful initially in cases of severe right-sided heart failure because of edema of the gastrointestinal tract, causing poor drug absorption. When this occurs, IV furosemide is frequently effective, especially when combined with aldactone or metolazone.

Primary disorders of the tricuspid valve associated with TR and severe right-sided heart failure are uncommon. Patients tolerate even an absent tricuspid valve (as has been surgically created for treatment of tricuspid endocarditis) for a considerable period of time as long as

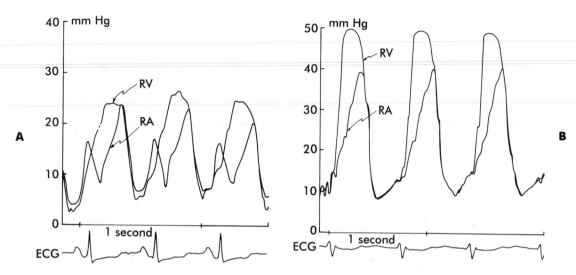

Fig. 59-15. Hemodynamic findings in tricuspid regurgitation documented by simultaneous recordings of right ventricular *(RV)* and right atrial pressures *(RA)*. *Panel A,* Severe tricuspid regurgitation with normal right ventricular systolic pressure from a patient with carcinoid involvement of the tricuspid valve. Note the large V wave in the right atrial pressure recordings *(arrow)* that nearly equals the magnitude of the right ventricular systolic pressure. *Panel B,* Severe tricuspid regurgitation in the patient with elevated right ventricular systolic pressure (the more common scenario). Again, note the large V wave in the right atrial pressure recording.

the pulmonary pressures are normal. Eventually, however, RV dilation and failure occur.

Tricuspid valve repair or replacement can be performed in patients with severe TR. Repair involves primarily ring annuloplasty. When valve replacement is required, porcine valves are preferred in the tricuspid position because of the possibility of valve thrombosis, which may occur despite adequate anticoagulation, with mechanical valves in this position.

Thus, the hemodynamic derangements in patients with valvular heart disease present unique diagnostic and therapeutic challenges in the CCU. Prompt recognition of these disorders and appropriate evaluation using echocardiographic, hemodynamic, and angiographic data allow for effective management of these complex patients.

REFERENCES

1. Harrison JK, Davidson CJ, Leithe ME, et al: Serial left ventricular performance evaluated by cardiac catheterization before, immediately after and at 6 months after balloon aortic valvuloplasty, *J Am Coll Cardiol* 16:1351-1358, 1990.
2. Roberts WC: The congenitally bicuspid aortic valve—a study of 85 autopsy cases, *Am J Cardiol* 26:72-83, 1970.
3. Sheikh KH, Davidson CJ, Honan MB, et al: Changes in left ventricular diastolic performance after aortic balloon valvuloplasty: acute and late effects, *J Am Coll Cardiol* 16:795-803, 1990.
4. Davidson CJ, Harrison JK, Pieper KS, et al: Determinants of one-year outcome from balloon aortic valvuloplasty, *Am J Cardiol* 68:75-80, 1991.
5. Gorlin R, Gorlin G: Hydraulic formula for calculation of area of stenotic mitral valve, other cardiac valves, and central circulatory shunts, *Am Heart J* 41:1-10, 1951.
6. Jacobs ML, Fowler BN, Vezeridis MP, et al: Aortic valve replacement: a nine year experience, *Ann Thorac Surg* 30:439-447, 1980.
7. Kirklin JW, Barratt-Boyes BG: Aortic valve disease. In *Cardiac surgery*, New York, 1986, John Wiley & Sons, pp 373-429.
8. Scott WC, Miller DC, Harerich A, et al: Determinants of operative mortality for patients undergoing aortic valve replacement. Discriminant analysis of 1479 operations, *J Thorac Cardiovasc Surg* 89:400-413, 1985.
9. Czer LSC, Matloff JM, Chaux A, et al: The St. Jude valve: analysis of thromboembolism, warfarin-related hemorrhage, and survival, *Am Heart J* 114:389-397, 1987.
10. Austen WG, Kastor JA, Sanders CA: Resolution of functional mitral regurgitation following surgical correction of aortic valvular disease, *J Thorac Cardiovasc Surg* 53:255-259, 1967.
11. Leithe ME, Harrison JK, Davidson CJ, et al: Surgical aortic valvuloplasty using the cavitron ultrasonic surgical aspirator: an invasive hemodynamic follow-up study, *Cathet Cardiovasc Diag* 24:16-21, 1991.
12. Wise JR Jr, Cleland WP, Hallidie-Smith KA: Urgent aortic valve replacement for acute aortic regurgitation due to infective endocarditis, *Lancet* 2:115-121, 1971.
13. Bonow RO, Lakatos E, Maron BJ, et al: Serial long-term assessment of the natural history of asymptomatic patients with chronic aortic regurgitation and normal left ventricular systolic function, *Circulation* 84:1625-1635, 1991.
14. Hegglin R, Scheu H, Rothlin M: Aortic insufficiency, *Circulation* 37(suppl):V77-V92, 1968.
15. Bonow RO, Picone AL, McIntosh CL, et al: Survival and functional results after valve replacement for aortic regurgitation from 1976 to 1983. Impact of preoperative left ventricular dysfunction, *Circulation* 72:1244-1256, 1985.
16. Borer JS, Herrold EM, Hochreiter C, et al: Natural history of left ventricular performance at rest and during exercise after aortic valve replacement for aortic regurgitation, *Circulation* 84(suppl III):III139, 1991.

17. Kirklin JW: Mitral valve repair for mitral incompetence, *Mod Concepts Cardiovasc Dis* 56:7-9, 1987.
18. Galloway AC, Colvin SB, Baumann FG, et al: A comparison of mitral valve reconstruction with mitral valve replacement. Immediate-term results, *Ann Thorac Surg* 47:655-662, 1989.
19. Cobanoglu A, Grunkenmeier GL, Aru GM, et al: Mitral replacement: clinical experience with the ball-valve prothesis; 25 years later, *Am J Surg* 202:376-382, 1985.
20. Magilligan DJ, Lewis JW, Tilley B, et al: The porcine bioprosthetic valve. Twelve years later, *J Thorac Cardiovasc Surg* 89:499-507, 1985.
21. Cohn LH, Allred EN, Cohn LA, et al: Early and late risk of mitral valve replacement. A 12 year concomitant comparison of the porcine bioprosthetic and prosthetic disk mitral valves, *J Thorac Cardiovasc Surg* 90:872-881, 1985.
22. Magovern JA, Pennock JL, Campbell DB, et al: Risks of mitral valve replacement and mitral valve replacement with coronary artery bypass, *Ann Thoracic Surg* 39:346-352, 1985.
23. Arcidi JM, Hebeler RF, Craver JM, et al: Treatment of moderate mitral regurgitation and coronary disease by coronary bypass alone, *J Thorac Cardiovasc Surg* 95:951-959, 1988.
24. Rankin JS, Livesey SA, Smith LR, et al: Trends in the surgical treatment of ischemic mitral regurgitation: effects of mitral valve repair on hospital mortality, *J Thorac Cardiovasc Surg* 1:149-163, 1989.
25. Harding MB, Harrison JK, Davidson CJ, et al: Critical mitral stenosis causing ischemic hepatic failure: successful treatment with percutaneous balloon mitral valvotomy, *Chest* 101:866-869, 1992.
26. Dean LS, Davis K, Feit F, et al: Complications and mortality of percutaneous balloon mitral commissurotomy, *Circulation* 82(suppl III):III545, 1990.
27. Esteves CA, Ramos AIO, Braga SLN, et al: Effectiveness of percutaneous balloon mitral valvotomy during pregnancy, *Am J Cardiol* 68:930-934, 1991.
28. Turi ZG, Reyes VP, Raju BS, et al: Percutaneous balloon versus surgical closed commissurotomy for mitral stenosis. A prospective, randomized trial, *Circulation* 83:1179-1185, 1991.
29. Salerno TA, Neilson IR, Charrette JP, et al: A 25-year experience with the closed method of treatment of 139 patients with mitral stenosis, *Ann Thorac Surg* 31:300-304, 1981.
30. Laschinger JC, Cunningham JN Jr, Baumann FG, et al: Early open radical commissurotomy: surgical treatment of choice for mitral stenosis, *Ann Thorac Surg* 34:287-296, 1982.
31. Ribeiro PA, Zaibag MA, Kasab SA, et al: Percutaneous double balloon valvotomy for rheumatic tricuspid stenosis, *Am J Cardiol* 61:660-662, 1988.

Chapter 60

RIGHT VENTRICULAR MYOCARDIAL INFARCTION

Vance E. Wilson
Eric R. Bates

The clinical importance of right ventricular dysfunction in patients with acute inferior MI was not recognized until 1974 when Cohn et al.[1] described six patients who presented with cardiogenic shock from predominantly right ventricular dysfunction. It is now known that the spectrum of right ventricular myocardial infarction (RVMI) is broad, ranging from asymptomatic minimal right ventricular involvement to major functional impairment producing death. Clinically, the presence of RVMI associated with inferior MI refers to the findings of systemic hypotension and venous congestion in the absence of left ventricular failure. Making the proper diagnosis is important because therapy is paradoxically different than for left ventricular MI complicated by hypotension and venous congestion.

INCIDENCE

The incidence of RVMI depends on the diagnostic criteria used. Andersen et al.[2] noted autopsy evidence for right ventricular involvement in 31 consecutive patients who died from posterior MI. About 40% of patients with acute inferoposterior MI have RVMI by imaging criteria that detect right ventricular ischemia or necrosis. Approximately 20% have hemodynamic evidence of right ventricular dysfunction. Fewer than 8% have cardiogenic shock.[2-4]

ANATOMY

Blood is supplied to the right ventricle predominantly by the right coronary artery (RCA). The proximal RCA courses in the atrioventricular groove, supplying blood to the right atrium and crista supraventricularis of the right ventricle. The crista supraventricularis is a muscle bundle extending from the top of the interventricular septum to the tricuspid annulus and the top of the free wall of the right ventricle (Fig. 60-1) and is essential to emptying the right ventricle and closing the tricuspid valve.[5] Acute marginal branches of the middle RCA supply the right ventricular free wall. In 85% of patients (right dominant coronary circulation), the distal RCA gives rise to the posterior descending artery supplying the posterior aspect of the interventricular septum and the right ventricle, and also gives origin to the AV nodal artery and one or more posterolateral branches supplying the posterior left ventricle. In 7% of patients (codominant circulation), the RCA supplies a posterior descending artery and then terminates. In 8% of patients (left dominant circulation), the posterior descending artery is supplied by the distal circumflex coronary artery.

Anatomically, clinically significant RVMI is almost always caused by occlusion of a dominant RCA before at least one of the major right ventricular branches, with transmural infarction involving predominantly the basal and posterior part of the right ventricular free wall near the atrioventricular groove in a triangular shape pointing toward the apex. The necrosis is rarely circumferential because usually a small part of the anterior right ventricular wall is supplied by the left anterior descending coronary artery.[2] The posterior interventricular septum is also frequently involved.[6] The more proximal the site of RCA occlusion, the larger the amount of RV

741

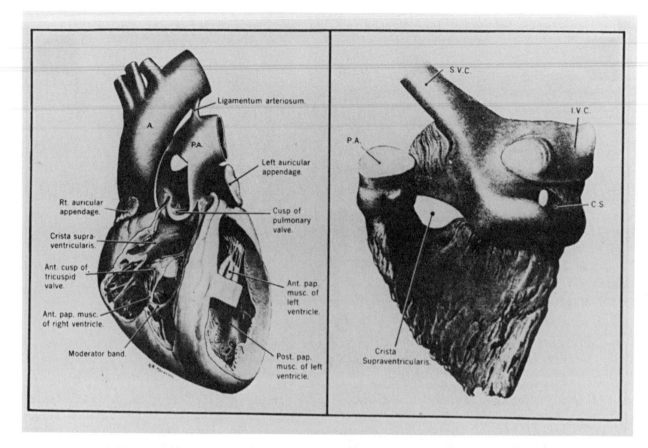

Fig. 60-1. Two illustrations demonstrating the location of the crista supraventricularis. During right ventricular systole this muscular structure narrows the tricuspid orifice and brings the free wall of the right ventricle toward the interventricular septum, thus assisting with stroke volume generation. (Reprinted by permission from James: *J Am Coll Cardiol* 6:1083, 1985.)

necrosis[2] and the more likely clinical features of RVMI will occur.[7,8] Figure 60-2 demonstrates one postmortem scheme used to grade the extent of right ventricular MI. Right ventricular function may be especially compromised when proximal RCA occlusion interrupts blood supply to the crista supraventricularis.[5] In addition, occlusion of the RCA proximal to the right atrial branches impairs right atrial function, which exacerbates hemodynamic compromise from RVMI by compromising preload.[9]

Rarely, isolated RVMI may result from occlusion of either a nondominant RCA[10,11] or a side branch of the RCA.[2,12] Occlusion of the circumflex coronary artery in left dominant patients may occasionally cause RVMI.[2,6,13] Autopsy studies have shown that some degree of RVMI also occurs in extensive anterior wall MI from contiguous extension.[2,14,15] These right ventricular infarcts tend to be small and involve the apical anterior third of the right ventricle.[2] In one echocardiographic study of 32 patients with anterior MI, 10 had evidence of right ventricular apical free wall motion abnormalities but no change in overall right ventricular function.[15]

RVMI in the absence of coronary artery disease is rare but has been reported in patients with right ventricular hypertrophy secondary to pulmonary hypertension,[16,17] acute pulmonary embolus,[18,19] or pulmonic stenosis.[20] Right ventricular hypertrophy predisposes patients with inferior AMI to RVMI independent of the site or extent of coronary artery disease[17,21] but is seldom present.[6]

PATHOPHYSIOLOGY

Differences in methodology have limited investigations in the pathophysiology of RVMI. Early experimental studies in open-chest dogs following pericardiotomy found little hemodynamic embarrassment produced by extensive right ventricular free wall cauterization.[22-25] Guiha et al.[23] produced a disproportionate rise in right ventricular filling pressure only with volume loading in this model. Donald and Essex[26] noted little effect from acute RCA and conus arteriosus branch ligation. However, when Goldstein et al.[27,28] left the pericardium intact and occluded the right coronary artery, equalization of right- and left-sided filling pressures was pro-

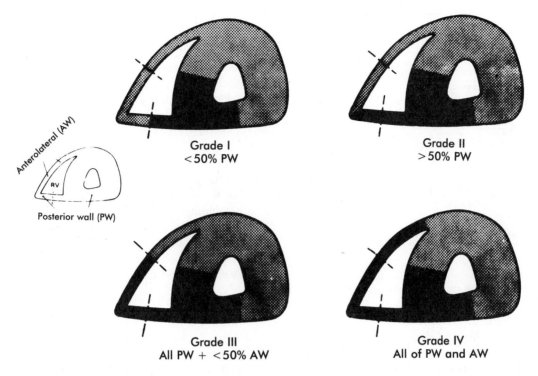

Anterolateral (AW)

RV

Posterior wall (PW)

Grade I
<50% PW

Grade II
>50% PW

Grade III
All PW + <50% AW

Grade IV
All of PW and AW

Fig. 60-2. Diagram of transverse slices of the right and left ventricles illustrating one grading scheme for measuring the extent of right ventricular infarction. AW = anterolateral wall; PW = posterior wall. (Reprinted by permission from Isner, Roberts: *Am J Cardiol* 42:885-894, 1978.)

duced and cardiac output decreased significantly. Volume loading increased cardiac output some, but pericardial incision significantly improved cardiac output and intracardiac volumes, suggesting that right ventricular enlargement and pericardial restraint were inhibiting left ventricular performance.

There is also a difference in right ventricular necrosis in experimental canine studies with nondominant RCA circulations compared with RVMI in humans. In most of the animal models, necrosis was limited to the right ventricular free wall by cauterization. In humans RVMI almost always involves the posterior interventricular septum. In addition, James[5] has argued that right ventricular dysfunction is more likely to be related to necrosis of the crista supraventricularis than that of the right ventricular free wall.

CLINICAL FINDINGS

Prompt recognition of clinically significant RVMI is important because therapy must frequently be started before invasive hemodynamic measurements or noninvasive testing can be performed. The diagnosis should be strongly considered in any patient with acute transmural inferior MI whose blood pressure decreases with morphine or nitrates[29] or who develops cardiogenic shock. Ferguson et al.[29] compared 20 patients with documented inferior MI and marked hypotension after nitrate

administration to 20 patients with inferior MI without hypotension after administration of nitroglycerin. Fifteen of the 20 patients who demonstrated a hypotensive response to nitroglycerin had evidence of RV involvement, whereas in 18 of the 20 patients without hypotension after nitrates there was no evidence of RV involvement. In a separate analysis of 28 patients with documented RV involvement in inferior MI, 20 patients developed hypotension after administration of nitroglycerin. Thus, in patients with inferior MI a hypotensive response to nitroglycerin suggests the presence of RV involvement.

The classic clinical triad for diagnosing RVMI is elevated jugular venous pressure, systemic hypotension, and clear lung fields[30] (See accompanying box). Kussmaul's sign, a late inspiratory increase in the jugular venous pressure, has also been reported in several series.[4,31-34] High-degree atrioventricular block or bradycardia are often present. Characteristic findings on physical examination may be absent despite noninvasive evidence of RV involvement.[13,33,35,36]

In a prospective study of 53 patients with inferior MI, physical examination findings were correlated with hemodynamic measurements.[33] Eight of the 53 patients had RVMI defined by hemodynamic criteria (right atrial pressure ≥ 10 and a right atrial:pulmonary artery wedge pressure ≥ 0.85). An elevated jugular venous pressure

---

Clinical findings in right ventricular infarction

Classic
  Elevated jugular venous pressure
  Systemic hypotension
  Absence of pulmonary congestion
Additional
  Kussmaul's sign
  Cannon "A" jugular venous waves
  Jugular venous "Y" ≥ "X" descent
  Right-sided S$_3$ or S$_4$
  Hepato-jugular reflux
  Tricuspid regurgitation
  Pulsus paradoxus
  Right pleural effusion

---

was found in 7 of the 8 patients but was also present in 14 of 45 patients without hemodynamic evidence of RVMI (sensitivity 88%, specificity 69%). Elevated jugular venous pressure *and* clear lung fields were more specific (82%) but less sensitive (50%). Only 2 patients with RVMI had the classic triad of hypotension, elevated jugular venous pressure, and clear lung fields, whereas 2 of the 45 patients without RVMI also had these findings (sensitivity 25%, specificity 96%). By contrast, Kussmaul's sign was observed and confirmed by hemodynamic monitoring in all 8 patients with RVMI and none of the patients without RVMI hemodynamics and elevated jugular venous pressure. Thus, elevated jugular venous pressure and Kussmaul's sign were found to be the most reliable predictors of RVMI defined by invasive hemodynamic measurements.

The jugular venous pressure waveform is abnormal with prominent "A" and "V" waves and a "Y" greater than or equal to "X" descent, reflecting a poorly compliant or stiff right ventricle. Cannon "A" jugular venous waves may occur from complete atrioventricular block. Right-sided gallops have been reported frequently.[37] Other physical exam findings sometimes seen include hepato-jugular reflux, tricuspid regurgitation, and pulsus paradoxus. Right pleural effusions have also been described.[4,6]

NONINVASIVE IMAGING
Electrocardiography

The classic electrocardiographic sign of RVMI is 1 mm or more ST-segment elevation in one of the right precordial leads, in particular V3R or V4R, in the setting of inferior MI. These changes have been shown to correlate with occlusion of the proximal RCA by angiography,[7] with autopsy evidence of right ventricular necrosis[38,39] and with hemodynamic and other noninvasive testing suggestive of RVMI,[40-47] with overall sensitivity and specificity of 80% to 90%. These changes may

be masked by large left ventricular infarction.[46] Greater predictive value has been claimed for changes in V6R and V7R.[48] Other cardiac conditions can cause right-sided ST-segment elevation, including acute pulmonary embolus, left ventricular hypertrophy, left bundle branch block, acute anteroseptal MI, pericarditis, and previous anterior MI with aneurysm formation. The sensitivity of a right-sided ECG in the diagnosis of RVMI is limited by the finding that ST-segment elevation in V4R disappears in 50% of patients by 10 to 18 hours and in nearly all patients by 72 hours.[7] Occasionally in patients with acute inferior MI, ST-segment elevation may be seen in lead V1, a finding that although very specific for RVMI is very insensitive.[40,49] Rarely, ST-segment elevation in leads V1 to V5 may be caused by RCA occlusion and acute RVMI.[50] In such cases, ST-segment elevation is maximal in V1 or V2 and decreases toward V6.

Echocardiography

Multiple studies have analyzed 2D-echocardiographic findings in the diagnosis of RVMI.[31,35,51-55] Right-ventricular wall motion abnormalities are common in RVMI. However, their presence is not specific for hemodynamic compromise, which is dependent more on the function of the crista supraventricularis. Involvement of the right ventricular diaphragmatic wall is most common,[35] in keeping with pathologic studies.[2,6] The number of asynergic right ventricular wall segments has been shown to correlate with right atrial pressure and the severity of the hemodynamic perturbation.[35] When hypotension with elevated right atrial pressure and absence of pulmonary rales are present, right-ventricular regional wall motion abnormalities typically exceed left ventricular wall motion abnormalities.[54]

Echocardiographic indices of hemodynamic compromise have been characterized in a retrospective study by Goldberger et al.[53] Descent of the right ventricular base (a measure of right ventricular ejection fraction previously described[56]) less than 1 cm with systole was 100% sensitive and 80% specific for hemodynamic compromise. A diminished respiratory caval index (percentage collapse of the inferior vena cava with inspiration) less than 50% was 100% sensitive and 33% specific for hemodynamic compromise. Finally, an increased ratio of right-ventricular to left-ventricular end-diastolic size (measured by single plane area-length method in the apical four-chamber view) greater than 0.9 was 56% sensitive and 87% specific for hemodynamic compromise. Other echocardiographic features sometimes seen in RVMI include tricuspid regurgitation,[52,57,58] right ventricular thrombus,[59] paradoxical septal motion, and localized anterior pericardial effusion.[52] In summary, 2D-echocardiography is useful in estimating the extent of RVMI and determining the need for hemodynamic monitoring.

Radionuclide Ventriculography

Abnormal radionuclide-determined RVEF has been reported in 20% to 48% of patients with acute inferior MI.[31,43,55,60-65] In a prospective study of 53 patients with acute inferior MI, right ventricular wall motion akinesis or dyskinesis alone or in combination with an RVEF less than 40% was found to be useful in the diagnosis of hemodynamically significant RVMI.[62] Patients with inferior MI who have RVMI have lower LVEF than patients without RVMI.[66]

Technetium pyrophosphate scanning

Technetium pyrophosphate scans have been reported to be positive for RVMI in as many as 38% of patients with inferior MI,[65] although a much lower incidence has also been reported.[31] There are limitations with using technetium pyrophosphate scans to diagnose RVMI. The study must be appropriately timed 48 to 72 hours after the infarct onset, when hemodynamic problems have often resolved. In addition, the interpretation of the images is made difficult by radioactivity in structures overlying the heart (chest wall, bone, and cartilage) and residual activity in the cardiac blood pool.

HEMODYNAMICS

Findings from invasive hemodynamic measurements in patients with RVMI reflect systolic and diastolic dysfunction of the right ventricle, including elevation of right atrial pressure and low cardiac output (Fig. 60-3). A stiff, noncompliant right ventricle causes an "M- " or "W-" shaped right atrial pressure waveform similar to constrictive pericarditis, with a deep "Y" descent. The right ventricular pressure waveform may have a diastolic dip-plateau pattern. A noncompliant atrial pressure waveform has been correlated with low cardiac output.[67] Right atrial function is critical to right ventricular preload and cardiac output in RVMI. The amplitude of the right atrial "A" wave is an indication of the status of right atrial function. A right atrial "M" pattern (characterized by depressed "A" waves) as opposed to a "W" pattern (characterized by augmented "A" waves) indicates more proximal RCA occlusion and greater hemodynamic compromise.[9]

The currently accepted hemodynamic criteria for the diagnosis of RVMI come from a combined hemodynamic/autopsy study of 60 patients.[68] Autopsy-proven right ventricular necrosis correlated with a right atrial pressure ≥ 10 mm Hg and a right atrial to pulmonary capillary wedge pressure pressure ratio ≥ 0.85. Several hemodynamic patterns were characterized. In the most severe forms of right ventricular dysfunction with shock, the right ventricle does not generate significant pressure. This causes a reduced difference between systolic and diastolic pulmonary artery pressure and similar pressure contours and mean pressures in the right atrium, right

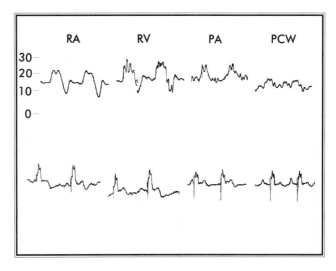

Fig. 60-3. Right atrial (RA), right ventricular (RV), pulmonary artery, (PA) and pulmonary capillary wedge (PCW) pressures in a patient with RVMI and cardiogenic shock. Note the similarities between RA, RV, and PA pressures. The PA pulse pressure is reduced. The RA pressure tracing has a prominent Y descent and the RA pressure exceeds PCW pressure.

ventricle, and pulmonary artery. When right atrial pressure is greater than pulmonary capillary wedge pressure, a severe noncompliant right atrial pressure waveform is present. In milder forms there is a normal difference between pulmonary artery systolic and diastolic pressure. In some patients the diagnosis of RVMI is supported only by a noncompliant right atrial pressure waveform. The close relationship between right atrial and pulmonary capillary wedge pressure may be lost if dysfunction of the left ventricle is greater than that of the right ventricle. In patients with low right atrial pressure, volume loading unmasks or increases the identification of patients with RVMI hemodynamics.[3,31,67]

Because of the constraining effects of the pericardium, right ventricular dilation may cause a dip-plateau or square-root sign on the right ventricular pressure tracing, aggravating the hemodynamic situation of a patient with RVMI.[69] Disproportionate elevation of right-sided filling pressures can lead to misdiagnosis, such as cardiac tamponade, constrictive pericarditis, restrictive myocardial disease, and acute pulmonary embolus.[4] Cardiac tamponade is unlikely in the presence of Kussmaul's sign and a noncompliant right atrial pressure pattern. Echocardiography is useful in excluding cardiac tamponade and assessing the extent of RVMI. Pulmonary embolus is unlikely in the absence of pulmonary hypertension.

CARDIAC ENZYMES

It has long been known that both early and late mortality are higher for anterior than inferior MI, even when equal infarct sizes are determined by cardiac

> **Complications of right ventricular infarction**
>
> Atrioventricular block
> Sinus node dysfunction
> Rupture
>   Free wall
>   Interventricular septum
>   Papillary muscle of the tricuspid valve
> Right-to-left intracardiac shunting via patent foramen
>   ovale
> Right ventricular thrombus with possible pulmonary
>   embolus
> Tricuspid regurgitation
> Cardiogenic shock
> Death

enzyme release. Right ventricular necrosis can be responsible for a considerable amount of the cardiac enzymes released into the blood during inferoposterior MI.[70,71] Weinshel et al.[72] suggested that a creatinine phosphokinase release >2000 IU in the setting of inferior MI strongly suggests coexistent RVMI. The better prognosis following inferior MI compared with anterior MI of equivalent enzymatic size may be the result of less left ventricular necrosis.

COMPLICATIONS (SEE ACCOMPANYING BOX)
AV Block

RVMI identifies a severalfold increased risk of developing atrioventricular block.[32,73,74] Braat et al.[32] reported that in 67 patients with inferior MI, high-degree atrioventricular block was seen in 48% of patients with RVMI, as opposed to only 13% in patients without RVMI. Atrioventricular block in the setting of acute RVMI has been associated with an excessively high mortality rate. Mavric et al.[75] analyzed 243 inferior MI patients and found that RVMI with complete atrioventricular block had a 41% mortality rate. The mortality rate for complete atrioventricular block without RVMI was 11% vs. 14% for RVMI alone without complete atrioventricular block.

Cardiac rupture

Rupture of the ventricular septum has been reported with RVMI.[76] Double rupture of the heart—the posterior ventricular septum and either the posterior free right ventricular or left ventricular wall—is a unique complication of RVMI.[77,78] Acute infarction complicated by rupture of the ventricular septum is associated with a 100% incidence of RV necrosis.[79] Several series have emphasized the profound importance of right ventricular function on the presence of shock and perioperative mortality for acute ventricular septal defects.[80-82] Grose et al.[81] described 8 patients who

underwent surgical repair of acute ventricular septal defect. Right ventricular dysfunction was the major cause of death in two cases and a contributing factor in three cases. In a 41-patient series by Radford et al.[82] mean pulmonary artery pressure was lower in patients with shock, suggesting that shock was produced mainly by right ventricular impairment.

Right-to-left interatrial shunting

A rare complication of RVMI is refractory hypoxemia caused by a right-to-left interatrial shunt through a patent foramen ovale or atrial septal defect.[83-90] Shunting occurs because right atrial pressure is elevated and may exceed left atrial pressure, especially during inspiration. Diagnosis can frequently be made by contrast two-dimensional echocardiography. Ventilation perfusion scans reveal radionuclide activity in the brain and kidneys. Recognition of this complication requires careful handling of intravenous lines to avoid systemic air or particulate emboli. Short-term percutaneous catheter closure can be performed by passing a balloon-tipped catheter through the patent foramen ovale into the left atrium, inflating the balloon, and then retracting the catheter against the interatrial septum.[84,86,90] Using a relatively large balloon such as a 5 F (4-cc) Rashkind balloon septostomy catheter[90] or Gensini catheter[86] may be more helpful than a standard 1.5-cc pulmonary artery balloon catheter. Maintaining the balloon position is critical and may be performed with a rubber band suture to provide continuous traction.[86] One reported patient has survived surgical closure.[83]

Tricuspid regurgitation

RVMI may rarely cause tricuspid regurgitation, acutely[91-95] or as a chronic sequela.[34,96,97] This may be the result of either right ventricular chamber dilatation or infarction of the right ventricular papillary muscle. This finding may be seen frequently by echocardiographic contrast study[52] but is infrequently evident on physical examination. Korr et al[93] described one case of RVMI with tricuspid regurgitation and shock unresponsive to fluid loading, dopamine, and nitroprusside. There was marked hemodynamic improvement after RCA grafting and tricuspid valve replacement.

Ventricular arrhythmias

Rechavia et al. found no increase in ventricular arrhythmias in patients during acute RVMI.[97] Patients with RVMI may be more susceptible to ventricular fibrillation during transvenous pacing[98] because of the proximity of the pacing lead to the infarcted region. In addition, the presence of RVMI increases the risk of developing ventricular fibrillation during insertion of a pulmonary artery balloon catheter. In one study involving 1138 patients with inferior MI, the risk was found to

Table 60-1. Mortality from cardiogenic shock complicating RVMI

Study	Number of patients	Mortality (%)
Lorell et al.[4]	12	3 (25)
Coma-Canella et al.[100]	10	4 (40)
Legrand et al.[102]	8	3 (38)
Judgutt et al.[56]	7	3 (43)
Cohn et al.[1]	6	2 (33)
Lloyd et al.[103]	6	1 (17)
Gewirtz et al.[101]	6	3 (50)
Rigo et al.[61]	3	1 (33)
Total	58	20 (34)

be 4.2% with evidence of RVMI as opposed to 0.28% in the absence of RVMI ($P < 0.00001$).[99] In patients in whom ventricular fibrillation occurred, attempts to reinsert the catheter produced ventricular fibrillation again in 5 of 23 patients. Isolated right ventricular infarction caused by occlusion of a nondominant RCA may result in ventricular tachycardia and sudden death.[11]

Cardiogenic shock

The incidence of right ventricular dysfunction producing cardiogenic shock can only be estimated from a few clinical studies. Cohn et al.[1] recognized 6 of 78 patients with this syndrome, an incidence rate of 8% that may have been high because of the tendency to select patients with evidence of heart failure for hemodynamic study. Lorell[4] found 8 patients in a retrospective analysis of 306 patients with inferior MI, providing an incidence rate of 3%. The incidence was probably underestimated because hemodynamic studies were not performed in all the patients. In a consecutive series of 53 patients with inferior MI,[3] 3 patients had this presentation, for an incidence of 6%. Thus, the overall incidence of RVMI with cardiogenic shock is 3% to 8%.

In-hospital mortality from RVMI is rare unless cardiogenic shock is present. Pooling the results of several studies in the prethrombolytic era* (Table 60-1), the mortality rate in the presence of RVMI and cardiogenic shock was 34%, approximately half that reported for left ventricular MI with shock.

TRADITIONAL MANAGEMENT OF RVMI COMPLICATED BY HEMODYNAMIC INSTABILITY (see accompanying box)
Fluid loading

The majority of patients with RVMI are hemodynamically stable and require no therapy. Nitroglycerin

---

*References 1, 4, 54, 61, 100-103.

> **Traditional management of right ventricular infarction**
>
> Avoidance of nitroglycerin or other vasodilators
> Judicious fluid loading
> Inotropic therapy
> Afterload reduction only for left ventricular dysfunction
> Maintenance of atrioventricular synchrony

and other agents that reduce preload, such as morphine and diuretics, should be withheld or administered cautiously to avoid hypotension. In the presence of hemodynamic instability from RVMI, fluid loading is the most recognized therapy to augment right ventricular preload and improve cardiac output.[1,103] The optimal value of right ventricular filling pressure has been well characterized in a prospective study of 41 patients with electrocardiographic and hemodynamic criteria for RVMI.[104] In most patients, raising mean right atrial pressure to 10 to 14 mm Hg was followed by an increase in right ventricular stroke work index and cardiac index. Raising mean right atrial pressure above 14 mm Hg was almost always accompanied by a decrease in right ventricular stroke work index and cardiac index. When the mean right atrial pressure was reduced by intravenous nitrates to less than 14 mm Hg, right ventricular stroke work index and cardiac index again increased. The mean optimal right atrial and pulmonary capillary wedge pressures were 11.7 and 16.5 mm Hg, respectively.

Several studies have shown that volume infusion does not uniformly raise cardiac output.[36,105,106] In all of these studies mean right atrial pressure was > 10 mm Hg before volume infusion, suggesting that RV filling pressure was already optimal. In the study by Dell'Italia et al.[105] 13 patients with RVMI were treated with volume infusion. Mean right atrial pressure was increased from 11 ± 2 to 15 ± 2 mm Hg, pulmonary capillary wedge pressure rose from 10 ± 4 to 15 ± 2 mm Hg, but cardiac index did not change significantly (1.9 ± 0.5 to 2.1 ± 0.4 L/min/m^2). Simultaneous radionuclide angiography demonstrated that right ventricular end-diastolic volume increased without any change in left ventricular end-diastolic volume. The pulmonary capillary wedge pressure, therefore, did not accurately reflect left ventricular preload in this hemodynamic situation.

Inotropic therapy

After appropriate volume loading to increase right atrial pressure to 10 to 14 mm Hg, inotropic agents may be added to augment cardiac output. Dobutamine or amrinone are theoretically preferred over dopamine because they do not raise pulmonary vascular resistance. Use of dobutamine for RVMI has been shown to

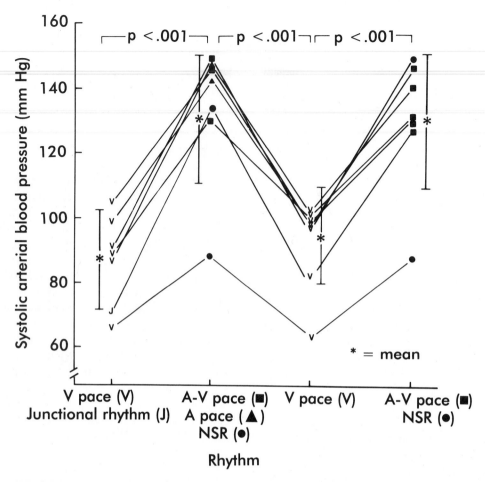

Fig. 60-4. Effects of restoring atrioventricular synchrony on systolic arterial blood pressure in 7 hypotensive patients with RVMI. (Reprinted by permission from Love et al: *Am Heart J* 1:10, 1984.)

augment cardiac index by 24%[57] and by 35%[105] in two studies.

Afterload reduction

Afterload reduction has not been extensively studied in RVMI. In one study nitroprusside was not found to improve right ventricular systolic performance or stroke volume index,[105] probably because right ventricular afterload does not present a significant obstacle to right ventricular ejection in this hemodynamic condition. Similar results have been found with intraaortic balloon counterpulsation.[4] If significant left ventricular dysfunction is present, however, decreasing afterload would be expected to be more beneficial.

Maintenance of atrioventricular synchrony

Augmentation of right ventricular preload by atrial systole is of critical importance when RVMI is severe. Consequently, atrial fibrillation is poorly tolerated and should be treated with electrical cardioversion when associated with hypotension. Similarly, accelerated junctional or idioventricular rhythm with intact atrioventricular conduction that fails to respond to atropine requires atrial pacing from either the atrial appendage or coronary sinus.[106] In patients with atrioventricular block and shock, atrioventricular sequential pacing may reverse hypotension and improve cardiac output. Ventricular pacing alone may not be effective[30,107-110] (Fig. 60-4).

REPERFUSION THERAPY

Several studies have examined the effects of early intracoronary thrombolytic therapy on the recovery of right ventricular function.[13,111-113] Braat et al.[111] reported on 54 patients with acute inferior MI caused by RCA occlusion randomized to intracoronary streptokinase vs. delayed catheterization. In the 12 patients with proximal RCA occlusion treated with intracoronary streptokinase, RVEF measured by radionuclide ventriculography performed on the second day was $36 \pm 7\%$ vs. $27 \pm 10\%$ in the 14 patients with proximal RCA occlusion treated conventionally ($P < 0.01$). This difference was maintained at 3 months (37 ± 12% vs. 30 10%, $P < 0.01$).

Heller et al.[114] studied 16 patients with acute proximal or mid-RCA occlusion treated with intracoronary thrombolytic therapy. RVEF was determined by radionuclide ventriculography at day 1, day 10, and day 70. In the 10 patients with unsuccessful reperfusion, RVEF was depressed initially at 24% but increased to 40% and then 46%. In the 6 patients with successful reperfusion, RVEF was much higher initially at 42% and increased to 49% and then 54%.

Schuler et al.[113] reported on 19 patients treated with intracoronary thrombolytic therapy for AMI secondary to proximal RCA occlusion. RVEF was measured by radionuclide ventriculography immediately after admission, 48 hours, and 4 weeks later. In the 7 patients in whom thrombolytic therapy failed, RVEF was 33 ± 5% initially and did not change significantly over time (33 ± 4% at 48 hours, 32 ± 6% at 4 weeks). However, in the 12 patients with successful recanalization, RVEF recovered significantly from 30 ± 9% to 39 ± 7% at 48 hours ($P < 0.01$) and improved further to 43 ± 5% by 4 weeks ($P < 0.01$).

Verani et al.[13] described 30 patients with acute inferior MI randomized to intracoronary nitroglycerin, intracoronary streptokinase, or conventional therapy. Radionuclide ventriculography was performed on admission before any intervention and 7 to 10 days later. Nineteen patients had an RVEF less than 40%, accompanied by right ventricular wall motion abnormalities. Mean RVEF increased from 26 ± 7% to 39 ± 14% in the 6 patients who achieved reperfusion; in 13 patients not treated with thrombolytic therapy or who did not achieve recanalization, RVEF increased from 20 ± 7% to 29 ± 7%.

These studies are limited by their small size. In patients achieving reperfusion, RVEF rapidly improved by 48 hours[113] or was markedly improved relative to controls by 24,[66] or 48 hours[111] after admission. Further late improvement in RVEF after reperfusion was noted in two studies,[112,113] but not in one.[111] In the TIMI-2 study the presence of right-ventricular wall motion abnormalities on predischarge radionuclide ventriculography was strongly associated with an occluded infarct-related artery at 18 to 48 hours (42% abnormal regional wall motion with occluded arteries vs. 13% abnormal regional wall motion with patent arteries),[66] suggesting that early patency facilitates early recovery of right ventricular function.

Rapid hemodynamic improvement in RVMI with shock has been reported in one patient after percutaneous transluminal coronary angioplasty.[115] The time course of hemodynamic improvement following reperfusion therapy for RVMI has been well characterized by Ajluni et al.[116] in a study of 27 RVMI patients, of whom

13 patients achieved reperfusion primarily by PTCA. Over the first 8 hours, mean RA pressure fell from 15.6 to 8 mm Hg in the group with successful reperfusion as opposed to no change (13.8 to 13.3 mm Hg) in the group without reperfusion ($P \leq 0.01$). Pulmonary capillary wedge pressure after 8 hours was 10.1 mm Hg with reperfusion, as opposed to 13 mm Hg without reperfusion ($P \leq 0.05$). There was an insignificant trend toward improved survival with reperfusion (92% vs. 64%).

It is important to note that right ventricular dysfunction in the setting of inferior MI is predominantly secondary to "stunned myocardium" rather than actual infarction.[63] In the absence of reperfusion therapy, most* but not all[60,111,113] studies have shown substantial improvement in RVEF in the majority of patients over a few days to several weeks. In patients not undergoing reperfusion therapy, RVEF probably improves because of the return of ischemic dysfunction secondary to spontaneous reperfusion or the development of collateral circulation. It has been shown that the right ventricle, as compared with the left ventricle, tolerates prolonged ischemia better with less necrosis. This was best demonstrated in an elegant study by Schofer et al.[120] Intracoronary thallium scintigraphy was performed before and after thrombolysis in 11 patients. Right ventricular thallium defects detected before thrombolysis were resolved after thrombolysis. In 8 of the 11 patients, intracoronary technetium-99m pyrophosphate scintigraphy was performed after thrombolysis to determine myocardial necrosis. Technetium-99m accumulation in the right ventricle was seen in only 3 of 8 patients vs. left ventricular accumulation in 7 of 8 patients.

There are several reasons why the right ventricle is less prone to infarction compared with the left ventricle. First the right ventricle has lower metabolic demands because of smaller myocardial mass and lower intracavity pressure.[121] Second, the thin-walled right ventricle has lower coronary vascular resistance, with minimal compression of the microvasculature during systole. Because of relatively higher coronary driving pressure (the difference between aortic pressure and right ventricular end-diastolic pressure), blood flow to the right ventricle occurs continuously throughout the cardiac cycle as opposed to only during diastole in the left ventricle.[122] Third, the RCA is frequently well collateralized by the left coronary artery.[123] Quantitative perfusion studies in human hearts have shown that potential collateral flow from the left coronary artery to the RCA is about three times that available in the opposite direction.[124] Also, the compressor effect of the contracting left ventricular myocardium tends to drive blood from the left coronary artery to the RCA during

*References 13, 63, 74, 113, 114, 117-119.

systole.[125] Finally, the view by Blumgart et al.[126] that the right ventricle is more immune to infarction because of direct perfusion from the right ventricular cavity through the *Thebesian* venous system is possible, but has been challenged.[127]

LONG-TERM PROGNOSIS

Several studies have examined the long-term prognostic significance of RVEF.[71,128-131] In the largest of these studies,[75] 21% of 168 patients with inferior MI had an RVEF by radionuclide ventriculography of 40% or less measured within 48 hours of admission. The 1-year survival was significantly worse (84 ± 6%) than in those with an RVEF > 40% (95 ± 2%). Multivariate analysis showed RVEF to be an independent predictor of survival. The prognostic effect of RVEF was marked in the presence of a reduced left ventricular ejection fraction. However, in the presence of a normal left ventricular ejection fraction, the prognostic effect of right ventricular dysfunction was decreased. Similarly, Shah et al.[131] found that an RVEF of 38% or less was an independent determinant of 1-year mortality by multivariate analysis. However, in the presence of LVEF > 30%, RVEF did not influence survival. Thus, LVEF is the major determinant of cardiac mortality. Pfisterer et al.[130] reported that RVEF was an independent predictor of complex ventricular arrhythmias in 127 patients followed for 1 year after AMI.

Two large studies failed to find a correlation between RVEF and survival.[128,129] Haines et al.[129] studied 74 patients 11 days after uncomplicated inferior MI who could perform predischarge exercise tests using a subjective analysis of right ventricular function. Gadsboll et al.[128] examined 134 patients but defined right ventricular dysfunction as RVEF < 57% by using a first-pass radionuclide technique. The lack of correlation between RVEF and survival in these two studies is probably related to assessment of low-risk cohorts.

Right ventricular infarction is commonly associated with inferior MI. The diagnosis may be made quickly by physical examination, electrocardiography, and other noninvasive imaging modalities. Prompt recognition is required so that appropriate therapy can be instituted if hypotension or shock develop. Traditional therapy involves avoiding nitrates and diuretics, fluid loading to maintain a right atrial pressure of 10-14 mm Hg, inotropic therapy with dobutamine, and maintenance of atrioventricular synchrony with either cardioversion or atrioventricular sequential pacing. Because the right ventricle tolerates prolonged ischemia without necrosis better than the left ventricle, reperfusion therapy may be especially effective in improving functional outcome and ameliorating hemodynamic compromise. Survival is adversely affected by rupture of the RV free wall or intraventricular septum or tricuspid valve papillary muscle, hypoxemia secondary to shunting across a patent foramen ovale or atrial septal defect, or cardiogenic shock. Long-term prognosis is excellent if right ventricular function improves. Persistent right or left ventricular dysfunction decreases long-term survival.

REFERENCES

1. Cohn JN, et al: Right ventricular infarction: clinical and hemodynamic features, *Am J Cardiol* 33:209-214, 1974.
2. Andersen HR, Falk E, Nielsen D: Right ventricular infarction: frequency, size, and topography in coronary heart disease: a prospective study comprising 107 consecutive autopsies from a coronary care unit, *J Am Coll Cardiol* 10:1223-1232, 1987.
3. Dell'Italia LJ, et al: Right ventricular infarction: identification by hemodynamic measurements before and after volume loading and correlation with noninvasive techniques, *J Am Coll Cardiol* 4:931-939, 1984.
4. Lorell B, et al: Right ventricular infarction. Clinical dignosis and differentiation from cardiac tamponade and pericardial constriction, *Am J Cardiol* 43:465-471, 1979.
5. James TN: Anatomy of the crista supraventricularis: its importance for understanding right ventricular function, right ventricular infarction and related conditions, *J Am Coll Cardiol* 6:1083-1095, 1985.
6. Isner JM, Roberts WC: Right ventricular infarction complicating left ventricular infarction secondary to coronary heart disease. Frequency, location, associated findings, and significance from analysis of 236 necropsy patients with acute or healed myocardial infarction, *Am J Cardiol* 42:885-894, 1978.
7. Braat SH, et al: Value of lead V4R for recognition of the infarct coronary artery in acute inferior myocardial infarction, *Am J Cardiol* 53:1538-1541, 1984.
8. Weinshel AJ, et al: The coronary anatomy of right ventricular myocardial infarction: relationship between the site of RCA occlusion and origin of the right ventricular free wall branches (abstract), *Circulation* 68:III-351, 1983.
9. Goldstein JA, et al: Determinants of hemodynamic compromise with severe right ventricular infarction, *Circulation* 82:359-368, 1990.
10. Nakahara K, et al: Isolated right ventricular infarction resulting from thrombotic occlusion of a hypoplastic RCA, *Jpn Heart J* 30:95-101, 1989.
11. Weiss AT, et al: Isolated right ventricular infarction with ventricular tachycardia, *Am Heart J* 108:425-426, 1984.
12. Forman MB, et al: Electrocardiographic changes associated with isolated right ventricular infarction, *J Am Coll Cardiol* 4:640-643, 1984.
13. Verani MS, et al: Effect of coronary artery recanalization on right ventricular function in patients with acute myocardial infarction, *J Am Coll Cardiol* 5:1029-1035, 1985.
14. Cabin HS, et al: Right ventricular myocardial infarction with anterior wall left ventricular infarction: an autopsy study, *Am Heart J* 113:16-23, 1987.
15. Chuttani K, Sussman H, Pandian NG: Echocardiographic evidence that regional right ventricular dysfunction occurs frequently in anterior myocardial infarction, *Am Heart J* 122:850-851, 1991.
16. Carlson EB, et al: Right ventricular subendocardial infarction in a patient with pulmonary hypertension, right ventricular hypertrophy, and normal coronary arteries, *Clin Cardiol* 8:499-502, 1985.
17. Forman MB, et al: Right ventricular hypertrophy is an important determinant of right ventricular infarction complicating acute inferior left ventricular infarction, *J Am Coll Cardiol* 10:1180-1187, 1987.

18. Case 42-1963, Case records of the Massachusetts General Hospital: Weekly clinicopathological exercises, *N Engl J Med* 268:1403-1410, 1963.

19. Coma-Canella I et al: Acute right ventricular infarction secondary to massive pulmonary embolism, *Eur Heart J* 9:534-540, 1988.

20. Franciosi RA, Blanc WA: Myocardial infarcts in infants and children. I. A necropsy study in congenital heart disease, *J Pediatr* 73:309-319, 1968.

21. Kopelman HA, et al: Right ventricular myocardial infarction in patients with chronic lung disease: possible role of right ventricular hypertrophy, *J Am Coll Cardiol* 5:1302-1307, 1985.

22. Bakos ACP: The question of the function of the right ventricular myocardium: an experimental study, *Circulation* 1:724-731, 1950.

23. Guiha NH, Limas CT, Cohn JN: Predominant right ventricular dysfunction after right ventricular destruction in the dog, *Am J Cardiol* 33:254-258, 1974.

24. Kagan A: Dynamic responses of the right ventricle following extensive damage by cauterization, *Circulation* 5:816-882, 1952.

25. Starr I, Jeffers WA, Meade RH, Jr: The absence of conspicuous increments of venous pressure after severe damage to the right ventricle of the dog, with a discussion of the relation between clinical congestive heart failure and heart disease, *Am Heart J* 26:291-301, 1943.

26. Donald DE, Essex HE: Pressure studies after inactivation of the major portion of the canine right ventricle, *Am J Physiol* 176:155-161, 1954.

27. Goldstein JA, et al: The role of right ventricular systolic dysfunction and elevated intrapericardial pressure in the genesis of low output in experimental right ventricular infarction, *Circulation* 65:513-522, 1982.

28. Goldstein JA, et al: Volume loading improves cardiac output in experimental right ventricular infarction, *J Am Coll Cardiol* 2:270-278, 1983.

29. Ferguson JJ, et al: Significance of nitroglycerin-induced hypotension with inferior wall acute myocardial infarction, *Am J Cardiol* 64:311-314, 1989.

30. Abraham KA, Brown MA, Norris RM: Right ventricular infarction, bradyarrhythmia, and cardiogenic shock: importance of atrial or atrioventricular sequential pacing, *Aust NZ J Med* 15:52-54, 1985.

31. Baigrie RS, et al: The spectrum of right ventricular involvement in inferior wall myocardial infarction: a clinical, hemodynamic and noninvasive study, *J Am Coll Cardiol* 1:1396-1404, 1983.

32. Braat SH, et al: Right ventricular involvement with acute inferior wall myocardial infarction identifies high risk of developing atrioventricular nodal conduction disturbances, *Am Heart J* 107:1183-1187, 1984.

33. Dell'Italia LJ, Starling MR, O'Rourke RA: Physical examination for exclusion of hemodynamically important right ventricular infarction, *Ann Intern Med* 99:608-611, 1983.

34. Zone DD, Botti RE: Right ventricular infarction with tricuspid insufficiency and chronic right heart failure, *Am J Cardiol* 37:445-448, 1976.

35. Lopez-Sendon J, et al: Segmental right ventricular function after acute myocardial infarction: two-dimensional echocardiographic study in 63 patients, *Am J Cardiol* 51:390-396, 1983.

36. Shah PK, et al: Scintigraphically detected predominantly right ventricular dysfunction in acute myocardial infarction: clinical and hemodynamic correlates and implications for therapy and prognosis, *J Am Coll Cardiol* 6:1264-1272, 1985.

37. Cintron GB, et al: Bedside recognition, incidence and clinical course of right ventricular infarction, *Am J Cardiol* 47:224-227, 1981.

38. Chou T, J Van Der Bel-Kahn, et al: Electrocardiographic diagnosis of right ventricular infarction, *Am J Med* 70:1175-1180, 1981.

39. Erhardt LR, Sjogren A, Wahlbert I: Single right-sided precordial lead in the diagnosis of right ventricular involvement in inferior myocardial infarction, *Am Heart J* 91:571-576, 1976.

40. Braat SH, et al: Value of electrocardiogram in diagnosing right ventricular involvement in patients with acute inferior wall myocardial infarction, *Br Heart J* 49:368-372, 1983.

41. Braat SH, et al: Right and left ventricular ejection fraction in acute inferior wall infarction with or without ST segment elevation in lead V4R, *J Am Coll Cardiol* 4:940-944, 1984.

42. Candall-Riera J, et al: Right ventricular infarction: relationships between ST segment elevation in V4R and hemodynamic, scintigraphic, and echocardiographic findings in patients with acute inferior myocardial infarction, *Am Heart J* 101:281-287, 1981.

43. Croft CH, et al: Detection of acute right ventricular infarction by right precordial electrocardiography, *Am J Cardiol* 50:421-427, 1982.

44. Klein HO, et al: The early recognition of right ventricular infarction: diagnostic accuracy of the electrocardiographic V4R lead, *Circulation* 67:558-565, 1983.

45. Lopez-Sendon J, et al: Electrocardiographic findings in acute right ventricular infarction: sensitivity and specificity of electrocardiographic alterations in right precordial leads V4R, V3R, V1, V2, and V3, *J Am Coll Cardiol* 6:1273-1279, 1985 .

46. Andersen HR, et al: Prognostic significance of right ventricular infarction diagnosed by ST elevation in right chest leads V3R to V7R, *Int J Cardiol* 23:349-356, 1989.

47. Morgera T, et al: Right precordial ST and QRS changes in the diagnosis of right ventricular infarction, *Am Heart J* 108:13-18, 1984.

48. Andersen HR, Falk E, Nielsen D: Right ventricular infarction: diagnostic accuracy of electrocardiographic right chest leads V3R to V7R investigated prospectively in 43 consecutive fatal cases from a coronary care unit, *Br Heart J* 61:514-520, 1989.

49. Coma-Canella I, et al: Electrocardiographic alterations in leads V1 to V3 in the diagnosis of right and left ventricular infarction, *Am Heart J* 112:940-946, 1986.

50. Geft IL, et al: ST elevations in leads V1 to V5 may be caused by RCA occlusion and acute right ventricular infarction, *Am J Cardiol* 53:991-996, 1984.

51. Cecchi F, et al: Echocardiographic features of right ventricular infarction, *Clin Cardiol* 7:405-412, 1984.

52. D'Arcy B, Nanda NC: Two-dimensional echocardiographic features of right ventricular infarction, *Circulation* 65:167-173, 1982.

53. Goldberger JJ, et al: Right ventricular infarction: recognition and assessment of its hemodynamic significance by two-dimensional echocardiography, *J Am Soc Echocardiogr* 4:140-146, 1991.

54. Jugdutt BI, et al: Right ventricular infarction: two-dimensional echocardiographic evaluation, *Am Heart J* 101:505-518, 1984.

55. Sharpe DN, et al: The noninvasive diagnosis of right ventricular infarction, *Circulation* 57:483-490, 1978.

56. Kaul S, et al: Assessment of right ventricular function using two-dimensional echocardiography, *Am Heart J* 107:526-531, 1984.

57. Dhainaut JF, et al: Role of tricuspid regurgitation and left ventricular damage in the treatment of right ventricular infarction-induced low cardiac output syndrome, *Am J Cardiol* 66:289-295, 1990.

58. Takeuchi M, et al: Role of right ventricular asynergy and tricuspid regurgitation in hemodynamic alterations during acute inferior myocardial infarction, *Jpn Heart J* 30:615-625, 1989.

59. Stowers SA, et al: Right ventricular thrombus in association with acute myocardial infarction: diagnosis by two-dimensional echocardiography, *Am J Cardiol* 52:912-913, 1983.

60. Reduto LA, et al: Sequential radionuclide assessment of left and

right ventricular performance after acute transmural myocardial infarction, *Ann Intern Med* 89:441-447, 1978.

61. Rigo P, et al: Right ventricular dysfunction detected by gated scintigraphy in patients with acute myocardial infarction, *Circulation* 52:268-274; 1975.

62. Starling MR, et al: First transit and equilibrium radionuclide angiography in patients with inferior myocardial infarction: criteria for the diagnosis of associated hemodynamically significant right ventricular infarction. *J Am Coll Cardiol* 4:923-930, 1984.

63. Tahara Y, et al: Evaluation with Fourier analysis on radionuclide angiography of viable but stunned myocardium in patients with right ventricular myocardial infarction, *Jpn Circ J* 55:543-552, 1991.

64. Tobinik E, et al: Right ventricular ejection fraction in patients with acute anterior and inferior myocardial infarction assessed by radionuclide angiography, *Circulation* 57:1078-1084, 1978.

65. Wackers FJ, et al: Prevalence of right ventricular involvement in inferior wall infarction assessed with myocardial imaging with thallium-201 and technetium-99m pyrophosphate, *Am J Cardiol* 42:358-362, 1978.

66. Berger PB, et al: Frequency and significance of right ventricular dysfunction during inferior wall left ventricular myocardial infarction treated with thrombolytic therapy (results from the Thrombolysis in Myocardial Infarction [TIMI] II trial), *Am J Cardiol* 71:1148-1152, 1993.

67. Coma-Canella I, Lopez-Sendon J: Ventricular compliance in ischemic right ventricular dysfunction, *Am J Cardiol* 45:555-561, 1980.

68. Lopez-Sendon J, Coma-Canella I, Gamallo C: Sensitivity and specificity of hemodynamic criteria in the diagnosis of acute right ventricular infarction, *Circulation* 64:515-525, 1981.

69. Coma-Canella I, et al: Hemodynamic findings in experimental right ventricular ischemia after right coronary arterial ligation, *Eur Heart J* 7:711-718, 1986.

70. Anderson HR, Nielsen D, Falk E: Right ventricular infarction: larger enzyme release with posterior than with anterior involvement, *Int J Cardiol* 22:347-355, 1989.

71. Strauss HD, Sobel BE, Roberts R: The influence of occult right ventricular infarction on enzymatically estimated infarct size, hemodynamics and prognosis, *Circulation* 62:503-508, 1980.

72. Weinshel AJ, et al: Peak CPK in transmural inferior wall infarction of the left ventricle: clue to presence or absence of coexistent right ventricular myocardial infarction (abstract), *Circulation* 68:II-391, 1983.

73. Barrillon A, et al: Premonitory sign of heart block in acute posterior infarction, *Br Heart J* 37:2-8, 1975.

74. Nistor-Hemmert D, Ciplea A: The predictive value of V3R-V4R precordial leads in the occurrence of conduction disturbances in inferior acute myocardial infarction (AMI), *Physiologie* 19:87-90, 1982.

75. Marwick TH, et al: Prognostic significance of right ventricular ejection fraction following inferior myocardial infarction, *Int J Cardiol* 31:205-211, 1991.

76. Kereiakes DJ, et al: Right ventricular myocardial infarction with ventricular septal rupture, *Am Heart J* 6:1257-1259, 1984.

77. Isner J, Roberts WC: Double rupture of the heart: a consequence of the unique pathology of right ventricular myocardial infarction (abstract), *Circulation* 68:II-392, 1983.

78. Van Tassel RA, Edwards JE: Rupture of heart complicating myocardial infarction: analysis of 40 cases including nine examples of left ventricular false aneurysm, *Chest* 61:104-116, 1972.

79. Cummings RG, et al: Quantitative analysis of right and left ventricular infarction in the presence of postinfarction ventricular septal defect, *Circulation* 77:33-42, 1988.

80. Fananapazir L, et al: Right ventricular dysfunction and surgical outcome in postinfarction ventricular septal defect, *Eur Heart J* 4:157-167, 1983.

81. Grose R, Spindola-Franco H: Right ventricular dysfunction in acute ventricular septal defect, *Am Heart J* 101:67-74, 1981.

82. Radford MJ, et al: Ventricular septal rupture: a review of clinical and physiologic features and an analysis of survival, *Circulation* 64:545-552, 1981.

83. Bansal RC, et al: Severe hypoxemia due to shunting through a patent foramen ovale: a correctable complication of right ventricular infarction, *J Am Coll Cardiol* 5:188-192, 1985.

84. Broderick TM, Dillon JC: Therapeutic balloon occlusion and pharmacologic therapy of a right-to-left atrial shunt produced by right ventricular infarction, *Am Heart J* 118:1044-1047, 1989.

85. Daubert JC, et al: Severe hypoxemia due to a right-to-left shunt at the atrial level caused by an infarction of the right ventricle, *Arch Mal Coeur* 78:563-568, 1985.

86. Krueger SK, Lappe DL: Right-to-left shunt through patent foramen ovale complicating right ventricular infarction: successful percutaneous catheter closure, *Chest* 94:1100-1101, 1988.

87. Manno BV, et al: Right ventricular infarction complicated by right to left shunt, *J Am Coll Cardiol* 2:554-557, 1983.

88. Rietveld AP, et al: Right to left shunt, with severe hypoxemia, at the atrial level in a patient with hemodynamically important right ventricular infarction, *J Am Coll Cardiol* 2:776-779, 1983.

89. Sterling I, et al: Refractory arterial hypoxemia and interatrial right-left shunt in myocardial infarction of the right ventricle, *Arch Mal Coeur* 83:425-427, 1990.

90. Uppstrom EL, et al: Balloon catheter closure of patent foramen ovale complicating right ventricular infarction: improvement of hypoxia and intracardiac venous shunting, *Am Heart J* 116:1092-1096, 1988.

91. Collins P, Daly JJ: Tricuspid incompetence complicating acute myocardial infarction, *Postgrad Med J* 53:51-52, 1977.

92. Eisenberg S, Suyemoto J: Rupture of a papillary muscle of the tricuspid valve following acute myocardial infarction, *Circulation* 30:588-591, 1964.

93. Korr KS, et al: Tricuspid valve replacement for cardiogenic shock after acute right ventricular infarction, *JAMA* 244:1958-1960, 1980.

94. McAllister RG Jr, Friesinger GC, Sinclair-Smith BC: Tricuspid regurgitation following inferior myocardial infarction, *Arch Intern Med* 136:95-99, 1976.

95. Raabe DS, Chester AC: Right ventricular infarction, *Chest* 73:96-99, 1978.

96. Case 3442: *N Engl J Med* 239:683-687, 1948.

97. Rechavia E, et al: The impact of right ventricular infarction on the prevalence of ventricular arrhythmias during acute inferior myocardial infarction, *Chest* 98:1207-1209, 1990.

98. Sclarovsky S, et al: Ventricular fibrillation complicating temporary ventricular pacing in acute myocardial infarction: significance of right ventricular infarction, *Am J Cardiol* 48:1160-1166, 1981.

99. Lopez-Sendon J, et al: Right ventricular infarction as a risk factor for ventricular fibrillation during pulmonary artery catheterization using Swan-Ganz catheters, *Am Heart J* 119:207-209, 1990.

100. Coma-Canella I, Lopez-Sendon J, Gamallo C: Low-output syndrome in right ventricular infarction, *Am Heart J* 98:613-620, 1979.

101. Gewirtz H, et al: Role of right ventricular infarction in cardiogenic shock associated with inferior myocardial infarction, *Br Heart J* 42:719-725, 1979.

102. Legrand V, et al: Right ventricular myocardial infarction diagnosed by 99m pyrophosphate scintigraphy: clinical course and follow-up, *Eur Heart J* 4:9-19, 1983.

103. Lloyd EA, Gersh BJ, Kennelly BM: Hemodynamic spectrum of

"dominant" right ventricular infarction in 19 patients, *Am J Cardiol* 48:1016-1022, 1981.

104. Berisha S, et al: Optimal valve of filling pressure in the right side of the heart in acute right ventricular infarction, *Br Heart J* 63:98-102, 1990.

105. Dell'Italia LJ, et al: Comparative effects of volume loading, dobutamine and nitroprusside in patients with predominant right ventricular infarction, *Circulation* 72:1327-1335, 1985.

106. Lopez-Sandon J, Coma-Canella I, Vinvelas Adanez J: Volume loading in patients with ischemic right ventricular dysfunction, *Eur Heart J* 2:329-338, 1981.

107. Isner JM, et al: Right ventricular infarction with hemodynamic decompensation due to transient loss of active atrial augmentation: successful treatment with atrial pacing, *Am Heart J* 102:792-794, 1981.

108. Love JC, et al: Reversibility of hypotension and shock by atrial or atrioventricular sequential pacing in patients with right ventricular infarction, *Am Heart J* 108:5-13, 1984.

109. Matangi MF: Temporary physiologic pacing in inferior wall acute myocardial infarction with right ventricular damage, *Am J Cardiol* 59:1027-1028, 1987.

110. Topol EJ, et al: Hemodynamic benefit of atrial pacing in right ventricular myocardial infarction, *Ann Intern Med* 96:594-597, 1982.

111. Braat SH, et al: Reperfusion with streptokinase of an occluded RCA: effects of early and late right and left ventricular ejection fraction, *Am Heart J* 113:257-260, 1987.

112. Heller GV, et al: Return of right ventricular function in patients with right coronary occlusion: the resilient right ventricle (abstract), *Circulation* 68:III-392, 1983.

113. Schuler G, et al: Effect of successful thrombolytic therapy on right ventricular function in acute inferior myocardial infarction, *Am J Cardiol* 54:951-957, 1984.

114. Steele P, et al: Prompt return to normal of depressed right ventricular ejection fraction in acute inferior infarction, *Br Heart J* 39:1319-1323, 1977.

115. Moreyra AE, et al: Rapid hemodynamic improvement in right ventricular infarction arter coronary angioplasty, *Chest* 94:197-199, 1988.

116. Ajluni SC, et al: The hemodynamic effects of coronary reperfusion in right ventricular infarction (abstract), *J Am Coll Cardiol* 17:186A, 1991.

117. Bellamy GR, et al: Value of two-dimensional echocardiography, electrocardiography, and clinical signs in detecting right ventricular infarction, *Am Heart J* 112:304-309, 1986.

118. Dell'Italia LJ, et al: Hemodynamically important right ventricular infarction: follow-up evaluation of right ventricular systolic function at rest and during exercise with radionuclide ventriculography and respiratory gas exchange, *Circulation* 75:996-1003, 1987.

119. Yasuda T, et al: Serial evaluation of right ventricular function with right ventricular infarction (abstract), *Am J Cardiol* 47:458, 1981.

120. Schofer J, et al: Scintigraphic evidence that right ventricular myocardium tolerates ischemia better than left ventricular myocardium (abstract), *Circulation* 68:III-392, 1983.

121. Henquell L, Honig CR: O$_2$ extraction of right and left ventricles, *Proc Soc Exp Biol Med* 152:52-53, 1976.

122. Hess DS, Bache RJ: Transmural right ventricular myocardial blood flow during systole in the awake dog, *Circ Res* 45:88-94, 1979.

123. Farrer-Brown G: Vascular pattern of myocardium of right ventricle of human heart, *Br Heart J* 30:679-686, 1968.

124. Prinzmetal M, et al: A quantitative method for determining collateral coronary circulation. Preliminary report on normal human hearts, *J Mt Sinai Hosp* 8:933-939; 1942.

125. Wiggers CJ: The interplay of coronary vascular resistance and myocardial compression in regulating coronary flow, *Circ Res* 2:271-279, 1954.

126. Blumgart HL, Schlesinger MJ, David D: Studies of relationship of clinical manifestations of angina pectoris, coronary thrombosis, and myocardial infarction to pathologic findings, with particular reference to significance of collateral circulation, *Am Heart J* 19:1-91, 1940.

127. Wade WG: The pathogenesis of infarction of the right ventricle, *Br Heart J* 21:545-554, 1957.

128. Gadsboll N, et al: Right and left ventricular ejection fractions: relation to one-year prognosis in acute myocardial infarction, *Eur Heart J* 8:1201-1209, 1987.

129. Haines DE, et al: A prospective clinical, scintigraphic, angiographic and functional evaluation of patients after inferior myocardial infarction with and without right ventricular dysfunction, *J Am Coll Cardiol* 6:995-1003, 1985.

130. Pfisterer M, et al: Prognostic significance of right ventricular ejection fraction for persistent complex ventricular arrhythmias and/or sudden cardiac death after first myocardial infarction: relation to infarct location, size and left ventricular function, *Eur Heart J* 7:289-298, 1986.

131. Shah PK, et al: Variable spectrum and prognostic implications of left and right ventricular ejection fractions in patients with and without heart failure after acute myocardial infarction, *Am J Cardiol* 58:387-398, 1986.

Chapter 61

DELIRIUM IN THE CORONARY CARE UNIT

K. Michael Zabel
William R. Hathaway

The development of acute confusional states and agitation in individuals admitted to intensive care units (ICUs) has been observed for more than 30 years. Patients who have no discernible cognitive deficits at the time of admission may rapidly develop restlessness, disorientation, hallucinations, and even paranoid ideation that often precipitates intense agitation and combativeness. Traditionally the term ICU psychosis has been used to describe such changes in mental status, especially when no organic cause could be readily identified. This is somewhat misleading, however, because the term psychosis generally refers to a functional disorder characterized by a loss of contact with reality in which the sensorium is normal, but thought processes are associated with abnormal perceptions and systematic delusions.[1] In contrast, cognitive impairment in the CCU patient often has an organic basis and typically is characterized by an abnormal sensorium with disorganized delusions.

Because of these discrepancies, we prefer the term ICU delirium to describe the temporary mental status changes seen in patients after admission to an ICU setting. Delirium can be defined as a "reversible, global impairment of cognitive processes, associated with disorientation, impaired short-term memory, short attention span, as well as altered perception, abnormal thought processes and inappropriate behavior."[2] This definition accurately reflects the manifestations most often attributed to "ICU psychosis" and encompasses both organic and functional causes for cognitive impairment.

INCIDENCE

The incidence of delirium in ICUs has been reported between 7%[3] and 57%.[4] This wide range results primarily from variability in the definition of delirium and in the specific patient population studied. The highest frequency of acute delirium appears to be seen in surgical ICUs, particularly those caring for large numbers of postsurgical cardiac patients. The observed incidence of delirium in medical CCUs is probably between 5% and 15%, although several studies have shown that a far greater proportion of patients (perhaps as high as 70%) experience transient symptoms of delirium or other psychologic disturbances that go unnoticed by ICU staff.[5,6]

CLINICAL FEATURES

The clinical manifestations of ICU delirium range from apprehension and mild disorientation to hallucinations, clouding of consciousness, and frankly paranoid delusions (Table 61-1). Although individuals with a prior history of psychosis or delirium are most susceptible,[7] the majority of patients that develop this syndrome have completely normal mental and psychologic profiles at the time of admission. In cases that do not involve a clearly definable etiology (e.g., alcohol withdrawal or physiologic disturbance), symptoms are most often noted between the third and seventh day after admission to the CCU.[5]

One of the most common manifestations of delirium in the CCU patient is alteration of the sleep-wake cycle. Patients may complain of nocturnal insomnia

Table 61-1. Manifestations of critical care unit delirium

Alterations of		
Mood	Labile affect	
	Depression	
	Mania	
	Euphoria	
	Anxiety	
Thought	Loose associations	Rambling speech
	Concrete thinking	Memory impairment
	Delusions	Disorientation
	Paranoia	Clouded sensorium
Perception	Illusions	
	Hallucinations	
	Auditory	
	Visual	
	Tactile	
Physiology	Tachycardia	Seizures
	Hypertension	Abnormal sleep patterns
	Diaphoresis	Combative behavior
	Nausea	

only to sleep for much of the day, or they may sleep in short 1- to 2-hour periods around the clock. A common observation is that the severity of delirium increases during the evening hours, a phenomenon sometimes termed "sundowning." Although the cause of sundowning is unclear, patients may display profound agitation and confusion during the evening and night hours only to recover a completely normal sensorium the next morning and then relapse again that night. Some investigators have suggested that abnormal sleep patterns are a cause rather than an effect of ICU delirium.[8]

The clinical consequences of delirium in the CCU patient may be profound and even lethal. For those with unstable angina or acute myocardial infarction (AMI), the hyperadrenergic state that usually accompanies delirium may adversely effect the tenuous balance between myocardial oxygen supply and demand, possibly resulting in AMI or infarct extension. Increased adrenergic tone contributes to the development of atrial or ventricular dysrhythmias and causes hypertension, increasing the risk of intracerebral bleeding in patients receiving thrombolytic agents. Agitated patients may harm themselves by traumatic removal of intravenous (IV) lines, arterial lines, femoral sheaths, or urethral catheters. Patients whose airways are intubated may displace the endotracheal tube, leading to extubation or selective right mainstem bronchus intubation with resultant left lung atelectasis or collapse. Seizures occurring in conjunction with alcohol withdrawal may lead to

pulmonary aspiration, respiratory arrest, or the adult respiratory distress syndrome.

ETIOLOGY

Recognition of risk and anticipation of the development of delirium are the initial steps in prevention of its onset. Although identifiable causes for the development of delirium in the CCU patient are sometimes found, this is not always the case. "Idiopathic" delirium, for lack of a better term, has been associated with a number of factors that should be considered by CCU personnel for all admitted patients. We have divided these risk factors into two categories: those related specifically to the individual patient, including certain disease states and the adverse effects of pharmacologic interventions, and those related to the CCU environment.

Patient factors

The most important patient factor correlating with the risk of developing CCU delirium is age. Studies show that patients more than 60 years of age are particularly vulnerable, with significantly less risk in younger individuals.[9] A fivefold increase in risk was observed for patients more than 80 years old compared with individuals aged 60 to 80 years.[10] This has been postulated to be related to a deficiency of acetylcholine in the aging brain, although convincing data to support this theory are lacking.[11] One study indicated that males may be more likely to develop delirium than females,[10] although others have found no sex predilection.[12] Individuals with a history of illicit drug use, previous episodes of delirium, and those with chronic cardiovascular, respiratory, renal, or metabolic illness are also at higher risk than the population as a whole.[5]

Patients with preexisting CNS dysfunction, secondary to chronic dementia or prior stroke for example, have less cognitive reserve and clearly are more vulnerable to developing delirium with stress.[7] Other authors have suggested that certain personality types may be prone to the development of delirium. There is little consensus in this matter, however, with some studies indicating dominant, aggressive individuals are the most likely to be affected,[12,13] whereas others indicate dependent, passive persons to be at the greatest risk for delirium.[14]

A number of organic disturbances can contribute to or mimic delirium. These include diseases that involve primarily the central nervous system (CNS) such as intracranial hemorrhage, encephalitis, meningitis, complex partial seizures, postictal state, stroke, CNS vasculitis, and normal pressure hydrocephalus. Frequent, careful neurologic examinations and the prompt use of appropriate radiologic (e.g., computed tomography and magnetic resonance imaging) and invasive (e.g., lumbar puncture) studies are essential in the early diagnosis of these entities, many of which are potentially treatable.

Table 61-2. Adverse effects of drugs commonly used in the coronary care unit

Drug	Hallucinations	Depression	Anxiety	Confusion	Other
Albuterol	✓				Paranoia
Antihistamines	✓		✓		
Anticholinergics	✓			✓	Memory loss, paranoia
Barbiturates	✓	✓			
β-Lactam Abx.	✓			✓	Seizures
Benzodiazepines	✓	✓			
β-Blockers	✓	✓		✓	
Corticosteroids	✓	✓		✓	Paranoia
Clonidine		✓	✓		Insomnia, nightmares
Digoxin	✓			✓	Paranoia, delusions, nightmares
Diltiazem				✓	Delusions
Disopyramide	✓			✓	Paranoia
Epinephrine					Fear, restlessness
H₂ blockers	✓		✓	✓	
Lidocaine	✓		✓	✓	Paranoia, seizures
Methyldopa	✓	✓			Paranoia
Morphine	✓			✓	
Nitroprusside	✓				Delusions
Procainamide	✓	✓			Psychosis
Quinidine	✓		✓		Delusions
Tocainine					Tremor, paranoia

The brain may also be adversely affected by disorders that primarily affect other organ systems. In the CCU patient with low cardiac output, the diminished flow of oxygen to the brain may result in restlessness, confusion, or agitation. As cerebral blood flow is further impaired, the patient may become increasingly somnolent, experience seizure activity, or become unresponsive. If treated promptly, the patient usually responds with complete recovery of brain function. Even a relatively short delay in correcting severe cerebral ischemia, however, can result in permanent neurologic deficits.

Metabolic and endocrine disorders are common in acutely ill patients, and many have been implicated as a cause of cerebral dysfunction. These include hypoxia, hypercapnia, hyponatremia or hypernatremia, hypercalcemia, hepatic failure, hypothyroidism, acid-base disturbances, hypoglycemia, renal failure, or deficiencies of thiamine or vitamin B₁₂. Because of the increased metabolic stress experienced by many CCU patients, acute adrenal insufficiency is a constant danger in predisposed patients and may present with symptoms of ICU delirium. Patients who are treated with chronic corticosteroids before admission are at increased risk for this disorder. A recent study indicated that more than 50% of patients receiving corticosteroid therapy for greater than 1 week had subnormal pituitary-adrenal function, even when receiving less than 5 mg of prednisone daily.[15]

Many drugs used in the CCU are capable of producing altered mental status and may contribute to the development of delirium (Table 61-2). Virtually all of the antiarrhythmic agents, including type II (β-blockers) and type IV (calcium channel blockers) agents, have been reported to cause psychiatric symptoms. In some cases (e.g., lidocaine) these effects are predictable and occur chiefly at high serum drug concentrations. Other agents such as quinidine and diltiazem exhibit idiosyncratic toxicity, with psychosis being demonstrated at subtherapeutic concentrations. Hepatic and renal dysfunction, common in the CCU patient, contribute to altered drug metabolism and excretion, further exacerbating potential CNS side effects.

A final common pathophysiologic factor in the development of CCU delirium is that of drug withdrawal. Although many drug classes cause unpleasant or adverse effects when discontinued (e.g., opiates, amphetamines), agents that depress the CNS elicit the most dangerous withdrawal responses. The sudden withdrawal of alcohol, benzodiazepines, or barbiturates leads to a rebound increase in CNS activity and adrenergic tone resulting in tremor, hyperactivity, tachycardia, diaphoresis, hyperpyrexia, insomnia, hallucinations, or seizures, including status epilepticus.[16] The treatment of acute abstinence syndromes seen with alcohol and other CNS depressants is discussed later on.

Environmental factors

The CCU, although indispensable in the care of acute cardiac disease, is not a comfortable place in which to reside. Noise,[17] constant artificial lighting,[5] and an unfamiliar environment[6] can contribute to disorientation and eventual delirium in patients hospitalized for more than a short time. A possible common denominator for many of these factors is their effect on the sleep-wake cycle. Patients in ICU settings spend more time in stage I sleep at the expense of deeper stages.[11] Healthy subjects undergoing sleep deprivation rapidly develop irritability, depression, disorientation, delusions, and illusions,[5,18] symptoms quite similar to those seen in patients with ICU delirium.

PREVENTION

Although there are few controlled studies demonstrating effective techniques for preventing acute delirium in the ICU setting, knowledge of predisposing and contributing factors suggests certain logical steps.

First, it is important to identify those patients at increased risk of delirium while in the CCU. As noted earlier, elderly patients fall into this group, and the risk increases with increasing age.[10] Patients with preexisting cognitive impairment (functional or organic) and those with a history of neuroleptic, alcohol, or illicit drug use are also at increased risk. Patients admitted to the CCU after cardiac surgery need to be monitored especially closely because the risk of transient delirium in the postcardiotomy patient may exceed 50%.[19] Factors believed to be associated with this increased incidence include decreased cerebral perfusion secondary to cardiac bypass, anesthetic agents, hypothermia, and relative hypotension.

Proper design and furnishing of the CCU may serve to decrease the incidence of acute delirium. Individual patient rooms are preferable to a common patient care area because the level of ambient noise at the bedside is minimized and patient privacy is enhanced. The provision of conference areas for CCU staff and the placement of monitoring alarms at a distance from the bedside also serve to decrease extraneous noise. Rooms should be equipped with windows or skylights and arranged to allow the patient an unobstructed view of the outside if possible. In one study, twice as many patients in ICU rooms without windows developed delirium when compared with those in rooms with windows.[20] Clocks and calendars visible to the patients provide valuable environmental orientation, as does the intermittent use of radio or television.[21] Periodic exposure to music may also be beneficial, especially when combined with a supervised relaxation program.[22]

Nursing interventions should be planned to allow for substantial periods of uninterrupted sleep. Appropriate day-night patterns should be encouraged by dimming artificial lights after evening hours and by maximizing cognitive stimulation during the day. Family members play an important role in this stimulation and also provide vital emotional support during times of stress. Their presence should be encouraged and facilitated to the degree that the individual's medical and nursing

requirements allow. In patients demonstrating increased confusion and agitation at night, we have found that the presence of a family member may markedly improve symptoms and can occasionally obviate the need for physical restraints or pharmacologic treatment. Long-term CCU patients may benefit from nursing staff schedules that provide for one or more "primary" caregivers, allowing the development of closer interpersonal relationships between patient and nurse.

One rather obvious but often overlooked solution to the problem of CCU delirium is to minimize the time spent in the CCU. Although it has been shown that perceived stress and urinary catecholamine excretion increase in patients after transfer out of the CCU,[23] in general, patients benefit from the decreased noise, increased privacy, and freedom found on nonunit wards. The widespread availability of telemetered cardiac monitoring and designated "step-down" units with a low patient/nurse ratio and specially trained staff give many patients the opportunity to transfer out of the CCU quickly. In patients without identifiable organic disturbances who develop acute delirium while in the CCU, symptoms generally improve within 48 hours of transfer.[5]

TREATMENT

The treatment of delirium in the CCU is guided by the following principles: (1) correct physiologic disturbances, (2) recognize adverse effects of administered drugs, (3) recognize and treat drug withdrawal, (4) provide adequate pharmacologic therapy when necessary.[1]

Physiologic causes of delirium

Any adverse change in the mental status of critically ill patients must first be attributed to physiologic disturbances, of which the potential causes are many. Initial evaluation begins with a careful physical examination paying close attention to the neurologic system (Fig. 61-1). Focal neurologic findings (e.g., motor or sensory disturbances, abnormalities in cranial nerve function, cerebellar signs) raise the suspicion of intracranial pathologic conditions such as hemorrhage, thromboembolism, or, much less commonly, tumor and provide indication for emergency cranial CT or MRI scanning. Patients without focal findings but who are anticoagulated or have received thrombolytic therapy should at a minimum receive a noncontrasted head CT to rule out intracranial hemorrhage when no other cause of the delirium is obvious.

Metabolic causes of delirium, generally characterized by a lack of focal findings on neurologic examination, are simultaneously investigated. Electrolyte abnormalities are common in the CCU population because of the frequent use of pharmacologic agents (e.g., diuretics)

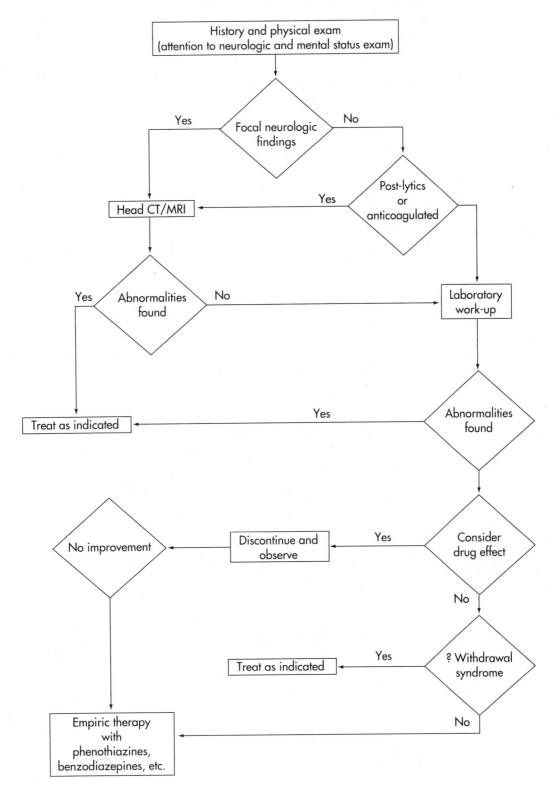

Fig. 61-1. Approach to the delirious coronary care unit patient. *CT,* Computed tomography; *MRI,* magnetic resonance imaging.

and physiologic states (e.g., heart failure) that can dramatically and rapidly affect regulatory homeostatic mechanisms. Measurement of serum sodium, potassium, bicarbonate, chloride, ionized calcium, and magnesium levels should be obtained on all patients with altered mental status. Serum creatinine and blood urea nitrogen (BUN) levels are obtained to assess renal function. Serum glucose measurement rules out diabetic ketoacidosis, hyperosmolar coma, or hypoglycemia. Serum ammonia levels may be elevated in some patients with hepatic encephalopathy, although the lack of sensitivity and specificity of this test makes it a poor screening test. Arterial blood gas analysis can reveal hypoxemia, hypercapnia, or profound acidosis, although there are generally other clues to these diagnoses.

Thyroid function studies, preferably including free thyroxine and thyroid-stimulating hormone, should be obtained in most CCU patients with altered mental status because the incidence of thyroid dysfunction is significant, especially in patients receiving amiodarone where it may exceed 30%.[24] Patients with a history of corticosteroid use or adrenal abnormalities who show other evidence of adrenal insufficiency, such as hypotension or hyponatremia, should be screened by measuring serum cortisol levels immediately before and 1 hour after IV administration of 0.25 mg of cosyntropin. The failure of the 1-hour cortisol to reach at least 18 μg/dl or to increase by at least 7 μg/dl over the baseline value suggests adrenal insufficiency and should prompt a trial of stress-dose glucocorticoid replacement.

Other commonly ordered studies are of questionable value in the routine evaluation of CCU patients with delirium. A urine drug screen may occasionally yield useful information, particularly in the patient who is admitted with an abnormal mental status. The yield of routine VDRL (Veneral Disease Research Laboratory), heavy metals, or B12 level is low except in patients who show specific symptoms or laboratory abnormalities suggesting one of these processes.

Adverse drug effects

If a physiologic abnormality is not obvious, the next consideration should be an adverse drug effect. As noted in Table 61-2, many drugs commonly used in the CCU have effects on the CNS and may induce or exacerbate delirium. Drugs with anticholinergic activity may be particularly likely to induce cognitive deficits in elderly patients.[6] In some cases where drug-induced delirium is suspected, the agent may be continued at a lower dose if thought to be crucial to the patient's medical care (e.g., lidocaine). Most agents, however, should be discontinued if they precipitate adverse CNS events. Often, an alternate agent, even one within the same class as the offending drug, can be substituted without recurrence of the adverse effect, but close observation and monitoring

are essential. Note that idiosyncratic reactions to medications used to sedate agitated patients (e.g., antihistamines or benzodiazepines) are not uncommon and should not be overlooked as potential contributing factors in the development of agitation or delirium.

Alcohol abstinence syndromes

Ethanol potentiates the action of γ-aminobutyric acid (GABA), an inhibitory neurotransmitter, on postsynaptic neurons in the CNS. Excess alcohol consumption results in a compensatory increase in neuronal activity. If the depressant effects of alcohol are removed suddenly (e.g., after an unexpected admission to the CCU), a state of generalized CNS arousal is produced.

Clinical manifestations. The most common symptoms resulting from acute alcohol abstinence can be grouped into four syndromes characterized by their manifestations, severity, time course, and degree of associated autonomic hyperactivity.[21]

The *alcohol withdrawal syndrome* is associated with tremor, insomnia, irritability, nausea, vomiting, and an intense craving for alcohol. These symptoms typically begin 8 to 12 hours after the last alcoholic drink and are of short duration, peaking after 24 to 48 hours. A coarse tremor and sleep abnormalities may last for weeks to months.[21]

Alcoholic hallucinosis occurs in approximately 25% of patients with withdrawal syndrome. It typically begins within 24 hours of the last drink and rarely lasts more than 48 hours. Visual hallucinations are the most common, although auditory and tactile hallucinations can also occur. This syndrome is distinguished from that of delirium tremens by its early onset, a relatively clear sensorium, and minimal autonomic hyperactivity. Because patients typically maintain cognitive function, alcoholic hallucinations can usually be treated with reassurance alone, especially within the controlled confines of the CCU. If pharmacologic therapy is required, haloperidol (Haldol) at a dose of 1 to 2 mg orally every 4 hours is often effective.

Alcohol withdrawal seizures can be seen alone or in combination with other withdrawal symptoms. They most commonly begin within 48 hours of the last drink and are typically self-limited.[25] Status epilepticus is rare in patients without a history of epilepsy.[21] Because of this, we do not recommend the routine use of phenytoin or phenobarbital in CCU patients undergoing alcohol withdrawal. In patients who have already experienced at least one seizure during the current admission or in the tenuous patient in whom even a limited seizure would be dangerous, we use IV diphenylhydantoin (Dilantin) at 25 to 50 mg/min, with a total loading dose of 18 mg/kg. This is followed by daily oral dosing to maintain serum levels of 10 to 20 μg/ml (approximately 100 mg every 6 hours).

The most feared syndrome in patients with cardiac

disease who are undergoing alcohol withdrawal is *delirium tremens*. This syndrome may develop 2 days to 2 weeks after the last ethanol intake and is usually preceded by early withdrawal symptoms such as agitation or hallucinosis. Delirium tremens is characterized by a clouded sensorium and signs of autonomic hyperactivity such as hypertension, tachycardia, fever, diaphoresis, and increased cardiac output. These signs and symptoms are often mistakenly attributed to complications of acute ischemic heart disease, such as heart failure or AMI. Approximately 80% of delirium tremens cases will resolve within 72 hours of symptom onset.

In 1908, the mortality rate for delirium tremens exceeded 35%.[26] By 1960, this figure had fallen to 12%.[27] Recent studies estimate the mortality between 1% and 5% in hospitalized patients.[25] Nonetheless, the profound increase in autonomic activity can be especially hazardous in the acutely ill cardiac patient, contributing to atrial and ventricular tachyarrhythmias and possibly resulting in ischemia or infarction in those patients with limited myocardial blood flow.

Wernicke's encephalopathy is another alcohol-related complication that may result in acute delirium. This syndrome is characterized by cognitive impairment, ataxia, and ocular dysfunction consisting of horizontal and vertical nystagmus with ophthalmoplegia. Many cases of Wernicke's syndrome do not demonstrate the typical symptoms and recognition may be difficult. In a study of 51 patients with a postmortem diagnosis of Wernicke's syndrome, only 7 had been diagnosed before death.[28] Administration of thiamine promptly reverses Wernicke's syndrome and given prophylactically can prevent its development. We recommend 100 mg of thiamine given either orally or intravenously daily for 5 days in patients with a history of heavy alcohol use or unexplained delirium.

Identification. Pharmacologic therapy for alcohol withdrawal is more effective as prophylaxis than for treatment of overt withdrawal, making the identification of patients at risk of withdrawal of utmost importance. Unfortunately, although the typical CCU population includes a substantial number of patients at risk for acute abstinence symptoms, prospective identification of these patients is often difficult. The risk of serious withdrawal symptoms, especially delirium tremens, is substantially increased in individuals who consume at least 80 g (six 12-oz beers or 1-oz drinks of 80-proof liquor) per day.[29] An accurate alcohol history, however, is frequently unavailable either because the individual is unresponsive or the patient's airway is intubated at the time of admission or because most alcoholics grossly underreport their consumption. The CAGE screening questionnaire (Table 61-3) has been shown to be a valid tool for identifying problem drinkers,[30] and a positive response to two or more of these questions should

Table 61-3. CAGE questions for alcohol abuse screening

1. Have you ever felt you should Cut down on your drinking?
2. Have people Annoyed you by criticizing your drinking?
3. Have you ever felt bad or Guilty about your drinking?
4. Have you ever had a drink first thing in the morning to steady your nerves or to get rid of a hangover (Eye-opener)?

prompt consideration of withdrawal prophylaxis. In addition, family members will occasionally volunteer a history of alcohol abuse even when this history has been minimized or withheld by the patient. Finally, although neither sensitive nor specific enough to be used for screening purposes, routine laboratory tests may suggest heavy ethanol use in some individuals. Findings that should prompt further investigation include an elevated erythrocyte mean corpuscular volume, elevated hepatocellular enzymes levels, hyperamylasemia, and hypoalbuminemia in an apparently healthy patient.

Treatment. Pharmacologic therapy for alcohol withdrawal is based on the administration of a substance that is cross-tolerant to the CNS depressant effects of ethanol. Several classes of drugs, including barbiturates, paraldehyde, and meprobamate, have historically been used for this purpose. The benzodiazepines, however, have largely supplanted these agents because of their increased margin of safety. The long-acting benzodiazepines chlordiazepoxide (Librium) and diazepam (Valium) are most commonly used for this purpose. Their active metabolites result in extended effective half-lives (40-80 hours), facilitating a smooth taper of effect as doses are decreased. In critically ill patients, however, a prolonged drug effect is often undesirable, especially in patients with rapidly changing hemodynamics or mental status. We prefer the use of lorazepam (Ativan) to treat most alcohol withdrawal syndromes because it has a relatively short half-life (10 hours), has no active metabolites, and can be given orally or intravenously. In addition, lorazepam is renally excreted and is not metabolized hepatically, a distinct benefit when patients with diminished cardiac output, as well as possible alcohol-induced hepatic dysfunction, are treated.

For prophylaxis of alcohol withdrawal, lorazepam may be given at a dose of 1 to 2 mg intravenously (or 3-5 mg orally) every 4 hours for the first day. Patients who have already begun to show signs of early alcohol withdrawal may require higher initial doses. In this population, we recommend giving 1 to 2 mg of lorazepam intravenously every 20 to 30 minutes until the patient is calm but awake. After 24 hours the dosage should be decreased by approximately 25% of the original amount each day, discontinuing use after 3 to 5 days. Although these doses must be individualized, we recommend using benzodiazepines at regular intervals rather than on an "as needed" basis.

Although not widely accepted as therapeutic agent, alcohol itself in modest doses is quite effective in preventing the symptoms of withdrawal during the period of acute illness. We routinely offer vodka or beer with each meal to patients admitted to the CCU at risk for withdrawal. Amounts administered vary, and patients are encouraged to request alcohol as they feel it is needed. Rarely we have used an IV alcohol drip in patients unable to take alcohol by mouth and in whom withdrawal would be particularly dangerous. The administration of alcohol is only a temporary measure, and the patient, as well as CCU staff, must understand this. Once the patient is stable, he or she must be offered the opportunity for long-term counseling and either inpatient or outpatient detoxification.

Patients undergoing alcohol withdrawal who show signs of increased adrenergic tone may benefit from the judicious use of β-blockers. These agents can decrease the heart rate and blood pressure, thereby decreasing cardiac work and the risk of myocardial ischemia. The centrally acting α_2-adrenergic agonist clonidine has also been used to control hyperadrenergic responses in patients undergoing alcohol withdrawal and may be effective alone or in conjunction with a benzodiazepine.[17] Because of the proven beneficial effects in unstable angina and AMI, β-blocking agents are the agents of choice in most patients with hyperadrenergic symptoms. In CCU patients in whom β-blockers are contraindicated, clonidine may be given at doses of 0.1 to 0.3 mg orally every 8 to 12 hours. Clonidine can, however, cause anxiety, insomnia, and depression, which may complicate alcohol withdrawal syndromes.

Electrolyte and nutritional deficiencies are commonly seen in patients with a history of heavy ethanol use and may be particularly dangerous in the CCU patient. Hypomagnesemia decreases the seizure threshold and increases the risk of ventricular arrhythmias, especially the polymorphic ventricular tachycardia known as torsade de pointes. In magnesium-depleted patients replacement therapy may be given with IV magnesium sulfate at 1 to 2 g every 6 hours as needed to maintain a serum magnesium of 2 to 3 mEq/L. We recommend checking serum magnesium concentrations every 24 hours in all CCU patients. More frequent monitoring is required in patients with renal insufficiency or receiving replacement therapy. Oral magnesium therapy is not recommended because of slow correction of hypomagnesemia and the side effect of diarrhea.

Malnutrition often accompanies alcohol abuse and may result in hypophosphatemia, which can exacerbate congestive heart failure or lead to rhabdomyolysis.

Supplementation consists of IV administration of 12 to 18 mmol of phosphate as either the sodium or potassium salt every 8 hours until normal serum levels are restored. The administration of thiamine (100 mg orally or intravenously daily), folate (1 mg orally daily), and a general purpose multivitamin are also recommended for the first 5 to 7 days in patients admitted with suspicion of alcohol abuse or malnutrition.

Though less common than alcohol withdrawal, other psychoactive agents also give rise to acute abstinence syndromes when discontinued abruptly. The pharmacologic management of acute withdrawal from barbiturates and related agents requires estimating the total daily dose of the abused drug, stabilizing the patient on an equivalent dose of a long-acting barbiturate (e.g., phenobarbital) and tapering the dose over 4 to 10 days. Patients who used benzodiazepines on a regular basis should be maintained on similar doses while in the hospital if possible, with a subsequent taper over several weeks as an outpatient. Details on the management of these and other acute abstinence syndromes can be found in a recent review by Milhorn.[16]

Pharmacologic therapy of CCU delirium

Even with the use of appropriate environmental and nursing modifications to diminish the incidence of delirium in the CCU population, a number of patients will nevertheless develop agitation, disorientation, and even frankly combative behavior. As previously mentioned, often no obvious cause is identified. When this occurs, it is imperative that effective symptom-oriented pharmacologic therapy be used to avoid further injury to the patient as a result of falls, self-extubation, or the traumatic removal of invasive monitoring or therapeutic devices. There are a number of agents that historically have been used to calm the agitated patient. Some of these are still useful, but others, such as paraldehyde and barbiturates, have no role in the modern CCU.

Haloperidol (Haldol), a butyrophenone neuroleptic agent, is ideally suited for the sedation of patients in the CCU. Its effects are similar to the phenothiazines that improve delirium, hallucinations, and disorganized cognition without disturbing higher intellectual functions. Unlike most phenothiazines, however, haloperidol has little anticholinergic and α-adrenergic antagonist effects and therefore causes minimal hypotension or CNS depression. Unlike barbiturates, opiates, or some benzodiazepines, haloperidol has little effect on respiratory drive or cardiac conduction, even when used in very high doses. Although it is available in oral form, we recommend IV administration for more rapid onset of action and because of the difficulty in giving oral medications to combative, delirious patients. When haloperidol is used intravenously, the line must be flushed thoroughly before and after administration because it may precipitate with a number of agents commonly used in the CCU, including heparin and phenytoin. Intramuscular administration may also be used, but it is painful and generally contraindicated in anticoagulated or postthrombolytic patients.

Haloperidol is approved by the Food and Drug Administration for oral and intramuscular use but as yet has not been approved for IV use. In spite of this, more than 20 years of experience has proven that the IV route is both effective and safe, even in the critically ill patient.[1,6,31-34] In one report, hospitalized patients were treated with up to 270 mg of IV haloperidol daily for a mean of 5 days without adverse cardiac or respiratory effects.[34] In another study, a continuous haloperidol drip at 25 mg per hour (600 mg/day) was used for 5 days in a severely agitated patient without complications.[33]

Rapid control of the acutely agitated patient can be gained with IV haloperidol because peak effects occur within 10 minutes of administration. We generally use a starting dose of 1 to 3 mg for mild agitation, 5 to 7 mg for moderate agitation, and 10 mg for severe agitation. If the patient has not had the desired response, the dose is doubled every 20 minutes until the patient is calm. Although the upper therapeutic range for haloperidol is unknown, IV boluses as high as 150 mg have been used without ill effect.[32] After the acute control of symptoms, maintenance therapy may be initiated with regular IV or oral doses given every 6 to 8 hours, with the dose tailored to the individual patient response. As in the case of alcohol withdrawal, maintenance doses should be given on a regular schedule rather than "as needed."

Because it antagonizes dopamine-mediated neurotransmission, haloperidol may cause extrapyramidal effects, including tremor, akathisia (a subjective feeling of restlessness), tortocollis (spasmodic contraction of the neck musculature), and oculogyria (uncontrolled rotation of the orbits). Fortunately, these effects are not common with oral haloperidol and may be even less common when used intravenously.[34] Extrapyramidal effects respond quickly to 25 to 50 mg of IV diphenhydramine and do not usually require discontinuation of the neuroleptic agent. Tardive dyskinesia, a serious problem with the long-term use of any neuroleptic, is not a consideration when these agents are used for short-term control of delirium in the CCU. The neuroleptic malignant syndrome is seen in patients treated chronically with neuroleptics and has also been reported in at least one case after a single injection of haloperidol.[35] Although haloperidol is a central dopamine antagonist, it seems to be safe in patients receiving IV dopamine for hemodynamic support. There is one report of transient hypotension after IV haloperidol in a critically ill patient receiving dopamine.[33] This patient responded promptly to an increased dopamine infusion rate. Haloperidol

may decrease the seizure threshold and has been shown to increase the incidence of alcohol withdrawal seizures in rats.[36] Therefore, patients requiring treatment for delirium while experiencing withdrawal seizures should avoid haloperidol and phenothiazines. Benzodiazepines are the sedatives of choice in this population.

Although less effective than haloperidol in acute delirium, benzodiazepines are excellent anxiolytic and hypnotic agents. They have minimal effects on the autonomic nervous or cardiovascular systems and cause little respiratory depression unless given rapidly in large doses or when used in conjunction with other respiratory depressants. We recommend lorazepam as the benzodiazepine of choice in critically ill patients because of the absence of both hepatic metabolism and active metabolites. The usual dose for control of anxiety associated with the critical care environment or for sleep is 1 to 2 mg intravenously or orally repeated every 4 to 6 hours as needed. Elderly patients may respond to doses as small as 0.25 mg. Midazolam, an ultra-short-acting benzodiazepine, is typically given as a constant infusion and may be useful in selected cases where the ability to titrate the level of sedation quickly is important. Midazolam is very expensive when used in this manner (more than $500.00 daily at our institution), and studies have revealed an unexpectedly high rate of respiratory arrest when used in elderly patients.[32]

Opiates and barbiturates have historically been some of the most frequently used sedatives in CCU settings. Neither can be recommended for routine sedation in the modern CCU because of their tendency for marked respiratory depression and adverse hemodynamic effects. Narcotics, of course, remain useful for many other roles in this setting, including the relief of pain associated with MI and the rapid decrease in right ventricular preload in cases of acute pulmonary edema.

Rarely, we have encountered acutely agitated patients who failed, at least initially, to respond to pharmacologic sedation, including high-dose IV haloperidol. In these cases, the physician must decide whether the patient's behavior represents enough of a risk to justify pharmacologic paralysis and mechanical ventilation. If this step is taken, it is imperative that the patients receive adequate concomitant sedation. This may be accomplished by administering large doses of lorazepam or morphine at 4- to 6-hour intervals.

ACKNOWLEDGMENT

We would like to thank Mr. Gary Dunham, Clinical Pharmacist, Duke University Medical Center for his thoughtful review of this chapter.

REFERENCES

1. Tesar GE, Stern TA: The diagnosis and treatment of agitation and delirium in the ICU patient. In Rippe J, Irwin J, Apert J, et al (eds): *Intensive care medicine*, Boston, 1991, Little, Brown.

2. Subcommittee of the Joint Commission on Public Affairs: *A psychiatric glossary of the American Psychiatric Association,* Boston, 1980, Little, Brown.
3. Hale M, Koss N, Kerstein M, et al: Psychiatric complications in a surgical ICU, *Crit Care Med* 5:199-203, 1977.
4. Blachy PH, Starr A: Post-cardiotomy delirium, *Am J Psychiatry* 121:371-375, 1964.
5. Easton C, MacKenzie F: Sensory-perceptual alterations: delirium in the intensive care unit, *Heart Lung* 17:229-237, 1988.
6. Weber RJ, Oszko MA, Bolender BJ, et al: The intensive care unit syndrome: causes, treatment, and prevention, *Drug Intell Clin Pharm* 19:13-20, 1985.
7. Levekoff SE, Evans DA, Liptzin B, et al: Delirium: the occurrence and persistence of symptoms among elderly hospitalized patients, *Arch Intern Med* 152:334-340, 1992.
8. Briggs D: Preventing ICU psychosis, *Nurs Times* 87:30-31, 1991.
9. Nadelson T: The psychiatrist in the surgical intensive care unit, *Arch Surg* 111:113-117, 1976.
10. Schor JD, Levkoff SE, Lipsitz LA: Risk factors for delirium in hospitalized elderly, *JAMA* 267:827-831, 1992.
11. Culpepper-Richards K, Bairnsfather L: Description of night sleep patterns in the critical care unit, *Heart Lung* 17:35-42, 1988.
12. Kornfield AS, Heller SS, Frank KA, et al: Personality and psychological factors in postcardiotomy delirium, *Arch Gen Psychiatry* 31:249-253, 1974.
13. Tesar GE, Stern TA: Evaluation and treatment of agitation in the intensive care unit, *Intensive Care Med* 1:137-148, 1986.
14. Rabiner CJ, Willner AE, Fishman J: Psychiatric complications following coronary bypass surgery, *J Nerv Ment Dis* 160:342-348, 1975.
15. Schlaghecke R, Kornely E, Santen RH, et al: The effect of long-term glucocorticoid therapy on pituitary-adrenal responses to exogenous corticotropin-releasing hormone, *N Engl J Med* 326: 226-230, 1992.
16. Milhorn HT: Pharmacologic management of acute abstinence syndromes, *Am Fam Phys* 45:231-239, 1992.
17. Hansel HN: The behavioral effects of noise on man: the patient with 'intensive care unit psychosis,' *Heart Lung* 13:59-65, 1984.
18. Finlay G: Sleep and intensive care, *Intensive Care Nurs* 7:81-88, 1991.
19. Dubin WR, Field HL, Gastfriend DR: Postcardiotomy delirium: a critical review, *J Thorac Cardiovasc Surg* 77:586, 1979.
20. Wilson LM: Intensive care delirium: the effect of outside deprivation in a windowless unit, *Arch Intern Med* 130:225-226, 1972.
21. Dootson S: Sensory imbalance and sleep loss, *Nurs Times* 86:26-29, 1990.
22. Guzzetta CE: Effects of relaxation and music therapy on patients in a coronary care unit with presumptive acute myocardial infarction, *Heart Lung* 18:609-616, 1989.
23. Klein RF, Kliner VA, Zipes DP, et al: Transfer from a coronary care unit: some adverse responses, *Arch Intern Med* 122:104-108, 1968.
24. Wilson JS, Podrid PJ: Side effects from amiodarone, *Am Heart J* 121:158-171, 1991.
25. Turner RC, Lichenstein PR, Peden JG, et al: Alcohol withdrawal syndromes; a review of pathophysiology, clinical presentation, and treatment, *J Gen Intern Med* 4:432-444, 1989.
26. Boston LN: Delirium tremens: statistical study of 156 cases, *Lancet* 1:18-19, 1908.
27. Tavel ME, Davidson W, Batterton TD: A critical analysis of mortality associated with delirium tremens: review of 39 fatalities in a nine-year period, *Am J Med Sci* 242:18-29, 1961.
28. Harper C: Wernicke's encephalopathy: a neuropathological study of 51 cases, *J Neurol Neurosurg Psychiatry* 42:226-231, 1979.
29. Chick J: Delirium tremens: try to spot it early, *Br Med J (Clin Res)* 289:3-4, 1989.
30. Mayfield D, McLeod G, Hall P: The CAGE questionnaire: validation of a new alcoholism screening instrument, *Am J Psychol* 131:1121-1123, 1974.
31. Clinton JE, Sterner S, Stelmachers Z, et al: Haloperidol for sedation of disruptive emergency patients, *Ann Emerg Med* 16:319-322, 1987.
32. Crippen DW: The role of sedation in the ICU patient with pain and agitation, *Crit Care Clin* 6:369-392, 1990.
33. Fernandez F, Holmes VF, Adams F, et al: Treatment of severe, refractory agitation with a haloperidol drip, *J Clin Psychiatry* 49:239-241, 1988.
34. Menza MA, Murray GB, Holmes VF, et al: Controlled study of extrapyramidal reactions in the management of delirious, medically ill patients: intravenous haloperidol versus intravenous haloperidol plus benzodiazepines, *Heart Lung* 17:238-241, 1988.
35. Konikoff F, Kuritzky A, Jerushalmii Y, et al: Neuroleptic malignant syndrome induced by a single injection of haloperidol [letter], *Br Med J (Clin Res)* 289:1228-1229, 1984.
36. Blum K, Eubanks JD, Wallace JE, et al: Enhancement of alcohol withdrawal convulsions in mice by haloperidol, *Clin Toxicol* 9:427-434, 1976.

Part IV

PREDISCHARGE PHASE

Chapter 62

EXERCISE TREADMILL TESTING AND AMBULATORY MONITORING

Daniel B. Mark
Victor F. Froelicher

As the patient recovering from an acute myocardial infarction (AMI) approaches hospital discharge, the physician must choose a plan for the predischarge evaluation. There are four general goals of this evaluation: (1) to estimate risk of major cardiac events after discharge; (2) based on this risk assessment, to decide what additional tests and therapies the patient should have before discharge; (3) to assess the patient's functional capacity and develop an exercise prescription as part of the post-MI rehabilitation effort; and (4) to provide the patient with the information and reassurances necessary to return to as full and productive a life-style as possible. To achieve these goals most effectively, the clinician needs to understand both the natural history of AMI, including the major prognostic factors, and the effect of early interventional therapy (thrombolytic agents, coronary angioplasty [PTCA]) on the natural history of the disease.

It is commonly stated that prognosis following AMI is determined primarily by the amount of myocardial damage present and the amount of noninfarct myocardium still in jeopardy.[1] In the early thrombolytic era it was believed that successful reperfusion therapy would substantially reduce the amount of myocardial damage from an infarct and consequently increase the amount of

myocardium in jeopardy.[2] As a result it was presumed that patients receiving thrombolytic therapy would have a higher rate of exercise-induced ischemia than comparable patients who did not receive this therapy. Recent studies, however, have not borne this expectation out.[3,4] Part of the explanation for this lies in the fact that reperfusion therapy has much more modest effects on left ventricular salvage than was initially expected. Although significant salvage definitely occurs in some patients and has major prognostic implications, for many treated patients the principal benefit of reperfusion comes from opening the infarct artery and keeping it open. As discussed in Chapter 7, the benefits of reperfusion therapy are more complicated than initially postulated and relate to myocardial healing, scar formation, and electrical stabilization as well as myocardial salvage.

It is important to recognize that the major goals of the predischarge evaluation of the AMI patient do not depend specifically on whether the patient has received reperfusion therapy. There are five general questions about the predischarge stress test that the clinician must answer:

1. Are any additional tests needed?
2. Which patients should receive a stress test?

Table 62-1. Reasons for predischarge exercise testing

Assess prognosis
 Multivessel disease
 Residual ischemia in infarct zone
 Need for predischarge catheterization/possible
  revascularization
 Suitability for early discharge
 Likelihood of death, MI, or angina after discharge
Assess functional status
 Basis for discharge "exercise prescription"
 Reassure patient, family, and physician
 Promote early return to work
 Assess adequacy of antianginal therapy
 Provide baseline for future elevation

Table 62-2. Factors against predischarge

Exercise testing
Congestive heart failure > Class I
Cardiogenic shock
Sustained VR or VF*
Advanced second- or third-degree AV block
Post-MI unstable angina
Severe (uncontrolled) hypertension

*VT = ventricular tachycardia, VF = ventricular fibrillation, AV = atrioventricular.

3. When should the stress test be done?
4. Which stress test should be used?
5. How should the results of the test be interpreted?

The purpose of this chapter is to examine the answers to these questions. We will be concerned largely with the treadmill test, whereas subsequent chapters will consider the exercise perfusion study and the exercise radionuclide angiogram. We will also examine the role of ambulatory ECG monitoring for detection of transient ischemia in the predischarge evaluation.

REASONS FOR PREDISCHARGE EXERCISE TESTING

The majority of exercise tests in nonacute patients who present with chest pain symptoms are performed for diagnosis of coronary artery disease (CAD). In the post-MI setting, however, the diagnosis of CAD is almost certain because the nonatherosclerotic causes of AMI are rare. The goal of exercise testing in this setting is therefore shifted from simple diagnosis (e.g., is CAD likely or unlikely?) to a variety of other objectives (Table 62-1). These objectives can be divided for discussion into two general categories: assessing prognosis (in order to select invasive studies and therapies appropriately) and assessing functional status. The use of the exercise test to satisfy these objectives is discussed later (see *Using the Information From the Exercise Test*).

SELECTION OF PATIENTS FOR EXERCISE TESTING

The reluctance to exercise a patient recovering from an MI stems, in part, from old concerns about the safety of the test.[5] For several decades after Levine and Lown proposed the "armchair treatment" for AMI (in 1952), the first step toward modern cardiac rehabilitation, most physicians would not exercise any MI patient for 3 to 6 months after the event because of safety concerns.[6-9] Any unnecessary stress prior to formation of a stable scar, it was feared, might lead to myocardial aneurysm formation or even rupture.

The first report of a low-level exercise test early after MI was published by Torkelson in 1964 and involved 10 patients tested 6 weeks after their MI.[10] Only in the last 15 years, however, has it become acceptable (if not standard practice) to do a predischarge or early postdischarge exercise test in patients with uncomplicated MI.[8,9] Cumulative experience with several thousand patients reported in the literature suggests that a properly performed predischarge (as well as an early postdischarge) exercise test carries a very low risk of serious complications in clinically uncomplicated patients.[11] Furthermore, it has been reasonably argued that if the patient is at increased risk for an exertion-related complication (e.g., serious arrhythmia, severe ischemia), the best place to discover this is in a properly supervised exercise laboratory setting.

With all the information potentially available from an exercise test (see Table 62-1), it might reasonably be asked not "Who should get an exercise test?" but "Who should *not* get an exercise test predischarge?" In general the patient with a "complicated" MI (Table 62-2) has not undergone early exercise testing. The occurrence of complicating factors defines a subset of MI patients with a high enough risk of future adverse cardiac events that a decision to proceed to cardiac catheterization can usually be made on clinical grounds alone.[12-16] For example, in a study of consecutive patients with AMI admitted to the Thoraxcenter in Rotterdam, 105 patients (26%) were judged ineligible for exercise after excluding in-hospital deaths and patients sent to surgery or PTCA. Of these, the 43 with cardiac limitations to exercise (mostly heart failure) had a 57% 1-year mortality rate, whereas the 62 with noncardiac limitations had an 8% 1-year mortality rate, similar to those in the exercise group.[17] Furthermore, in the Multicenter Postinfarction Study, the 24% of patients surviving to coronary care unit discharge who were not sent for an exercise test had a 1-year mortality almost three times that of the patients who did complete an exercise test (17% vs. 6%).[18] These high-risk post-MI patients, who are largely excluded from early exercise testing, are among the patients most likely to benefit from revascularization therapy (PTCA, bypass surgery).[19]

Several recent observations suggest that some of the traditional rules about who not to exercise may need to be reevaluated, as the benefits of acute interventional therapy, particularly for the complicated patient, become more well defined. For example, in a recent large series of patients treated with intravenous thrombolytic therapy and acute PTCA, we noted that high-risk patients (e.g., those in cardiogenic shock, of an older age, or women) who survived to hospital discharge had a remarkably low first-year mortality rate (2% to 5%).[20] These observations suggest that after successful reperfusion and revascularization with aggressive interventional therapy, a patient with a "complicated" MI may have a prognosis approaching that of the low-risk patient.[21] We believe that if such patients have no major noncardiac limitations, they can be exercised predischarge with the goal of assessing functional capacity and formulating a postdischarge rehabilitation program (see further).

TIMING OF THE EXERCISE TEST

Exercise tests "early" after an AMI can be performed either before discharge (i.e., days 4 to 10) or during an early follow-up visit after discharge (i.e., 3 to 6 weeks). The objectives listed in Table 62-1 for exercise testing generally favor predischarge testing, especially in the clinically uncomplicated MI patient. In addition, it appears that a predischarge test has the at least theoretical advantage of identifying patients who will develop complications before they can return for a postdischarge test. On the other hand a predischarge test is usually done with a preselected submaximal target heart rate or workload (because it is believed to be safer), whereas an early postdischarge test is often maximal and symptom-limited.[11] DeBusk and Haskell observed that there were no differences between a heart-rate-limited (130 beats/minute) and a symptom-limited exercise test 3 weeks after MI in the prevalence of ST-segment depression, premature ventricular complexes, or exercise angina.[22] Furthermore the average maximal ST-segment depression observed was no different between the two testing protocols.

However, two recent studies have contradicted these observations. Juneau et al. compared a low level (5 METs) and a symptom-limited treadmill test in 202 uncomplicated MI patients.[4] The modified Naughton protocol was used in both tests. The symptom-limited test averaged 2 minutes and 45 seconds longer and the peak workload achieved was 5.7 vs. 4.2 METs for the low-level test. The percentage of patients who developed ≥1 mm of exercise-induced ST depression increased from 28% to 44% ($P < .0001$). In addition, twice as many patients developed ST depression ≥2 mm with the

symptom-limited test. Overall, angina or ST depression occurred in 33% of the low-level tests and 52% of the symptom limited tests ($P < .0001$). This well-done study tested patients an average of 7.4 days after MI and administered the two tests in random order on consecutive days to each patient. Jain et al. performed a symptom-limited modified Bruce protocol test in 150 consecutive uncomplicated patients at a mean of 6.4 days after MI.[23] These investigators compared the ST response of each patient at a point representing 70% of the age-predicted maximum with the symptom-limited endpoint. They found that 23% of patients had ST depression ≥1 mm at the low-level endpoint and 40% had such ST changes with the continuation of exercise to the symptom-limited endpoint ($P < .0001$). These results are remarkably similar to those of the study by Juneau et al. and together these two studies strongly suggest that a symptom-limited test is more informative (at least in terms of abnormal findings) than a low-level test. What remains uncertain, however, is whether the *extra information* provided by moving to the symptom-limited endpoint has prognostic significance. Jain et al. attempted to address this question but had no cardiac deaths in their population during a 15-month follow-up.[23] In fact, the excellent prognosis of this study population calls into question the added value of exercise ischemia evident only at a high workload. Data from the literature on exercise testing involving stable CAD suggests that most patients who develop exercise-induced ischemia only at a high workload will fall into the intermediate-risk group and only very infrequently would have enough exercise-induced ischemia to receive a high-risk designation.[24,25]

Caru et al. compared the utility of a symptom-limited Bruce protocol performed at a mean of 8.6 days following AMI with an identical test performed 20 days after the MI in 25 patients.[26] Unlike most of the studies in this area, these patients were taken off their cardiac medications before each test. An ischemic ST response was seen in approximately 50% of both treadmill tests. In addition, 76% of patients with an ischemic response on one of the two tests had a repeat ischemic response on the second test. At the second test, exercise time increased by 1 minute and 45 seconds ($P < .001$) and the maximum heart rate attained increased from 141 to 155 ($P < .001$). This is similar to the improvements noted by Williams et al. between predischarge and 3-month exercise tests.[27] Given the small sample size of this study, the prognostic implications of these differences could not be determined.

DeBusk and Dennis have suggested that the predischarge submaximal test (rather than a postdischarge symptom-limited test) is preferred by physicians in academic medical centers because they generally wish to complete the patient evaluation before returning the patient to the care of the referring physician.[28] They argue that such considerations need not dictate clinical practice patterns at the community hospital because the local physician can just as easily follow a patient after discharge and perform a maximal, symptom-limited exercise test at 3 weeks. This argument, however, does not take into account the fact that a negative exercise test before discharge can be quite reassuring to the physician (as well as the patient), particularly the primary care physician who does not care for many cardiac patients.

Although a randomized trial with long-term follow-up would be the ideal method by which to evaluate the optimal timing and endpoints of the exercise test following an MI, such a trial is unlikely to ever be performed. We believe that the available data are not strong enough to dictate one strategy dogmatically. Thus the physician should choose the timing most suitable to his or her practice and the evaluation of the patient's predischarge prognosis based on clinical data. It is likely that this decision, in the absence of definitive data, will be increasingly influenced by reimbursement rules. The most recent guidelines from the American College of Cardiology/American Heart Association for early management of AMI recommend that clinically low-risk patients who are being discharged at 6 to 10 days undergo a low-level (5 MET) exercise test before discharge and a symptom-limited exercise test 3 to 8 weeks later.[29]

SELECTION OF THE EXERCISE TEST

Once the decision has been made to exercise a post-MI patient, the physician must decide which exercise test to perform. Usually the decision centers around whether to do a treadmill or a pharmacologic stress test, and if a treadmill is selected what exercise protocol to use and whether to add an imaging component to the test. The added benefits of an imaging stress test are discussed in subsequent chapters. Although much has been written about the relative merits of the bicycle vs. the treadmill, the preference for the treadmill test in the United States and the bicycle test in Europe seems largely nonmedical.[30] Other forms of exercise, such as arm ergometry, have been used in selected situations (e.g., a patient unable to exercise with his or her legs) but remain largely research tools and have generally been supplanted by pharmacologic stress tests.

The most popular treadmill protocols all use continuous, progressive stages and differ mainly in the rate and severity of progression represented by each subsequent stage. Some protocols are "modified," meaning that they have one or two very easy stages added on at the beginning to give the patient a chance to warm up. The three most commonly used protocols are the modified Bruce, the standard Bruce, and the Naughton (Table 62-3).[11] If these protocols are used in symptom-limited

Table 62-3. Common post-MI treadmill protocols

Stage	Speed (mph)	Grade (%)	Mets
Modified Bruce*			
(3-min stages)			
0	1.7	0	2.3
½	1.7	5	3.5
1	1.7	10	5
2	2.5	12	7
3	3.4	14	9.7
4	4.2	16	13
Modified Naughton†			
(2-min stages)			
1	2	0	2
2	2	3.5	3
3	2	7	4
4	2	10.5	5
5	2	14	6

MPH = miles per hour, METS = metabolic equivalents, where 1 MET is the rate of oxygen consumption required for sitting quietly (figures are approximations).
*The standard Bruce protocol does not include the two warm-up stages (0 and ½).[34]
†Several different versions of the Naughton protocol have been published.

testing, they all achieve the same ultimate workloads but at different rates.[31] Thus, patients exercising on the Bruce protocol tend to reach their peak workload faster than with the Naughton protocol. In a busy exercise laboratory the Bruce protocol is often preferred for this reason. The few comparisons of protocols available in post-MI patients suggest they are equally effective for achieving the goals in Table 62-1.[32] One reasonable alternative to these protocols in post-MI patients is to start at a low level (e.g., 2 METs) and gradually increase the difficulty in 1 to 2 MET increments based on patient tolerance.[33] On the other hand, an advantage of using a standard protocol is that it provides results that can be related to published outcomes in similar patients.

As noted above, for predischarge testing there is still no consensus on whether to use a heart-rate- (or workload-) limited or a symptom-limited test. There does not appear to be any difference in safety between the two approaches (see Timing of the Exercise Test), although none of the studies of this question has been large enough to detect small differences in an uncommon or rare complication. DeBusk and Haskell have pointed out that heart-rate targets that are "submaximal" for healthy adults or even patients with chronic CAD may be maximal or near maximal for many patients 1 week after an AMI.[22] This may be particularly true for patients on full-dose beta blockers for secondary prevention. At present most institutions continue to use a predischarge exercise test that is submaximal and heart-rate (or workload-) limited.[11] At Duke we generally use a modified Bruce protocol with a target heart

Table 62-4. The Borg perceived exertion scale

6	
7	Very, very light
8	
9	Very light
10	
11	Fairly light
12	
13	Somewhat hard
14	
15	Hard
16	
17	Very hard
18	
19	Very, very hard
20	

rate of 130 beats/min (or a MET level of 5) in patients age 50 or older and 140 beats/min (or a MET level of 7) in patients younger than 50. In patients who have had successful revascularization, however, we often use a standard Bruce protocol. In patients who are on effective doses of beta blockers, an alternative endpoint is to use the Borg-perceived exertion scale, with a target exertion level of around 16 (Table 62-4). At the Palo Alto VA Hospital we generally use a "ramp" protocol, in which work is continuously increased by very small increments.[31] This protocol avoids the sudden stresses on the cardiovascular system produced by changing stages and appears to have a more predictable relationship to VO_2 max than multistage protocols such as the Bruce.

RISK STRATIFICATION USING THE EXERCISE TEST
Methodologic considerations

There are four important methodologic issues that should be considered by a clinician when evaluating the results of a prognostic exercise test study in the literature. First, a large sample size is generally needed. For prognostic studies the total number of outcome events (e.g., cardiac deaths, MIs) is more important than the total number of patients enrolled. The number of cardiac events observed in a study population increases with a larger sample size and a longer length of follow-up. There is very little that can be learned about prognosis from a small study with a short follow-up because there will not be enough outcome events to describe *with precision* the relationship of any treadmill variable with prognosis. Similarly, a larger study of low-risk patients followed for a longer interval but with only, for instance, eight cardiac deaths is too small to identify more than one prognostically important factor. As a rough guide to sample-size requirements in prognostic studies, we use the rule that there should be *five to ten outcome events for every candidate variable tested* for its relationship with outcome.

The second methodologic requirement is that the study endpoint(s) should preferably be a "hard" objectively verifiable event, such as death or MI. It is common for investigators to increase the number of outcome events by including softer endpoints, such as the need for bypass surgery or angioplasty. Revascularization, however, is an event that is often decided more by the clinician than by the natural history of the disease, and different clinicians make these decisions differently.[35] Furthermore, the decision for revascularization may be based, in part, on the results of the exercise test, creating the potential for a self-fulfilling prophecy. In other words, if a markedly abnormal treadmill test makes the clinician more likely to send a patient for surgery, then it should be no surprise that treadmill abnormalities predict future cardiac events (including surgery).

The third methodologic requirement is for proper adjustment for unequal follow-up times. In most prognostic studies, some patients have been followed for a few months, some have been observed for several years, whereas others may be lost to follow-up. Most investigators have taken such a population and examined the relationship of treadmill variables with survival to some arbitrary follow-up point, typically 1 year. There are three important problems with this approach. First, all patients followed less than 1 year must be dropped from the study (because their 1-year outcome is not known), thereby reducing the sample size. Second, a death occurring the day after the exercise test is counted equal to a death at exactly 1 year, which certainly does not reflect the way clinicians (and patients) value survival. Finally, all deaths after 1 year are ignored in the analysis, again reducing the sample size and the power of the analysis. There are excellent techniques for handling unequal follow-up times and losses to follow-up, such as Kaplan-Meier lifetables, the log rank test, and the Cox proportional hazards regression model.

The final methodologic point is that the prognostic value of the stress test should not be analyzed in isolation from other, more readily available information. The analysis should first adjust for important clinical variables (e.g., age, sex, history of previous MI, heart failure), because these are already known to the clinician, and then consider what independent prognostic information can be added by the stress test. Furthermore, many stress test variables may actually be redundant (in terms of their prognostic message), and it may be possible to identify the subset of variables containing all the prognostic information available from the test using multivariable analysis (e.g., the Cox regression model). The alternative is that one investigator concentrates on one treadmill variable (e.g., ST depression) and reports how important it is, while a second investigator

Table 62-5. Measurements available from the exercise treadmill test

---

Electrocardiographic
    Maximum net ST depression
    Maximum net ST elevation
    ST slope (downsloping vs. horizontal vs. upsloping)
    Leads showing ST changes
    Time to "significant" exercise ST deviation
    Duration of ST deviation
    ST/HR* indexes
    Exercise-induced ventricular arrhythmias
    Other (R-wave changes, U-wave changes)
Hemodynamic
    Peak exercise heart rate
    Peak exercise blood pressure
    Peak exercise double product (heart rate × blood
      pressure)
    Exercise duration
    Exertional hypotension
    "Chronotropic incompetence"
Symptomatic
    Exercise-induced angina
    Exercise-limiting symptom(s)

---

*HR = heart rate.

does the same for another treadmill variable (e.g., exercise angina). Neither investigator has answered the more important clinical question, "Which treadmill variables out of all that are available should I measure, and what do they mean prognostically?"[36]

Clinical considerations

Measurements made during and immediately following an exercise treadmill test can be divided into three general categories (Table 62-5): electrocardiographic, hemodynamic, and symptomatic. In the traditional conceptual model proposed for interpretation of these measures, exercise-induced electrocardiographic abnormalities and angina are indicative of myocardial ischemia, whereas certain hemodynamic parameters, such as exercise duration and peak rate-pressure product, and symptoms such as fatigue and dyspnea are correlated with left ventricular dysfunction.[37] Exercise-induced ischemia in this model is the result of one or more flow-limiting coronary stenosis which, in turn, is the presumed substrate for future cardiac events (MI, cardiac death). Left ventricular dysfunction is presumed to result from either exercise-induced ischemia or preexisting left ventricular damage and indicates compromise of a certain critical mass of the left ventricle.

We are now increasingly aware, however, that this model provides a somewhat misleading view of the value of the stress test for predicting prognosis. From pathologic data it appears that most MIs and sudden cardiac deaths are the result of small tears or fissures in a coronary atherosclerotic plaque, with subsequent devel-

opment of a propagating and eventually occlusive thrombus (see Chapter 1). The plaques most likely to rupture and cause a major cardiac event are not the chronic subtotal stenoses that receive so much attention at angiography but rather are frequently angiographically "insignificant" plaques with an extracellular cholesterol gruel core and a thin fibrous cap. Tears most often develop at stress points in the shoulders of the plaque cap. Unfortunately, plaque events are still not predictable. In addition, because the future culprit lesion is often angiographically insignificant, it is unlikely to be responsible for an ischemic response during a stress test. Because MIs and sudden deaths result from local "plaque events" that often occur in noncritical atherosclerotic lesions, the treadmill (or any exercise) test will not be able to predict them accurately. Instead, it appears that the likelihood of a cardiac event (plaque rupture) is generally proportional to the total coronary tree atherosclerotic burden (i.e., more extensive atherosclerosis indicates an individual with more "insignificant" high-risk lesions that may rupture, as well as more high-grade obstructive lesions), whereas the traditional prognostic measures describing the left ventricular function and number of diseased vessels relate to the likelihood of survival if a clinically significant plaque event does develop. These issues have been recently reviewed.[1]

Despite all these limitations the treadmill test has been shown repeatedly to provide important prognostic information. Froelicher, in a comprehensive review of the literature on exercise testing, found that five exercise test parameters have been most often linked with prognosis in the post-MI patient[33]: exercise-induced ST-segment deviation (usually depression), exercise angina, exercise capacity (ability to reach target heart rate or workload), exercise ventricular arrhythmias, and an inadequate blood pressure response to exercise. However, interpretation of most of these studies is hampered by their methodologic limitations.

There is, unfortunately, no study that fulfills all the desirable methodologic criteria outlined previously, although some come a lot closer than others. Examination of several of the best studies provides at least a partial response to the clinical question posed in the previous section. Theroux, Waters, et al. from the Montreal Heart Institute studied 225 uncomplicated post-MI patients before discharge using a heart–rate- or workload-limited Naughton protocol.[38,39] Patients were followed for 5 to 7 years, and clinical variables were considered in addition to treadmill variables. Exercise-induced ST-segment deviation (depression or elevation) was the single most powerful prognostic variable, followed by a history of previous MI, failure to reach the target heart rate/workload, ventricular arrhythmias during exercise, and the QRS score. All five of these variables remained significant in a Cox regression analysis, which revealed that the risk of death was independently doubled by each of the three exercise test variables.

Weld et al. studied 236 patients with a predischarge, 9-minute modified Bruce protocol.[40] Logistic regression analysis was used to examine clinical and exercise predictors of 1-year survival. These investigators found that the major independent predictors of 1-year survival were exercise duration, frequency of ventricular premature beats during exercise, and vascular congestion on the predischarge chest radiograph. Exercise ST-segment depression and exercise angina were not independently significant in this study.

In their study of 665 post-MI patients who had survived for at least 3 weeks after the event, DeBusk et al. used a risk stratification algorithm that parallels the reasoning of many clinicians.[41] They first identified three independent historic predictors of prognosis, using the Cox regression model: history of previous angina, history of previous MI, and recurrent angina post-MI. Patients with at least two of these characteristics (9% of the study group) had a 6-month risk of cardiac death or nonfatal MI of 18%. Next, they stratified the remaining 603 patients into those not undergoing an exercise test (because of contraindications, noncardiac limitations, and refusal) and those referred for the test. The 265 patients who did not exercise (40% of the study group) had a 6-month cardiac event rate of 6%. The remaining 338 patients underwent a symptom-limited Naughton treadmill test at 3 weeks after MI. The 31 patients (5% of the study group) with a positive treadmill test (defined as ≥ 0.2 mV ST-segment depression and a peak heart rate ≤ 135 beats/minute) had a 6-month cardiac event rate of 10%, compared with 4% in the remaining patients. The sequential use of historic, clinical, and treadmill data thus identified as "high risk" 72% of patients, who actually had a cardiac event in the interval between day 21 and 6 months.

Madsen et al. pooled the results of exercise tests in 466 patients from four medical centers.[42] The exercise test was conducted before discharge in 80% and within 6 weeks of discharge in the remainder, and several exercise protocols were used. Ninety-two patients (20%) were excluded from the analysis because of indeterminate test results, and 79 (17%) were excluded because of < 1 year of follow up. Linear discriminant analysis was used to identify predictors of the 19 cardiac deaths or nonfatal MIs within the first year. Considered individually, only the functional capacity in METs and the occurrence of exercise-induced ST-segment depression predicted the 1-year cardiac event rate, and only the former was an independent predictor in a multivariable analysis.

Krone et al. reported results from the Multicenter Postinfarction Research Group in 667 patients who underwent a predischarge, 9-minute modified Bruce test.[18] Analysis with the logistic regression model revealed that an inadequate blood pressure rise during exercise, exercise-induced ventricular couplets, and exercise-induced angina were independently associated with 1-year survival probability. When combined with clinical variables, the independent prognostic factors were pulmonary congestion on the chest radiograph, inadequate blood pressure response to exercise, exercise-induced angina, and a resting heart rate ≥ 90 beats/minute.

Some studies have shown that an indicator of exercise-induced ischemia (e.g., ST-segment depression, angina) is the most powerful predictor of prognosis, whereas other studies have found indicators of exercise-induced left ventricular dysfunction (e.g., exercise duration, peak workload) to be most important. The reason for this discrepancy is unclear. Froelicher has applied the technique of metaanalysis to the available studies in an attempt to resolve this issue; however, metaanalysis is not a remedy for deficiencies in the original reported data.[33] One interesting result of his analysis was the finding that ST-segment deviation was more strongly related to prognosis in studies that included fewer patients with anterior MI. This observation was examined further by Froelicher et al. in 198 veterans who had a submaximal predischarge treadmill test. The 55 patients who did not have Q waves had a much stronger relationship between exercise-induced ST depression and subsequent prognosis than did patients with Q waves.[43] Ellestad et al. previously reported that in patients with extensive precordial Q waves, the treadmill test gave a lowered sensitivity for detecting significant CAD.[44] Similar results were observed by Ahnve et al. in 76 patients with stable CAD and prior Q-wave MI who underwent exercise thallium testing.[45] On the other hand, Miranda et al. found that the ability of a post-MI exercise test to identify severe coronary artery disease did not depend on whether the patient had Q waves or not.[46] Finally, at a low-level exercise (70% of predicted heart rate) endpoint, Jain et al. found a higher rate of exercise-induced ST-segment depression in Q-wave infarct patients than in non–Q-wave patients, although this difference was not evident at a symptom-limited endpoint. They also found that anterior Q waves had a much lower rate of positive ST response than those with inferior Q waves (17% vs. 57%, $P < .01$).[23]

These data suggest that one reason the available studies do not agree on the relative prognostic significance of exercise test findings is that their patient populations differed in the prevalence of factors that can affect the outcome of the test. Thus a higher prevalence of patients with large anterior Q-wave MIs, with their associated QRS distortion (decreased R-wave amplitude, intraventricular conduction delay) and masking of ischemic electrocardiographic changes, would be expected to increase the apparent prognostic importance of left ventricular dysfunction measures (e.g., exercise duration) relative to ischemia measures.[23,43] Conversely, a higher prevalence of inferior Q-wave MIs and non–Q-wave MIs, with their more preserved QRS complexes and better left ventricular function, would tilt the balance toward ischemic endpoints (e.g., ST depression, angina) as the primary predictor of prognosis.

Most of the studies referred to previously were done in the prethrombolytic era. There is substantially less data available on the utility of risk stratification with exercise testing following reperfusion therapy. In the TIMI II trial 77% of patients had a predischarge submaximal supine bicycle exercise radionuclide angiogram.[47] During the initial hospitalization (before exercise testing), one third of the conservative group had coronary angiography and approximately 20% had PTCA or CABG. In the invasive group 93% had cardiac catheterization and approximately two thirds of the patients had PTCA or CABG before exercise testing. Despite a presumably much higher prevalence of residual severe subtotal stenoses in the conservative group, these patients showed only a slightly higher rate of positive exercise tests than the deferred invasive group (18% vs. 13%, $P < .001$). At 6 weeks a maximal supine bicycle radionuclide angiogram was performed in approximately 75% of the study population. A positive test was seen in 19% of the conservative arm and 17% of the invasive arm ($P = .09$).

Sutton and Topol found that approximately half of patients with a 70% or more residual stenosis after thrombolytic therapy had a negative submaximal exercise thallium-201 tomogram.[48] In this study, patients with higher peak CK levels, reflecting larger infarcts, had a higher likelihood of a negative exercise test.

In a study from Italy, 157 (57%) of 275 consecutive hospital survivors receiving thrombolytic therapy underwent predischarge maximal exercise treadmill testing off antianginal therapy.[49] One third of these patients had a positive test (defined as exercise ST depression or angina). During the 6-month follow-up period no deaths occurred. A positive exercise test was unrelated to the likelihood of reinfarction but was predictive of the development of postinfarction angina and need for revascularization. In a similar study from England, 256 consecutive patients receiving thrombolytic therapy underwent predischarge symptom-limited treadmill testing.[3] Exercise ST depression occurred in 49% of patients overall, and 30% of patients had ST depression at a low workload (≤ 7 METs). There was a trend toward increased risk of future cardiac events (death, MI, unstable angina) in patients with a positive test ($P < .10$), but this only reached statistical significance for patients who had ischemic ST changes at a low workload ($P < .01$). Another very small study by Melin et al.

found that exercise ST-segment depression was more common in patients with either a reperfused infarct artery or an occluded infarct artery and multivessel disease than in patients with single-vessel disease and occluded infarct artery.[50] Thallium scans in these patients showed that reperfusion was associated with a larger amount of exercise-induced ischemia.

Thus although the data on the prognostic value of exercise testing in thrombolytic-treated patients is not as extensive as the prethrombolytic data, it seems reasonably consistent. In interpreting these data it should be kept in mind that thrombolytic-eligible patients represent a low-risk subset of AMI patients.[51] Thus in any series of these patients, hard cardiac event rates will be low and many studies will have inadequate statistical power for testing prognostic relationships with exercise testing data.

The issue of how well a predischarge exercise test predicts future complications in patients treated with early PTCA for AMI also remains largely unstudied. Because restenosis following PTCA is still not well understood, it is not surprising that the utility of the exercise test in predicting restenosis, even following elective PTCA, remains unclear. In a very small study Fung et al. from the University of Michigan reported that MI patients treated with PTCA had less periinfarct ischemia on an exercise thallium test and a smaller residual stenosis in the infarct vessel than patients treated with streptokinase alone.[52] In the Primary Angioplasty in Myocardial Infarction (PAMI) study comparing primary angioplasty and t-PA, a predischarge modified Bruce protocol treadmill was positive in 9% of t-PA patients and 3% of PTCA patients ($P = .04$).[53] There was also more ischemic redistribution on the accompanying SPECT thallium in the t-PA group (38% vs. 27%, $P = .06$). A 6-week rest-exercise radionuclide ventriculogram showed equivalent exercise times and exercise ejection fraction responses in these two groups. These data plus the results of the TIMI II study described earlier suggest that aggressive reperfusion with PTCA is associated with a low likelihood of a positive predischarge exercise test ($\leq 15\%$). Use of thrombolytic therapy with selective cardiac catheterization and revascularization (the TIMI-II conservative strategy) appears to be associated with only a modest increase in the likelihood of a positive predischarge exercise test, which is of uncertain prognostic significance.[54] Because most of the work referred to relied on exercise radionuclide imaging, additional studies will be required to define the value of the exercise treadmill test in this area.

ASSESSING FUNCTIONAL CAPACITY

A major role of the predischarge (and early postdischarge) exercise test is to discover how much of a workload the patient can tolerate without developing evidence of ischemia or hemodynamic compromise. Treadmill performance can thus provide the basis for the physician's instructions about home activities and the exercise prescription. Psychologic well-being and early return to work can also be promoted by the results of exercise testing. In fact, the demonstration that the patient can tolerate mild to moderate exercise without angina or adverse events may, for many patients, be the single largest contribution of the treadmill test to the predischarge evaluation.

The workload achieved by the patient during exercise provides the physician with an objective measure of the level of physical activity that can safely be undertaken after hospital discharge. The workload imposed by common daily activities can be related to the patient's maximum workload; MET units are often used as measures of equivalent workload. Exercise capacity usually increases after discharge even in patients not in a formal rehabilitation program so that repeat exercise testing at 6 to 8 weeks may be used to modify the patient's list of acceptable activities. The subject of cardiac rehabilitation is beyond the scope of this chapter (see Chapters 65 and 67), except to note that predischarge and follow-up exercise testing can be used to prescribe a home exercise program (e.g., walking briskly on level ground for 15 to 20 minutes, fast enough to keep heart rate at 70% to 85% of peak heart rate achieved on the predischarge treadmill test).

After an MI, psychologic disorders are common and can affect functioning in all portions of a patient's daily life as well as his or her family interactions (see Chapter 16 on quality of life). It is vital for the physician to recognize the tendency for anxiety and depression to develop in a post-MI patient and to deal with them preemptively. DeBusk et al. have found that the exercise test can be a valuable tool in this process by showing patients that they can exert themselves without having recurring chest pain, provoking another MI, or otherwise decompensating.[55] They have also shown that the patient's spouse can develop increased confidence in the patient's cardiac and physical capabilities by observing the exercise test and exercising briefly at the patient's maximum workload.[56]

One of the most tangible markers of recovery after an MI is return to work, and one of the questions the physician must answer is whether it is safe for the patient to return to his or her pre-MI job. The exercise test can aid the physician in making this determination.[57] For example, a construction worker needs to be able to tolerate a much higher workload without limiting symptoms or ischemia before returning to work than an office worker. Although the patient's functional capacity is certainly not the only determinant of returning to work,[58] perceived or real physical limitations can be important.

Functional capacity assessed for purposes of cardiac

rehabilitation has also recently been shown to provide important information regarding long-term prognosis.[59] A group of 527 post-MI and post-CABG patients entered a rehabilitation program an average of 13 weeks after their cardiac event and performed a maximal bicycle stress test with measurement of peak oxygen uptake by expired gas analysis. Maximum exercise capacity in this group, exercised to exhaustion, averaged 6.8 METs. Peak oxygen uptake was an independent predictor of long-term (average follow-up 6 years) mortality in this population: patients able to exercise to 8 METs or more had no deaths in follow-up, whereas patients unable to exceed 5 METs had the highest mortality rate (average of approximately 3% per year).[59]

AMBULATORY ELECTROCARDIOGRAPHIC MONITORING

Ambulatory electrocardiographic monitoring was introduced by Holter in 1961 for detection of arrhythmias. Over the last 15 years much data has been accumulated using this technology for detection of ischemic episodes.[60] Cohn was the first to develop the concept that clinically significant ischemia could occur in the absence of anginal symptoms.[61] In recent years debate in this area has shifted from the question of whether silent ischemia is a real phenomenon (it clearly is) to issues relating to its prognostic and therapeutic importance. In 1986 Gottlieb et al. reported that silent myocardial ischemia detected in 37 out of 70 unstable angina patients predicted a significantly higher rate of subsequent MI (16% vs. 3%, $P = .005$).[62] These findings, which were independently confirmed,[63] stimulated interest in using ambulatory monitoring for risk stratification and management of acute ischemic heart disease. In 103 high-risk AMI patients, Gottlieb et al. found that silent ischemia detected on a predischarge 24-hour monitoring study (in 29% of the patients) was a significant independent predictor of 1-year mortality (30% vs. 11% mortality for patients without silent ischemia, $P < .05$).[64] Further analysis showed that inability (or contraindications) to perform an exercise test was an even stronger prognostic factor: 18 of the 19 patients who died or had a recurrent MI in the follow-up year fell into this subgroup. When these two variables were combined in multivariable analysis, inability to exercise was the principal prognostic variable ($P < .001$) followed by silent ischemia ($P < .02$), suggesting that these two characteristics provided complementary prognostic information. In a separate study of 52 MI patients able to perform a predischarge exercise test, these investigators found that of the 14 patients with ischemic changes on ambulatory monitoring 64% had a positive treadmill test.[65] A similar study in 173 AMI patients with both ambulatory monitoring and bicycle exercise testing reported that each test showed ischemic changes in about one quarter of the tested population and both tests were positive in 11%.[66] Because of the overall low event rate in this population (3.5% mortality and 4% recurrent infarction at 1 year), this study was unable to define the relative prognostic importance of these two tests.

Langer et al. found that ambulatory ischemia was associated with a reduced cross-sectional area of the infarct-related artery (0.59 vs. 1.04 mm^2, $P < .05$) and with a failure of global left ventricular function to improve during the acute hospitalization.[67] In this study ambulatory ischemia was associated with a higher death and recurrent infarction rate (27% vs. 6% at 18 months, $P = .03$). Patients with ambulatory ischemia have also been reported to have more three-vessel CAD in some[65,67] but not all of the studies that have looked at this issue.

In contrast to these studies, in the Multicenter Study of Myocardial Ischemia, which enrolled 936 patients 1 to 6 months after an acute ischemic event (44% Q-wave MI, 26% non–Q-wave MI, 30% unstable angina), neither the ambulatory monitor nor the exercise thallium test provided independent prognostic information.[68] However, this study had a low cardiac event rate (1.3% average annual mortality) and tested patients after the acute phase of their illness had largely resolved.

Thus the proper role of ambulatory monitoring for detection of transient ischemic events after AMI remains undefined. The occurrence of transient ischemia in the early post-MI phase appears to correlate with a more severe coronary stenosis in the culprit vessel, possibly with more three-vessel disease, and with other markers of high risk (i.e., inability to exercise, a positive treadmill test). One significant limitation shared by the ambulatory monitor and the exercise treadmill is the inability to make an interpretable recording in patients with significant distortion of the resting ECG (e.g., bundle branch block, left ventricular hypertrophy, digitalis therapy, pacemaker). We do not use ambulatory monitoring as part of our post-MI risk stratification program. In addition, a recent national survey suggests that routine use of this technology for uncomplicated MI patients is currently quite uncommon.[69]

CLINICAL MANAGEMENT STRATEGIES

Although far from an ideal test, the exercise treadmill still provides much useful information, is substantially cheaper than its nuclear imaging alternatives such as thallium scintigraphy or radionuclide angiography, and remains the test most clinicians (over 75% in a recent national survey) use in their predischarge evaluation of the AMI patient.[70]

The goals and basic principles of the predischarge evaluation have not been changed by the advent of reperfusion therapy. In each patient the need for and value of additional testing (either invasive or noninva-

Table 62-6. Factors assessed at presentation that are predictive of six-week mortality following AMI*

Risk factor	Six-week mortality rate
Cardiogenic shock/pulmonary edema	33%
Rales >one third way up	12%
Age ≥70	11%
Atrial fibrillation	11%
Hypotension and sinus tachycardia	10%
Diabetes mellitus	9%
Previous infarction	8%
Female gender	7%
Anterior infarction	6%

Number of risk factors	Prevalence	Six-week mortality rate
0	26%	1.5%
1	41%	2.3%
2	21%	7%
≥3	10%	14.2%

*Data from 3339 patients enrolled in TIMI II trial.[71]

sive) must be judged in light of what is already known about the patient. Aside from the presenting characteristics (Table 62-6)[71] and the clinical course during the first several days of hospitalization (Table 62-7)[72] (i.e., looking specifically at the presence or absence of complicating shock, heart failure, recurrent ischemia, advanced AV block, or high-grade ventricular arrhythmia), many patients will have had an assessment of left ventricular function. Patients with an uncomplicated course and well preserved left ventricular function are low risk, and exercise testing will add relatively modest additional prognostic information in this setting. Patients with significant left ventricular dysfunction, even if they have a clinically uncomplicated course, are relatively high risk and in many cases should be considered for angiography. In fact recent estimates are that among clinically uncomplicated patients, up to 80% will require angiography either because of significant resting left ventricular dysfunction, inability to exercise or an abnormal or inconclusive exercise test result.[14,15]

Although we initially expected that patients treated with intravenous thrombolytic therapy alone would more often have ischemic treadmill responses (e.g. ST-segment depression, angina) than patients not receiving these agents, recent data shows that among uncomplicated MI patients undergoing predischarge exercise testing, those who had received thrombolytic therapy had a longer exercise duration and less frequent exercise-induced ST depression than patients who did not receive this therapy.[4] In addition, early revascularization with PTCA or bypass surgery further

Table 62-7. Predictors of complications between day 4 and day 30 following AMI*

Risk score components	Points
Sustained VT or VF	1
Sustained hypotension or shock	1
Number of diseased vessels	1
Baseline ejection fraction	1

Late complication risk score	Late complications	Late death or reinfarction
0	5%	0.5%
1	12%	3%
≥2	28%	8%

*Risk score based on first 3 hospital days. "Late" complications refer to shock, new pulmonary edema, sustained VT, VF, sustained hypotension, advanced AV block, or reinfarction occurring between day 4 and day 30 after MI. Based on analysis of 580 TAMI study patients.[72]

reduces the incidence of exercise ischemia in patients so treated.

In general, we feel that patients who are asymptomatic after intravenous thrombolytic therapy and who have not already undergone cardiac catheterization should at least have a predischarge (or early postdischarge) exercise test. Evidence of ischemia, such as typical angina or exercise ST-segment depression ≥ 0.10 mV that is horizontal or downsloping at a low workload, should prompt early referral for cardiac catheterization. Most studies agree that if a patient can exercise ≥ 9 minutes or achieve a heart rate ≥ 135 beats/min or a workload ≥ 5 to 7 METs, then he or she is at "low risk." The decision of how low the risk must be to defer cardiac catheterization must be determined by the clinician designing the predischarge testing strategy.

One frequent question about the predischarge exercise test is whether to withhold antianginal therapy (particularly beta blockers). Our approach is to exercise the patient on medicine if the primary goal of the test is to evaluate the patient's functional and symptom status on their medical regimen. On the other hand, if the goal is to discover if the patient has exercise-inducible ischemia, then we withhold the medicine for an appropriate period.

Patients who undergo acute reperfusion therapy with PTCA already have a great deal known about their prognosis (left ventricular function, extent of coronary disease, completeness of revascularization). In this setting the predischarge exercise test serves to define the patient's functional status, as part of the post-MI rehabilitation process, and to detect any residual ischemia from incomplete revascularization (including that caused by restenosis or reocclusion of the infarct vessel). It may be that in the near future such patients will routinely undergo very early exercise testing, day 3 discharge, and aggressive cardiac rehabilitation.[73,74]

REFERENCES

1. Mark DB: Assessment of prognosis in patients with coronary artery disease. In Roubin GS, Califf RM, O'Neill WW, et al (eds): *Interventional cardiovascular medicine: principles and practice,* New York, 1994, Churchill Livingstone.
2. Mark DB, Hlatky MA, Pryor DB: The exercise treadmill test in patients recovering from an acute myocardial infarction. In: Califf RM, Mark DB, Wagner GS, (eds): *Acute coronary care in the thrombolytic era,* Chicago, 1988, Year Book.
3. Stevenson R, Umachandran V, Ranjadayalan K, et al: Reassessment of treadmill stress testing for risk stratification in patients with acute myocardial infarction treated by thrombolysis, *Br Heart J* 70:415-420, 1993.
4. Juneau M, Colles P, Theroux P, et al: Symptom-limited versus low-level exercise testing before hospital discharge after myocardial infarction, *J Am Coll Cardiol* 20(4):927-933, 1992.
5. Mallory GK, White PD, Salcedo-Salgar J: The speed of healing of myocardial infarction. A study of the pathologic anatomy in seventy-two cases, *Am Heart J* 18(6):647-671, 1939.
6. Levine SA, Lown B: "Armchair" treatment of acute coronary thrombosis, *JAMA* 148(16):1365-1369, 1952.
7. Lown B, Sidel VW: Duration of hospital stay following acute myocardial infarction, *Am J Cardiol* 23(1):1-3, 1969.
8. Hamm LF, Stull GA, Crow RS: Exercise testing early after myocardial infarction: historic perspective and current uses, *Progr Cardiovasc Dis* 28(6):463-476, 1986.
9. Pryor DB, Hindman MC, Wagner GS, et al: Early discharge after acute myocardial infarction, *Ann Intern Med* 99(4):528-538, 1983.
10. Torkelson LO: Rehabilitation of the patient with acute myocardial infarction, *J Chronic Dis* 17:685-704, 1964.
11. Hamm LF, Crow RS, Stull GA, et al: Safety and characteristics of exercise testing early after acute myocardial infarction, *Am J Cardiol* 63:1193-1197, 1989.
12. DeBusk RF, Blomqvist CG, Kouchoukos NT, et al: Identification and treatment of low-risk patients after acute myocardial infarction and coronary-artery bypass graft surgery, *N Engl J Med* 314(3):161-166, 1986.
13. DeBusk RF: Specialized testing after recent acute myocardial infarction, *Ann Intern Med* 110(6):470-481, 1989.
14. Ross J Jr, Gilpin EA, Madsen EB, et al: A decision scheme for coronary angiography after acute myocardial infarction, *Circulation* 79(2):292-303, 1989.
15. Kulick DL, Rahimtoola SH: Risk stratification in survivors of acute myocardial infarction: routine cardiac catheterization and angiography is a reasonable approach in most patients, *Am Heart J* 121(2):641-656, 1991.
16. Krone RJ: The role of risk stratification in the early management of a myocardial infarction, *Ann Intern Med* 116(3):223-237, 1992.
17. Fioretti P, Brower RW, Simoons ML, et al: Prediction of mortality during the first year after acute myocardial infarction from clinical variables and stress test at hospital discharge, *Am J Cardiol* 55:1313-1318, 1985.
18. Krone RJ, Gillespie JA, Weld FM, et al: Low-level exercise testing after myocardial infarction: usefulness in enhancing clinical risk stratification, *Circulation* 71:80-89, 1985.
19. Califf RM, Harrell FE Jr, Lee KL, et al: The evolution of medical and surgical therapy for coronary artery disease: a 15-year perspective, *JAMA* 261:2077-2086, 1989.
20. Stack RS, Califf RM, Hinohara T, et al: Survival and cardiac event rates in the first year following emergency angioplasty for acute myocardial infarction, *J Am Coll Cardiol* 11:1141-1148, 1988.
21. McCallister BD, Christian TF, Gersh BJ, et al: Prognosis of

myocardial infarctions involving more than 40% of the left ventricle after acute reperfusion therapy, *Circulation* 88(1):1470-1475, 1993.

22. DeBusk RF, Haskell W: Symptom-limited vs. heart-rate-limited exercise testing soon after myocardial infarction, *Circulation* 61:738-743, 1980.

23. Jain A, Myers GH, Sapin PM, et al: Comparison of symptom-limited and low level exercise tolerance tests early after myocardial infarction, *J Am Coll Cardiol* 22(7):1816-1820, 1993.

24. Mark DB, Hlatky MA, Harrell FE Jr, et al: Exercise treadmill score for predicting prognosis in coronary artery disease, *Ann Intern Med* 106:793-800, 1987.

25. Mark DB, Shaw L, Harrell FE, et al: Prognostic value of a treadmill exercise score in outpatients with suspected coronary artery disease, *N Engl J Med* 325:849-853, 1991.

26. Caru B, Bossi M, Bonelli R, et al: Functional evaluation 10 days and 3 weeks after acute myocardial infarction: comparative significance and prognostic value, *Eur Heart J* 13:201-206, 1992.

27. Williams WL, Nair RC, Higginson LAJ, et al: Importance of timing of treadmill predictors for risk stratification after myocardial infarction: a five-year follow-up study, *Can J Cardiol* 7(2):65-73, 1991.

28. DeBusk RF, Dennis CA: "Submaximal" predischarge exercise testing after acute myocardial infarction: who needs it? *Am J Cardiol* 55:499-500, 1985.

29. American College of Cardiology, American Heart Association Task Force on Assessment of Diagnostic and Therapeutic Cardiovascular Procedures: ACC/AHA guidelines for the early managment of patients with acute myocardial infarction, *Circulation* 82:664-707, 1990.

30. Froelicher VF, Myers J, Follansbee WP, (eds): *Exercise and the heart,* ed 3, St Louis, 1993, Mosby.

31. Froelicher VF, Myers J, Follansbee WP, et al (eds): Exercise testing methodology. In *Exercise and the heart,* ed 3, St Louis, 1993, Mosby, pp 10-31.

32. Handler CE, Sowton E: A comparison of the Naughton and modified Bruce treadmill exercise protocols in their ability to detect ischemic abnormalities six weeks after myocardial infarction, *Eur Heart J* 5:752-755, 1984.

33. Froelicher VF, Myers J, Follansbee WP, et al (eds): Exercise testing of patients recovering from myocardial infarction. In *Exercise and the heart,* ed 3, St Louis, 1993, Mosby, pp 175-207.

34. McInnis KJ, Balady GJ, Weiner DA, et al: Comparison of ischemic and physiologic responses during exercise tests in men using the standard and modified Bruce protocols, *Am J Cardiol* 69:84-89, 1992.

35. Every NR, Larson EB, Litwin PE, et al for the Myocardial Infarction Triage and Intervention Project Investigators: The association between on-site cardiac catheterization facilities and the use of coronary angiography after acute myocardial infarction, *N Engl J Med* 329:546-551, 1993.

36. Froelicher VF, Myers J, Follansbee WP, et al (eds): Prognostic applications of the exercise test. In *Exercise and the heart,* ed 3, St Louis, 1993, Mosby, pp 148-174.

37. Juneau M: Updating concepts of exercise testing after myocardial infarction, *Prim Cardiol* 19(11):21-25, 1993.

38. Theroux P, Waters DD, Halphen C, et al: Prognostic value of exercise testing soon after myocardial infarction, *N Engl J Med* 301:341-345, 1979.

39. Waters DD, Bosch X, Bouchard A, et al: Comparison of clinical variables and variables derived from a limited predischarge exercise test as predictors of early and late mortality after myocardial infarction, *J Am Coll Cardiol* 5:1-8, 1985.

40. Weld FM, Chu KL, Bigger TJ Jr, et al: Risk stratification with low-level exercise testing 2 weeks after acute myocardial infarction, *Circulation* 64:306-314, 1981.

41. DeBusk RF, Kraemer HC, Nash E, in cooperation with Berger WE III, Lew H: Stepwise risk stratification soon after acute myocardial infarction, *Am J Cardiol* 52:1161-1166, 1983.

42. Madsen EB, Gilpin E, Ahnve S, et al: Prediction of functional capacity and use of exercise testing for predicting risk after acute myocardial infarction, *Am J Cardiol* 56(13):839-845, 1985.

43. Klein J, Froelicher VF, Detrano R, et al: Does the rest electrocardiogram after myocardial infarction determine the predictive value of exercise-induced ST depression? A 2-year follow-up study in a veteran population, *J Am Coll Cardiol* 14(2):305-311, 1989.

44. Castellanet M, Greenberg PS, Ellestad MH: Comparison of S-T segment changes on exercise testing with angiographic findings in patients with prior myocardial infarction, *Am J Cardiol* 42:24-35, 1978.

45. Ahnve S, Savvides M, Abouantoun S, et al: Can myocardial ischemia be recognized by the exercise electrocardiogram in coronary disease patients with abnormal resting Q waves? *Am Heart J* 111:909-916, 1986.

46. Miranda CP, Herbert WG, Dubach P, et al: Post-myocardial infarction exercise testing. Non-Q wave versus Q wave correlation with coronary angiography and long-term prognosis, *Circulation* 84(6):2357-2365, 1991.

47. TIMI Study Group: Comparison of invasive and conservative strategies after treatment with intravenous tissue plasminogen activator in acute myocardial infarction. Results of the Thrombolysis in Myocardial Infarction (TIMI) Phase II Trial, *N Engl J Med* 320:618-627, 1989.

48. Sutton JM, Topol EJ: Significance of a negative exercise thallium test in the presence of a critical residual stenosis after thrombolysis for acute myocardial infarction, *Circulation* 83:1278-1286, 1991.

49. Piccalo G, Pirelli S, Massa D, et al: Value of negative predischarge exercise testing in identifying patients at low risk after acute myocardial infarction treated by systemic thrombolysis, *Am J Cardiol* 70:31-33, 1992.

50. Melin JA, De Coster PM, Renkin J, et al: Effect of intracoronary thrombolytic therapy on exercise-induced ischemia after acute myocardial infarction, *Am J Cardiol* 56:705-711, 1985.

51. Cragg DR, Friedman HZ, Bonema JD, et al: Outcome of patients with acute myocardial infarction who are ineligible for thrombolytic therapy, *Ann Intern Med* 115:173-177, 1991.

52. Fung AY, Lai P, Juni JE, et al: Prevention of subsequent exercise-induced periinfarct ischemia by emergency coronary angioplasty in acute myocardial infarction: comparison with intracoronary streptokinase, *J Am Coll Cardiol* 8:496-503, 1986.

53. Grines CL, Browne KF, Marco J, et al: A comparison of immediate angioplasty with thrombolytic therapy for acute myocardial infarction, *N Engl J Med* 328:673-679, 1993.

54. Zaret BL, Wackers FJT, Terrin ML, et al for the TIMI Investigators: Assessment of global and regional left ventricular performance at rest and during exercise after thrombolytic therapy for acute myocardial infarction: results of the Thrombolysis in Myocardial Infarction (TIMI) study, *Am J Cardiol* 69:1-9, 1992.

55. Ewart CK, Taylor CB, Reese LB, et al: Effects of early postmyocardial infarction exercise testing on self-perception and subsequent physical activity, *Am J Cardiol* 51:1076-1080, 1983.

56. Taylor CB, Bandura A, Ewart CK, et al: Exercise testing to enhance wives' confidence in their husbands' cardiac capability soon after clinically uncomplicated acute myocardial infarction, *Am J Cardiol* 55:635-638, 1985.

57. Working Group on Rehabilitation of the European Society of Cardiology: Risk of poor quality of life, *Eur Heart J* 13(suppl C):20-34, 1992.

58. Mark DB, Lam LC, Lee KL, et al: Identification of patients with coronary disease at high risk for loss of employment: a prospective validation study, *Circulation* 86:1485-1494, 1992.

59. Vanhees L, Fagard R, Thijs L, et al: Prognostic significance of peak exercise capacity in patients with coronary artery disease, *J Am Coll Cardiol* 23(2):358-363, 1994.

60. Cohn PF: Silent myocardial ischemia in patients with a defective anginal warning system, *Am J Cardiol* 45:697-702, 1980.

61. Cohn PF, Harris P, Barry WH, et al: Prognostic importance of anginal symptoms in angiographically defined coronary artery disease, *Am J Cardiol* 47:233-237, 1981.

62. Gottlieb SO, Weisfeldt ML, Ouyang P, et al: Silent ischemia as a marker for early unfavorable outcomes in patients with unstable angina, *N Engl J Med* 314:1214-1219, 1986.

63. Nademanee K, Intarachot V, Josephson MA, et al: Prognostic significance of silent myocardial ischemia in patients with unstable angina, *J Am Coll Cardiol* 10(1):1-9, 1987.

64. Gottlieb SO, Gottlieb SH, Achuff SC, et al: Silent ischemia on Holter monitoring predicts mortality in high-risk postinfarction patients, *JAMA* 259(7):1030-1035, JAMA.

65. Chandra NC, Ouyang P, Abell RT, et al: Assessment of early post-infarction ischemia:correlation between ambulatory electro-cardiographic monitoring and exercise treadmill testing, *Am J Med* 95:371-376, 1993.

66. Jereczek M, Andresen D, Schroder J, et al: Prognostic value of ischemia during Holter monitoring and exercise testing after acute myocardial infarction, *Am J Cardiol* 72:8-13, 1993.

67. Langer A, Minkowitz J, Dorian P, et al for the Tissue Plasminogen Activator: Pathophysiology and prognostic significance of Holter-detected ST segment depression after myocardial infarction, *J Am Coll Cardiol* 20(6):1313-1317, 1992.

68. Moss AJ, Goldstein RE, Hall J, et al: Detection and significance of myocardial ischemia in stable patients after recovery from an acute coronary event, *JAMA* 269(18):2379-2385, 1993.

69. Pilote L, Mark DB, Hlatky MA: Changes in the treatment of uncomplicated acute myocardial infarction in the United States between 1987 and 1992, *Arch Int Med,* 1994 (in press).

70. Hlatky MA, Cotugno HE, Mark DB, et al: Trends in physician management of uncomplicated acute myocardial infarction, *Am J Cardiol* 61:515-518, 1988.

71. Hillis LD, Forman S, Braunwald E, and the TIMI Phase II Co-Investigators: Risk stratification before thrombolytic therapy in patients with acute myocardial infarction, *J Am Coll Cardiol* 16(2):313-315, 1990.

72. Mark DB, Sigmon K, Topol EJ, et al: Identification of acute myocardial infarction patients suitable early discharge after aggressive interventional therapy. Results from the Thrombolysis and Angioplasty in Acute Myocardial Infarction Registry, *Circulation* 83:1186-1193, 1991.

73. Topol EJ, Juni JE, O'Neill WW, et al: Exercise testing three days after onset of acute myocardial infarction, *Am J Cardiol* 60:958-962, 1987.

74. Topol EJ, Burek K, O'Neill WW, et al: A randomized controlled trial of hospital discharge three days after myocardial infarction in the era of reperfusion, *N Engl J Med* 318(17):1083-1088, 1988.

Chapter 63

MYOCARDIAL PERFUSION IMAGING FOLLOWING ACUTE MYOCARDIAL INFARCTION

Joseph M. Sutton

In current medical practice, radionuclide myocardial perfusion imaging is most frequently used for diagnostic and prognostic assessment of patients with suspected or known obstructive coronary artery disease (CAD). For this application, these tests may be performed at rest only or, more commonly, at rest and following physiologic or pharmacologic stress. Other applications that have been studied in recent years include localization and sizing of acute myocardial infarction (AMI) and evaluation of reperfusion following thrombolytic therapy. There are three major options for assessing myocardial blood flow with radionuclide imaging techniques: planar imaging, which is used principally with thallium-201 (^{201}Tl); single photon emission computed tomography (SPECT), which can be performed using either Tl^{201} or technetium-99m (^{99m}Tc) sestamibi; and positron emission tomography (PET) with either rubidium-82 (^{82}Rb) or nitrogen-13 (^{13}N) ammonia.

This chapter will begin with an overview of the techniques of radionuclide myocardial perfusion imaging. Following this, we will review the use of these techniques for diagnostic and prognostic risk stratification; the assessment of myocardial viability is then evaluated. The use of radionuclide imaging techniques to detect coronary reperfusion following thrombolysis is discussed in Chapter 37.

TECHNIQUES OF RADIONUCLIDE PERFUSION IMAGING
Radionuclide agents
Thallium-201
^{201}**Thallium perfusion kinetics.** ^{201}Thallium, a metallic element from group IIIA of the periodic table, has been the principal radionuclide myocardial perfusion agent for over a decade. Both ^{201}Tl and the other radionuclide isotopes of the group IIIA elements (^{43}potassium and ^{81}rubidium) emit a single photon upon degradation and are suitable for perfusion and viability imaging because, as potassium analogues, they are actively moved across the cellular membrane by ATP-dependent sodium-potassium exchange mechanisms. The earliest perfusion studies of the heart were done with ^{43}potassium; they demonstrated the ability of such scans to accurately define and localize exercise-induced regions of myocardial hypoperfusion and to distinguish regions of transient ischemia from necrosis.[1] The clinical usefulness of ^{43}potassium was limited, however, by its high-energy photon peak of 373 keV, prohibiting imaging with a standard gamma scintillation camera, and by its concomitant beta emission, which resulted in high radiation doses to the patient. Subsequent studies with ^{81}rubidium perfusion imaging demonstrated an 88% sensitivity in the detection of significant coronary artery

781

lesions.[2] Imaging this element with a standard gamma camera required a pinhole collimator, however, to limit scatter from adjacent, high-energy photons, reducing sensitivity and making accurate image acquisition difficult.[1,3] The related isotope [82]rubidium is still used as a perfusion tracer in conjunction with positron emission tomography.

Thallium has supplanted both [81]rubidium and [43]potassium as the perfusion agent of choice because of its lower radiation per unit dose and the suitability of the agent for either planar imaging with a standard gamma scintillation camera or single photon emission computed tomography. Planar images of the heart can be acquired with a high-resolution gamma camera using a low-energy collimator (a type of filter) to collect the 80 keV mercury x-rays emitted by thallium upon radioactive decay. Although this radiation energy is actually at the low end of the resolution spectrum for a standard gamma scintillator and tissue attenuation of the photon energy may be a significant problem in some patients, thallium overcomes several important technical difficulties involved in imaging with the earlier higher-energy isotopes. Thallium also significantly lowers the radiation exposure of the patient relative to the other group IIIA isotopes.

Following the intravenous administration of thallium, uptake by viable myocardium is quite rapid, with a first-pass coronary blood extraction fraction of approximately 85%.[4,5] Although cardiac glycosides such as digitalis may impair active sarcolemmal uptake of the group IIIA cationic potassium analogues by the active sodium potassium ATPase transport enzyme, clinically useful doses of these agents have been shown to have little impact on thallium imaging.[5,6] Myocardial uptake is directly proportional to the extraction fraction and to regional myocardial blood flow and appears essentially unaltered by the clinical use of drugs (such as beta blockers) that alter coronary flow.[5,6] With increasing heart rate at the time of thallium injection, the accompanying increase in coronary blood flow results in a higher initial uptake and more rapid clearance of the tracer from normally perfused myocardium. In general, decreasing peak exercise heart rate by one beat per minute slows thallium clearance by 0.05 hours.[7] An optimal thallium stress test should therefore approximate peak target heart rate as closely as possible to promote optimal, rapid tracer uptake by the normal, hyperemic myocardial segment relative to any ischemic zones present to maximize detection of hypoperfused areas.[8]

The development of local hypoxemia and lactic acidosis accompanying myocardial ischemia may independently diminish thallium extraction; however, this modest effect is difficult to separate from a primary ischemic-related diminution in coronary blood flow.[9]

These physical sequelae of myocardial ischemia do not affect thallium uptake in an isolated rabbit heart model when coronary blood flow is held constant.[10] Experimental ischemia in the canine model does not alter thallium uptake in the absence of cellular necrosis; even when repeated ischemia and reflow results in a reversible regional wall motion defect ("stunned" myocardium), thallium uptake by the viable but akinetic myocardial segment is unaltered and directly parallels coronary blood flow.[11,12] Thus, [201]thallium active transport across the myocellular sarcolemmal membrane remains unaltered in the absence of necrosis and varies directly with coronary blood flow. This characteristic makes thallium well suited to be used in assessment of regional myocardial blood flow.

[201]**Thallium redistribution.** Following injection into the blood at peak exercise, there is an initial distribution phase in which myocardial regions with normal perfusion take up large amounts of ^{201}Tl, hypoperfused areas take up proportionally less, and areas of infarction take up little or no [201]Tl. Following the initial distribution phase, which occurs quite rapidly, there is a prolonged redistribution phase made possible by the 74-hour half-life of [201]thallium. After initial distribution, a continuous exchange or recirculation is established between blood pool ^{201}Tl and myocardial [201]Tl. As myocardial ^{201}Tl is washed out, it is replaced by ^{201}Tl from the blood pool. The amount of thallium detectable in normally perfused myocardium diminishes significantly by 4 to 6 hours following injection. However, uptake in myocardium perfused by a severely stenotic coronary artery, which is initially abnormally low, increases over this same period as ^{201}Tl is redistributed to the hypoperfused segments of myocardium (Fig. 63-1). As a consequence, initial postexercise images in a patient with a significant coronary stenosis will show a significant difference in tracer uptake between normal and hypoperfused myocardial regions, whereas repeat images at 4 hours will show comparable thallium image intensity in the two regions as a result of redistribution (Fig. 63-2). An area of infarcted myocardium will show little or no thallium uptake on the initial images and no redistribution on the delayed images. Areas of partial redistribution may also be seen, especially in patients with non–Q-wave MI.[13]

Coadministration of intravenous dipyridamole or adenosine in patients with significant CAD can produce an initial inhomogeneity of myocardial blood flow with late redistribution similar to that seen after exercise by producing marked vasodilation and hyperperfusion in normal coronary arteries with an attenuated relative increase, or even an absolute decrease caused by "steal" through parallel capacitance vessels, in coronary flow in arteries with significant stenoses.[14] These agents are now used commonly with perfusion imaging in lieu of exercise stress in patients with limited physical capacity.

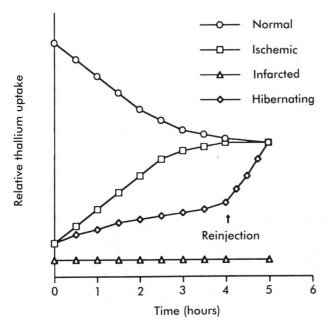

Fig. 63-1. Relative thallium uptake over the 6 hours following injection for 4 types of myocardial perfusion. Normally perfused myocardium *(circles)* demonstrates the highest thallium uptake initially after injection with a progressive decrease over the following 6 hours. Severely ischemic myocardium *(boxes)* demonstrates little or no early thallium uptake and a progressive rise over the ensuing 6 hours due to redistribution. Infarcted myocardium *(triangles)* shows no uptake initially and no uptake during the following 5- to 6-hour imaging period. Hibernating myocardium is intermediate between infarcted and severely ischemic myocardium in that there is a small amount of redistribution. This is augmented by a 4-hour reinjection, which equalizes the uptake of thallium between the hibernating myocardial region and the normal myocardial regions. (From Cerqueira MD, (ed): *Nuclear cardiology,* Boston, 1994, Blackwell Scientific.)

²⁰¹Thallium late redistribution and reinjection. A lack of redistribution indicates either persistent, complete obstruction of blood flow into the defective region or the presence of nonviable myocardium or "scar" from prior infarction within the region of persistent defect — the segment is either incapable of thallium uptake because of lack of access to the isotope, or there is an inability to actively "pump" the tracer into the cell because of injury and physical disruption of the sarcolemma. In the presence of a critically severe coronary artery stenosis, the disparity between early "wash-out" from normal segments and ongoing, markedly delayed uptake within the especially ischemic zone may not demonstrate redistribution until 12 to 24 hours after the initial injection of thallium.[15,16] This exaggerated delay in redistribution will incline the observer to diagnose the abnormal region as nonviable scar on the standard 2½- to 4-hour postinjection images. Delayed redistribution at 12 to 24 hours has been interpreted as evidence for viable but hibernating myocardium. Injection of a second

dose of ²⁰¹Tl at 4 hours has been proposed as a more efficient method of identifying this same phenomenon (see Fig. 63-1). Thus, diagnostic accuracy may be enhanced by late reimaging in subsets of patients with severe coronary disease or extensive prior infarction.

Technetium-99m perfusion agents. Although thallium has been used extensively over the last decade, it has several important limitations that make it a less than ideal perfusion imaging agent.[17] As noted earlier, its low photon energy results in significant attenuation of the radioactive signal because of absorption by the patient's body tissues, with a resulting decrease in the number of counts reaching the gamma camera. In some patients (e.g., obese subjects, women with large breasts), this problem may cause significant attenuation artifacts that can mimic regional myocardial hypoperfusion. A second problem with thallium is its relatively long half-life, which limits the total dose that can be given for a single study to 4 mCi (in order to keep the patient's total radiation exposure at an acceptable level). The lower thallium dose results in lower image acquisition counts and images that may be more difficult to interpret. The final major limitation of thallium-201 is its need to be produced in a cyclotron, a device that collides different nuclei together at high speeds to produce the desired isotopes. Because most hospitals do not have such equipment, the agent must usually be shipped to the hospital from a remote production site. Therefore, if the hospital runs out of thallium on any particular day there is usually no readily available replacement source.

To address the limitations of thallium, several new technetium-based perfusion imaging agents have been developed. To date, two have been approved by the Food and Drug Administration for routine clinical use: ⁹⁹ᵐTc-sestamibi and ⁹⁹ᵐTc-teboroxime. A comparison of these two agents with ²⁰¹Tl is shown in Table 63-1. Of the two new agents, much more experience has been acquired to date with ⁹⁹ᵐTc-sestamibi. Technetium-99m has a higher photon energy (140 keV) than thallium and is therefore about twice as bright to the gamma camera and produces correspondingly higher-quality images. It has a shorter half-life than thallium (6 hours) and can thus be given in a significantly higher dose. Like thallium, this agent distributes into the myocardium after injection in proportion to regional blood flow. Unlike thallium, however, ⁹⁹ᵐTc-sestamibi is bound within mitochondria in the myocardial cytoplasm and, in most patients, does not undergo a significant redistribution phase. After the initial distribution phase, sestamibi is cleared rapidly from the blood. The cellular binding of the isotope allows for imaging at a convenient time without concern for image degradation or early recirculation. Because of the absence of redistribution, sestamibi protocols require two separate injections to differentiate ischemia

Exercise

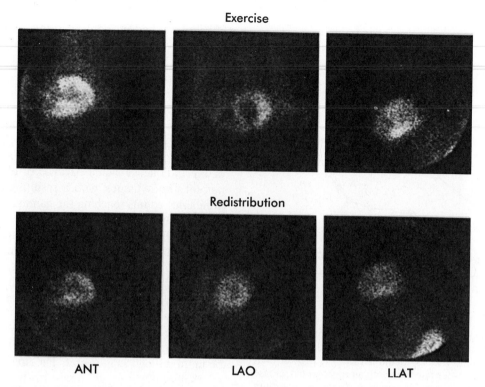

Redistribution

ANT   LAO   LLAT

Fig. 63-2. This figure shows a planar exercise thallium study in a patient with transient myocardial ischemia. The top three images show the anterior LAO and left lateral projections during exercise, and the bottom three figures show the same projections in the 4-hour redistribution images. This study shows a perfusion defect during exercise in the anteroseptal region, seen best on the left anterior oblique projection during exercise. At the 4-hour images, this defect is completely filled in, consistent with redistribution due to ischemia. (From Zaret BL, Berger HJ: *Techniques of nuclear cardiology.* In Hurst JW, Logue KB, Rackley CE, et al, (eds): *The heart: arteries and veins,* ed 6, New York, 1986, McGraw-Hill.)

Table 63-1. Characteristics of various agents used in myocardial perfusion imaging

Characteristics	201Thallium	99mTechnetium sestamibi	99mTechnetium teboroxime
Energy emitted (keV)	69-83, 135, 165, 167	140	140
Physical half-life (hr)	74	6	6
Dose (mCi)	2.5-3.5	30	30
Radiation dose (rad/mCi)			
Whole body	0.21	0.02	0.02
Intestines	0.54	0.18	0.11
Variables displayed			
Blood flow	Yes	Yes	Yes
Viability	Yes (delayed image)	Yes	No
Redistribution	Yes	Yes (minimal)	No
Imaging time (min)			
Planar (per view)	10	5	1-2
Tomography	21	13-21	

From Zaret BL, Wackers FJ: Nuclear cardiology, *N Engl J Med* 329(11):775-783, 1993.

from myocardial scar. Several different protocols have been devised for this purpose involving either two injections on the same day or injections on 2 successive days (Fig. 63-3). The separate-day protocol allows use of a full 20 to 30 mCi dose for each set of images (with better resulting image quality), but is somewhat less convenient, particularly when the results of the study are being used for predischarge risk stratification and planning. Thus the separate-day protocol is often used primarily in patients in whom tissue attenuation is likely

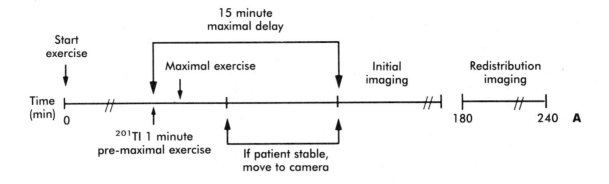

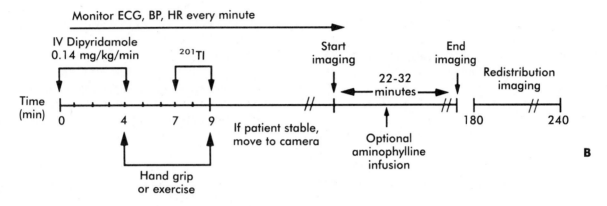

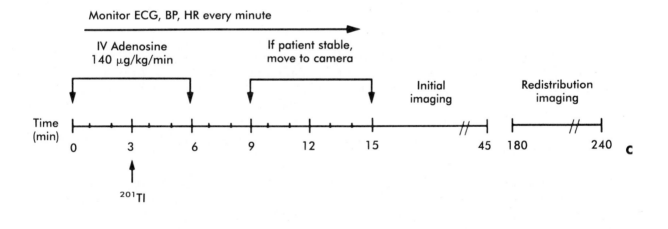

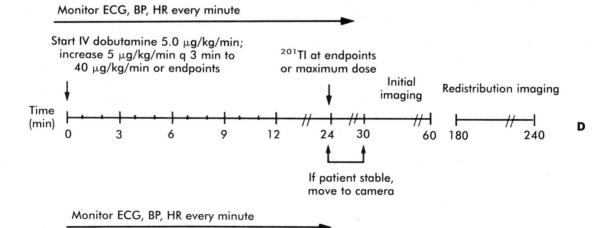

Fig. 63-3. Representative same-day and separate-day ^{99m}Tc-sestamibi imaging protocols. (From Cerqueira MD, (ed): *Nuclear cardiology,* Boston, 1994, Blackwell Scientific.)

to be a problem (e.g., obese patients, women with large breasts).

One other feature differentiating thallium and technetium-based perfusion imaging is that the latter can perform first-pass ventriculography. When the ^{99m}Tc-sestamibi dose is injected, the initial transit of the radionuclide bolus through the right and left ventricles can be recorded in the anterior projection, using an appropriate type of gamma camera (such as a multi-crystal camera that can record three times as many counts per second as a standard gamma camera). When these first-pass studies are performed as part of a rest-exercise examination, the exercise is typically done using an upright or supine bicycle ergometer, rather than a treadmill, to minimize motion artifact during the brief acquisition period.

Imaging technique

Planar imaging. Scintigraphy refers to the process of converting ionizing radiation into visible light.[18] Photons produced by the radioactive decay of radionuclide agents (thallium-201, technetium-99) pass through the patient's body and interact with a scintillator medium that detects incoming gamma rays (technetium-99) and x-rays (thallium-201) and gives off an equivalent pattern but a much larger number of visible light photons. The scintillation medium used in current gamma cameras is an inorganic crystal composed of sodium iodide mixed with a very small amount of thallium-201. This material is preferred because it generates the largest amount of visible light per incoming photon of all available scintillators.

Once visible light photons are generated by the scintillation medium, photomultiplier tubes in the gamma camera are used to detect this light, convert the relevant information about it (energy level, position) to electrons, and amplify the resulting electron signal.[18] After further amplification steps, the signal is passed to an analogue-to-digital converter, which converts the position information into a two-dimensional image matrix, with each possible location point represented as a pixel (picture element). The number of pixels created (and consequently the resolution of the final images) is determined by the type of analogue to digital converter used (e.g., 8-bit conversion yields a 256 × 256 pixel matrix). The final aspect of image generation with a gamma camera is computer processing. The computer plots the detected photons into the image matrix. The final display for a planar image uses either grey scale (black to white) or color to represent the number of counts detected at each location. Neither planar nor SPECT perfusion imaging can be used to determine absolute levels of blood flow because of problems with radiation scatter and attenuation. Thus, the computer processing of a gamma camera image will

assign a normal intensity display to the area of highest detected counts. If blood flow is uniformly reduced to all segments of the myocardium (e.g., severe three-vessel disease), the computer may (incorrectly) generate a perfusion scan that looks normal because the computer cannot evaluate whether the overall count intensity detected is abnormally low.

Sophisticated algorithms are often used in image processing to smooth the obtained image and reduce random variations in image intensity from one pixel to the next. Smoothing can make images somewhat easier to interpret but also tends to blur the image slightly.[19,20]

Planar ^{201}Tl imaging has been used substantially longer than SPECT ^{201}Tl and continues to be used at many centers. It requires less sophisticated equipment (which is consequently less expensive) and is somewhat simpler to perform and interpret. Representative protocols for exercise thallium, dipyridamole thallium, and adenosine thallium are shown in Fig. 63-4. The common features are injection of the thallium dose (typically 2.5 to 3.5 mCi) at the time of peak exercise or drug effect, initial imaging as soon as possible thereafter, and redistribution imaging at 3 to 4 hours. For each set of images, three views are typically obtained: 45-degree left anterior oblique (LAO), anterior, and steep (70-degree) LAO or left lateral (Fig. 63-5). Imaging is performed for 8 to 10 minutes in each view.

The simplest interpretation of a planar stress thallium study involves visual analysis.[17] The reader may employ various ordinal scoring methods that have been proposed in this interpretation (e.g., 0 = normal, 4 = no uptake of tracer). The essence of visual interpretation is identification of at least one myocardial segment with presumed normal ^{201}Tl uptake and comparison of all other myocardial segments in each image with this reference segment. Planar images can also be analyzed quantitatively by additional computer processing of the thallium image data. Several different approaches have been used for quantitative planar analysis.[20]

One distinct advantage of planar imaging over SPECT is the ability to determine thallium lung activity as a percentage of myocardial activity.[21] This is accomplished by obtaining an activity count per pixel within a region overlying only lung in an initial image, and comparing the count with that obtained from an area overlying the most active myocardial segment. The presence of an increased lung-to-heart thallium distribution ratio has a high correlation with the presence of left ventricular dysfunction at the time of imaging. Centers using SPECT thallium now commonly obtain a 10-minute planar anterior image for this determination before beginning SPECT acquisition.

Emission computed tomography. Planar myocardial perfusion imaging is analogous to a conventional chest radiograph in that a three-dimensional structure is pro-

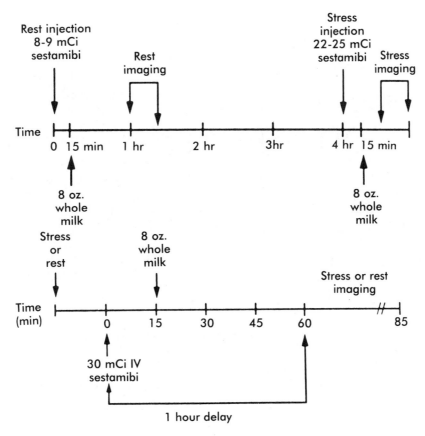

Fig. 63-4. Representative protocols for exercise thallium, dipyridimole thallium, adenosine thallium, and dobutamine thallium imaging studies. (From Cerqueira MD (ed): *Nuclear cardiology,* Boston, 1994, Blackwell Scientific.)

jected onto a two-dimensional image. Overlying structures are superimposed on such an image and cannot readily be distinguished. Emission computed tomography is analogous to an x-ray computed tomograph (CT scan).[22] The three-dimensional nature of the imaged structure is reconstructed mathematically from multiple sequential planar projection images. Nuclear tomographic studies can be performed with the single photon emitting radionuclides [201]thallium or [99m]technetium (and is then referred to as *SPECT*) or with positron emitting agents such as [82]rubidium (and is then referred to as *PET*). The basics of tomographic image reconstruction are similar regardless of the isotope used. For cardiac SPECT studies, tomographic slices are made through a 180-degree arc between 45-degree right anterior oblique and 45-degree left posterior oblique using one (or more) gamma cameras that are rotated on a gantry around the patient. The camera head makes a predetermined number of stops (e.g., 32 stops at 6-degree intervals) and acquires an image for a selected time interval (e.g., 40 seconds for thallium, 20 to 30 seconds for sestamibi) at each stop. For cardiac PET scans, a circumferential array of detectors is used. In both cases, complex computer processing of the raw im-

age data (i.e., filtered backprojection) is used to reconstruct three-dimensional tomographic representations of myocardial perfusion. Many professionals in nuclear cardiology believe that SPECT perfusion imaging with technetium-99m-labeled agents will be the standard myocardial perfusion method in the near future.[22] Because of cost and complexity issues, however, the use of PET scanning is likely to remain restricted for the foreseeable future.

Although there are many possible ways that SPECT data can be presented for clinical interpretation, standards have recently been developed by a joint committee of the American College of Cardiology, the American Heart Association, and the Society for Nuclear Medicine; these standards are likely to become widely (if not universally) adopted in the next few years.[17] The three major display orientations are shown schematically in Figure 63-6; an example patient study is shown in Figure 63-7.

Compared with planar images, SPECT improves localization of defects to specific coronary vascular territories and increases the sensitivity for detection of small defects.[17,22] As with planar imaging, SPECT studies can be interpreted visually (semiquantitatively)

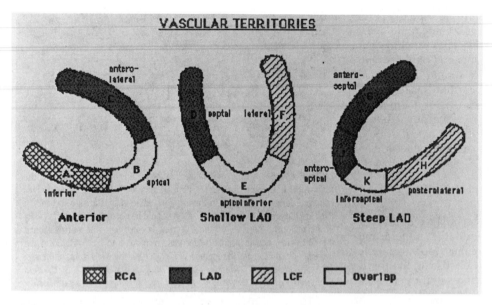

Fig. 63-5. Schematic of the three views typically obtained in a planar thallium study: anterior, shallow left anterior oblique, and steep left anterior oblique or left lateral. Specific myocardial segments are indicated on this figure along with the typical coronary artery supply to that myocardial segment. LAD = left anterior descending; LCF = left circumflex; RCA = right coronary artery. (From Johnson LL, Pohost GM: *Nuclear cardiology.* In Schlant RC, Alexander RW, (eds): *Hurst's The heart: arteries and veins,* ed 8, New York, 1994, McGraw-Hill.)

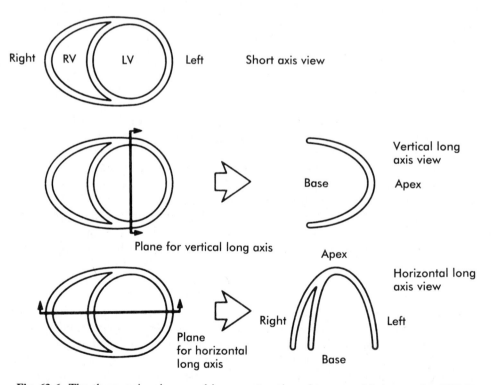

Fig. 63-6. The three major views used in reconstruction of tomographic images for SPECT perfusion studies. (From Cerqueira MD, (ed): *Nuclear cardiology,* Boston, 1994, Blackwell Scientific.)

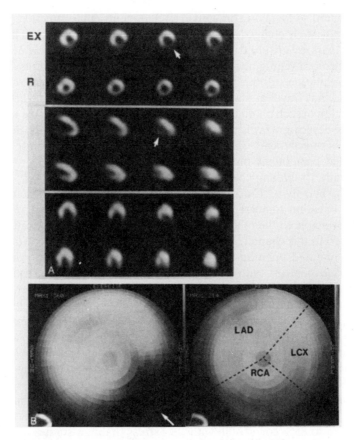

Fig. 63-7. A sample SPECT exercise perfusion study in a patient with a reversible anterolateral perfusion defect. Panel A shows the standard three SPECT views: short axis, vertical long axis, and horizontal long axis. Each set of tomographic slices is paired with the exercise image on top and the redistribution image below it. The arrows show the anterolateral perfusion defect. Panel B shows the bullseye or polar coordinate display of an exercise perfusion study. The left image shows the exercise data, and the arrow indicates a perfusion defect in the inferolateral region. The redistribution image (right panel) shows no defect. Superimposed on this latter figure are the approximate corresponding distributions of the three main coronary arteries. LAD = left anterior descending; RCA = right coronary artery; LCX = left circumflex artery. (From Zaret BL, Wackers FJ, Soufer R: *Nuclear cardiology.* In Braunwald E, (ed): *Heart disease: a textbook of cardiovascular medicine,* ed 4, Philadelphia, 1992, WB Saunders Company.)

or quantitatively. Visual analysis typically involves grading tracer uptake in each defined myocardial segment using an ordinal score as described above for planar image interpretation. The most common quantitative analysis protocol for SPECT involves the short axis and vertical long axis images (see Fig. 63-6). The series of short axis slices are aligned from apex to base, the center of the ventricle and epicardial border for each slice is then defined, and each slice is divided into 30 to 60 circumferential segments or radians extending from the center of the ventricle to the epicardium. Count profiles are constructed for each radian and used to create circumferential count profiles for each short axis slice. Similar profiles are created for the apex from the vertical long axis images. One common display mode for these data involves showing circumferential count profiles in a

"bull's-eye" or polar coordinate format with the apex at the center and the base at the periphery (see Fig. 63-7, *B*). This figure provides a convenient two-dimensional representation of the three-dimensional SPECT data.[23] The final step in quantitative analysis involves mathematical comparisons of count profiles for a given patient with an appropriate reference file of normal count data. SPECT images are subject to the same attenuation artifacts as planar images. In addition, the computer reconstruction process can create artifacts (e.g., from patient motion during image acquisition) that may be difficult to detect. Such reconstruction artifacts may, in part, be responsible for the lower specificity reported with this technique (see next section).

Positron emission tomography (PET). Radionuclides used in PET scans differ importantly from the single photon emitting agents discussed so far. Positron emitting radionuclides give off a positively charged antimatter particle with the same mass as an electron. This particle collides with an electron, resulting in a matter-antimatter reaction with annihilation of both particles and emission of two photons that travel at 180-degree paths from each other. Detection of such photon pairs by a circumferential scintillation detector array is the basis of PET scanning. Radiopharmaceuticals that emit positrons are complex labeled compounds that determine either perfusion (typically [82]rubidium chloride or ^{13}N-ammonia) or metabolic activity (^{11}C-acetate or ^{18}F-deoxyglucose). Positron emission tomography perfusion imaging is similar in principle to the other forms of perfusion imaging discussed in this chapter. Because of the high-energy photons released upon antiparticle annihilation (511 keV), image contrast with PET is improved, and the problems of attenuation involving the inferoposterior ventricular wall and from overlying soft tissues seen with the single photon agents are overcome and a clear image is produced. However, the advantages of PET are not currently sufficient to justify its routine clinical use in myocardial perfusion imaging.

Use of PET imaging to study the metabolism of ischemic and infarcted myocardium has been an area of much recent investigation. Although PET-determined myocardial viability has a 75% to 85% correlation with regional wall motion recovery (sensitivity) in patients undergoing surgical revascularization,[24,25] tissue recovery determined by thallium viability assessment after late (8 to 24 hour)[15,16] redistribution imaging and reinjection[26,27] is comparable. Further, the ongoing development of labeled fatty acids such as ^{123}I-iodo-phenylpentadecanoic acid, which can be imaged with less expensive SPECT equipment, has been suggested to have a similar predictive value for functional recovery after surgical revascularization.[28] Thus the superior spatial imaging afforded by the more expensive PET technique does not necessarily translate into more accurate viability determination compared with SPECT imaging, except perhaps in the presence of extremely severe dysfunction, where very little viable myocardium remains.

CLINICAL APPLICATIONS OF PERFUSION SCINTIGRAPHY

The coupling of perfusion scintigraphy with an exercise ECG not only increases the sensitivity of the test to detect myocardial ischemia that can be provoked but also conveys important localizing information to implicate a specific vascular territory. This additional information is invaluable when the study is performed to determine the functional significance of a known coronary artery lesion, or in the presence of multiple lesions when the "culprit lesion" is not apparent. Thallium stress testing may also convey indirect information about

left ventricular function by identifying patients with abnormal lung uptake. The sensitivity and specificity of the test remains largely dependent upon the prevalence of coronary artery disease within the population undergoing the study. However, results available to date suggest that the choice of radioisotope (thallium, sestamibi) does not affect the accuracy of detection of CAD. In addition, pharmacologic stress tests appear to provide equivalent information to exercise tests.

Diagnosis of coronary artery disease

To use perfusion scintigraphy to determine if a patient has segmental reduction in myocardial blood flow caused by obstructive CAD, it is important to maximize the degree of inhomogeneity present in myocardial blood flow. Where possible, dynamic exercise remains the preferred method of stressing the myocardial circulation. However, some patients are not physically able to perform a bicycle or treadmill stress test. For these subjects, pharmacologic stress testing provides a valuable alternative. As noted earlier, dipyridamole and adenosine maximize inhomogeneities in myocardial blood flow by increasing flow through vasodilation of nondiseased coronary segments. In contrast, dobutamine increases myocardial contractility and heart rate. Representative protocols for use of these three agents in stress thallium studies are shown in Figure 63-4.

Like exercise treadmill testing, stress perfusion studies can be used to diagnose the presence of obstructive CAD, assess its severity, and stratify the risk of future cardiac events (see Chapter 62). Much of the work defining the accuracy of stress thallium or sestamibi has been carried out in patients with stable CAD. The literature evaluating the use of these techniques for assessing disease severity in acute ischemic heart disease and predicting prognosis is still relatively small, especially that literature dealing with patients who have undergone successful reperfusion therapy.

Accuracy of stress perfusion imaging for diagnosis of CAD

In a recent review, Kotler and Diamond reported that the average sensitivity of thallium testing when analyzed visually was 84% with a specificity of 87%.[29] The accuracy of [201]thallium SPECT stress test imaging remains controversial. Although comparative studies have reported the superiority of tomographic over planar imaging technique,[30,31] SPECT imaging is still limited by overlying soft tissue and inferoposterior signal attenuation. Iskandrian et al.[32] found the sensitivity for exercise thallium stress testing to be 88% in a study of 164 patients; however, the specificity of the method was low (62%). Subsequent cardiac catheterization demonstrated at least one significant lesion ($\geq 50\%$) in 22 of the 58 patients with a negative stress result.

In a multicenter study, Van Train et al. reported an even lower (44%) specificity for thallium stress testing as a screen for significant coronary artery lesions.[33] These investigators pointed out the referral bias that may evolve when evaluating a more sensitive diagnostic technique. The study cohort consisted mainly of patients in whom there was a strong pretest clinical suspicion for coronary disease; many of these patients had negative or equivocal stress ECGs before entry into the study. Thus the patients had a skewed higher disease prevalence, increasing the possibility of an erroneous negative response. Diamond[34] illustrated this effect in a report of 248 patients whose planar thallium results were correlated with angiographic findings. Planar stress thallium imaging had a sensitivity and specificity of 91% and 34% respectively. After correcting for referral bias, the specificity of the test increased to 71%, but the sensitivity among the cohort of patients with a lower pretest likelihood of coronary disease fell significantly to 68%. Gould[35] later suggested that in addition to the biased disease prevalence in the select referral population, overly aggressive interpretation of the images further contributed to the low specificity of stress thallium testing found in the literature.

Visual interpretation of SPECT thallium images has been reported to be more accurate than planar imaging in the detection and localization of coronary artery lesions.[23,30,36] In a study of 112 patients undergoing cardiac catheterization, Fintel et al. visually analyzed the paired planar and SPECT thallium images acquired at the time of stress testing and found that SPECT was more accurate in the detection of significant coronary artery lesions compared with the planar technique.[30] Quantitative computer analysis of planar images enhances diagnostic accuracy.[37,38] When comparing exercise and delayed images, quantitative analysis of the washout rate characteristics of a persistent but partially redistributing thallium defect can enhance the detection of viable, ischemic myocardium. The identification of myocardial segments with abnormal thallium clearance has the same diagnostic significance as redistribution and has increased the sensitivity and specificity of even planar image interpretation to nearly 90%.[37,39] Only one of the studies pooled in the metaanalysis of Diamond[34] used quantitative planar thallium imaging; there have been no large prospective randomized trials comparing quantitative planar analysis with SPECT imaging.

Thus, visual interpretation of SPECT thallium images for detecting ischemia related to CAD remains superior to visual interpretation of planar imaging; however, the accuracy of both methods may be similar when quantitative methods of planar image analysis are used. Serial studies are exceedingly reproducible in the same patient over time,[40] and images obtained with pharmacologic vs. exercise stress provide similar diagnostic information, although pharmacologic defect sizes may be slightly overestimated compared with those defined by exercise.[41,42]

Thallium stress imaging remains particularly useful in distinguishing true- from false-positive exercise ECG changes, especially when the baseline ECG is obscured by the presence of a baseline Q-wave infarction pattern, preexcitation, or ST-segment abnormalities associated with left ventricular hypertrophy or digitalis use[43] (see Chapter 62).

For most patients with a well-documented AMI the diagnosis of CAD is not in question. What the clinician wants to learn from stress testing in such patients is rather the extent of CAD and the associated prognosis. The distribution of the underlying coronary artery disease has an impact on the sensitivity of both planar and SPECT thallium stress results. Ischemia in the posterolateral distribution resulting from left circumflex artery disease can be more difficult to detect when compared with left anterior descending and right coronary artery lesions.[30,37] Similarly, disease limited to branch vessels of the left anterior descending (diagonal) or circumflex (obtuse marginal) arteries supplying the high lateral wall are more difficult to identify than more proximal lesions in the main left coronary system.[44] Single-vessel disease is more difficult to detect than multivessel disease.[34,38] A limited 78% sensitivity of thallium scintigraphy to discern single-vessel disease has been observed, compared with an 89% sensitivity when studying patients with at least two diseased coronary arteries. Further, stress-induced thallium defects are more common in the presence of severe ($\geq 90\%$) coronary stenoses than with less severe lesions.

^{201}Thallium vs. positron emission tomographic imaging. The improved sensitivity and specificity of thallium image interpretation for the diagnosis of CAD that accompanies computed tomographic and quantitative analysis rivals that achieved with the higher-resolution PET perfusion methods. A persistent limitation common to both planar and SPECT thallium imaging remains the high false-positive interpretation rate of the inferoposterior wall that results from attenuation of the signal by overlying tissue. Some smaller studies suggest that positron emission tomography may not be subject to this limitation. Stewart et al. studied 81 patients: 60 with CAD and 21 without CAD at subsequent catheterization.[45] Visual interpretation of the SPECT thallium images yielded a sensitivity of 84% (50 of 60 patients), and a specificity of 53% (11 of 21 patients), results which are similar to previous reports. ^{82}Rubidium PET perfusion imaging yielded a sensitivity and specificity in the detection of coronary artery lesions of 84% (50 of 60 patients) and 81% (18 of 21 patients) respectively.

Use of stress perfusion imaging for risk stratification

Many studies of the prognostic value of exercise perfusion imaging (largely exercise ^{201}Tl) have used the extent of CAD or "myocardium in jeopardy" as a surrogate for a direct assessment of prognosis. One of the difficulties in studying the prognostic value of exercise perfusion scans in predischarge risk stratification has been the relatively low-risk nature of the tested population. Traditionally only uncomplicated patients have been tested[46,47] (see Chapter 62). Thus the test has the relatively difficult task of picking the few high-risk patients out from the much larger number of truly low-risk subjects. Compounding this difficulty has been the fact that most prognostic studies of exercise thallium have had sample sizes and/or follow-up times that were not adequate enough to have the statistical power needed to evaluate the issue properly.

In the prethrombolytic era, Gibson et al. at the University of Virginia examined the value of predischarge planar exercise thallium for stratifying the risk of future cardiac events in patients age ≤ 65 with recent uncomplicated AMI.[48] Over a mean follow-up of 16 months, 50 cardiac events were recorded: 7 deaths, 9 nonfatal MIs, and 34 unstable angina hospitalizations. Comparison with the exercise ECG and the coronary angiogram revealed that all three studies predicted mortality with equivalent accuracy (this may be a problem of inadequate statistical power), but thallium was the best test for predicting nonfatal MI or unstable angina. The presence of a multivessel disease thallium pattern and/or abnormal lung thallium uptake identified 94% of patients who died or had a nonfatal MI, compared with a 50% detection rate by the exercise ECG. Of the 13 single-vessel disease patients in this population who experienced a follow-up event, 12 (92%) demonstrated thallium redistribution within the infarct zone.

Comparison of the 154 Q-wave MIs with the 87 non–Q-wave MIs in this population showed that quantitatively determined ^{201}Tl redistribution in the infarct zone was greater in the non-Q MI patients.[13] Although the mortality rate was not different between the two groups, the non-Q MI patients had a higher reinfarction rate and a higher rate of follow-up hospitalization for AMI. This prethrombolytic study suggested that the pathophysiology of non-Q MI might represent spontaneous reperfusion and thus that the natural history of these patients might resemble those receiving thrombolytic therapy.

In a prospective comparative study of symptom-limited treadmill testing, planar exercise thallium testing, and rest and exercise-gated blood pool scans in 117 men 3 weeks after AMI, Hung et al. found that peak exercise treadmill work load and change in radionuclide left ventricular ejection fraction during exercise were the only two independent predictors of hard cardiac events in follow-up.[49] However, like the study by Gibson et al.,[48] the statistical power of this analysis was limited by the small number (i.e., 8) of "hard" cardiac events.

A few studies of predischarge exercise thallium testing have now been reported following reperfusion therapy. Tilkemeier et al. found that 64 AMI patients who received thrombolysis and/or angioplasty had a 15% prevalence of exercise ST depression and a 42% prevalence of ^{201}Tl redistribution.[50] Thallium scintigraphy had a 55% sensitivity for detecting cardiac events in the post-MI year in these 64 thrombolysis patients, compared with an 81% sensitivity in 107 MI patients who did not receive thrombolytic therapy. In 88 consecutive post-MI patients who had received thrombolytic therapy and were subsequently referred for predischarge testing at the University of Virginia, exercise ST depression occurred in 14% whereas exercise-induced thallium redistribution occurred in 48%.[51] However, in this latter study the sensitivity and specificity of exercise thallium for detection of a multivessel CAD pattern was not significantly better than that seen with exercise ST depression alone.

Sutton and Topol studied 101 consecutive thrombolysis patients with an uncomplicated AMI and at least 70% residual stenosis of the infarct artery.[52] Forty-nine percent of these patients had a negative submaximal SPECT thallium. Comparison with the patients who had a positive thallium test revealed only two significant differences. First, the higher the peak CK level, the more likely the test was to be negative. Second, the presence of exercise-induced angina was a strong predictor of a positive exercise thallium test. These results are important because they pose the apparent paradox of a negative post-MI thallium test associated with larger infarcts and, possibly, a poorer prognosis.

Several studies have recently investigated pharmacologic stress thallium testing for predischarge risk stratification in AMI patients. Brown et al. studied intravenous dipyridamole and quantitative planar thallium in 50 MI patients (50% of whom had received thrombolytics).[53] Thallium redistribution occurred in 20 patients (40%) and was associated with late in-hospital recurrent angina and postdischarge recurrent angina or MI. However, this study is limited by the lack of hard follow-up events (0 deaths, 3 AMIs). Gimple et al. compared predischarge dipyridamole thallium testing with submaximal exercise treadmill testing and with 6-week maximal exercise testing.[54] Of the 40 patients studied, 8 had cardiac events in the 6-month follow-up (including 4 unstable angina hospitalizations). In this evaluation stress thallium and exercise ECG testing had equivalent accuracy in predicting future cardiac events.

Viability determination

Modified ^{201}*thallium techniques.* Although metabolic PET imaging with either ^{11}C-acetate or ^{18}F-deoxyglucose remains the standard for viability determination within a region of left ventricular asynergy following MI, results with modified ^{201}thallium imaging protocols have rivaled the predictive value of PET to define myocardial segments that will exhibit improved wall motion upon revascularization. The identification of thallium uptake in excess of 50% on delayed resting images can identify viable myocardial wall segments that have a greater than 70% chance of demonstrating improved function after revascularization. Ragosta et al. have described a direct correlation between the number of preoperative viable asynergic wall segments defined by standard resting thallium scintigraphy and the magnitude of increase in the global left ventricular ejection fraction observed after coronary bypass surgery.[55]

Several studies have shown that severe regional wall motion abnormalities may improve after successful revascularization, despite the preoperative observation of a fixed thallium defect using standard single-injection and 4-hour redistribution planar or SPECT imaging.[56,57] Thallium uptake within a previously defined fixed region of presumed myocardial scarring after Q-wave infarction has also been improved with percutaneous balloon angioplasty.[58] Thus, fixed thallium defects using standard imaging protocols do not necessarily indicate nonviability of the asynergic myocardial segment accompanying MI.

Modifying thallium imaging techniques by performing delayed reimaging as late as 72 hours has shown late redistribution to be a more sensitive marker for myocardial tissue viability compared with standard imaging protocols.[16] Using a 1.5-mCi thallium reinjection before the 4-hour redistribution image, Dilsizian et al.[26,27] have shown that viability determination can be made that is equivalent to results obtained with additional reimaging as late as 24 hours.[59] Most investigators now consider 4 hours the optimal time for reinjection of thallium for viability screening, although early reinjection immediately after the stress image acquisition and even a rest-injected thallium study with 4-hour reimaging have been proposed for studying viability.[16,59,60]

There has been excellent correlation between these modified thallium imaging protocols and PET-determined viability in comparative studies. Bonow et al. compared thallium reinjection at the time of 4-hour reimaging with ^{18}F-deoxyglucose PET imaging to distinguish viable from nonviable myocardial segments. These investigators found that the results of thallium reinjection correlated with PET metabolic imaging in 88% of the segments studied, with 45% identified as viable and 43% identified as scar.[61,62] The correlation between

PET-defined viability and thallium reinjection analysis may be even greater when the differential uptake of the tracer between the baseline and delayed image is carefully quantitated.[63,64] Additional tracer uptake in excess of 50% of baseline may define viability in apparently fixed thallium defects that are still metabolically active by PET determination. Thus the thallium reinjection technique or delayed reimaging appears to differentiate viable myocardium from scar about as well as the more elaborate PET technique.

Viability and ^{99m}*Tc-sestamibi.* Because of the marked cost differential between thallium and PET imaging and the widespread availability of standard scintigraphy equipment, reinjection thallium scintigraphy remains an important method of viability assessment. Widespread use of PET viability imaging remains limited by the requirement of an on-site cyclotron and expensive imaging equipment. Any competing method for viability determination will need to be inexpensive, convenient, and compatible with common scintigraphic equipment readily available at a large number of institutions.

Initial clinical studies of this issue have reported results with ^{99m}Tc-sestamibi similar to thallium imaging in the determination of viability and residual ischemia after MI. Dilsizian et al.[65] found that over a third of irreversible sestamibi defects were determined viable by thallium reinjection and PET imaging. This disparity resulted mainly from overly aggressive interpretation of the images, with lesions having only mild to moderate reduction in sestamibi uptake being considered initially to be nonviable. When the images were reanalyzed quantitatively according to the severity of the defects, concordance between thallium and sestamibi increased to 93%. Some data has now been presented to suggest that at least in certain circumstances, sestamibi does redistribute in a manner similar to thallium.[65] Agreement between sestamibi, thallium, and PET also improved when a delayed 4-hour sestamibi image was acquired to detect this redistribution. However, additional confirmatory studies of the equivalence of thallium and sestamibi for determination of myocardial viability are needed.

REFERENCES

1. Zaret BL, Strauss HW, Martin ND, et al: Noninvasive regional myocardial perfusion with radioactive potassium. Study of patients at rest, with exercise, and during angina pectoris, *N Engl J Med* 288(16):809-812, 1973.
2. Botvinick EH, Shames DM, Gershengorn KM, et al: Myocardial stress perfusion scintigraphy with rubidium-81 versus stress electrocardiography, *Am J Cardiol* 39(3):364-371, 1977.
3. Berman DS, Salel AF, DeNardo GL, et al: Noninvasive detection of regional myocardial ischemia using rubidium-81 and the scintillation camera: comparison with stress electrocardiography in patients with arteriographically documented coronary stenosis, *Circulation* 52(4):619-626, 1975.

4. Strauss HW, Harrison K, Langan JK, et al: Thallium-201 for myocardial imaging. Relation of thallium-201 to regional myocardial perfusion, *Circulation* 51(4):641-645, 1975.

5. Weich HF, Strauss HW, Pitt B: The extraction of thallium-201 by the myocardium, *Circulation* 56:188, 1975.

6. Nielson AT, Morris KG, Murdock R, et al: Linear relationship between the distribution of thallium-201 and blood flow in ischemic and non-ischemic myocardium during exercise, *Circulation* 61:797, 1980.

7. Kaul S, Chesler DA, Pohost GM, et al: Influence of peak exercise heart rate on normal 201 thallium clearance, *J Nucl Med* 27:26, 1986.

8. Iskandrian AS, Heo J, Kong B, et al: Effect of exercise level on the ability of thallium-201 tomography for identifying and localizing coronary artery disease, *Circulation* 77:316-327, 1988.

9. Leppo JA: Myocardial uptake of thallium and rubidium during alterations in perfusion and oxygenation in isolated rabbit hearts, *J Nucl Med* 28:878, 1987.

10. Leppo JA: MacNeil PB, Moring AF, et al: Separate effects of ischemia, hypoxia and contractility on thallium-201 kinetics in rabbit myocardium, *J Nucl Med* 27:66, 1986.

11. Grunwald AM, Watson DD, Holzgrefe HH, et al: Myocardial thallium-201 kinetics in normal and ischemic myocardium, *Circulation* 64:610, 1981.

12. Moore CA, Cannon J, Watson DD, et al: Thallium 201 kinetics in stunned myocardium characterized by severe postischemic systolic dysfunction, *Circulation* 81(5):1622-1632, 1990.

13. Gibson RS, Beller GA, Gheorghiade M, et al: The prevalence and clinical significance of residual myocardial ischemia 2 weeks after uncomplicated non-Q wave infarction: a prospective natural history study, *Circulation* 73(6):1186-1198, 1986.

14. Beller GA, Holzgrefe HH, Watson DD: Effects of dipyridamole-induced vasodilation on myocardial uptake and clearance kinetics of thallium-201, *Circulation* 68:1328, 1983.

15. Cloninger KG, DePuey EG, Garcia EV, et al: Incomplete redistribution in delayed thallium-201 single photon emission computed tomography (SPECT) images: an overestimation of myocardial scarring, *J Am Coll Cardiol* 12:955-963, 1988.

16. Kiat H, Berman DS, Maddahi J, et al: Late reversibility of tomographic myocardial thallium-201 defects: an accurate marker of myocardial viability, *J Am Coll Cardiol* 12:1456-1463, 1988.

17. Cerqueira MD: Assessment of myocardial perfusion and viability. In Cerqueira MD, (ed): *Nuclear cardiology,* Boston, 1994, Blackwell Scientific Publications.

18. Mankoff DA: Basics of physics for nuclear cardiology. In Cerqueira MD, (ed): *Nuclear cardiology,* Boston, 1994, Blackwell Scientific Publications.

19. Goris ML, Daspit SG, McLaughlin P, et al: Interpolative background subtraction, *J Nucl Med* 17:744, 1976.

20. Watson DD, Campbell NP, Read EK, et al: Spatial and temporal quantitation of plane thallium myocardial images, *J Nucl Med* 22:577, 1981.

21. Homma S, Kaul S, Boucher CA: Correlates of lung/heart ratio of thallium-201 and coronary artery disease, *J Nucl Med* 28:1531, 1987.

22. Zaret BL, Wackers FJ: Nuclear cardiology, *N Engl J Med* 329(11):775-783, 1993.

23. DePasquale EE, Noby AC, DePuey EG, et al: Quantitative rotational thallium-201 tomography for identifying and localizing coronary artery disease, *Circulation* 77:316, 1988.

24. Tillisch J, Brunken R, Marshall R, et al: Reversibility of cardiac wall-motion abnormalities predicted by positron tomography, *N Engl J Med* 314:884-888, 1986.

25. Gropler RJ, Geltman EM, Sampathkumaran K, et al: Functional recovery after coronary revascularization for chronic coronary artery disease is dependent on maintenance of oxidative metabolism, *J Am Coll Cardiol* 20(3):569-577, 1992.

26. Dilsizian V, Rocco TP, Freedman NM, et al: Enhanced detection of ischemic but viable myocardium by the reinjection of thallium after stress-redistribution imaging, *N Engl J Med* 323(3):141-146, 1990.

27. Rocco TP, Dilsizian V, McKusick KA, et al: Comparison of thallium redistribution with rest "reinjection" imaging for the detection of viable myocardium, *Am J Cardiol* 66:158-163, 1990.

28. Murray G, Schad N, Ladd W, et al: Metabolic cardiac imaging in severe coronary disease: assessment of viability with iodine-123-iodophenylpentadecanoic acid and multicrystal gamma camera and correlation with biopsy, *J Nucl Med* 33:1269-1277, 1992.

29. Kotler TS, Diamond GA: Exercise thallium-201 scintigraphy and the diagnosis and prognosis or coronary artery disease, *Ann Intern Med* 113(9):684-702, 1990.

30. Fintel DJ, Links JM, Brinker JA, et al: Improved diagnostic performance of exercise thallium-201 single photon emission computed tomography over planar imaging in the diagnosis of coronary artery disease: a receiver operating characteristics analysis, *J Am Coll Cardiol* 13:600-612, 1989.

31. Kiat H, Maddahi J, Roy LT, et al: Comparison of technetium 99m methoxy isobutyl isonitrile and thallium-201 for evaluation of coronary artery disease by planar and tomographic methods, *Am Heart J* 117:1-11, 1989.

32. Iskandrian AS, Heo J, Kong B, et al: Effect of exercise level on the ability of thallium-201 tomographic imaging in detecting coronary artery disease: analysis of 461 patients, *J Am Coll Cardiol* 14:1477-1486, 1989.

33. Van Train KF, Maddahi J, Berman DS, et al: Quantitative analysis of tomographic stress thallium-201 myocardial scintigrams: a multicenter trial, *J Nucl Med* 31(7):1168-1179, 1990.

34. Diamond GA: How accurate is SPECT thallium scintigraphy? *J Am Coll Cardiol* 16:1017-1021, 1990.

35. Gould KL: Agreement on the accuracy of thallium stress testing, *J Am Coll Cardiol* 16:1022-1023, 1990.

36. Tamaki N, Yonekura Y, Mukai T, et al: Stress thallium-201 transaxial emission computed tomography: quantitative versus qualitative analysis for evaluation of coronary artery disease, *J Am Coll Cardiol* 4:1213, 1984.

37. Berger BC, Watson DD, Taylor GJ, et al: Quantitative thallium-201 exercise scintigraphy for detection of coronary artery disease, *J Nucl Med* 22:585, 1981.

38. Wackers FJT, Fetterman RC, Mattera JA, et al: Quantitative planar thallium-201 stress scintigraphy: a critical evaluation of the method, *Semin Nucl Med* 15:46, 1985.

39. Garcia E, Maddahi J, Berman DS, et al: Space/time quantitation of thallium-201 myocardial scintigraphy, *J Nucl Med* 22:309, 1981.

40. Prigent FM, Berman DS, Elashoff J, et al: Reproducibility of stress redistribution thallium-201 SPECT quantitative indexes of hypoperfused myocardium secondary to coronary artery disease, *Am J Cardiol* 70:1255-1263, 1992.

41. Nishimura S, Mahmarian JJ, Boyce TM, et al: Equivalence between adenosine and exercise thallium-201 myocardial tomography: a multicenter, prospective, crossover trial, *J Am Coll Cardiol* 20:265-275, 1992.

42. Gupta NC, Esterbrooks DJ, Hilleman DE, et al: Comparison of adenosine and exercise thallium-201 single-photon emission computed tomography (SPECT) myocardial perfusion imaging. The GE SPECT Multicenter Adenosine Study Group, *J Am Coll Cardiol* 19:248-257, 1992.

43. Guiney TE, Pohost GM, McKusick KA, et al: Differentiation of false- from true-positive ECG responses to exercise stress by thallium-201 perfusion imaging, *Chest* 80:4, 1981.

44. Iskandrian AS, Scherer H, Croll MN, et al: Exercise thallium-201 myocardial scans in patients with disease limited to the secondary

branches of the left coronary system, *Clin Cardiol* 2:121-125, 1979.

45. Stewart RE, Schwaiger M, Molina E, et al: Comparison of rubidium-82 positron emission tomography and thallium-201 SPECT imaging for detection of coronary artery disease, *Am J Cardiol* 67:1303-1310, 1991.

46. Krone RJ: The role of risk stratification in the early management of a myocardial infarction, *Ann Intern Med* 116(3):223-237, 1992.

47. American College of Cardiology, American Heart Association Task Force on Assessment of Diagnostic and Therapeutic Cardiovascular Procedures: ACC/AHA guidelines for the early management of patients with acute myocardial infarction, *Circulation* 82:664-707, 1990.

48. Gibson R, Watson D, Craddock G, et al: Prediction of cardiac events after uncomplicated myocardial infarction: a prospective study comparing predischarge exercise thallium-201 scintigraphy and coronary angiography, *Circulation* 68:321-336, 1983.

49. Hung J, Goris ML, Nash E, et al: Comparative value of maximal treadmill testing, exercise thallium myocardial perfusion scintigraphy and exercise radionuclide ventriculography for distinguishing high- and low-risk patients soon after myocardial infarction, *Am J Cardiol* 53:1221-1227, 1984.

50. Tilkemeier PL, Guiney TE, LaRaia PJ, et al: Prognostic value of predischarge low-level exercise thallium testing after thrombolytic treatment of acute myocardial infarction, *Am J Cardiol* 66(17): 1203-1207, 1990.

51. Haber HL, Beller GA, Watson DD, et al: Exercise thallium-201 scintigraphy after thrombolytic therapy with or without angioplasty for acute myocardial infarction, *Am J Cardiol* 71(15):1257-1261, 1993.

52. Sutton JM, Topol EJ: Significance of a negative exercise thallium test in the presence of a critical residual stenosis after thrombolysis for acute myocardial infarction, *Circulation* 83:1278-1286, 1991.

53. Brown KA, O'Meara J, Chambers CE, et al: Ability of dipyridamole-thallium-201 imaging one to four days after acute myocardial infarction to predict in-hospital and late recurrent myocardial ischemic events, *Am J Cardiol* 65:160-167, 1990.

54. Gimple LW, Hutter AM Jr, Guiney TE, et al: Prognostic utility of predischarge dipyridamole-thallium imaging compared to predischarge submaximal exercise electrocardiography and maximal exercise thallium imaging after uncomplicated acute myocardial infarction, *Am J Cardiol* 64:1243-1248, 1989.

55. Ragosta M, Beller GA, Watson DD, et al: Quantitative planar rest-redistribution 201 T1 imaging in detection of myocardial viability and prediction of improvement in left ventricular function after coronary bypass surgery in patients with severely depressed left ventricular function, *Circulation* 87(5):1630-1641, 1993.

56. Gibson RS, Watson DD, Taylor GJ, et al: Prospective assessment of regional myocardial perfusion before and after coronary revascularization surgery by quantitative thallium-201 scintigraphy, *J Am Coll Cardiol* 1:804-815, 1983.

57. Colininger KG, DePuey EG, Garcia EV, et al: Incomplete redistribution in delayed thallium-201 single photon emission tomography (SPECT) images: an overestimation of myocardial scarring, *J Am Coll Cardiol* 12:955-963, 1988.

58. Montalescot G, Faraggi M, Drobinski G, et al: Myocardial viability in patients with Q-wave myocardial infarction and no residual ischemia, *Circulation* 86:47-55, 1992.

59. Ohtani H, Tamaki N, Yonekura Y, et al: Value of thallium-201 reinjection after delayed SPECT imaging for predicting reversible ischemia after coronary artery bypass grafting, *Am J Cardiol* 66:394-399, 1990.

60. Mori K, Minamigi K, Kurogane H, et al: Rest-injected thallium-201 imaging for assessing viability of severe asynergic regions, *J Nucl Med* 32:1718-1724, 1991.

61. Bonow RO, Dilsizian V, Cuocolo A, et al: Identification of viable myocardium in patients with chronic coronary artery disease and left ventricular dysfunction: comparison of thallium scintigraphy with reinjection and PET imaging with F-Fluorodeoxyglucose, *Circulation* 83:26-37, 1991.

62. Bonow RO, Dilsizian V: Thallium-201 for assessment of myocardial viability, *Semin Nucl Med* 21:230-241, 1991.

63. Dilsizian V, Freedman N, Bacharach SL, et al: Regional thallium uptake in irreversible defects. Magnitude of change in thallium activity after reinjection distinguishes viable from nonviable myocardium, *Circulation* 85:627-634, 1992.

64. Dilsizian V, Bonow RO: Differential uptake and apparent thallium-201 washout after thallium reinjection. Options regarding early redistribution imaging before reinjection or late redistribution imaging after reinjection, *Circulation* 85:1032-1038, 1992.

65. Dilsizian V, Arrighi JA, Diodati JG, et al: Myocardial viability in patients with chronic coronary artery disease: comparison of 99mTc-sestamibi with thallium reinjection and 18-fluorodeoxyglucose, *Circulation* 89:578-587, 1994.

Chapter 64

USE OF RADIONUCLIDE ANGIOGRAPHY FOLLOWING ACUTE MYOCARDIAL INFARCTION

Kenneth G. Morris

Radionuclide ventricular function imaging, also known as radionuclide angiography (RNA), can be very useful in answering questions about the extent of myocardial damage, appropriate forms of therapy, and the short- and long-term prognosis of patients with AMI. There are two main types of radionuclide angiography, *first pass* and *gated equilibrium* methods. Both methods provide accurate and reproducible measurements.[1,2] RNA is the most widely applied method for the construction of ventricular volume curves in human subjects. From these curves, an example of which is shown in Figure 64-1, a variety of quantifiable indices can be derived. These include left ventricular ejection fraction, right ventricular ejection fraction, regional ejection fraction, peak and average systolic ejection rates, and peak and average diastolic filling rates. In addition, left ventricular volume information, including assessment of relative changes and absolute measurements, can be obtained using this technology.[3] All these measurements can be made both at rest and at various levels of exercise. Exercise studies also return important information regarding changes in heart rate, blood pressure, exercise duration, and work load. Visual assessment of radionuclide angiograms can provide subjective wall motion information either at rest or at exercise, which combined with changes in global and regional ejection fraction and other quantifiable mea-

sures, can be used to diagnose and quantify exercise-induced ischemia.[4] Thus the versatility of radionuclide angiography provides many potentially useful roles for its use in the evaluation of patients with AMI.

RADIONUCLIDE ANGIOGRAPHY IN EXPERIMENTAL INFARCTION AND ISCHEMIA

Permanent coronary artery occlusion in a canine model produces an MI that is directly proportional in size to the size of the vascular bed at risk, as determined by radioactive microsphere methods.[5] Collateral flow and occlusion duration are the other major determinants of infarct size. In a study of 41 dogs with permanent coronary occlusion, the change in ejection fraction as assessed by radionuclide angiography from the preocclusion value to a second value obtained 30 to 60 minutes after occlusion has been shown to be directly proportional to the size of the MI as determined 3 days later by standard histologic methods.[6] Although there is a significant correlation overall, the slopes of the relationship are different for LAD and circumflex occlusions, as demonstrated in Figure 64-2. The lower slope in the circumflex occlusions can be partially explained by differences in attenuation and counting geometry between the more superficial anterior wall and the deeper inferoposterior wall. In the experimental animal, however, anterior wall infarction has a greater effect on

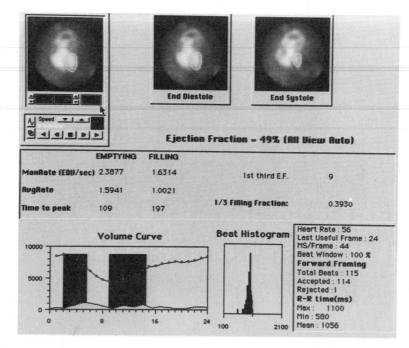

Fig. 64-1. Left ventricular volume curve from multigated radionuclide angiogram with derived indices of ventricular function.

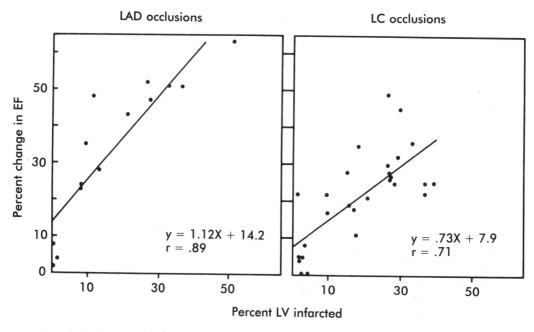

Fig. 64-2. Relationship between percent change in ejection fraction and percent left ventricular infarction for LAD and left circumflex occlusions in the canine model. (From Schneider RM, Chu A, Akaishi M, et al: *Circulation* 72:632-638, 1985.)

ejection fraction than inferoposterior infarctions, even after adjusting for size of the infarct. However, ejection fraction can serve as a reasonable marker of infarct size, especially when the site of the infarction is known.[7] Figure 64-3 demonstrates the linear relationship be-

tween percent change in ejection fraction from before coronary occlusion to that measured 10 minutes after occlusion, as compared with the percent reduction in total left ventricular blood flow. As can be seen, there is a significant difference in the slope of the relationship

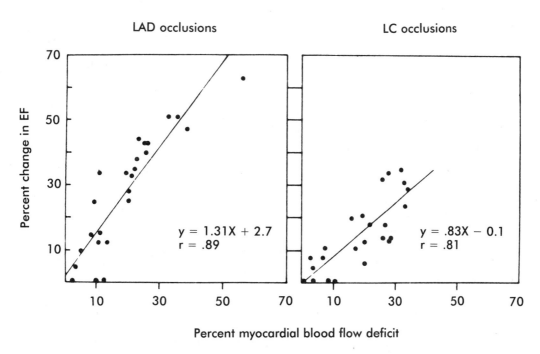

Fig. 64-3. Percent change in ejection fraction vs. percent reduction in total left ventricular blood flow for left anterior descending and left circumflex occlusions. (From Schneider RM, Morris KG, Chu A, et al: *Circ Res* 60:60-71, 1987.)

for LAD and left circumflex occlusions. About half of this difference can be accounted for by differences in attenuation and counting geometry. Nonetheless it is clear that there is a good correlation between the amount of reduction in myocardial blood flow and changes in ejection fraction with coronary occlusion. These experimental models using radionuclide angiography demonstrate the relationship between infarct size and ejection fraction following infarction, and between changes in ejection fraction that might occur between rest and exercise and the severity of ischemia being experienced by a patient during exercise.

EVALUATION OF CONGESTIVE HEART FAILURE

Congestive heart failure is among the most frequent complications of AMI, and its occurrence raises the possibility that certain drugs such as ACE inhibitors may be indicated and concern that other agents such as calcium channel blockers and beta blockers may be relatively contraindicated. The pathophysiology of congestive heart failure in MI is complex and includes acute left ventricular systolic dysfunction, diastolic dysfunction, and ultimately dilation associated with left ventricular remodeling (see Chapter 68).

Assessment of left ventricular systolic function

Nicod et al.[8] examined the relationship between left ventricular ejection fraction as determined by radionuclide angiography and clinical and x-ray evidence of congestive heart failure in 2089 patients with AMI. In this study the criteria for clinical heart failure were a third heart sound and/or rales to the scapulae on physical examination, and chest x-ray evidence of interstitial or alveolar pulmonary edema. The presence of any two of the three criteria were considered diagnostic of CHF. Fifty-seven percent of patients meeting two of these criteria had ejection fractions greater than 40%, and 33% of these patients had ejection fractions greater than 50%. Of patients with ejection fractions less than 40%, nearly 36% did not have two of the criteria. Using radiographic criteria alone, 54% of patients with interstitial, local perihilar, or diffuse alveolar pulmonary edema had ejection fractions greater than 40%, and 33% of patients with these x-ray findings had ejection fractions greater than 50%. Only 33% of patients with ejection fractions less than 40% had radiographic congestive heart failure while in the cardiac care unit. More recently, Gottlieb et al.[9] reported very similar findings regarding radiographic CHF in another large series of patients from the Multicenter Post-Infarction Program (MPIP) and Multicenter Diltiazem Post-Infarction Trial (MDPIT). Figure 64-4 is a histogram relating the presence and severity of pulmonary congestion on chest x-ray to RNA ejection fraction. Mild pulmonary congestion was defined as venous congestion, moderate pulmonary congestion as interstitial congestion, and severe pulmonary congestion as pulmonary edema. Very broad ranges of RNA ejection

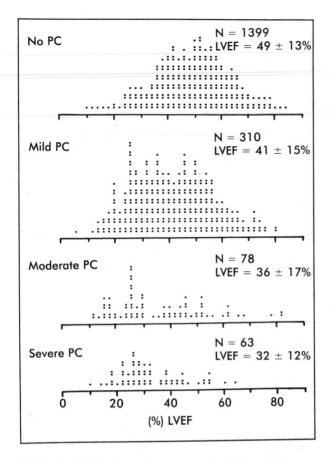

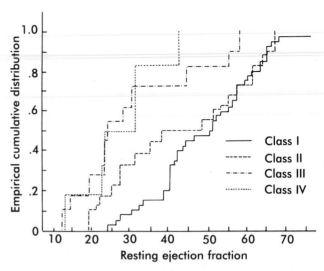

Fig. 64-5. Relationship between clinical class for congestive heart failure and rest ejection fraction. The cumulative distribution function demonstrates the proportion of patients in each functional class with a given level of ejection fraction. Although significant correlation between clinical class and ejection fraction is seen, significant numbers of patients with low rest ejection fractions are found in each clinical class.

Fig. 64-4. Distribution of predischarged RNA EF by four grades of radiographic pulmonary congestion (PC) in patients with no pulmonary congestion; each dot represents 6 cases. Each dot represents one case for mild PC (interstitial edema), moderate PC (perihilar edema), and severe PC (diffuse pulmonary edema). (From Gottlieb S, Moss AJ, McDermott M, et al: *Am J Cardiol* 69:977-984, 1992.)

fraction are seen for each radiographic level of congestion. Many patients with normal chest x-rays had reduced RNA ejection fraction. Thus, in the CCU phase of AMI, clinical and x-ray evidence of heart failure are poor predictors of left ventricular ejection fraction.

Assessing ventricular function clinically after hospital discharge can be fraught with error as well. In Figure 64-5 the cumulative distribution function of resting ejection fraction for each NYHA functional class of CHF is shown in a consecutive series of 105 survivors of MI from the Durham VA Medical Center. It can be seen that, whereas the median ejection fraction of Class III and IV patients is less than 30%, approximately 20% of patients with Class III or IV heart failure 3 weeks after MI have ejection fractions greater than 40. An equal number of patients suffering Class II heart failure symptoms have ejection fractions above or below 40%, and 20% of patients with no symptoms of heart failure in the recovery phase of infarction have ejection

fractions less than 40. Thus, symptoms of heart failure alone are not a reliable means to assess systolic left ventricular function in individual patients, despite a significant association between functional class for heart failure and ejection fraction in population studies. This discrepancy probably reflects the less-than-specific nature of dyspnea as a complaint and the potential for diastolic dysfunction as a cause for heart failure in this population.

Knowledge of a patient's left ventricular function is often important in guiding therapy and therefore an objective measurement is frequently useful. For instance, the SAVE trial[10] demonstrated significant reduction in long-term mortality and congestive heart failure symptoms in survivors of MI with asymptomatic left ventricular dysfunction treated with captopril. An ejection fraction by radionuclide angiography of less than or equal to 40% was required for admission to the study. The SOLVD investigators demonstrated an improved survival in patients with symptomatic congestive heart failure and ejection fractions less than or equal to 35% treated with enalapril.[11] In a subsequent publication a reduction in late CHF morbidity and a trend towards improved survival was demonstrated for asymptomatic patients with ejection fractions of less than or equal to 35% who were receiving enalapril therapy.[12] In contrast to the beneficial effects of ACE inhibitors in patients with left ventricular dysfunction, the Multicenter Diltiazem Postinfarction Trial Research Group[13] reported a significant increase in cardiac event rates in patients receiving diltiazem with ejection fractions less than 40%. Finally, although the role of beta blockers in these patients is still controversial, these agents are frequently avoided in patients with profoundly reduced left ventricular ejection fractions. Thus, a postinfarct patient for whom no prior quantitative assessment of left ventricular systolic performance has been obtained may benefit from the use of radionuclide angiography as a guide to selection of medical therapy.

Assessment of diastolic dysfunction

The left ventricular volume curve can be used to assess filling (diastole) as readily as ejection (systole). Parameters such as the average and peak filling rates and time-to-peak filling rate can be used to evaluate left ventricular diastolic function, using either first pass or equilibrium-gated radionuclide angiographic methods. Reduto et al.[14] found abnormalities of left ventricular diastolic performance at rest and during exercise in patients with coronary disease without resting wall motion abnormalities or prior MI, and even more profound abnormalities in patients with prior MI. Subsequently, Bonow et al.[15] reported a decrease in peak left ventricular diastolic filling rate in coronary disease patients with normal resting wall motion and normal global ejection fractions, and even more profound abnormalities in patients with reduced ventricular performance and wall motion abnormalities suggesting prior MI (Fig. 64-6). Although some of these abnormalities are caused by irreversible factors such as myocardial tissue fibrosis, patients treated with verapamil exhibit improvement in peak filling rates. Thus, the identification of diastolic dysfunction in patients with adequate systolic performance can serve as a guide to potential medical therapy of this abnormality as well.

Evaluation of left ventricular remodeling

Using contrast angiography, White et al.[16] identified left ventricular end-systolic and end-diastolic volumes as significant determinants of survival after recovery from AMI. Changes in left ventricular volume, as well as absolute measurements of volume, can also be assessed using radionuclide methods. Jeremy et al.[17] reported a series of 40 patients surviving their first MI. None of their patients were treated with thrombolytic therapy. Left ventricular volume was assessed using radionuclide angiography within 48 hours of infarction and after 1 month of follow-up. Before being discharged, all patients underwent coronary angiography to assess coronary patency. There was no significant change in left ventricular volume over the month of follow-up in those 16 patients who had patent vessels before discharge. Nor was there any significant change in those 10 patients who had total occlusion, but significant collateralization of

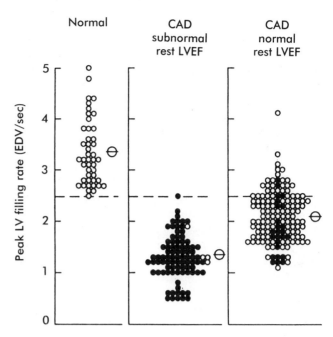

Fig. 64-6. Gated RNA peak LV filling rates for normal patients, patients with coronary disease and reduced left ventricular ejection fraction, and patients with coronary artery disease and normal left ventricular ejection fraction. Closed circles indicate the presence of resting wall motion abnormalities. (From Bonow RO, Bacharach SL, Green MV, et al: *Circulation* 64:315-323, 1981.)

the distal bed. However, in 14 patients with total occlusion and no significant collateral flow, there was a median increase in end-diastolic volume of 28%. Increases in ventricular volume were related to infarct size as assessed by peak CK levels or QRS scores and were also much more frequently seen in anterior as compared with inferior infarction. This study was among the earliest to assess the impact of coronary patency on left ventricular remodeling in human subjects. Since then Ertl et al.[18] have performed a series of studies of left ventricular remodeling using gated SPECT radionuclide angiography. In a series of 78 patients, 37 of whom had large infarcts by creatine kinase criteria, left ventricular volume was increased by greater than 27% after 3 to 5 weeks relative to the early postinfarct period. This resulted in a restoration of stroke volume via the Starling mechanism despite a persistently depressed ejection fraction. However, continuing dilation was seen in this group over the subsequent 5 to 8 months and was not associated with further improvements in left ventricular stroke volume. Thus, this late left ventricular dilation was noncompensatory and frequently preceeded the development of clinical heart failure.

ASSESSMENT OF PROGNOSIS

A variety of clinical and laboratory variables have prognostic significance in survivors of AMI.[19-23] An analysis of these variables suggests that they may reflect three separate but interrelated pathophysiologic conditions: left ventricular dysfunction, residual potential for ischemia, and electrical instability (see Chapter 62). Among clinical and cardiac catheterization variables, ejection fraction at rest, a direct measure of left ventricular function, is the most important predictor of mortality after AMI.[24-26] Variables such as Killip class, cardiomegaly, infarct location, and exercise duration may be prognostically significant because they also reflect the severity of left ventricular dysfunction produced by the infarction. The second most important prognostic variable among clinical and angiographic parameters is the angiographic severity of the coronary artery disease.[25] Variables, such as recurrent angina pectoris and evidence of ischemia on exercise testing or Holter monitoring, may also be prognostically useful because they are indicators of residual potentially ischemic myocardium.[27,28] A third group of variables that may suggest myocardial electrical instability includes the late occurrence of ventricular tachycardia or fibrillation,[29] evidence of significant ventricular arrhythmias on Holter monitoring,[30] the presence of delayed potentials on signal-averaged ECG studies,[31] or provoked ventricular arrhythmias on electrophysiologic testing. Although these variables correlate strongly with the presence and severity of left ventricular dysfunction, they also appear to have some independent prognostic significance[31,32] (see Chapter 66).

The ability of radionuclide angiography to assess left ventricular function accurately and noninvasively makes it a potentially very useful prognostic tool. The relationships demonstrated between infarct size, location, and changes in ejection fraction in experimental models provide useful clinical guidelines for interpretation of the results of radionuclide angiographic studies.

Relationship between RNA ejection fraction and arrhythmias

Several studies have noted correlations between RNA parameters and clinical or laboratory parameters related to ventricular arrhythmias. Schulze et al.[30] reported a highly significant correlation between multiform and repetitive PVCs on Holter monitoring and a RNA rest ejection fraction of less than 40%. Borer et al.[29] observed that patients with these high-grade ventricular arrhythmias not only had lower rest ejection fractions but lower exercise ejection fractions as well.

There have been three studies comparing signal-averaged ECG, Holter monitoring, and radionuclide angiography in the prediction of arrhythmic events in survivors of AMI. Kuchar et al. studied 210 survivors of MI with Holter monitoring, signal-averaged ECG, and radionuclide angiography.[31] A stepwise logistic regression model comparing these techniques revealed that

each was significant in predicting arrhythmic events, with an ejection fraction of <40% being the best single predictor of sustained ventricular tachycardia or sudden death. An abnormal signal-averaged ECG was next in importance and complex ventricular ectopy on Holter monitoring third in significance. Abnormalities on the signal-averaged ECG correlated with an ejection fraction <40%, and when both abnormalities were present, they were associated with a 34% rate of subsequent sustained ventricular tachycardia or sudden death. When neither abnormality was present, the event rate was 0, and when only one was found, the event rate was 4%. Gomes et al.[33] made very similar observations using stepwise Cox model regression analysis. They found that ejection fraction, abnormal signal-averaged ECG variables, and the occurrence of nonsustained ventricular tachycardia on Holter were all predictive of subsequent sustained ventricular tachycardia, ventricular fibrillation, or sudden death. Finally, McClements and Adgey[34] compared the same three methods in the evaluation of 301 survivors of MI, 68% of whom had received thrombolytic therapy. Using a multivariate stepwise regression analysis of the three procedures, once again an ejection fraction < 40% by RNA was the first selected variable, followed by the signal-averaged ECG at the time of discharge. Together the two methods selected a high-risk group comprising only 12% of the study patients with an event rate of 26%, as compared with a rate of only 0.8% in the remaining 88% of patients who comprised the low-risk group.

Predictive value of RNA rest ejection fraction for mortality

Several studies have reported that rest ejection fraction as measured by RNA provides significant prognostic information regarding subsequent mortality. Shah et al.[35] reported an in-hospital mortality of 55% in patients with acute infarction and rest ejection fractions of less than 30%. Different levels of rest ejection fraction have been considered important by various investigators. Schulze et al.[30] reported a 30% 1-year mortality in patients with ejection fractions of less than 40% at the time of discharge. Borer et al.[29] reported that all deaths occurring in the first year of follow-up occurred in patients with ejection fractions less than 35%. Battler et al.[36] noted a 24% 1-year mortality in patients with ejection fractions less than 52% as compared to 10% for patients with higher values. The Multicenter Postinfarction Research Group[37] has determined, in a series of 799 patients, that a rest ejection fraction of less than 40% was the most important of the variables they studied for predicting subsequent mortality.

Califf et al.[38] have observed, however, that the predictive value of rest ejection fraction (treated dichotomously) and its value vis-à-vis other parameters changes significantly depending on the level of ejection fraction that is assumed to be important. They observed in a population with chronic stable coronary artery disease that rest ejection fraction greater or less than 50% was not significantly related to mortality. However, when the critical level of rest ejection fraction was considered to be 40%, it was the third most important variable. When considered in a continuous fashion, however, rest ejection fraction was the most important predictor of mortality.

In a Duke/Durham VA RNA prognosis study,[39] the rest ejection fraction analyzed in a continuous fashion was significantly associated with 2-year mortality; mortality increased sharply as ejection fraction fell below 40%. Rest ejection fraction was more powerful than clinical variables and provided independent prognostic information in a multivariable model. Rollag et al.[40] studied 485 patients with a first MI and found that of all routine clinical laboratory and radionuclide angiographic variables acquired during hospitalization, only age and ejection fraction were predictive of 5-year survival.

In addition to the measurement of left ventricular ejection fraction, radionuclide angiography is one of the few methods that can be used to estimate right ventricular ejection fraction. Marwick et al.[41] studied the prognostic significance of right ventricular ejection fraction following inferior MI. In their multivariate Cox model analysis of 168 consecutive patients recovering from inferior infarction, left ventricular ejection fraction, right ventricular ejection fraction, and age were the only significant variables in the model. Dell Italia et al.[42] found that in 27 patients with hemodynamically significant right ventricular infarction, right ventricular ejection fraction at rest improved at late follow-up and rose during exercise testing performed just before hospital discharge. In addition, anaerobic threshold was significantly correlated with peak right ventricular ejection fraction but was not significantly correlated with peak left ventricular ejection fraction. Thus, radionuclide angiography was able to assess the impact of right ventricular function on exercise capacity.

Prognostic value of exercise RNA parameters

Myocardial ischemia during exercise has long been considered to be clinically and prognostically important. The relationship between changes in ejection fraction and the severity of residual ischemia in the experimental model make RNA an interesting method for assessing the potential for recurrent ischemia in patients. Both the change in ejection fraction from rest to exercise and the exercise ejection fraction correlate with the severity of the underlying coronary artery disease[43] and are more sensitive than ST-segment changes for the detection of abnormalities resulting from exercise-induced myocar-

dial ischemia.[44] Evidence of ischemia during exercise may be predictive of events such as recurrent nonfatal infarction, unstable angina, and disabling angina requiring revascularization. Thus, exercise RNA is an attractive procedure for risk assessment after AMI.

Corbett et al.[45] reported the first study to analyze the prognostic value of exercise RNA parameters. Their 6-month follow-up study of 61 patients surviving AMI was also the first study that analyzed events other than death in the follow-up period. Discriminate function analysis of multiple RNA parameters (treated dichotomously) was used to assess their prognostic value with regard to major and minor cardiac events. The majority of major events (75%) were ischemic (recurrent MI and medically refractory angina). Approximately half the minor events were persistent angina. These investigators found the change in left ventricular ejection fraction with submaximal exercise to be the most important variable for identifying patients who would subsequently suffer any cardiac event. They also found rest ejection fraction, left ventricular wall motion score, and left ventricular end-systolic volume index to have significant associations with subsequent events. In an extension of this work,[46] the authors noted that the peak left ventricular ejection fraction during exercise was the most important variable in distinguishing between these groups if the left ventricular ejection fraction at rest was less than 40%. This variable was also the most significant in those patients with an anterior MI. The discriminate function using the change in the left ventricular ejection fraction with exercise was less capable of separating patients who would have major rather than minor cardiac events.

In studies of 117 men recovering from AMI, Hung et al.[47] found the change in ejection fraction from rest to exercise to be the best variable for predicting a combination of cardiac events. "Hard events" included two patients with sudden cardiac death or nonfatal ventricular fibrillation and six recurrent MIs. Patients with congestive heart failure or chest pain refractory to medical treatment were excluded from evaluation. The left ventricular ejection fraction during exercise was also a significant predictor of "hard events" and other events that included hospitalization for unstable angina pectoris, congestive heart failure, or coronary bypass surgery.

The studies by Corbett et al.[45] and Hung et al.[47] clearly demonstrate the ability of exercise RNA variables to predict cardiac events during follow-up. However, it is unclear from their analyses which events are actually being predicted and which RNA variable is most closely associated with each specific event. The Duke/Durham VA study[39] was performed in an attempt to associate specific cardiac events with rest and exercise RNA parameters. One hundred and six survivors of AMI were studied. Patients were recruited from a consecutive series of patients with well-documented MIs admitted to the cardiac care unit at the Durham VA Medical Center. Patients were excluded from the study if they had serious comorbid disease or were unable to perform the bicycle exercise. Clinical characteristics such as age, history of previous infarction, infarct location, worst Killip class, infarct extension, cardiomegaly on chest radiograph, interventricular conduction defects, atrioventricular block, and ventricular and atrial arrhythmias were recorded. All patients underwent a heart rate–limited rest and exercise RNA 3 weeks following MI. Antianginal therapy had been previously discontinued. The patients were exercised to the onset of significant symptoms, ST-segment depression, or heart rate of 120 beats/minute. The patient's functional class for angina and/or heart failure, and the occurrence of ST-segment changes and/or angina during exercise were recorded.

The prognostic significance of the rest and exercise RNA measurements was analyzed for four specific events in follow-up. These included death, recurrent nonfatal MI, coronary artery bypass grafting for medically refractory disabling angina pectoris, and admission to the coronary care unit for unstable angina. The analysis of nonfatal events included the censoring of follow-up of patients at the time of their death. The four RNA variables examined for significance were rest ejection fraction, exercise ejection fraction, change in ejection fraction from rest to exercise, and exercise-induced wall motion abnormalities. Associations between each RNA variable and the time to an event were determined using a Cox proportional hazards regression model. A model chi-square statistic was used to assess the significance of the relationship between each RNA variable and the time to an event both before and after adjustment for the significance of clinical descriptors. Clinical variables included age, history of previous infarction, infarct location, worst Killip class, infarct extension, cardiomegaly, serious arrhythmias, New York Heart Association functional classes for angina and congestive heart failure (at 3 weeks), and ST-segment depression > 0.1 mV with exercise.

The results of the Cox model analysis are summarized in Table 64-1. Both rest and exercise ejection fractions were inversely correlated with subsequent mortality. Exercise ejection fraction had a higher chi-square value. The association of both rest and exercise ejection fraction with the time to death remains significant after adjustment for the clinical variables. Change in ejection fraction from rest to exercise and the occurrence of exercise-induced wall motion abnormalities were not significantly related to death. Two-year mortality predicted by the Cox regression model from rest or exercise ejection fraction alone is demonstrated in Figure 64-7. Mortality increases dramatically for both variables, as ejection fractions fall below 40%. Kaplan-Meier survival curves for the entire period of follow-up are shown in

Figure 64-8. Patients with exercise ejection fraction less than 40% had a significantly higher mortality rate throughout the period of follow-up. In a later study, Abraham et al.[48] also evaluated the prognostic value of exercise RNA 1 month after MI. As with the Duke/Durham VA study, rest and exercise ejection fraction were predictive of 2-year mortality, with the exercise value having the stronger relationship.

In the Duke/Durham VA study,[39] of the four RNA variables, only exercise-induced wall motion abnormalities were significantly associated with subsequent nonfatal MI. This relationship was not significant after adjustment for the clinical variables. No RNA variable was significantly associated with the time to readmission to the coronary care unit for unstable angina pectoris. There was, however, a very strong relationship between the change in ejection fraction from rest to exercise and the time to coronary artery bypass grafting for medically refractory and disabling angina pectoris. This relationship remained strong, even after adjustment for other clinical descriptors, which included ST-segment changes and functional class for angina. These data demonstrate that different RNA angiographic parameters have significant prognostic value for specific events in follow-up and that the prognostic information is greater than that available in the clinical descriptors.

The Duke/Durham VA study also analyzed the independent prognostic value of serial rest and exercise RNA 3 and 8 weeks following MI.[49] There is additional independent prognostic value to a second exercise test 8 weeks following infarction. Exercise ejection fraction at 8 weeks provided additional information regarding mortality to that available at 3 weeks, although most of the prognostic information was available in the 3-week study. More importantly, however, the change in ejection fraction from rest to exercise on RNA 8 weeks following MI was a highly significant predictor of nonfatal MI in the subsequent follow-up period. This relationship remained significant even after adjustment for clinical descriptors. The additional prognostic information provided at 8 weeks was due in part to significant changes in rest ejection fraction as well as changes in exercise performance. Some patients had improvement in their left ventricular function while at rest but had similar exercise ejection fractions at both 3 and 8 weeks. Other patients who initially had good exercise function had significant declines in their exercise ejection fractions at 8 weeks without any change in their left ventricular performance while at rest. This suggests that either the coronary stenoses in the epicardial vessel or flow regulation in the resistance bed are undergoing significant changes in the first few weeks postinfarction.

These studies of rest and exercise radionuclide angiography in postinfarct patients suggest that mortality can be assessed by rest EF, which is a function of the

Table 64-1. Prognostic significance of RNA variables for specific subsequent events

RNA variable	Death (N = 24) Univariable		Death (N = 24) Multivariable		Nonfatal MI (N = 20) Univariable		Nonfatal MI (N = 20) Multivariable		Unstable angina (N = 21) Univariable		Unstable angina (N = 21) Multivariable		Refractory angina (N = 10) Univariable		Refractory angina (N = 10) Multivariable	
	X^2	P	X^2	P	X^2	P	X^2	P	X^2	P	X^2	P	X^2	P	X^2	P
Rest EF	11.1	0.001*	4.3	0.04*	0.0	0.84	0.00	1.00	0.4	0.53	1.7	0.19	0.4	0.55	0.1	0.82
Exercise EF	14.0	0.001*	5.7	0.02*	0.1	0.76	0.1	0.76	1.5	0.22	0.9	0.35	2.1	0.15	3.8	0.05*
ΔEF	1.1	0.29	0.3	0.60	1.6	0.21	0.5	0.49	2.2	0.13	0.1	0.82	21.1	0.001*	13.2	0.001*
Exercise wall motion Δ	0.2	0.64	0.1	0.76	4.1	0.04*	3.3	0.07	2.2	0.14	0.1	0.79	4.2	0.04*	2.0	0.15
Clinical variables	—	—	24.9 (12 d.f.)	0.02*			9.2 (12 d.f.)	0.68			24.5 (12 d.f.)	0.02*			8.3 (4 d.f.)	0.08

N = number of events; X^2 = likelihood ratio chi-square with 1 degree of freedom except where indicated (the multivariable X^2 for each parameter is an assessment of prognostic significance, adjusted for clinical variables).
*$P \leq .05$.
(Adapted from Morris KG, Palmeri ST, Califf RM, et al: Value of radionuclide angiography for predicting specific cardiac events after acute myocardial infarction, *Am J Cardiol* 53:318-324, 1985.)

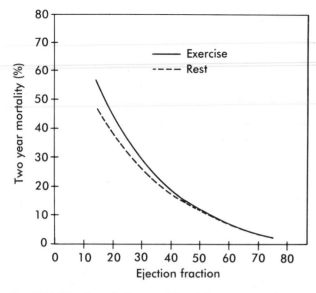

Fig. 64-7. Unadjusted Cox models of 2-year mortality as a function of rest and exercise ejection fraction.

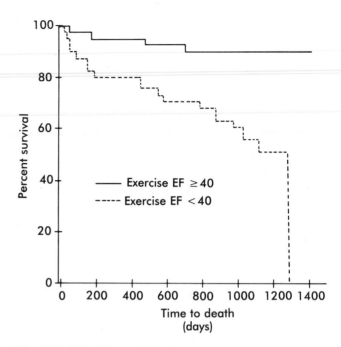

Fig. 64-8. Life table survival of patient population by exercise ejection fraction (EF). Seventy-two patients had EFs ≥ 40%; 34 had EFs < 40%. (From Morris KG, Palmeri ST, Califf RM, et al: *Am J Cardiol* 55:318-324, 1985.)

size and location of the infarction. However, exercise EF, which reflects both the size of the infarction and the amount of potentially ischemic myocardium, is a more powerful predictor of subsequent mortality. The change in EF with exercise, a measure of ischemia alone, is predictive of recurrent ischemic events such as nonfatal infarction, medically refractory angina requiring revascularization, or unstable angina.

Comparative prognostic value of RNA with other clinical and laboratory parameters

The results of the Duke/Durham VA study and those by Corbett et al.[45] and Dewhurst and Muir[50] all suggest that the RNA variables are more potent predictors of subsequent events than those available through history, physical examination, or electrocardiogram. In the discriminate function analyses used by Corbett et al.[45] for combined events, the RNA variables were ranked higher than other clinical variables. In the multivariable Cox models used for the Duke/Durham VA series, a similar result was obtained. Dewhurst and Muir found the RNA variables to be superior to any of the traditional prognostic indices, such as those described by Norris or Luria.[21,23]

Exercise electrocardiography has been extensively studied as a prognostic procedure after MI. Exercise-induced ST-segment changes were not as potent predictors of subsequent cardiac events as the RNA variables in the Duke/Durham VA series. In the combined event analysis of Corbett, Hung, and their co-workers,[45,47] submaximal exercise test variables such as maximal heart rate, blood pressure, workload, angina, ST segment changes, and arrhythmias were compared with the RNA

variables for prognostic significance; the RNA variables were found to be more significantly related to subsequent events.

Thallium-201 myocardial scintigraphy has also been used prognostically in survivors of AMI. Hung et al.[47] specifically compared thallium-201 myocardial perfusion scintigraphy with rest and exercise radionuclide ventriculography. Although they found that the results of thallium scintigraphy were significantly related to subsequent combined events, they determined that the RNA variables were superior to thallium scintigraphy for predicting events in patients recovering from MI.

The power of the RNA variables is clear from the available literature, but it must be asked what value they add to basic clinical information and other technologies in a variety of clinical scenarios in order to ultimately assess when they are worth the cost. Griffin et al.[51] used a stepwise model to assess the additional value of resting left ventricular ejection fraction determined by RNA and by right heart catheterization compared with clinical evaluation in the acute phase of MI. The significant clinical variables that were forced into each model included age, history of prior infarction, and heart rate and mean arterial pressure at the time of hemodynamic evaluation. Including either left ventricular ejection fraction or invasively determined left ventricular stroke work as a second step added additional prognostic information, with the left ventricular stroke work adding more information but requiring greater risk and expense.

They emphasized the importance of the clinical variables and that further procedures be performed only if the resultant information was considered clinically indicated for patient management.

Tibbets et al.[52] from the Multicenter Postinfarction Group followed 866 patients less than 70 years of age with documented MI. Among 150 variables from the history, physical examination, electrocardiogram, chest x-ray, Holter monitoring, rest radionuclide angiography, and exercise treadmill testing, 69 variables were univariately significant at <.01 level for 1-year follow-up using a logistic regression analysis. Sequential analysis of the significance of these variables in a multivariate model, which included first the history, physical examination, ECG, and chest x-ray variables, found that the Holter monitoring results were of no additional significance, but that radionuclide ejection fraction and the completion of an exercise treadmill test were highly significant in predicting 1-year cardiac mortality. Most of the additional predictive information beyond the history, physical examination, initial ECGs, and chest x-rays was provided by the radionuclide variables. Events other than mortality were not evaluated, and exercise RNA was not performed. They concluded, however, that testing for prognostic reasons was probably not indicated in all patients and should be based on significant symptoms or signs of electrical, mechanical, or metabolic dysfunction.

Coronary angiography has been used widely for prognostic purposes. The number of significantly diseased coronary vessels is second only to ejection fraction among clinical and angiographic variables as a predictor of subsequent mortality in patients recovering from MI. It is a reasonable hypothesis that the functional information obtained from rest and exercise RNAs might offer information in addition to that available in an anatomic evaluation. Mazzotta et al.[53] studied 53 consecutive patients with one- or two-vessel coronary artery disease and ejection fractions between 20% and 40%. Nearly all of their patients had well documented prior MIs, but none of them were in the immediate recovery phase from MI. The patients had at worst Canadian Class II angina pectoris and thus were minimally symptomatic. Follow-up events included eight deaths, five patients with significant heart failure, two MIs, and three patients with subsequent bypass surgery. They found that an exercise ejection fraction less than or equal to 30% and failure to increase ejection fraction during exercise were predictive of subsequent events in this minimally symptomatic group of patients with known coronary anatomy.

Lee et al.[54] have studied a large population of patients with medically treated stable coronary artery disease with exercise radionuclide angiography and compared it with clinical and catheterization variables. Although their study does not focus specifically on patients

recovering from MI, it defines the overall relationship between radionuclide angiography and clinical and catheterization information. When exercise radionuclide variables were studied alone, exercise ejection fraction was predictive of cardiovascular death, with the change in heart rate during exercise and resting end-diastolic volume index being of additional significance in the RNA model. In the prediction of cardiovascular deaths, clinical, catheterization, and radionuclide angiographic variables combined together provided the greatest total model chi-square. Approximately half of the total predictive value was available in the clinical information. Approximately 70% of the predictive information was available in either the catheterization or the RNA models. However, in a model containing radionuclide, clinical, and catheterization variables, exercise RNA ejection fraction was the most important variable; the number of diseased vessels was of secondary importance. They concluded that by characterizing the functional significance of underlying coronary artery stenoses described by cardiac catheterization, radionuclide angiography contributed prognostic information beyond that contained in both clinical and catheterization variables. Although this study was performed in the general population of coronary artery disease patients, there is no reason to believe the conclusions are not valid in a postinfarct population.

RADIONUCLIDE ANGIOGRAPHY AND THROMBOLYTIC THERAPY

In animal models of infarction, reperfusion of the ischemic bed results in a reduction in infarct size. The shorter the duration of occlusion the smaller the percentage of the bed at risk that becomes infarcted. This, in theory, should translate into less LV dysfunction and an improved prognosis for patients receiving thrombolytic therapy. Most of the studies reported to date regarding the value of RNA after MI have been performed in populations of patients who have not received thrombolytic therapy. Some contrast angiographic studies of the effect of thrombolytic agents on rest left ventricular ejection fraction after MI have shown improved ejection fractions in patients receiving these drugs compared with those receiving placebo, but others have shown no significant effect on global ejection fraction. Despite this variable effect on EF, thrombolytic therapy has been convincingly shown to improve mortality following MI,[55-57] and this has raised some question regarding the mechanism by which the mortality reduction is achieved. As shown in Figure 64-7, there is a highly significant relationship between both resting ejection fraction and exercise ejection fraction and mortality in patients recovering from MI who have not been treated with thrombolytic agents. Thrombolytic therapy could reduce mortality in patients recovering

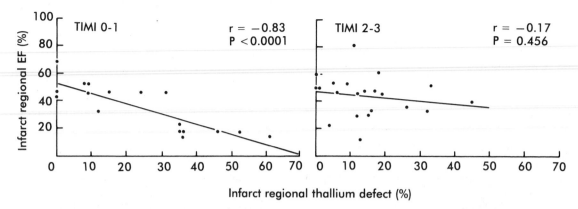

Fig. 64-9. Plots of regression analysis between infarct region LVEF and infarct region fixed thallium defect for patients with TIMI 0-1 flow and TIMI 2-3 flow. The significant relationship between infarct regional EF and infarct regional thallium defect in patients without reperfusion is not seen in patients with TIMI 2-3 reperfusion. (From Morgan CD, Roberts RS, Haq A, et al: *J Am Coll Cardiol* 17:1451-1457, 1991.)

from infarction, either by salvaging myocardium and improving ejection fraction, thereby moving the patient along the curve, or by altering the relationship between mortality and ejection fraction, thereby shifting the curve. Either or both of these effects may be important in the improvement of mortality after reperfusion therapy for MI. Early in the thrombolytic era, Stadius et al.[58] confirmed that rest ejection fraction as determined by contrast angiography remained an excellent predictor of mortality in the first year following MI in patients treated with thrombolytic therapy.

Radionuclide angiography's ability to measure ejection fraction, regional function, and volume have made it a useful tool in a large number of trials studying the efficacy of thrombolysis and/or angioplasty in the treatment of MI. As with the thrombolytic literature using contrast angiography, changes in global left ventricular function observed after thrombolytic therapy by radionuclide angiography have been highly variable. Res et al.[59] reported that patients receiving thrombolytic therapy for anterior MIs had higher ejection fractions at 2 days, 2 weeks, and 3 months following MI than control patients, with progressive improvement in the thrombolytic patients over time. Similar trends were seen with inferior MI; however, the magnitude of change was much lower. There was no significant change in ejection fraction in the control populations.

Morgan et al.[60] reporting for the TPAT trial noted no significant change in global ejection fraction in patients with reperfusion documented at 18 hours. However, analysis of infarct regional ejection fraction by RNA showed significant improvement compared with nonreperfused patients. There was no significant change in regional function of the noninfarct region. Furthermore, as shown in Figure 64-9, they observed a relationship between infarct regional ejection fraction as measured by RNA and infarct regional thallium defect size in the patients who were not reperfused. However, this relationship between regional function and regional defect size was not found in patients who had angiographically documented reperfusion. In a trial of early APSAC therapy, Bassand et al.[61] found higher global and regional ejection fractions as determined by RNA in the APSAC patients compared with those receiving placebo. Marzoll et al.[62] analyzed factors determining improvement in left ventricular function after reperfusion therapy for MI. They noted that the most important factor predicting improvement in ejection fraction as measured by paired RNA measurements in the first 24 hours and at discharge was a low baseline ejection fraction. Vessel patency was the next important factor. Harrison et al.,[63] using contrast angiography, also found that a low initial ejection fraction was the critical factor in having subsequent improvement in global ejection fraction. The timing of reperfusion has also been established to be an important factor in achieving improvement in global ejection fraction. Belenkie et al.[64] noted that treatment within 2 hours was associated with an ejection fraction increase of 6% in patients achieving reperfusion, whereas patients treated more than 5 hours after the onset of symptoms had no change in ejection fraction, even if patency was reestablished. Little et al.,[65] in a study of the effect of thrombolytic therapy on exercise ejection fraction, found an inverse correlation between the time to reperfusion and exercise ejection fraction in patients with anterior infarction. This relationship, shown in Figure 64-10, was found to be significant by linear regression analysis. Using contrast angiography, the GUSTO trial has recently made very similar observations with progressive improvement in ejection fraction as the time from onset of symptoms to thrombolytic administration shortens.[66] This improvement in ejection

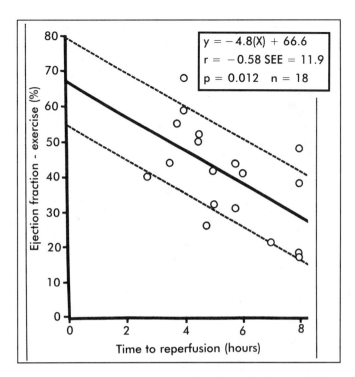

Fig. 64-10. Relationship between global ejection fraction at discharge and 1-month follow-up and TIMI grade of reperfusion. (From Anderson JL, Karagounis LA, Becker LC, et al: *Circulation* 87:1829-1839, 1993.)

fraction at shorter intervals of therapeutic administration was also associated with lower mortality.

The effects of reperfusion on ventricular function, as assessed by RNA, are also importantly related to the completeness of reperfusion. Anderson et al.[67] reported that angiographic TIMI perfusion grade 3 but not grade 2 or lower grades of reperfusion were associated with improvement in global ejection fraction (Fig. 64-11). They made identical observations regarding infarct zone regional ejection fraction. The GUSTO investigators reported similar results with global ejection fraction as measured by contrast angiography.[66] These results suggest that early and complete reperfusion is associated with a significant improvement in LVEF and improved survival; that is, the patient will be moved along the curve shown in Figure 64-7.

It is also possible that the curve may be shifted by thrombolytic therapy in some patients. One mechanism would be via a favorable effect on remodeling and resulting LV volumes instead of a favorable effect on LVEF. Lavie et al.[68] evaluated ventricular dilation after AMI in patients receiving successful thrombolytic reperfusion. They used radionuclide angiography performed within 12 hours of thrombolysis and at 1 and 6 weeks following thrombolytic therapy in 34 patients from the TIMI trial (Fig. 64-12). In successfully reperfused patients there was a small but significant decrease in end-diastolic volume index (EDVI) between the acute

phase and 1 week not seen in the unreperfused patients. This was followed by a small but significant increase in EDVI. However, in the nonreperfused subjects, there was a marked degree of dilation (35%) in the nonreperfused group. By 6 weeks both end-diastolic volume index and end-systolic volume index were significantly greater in the nonreperfused group. The reperfused group also had significantly higher global ejection fractions at both 1 and 6 weeks. These investigators concluded that significant left ventricular dilation occurred between 1 and 6 weeks after infarction and that this may be largely prevented by successful thrombolytic reperfusion. Earlier studies have shown that this benefit on EDVI may extend even to late reperfusion, thereby favorably affecting mortality without improving ejection fraction.

Several studies have found an increase in the incidence of recurrent infarction and unstable angina in patients receiving thrombolytic therapy, suggesting that salvaged myocardium may remain jeopardized.[69-71] Melin et al.[72] studied a small group of patients who received randomized treatment with streptokinase or placebo with rest and exercise radionuclide angiography. The exercise-induced increase in ejection fraction was significantly smaller in patients with patent vessels than in those with occluded vessels, despite the fact that patients treated with streptokinase demonstrated an improvement in rest left ventricular ejection fraction between

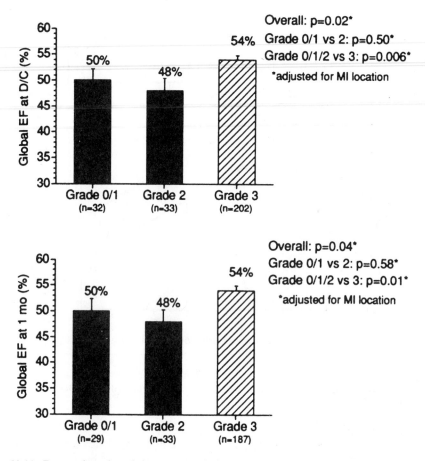

Fig. 64-11. Regression plot of time to reperfusion vs. exercise ejection fraction. (From Little T, Crenshaw M, Liberman HA, et al: *Am J Cardiol* 67:797-805, 1991.)

their admission and follow-up RNA. In this small study, RNA demonstrated myocardial salvage (as suggested by improved rest ventricular performance) but an increase in residual ischemic myocardium (as demonstrated by the change in ejection fraction from rest to exercise). In another small series of patients, Lim et al.[73] using first-pass radionuclide angiography, evaluated the value of exercise radionuclide angiography. These subjects had events primarily related to ischemia in follow-up. Three patients required revascularization for progressive angina pectoris, one patient was admitted for unstable angina, and one patient suffered a follow-up nonfatal MI. In 31 patients the change in ejection fraction from rest to exercise was the best predictor of these subsequent events. Roig et al.[74] studied 93 survivors of AMI who were free of postinfarct angina, able to exercise, and who had no severe left ventricular failure at the time of presentation. Of their patient population 24% had been treated with thrombolytic therapy. During the period of follow-up there were two deaths and four MIs, and eight patients developed Class III or IV angina pectoris. Multivariant analysis of resting RNA variables found an association of severity of resting wall motion abnormali-

ties and end-diastolic volume index to be predictive of events in follow-up. Multivariable analysis of exercise variables showed a drop in ejection fraction of >5% and an end-systolic volume index at rest to be most predictive of events in follow-up. It is important to note that MI and angina pectoris, both ischemic events, made up the overwhelming majority of events in follow-up. An increase in the prevalence of residual jeopardized myocardium after infarction would increase the relevance of predischarge exercise testing. This can be assessed by the inclusion of prognostic tests such as rest and exercise RNA in the evaluation of postinfarction patients in whom intervention is neither already indicated clinically nor irrelevant because of comorbidity or other factors.

Because of its ability to assess a variety of parameters of cardiac function noninvasively both at rest and during exercise, radionuclide angiography can be a versatile and robust technology for the evaluation of patients recovering from MI. Most patients following MI should have some assessment of their left ventricular performance to assist in the selection of medical therapy following infarction. For patients whose left ventricular function

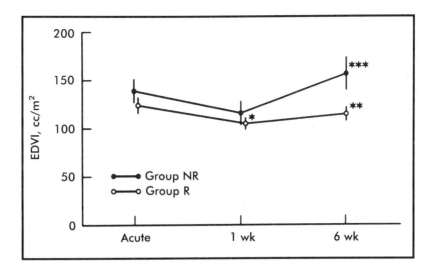

Fig. 64-12. Changes in left ventricular end-diastolic volume index (EDVI) with respect to time in patients with reperfusion (Group R) and those without successful reperfusion (Group NR). *P = 0.02 for short term vs. 1 week in Group R. **P = 0.01 for 1 week vs. 6 weeks. ***P = 0.01 for 1 week vs. 6 weeks in Group NR. (From Lavie CJ, OKeefe JH Jr, Chesebro JH, et al: *Am J Cardiol* 66:31-36, 1990.)

has not been assessed by contrast angiography during the acute phase of infarction, radionuclide angiography is perhaps the best method for making these assessments. In addition, patients whose clinical course has not required earlier intervention and who do not suffer comorbid illness that would prohibit intervention should be assessed for residual potential for ischemia by some form of exercise testing. Exercise radionuclide angiography is well adapted to this task and thus can serve as a guide for revascularization therapy as well. Finally, rest and exercise radionuclide angiography remains a potent tool for clinical investigation in the evaluation and treatment of patients recovering from MI.

REFERENCES

1. Burow RD, Strauss HW, Singleton R, et al: Analysis of left ventricular function from multiple gated acquisition cardiac blood pool imaging: comparison to contrast angiography, *Circulation* 56:1024, 1977.

2. Upton MT, Rerych SK, Newman GE, et al: The reproducibility of radionuclide angiographic measurements of left ventricular function in normal subjects at rest and during exercise, *Circulation* 62:126-132, 1980.

3. Massando T, Rami AG, Grenier RP, et al: Left ventricular volume calculation using a count-based ratio method applied to multigated radionuclide angiography, *J Nuc Med* 31:450, 1990.

4. Okada RD, Kirshenbaum HD, Kushner FR, et al: Observer variance in the qualitative evaluation of left ventricular wall motion and the quantitation of left ventricular ejection fraction using rest and exercise multigated blood pool imaging, *Circulation* 61:128-136, 1980.

5. Rivas F, Cobb F, Bache RJ, et al: Relationship between blood flow to ischemic regions and extent of myocardial infarction: serial measurement of blood flow to ischemic regions in dogs, *Circ Res* 38:439-447, 1976.

6. Schneider RM, Chu A, Akaishi M, et al: Left ventricular ejection

fraction after acute coronary occlusion in conscious dogs: relation to the extent and site of myocardial infarction, *Circulation* 72:632-638, 1985.

7. Schneider RM, Morris KG, Chu A, et al: Relation between myocardial perfusion and left ventricular function folowing acute coronary occlusion: disproportionate effects of anterior vs. inferior ischemia, *Circ Res* 60:60-71, 1987.

8. Nicod P, Gilpin E, Dittrich H, et al: Influence on prognosis and morbidity of left ventricular ejection fraction with and without signs of left ventricular failure after acute myocardial infarction, *Am J Cardiol* 61:1165-1171, 1988.

9. Gottlieb S, Moss AJ, McDermott M, et al: Interrelation of left ventricular ejection fraction, pulmonary congestion, and outcome in acute myocardial infarction, *Am J Cardiol* 69:977-984, 1992.

10. Pfeffer MA, Braunwald E, Moye LA, et al: Effect of captopril on mortality and morbidity in patients with left ventricular dysfunction after myocardial infarction, *New Engl J Med* 327:669-677, 1992.

11. SOLVD Investigators: Effect of enalapril on survival in patients with reduced left ventricular ejection fractions and congestive heart failure, *New Engl J Med* 325:293-302, 1991.

12. SOLVD Investigators: Effect of enalapril on mortality and the development of heart failure in asymptomatic patients with reduced left ventricular ejection fractions, *New Engl J Med* 327:685-691, 1992.

13. The Multicenter Diltiazem Postinfarction Trial Research Group: The effect of diltiazem on mortality and reinfarction post myocardial infarction, *New Engl J Med* 319:385-392, 1988.

14. Reduto LA, Wickemeyer WJ, Young JB et al: Left ventricular diastolic performance at rest and during exercise in patients with coronary artery disease: assessment with first-pass radionuclide angiography, *Circulation* 63:1228-1237, 1981.

15. Bonow RO, Bacharach SL, Green MV, et al: Impaired left ventricular diastolic filling in patients with coronary artery disease: assessment with radionuclide angiography, *Circulation* 64:315-323, 1981.

16. White HD, Norris RM, Brown MA, et al: Left ventricular end-systolic volume as the major determinant of survival after recovery from myocardial infarction, *Circulation* 76:44-51, 1987.

17. Jeremy RW, Hackworthy RA, Bautovich G, et al: Infarct artery perfusion and changes in left ventricular volume in the month after acute myocardial infarction, *J Am Coll Cardiol* 9:989-995, 1987.

18. Ertl G, Gaudron P, Eilles C, et al: Serial changes in left ventricular size after acute myocardial infarction, *Am J Cardiol* 68:116D-120D, 1991.

19. Battler A, Karliner JS, Higgins CB, et al: The initial chest x-ray and acute myocardial infarction: prediction of early and late mortality and survival, *Circulation* 60:1004-1009, 1980.

20. Harris PH, Harrell FE Jr, Lee KL, et al: Survival in medically treated coronary artery disease, *Circulation* 60:1259-1269, 1979.

21. Luria MH, Knoke JD, Wachs JS, et al: Survival after recovery from acute myocardial infarction: two- and five-year prognostic indices, *Am J Med* 67:7-14, 1979.

22. McNeer JF, Wallace AG, Starmer CF, et al: The course of acute myocardial infarction: the feasibility of early discharge of the uncomplicated patient, *Circulation* 51:410-413, 1975.

23. Norris RM, Caughey DE, Deeming LW, et al: Coronary prognostic index for predicting survival after recovery from acute myocardial infarction, *Lancet* 2:485-488, 1970.

24. DeFeyter PJ, Van Eenige MJ, Dighton DH, et al: Prognostic value of exercise testing, coronary angiography and left ventriculography 6-8 weeks after myocardial infarction, *Circulation* 66:527-536, 1982.

25. Sanz G, Castaner A, Betriu A, et al: Determinants of prognosis in survivors of myocardial infarction: a prospective clinical angiography study, *New Engl J Med* 306:1065-1079, 1982.

26. Taylor GJ, Humphries JO, Mellits ED, et al: Predictors of clinical course, coronary anatomy, and left ventricular function after recovery from acute myocardial infarction, *Circulation* 62:960-970, 1980.

27. DeBusk RF, Davidson DM, Houston N, et al: Serial ambulatory electrocardiography and treadmill exercise testing after uncomplicated myocardial infarction, *Am J Cardiol* 45:547-554, 1980.

28. Théroux P, Waters DD, Halphen C, et al: Prognostic value of exercise testing soon after myocardial infarction, *New Engl J Med* 301:341-345, 1979.

29. Borer JS, Rosing DR, Miller RH, et al: Natural history of left ventricular function during 1 year after acute myocardial infarction: comparison with clinical, electrocardiographic and biochemical determinations, *Am J Cardiol* 46:1-12, 1980.

30. Schulze RA Jr, Strauss HW, Pitt B: Sudden death in the year following myocardial infarction: relation to ventricular premature contractions in the late hospital phase and left ventricular ejection fraction, *Am J Med* 62:192-199, 1977.

31. Kuchar DL, Throburn CW, Neville LS: Prediction of serious arrhythmic events after myocardial infarction: signal averaged electrocardiogram, Holter monitoring, and radionuclide ventriculography, *J Am Coll Cardiol* 9:531, 1987.

32. Mukharji J, Rude RE, Poole K, et al: Risk factors for sudden death after acute myocardial infarction: two-year follow-up, *Am J Cardiol* 54:31-36, 1984.

33. Gomes JA, Winters SL, Stewart D, et al: A new noninvasive index to predict sustained ventricular tachycardia and sudden death in the first year after myocardial infarction: based on signal-averaged electrocardiogram, radionuclide ejection fraction, and Holter monitoring, *J Am Coll Cardiol* 10:349-357, 1987.

34. McClements BM, Adgey AA: Value of signal-averaged electrocardiography, radionuclide ventriculography, Holter monitoring, and clinical variables for prediction of arrhythmic events in survivors of acute myocardial infarction in the thrombolytic era, *J Am Coll Cardiol* 21:1419-1427, 1993.

35. Shah PK, Pichler M, Berman DS, et al: Left ventricular ejection fraction determined by radionuclide ventriculography in early stages of first transmural myocardial infarction: relation to short-term prognosis, *Am J Cardiol* 45:542-546, 1980.

36. Battler A, Slutsky R, Karlin JS, et al: Left ventricular ejection fraction and first third ejection fraction early after acute myocardial infarction: value for predicting mortality and morbidity, *Am J Cardiol* 45:197-202, 1980.

37. The Multicenter Postinfarction Research Group: Risk stratification and survival after myocardial infarction, *New Engl J Med* 309:331-336, 1983.

38. Califf RM, Harrell FE, Pryor DB, et al: Prognostic stratification using ejection fraction. *Circulation* 68:III-413, 1983.

39. Morris KG, Palmeri ST, Califf RM, et al: Value of radionuclide angiography for predicting specific cardiac events after acute myocardial infarction, *Am J Cardiol* 55:318-324, 1985.

40. Rollag A, Abdelnoor M, Mangschau A, et al: First myocardial infarction: 5-year survival predicted from routine clinical, laboratory, and radionuclide findings during the acute stage, *Eur Heart J* 12:968-973, 1991.

41. Marwick TH, Birbara TM, Allman KC, et al: Prognostic significance of right ventricular ejection fraction following inferior myocardial infarction, *Int J Cardiol* 31:205-211, 1991.

42. Dell Italia LJ, Lembo NJ, Starling MR, et al: Hemodynamically important right ventricular infarction: follow-up evaluation of right ventricular systolic function at rest and during exercise with radionuclide ventriculography and respiratory exchange, *Circulation* 75:996-1003, 1987.

43. Jones RH, McEwan P, Newman GE, et al: Accuracy of diagnosis of coronary artery disease by radionuclide measurement of left ventricular function during rest and exercise, *Circulation* 64:586-601, 1981.

44. Upton MT, Rerych SK, Newman GE, et al: Detecting abnormalities in left ventricular function during exercise before angina and ST segment depression, *Circulation* 62:341-349, 1980.

45. Corbett JR, Dehmer GJ, Lewis SE, et al: The prognostic value of submaximal exercise testing with radionuclide ventriculography before hospital discharge in patients with recent myocardial infarction, *Circulation* 64:535-544, 1981.

46. Corbett JR, Nicod P, Lewis SE, et al: Prognostic value of submaximal exercise radionuclide ventriculography after myocardial infarction, *Am J Cardiol* 52:82A, 1983.

47. Hung J, Goris ML, Nash E, et al: Comparative value of maximal treadmill testing, exercise thallium myocardial perfusion scintigraphy, and exercise radionuclide ventriculography for distinguishing high- and low-risk patients soon after myocardial infarction, *Am J Cardiol* 53:1221-1227, 1984.

48. Abraham RD, Harris PJ, Roubin CS, et al: Usefulness of injection fraction response to exercise 1 month after acute myocardial infarction in predicting coronary anatomy and prognosis, *Am J Cardiol* 60:225-230, 1987.

49. Morris KG, Califf RM, Palmeri ST, et al: Independent prognostic value to rest and exercise radionuclide angiography 3 and 8 weeks after infarction, *Circulation* 68:III-118, 1983.

50. Dewhurst NG, Muir AL: Comparative prognostic value of radionuclide ventriculography at rest and during exercise in 100 patients after first myocardial infarction, *Br Heart J* 49:111-121, 1983.

51. Griffin BP, Shah PK, Diamond GA, et al: Incremental prognostic accuracy of clinical, radionuclide, and hemodynamic data in acute myocardial infarction, *Am J Cardiol* 68:707-712, 1991.

52. Tibbits PA, Evaul JE, Goldstein RE, et al: Serial acquisition of data to predict one-year mortality rate after acute myocardial infarction, *Am J Cardiol* 60:451-455, 1987.

53. Mazzotta G, Bonow RO, Pace L, et al: Relation between exertional ischemia and prognosis in mildly symptomatic patients with single or double vessel coronary artery disease and left ventricular dysfunction at rest, *J Am Coll Cardiol* 13:567-573, 1989.

54. Lee KL, Pryor DB, Pieper KS, et al: Prognostic value of radionuclide angiography in medically treated patients with

coronary artery disease: a comparison with clinical and catheterization variables, *Circulation* 82:1705-1717, 1990.

55. Reduto LA, Smalling RW, Freund GC, et al: Intracoronary infusion of streptokinase in patients with acute myocardial infarction: effects of reperfusion on left ventricular performance, *Am J Cardiol* 48:403-409, 1981.

56. Rentrop P, Blanke H, Karsch KR: Changes in left ventricular function after intracoronary streptokinase infusion in clinically evolving myocardial infarction, *Am Heart J* 102:1188-1192, 1981.

57. Serruys PW, Simoons ML, Suryapranata H, et al: Preservation of global and regional left ventricular function after early thrombolysis in acute myocardial infarction, *J Am Coll Cardiol* 7:729-742, 1986.

58. Stadius ML, Davis K, Maynard C, et al: Risk stratification for 1-year survival based on characteristics identified in the early hours of acute myocardial infarction. The Western Washington intracoronary streptokinase trial, *Circulation* 74:703-711, 1986.

59. Res JC, Simoons ML, van der Wall EE, et al: Long term improvement in global left ventricular function after early thrombolytic treatment in acute myocardial infarction. Report of a randomised multicentre trial of intracoronary stretokinase in acute myocardial infarction, *Br Heart J* 56:414-421, 1986.

60. Morgan CD, Roberts RS, Haq A, et al: Coronary patency, infarct size and left ventricular function after thrombolytic therapy for acute myocardial infarction: results from the tissue plasminogen activator Toronto (TPAT) placebo-controlled trial. TPAT Study Group, *J Am Coll Cardiol* 17:1451-1457, 1991.

61. Bassand JP, Machecourt J, Cassagnes J, et al: Limitation of myocardial infarct size and preservation of left ventricular function by early administration of APSAC in myocardial infarction, *Am J Cardiol* 64:18A-23A, 1989.

62. Marzoll U, Kleiman NS, Dunn JK, et al: Factors determining improvement in left ventricular function after reperfusion therapy for acute myocardial infarction: primacy baseline ejection fraction, *J Am Coll Cardiol* 17:613-620, 1991.

63. Harrison JK, Califf RM, Woodlief LH, et al: Systolic left ventricular function after reperfusion therapy for acute myocardial infarction. Analysis of determinants of improvement. The TAMI Study Group, *Circulation* 87:1531-1541, 1993.

64. Belenkie I, Thompson CR, Manyari DE, et al: Improtance of effective, early and sustained reperfusion during acute myocardial infarction, *Am J Cardiol* 63:912-916, 1989.

65. Little T, Crenshaw M, Liberman HA, et al: Effects of time required for reperfusion (thrombolysis or angioplasty, or both) and location of acute myocardial infarction on left ventricular functional reserve capacity several months later, *Am J Cardiol* 67:797-805, 1991.

66. The GUSTO Angiographic Investigators: The effects of tissue plasminogen activator, streptokinase, or both on coronary artery patency, ventricular function, and survival after acute myocardial infarction, *N Engl J Med* 329:1615-1622, 1993.

67. Anderson JL, Karagounis LA, Becker LC, et al: TIMI perfusion grade 3 but no grade 2 results in improved outcome after thrombolysis for myocardial infarction. Ventriculographic, enzymatic, and electrocardiographic evidence from the TEAM-3 Study, *Circulation* 87:1829-1839, 1993.

68. Lavie CJ, OKeefe JH Jr, Chesebro JH, et al: Prevention of late ventricular dilatation after acute myocardial infarction by successful thrombolytic reperfusion, *Am J Cardiol* 66:31-36, 1990.

69. Kennedy JW, Ritchie JL, Davis KB, et al: Western Washington randomized trial of intracoronary streptokinase in acute myocardial infarction: a 12-month follow-up report, *New Engl J Med* 312:1073-1078, 1985.

70. Gruppo Italiano per lo Studio della Streptochinasi nell'Infarto Miocardico (GISSI): Effectiveness of intravenous thrombolytic treatment in acute myocardial infarction, *Lancet* 1:397-402, 1986.

71. Schauer DH, Lerkoff RH, Katz RJ, et al: Recurrent early ischemic events after thrombolysis for acute myocardial infarction, *Am J Cardiol* 59:788, 1987.

72. Melin J, Coster P, Renkin J, et al: Effect of intracoronary thrombolytic therapy on exercise-induced ischemia after acute myocardial infarction, *Am J Cardiol* 56:705-711, 1985.

73. Lim R, Dyke L, Dymond DS: Early prognosis after thrombolysis: value of exercise radionuclide ventriculography performed on antiischaemic medication, *Int J Card Imaging* 7:125-131, 1991.

74. Roig E, Magrina J, Garcia A, et al: Prognostic value of exercise radionuclide angiography in low-risk acute myocardial infarction survivors, *Eur Heart J* 14:213-218, 1993.

Chapter 65

EARLY CARDIAC REHABILITATION

Margaret B. Munster
Debra Eckart
Leigh Rogers

A myocardial infarction (MI), though acute in nature, is one event in a chronic disease with lifelong implications. The initial phase of an MI is marked by chaos for both the patient and family because the treatment is increasingly aggressive and highly technologic. "Cardiac rehabilitation is the process of restoring physical, psychological and social functions to optimal levels in persons with coronary heart disease."[1] Specific goals of cardiac rehabilitation include risk stratification, limitation of potential adverse psychologic and emotional consequences of cardiovascular disease, modification of cardiac risk factors, reduction in morbidity and mortality, alleviation of symptoms, and improvement of physical functioning.[1]

Cardiac rehabilitation occurs in four phases: acute illness in the coronary care unit (CCU), recovery in the intermediate unit, convalescence at home, and long-term conditioning or maintenance.[2] A rehabilitation program generally consists of four components: patient education, risk factor modification, activity progression, and psychologic support. Rehabilitation after an MI requires the active participation of the patient and family with all components and throughout the four phases. Providing information is the first step in fostering this participation.

PATIENT EDUCATION

Patient education has become a patient right and a health professional's legal responsibility. Numerous major professional organizations, including the American Medical Association (AMA), American Nurses Association (ANA), and Joint Commission of Accreditation of Hospitals (JCAH), have published statements recognizing patient education as a fundamental component of quality health care. According to JCAH guidelines, the patient "has the right . . . to receive from persons responsible for his care adequate information concerning the nature and extent of his medical problem, the planned course of treatment and the prognosis."[3] The following topics should be included in the teaching plan for the recovering MI patient: an individualized diagnosis and treatment plan, risk factors of coronary artery disease, signals for use of nitroglycerin and seeking of medical assistance, information on medications, and activity progression.

During the acute and recovery phases of an MI, many factors impede learning, retention, and use of information. The emotionalism of the event, sleeplessness, and the medications used to alleviate pain often interfere with the patient's ability to concentrate. The cardiac care unit (CCU) is usually not an environment conducive to patient learning, but the CCU waiting room can provide a useful place for family education. A slide-tape or video presentation, followed by a discussion period, encourages the families to ask questions and have dialogue with others experiencing similar events. Group classes for patients after transfer from CCU can be time efficient for the educator and psychologically beneficial for the participants. To reach as many people as possible, the classes should be offered several times during the week at varying times during the day.

Written materials can be helpful aids for retention and clarification, particularly after discharge. However, with 20% of the population and 35% of people more than age 60 years considered functionally illiterate,[4] educators should be cautioned against just handing out a booklet.

Audiovisual aids, booklets, and group sessions should be used only as supplements to individualized teachings at the patient's bedside. Interaction with the same staff member should include the opportunity to express concerns and anxieties and may be as important as the educational material itself.[5] The patient should be given the telephone number of a member of the health care team who can answer questions that inevitably arise after the patient returns home.

The shortened length of hospitalization demands that a great deal of information be prioritized and simplified. Instructions are most effective if personalized, repeated frequently during hospitalization and reinforced during postdischarge office visits and in an outpatient cardiac rehabilitation program.

RISK FACTOR MODIFICATION

Epidemiologic research has repeatedly shown the multifactorial etiology of coronary artery disease. Having the patient fill out a risk factor profile can be a useful exercise in helping the patient identify his or her particular risk factors. Therapies are then instituted to promote changes that will decrease the patient's risks for further cardiac events. The three major modifications to be incorporated into a cardiac patient's lifestyle are smoking cessation, healthy eating, and regular exercise.

Patient education regarding risk factor modification is seen as a responsibility of the health professional and also of the patient, with the expectation of some degree of change in the patient's behavior.[6] However, the association between information given and extent to which instructions are followed is not always strong. Though reports of compliance rates vary widely, on the average one third to one half of all patients studied are classified as noncompliant.[7] Furthermore, the most difficult regimens to adhere to are those that do not produce an immediately obvious positive result, namely, quitting smoking, moderating drinking, and making dietary changes—behaviors particularly relevant to the recovering MI patient. Compliance has also been shown to decrease over time.

Compliance is heightened when a patient senses a genuine concern by the health care professional.[6] Friendliness, warmth, interest, and empathy have been shown to be professional qualities that increase patient compliance.[8] Consistency should also be on this list. The information given gains credibility only if the patient hears concordance among the members of the health team. Further, the health team should emulate the doctrine of the program: an overweight cardiologist, a cardiology nurse who smokes, and a fat-laden hospital meal do little to promote patient cooperation with risk-factor modification.

Smoking

Cigarette smoking is probably "the most addictive and dependence-producing form of self-administered gratification known to man."[9] One fourth of the American population smoke and smokers have a twofold to fourfold higher incidence of coronary artery disease and risk for sudden death than nonsmokers.[10]

The process of smoking cessation is a dynamic one with many smokers attempting to quit then relapsing on several occasions before they are able to stop. Annually 17 million adults try, but only 1.3 million succeed in breaking the habit.[11] Smokers generally associate cigarettes with pleasureable events, such as eating, having a coffee break, having sex, or relaxing. Conversely, cigarette cessation instills fears of weight gain, withdrawal symptoms, and inability to cope with stress. Males have been shown to be more successful than females and married people more than single or divorced in permanently withdrawing from cigarette use.[12]

Evidence suggests that stopping smoking is the single most effective action in the management of coronary artery disease (CAD).[13] Comparison of post-MI patients who continue to smoke and those who stopped reveals a reduction in recurrent MI[14] and a 62% reduction in mortality among the exsmokers.[15]

A heart attack and all its ramifications often provide the patient with the motivation needed to quit, yet misconceptions and knowledge deficits may cloud the process. For example, a "deed is done" mentality may give the patient the false impression that there is no benefit to quitting once CAD has developed. Emphasis on the importance of quitting should begin during the acute convalescent period and be reaffirmed frequently after discharge.

The patient should be instructed in skills needed to help break the smoking habit. The patient is encouraged to capitalize on the time spent in the hospital to abstain from cigarettes. After 3 to 6 days, the nicotine withdrawal symptoms usually subside, and the craving to light up generally lasts only 3 to 5 minutes.[16] Cigarette substitutes such as gum, mints, ice chips, tooth picks, low-calorie snacks, frequent tooth brushing, relaxation techniques, and brief walks are simple and useful interventions. A new approach to smoking cessation is a transdermal nicotine replacement patch. Although the once-daily patch does provide the smoker with nicotine, plasma levels are lower than with cigarettes, absorption rates are slower, and fluctuations in blood levels are smaller. Abstinence rates have been shown to be promising.[17]

Stimulus control strategies are important as a patient struggles to remain a nonsmoker after discharge. These include removing cues for smoking (e.g., ashtrays), avoiding "trigger" situations (e.g., alcohol intake), or setting up barriers to smoking (e.g., sitting in a no smoking area). Clinicians and patients should anticipate relapses, particularly within the first 3 months, and be attuned to the physical, psychologic, and social components of cigarette dependence.

Diet

More questions are asked and more concern is voiced by the patient and spouse about dietary changes than any other topic during the post-MI period. A dietition should be consulted to assist the family with menu planning and cooking tips in accordance with the American Heart Association guidelines of 100 mg of cholesterol per 1,000 calories consumed, and fat intake of 20% to 30% of the total calories.[18] Cholesterol levels decrease during the course of an MI and do not stabilize for 6 to 8 weeks after MI. Educators must be aware of the possibility of an inappropriately low reading in a sample obtained beyond the first 24 hours of the MI[19] and avoid the tendency to minimize the need for dietary modifications in the patient with an apparent "normal" lipid panel. The cardiac disease patient with hypercholesterolemia warrants close follow-up after discharge and the institution of medical therapy if dietary restrictions alone do not result in an improved cholesterol panel after 2 to 3 months.

In the presence of hypertension, poor ventricular function, or congestive heart failure, strict sodium restrictions should be included. Caloric limitations should be calculated for obese patients to promote weight loss of 1 to 2 lb per week until established ideal weight is achieved. The emphasis should, however, focus on counting fat grams and not calories. If the patient monitors fat consumption, he or she will simultaneously control the caloric intake. This shift in focus can often help patients realize they are improving their nutritional pattern and not just endlessly dieting.

Education should include the distinction between cholesterol and fat and the difference in types of fat. A food low in cholesterol does not necessarily mean it is low in fat. Patients must be able to read and understand food labels if they are to adhere to their prescribed diet in the prepackaged world of the 1990s.

Eating is a very important American social pasttime, and changing dietary habits can be difficult for many patients and their families. Being instructed to change to a low-fat, low-cholesterol diet in the hospital and then going home and cooking it are two very different concepts. The continued support from an outpatient dietition can be particularly helpful in making this change a more palliative one.

ACTIVITY PROGRESSION

The physical and psychologic benefits of mobility after MI have been well documented and generally accepted. Early successful thrombolysis results in less myocardial necrosis, less residual ischemia, and less ventricular dysfunction.[20] Consequently, exercise rehabilitation can be initiated earlier and many times at a higher intensity. Unfortunately, the frequent use of indwelling femoral sheaths after catheterizations, angioplasty, and other invasive devices require that patients not only remain in bed but also remain supine. Complaints of back pain are as common in CCUs as complaints of chest pain.

The patient without hardware restrictions or post-MI complications should begin activity progression within the first 24 hours. While in the CCU, the patient should be assisting the staff with his or her bath and sitting in a chair. On transfer to an intermediate floor, the patient is permitted to shower and engage in frequent walks in the halls. Before discharge, the patient is generally walking more than 1 mile daily in one-fourth to one-half mile increments and climbing one to two flights of stairs. Nurses supervise the patient during ambulation and assess for the presence of chest pain, dizziness, dyspnea, palpitations, or excessive fatigue. After thrombolytic therapy and interventional catheterization, the patient's access site should be assessed for hematoma formation and the affected extremity assessed for signs of circulatory and neurologic compromise. Blood pressure and pulse readings are taken before and after ambulation, and abnormal responses are reported so that their causes can be investigated. An appropriate response to exertion includes no decrease in systolic blood pressure of more than 10 to 20 mm Hg and no increase in heart rate greater than 20 beats/min.[21]

Before discharge, a home exercise program is outlined, as well as specific guidelines for resumption of sex, work, driving, and leisure activities. Vague instructions such as "take it easy" or "do what you feel up to" are unacceptable and set the stage for unnecessary anxiety and confusion during and after hospitalization. The patient with a limited infarct should not be deconditioned by an overly conservative exercise program. This type of patient can be appropriately progressed by entering a medically supervised outpatient rehabilitation program where the staff can prod the tentative patient and curtail the overzealous one.

If an outpatient program is not available, the results of a predischarge exercise test are used to prescribe the intensity and duration of a daily home exercise plan. Within 4 weeks after discharge, many patients advance to walking 2 miles in 30 minutes. Walking is the most commonly prescribed exercise, but other types of aerobic exercise may better compliment the patient's condition and interests. Swimming is particularly beneficial for the patient with claudication, orthopedic disorders, or obesity. Stationary biking skirts the problems posed by inclement weather. The patient should be advised regarding proper footwear or equipment, the importance of warm-up and cool-down sessions, and the benefits of an "exercise buddy."[7]

Sexual counseling is often omitted because of embarrassment on the part of the patient, partner, or health care personnel. The lack of communication can result in unnecessary delay in the patient returning to sexual activity. The cardiac demand of intercourse with a usual partner is comparable with climbing two flight of steps, and most patients safely resume their usual pattern of activity within 2 to 4 weeks after MI. Nitroglycerin should be kept at the bedside, and the patient is advised to avoid excessive amounts of food or alcohol before engaging in sex. Decreased sexual performance should be reported to the physician and the cause investigated.

The timing of the patient's return to work depends on his or her physical condition and the energy requirements of the job. Published energy expenditures tables can be used as a frame of reference for counseling the patient on return to work and other desired activities. Sedentary occupations can usually be resumed within 1 month after MI, whereas those involving travel, heavy lifting, use of heavy equipment, or outdoor work generally require a few additional weeks. Likewise, light household chores such as dusting, making a bed, and watering plants may be resumed almost immediately; vacuuming, car washing, and lawn cutting should be delayed 2 to 4 weeks.

PSYCHOLOGIC SUPPORT

For the patient surviving an MI, the experience can be traumatic and frightening. Grief is a normal response to the real and potential loss resulting from the event and may be characterized by denial, anxiety, depression, hostility, or withdrawal. Denial helps to minimize the seriousness of the situation and may increase feelings of competence and control. The anxious patient may need to recount his or her story and verbalize its impact and possible negative consequences. The patient is often concerned about financial problems, employment, and social circumstances at home. Depression is nearly universal in the post-MI patient and ranges from mild to severe. Depression is typically more prominent after discharge from the hospital and may be associated with hostility or withdrawal.[2] These feelings resolve spontaneously within the first 3 to 4 weeks after discharge, but persistent symptoms should be further evaluated.[22] Prolonged depression or anxiety may be caused by the severity of the cardiac event, medications such as β-blockers, or a preexisting state. These disorders can

affect the patient's ability to return to work, as well as to optimal physical and social functioning.

Although patients directly experience the MI, spouses live through a parallel experience of their own that may equal the patients' in its intensity.[2] Spouses are likely to be in a state of shock and are confronted with the threat of the loss of a partner, changes in child and household care, financial strains, and an uncertain future. Reactions include sleep and appetite disturbances, headaches, poor concentration, anxiety, fear, and self-blame for their partner's illness.[23]

The four most important needs of families in the acute phase of hospitalization are to receive information about the patient's condition, to be kept informed as honestly as possible, to have a chance to speak to the physician, and to know that their relative is receiving the best possible care.[24] The family should be given a simple explanation of what has happened and what to expect. Most important but often most neglected is allowing ample opportunity for the patient and family to express their feelings and concerns. Hospital volunteers may be enlisted to provide companionship to lonely spouses.

Transfer from the highly visible CCU to an intermediate care unit often brings on fear and trepidation. The patient and family should be encouraged to view this as a step up toward recovery and discharge. Mood swings, fatigue, sleep disturbances, and hypersensitivity to symptoms are to be expected during the early convalescent period, and the patient and family should be aware that these are normal responses.

The convalescent time may seem restrictive and frustrating, particularly if the patient was healthy and active before the MI. The patient may need suggestions for hobbies or other ways to effectively use the recovery time. Oversolicitousness of the spouse after an MI is a frequent complaint, and reports of marital conflict are usually found in activity instruction. Conversely, strong spouse support is instrumental in a patient's successful rehabilitation and adjustment to lifestyle changes.

SUMMARY

The decline in cardiovascular deaths over the past 20 years is attributed in part to public education efforts regarding risk factors, symptom recognition, and cardiopulmonary resuscitation, as well as medical and technologic advances. Despite these efforts, MI remains the leading cause of death in the United States today. The treatment of a patient with an MI is a rapid, high-technology process lending itself to only brief encounters between many busy clinicians and a frightened patient. The patient and family must be given the relevant information and skills needed to cope with a cardiac event and the changes in their lives that this event demands. Rapid "time to treatment" should encompass early rehabilitation and early interventions aimed at artery patency. The limiting of infarct size must not be the limit of our care of the MI patient.

REFERENCES

1. Squires RW, Gau GT, Miller TD, et al: Cardiac rehabilitation: status 1990, *Mayo Clin Proc* 65:731-755, 1990.
2. King SC, Froelicher ES: Cardiac rehabilitation: activity and exercise program. In Underhill S, et al (eds): Cardiac nursing, ed 2, Philadelphia, 1989, JB Lippincott.
3. American Hospital Association: *Professional, accreditation and legal statement supporting patient education,* AHA catalog no PO14, Dallas, 1977, American Hospital Association.
4. Dixon E, Park R: Do patients understand written health information? *Nurs Outlook* 38(6):278-281, Nov-Dec 1990.
5. Pryor DB, et al: Early discharge after acute myocardial infarction, *Ann Intern Med* 99:528-538, 1983.
6. Falvo DR: *Effective patient education,* Rockville, Md, 1985, Aspen.
7. Dehn MM, Mullins CB: Design and implementation of exercise training regimens. In Wenger NK, Hellerstein HK (eds): *Rehabilitation of the coronary patient,* ed 2, New York, 1984, John Wiley & Sons.
8. Chatham MAH, Knapp BL: *Patient education handbook,* Bowie, Md, 1982, Brady.
9. Schwartz JL: Methods for smoking cessation, *Clin Chest Med* 12:737-753, 1991.
10. Sherman CB: Health effects of cigarette smoking, *Clin Chest Med* 12:643-658, 1991.
11. National Institutes of Health: *Nurses: help your patients stop smoking,* NIH publ no 92-2962, February 1992.
12. DiTullio M, Granata D, Taioli E, et al: Early predictors of smoking cessation after myocardial infarction, *Clin Cardiol* 14:809-812, 1991.
13. Marshall P: "Just one more...!" A study into the smoking attitudes and behaviors of patients following first myocardial infarction, *Int J Nurs Stud* 27(4):375-387, 1990.
14. Wilhelmsson C, Vedin JA, Elmfeldt D, et al: Smoking and myocardial infarction, *Lancet* 1:415-420, 1975.
15. Sparrow D, Dawber TR, Colton T: The influence of cigarette smoking on prognosis after a first myocardial infarction, *J Chronic Dis* 31:425-432, 1978.
16. Shipley RH: *Quit smart,* Durham, NC, 1985, JB Press.
17. Sachs D, Leischow SJ: Pharmacologic approaches to smoking cessation, *Clin Chest Med* 12:769-791, 1991.
18. American Heart Association: *The Heart Association cookbook,* ed 4, New York, 1984, David McKay, 1984.
19. Gore JM, Goldberg RJ, Matsumoto AS, et al: Validity of serum total cholesterol level obtained within 24 hours of acute myocardial infarction, exercise program. In Underhill S, et al (eds): *Cardiac nursing,* ed 2, Philadelphia, 1989, JB Lippincott.
20. Wenger NK: Rehabilitation of the coronary patient: a preview of tomorrow, *J Cardiopulmonary Rehabil* 11:93-98, 1991.
21. Wenger NK: Early ambulation after myocardial infarction: rationale, program components and results. In Wenger NK, Hellerstein HK (eds): *Rehabilitation of the coronary patient,* ed 2, New York, 1984, John Wiley & Sons.
22. Miller NH, Taylor CB, Davidson DM, et al: The efficacy of risk factor intervention and psychological aspects of cardiac rehabilitation, *J Cardiopulmonary Rehabil* 10:198-209, 1990.
23. Nyamathi AM: Perspectives of factors influencing the coping of wives of myocardial infarction patients, *J Cardiovasc Nurs* 2:65-74, 1988.
24. Caplin M, Sexton DL: Stress experienced by spouses of patients in a coronary care unit with myocardial infarction, *Focus Crit Care* 15(5):31-40, 1988.

Part V

REHABILITATION AND PROGNOSIS

Chapter 66

VENTRICULAR TACHYARRHYTHMIAS AFTER ACUTE MYOCARDIAL INFARCTION

J. Marcus Wharton
Robert A. Sorrentino
Ruth Ann Greenfield
James J. Merrill

Sudden cardiac death (SCD) is responsible for over 300,000 deaths per year in the United States and remains the major cause of death in industrialized nations. Although most patients who have SCD have underlying coronary artery disease, clinical or pathologic evidence of acute myocardial infarction (AMI) is present in less than 25%.[1] In patients who have sustained an AMI, SCD accounts for approximately 50% of total mortality during long-term follow-up.[1,2] Even though overall cardiovascular mortality has been decreasing in the United States, the rate of SCD has remained unchanged.[3]

Early thrombolytic therapy has been shown to decrease the risk of ventricular fibrillation (VF) during the initial hospitalization, especially VF secondary to severe left ventricular dysfunction.[4] There are suggestions that successful early reperfusion therapy also decreases the long-term risk of SCD after myocardial infarction, although there are no prospectively acquired data to confirm this. In a retrospective analysis, patients with either spontaneous or thrombolytic-induced successful reperfusion documented by cardiac catheterization had no SCD, compared with 18% SCD mortality in patients who were not or were unsuccessfully reperfused.[5] In prospective trials comparing thrombolytic therapy with conventional care, specific effects on SCD have not been examined. Because further prospective trials of acute reperfusion vs. conservative care cannot be performed ethically, given the marked improvement in survival seen with thrombolytic therapy, it is unlikely that further data will be forthcoming on the effect of reperfusion therapy relative to no intervention on the prevention of SCD.

The risk of developing SCD from VF or sustained ventricular tachycardia (VT) after MI is related to a number of complex interacting factors (Fig. 66-1). These include myocardial necrosis with resulting ventricular dysfunction, myocardial ischemia, electrical instability, as well as autonomic tone, electrolyte imbalance, and antiarrhythmic drugs.[6] These factors interact to cause variable risks for developing arrhythmic complications after MI or with other types of heart disease. The highest risk occurs when all these adverse factors are present, with shades of gray existing when only two or three are present. Of course the factors are not necessarily independent of each other. For instance, large MIs have a greater probability of providing electrically unstable substrate, of having areas of residual ischemia, and of being associated with enhanced sympathetic tone as compensation for the left ventricular dysfunction. The

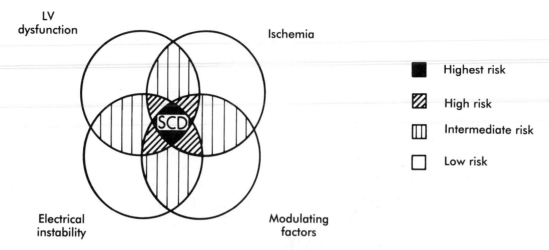

Fig. 66-1. Venn diagram showing the relationships between risk factors for developing SCD after MI. As indicated by the cross-hatching, the risk of SCD increases progressively as the number of risk factors increases. However, the risk factors are not necessarily independent of each other (see text for discussion). (From Wharton JM et al: *Trends Cardiovasc Med* 2:65-71, 1992.)

complexity of the interactions of these factors has made the basic and clinical study of SCD very difficult. Despite this complexity, great progress has been made in recent years in defining clinical risk factors for SCD in patients with ischemic heart disease. Unfortunately, however, little progress has been made in diminishing this risk in the patient who has not had a prior episode of SCD.

PREDICTORS OF SCD
Left ventricular dysfunction

As was shown in the Multicenter Post-Infarction Program (MPIP), the risk of death, 50% of which is SCD, is inversely related to ejection fraction in a nonlinear fashion[7] (Fig. 66-2). Reperfusion therapy, by limiting infarct size, should decrease the subsequent risk of total and arrhythmic mortality. However, not all studies have demonstrated significant improvements in global ejection fraction despite reperfusion within 6 hours of onset of symptoms, although reperfusion within 60 to 90 minutes of symptom onset has had a more consistent effect on increasing ejection fraction.[8,9] The marked improvement in survival despite little change in ejection fraction and even with reperfusion as late as 6 to 24 hours after symptom onset suggests that other factors may be responsible for the improved survival.[10]

Larger infarct size presumably is associated with a higher risk for the development of ventricular arrhythmias because there is greater probability of generation of arrhythmogenic substrate, that is, areas bordering the infarct zone that are capable of sustaining reentrant circuits. Clearly an infarct of any size could generate arrhythmogenic substrate, but the probability is greater with larger infarcts. Thus, measures of infarct size such

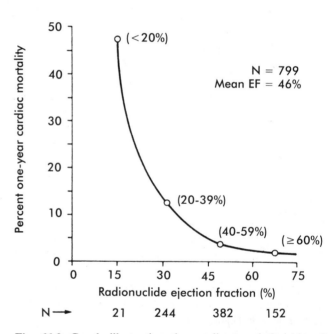

Fig. 66-2. Graph illustrating the nonlinear relationship of mortality to ejection fraction in patients recovering from AMI. Note the marked increase in mortality as the ejection fraction decreases below 30%. (From The Multicenter Post-Infarction Research Group: *N Engl J Med* 309:331-336, 1983.)

as ejection fraction serve as only indirect measures of arrhythmogenic potential. In the last decade there has been a search for noninvasive and invasive tools that would more precisely identify electrically unstable, or potentially unstable, myocardium. These tools include the Holter monitor, signal-averaged electrocardiography, and the electrophysiological study (EPS).

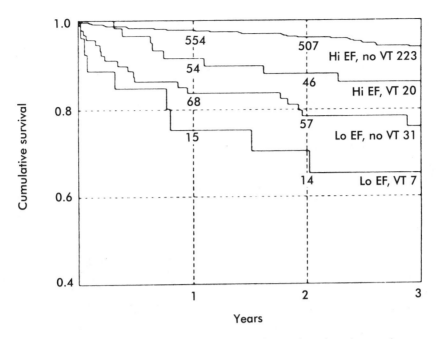

Fig. 66-3. Kaplan-Meier survival curves for postinfarction patients based upon the presence or absence of nonsustained ventricular tachycardia (VT) on a Holter recording and upon an ejection fraction < 30% (Lo EF) or ≥ 30% (Hi EF). Note the significantly worse prognosis in patients with nonsustained VT in both EF classifications. (From Bigger JT et al: *Am J Cardiol* 58:1151-1160, 1986.)

Holter monitoring

Several studies have shown that frequent premature ventricular contractions (PVC) and nonsustained ventricular tachycardia (NSVT) are associated with increased risks of total mortality and SCD after MI. Although results have been variable, recent studies have suggested that as few as a mean of 10 PVCs/hr on a Holter monitor recording were predictive of increased risk.[11,12] PVC frequency is strongly associated with the amount of myocardial damage present, and there has been an ongoing debate in the literature about whether PVCs predict SCD *independent* of measures of left ventricular function. The majority of studies have reported that frequent ectopy is independent of ejection fraction as a prognostic factor, although results from the Duke Databank contradict this finding.[11-15] The advocates of the PVC risk-factor theory have postulated that frequent PVCs serve as a marker of electrical instability, either as an agent for inducing or triggering sustained VT or VF in susceptible patients or as a direct marker of myocardium capable of sustaining a reentrant circuit. The alternative theory is that damaged myocardium is commonly associated with frequent PVCs and separately with the risk of SCD (e.g., via plaque events). Thus, PVCs are not necessarily in the causal chain for SCD.

Three or more consecutive ventricular ectopic complexes at a rate of > 100 bpm is defined as NSVT if the run does not last greater than 30 seconds. An episode of ventricular tachycardia lasting greater than 30 seconds is arbitrarily considered sustained VT even though the episode may be self-terminating. The presence of one or more episodes of NSVT on a 24-hour Holter recording has been shown to be an even more powerful predictor of subsequent arrhythmic risk and total mortality after MI than the presence of frequent PVCs. In the Multicenter Post Infarction Program (MPIP), the 3-year survival rate was 0.85 for patients without NSVT and 0.67 for those with NSVT ($P < .0001$).[13] Three-year freedom from arrhythmic death rates adjusted for ejection fraction, age, and other independent prognostic factors, were 0.93 and 0.87 respectively. If the ejection fraction was < 30%, the 3-year freedom from arrhythmic death rates were 0.77 and 0.65 for those without and with NSVT, respectively, compared with 0.94 and 0.86, respectively, if the EF was ≥ 30%.[13] (Fig. 66-3). (Note that this widely cited MPIP analysis included two patients with sustained VT and a number of patients with accelerated idioventricular rhythm in the VT group.) Although the presence of NSVT is strongly correlated with PVC frequency, it appears to be a stronger predictor for worse prognosis. Presumptively NSVT demonstrates that myocardial substrate for repetitive reentrant beats is present and that under appropriate modulatory influences sustained VT may occur. This is unlike isolated PVCs, which serve as a marker for the presence of damaged myocardial substrate but not necessarily of sustainable reentrant cir-

cuitry. One recent study suggested that the first beat of
VT is usually identical to all subsequent beats, suggesting
that in most cases VT arises *de novo* and not from induction with a premature beat from a distant site.[16] Thus,
NSVT detected on random Holter monitoring may be a
more specific marker than isolated PVCs of underlying
substrate capable of sustaining reentry. Unfortunately,
the large day-to-day variability of both PVC frequency
and NSVT decreases the probability of their detection by
random Holter monitoring and underscores the importance of other modulating factors.

Successful reperfusion therapy of AMI may decrease
the frequency of high-grade ventricular ectopy on Holter
monitoring. In a canine study by Arnold et al., reperfusion 1 to 4 hours after LAD occlusion resulted in
markedly less frequent PVCs and VT on Holter recordings 4 days later than did reperfusion 6 hours after
occlusion or no reperfusion.[17] In humans Theroux et al.
found that the mean hourly number of PVCs was
significantly lower in patients successfully reperfused
with streptokinase (21 ± 64/hr) and streptokinase with
PTCA (17 ± 61/hr), as compared with a control group
of patients who were not reperfused (40 ± 123/hr).[18]
However, other investigators have not found these
differences.[19,20] Turitto et al. showed that the mean
hourly PVC frequency was lower in patients receiving
thrombolytic agents compared with controls and that
the PVC frequency was lower in patients successfully
reperfused compared with those who were not;
however, the frequency of complex ventricular ectopy
including NSVT was not significantly altered between
groups.[21] Thus, at the present time the data are
inconclusive as to whether successful reperfusion
therapy limits electrical instability as manifested by
frequent and complex ventricular ectopy. In addition,
less is known about the predictive value of complex
ventricular ectopy in the thrombolytic era compared
with the prethrombolytic era. GISSI-2 demonstrated
that frequent PVCs (≥ 10/hour) were still an independent predictor of total and sudden cardiac mortality;
however, nonsustained ventricular tachycardia was not
associated with a worse prognosis in the multivariate
analysis.[22]

Signal-averaged electrocardiography

The signal-averaged electrocardiogram (SAECG)
was developed to detect potentially arrhythmogenic
myocardial substrate. The SAECG creates a highly amplified ECG from the Frank X, Y, and Z leads; the ECG
is then digitized. Because amplification of electrocardiographic signals on the body surface also amplifies random noise and the signal of interest is low-amplitude
with a high frequency, temporal averaging signals are
used to remove noise. By overlaying many consecutive
electrocardiographic signals the computer preserves re-

petitive processes (the QRS complex) and eliminates
random processes (noise) caused by the cancellation of
equally probable positive and negative deflections from
noise over time. The process of signal-averaging allows
high-amplification electrocardiography with very low
noise, typically < 0.4 μV. Thus, electrocardiographic signals of a couple of microvolts can be readily detected on
the SAECG.

Areas of slow, fractionated (i.e., irregular progression,
rather than a uniform wavefront) conduction of the
cardiac impulse at the border zone of an MI have been
shown to provide the critical substrate for reentrant
circuits[23,24]; these sites generate low-amplitude, fractionated, and delayed electrical signals known as "late
potentials." On the SAECG they appear as low-
amplitude, high-frequency waveforms occurring after
the main portion of the QRS complex (Fig. 66-4). The
presence of late potentials on the SAECG suggests that
there are areas of myocardium potentially capable of
generating and maintaining a reentrant circuit. However, questions remain as to whether the late potentials
detected by SAECG are generated by the myocardium
critically necessary for VT maintenance or by adjacent
uninvolved areas.[25]

A number of quantitative definitions of late potentials
have been suggested by different investigators. Three
quantitative components of the terminal QRS complex
have generally been used: the root mean square voltage
of the terminal 40 msec (RMS-V40) of the filtered QRS,
the total filtered QRS duration (QRSd), and the
duration of low-amplitude signal (LAS) in the terminal
QRS, which is less than 40 μV (Fig. 66-4). The limit of
normal values varies with the high-pass filter setting
used, as is shown in Table 66-1. Gomes et al. have
suggested that data processing at a 40-Hz cutoff provides
the best overall sensitivity and specificity, whereas 25 Hz
has the best specificity and 80 Hz the best sensitivity.[26]
For general screening purposes a 40-Hz high-pass filter
is probably optimal.

Multiple studies have shown that the prevalence of
late potentials in patients recovering from a nonreperfused MI is relatively high (25% to 45%) and that such
late potentials are predictive of an increased risk of
developing an arrhythmic event or of having inducible
sustained VT at EPS.[27-30] In a study by Gomes et al., 102
patients with recent MIs were studied with Holter monitoring, radionuclide ventriculography, and signal-
averaged electrocardiography and followed for 12 ± 6
months.[29] An abnormal Holter monitor was considered
present if frequent PVCs (> 10/hr) and/or NSVT were
present. The ejection fraction was abnormal if it was
< 40%, and the SAECG was abnormal if late potentials
were present. Twenty-five percent of patients with abnormal results on any one of the three tests had an
arrhythmic event, 35% if two of the three tests yielded

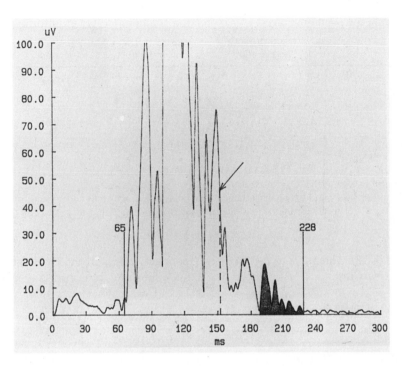

Fig. 66-4. Signal-averaged electrocardiogram (SAECG) recorded with a high-pass filter of 25 Hz in a patient several days after an AMI. The total filtered QRS duration on the SAECG is markedly prolonged at 163 msec (from 65 to 228 msec as marked by the solid vertical lines). The shaded area under the terminal 40 msec of the filtered QRS complex is abnormally low, with a root mean square of 8 μV. Lastly, the duration of the terminal filtered QRS complex that is < 40 μV (from the dashed vertical line to the end of the filtered QRS) is markedly prolonged at 76 msec. All of these parameters represent criteria for the presence of late potentials. See Table 66-1 for normal values.

Table 66-1. Definition of late potentials by high pass filter setting

	25 Hz	40 Hz	80 Hz
RMS-40 (μV)	≤ 25	≤ 20	≤ 17
LAS (msec)	≥ 32	≥ 38	≥ 42
QRSd (msec)	≥ 114	≥ 114	≥ 107

RMS-40 = root mean square voltage in terminal 40 msec; LAS = low-amplitude signal; QRSd = duration of QRS complex.
(From Gomes JA, et al: Optimal bandpass filters for time-domain analysis of the signal-averaged electrocardiogram, *Am J Cardiol* 60:1290-1298, 1987.)

abnormal results, and 50% of patients with abnormal results on all 3 tests had an arrhythmic event during follow-up[29] (Table 66-2). Furthermore, if one or more of the tests were normal, the risk of an arrhythmic event was less than 10%. In a prospective study by Kuchar et al. of 165 patients with MI, 17% of patients with late potentials had an arrhythmic event, compared with 1% without late potentials.[28] The SAECG has predictive value independent of ejection fraction, wall-motion abnormalities, frequent ventricular ectopy, and exercise testing.[28,29,31-35] Studies that have examined the value of SAECG in predicting whether sustained VT will be induced during EPS have reported a positive predictive value of 15% to 60% and a negative predictive value greater than 85%.[27,30,31,36,37] The relatively high negative predictive value is reassuring in terms of arrhythmic outcome. However, because of the high number of false positives, the positive predictive accuracy is relatively poor. The high incidence of false-positive studies presumably represents the fact that areas of slowed and fractionated conduction can be present and can generate late potentials on the SAECG but are not adequate for maintaining sustained reentry, or that sufficient modulating factors are not present to make the substrate arrhythmogenic.

Successful reperfusion therapy dramatically decreases the incidence of late potentials on the SAECG.[19,21,38-40] In the study by Gang et al.,[38] no patient with a patent infarct-related artery after t-PA therapy had late potentials, whereas 33% of patients with a closed infarct-related artery had evidence of late potentials (Table 66-3). Less dramatic and nonsignificant differences in the prevalence of late potentials were seen in patients not receiving thrombolytic therapy

Table 66-2. Relation among the signal-averaged ECG, ejection fraction, Holter monitoring, and arrhythmic events

	Normal (%)	Abnormal (%)	*P* value	Odds ratio
SA-ECG	2/57 (4)	13/45 (29)	0.003	11
EF	3/47 (6)	12/50 (24)	0.01	4.6
Holter	3/32 (9)	12/52 (23)	0.09	2.9
SA-ECG + EF	0/26 (0)	10/28 (36)	0.0007	30.1
SA-ECG + Holter	0/14 (0)	9/26 (35)	0.01	15.7
EF + Holter	1/16 (6)	11/30 (37)	0.025	8.68
SA-ECG + EF + Holter	0/9 (0)	8/16 (50)	0.01	19

SA-ECG = signal-averaged electrocardiogram; ECG = electrocardiogram; EF = ejection fraction.
(From Gomes JA et al: A new noninvasive index to predict sustained ventricular tachycardia and sudden death in the first year after myocardial infarction: based on signal-averaged electrocardiogram, radionuclide ejection fraction and Holter monitor, *J Am Coll Cardiol* 10:349-357, 1987.)

Table 66-3. Relationship of late potentials to patency of the infarct-related coronary artery

	No. with late potentials *N* (%)		
Treatment group	Artery patent	Artery closed	*P* value
t-PA	0/38 (0)	2/6 (33)	0.02
Comparison	4/29 (14)	7/22 (32)	NS
Total	4/67 (6)	9/28 (32)	<0.01

t-PA = tissue plasminogen activator; NS = not significant. The comparison group received conventional treatment without t-PA.
(From Gang et al: Decreased incidence of ventricular late potentials after successful thrombolytic therapy for acute myocardial infarction, *N Engl J Med* 321:712-716, 1989.)

based upon patency of the infarct-related artery. Tranchesi et al. showed that the incidence of late potentials was decreased from 46% before administration of thrombolytic agents to 23% 2 hours after successful reperfusion.[41] On the other hand, Eldar et al. demonstrated equal incidence of late potentials (14% vs. 12%) in patients receiving thrombolytic agents and controls within the first 2 days of infarction, which became significantly different (14% vs. 23%) between 7 and 10 days.[42] Differences in the time course for development and loss of late potentials may depend upon the thrombolytic agent used, time before drug administration, frequency of successful reperfusion, and other factors. Two recent studies have shown that the single strongest determinant of the presence (or absence) of late potentials after MI is the patency status of the infarct-related artery.[39,40] The decreased incidence of late potentials soon after successful reperfusion may be secondary to salvage of severely ischemic border zones that create slow and fractionated conduction manifested as late potentials on the SAECG. Conversely, reperfusion may result in death of such severely ischemic cells, perhaps from calcium overload. In addition, successful reperfusion alters infarct healing and remodeling and may make areas of slow and fractionated

conduction less likely. By decreasing the probability of such substrate, reperfusion therapy should decrease the risk of developing ventricular arrhythmias.

Electrophysiological testing

Electrophysiological studies (EPS) have been suggested as a method to determine if clinically important reentrant substrate is available in the myocardium. If areas of slow conduction are present, premature extrastimuli during EPS can lead to further slowing of conduction and unidirectional block in areas surrounding the infarct, conditions necessary for the initiation and maintainance of sustained VT. Thus, if EPS in patients recovering from a MI demonstrates inducible monomorphic VT, we assume that stable substrate is presumptively present for the spontaneous development of VT. Initiation of polymorphic VT or VF with EPS in post-MI patients who do not have a history of SCD is generally thought not to carry specific prognostic information because aggressive stimulation protocols can induce these arrhythmias in even normal hearts, independent of any fixed arrhythmogenic substrate.

A number of studies have evaluated the usefulness of EPS in predicting arrhythmic events after MI. Most have shown that inability to induce sustained monomorphic VT predicted a low risk of development of VT or other arrhythmic events and a low overall mortality and that inducibility of VT predicted an increased risk.[43-45] However, a relatively large number of patients with inducible VT do not subsequently develop arrhythmic events. Thus, although the negative predictive accuracy of the test is high (>90%), the positive predictive accuracy is low (<30%) because of the large number of false-positive studies.[43-45] This observation again suggests, as does the low positive predictive accuracy of the SAECG, that substrate may be present but may never be utilized spontaneously, perhaps because appropriate triggers or modulating factors are not available. More importantly, given the relatively low incidence of inducible sustained VT in unselected infarction patients, the

Table 66-4. Relative risk of an electrical event after acute myocardial infarction by various tests

	Risk	***P***
Univariate analysis		
EPS	15.2	< 0.001
LVEF	4.8	0.002
Cardiomegaly	4.5	0.002
SAECG	4.4	0.003
Holter	3.1	0.08
Aneurysm	1.8	0.4
Exercise test	1.0	1.0
Failure	2.0	0.2
Previous AMI	2.0	0.2
Female sex	1.0	1.0
Multivariate analysis		
EPS	10.4	< 0.001
LVEF	3.2	0.05

(From Richards DAB et al: What is the best predictor of spontaneous ventricular tachycardia and sudden death after myocardial infarction? *Circulation* 83:756-763, 1991.)

low positive predictive accuracy of EPS, and the invasive nature and expense of the test, the routine use of EPS in infarction patients cannot be recommended.[46]

One recent study compared the utility of EPS with other noninvasive tests and historical factors in patients recovering from MI.[45] Inducibility of at least 10 seconds of monomorphic VT with a cycle length of $\geq$ 230 msec was compared with an ejection fraction $\leq$ 40% and presence of aneurysm on radionuclide gated heart pool scans, late potentials on the SAECG, ventricular ectopy of Lown grades 3 to 5 on Holter monitoring, and evidence of ischemia on exercise treadmill testing. The results are shown in Table 66-4. As defined in this study, inducibility of VT was a much stronger predictor of an arrhythmic event after MI than were the other noninvasive studies in both the univariate and multivariate analysis. In the multivariate analysis only EPS and ejection fraction were independent predictors of an arrhythmic event after MI, with relative risks of 10.4 and 3.2, respectively.[45] However, the stimulation protocol used by this group was not a standard protocol nor was the endpoint of only nonsustained VT. Other investigators have not found such dramatic predictive value from EPS.[44] In any event, given the absence of proven interventions to decrease this risk once identified, EPS can be considered only an investigational form of risk stratification at the present time.

The effect of reperfusion on inducibility of arrhythmias after MI has also been evaluated. Kersschot et al. studied 36 patients randomly assigned to therapy with streptokinase (21 patients) or placebo (15 patients).[47] Induction of a sustained ventricular tachyarrhythmia occurred in 10 (48%) of the patients receiving streptokinase and 15 (100%) of the patients randomized to placebo. Sustained monomorphic VT was induced in 6 (29%) and 10 (67%), respectively. When patients were divided into groups successfully reperfused vs. nonreperfused (whether because of placebo therapy or lack of efficacy with streptokinase), the results of EPS became even more impressive. Inducible sustained ventricular tachyarrhythmias were seen in 6 (35%) of 17 reperfused patients and in 19 (100%) of 19 nonreperfused patients; sustained VT was induced in 2 (12%) and 14 (74%), respectively. Mean ejection fraction was significantly higher in the reperfused group (62 $\pm$ 14%) compared with the nonreperfused group (45 $\pm$ 16%). The results of this relatively small study suggest that successful early reperfusion decreases the amount of arrhythmogenic substrate by limiting overall infarct size.[47] However, in an uncontrolled evaluation of EPS in patients recovering from an AMI after treatment with streptokinase, t-PA, or both, successful reperfusion, time to reperfusion, and degree of residual stenosis of the infarct-related artery were not predictive of inducible sustained VT in a multivariate analysis.[48]

In a small series of patients with ventricular aneurysm resulting from MI and a mean ejection fraction of 28% to 30%, Sager et al. showed that the patency of the infarct-related artery predicted both the frequency of inducible VT and the subsequent risk of developing arrhythmic events.[20] Of the patients with an aneurysm and an occluded infarct-related artery, 7 (88%) of 8 patients had inducible VT at EPS, compared with 1 (8%) with a patent infarct-related artery. After a mean follow-up of 11 months, 8 (50%) of 16 patients with an occluded infarct-related artery, compared with 0 of 16 patients without an occluded infarct-related artery, had SCD. Prior studies in patients with ventricular aneurysms, like the group with occluded infarct-related arteries in the study by Sager et al., have shown arrhythmic mortalities of approximately 50% at 1 to 2 years.[20] Although needing to be confirmed in a prospective fashion, the data suggest that successful reperfusion decreases the risk of sudden death and arrhythmia development after MI. This effect may be related to altered infarct healing.

MODULATING FACTORS

As shown in Figure 66-1 a number of modulating factors may determine if VT develops, assuming availability of arrhythmogenic substrate. The two most important of these modulating factors are concomitant ischemia and autonomic tone. As will be seen later, the presence of Class I antiarrhythmic drugs may be another modulating factor.

Ischemia

The role of ischemia in generating polymorphic VT and VF is well known, given the frequent occurrence of these arrhythmias in the setting of AMI or severe ischemia. In the absence of fixed coronary artery disease, polymorphic VT and VF can occur in the setting of coronary artery spasm.[49] Acute, severe ischemia is thought to generate polymorphic VT and VF because the ischemic substrate is evolving constantly over time and is not "fixed," as is the setting with a prior healed infarct. Indeed, some have suggested that the occurrence of monomorphic VT during AMI may herald a high risk of developing the arrhythmia in the absence of acute severe ischemia because the same morphological VT is usually inducible during baseline EPS.[50] The occurrence of VF in the first 48 hours following AMI requires no chronic treatment because most studies have shown that it does not predict subsequent recurrence after discharge from the hospital (see Chapter 50). Acute reperfusion therapy has been shown to decrease the in-hospital risk of VF.[4] Revascularization procedures may be all that are necessary to prevent recurrence of VF clearly associated with ischemia,[51] but it is frequently difficult to ascertain whether ischemia was the initiating event or whether the VF was a primary electrical event in a patient with severe coronary artery disease. In reports of cases of VF occurring in patients wearing Holter monitors, ST-segment changes are infrequently seen preceding VF.[52] When distinction between a primary or secondary electrical instability is blurred, then an aggressive approach including revascularization and electrophysiologically guided antiarrhythmic therapy should be pursued.

The role of ischemic modulation of substrate in the initiation of monomorphic VT is poorly understood. Monomorphic VT implies a fixed or stable substrate, but subtle degrees of functional change induced by ischemia could increase its arrhythmogenic potential. However, Holter monitoring studies of patients developing monomorphic VT have generally not shown a high incidence of ischemic ST-segment changes preceding the onset of VT.[52] Nonetheless, it is possible for undetectable ischemia to modify the substrate to allow monomorphic VT to occur. Most studies have reported that CABG does not eliminate monomorphic VT (or late potentials); thus, revascularization procedures should not be the primary form of therapy for monomorphic VT.[51,53] Exercise testing has been shown to be a rather limited means of precipitating monomorphic VT in patients with ischemic heart disease.[54] Although revascularization procedures remain a important adjunct to the care of these patients at the present time, electrophysiologically guided therapy still remains the most appropriate therapy for patients with sustained monomorphic VT.

Autonomic factors

Fluctuations in autonomic tone are also potent modulating factors. In general, sympathetic tone facilitates and parasympathetic tone protects against ventricular arrhythmia formation.[6] Recently tests have been developed to measure indirectly various aspects of autonomic tone. The most widely applicable is measurement of heart rate variability from standard electrocardiographic recordings. Wide variation in spontaneous heart rate suggests preservation of parasympathetic tone (and decreased sympathetic tone) to the heart. Thus, wide variation in heart rate would be anticipated to indicate a good prognosis, whereas little heart rate variability (i.e., little parasympathetic tone and typically higher sympathetic tone) would indicate a worse prognosis. Measures of heart rate variability, such as the standard deviation of the mean cycle length, mean of all 5-minute standard deviations of cycle length, proportion of adjacent RR intervals that differ by > 50 msec, or root mean square of successive differences (all of which are time domain measures), have been useful predictors of mortality.[55-59] These measures are clearly related to each other,[58] but it is presently not known which one or combination of these is the best predictor of survival. In a large Holter monitor study of MI patients, Kleiger et al.[55] found that patients with low heart rate variability as indicated by a mean standard deviation of all normal RR intervals of less than 50 msec had an approximate 60% 3-year survival, which was much lower than survival of patients with mean standard deviations greater than this (Fig. 66-5). The prognostic value of heart rate variability was independent of ejection fraction or frequent ventricular ectopy.[55,60] Farrell et al. performed a multivariate analysis of various predictors of arrhythmic complications after infarction, including impaired heart rate variability, late potentials, frequent PVCs, couplets and NSVT (repetitive forms), depressed ejection fraction, and heart failure.[61] Impaired heart rate variability was the strongest single predictor, followed by late potentials and repetitive ventricular ectopy. The positive predictive accuracy for the prediction of arrhythmic events by impaired heart rate variability alone was only 17% but increased to 43% when combined with repetitive ventricular ectopy and 58% with further addition of late potentials. The negative predictive accuracy of impaired heart rate variability, repetitive ventricular ectopy, and late potentials was 95%.[61] Thus, measures of heart rate variability provide an additional tool to risk-stratify patients after AMI.

Spectral analysis of heart rate variability (frequency domain measures) along with assessment of heart rate changes induced by infusion of phenylephrine (which increases blood pressure and reflexively decreases heart rate) have also shown promise in predicting arrhythmic complications after infarction.[58-60,62-64] These data indirectly support the role of the autonomic nervous system in the genesis of arrhythmias after MI, as does the improvement in survival with the use of beta-adrenergic

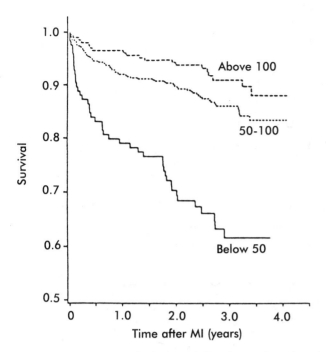

Fig. 66-5. Actuarial survival of postinfarction patients based upon stratification of mean standard deviation of all normal RR intervals from a Holter monitor into three groups—above 100 msec, 50 to 100 msec, and below 50 msec. Note the poor survival in patients having a decreased heart rate variability of < 50 msec, which was significantly worse than in the other two groups. The survival of groups with heart rate variability between 50 to 100 msec and >100 msec were not significantly different from each other. (From Kleiger RE et al: *Am J Cardiol* 59:256-262, 1987.)

blocking agents. However, little is presently known about the mechanisms underlying the modulating influences of the autonomic nervous system on the genesis of ventricular arrhythmias.

PREVENTION OF ARRHYTHMIC EVENTS

If frequent PVCs are associated with an increased mortality after MI, it would seem logical that decreasing PVC frequency with antiarrhythmic drugs would decrease SCD mortality (the so-called PVC suppression hypothesis). Earlier studies aimed at decreasing PVC and NSVT frequency with Class I antiarrhythmic drugs in patients recovering from MI have, contrary to expectations, demonstrated either no change in survival or actually a worse prognosis with these agents.[65] Most of these trials were flawed by small sample size and other methodological problems. The recent large scale Cardiac Arrhythmia Suppression Trial (CAST) has definitively shown the potential risk of Holter-guided antiarrhythmic drug suppression of frequent ventricular ectopy in patients recovering from an AMI. In this study the rates of SCD and other arrhythmic events were increased during long-term follow-up in patients treated with flecainide and encainide (both Class IC agents).[66]

These increased risks were seen throughout the treatment period with encainide and flecainide and not just during the initiation of the drugs. This important observation suggests that some antiarrhythmic drugs, such as the Class IC agents, may have both acute and long-term proarrhythmic effects. Interestingly, the risk of fatal MI was also increased with flecainide and encainide, although the total incidence of fatal and nonfatal ischemic events was not changed relative to the placebo arm.[67] This suggests that some attribute of therapy with flecainide and encainide increases the risk of fatal ischemic events, possibly by increasing the risk of ventricular fibrillation at the time of severe ischemia. Mortality and proarrhythmic events were increased during the loading phase with moricizine, which was the other Class I drug used in CAST.[68] However, moricizine did not cause any clear-cut long-term adverse (or beneficial) effect. There are no definitive data as to the long-term safety of Class IA drugs such as quinidine and Class IB drugs such as mexiletine, although some studies have at least raised questions concerning their long-term safety in patients with heart disease.[69,70]

A number of other Class III antiarrhythmic drugs are being evaluated for clinical use, but very little data are available on their efficacy in preventing SCD in patients with ischemic heart disease. One study of 1456 infarction patients treated with sotalol (a new Class III antiarrhythmic drug with beta-adrenergic blocking properties) revealed an 18% reduction in mortality in patients treated with sotalol (7.3%) compared with placebo (8.9%).[71] However, this difference was not statistically significant. Further studies are needed with sotalol and newer Class III agents to see if any of these agents can render benefits similar to amiodarone but with less risk of toxicity.

Although Class I antiarrhythmic agents have failed to show benefit in the prevention of SCD, four recent small studies have shown a beneficial effect of low dosages (e.g., 200 mg to 400 mg per day) of amiodarone for prevention of sudden death in postinfarction patients with high-grade ventricular ectopy.[72-75] These trials include the Basel Antiarrhythmic Study on Infarct Survival (BASIS), the Canadian Amiodarone Myocardial Infarction Arrhythmia Trial (CAMIAT) pilot study, the Polish Amiodarone Trial (PAT), and the Spanish Study of Sudden Death (SSSD). An overview of these studies showed statistically significant decreases in sudden death and total mortality with amiodarone compared with placebo (or compared with empiric metoprolol in SSSD).[76] Toxicity was acceptably low, but follow-up for each study was between 12 and 24 months. Clearly, a large-scale study is needed to confirm the results of these four small studies before routine use of low-dose amiodarone post-MI can be recommended.

A recent subgroup analysis of BASIS demonstrated

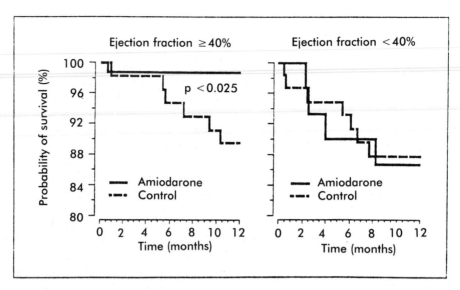

Fig. 66-6. Probability of survival after MI in amiodarone- and placebo-treated patients in the BASIS trial based upon whether the ejection fraction was ≥ or < 40%. (From Pfisterer M et al: *Am J Cardiol* 69:1399-1402, 1992.)

that the favorable impact of amiodarone on survival was seen only in patients with an ejection fraction of greater than 40%[77] (Fig. 66-6). However, a metaanalysis of BASIS and SSSD data showed that 145 patients with decreased ejection fractions < 45% treated with low-dose amiodarone (200 mg/day) had nonsignificantly lower total mortality than 181 placebo patients (5.5% vs. 9.4%, respectively).[76] The ongoing European Myocardial Infarct Amiodarone Trial (EMIAT) is comparing 200 mg/day of amiodarone vs. placebo in patients 5 to 21 days after MI who have an ejection fraction ≤ 40% by MUGA (but not requiring high-grade ventricular ectopy) to help resolve this issue.[78] This study plans to enroll 1500 patients and has projected a 15% 2-year mortality in the placebo group and a 35% mortality reduction for amiodarone. Follow-up will finish in October 1995, so results should be available by 1996. No data are currently available to address the issue of whether the favorable impact of amiodarone in postinfarction patients is comparable in patients who were successfully reperfused vs. those who were not.

Another unresolved issue concerns how long the beneficial effect of amiodarone persists. BASIS demonstrated that improvements in survival persisted even after the drug was discontinued after 1 year of therapy when amiodarone was stopped by study design.[79] Thus there was no "rebound" effect on mortality after discontinuation of the drug, and survival curves of patients treated with placebo or with 1 year of amiodarone parallel each other after 1 year. However, whether longer durations of treatment with amiodarone would exert additional benefits on mortality is presently unknown. Any benefits for longer courses of amiodarone

would need to be balanced against the risk of toxicity with low-dose amiodarone. In a recent prospective study of low-dose amiodarone in sudden-death survivors, toxicity necessitating discontinuation of amiodarone occurred in 25% of patients at 2 years of follow-up and pulmonary toxicity occurred in 10%, despite a mean daily dose of 158 mg.[80]

The results of all of these studies suggest that any benefit afforded by an antiarrhythmic drug must be weighed carefully against its risk of toxicity, especially acute and late proarrhythmia. A drug may at one time decrease the probability of PVCs initiating VT and/or suppress arrhythmia circuitry and at another time increase PVCs and/or facilitate arrhythmia circuitry. The difference in this effect may be the result of ischemia, fluctuations in autonomic tone, electrolyte shifts, etc. The long-term effects on survival and arrhythmia recurrence of a drug will depend upon the balance of its antiarrhythmic and proarrhythmic effects over many years.

In CAST the placebo group mortality was relatively low (3%) compared with the anticipated 8% to 10% from historical controls.[66] This may be because of a number of factors, including selection bias to enroll lower-risk patients, antiarrhythmic drug response in the open-label phase predicting a more favorable prognosis, and the effect of confounding factors such as successful reperfusion. Regardless of the reason for the low mortality in the control group in CAST, the observation raises the question of whether higher-risk patients can be identified using methods separate from or additive to measuring ventricular ectopy. Whether inclusion in CAST of more patients with NSVT or other risk factors

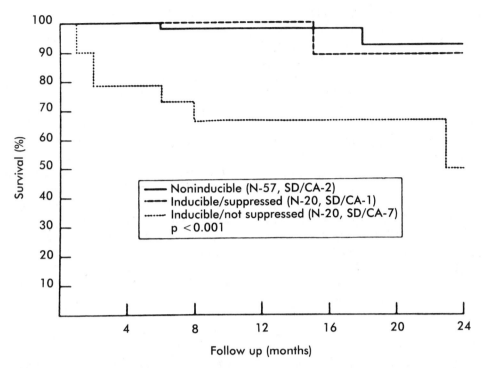

Fig. 66-7. Actuarial survival from sudden death (SD) and cardiac arrest (CA) in 97 patients with asymptomatic nonsustained ventricular tachycardia, stratified by their response to electrophysiological testing (EPS). Noninducible patients had no ventricular tachycardia initiated by EPS at baseline. Inducible/suppressed patients had ventricular tachycardia induced during baseline EPS, but initiation of VT by EPS was subsequently prevented by antiarrhythmic drug therapy. Patients with inducible ventricular tachycardia that could still be initiated with EPS despite multiple drug attempts (inducible/not suppressed) were discharged on the antiarrhythmic drug that caused the greatest slowing of the ventricular tachycardia rate. Note the poor survival in the inducible/not suppressed group. (From Wilber DJ et al: *Circulation* 82:350-358, 1990.)

mentioned above would have identified a higher-risk group in whom the balance of risk vs. benefit of antiarrhythmic drug therapy could have been favorably altered is not known.

Several studies have suggested that patients with NSVT who have inducible monomorphic VT in the EP laboratory and who have successful arrhythmia suppression with medical therapy have a markedly improved survival compared with patients who remain inducible on drug therapy.[81-83] In the study by Wilber et al. 100 consecutive patients with NSVT underwent baseline EPS.[83] Fifty-seven patients were not inducible in the baseline state and were not treated with antiarrhythmic drugs. Forty-three patients were inducible at baseline and underwent serial EPS with several Class I antiarrhythmic drugs or amiodarone. Twenty patients were rendered noninducible by drug therapy and were discharged on that drug. Twenty patients remained inducible on all drugs tested and were discharged on the drug that resulted in the slowest induced VT. Three patients had severe proarrhythmia and were withdrawn from the study. Actuarial incidence of SCD at 2 years was low in

patients who were not inducible at baseline (6%) or who were inducible but suppressed (11%), whereas persistently inducible patients who were discharged on the drug that cause the maximal slowing of VT had a 50% risk of an arrhythmic event[83] (Fig. 66-7). One possible interpretation of these data is that pharmacologic suppression of inducible VT in this patient group normalizes survival to that of those who are not inducible. However, another possible interpretation is that patients who have drug-suppressible VT have less severe left ventricular damage and/or coronary disease and are at lower risk compared with the patients who remain inducible regardless of the therapy administered. Furthermore, the question remains as to whether use of implantable cardioverter defibrillators (ICDs) would have improved long-term survival in the group of patients who remained inducible despite drugs.

Several studies are presently under way to evaluate the effect of electrophysiologically guided therapy and ICDs as a means of improving survival in high-risk patients. One of the most important of these is the Multicenter Unsustained Tachycardia Trial (MUSTT), which is comparing electrophysiologically guided therapy to no therapy for patients with ischemic heart disease, a depressed ejection fraction (<0.40), and asymptomatic NSVT.[84] All patients who meet these criteria undergo EPS off all antiarrhythmic drugs. Patients who are not inducible are not treated. Patients with inducible sustained VT at baseline EPS are randomized to electrophysiologically guided therapy vs. no therapy. Patients randomized to therapy undergo serial EPS on different drugs and, if this is not effective, therapy with an ICD. Thus, the most aggressive therapeutic approach to prevention of SCD is compared with no therapy.

Other ongoing trials evaluating ICD therapy for prevention of SCD include the Multicenter Automatic Defibrillator Implantation Trial (MADIT) and the Coronary Artery Bypass Graft (CABG) Patch Trial.[85,86] MADIT is comparing the effect on survival of convention EPS-guided medical therapy with initial ICD implantation in patients with a prior Q-wave MI, an ejection fraction < 36%, asymptomatic NSVT, and inducible sustained ventricular tachycardia not suppressed by intravenous procainamide.[85] The CABG-Patch trial looks at the impact on survival of prophylactic ICD placed at the time of CABG in patients with an ejection fraction < 36% and an abnormal SAECG.[86] Both trials will help to determine if the most aggressive intervention available can improve survival in asymptomatic, high-risk patients with coronary artery disease. Nonetheless, the feasibility of these approaches for widespread application must be seriously questioned, given the requirements of specialized manpower, invasive procedures, and potentially lengthy hospitalizations. Even if these approaches are shown to be effective, their high costs may greatly limit their application in the current era of cost containment.

At the present time, given the lack of available data on how to safely approach patients with coronary artery disease who are at high risk for SCD, we recommend treating these patients with beta-adrenergic blocking agents, given the wealth of data supporting their efficacy and safety. Even small, tolerated dosages of beta blockers may be helpful in patients who have heart failure or are intolerant to higher dosages. Furthermore, as discussed in other chapters, prompt reperfusion at the time of initial presentation, appropriate use of revascularization, and treatment of heart failure with ACE inhibitors are all important therapeutic interventions in these patients.

TREATMENT OF SUSTAINED VENTRICULAR TACHYCARDIA OR FIBRILLATION

As mentioned at the beginning of the chapter, SCD is the most common cause of death in the United States. Unfortunately, few patients survive the initial episode.

For patients who are successfully resuscitated or who have sustained ventricular tachycardia, recurrence rates for death and arrhythmias are very high. Thus, therapy in these individuals is necessary. Empiric antiarrhythmic therapy with Class I antiarrhythmic drugs may be associated with a decreased survival.[87] In order to improve survival, two means of guiding antiarrhythmic drug therapy, Holter monitoring and serial electrophysiologic testing, have evolved. Controversy exists as to which means of guiding therapy is better. Most of the retrospective studies have suggested that rendering a patient noninducible on therapy during electrophysiologic testing predicted a better prognosis in terms of arrhythmia recurrence and possibly mortality than suppression of ectopy on Holter monitoring.[88,89] However, many patients who remain inducible may still do well. Conversely, many patients who have suppression of ectopy on Holter monitoring have recurrent ventricular tachycardia. There have been several prospective studies designed to examine the utility of EPS for guiding medical treatment of ventricular tachyarrhythmias.[90-92] Unfortunately, methodological problems limit the application of results from these studies. Two of the three trials have shown that noninducibility on therapy predicted a marked reduction in risk of recurrent arrhythmia compared with Holter-guided therapy[90] and in the risk of recurrent ventricular tachycardia or sudden death compared with empiric beta blockers.[91] However, the two trials comparing EPS vs. Holter-guided therapy had insufficient statistical power to address whether mortality, not just recurrence of arrhythmia, is improved by EPS guided therapy.[90,92]

The Electrophysiologic Study vs. Electrocardiographic Monitoring (ESVEM) trial was designed to address definitively the issue of whether EPS or Holter were superior for guiding medical therapy.[93] This study randomized 486 patients who had been resuscitated from SCD or had documented sustained VT into an EPS-guided strategy or a Holter- and exercise test–guided strategy. The results of ESVEM have generated a substantial controversy among electrophysiologists about whether the study appropriately answers the question it set out to address. Our opinion is that it does not. ESVEM reported that there was no difference during follow-up in the risk of recurrent ventricular tachyarrhythmia in patients having no inducible arrhythmia on therapy during EPS vs. those who had ventricular ectopy suppressed on Holter monitoring[92] (Fig. 66-8). Importantly, ESVEM was not designed with sufficient population size to detect possible survival differences. The results of ESVEM are particularly surprising in terms of the risk of recurrent arrhythmia in the EPS limb. Previous retrospective and prospective studies indicate that the risk of recurrent ventricular tachycardia at 1 to 2 years is approximately 10% in patients rendered

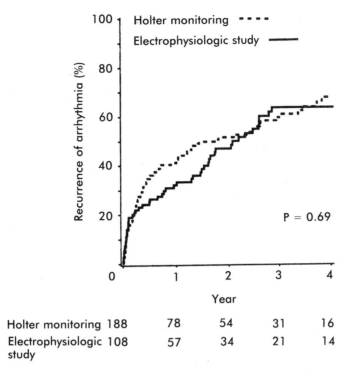

Holter monitoring 188   78   54   31   16

Electrophysiologic 108   57   34   21   14
study

Fig. 66-8. Probability of recurrent arrhythmia in the ESVEM trial in patients who had efficacy prediction by Holter monitoring (188 patients) and electrophysiological study (108 patients). (From Mason JW et al: *N Engl J Med* 329:445-451, 1993.)

noninducible using a stimulation protocol of three extrastimuli on therapy.[90,91,94-96] The risk at 1 year in ESVEM patients rendered noninducible was 32%, three times higher than anticipated from prior studies.[92] This high rate of recurrent arrhythmias observed in patients rendered noninducible on therapy may be the result of a number of factors, but principal among them is the stimulation protocol used on therapy in ESVEM. At the present time noninducibility on therapy is defined as no inducible sustained arrhythmia with three extrastimuli at two right ventricular sites of stimulation and delivered after constant pacing at several different rates.[97] In ESVEM, noninducibility on therapy was defined as no inducible arrhythmia with up to the same number of extrastimuli that induced the arrhythmia at baseline.[93] Thus, if two extrastimuli were used to induce ventricular tachycardia at baseline then a patient was called noninducible if only two extrastimuli failed to induce ventricular tachycardia on therapy. This protocol reflects how serial EPS was performed in the early 1980s when ESVEM was designed. However, day-to-day reproducibility of EPS induction of ventricular tachycardia off therapy have shown that up to 25% of patients require an additional extrastimulus to induce tachycardia when EPS is repeated on the following day in the absence of any other intervention.[98-100] Thus, using a protocol on therapy that only goes to the same number of extrastimuli as required to induce tachycardia at baseline runs

about a 25% chance of classifying a patient as a responder when in fact all that was being measured was day-to-day variability in EPS testing. This design feature of ESVEM may explain the unexpectedly high recurrent arrhythmia rate seen in the patients rendered "noninducible" during serial EPS. Studies using the more rigorous serial EPS testing protocols have demonstrated much lower risk of recurrent arrhythmia at the expense of fewer patients being classified as responders.

Another concern about ESVEM relates to the patient group enrolled. Although only > 10 PVCs per hour were required for inclusion, the mean PVC count was > 300 PVCs per hour (approximately 8000 PVCs per day).[92,101] Patients with this high degree of ventricular ectopy may be at greater risk of recurrent arrhythmia despite medical therapy; however, patients in the study by Mitchell et al. had a similar amount of ectopy but only a 11% ventricular tachycardia recurrence rate when rendered noninducible on therapy using an aggressive stimulation protocol.[90] Finally, beta-adrenergic blockers may have a significant impact on arrhythmia occurrence, and the Holter monitoring group in ESVEM was treated significantly more often with beta blockers than were EPS-guided patients.[101]

ESVEM did demonstrate a significantly greater suppression rate with the Class III antiarrhythmic drug, sotalol, compared with several Class I agents— imipramine, quinidine, procainamide, mexiletine, pirme-

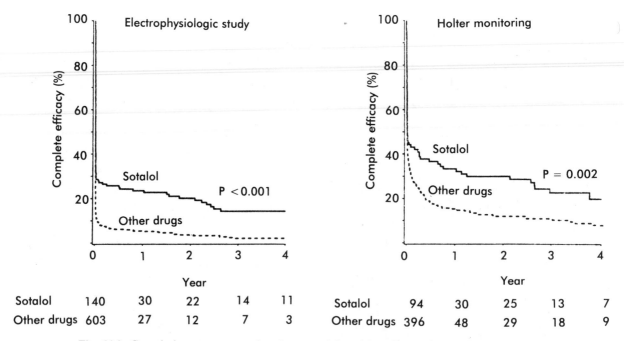

Fig. 66-9. Cumulative percentage of patients receiving either Class I drugs (other drugs) or sotalol in ESVEM who had efficacy predictions by electrophysiologic testing (Panel A) or Holter monitoring (Panel B) and who remained on therapy during follow-up. Although sotalol was superior to Class I drugs in both panels, note that a large percentage of patients were not successfully treated by either sotalol or Class I drugs and required alternative therapies. (From Mason JW et al: *N Engl J Med* 329:452-458, 1993.)

nol, and propafenone[102] (Fig. 66-9). Furthermore, sotalol has been shown to be safe over the long term in postinfarction patients with complex ventricular ectopy,[80] although the acute risk of proarrhythmia (principally torsades de pointes) appears similar to quinidine. The other available oral Class III agent, amiodarone, is also thought to be more efficacious than Class I antiarrhythmic agents. The Cardiac Arrest in Seattle: Conventional versus Amiodarone Drug Evaluation (CASCADE) compared the efficacy of Class I agents singularly or in combination with low-dose amiodarone in 224 out of hospital VF survivors.[80] During the first half of the study a high 1-year mortality of 17% was seen, and the protocol was changed to include implantation of ICDs in all eligible patients.[103] CASCADE demonstrated a decreased mortality and arrhythmic event rate in patients treated with low-dose amiodarone compared with conventional agents; however, recurrent arrhythmias were still frequent in patients treated with amiodarone, with approximately one quarter and one half having arrhythmic events at 2 and 4 years, respectively.[80]

These observations suggest that Class III antiarrhythmic drugs may be more efficacious and safer than the Class I antiarrhythmic drugs. The only direct long-term comparison of sotalol and amiodarone, both given empirically to patients with SCD, showed no difference in terms of efficacy or toxicity, with only about 50% of patients in either group remaining on therapy at the end of 1 year.[104] A recent cross-over design study comparing

the electrophysiologic properties of amiodarone and sotalol demonstrated a high concordance rate of 87% between the two drugs for suppressing or not suppressing arrhythmia induction.[105] Further data from larger trials are needed before sotalol and amiodarone can be considered to be equivalent. Furthermore, although sotalol and amiodarone are effective and safe, it cannot be assumed that all Class III agents behave similarly. Because sotalol and amiodarone have significant beta-adrenergic blocking properties, much of their efficacy and safety may be caused by beta blockade rather than their Class III effect. Some investigational pure Class III agents have had undue late proarrhythmia. Commercial sotalol is a racemic mixture of D- and L-sotalol. D-sotalol is a pure Class III agent without beta-blocking properties. Studies comparing D-sotalol to racemic sotalol will hopefully clarify the role of beta blockade in producing the benefits of Class III drug therapy.

Regardless of the antiarrhythmic drug used, efficacies remain low in terms of arrhythmia recurrence and possibly in terms of prevention of SCD or improvement in overall mortality. ESVEM highlights the overall poor results with treatment with conventional antiarrhythmic agents (Fig. 66-9). Because 50% to 90% of patients remain inducible despite multiple drug trials and arrhythmia recurrence rates are high in this group, alternative approaches to therapy are needed. Even a 10% 1-year arrhythmia event rate, as seen in noninducible patients, could be considered too high. In addition,

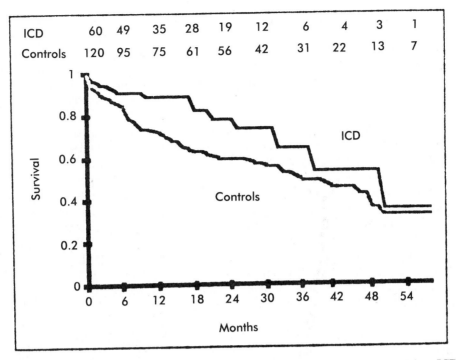

Fig. 66-10. Survival of patients with sustained ventricular tachycardia receiving ICDs compared with case controls from a database of patients treated with amiodarone. Note the improvement in survival during the first 3 years, which is the result of a decrease in the risk of sudden cardiac death. However, survival curves converge at 4 years of follow-up. (From Newman D et al: *Am J Cardiol* 69:899-903, 1992.)

amiodarone may not be a panacea, especially in patients who present with sudden death or who remain inducible with hemodynamically unstable arrhythmias despite amiodarone loading, because sudden cardiac death rates during follow-up are high.[106-108] Furthermore, antiarrhythmic drugs are associated with loss of efficacy over time, acute and late proarrhythmic potentials, decreased efficacy and enhanced proarrhythmia with ischemia, electrolyte disturbances, other drugs, etc., negative inotropic effects, manifest and subclinical toxicities, and high cost (the average cost per month of sotalol or amiodarone is approximately $160 to 180).

Alternative strategies for treatment of ventricular tachycardia include surgical ablation, catheter ablation, and implantable cardioverter-defibrillators (ICDs). In carefully selected patients with discrete aneurysms and otherwise well-preserved left ventricular function, surgical ablation is an excellent alternative with success rates greater than 85% and operative mortalities less than 10%.[109,110] However, few patients are candidates for this procedure. Catheter ablation of ventricular tachycardia in the setting of ischemic heart disease is evolving rapidly, but rates of success for eradicating all inducible ventricular tachycardias are still relatively low.[111,112] However, with continued development in catheter-based mapping technologies and use of alternative energy sources, greater success rates may be possible. A problem that must be addressed with

catheter ablation is whether short-term results are sustained over the long term.

Given the limitations of drug therapy and of the nonpharmacologic alternatives just mentioned, ICDs have become the standard form of therapy for most patients who are resistant to medical treatment. Retrospective analyses suggest that ICD therapy is better than medical therapy based upon historical controls,[113,114] medically treated case controls,[115] and analyses of shock frequency for potentially malignant arrhythmias.[116-118] The latter analyses assume that death would have occurred if a shock had not been given by the ICD for an arrhythmic episode associated with presyncope or syncope (thus a presumptively hemodynamically unstable ventricular tachyarrhythmia). More recent studies using tiered-therapy devices (ICDs capable of discriminating different types of arrhythmias and delivering antitachycardia pacing, low-energy cardioversion, or defibrillation shocks) demonstrated similar beneficial effects on survival when only ventricular fibrillation therapy delivery was analyzed.[118] However, although total survival may be improved by ICD therapy for the first 2 to 3 years, the one published case-control study demonstrated convergence of survival curves at 4 years because of increased late rates of nonsudden cardiac and noncardiac mortality in ICD-treated patients[115] (Fig. 66-10). Thus, the benefits of ICD therapy may be sustained for only a few years, especially in patients with depressed left ventricular function and/or ischemic disease that cannot be revascularized.

The three major disadvantages of ICD therapy are pain associated with shocks, requirement for surgical implantation, and high cost. Newer tiered-therapy devices offer antitachycardia pacing for termination of hemodynamically stable ventricular tachycardia, thus limiting the number of painful shocks most patients will need to receive. This should result in improved patient acceptance of ICD therapy. With presently available ICDs attached to intravascular shock electrodes solely or in conjunction with a left lateral chest subcutaneous patch electrode, most patients no longer require an open chest procedure for ICD implantation. This has greatly increased the applicability of ICD therapy to a larger number of patients because many SCD patients are too ill for open chest procedures. The large size of the ICD generator requires implantation in the abdominal wall with leads tunneled subcutaneously to insertion sites. Newer ICDs presently undergoing clinical evaluation are substantially smaller and may be implanted subcutaneously or submuscularly in the infraclavicular region. These new devices can easily be implanted in catheterization laboratories by cardiologists and require only mild sedation. All these innovations will have a dramatic impact on the third problem of ICD therapy—cost. By eliminating open chest procedures, prolonged recovery times, and operating room costs, the cost of ICD therapy can be substantially decreased. Kuppermann et al. estimated that ICD therapy (using devices requiring open chest procedures for implantation) cost $17,100 per life-year saved in 1986 dollars.[119] They estimated that nonthoracotomy systems would cost $7400 per life-year saved, a cost similar to that encountered for coronary artery bypass surgery for triple-vessel disease.[119] Earlier implantation may result in further savings.

Larsen et al. used a Markov decision analytic model to examine the cost effectiveness of ICD, amiodarone, and conventional therapy in reducing SCD in patients with recurrent sustained VT or VF who fail conventional antiarrhythmic therapy.[120] Using data published through 1989, these investigators assumed that amiodarone would decrease SCD rates by 69% and ICD would decrease SCD by 91%. They also assumed an operative morbidity of 2.9% for ICD implantation and an average 2-year battery life. Severe amiodarone side effects requiring discontinuation were assumed to occur in 8% of patients per year (with 2.8% of the 8% dying from these side effects). With these assumptions, Larsen et al. estimated the cost effectiveness of amiodarone over conventional therapy at $6600 and that of ICD over amiodarone at $29,200 per quality-adjusted life year added. The cost-effectiveness ratio for ICD vs. conventional care was $40,300 per quality-adjusted life year added.

The Kuppermann and Larsen cost-effectiveness models demonstrate two important concepts. First, despite its substantial expense (currently equivalent to coronary bypass surgery at many centers), ICD placement may be cost effective in high-risk patients relative to other commonly accepted medical interventions (see Chapter 15). Second, these models are critically dependent on key assumptions about cost and effectiveness. Over the next few years we should see the cost of ICDs come down as a result of these innovations. In addition, we should have the results of important ongoing randomized trials investigating the benefits of amiodarone and ICDs that will allow refinement of these models.

Three prospective randomized trials comparing ICDs to medical therapy are presently in progress. The Cardiac Arrest Study Hamburg (CASH), which started in 1987, is comparing ICD therapy with empirically given amiodarone, metoprolol, or propafenone in 400 patients resuscitated from SCD.[121] The primary endpoint is total mortality. The propafenone treatment limb was prematurely discontinued in March 1992 when mortality was shown to be significantly greater in this arm compared with ICD therapy during an interim safety analysis. Patient enrollment continues in the other three arms, and as of December 1991, 230 patients had been enrolled. The results of CASH may be somewhat limited in their application because the mean ejection fraction of the study group is about 40% (approximately 10% higher than usual in SCD studies, possibly related to their need to tolerate metoprolol).[121] The second study is the Canadian Implantable Defibrillator Study (CIDS), which compares ≥ 300 mg/day of amiodarone with ICDs in patients with prior cardiac arrest or hemodynamically unstable VT.[122] The primary endpoint consists of either arrhythmic death or any death occurring within 30 days of initiation of study-assigned therapy. The study hypothesis is that ICDs will decrease this endpoint by at least 58% relative to amiodarone. The target sample size is 400 patients. Enrollment began in October 1990, and as of September 1993, 249 patients had been enrolled. The study is currently projected to complete enrollment and follow-up by December 1995. CIDS is collecting economic and quality-of-life data in addition to the medical outcome data. Lastly, there is the NIH-sponsored Antiarrhythmic Drugs Versus Implantable Defibrillator (AVID) trial that is randomizing patients with hemodynamically unstable ventricular arrhythmias to ICD therapy vs. medical therapy with empirically given amiodarone or sotalol therapy guided either by Holter monitoring or EPS. AVID is currently completing a pilot phase and should initiate a 1000-patient mortality trial within the next year. Besides comparing the impact of therapy on total mortality, AVID also seeks to analyze the impact on the quality of life and cost of medical and ICD therapy.

RECOMMENDATIONS

Given the controversies regarding therapy, how should the patient with ventricular tachycardia or fibrillation be approached at the present time? We strongly feel that all patients with documented or suspected sustained ventricular tachycardia or aborted sudden cardiac death should undergo intensive evaluation to define the nature and extent of their underlying cardiac disease. Furthermore, all patients should undergo baseline electrophysiologic testing to define the mechanism and nature of their underlying arrhythmia. Patients with inducible, sustained ventricular tachycardia should undergo serial drug testing using EPS. Given the methodological limitations of ESVEM, we feel that this single study does not invalidate the larger body of both retrospective and prospective data supporting the utility of EPS-guided therapy. At greater issue is how many conventional antiarrhythmic drugs should be evaluated before pursuing amiodarone or nonpharmacologic therapy. After demonstrating lack of efficacy with two or three drugs, the probability of any agent being effective in rendering a patient noninducible is probably less than 5% and not justifiable in terms of prolonging the patient's hospitalization. We presently recommend using two drugs, a Class I drug and sotalol if tolerated. If these drugs do not prevent induction of ventricular tachycardia, available options at that point include (1) discharging the patient home on a drug that slows ventricular tachycardia to the point that it is well tolerated hemodynamically, (2) amiodarone, or (3) ICD. The first option is reasonable in terms of mortality, but the patient must accept a high risk of recurrent ventricular tachycardia that may require medical or electrical termination in the emergency department or hospital.[94] Given the significant toxicity of amiodarone and the uncertain long-term efficacy of the drug, we currently prefer to reserve this option for debilitated or elderly patients whose survival is thought to be markedly limited for nonarrhythmic reasons. In addition, amiodarone is possibly the best form of therapy for patients refractory to conventional agents who do not want ICD therapy. However, young or active patients are probably better treated with ICD therapy, especially if left ventricular function is relatively well preserved. Patients with only a single inducible ventricular tachycardia morphology should also be considered for catheter ablation, and patients with well-defined aneurysms and normally functioning nonaneurysmal segments should be considered for surgical ablation.

REFERENCES

1. Akhtar M, Garan H, Lehmann MH, et al: Sudden cardiac death: management of high-risk patients, *Ann Int Med* 114:499-512, 1991.
2. Marcus FI, Cobb LA, Edwards JE, et al, the Multicenter Post Infarction Research Group: Mechanism of death and prevalence of myocardial ischemic symptoms in the terminal event after acute myocardial infarction, *Am J Cardiol* 61:8-15, 1988.
3. Sytkowski PA, Kannel WB, D'Agostino RB: Changes in risk factors and the decline in mortality from cardiovascular disease: the Framingham Heart Study, *N Engl J Med* 322:1635-1641, 1990.
4. Volpi A, Cavalli A, Santoro E, et al, the GISSI Investigators: Incidence and prognosis of secondary ventricular fibrillation in acute myocardial infarction: evidence for a protective effect of thrombolytic therapy, *Circulation* 82:1279-1288, 1990.
5. Cigarroa RG, Lange RA, Hillis LD: Prognosis after acute myocardial infarction in patients with and without residual anterograde coronary blood flow, *Am J Cardiol* 64:155-160, 1989.
6. Wharton JM, Coleman RE, Strauss HC: The role of autonomic nervous system in sudden cardiac death, *Trends in Cardiovasc Med* 2:65-71, 1992.
7. The Multicenter Post-Infarction Research Group: Risk stratification and survival after myocardial infarction, *N Engl J Med* 309:331-336, 1983.
8. Kennedy JW, Martin GV, Davis KB, et al: The Western Washington Intravenous Streptokinase in Acute Myocardial Infarction randomized trial, *Circulation* 77:345-352, 1988.
9. Selzer A: Does thrombolytic therapy reduce infarct size? *J Am Coll Cardiol* 13:1431-1434, 1989.
10. Braunwald E: Myocardial reperfusion, limitation of infarct size, reduction of left ventricular dysfunction, and improved survival. Should the paradigm be expanded? *Circulation* 79:441-444, 1989.
11. Moss AJ, Bigger JT, Odoroff CL: Postinfarct risk stratification, *Prog Cardiovasc Dis* 29:389-412, 1987.
12. Mukharji J, Rude RE, Poole WK, et al. and the MILIS Study Group: Risk factors for sudden death after acute myocardial infarction: two-year follow-up, *Am J Cardiol* 54:31-36, 1984.
13. Bigger JT Jr, Fleiss JL, Rolnitzky LM, the Multicenter Post-Infarction Research Group: Prevalence, characteristics and significance of ventricular tachycardia detected by 24-hour continuous electrocardiographic recordings in the late hospital phase of acute myocardial infarction, *Am J Cardiol* 58:1151-1160, 1986.
14. Schulze RA, Strauss HW, Pitt B: Sudden death in the year following myocardial infarction. Relation to ventricular premature contrations in the late hospital phase and left ventricular ejection fraction, *Am J Med* 62:192-198, 1977.
15. Califf RM, McKinnis RA, Burks J, et al: Prognostic implications of ventricular arrhythmias during 24-hour ambulatory monitoring in patients undergoing cardiac catheterization for coronary artery disease, *Am J Cardiol* 50:23-31, 1982.
16. Bardy GH, Olson WH: Clinical characteristics of spontaneous-onset sustained ventricular tachycardia and ventricular fibrillation in survivors of cardiac arrest. In Zipes DP, Jalife J (eds): *Cardiac electrophysiology*, Philadelphia, 1990, WB Saunders Co, pp. 778-790.
17. Arnold JMO, Antman EM, Przyklenk K, et al: Differential effects of reperfusion on incidence of ventricular arrhythmias and recovery of ventricular function at 4 days following coronary occlusion, *Am Heart J* 113:1055-1065, 1987.
18. Theroux P, Morissette D, Juneau M, et al: Influence of fibrinolysis and percutaneous transluminal coronary angioplasty on the frequency of ventricular premature complexes, *Am J Cardiol* 63:797-801, 1989.
19. Leor J, Hod H, Rotstein Z, et al: Effects of thrombolysis on the 12-lead signal-averaged ECG in the early postinfarction period, *Am Heart J* 120:495-502, 1990.
20. Sager PT, Perlmutter RA, Rosenfeld LE, et al: Electrophysiologic effects of thrombolytic therapy in patients with a transmural anterior myocardial infarction complicated by left ventricular aneurysm formation, *J Am Coll Cardiol* 12:19-24, 1988.
21. Turitto G, Risa AL, Zanchi E, et al: The signal-averaged electrocardiogram and ventricular arrhythmias after thromboly-

sis for acute myocardial infarction, *J Am Coll Cardiol* 15:1270-1276, 1990.

22. Maggioni AP, Zuanetti G, Franzosi MG, et al., and the GISSI-2 Investigators: Prevalence and prognostic significance of ventricular arrhythmias after acute myocardial infarction in fibrinolytic era, *Circulation* 87:312-322, 1993.

23. Gardner PI, Ursell PC, Fenoglio JJ, et al: Electrophysiologic and anatomic basis for fractionated electrograms recorded from healed myocardial infarcts, *Circulation* 72:596-611, 1985.

24. Vassallo JA, Cassidy D, Simson MB, et al: Relation of late potentials to site of origin of ventricular tachycardia associated with coronary artery disease, *Am J Cardiol* 55:985-989, 1985.

25. Hood MA, Pogwizd SM, Peirick J, et al: Contribution of myocardium responsible for ventricular tachycardia to abnormalities detected by analysis of signal-averaged ECGs, *Circulation* 86:1888-1901, 1992.

26. Gomes JA, Winters SL, Stewart D, et al: Optimal bandpass filters for time-domain analysis of the signal-averaged electrocardiogram, *Am J Cardiol* 60:1290-1298, 1987.

27. Denniss AR, Richards DA, Cody DV, et al: Prognostic significance of ventricular tachycardia and fibrillation induced at programmed stimulation and delayed potentials detected on the signal-averaged electrocardiograms of survivors of acute myocardial infarction, *Circulation* 74:731-745, 1986.

28. Kuchar DL, Thorburn CW, Sammel NL: Late potentials detected after myocardial infarction: natural history and prognostic significance, *Circulation* 74:1280-1289, 1986.

29. Gomes JA, Winters SL, Stewart D, et al: A new noninvasive index to predict sustained ventricular tachycardia and sudden death in the first year after myocardial infarction: based on signal-averaged electrocardiogram, radionuclide ejection fraction and Holter monitoring, *J Am Coll Cardiol* 10:349-357, 1987.

30. Denniss AR, Richards DA, Cody DV, et al: Correlation between signal-averaged electrocardiogram and programmed stimulation in patients with and without spontaneous ventricular tachyarrhythmias, *Am J Cardiol* 59:586-590, 1987.

31. Buckingham TA, Ghosh S, Homan SM, et al: Independent value of signal-averaged electrocardiography and left ventricular function in identifying patients with sustained ventricular tachycardia with coronary artery disease, *Am J Cardiol* 59:568-572, 1987.

32. Kanovsky MS, Falcone RA, Dresden CA, et al: Identification of patients with ventricular tachycardia after myocardial infarction: signal-averaged electrocardiogram, Holter monitoring, and cardiac catheterization, *Circulation* 70:264-270, 1984.

33. Pollak SJ, Kertes PJ, Bredlau CE, et al: Influence of left ventricular function on signal-averaged late potentials in patients with coronary artery disease with and without ventricular tachycardia, *Am Heart J* 110:747-752, 1985.

34. Gomes JA, Horowitz SF, Millner M, et al: Relation of late potentials to ejection fraction and wall motion abnormalities in acute myocardial infarction, *Am J Cardiol* 59:1071-1074, 1987.

35. Cripps T, Bennett D, Camm J, et al: Prospective evaluation of clinical assessment, exercise testing and signal-averaged electrocardiogram in predicting outcome after acute myocardial infarction, *Am J Cardiol* 62:995-999, 1988.

36. Turitto G, Fontaine JM, Ursell SN, et al: Value of signal-averaged electrocardiogram as a predictor of the results of programmed stimulation in nonsustained ventricular tachycardia, *Am J Cardiol* 61:1272-1278, 1988.

37. Winters SL, Stewart D, Gomes JA: Signal averaging of the surface QRS complex predicts inducibility of ventricular tachycardia in patients with syncope of unknown origin: a prospective study, *J Am Coll Cardiol* 10:775-781, 1987.

38. Gang ES, Lew AS, Hong M, et al: Decreased incidence of ventricular late potentials after successful thrombolytic therapy for acute myocardial infarction, *N Engl J Med* 321:712-716, 1989.

39. Vatterott PJ, Hammill SC, Bailey KR, et al: Late potentials on signal-averaged electrocardiograms and patency of the infarct-related artery in survivors or acute myocardial infarction, *J Am Coll Cardiol* 17:330-337, 1991.

40. De Chillou C, Sadoul N, Briancon S, et al: Factors determining the occurrence of late potentials on the signal-averaged electrocardiogram after a first myocardial infarction: a multivariate analysis, *J Am Coll Cardiol* 18:1638-1642, 1991.

41. Tranchesi B, Verstraete M, Van de Werf F, et al: Usefulness of high-frequency analyisis of signal-averaged surface electrocardiograms in acute myocardial infarction before and after coronary thrombolysis for assessing coronary reperfusion, *Am J Cardiol* 66:1196-1198, 1990.

42. Eldar M, Lear J, Hod H, et al: Effect of thrombolysis on the evaluation of late potentials within 10 days of infarction, *Br Heart J* 63:273-276, 1990.

43. Uther JB, Richards AB, Denniss AR, et al: The prognostic significance of programmed ventricular stimulation after myocardial infarction: a review, *Circulation* 75(suppl III):III-161-III-165, 1987.

44. Bhandari AK, Rahimtoola SH: Indications for intracardiac electrophysiologic testing in survivors of acute myocardial infarction, *Circulation* 75(suppl III):III-166-III-168, 1987.

45. Richards DAB, Byth K, Ross DL, et al: What is the best predictor of spontaneous ventricular tachycardia and sudden death after myocardial infarction? *Circulation* 83:756-763, 1991.

46. Goldman L: Electrophysiological testing after myocardial infarction. A paradigm for assessing the incremental value of a diagnostic test, *Circulation* 83:1090-1092, 1991.

47. Kersschot IE, Brugada P, Ramentol M, et al: Effects of early reperfusion in acute myocardial infarction on arrhythmias induced by programmed stimulation: a prospective, randomized study, *J Am Coll Cardiol* 7:1234-1242, 1986.

48. McComb JM, Gold HK, Leinbach RC, et al: Electrically induced ventricular arrhythmias in acute myocardial infarction treated with thrombolytic agents, *Am J Cardiol* 62:186-191, 1988.

49. Myerburg RJ, Kessler KM, Mallon SM, et al: Life-threatening ventricular arrhythmias in patients with silent myocardial ischemia due to coronary artery spasm, *N Engl J Med* 326:1451-1455, 1992.

50. Welch WJ, Blackwell WH, Whitlock RA, et al: Sustained monomorphic ventricular tachycardia with acute myocardial necrosis, *Circulation* 78(suppl):II-236, 1988.

51. Kelly P, Ruskin JN, Vlahakes GJ, et al: Surgical coronary revascularization in survivors of prehospital cardiac arrest: its effect on inducible ventricular arrhythmias and long-term survival, *J Am Coll Cardiol* 15:267-273, 1990.

52. Bayes de Luna A, Coumel P, Leclercq JF: Ambulatory sudden cardiac death: mechanisms of production of fatal arrhythmia on the basis of data from 157 cases, *Am Heart J* 117:151-159, 1989.

53. Borbola J, Serry C, Goldin M, et al: Short-term effect of coronary artery bypass grafting on the signal-averaged electrocardiogram, *Am J Cardiol* 61:1001-1005, 1988.

54. Allen BJ, Casey TP, Brodsky MA, et al: Exercise testing in patients with life-threatening ventricular tachyarrhythmias: results and correlation with clinical and arrhythmia factors, *Am Heart J* 116:997-1002, 1988.

55. Kleiger RE, Miller JP, Bigger JT, et al, the Multicenter Post-Infarction Research Group: Decreased heart rate variability and its association with increased mortality after acute myocardial infarction, *Am J Cardiol* 59:256-262, 1987.

56. Martin GJ, Magid NM, Myers G, et al: Heart rate variability and sudden death secondary to coronary artery disease during ambulatory electrocardiographic monitoring, *Am J Cardiol* 60:86-89, 1987.

57. Bigger JT Jr, Kleiger RE, Fleiss JL, et al., and the Multicenter

Post-Infarction Research Group: Components of heart rate variability measured during healing of acute myocardial infarction, *Am J Cardiol* 61:208-215, 1988.

58. Bigger JT Jr, La Rovere MT, Steinman RC, et al: Comparison of baroreflex sensitivity and heart period variability after myocardial infarction, *J Am Coll Cardiol* 14:1511-1518, 1989.

59. Bigger JT Jr, Fleiss JL, Rolnitzky LM, et al., and CAPS and ESVEM Investigators: Stability over time of heart period variability in patients with previous myocardial infarction and ventricular arrhythmias, *Am J Cardiol* 69:718-723, 1992.

60. Kienzle MG, Ferguson DW, Birkett CL, et al: Clinical, hemodynamic and sympathetic neural correlates of heart rate variability in congestive heart failure, *Am J Cardiol* 69:761-767, 1992.

61. Farrell TG, Bashir Y, Cripps T, et al: Risk stratification for arrhythmic events in postinfarction patients based on heart rate variability, ambulatory electrocardiographic variables and the signal-averaged electrocardiogram, *J Am Coll Cardiol* 18:687-697, 1991.

62. Lombardi F, Sandrone G, Pernpruner S, et al: Heart rate variability as an index of sympathovagal interaction after acute myocardial infarction, *Am J Cardiol* 60:1239-1245, 1987.

63. La Rovere MT, Specchia G, Mortara A, et al: Baroreflex sensitivity, clinical correlates, and cardiovascular mortality among patients with a first myocardial infarction: a prospective study, *Circulation* 78:816-824, 1988.

64. Farrell TG, Paul V, Cripps TR, et al: Baroreflex sensitivity and electrophysiologic correlates in patients after acute myocardial infarction, *Circulation* 83:945-952, 1991.

65. Hine LK, Laird NM, Hewitt P, et al: Metaanalysis of empirical long-term antiarrhythmic therapy after myocardial infarction, *JAMA* 262:3037-3040, 1989.

66. The Cardiac Arrhythmia Suppression Trial (CAST): Effect of encainide and flecainide on mortality in a randomized trial of arrhythmia suppression after myocardial infarction, *N Engl J Med* 321:406-412, 1989.

67. Echt DS, Liebson PR, Mitchell LB, et al: Mortality and morbidity in patients receiving encainide, flecainide, or placebo: the Cardiac Arrhythmia Suppression Trial, *N Engl J Med* 324:781-788, 1991.

68. The Cardiac Arrhythmia Suppression Trial II Investigators: Effect of the antiarrhythmic agent moricizine on survival after myocardial infarction, *N Engl J Med* 327:227-233, 1992.

69. Morganroth J, Goin JE: Quinidine-related mortality in the short to medium-term treatment of ventricular arrhythmias. A meta-analysis, *Circulation* 84:1977-1983, 1991.

70. Impact Research Group: International mexiletine and placebo antiarrhythmic coronary trial: I. Report on arrhythmia and other findings, *J Am Coll Cardiol* 4:1148-1163, 1984.

71. Julian DG, Jackson FS, Prescott RJ, et al: Controlled trial of sotalol for one year after myocardial infarction, *Lancet* 1: 1142-1147, 1982.

72. Cairns JA, Connolly SJ, Gent M, et al: Postmyocardial mortality in patients with ventricular premature depolarizations. Canadian Amiodarone Myocardial Infarction Arrhythmia Trial pilot study, *Circulation* 84: 550-557, 1991.

73. Ceremuzynski L, Kleczar E, Krzeminska-Pakula M, et al: Effect of amiodarone on mortality after myocardial infarction: a double-blind, placebo-controlled, pilot study, *J Am Coll Cardiol* 20:1056-1062, 1992.

74. Navarro-Lopez F, Cosin J, Marrugat J, et al, SSSD Investigators: Comparison of the effects of amiodarone versus metoprolol on the frequency of ventricular arrhythmias and on mortality after acute myocardial infarction, *Am J Cardiol* 72:1243-1248, 1993.

75. Burkart F, Pfisterer M, Kiowski W, et al: Effect of antiarrhythmic therapy on mortality in survivors of myocardial infarction with asymptomatic complex ventricular arrhythmias: Basel Antiar-

rhythmic Study of Infarct Survival (BASIS), *J Am Coll Cardiol* 16:1711-1718, 1990.

76. Zarembski DG, Nolan PE, Slack MK, et al: Empiric long-term amiodarone prophylaxis following myocardial infarction, *Arch Intern Med* 153:2661-2667, 1993.

77. Pfisterer M, Kiowski W, Burckhardt D, et al: Beneficial effect of amiodarone on cardiac mortality in patients with asymptomatic complex ventricular arrhythmias after acute myocardial infarction and preserved but not impaired left ventricular function, *Am J Cardiol* 69:1399-1402, 1992.

78. Camm AJ, Julian D, Janse G, et al., and the EMIAT Investigators: The European Myocardial Infarct Amiodarone Trial (EMIAT), *Am J Cardiol* 72:95F-98F, 1993.

79. Pfisterer ME, Kiowski W, Brunner H, et al: Long-term benefit of 1-year amiodarone treatment for persistent complex ventricular arrhythmias after myocardial infarction, *Circulation* 87:309-311, 1993.

80. The CASCADE Investigators: Randomized antiarrhythmic drug therapy in survivors of cardiac arrest (the CASCADE Study), *Am J Cardiol* 72:280-287, 1993.

81. Buxton AE, Marchlinski FE, Flores BT, et al: Nonsustained ventricular tachycardia in patients with coronary artery disease: role of electrophysiologic study, *Circulation* 75:1178-1185, 1987.

82. Klein RC, Machell C: Use of electrophysiologic testing in patients with nonsustained ventricular tachycardia: prognostic and therapeutic implications, *J Am Coll Cardiol* 14:155-161, 1989.

83. Wilber DJ, Olshansky B, Moran JF, et al: Electrophysiological testing and nonsustained ventricular tachycardia. Use and limitations in patients with coronary artery disease and impaired left ventricular function, *Circulation* 82:350-358, 1990.

84. Buxton AE, Fisher JD, Josephson ME, et al. and the MUSTT Investigators: Prevention of sudden death in patients with coronary artery disease: the Multicenter Unsustained Tachycardia Trial (MUSTT), *Prog Cardiovasc Dis* 36:215-226, 1993.

85. MADIT Executive Committee: Multicenter automatic defibrillator implantation trial (MADIT): design and clinical protocol, *PACE* 14:920-927, 1991.

86. The CABG Patch Trial Investigators and Coordinators: The coronary artery bypass graft (CABG) patch trial, *Prog Cardiovasc Dis* 36:97-114, 1993.

87. Moosvi AR, Goldstein S, VanderBrug Medendorp S, et al: Effect of empiric antiarrhythmic therapy in resuscitated out-of-hospital cardiac arrest victims with coronary artery disease, *Am J Cardiol* 65:1192-1197, 1990.

88. Kim SG, Seiden SW, Felder SD, et al: Is programmed stimulation of value in predicting the long-term success of antiarrhythmic therapy for ventricular tachycardias? *N Engl J Med* 315:356-362, 1986.

89. Kim S: The management of patients with life-threatening ventricular tachyarrhythmias: programmed stimulation or Holter monitoring (either or both)? *Circulation* 76:1-5, 1987.

90. Mitchell LB, Duff HJ, Manyari DE, et al: A randomized clinical trial of the noninvasive and invasive approaches to drug therapy of ventricular tachycardia, *N Engl J Med* 317:1681-1687, 1987.

91. Steinbeck G, Andresen D, Bach P, et al: A comparison of electrophysiologically guided antiarrhythmic drug therapy with beta-blocker therapy in patients with symptomatic, sustained ventricular tachyarrhythmias, *N Engl J Med* 327:987-992, 1992.

92. Mason JW, The Electrophysiologic Study versus Electrocardiographic Monitoring Investigators: A comparison of electrophysiologic testing with Holter monitoring to predict antiarrhythmic-drug efficacy for ventricular tachyarrhythmias, *N Engl J Med* 329:445-451, 1993.

93. The ESVEM Investigators: The ESVEM Trial. Electrophysiologic Study versus Electrocardiographic Monitoring for Selec-

tion of Antiarrhythmic Therapy of Ventricular Tachyarrhythmias, *Circulation* 79:1354-1360, 1989.

94. Waller TJ, Kay HR, Spielman SR, et al: Reduction in sudden death and total mortality by antiarrhythmic therapy evaluated by electrophysiologic drug testing: criteria of efficacy in patients with sustained ventricular tachyarrhythmia, *J Am Coll Cardiol* 10:83-89, 1987.

95. Freedman RA, Swerdlow CD, Soderholm-Difatte V, et al: Prognostic significance of arrhythmia inducibility or noninducibility at initial electrophysiologic study in survivors of cardiac arrest, *Am J Cardiol* 61:578-582, 1988.

96. Wilber DJ, Garan H, Finklestein D, et al: Out-of-hospital cardiac arrest. Use of electrophysiologic testing in the prediction of long-term outcome, *N Engl J Med* 318:19-24, 1988.

97. Wellens HJJ, Brugada P, Stevenson WG: Programmed electrical stimulation of the heart in patients with life-threatening ventricular arrhythmias: what is the significance of induced arrhythmias and what is the correct stimulation protocol? *Circulation* 72:1-7, 1985.

98. Cooper MJ, Hunt LJ, Palmer KJ, et al: Quantitation of day to day variability in mode of induction of ventricular tachyarrhythmias by programmed stimulation, *J Am Coll Cardiol* 11:101-108, 1988.

99. McPherson CA, Rosenfeld LE, Batsford WP: Day-to-day reproducibility of responses to right ventricular programmed electrical stimulation: implications for serial drug testing. *Am J Cardiol* 55:689-695, 1985.

100. Lombardi F, Stein J, Podrid PJ, et al: Daily reproducibility of electrophysiologic test results in malignant ventricular arrhythmia, *Am J Cardiol* 57:96-101, 1986.

101. The ESVEM Investigators: Determinants of predicted efficacy of antiarrhythmic drugs in the electrophysiologic study versus electrocardiographic monitoring trial, *Circulation* 87:323-329, 1993.

102. Mason JW, The Electrophysiologic Study versus Electrocardiographic Monitoring Investigators: A comparison of seven antiarrhythmic drugs in patients with ventricular tachyarrhythmias, *N Engl J Med* 329:452-458, 1993.

103. The CASCADE Investigators: Cardiac arrest in Seattle: conventional versus amiodarone drug evaluation (The CASCADE Study), *Am J Cardiol* 67:578-584, 1991.

104. Amiodarone vs. Sotalol Study Group: Multicentre randomized trial of sotalol vs. amiodarone for chronic malignant ventricular tachyarrhythmias, *Eur Heart J* 10:685-694, 1989.

105. Martinez-Rubio A, Shenasa M, Chen X, et al: Response to sotalol predicts the response to amiodarone during serial drug testing in patients with sustained ventricular tachycardia and coronary artery disease, *Am J Cardiol* 73:357-360, 1994.

106. Dicarlo LA, Morady F, Sauve MJ, et al: Cardiac arrest and sudden death in patients treated with amiodarone for sustained ventricular tachycardia or ventricular fibrillation: risk stratification based on clinical variables, *Am J Cardiol* 55:372-374, 1985.

107. Horowitz LN, Greenspan AM, Spielman SR, et al: Usefulness of electrophysiologic testing in evaluation of amiodarone therapy for sustained ventricular tachyarrhythmias associated with coronary heart disease, *Am J Cardiol* 55:367-371, 1985.

108. Kadish AH, Buxton AE, Waxman HL, et al: Usefulness of electrophysiologic study to determine the clinical tolerance of arrhythmia recurrences during amiodarone therapy, *J Am Coll Cardiol* 10:90-96, 1987.

109. Haines DE, Lerman BB, Kron IL, et al: Surgical ablation of ventricular tachycardia with sequential map-guided subendocardial resection: electrophysiologic assessment and long-term follow-up, *Circulation* 77:131-141, 1988.

110. Krafchek J, Lawrie GM, Roberts R, et al: Surgical ablation of ventricular tachycardia: improved results with a map-guided regional approach, *Circulation* 73:1239-1247, 1986.

111. Gonska BD, Brune S, Bethge KP, et al: Radiofrequency catheter ablation in recurrent ventricular tachycardia, *Eur Heart J* 12:1257-1265, 1991.

112. Morady F, Harvey M, Kalbfleisch SJ, et al: Radiofrequency catheter ablation of ventricular tachycardia in patients with coronary artery disease, *Circulation* 87:363-372, 1993.

113. Mirowski M, Reid PR, Winkle RA, et al: Mortality in patients with implanted automatic defibrillators, *Ann Int Med* 98:585-588, 1983.

114. Powell AC, Fuchs T, Finkelstein DM, et al: Influence of implantable cardioverter-defibrillators on the long-term prognosis of survivors of out-of-hospital cardiac arrest, *Circulation* 88:1083-1092, 1993.

115. Newman D, Sauve MJ, Herre J, et al: Survival after implantation of the cardioverter defibrillator, *Am J Cardiol* 69:899-903, 1992.

116. Fogoros RN, Elson JJ, Bonnet CA, et al: Efficacy of the automatic implantable cardioverter-defibrillator in prolonging survival in patients with severe underlying cardiac disease, *J Am Coll Cardiol* 16:381-386, 1990.

117. Tchou PJ, Kadri N, Anderson J, et al: Automatic implantable cardioverter defibrillators and survival of patients with left ventricular dysfunction and malignant ventricular arrhythmias, *Ann Int Med* 109:529-534, 1988.

118. Fromer M, Brachmann J, Block M, et al: Efficacy of automatic multimodal device therapy for ventricular tachyarrhythmias as delivered by a new implantable pacing cardioverter-defibrillator, *Circulation* 86:363-374, 1992.

119. Kuppermann M, Luce BR, McGovern B, et al: An analysis of the cost effectiveness of the implantable defibrillator, *Circulation* 81:91-100, 1990.

120. Larsen GC, Marcolis AS, Sonnenberg FA, et al: Cost effectiveness of the implantable cardioverter-defibrillator: effect of improved battery life and comparison with amiodarone therapy, *J Am Coll Cardiol* 1323-1334, 1992.

121. Siebels J, Cappato R, Ruppel R, et al, the CASH Investigators: Preliminary results of the cardiac arrest study Hamburg (CASH), *Am J Cardiol* 72:109F-113F, 1993.

122. Connolly SJ, Gent M, Roberts RS, et al., and the CIDS Co-Investigators: Canadian Implantable Defibrillator Study (CIDS): study design and organization, *Am J Cardiol* 72:103F-108F, 1993.

Chapter 67

CARDIAC REHABILITATION: CONTROL OF ATHEROSCLEROSIS PROGRESSION

Martin J. Sullivan
Matthew Flynn
Meg Molloy
Frederick R. Cobb
Carola C. Ekelund
Leslie Domalik
James Spira
Mitchell Mroz
Lars G. Ekelund

In the 1940s and 1950s physicians usually treated myocardial infarction (MI) patients with 4 to 8 weeks of bed rest, oxygen, and sedation. Return to work was often delayed for 4 to 6 months, with progressive ambulation being started 1 week after hospital admission and heavier activities such as stair climbing allowed after about 1 month of recovery. In a 1970 survey less than one fourth of the 2491 responding physicians, who managed 70,000 patients, employed any standardized exercise test to gauge their patient's functional work capacity.[1] In this conservative climate cardiac rehabilitation efforts in patients with MI in the 1960s and 1970s focused on early mobilization, gradual increases in activity, and then aerobic exercise training. With the use of widespread exercise testing to identify patients with ongoing ischemia, a number of studies identified that exercise after MI was safe and could lead to improved aerobic fitness and delay in the onset of angina during exercise.[2-4] In

addition, the results of metaanalyses using large patient populations have demonstrated that exercise may reduce mortality and fatal reinfarction by approximately 20% in post-MI patients.[5-7]

From the 1960s to the early 1980s, cardiac rehabilitation efforts focused primarily on exercise training for patients who had had a MI. Over the last 10 years, the emphasis has shifted to include a multidisciplinary approach to reduce risk factors, alter diet, improve psychosocial functioning, and increase exercise performance. Today at least nine clinical trials[8-21] using serial angiography have demonstrated delayed progression or regression of coronary artery atherosclerotic lesions in patients who have undergone intensive risk factor modification interventions. These studies have heightened interest in medically modifying the progression of atherosclerosis. This may be accomplished by lowering serum low-density lipoprotein cholesterol (LDL-C) and

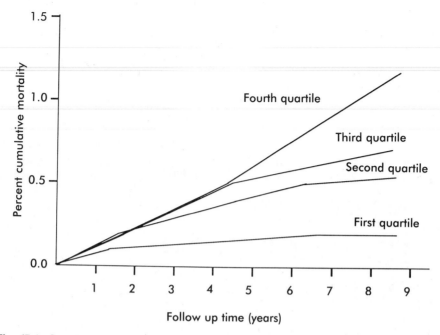

Fig. 67-1. Cumulative mortality as a function of fitness. (From Ekelund LG, Ekelund CC: Cardiac rehabilitation today: programs, their effects and practical guidelines, *Scand J Med Sci Sports* 2:190-196, 1992. Used by permission.)

raising serum high-density lipoprotein cholesterol (HDL-C) through use of cholesterol-altering drugs,[8-14] partial ileal bypass surgery,[15,16] and programs that increase exercise, change diet, and modify lifestyle.[17-21] Although the change in percent diameter stenosis with treatment has been small in these studies, it is important to note that these small changes are associated with a reduction in angina frequency,[17-19] stress-induced ischemia,[18,21] and cardiac morbidity, including the occurrence of unstable angina.[13,19,22] The finding that lifestyle changes, exercise, and antihyperlipidemic therapy can be used to improve both coronary anatomy and outcome when compared with usual care suggests that with the incorporation of intensive risk factor management programs, cardiac rehabilitation in the 1990s not only will offer the benefits of aerobic exercise but will also aim at the stabilization or reversal of coronary artery disease.

EXERCISE IN CARDIAC REHABILITATION
Exercise physiology

There is now clear evidence that a sedentary lifestyle is an independent risk factor for coronary artery disease.[23-26] In a study by Ekelund et al.,[25] the relative risk of a coronary heart disease death during 8.5 years of follow-up was 4.3 (least fit quartile compared with most fit quartile), adjusted for other risk factors (Fig. 67-1). This risk can be compared with relative risks of 4.3, 1.5, and 2.4 for current smokers, high blood pressure, and 1 mmol/L higher LDL-C, respectively. In this study, the mortality curves continue to diverge after 12.5 years of follow-up, indicating the long-term consequences of

fitness. In an 8-year follow-up study, Blair et al.[23] examined physical fitness and the risk of all-cause and cause-specific mortality in a group of 10,224 men and 3120 women. Fitness quintiles were established based on a maximal treadmill test time and adjusted for age and gender. The results showed a decline in age-adjusted all-cause mortality rates across fitness quintiles, low fit to high fit, for both men and women. These trends remained after adjustment for other potentially confounding variables. Lower mortality rates for cardiovascular disease and cancer were also observed in the higher fitness quintiles. It is important to note that most of the reduction in all-cause mortality was exhibited between the first and second quintiles, suggesting that even mild to moderate physical activity has a marked benefit on outcome. In addition to reducing mortality, some studies have shown that exercise decreases blood pressure at rest and during exercise, reduces triglycerides levels, and also may decrease the risk of developing thrombosis.[27,28] Exercise also leads to an increase in HDL-C,[29,30] an improvement in glucose tolerance,[31] and weight loss, which may lower LDL-C.

In patients with coronary artery disease, several studies have shown that exercise in a cardiac rehabilitation program decreases depression and anxiety, which in turn is associated with an improved quality of life.[32,33] Exercise training also leads to an increase in peak oxygen consumption, a training bradycardia, and an increase in peak arteriovenous oxygen difference.[34-37] Although exercise stroke volume may improve in selected patients after 12 months of intense exercise training,[38] most studies have not demonstrated an improvement in stroke volume, left ventricular (LV) ejection fraction, or intracardiac filling pressures after long-term exercise.[34-37,39,40] Thus, peripheral adaptations, including an increase in peak muscle blood flow[37] and increased aerobic enzyme content in skeletal muscle,[41] which lead to more efficient oxygen extraction, play an important role in the response to training in patients with coronary artery disease. It appears that elderly cardiac patients can also benefit from exercise training. Williams et al.[42] studied patients 65 years of age or older before and after a 12-week exercise program, which was initiated within 6 weeks of acute MI (AMI) or coronary artery bypass grafting (CABG). These elderly patients increased their physical work capacity 53% compared with 48% for patients 40 to 64 years of age.

Exercise training in patients with coronary artery disease also leads to an increase in the work rate at which myocardial ischemia or angina occurs.[43-51] Although some studies have demonstrated an increase in the rate-pressure product at which ischemia occurs after intensive training,[43,47-49] many have found that the onset of ischemia occurs at the same rate-pressure product but at a higher work rate after training.[44-46] Although a previous study at Duke by Cobb et al.[40] did not demonstrate an improvement in exercise-induced wall motion abnormalities with exercise training, studies by Froelicher et al.[50] and Sebrechts et al.[51] have suggested that thallium perfusion defects during stress testing tended to improve in patients after long-term exercise, especially if they had angina. However, these differences could be detected in only a subset of patients using computerized analysis of scintigrams. Although these results suggest that exercise conditioning in certain patients may improve myocardial perfusion during exercise, possibly because of improved collateral flow, increased coronary artery diameter, or improved coronary vasomotor tone,[47] it is generally believed that exercise alone does not improve myocardial oxygen delivery in most patients with coronary artery disease.

Effects on morbidity and mortality

In addition to increasing the work rate threshold at which myocardial ischemia occurs, there is evidence that cardiac rehabilitation may decrease overall mortality in patients who have had an MI.[5-7,52,53] Because of the large sample size that would be needed to test the effects of exercise on mortality in post-MI patients, most single-center studies have not shown a statistically significant treatment effect from cardiac rehabilitation. Early reports by Collins et al.[5] and Shephard et al.,[53] which pooled the results from several studies, found a 20% to 29% reduction in mortality in patients who exercised when compared with controls who did not exercise.

O'Connor et al.[7] examined morbidity and mortality from a metaanalysis of 22 randomized trials of rehabilitation of 4544 post-MI patients. As illustrated in Fig. 67-2, most studies had an overall beneficial effect on survival, although the confidence intervals for individual studies were wide. In treated patients during a 3-year follow-up period, the overall odds ratio was 0.80 for total mortality, 0.78 for cardiovascular mortality, and 0.75 for fatal reinfarction. These results are supported by Oldridge et al.,[6] who found a similar reduction in mortality in pooled data from ten studies. A recent study,[54] not included in these metaanalyses, involved 182 post-MI patients less than age 65 years who were placed into three groups: exercise training, risk factor counseling, and usual care. The number of deaths at 2 years was 0, 5, and 4 in the training, counseling, and usual care groups, respectively. If counseling and usual care were combined and tested against the training group, the difference in mortality was statistically significant ($P < 0.03$). These results support the findings from pooled analyses that cardiac rehabilitation with a focus on exercise training decreases mortality by about 20% in patients who have had an MI. This is similar to the reduction in mortality seen with β-blocker therapy.

Cardiac rehabilitation in patients with severe LV dysfunction

Patients with severe LV dysfunction caused by large infarctions have often been excluded from cardiac rehabilitation because it was feared that exercise might exacerbate chronic heart failure and worsen LV dilation. Although a small number of patients with severe systolic LV dysfunction have been included in earlier training studies,[38,40,55-57] it has been only in the last 10 years that research has been directed specifically at examining the training response in this group of patients. These studies have demonstrated an increase in peak exercise performance after training in patients with LV dysfunction with no change in LV ejection fraction or alterations in wall motion abnormalities,[58-69] and with few reports of exercise-related morbidity.

Studies in our laboratory have examined the effects of 4 to 6 months of exercise conditioning in patients with class I to III chronic heart failure caused by systolic LV dysfunction (LV ejection fraction 24% ± 10%).[59,60] Before and after 4 to 6 months of exercise training, patients underwent maximal graded bicycle exercise tests with measurement of expired gases and hemodynamics. Patients improved functional class from 2.4 ± 0.6 to 1.3 ± 0.7 ($P < 0.01$) and peak oxygen uptake (VO_2) from 1.11 ± 0.33 L/min (16.8 ± 3.7 ml/kg/min) to 1.40 ± 0.40 L/min (20.6 ± 4.7 mL/kg/min) (both $P < 0.01$) after training (Fig. 67-3, *A*). Cardiac output was unchanged during submaximal exercise (Fig. 67-3, *B*) but demonstrated a tendency to increase at maximal exercise

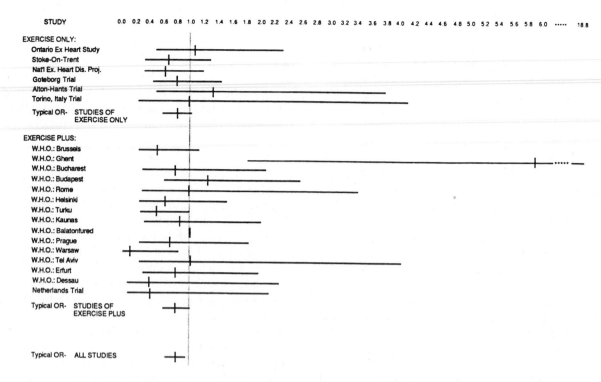

Fig. 67-2. Chart of effects of pooling from randomized trials of cardiac rehabilitation on the estimate of mortality 3 years after randomization. Short vertical lines indicate the point estimates; horizontal lines depict the 95% confidence intervals. (From O'Connor GT, Buring JE, Yusuf S, et al: An overview of randomized trials of rehabilitation with exercise after myocardial infarction, *Circulation* 80:235-244, 1989. Used by permission.)

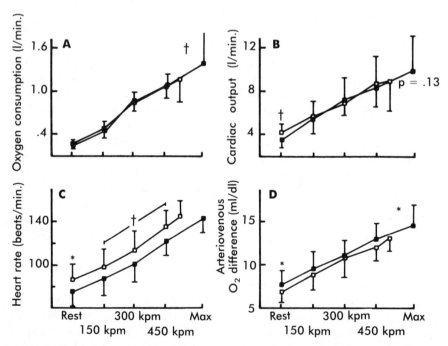

Fig. 67-3. Plots of resting and exercise (**A**) oxygen consumption, (**B**) cardiac output, (**C**) heart rate, and (**D**) systemic arteriovenous oxygen difference in patients before *(open boxes)* and after *(closed boxes)* training. *$P < 0.05$; †$P < 0.01$ by Wilcoxon signed rank test. (From Sullivan MJ, Higginbotham MB, Cobb FR: Exercise training in patients with severe left ventricular dysfunction: hemodynamic and metabolic effects, *Circulation* 78:506-515, 1988. Used by permission.)

from 8.9 ± 2.9 to 9.9 ± 3.2 L/min ($P = 0.13$). Heart rate (Fig. 67-3, *C*) was reduced at rest and during submaximal exercise but did not change at maximal exercise. Systemic arteriovenous oxygen (AVO_2) difference (Fig. 67-3, *D*) increased at rest, was unchanged during submaximal exercise, and increased at peak exercise from 13.1 ± 1.4 to 14.6 ± 2.3 mL/dL ($P < 0.05$). There were no differences in intracardiac pressures, LV ejection fraction, or cardiac volumes at rest or during exercise after training. Blood flow to a single leg increased at peak exercise from 2.5 ± 0.7 to 3.0 ± 0.8 L/min ($P < 0.01$). Arterial and femoral venous lactate concentrations were markedly reduced during submaximal exercise, suggesting that peripheral adaptations in skeletal muscle played a major role in improving exercise tolerance in our patients. This concept is supported by a recent study by Minotti et al.,[61] which demonstrated improved forearm metabolism, by phosphorus-31 nuclear magnetic resonance, before and after one-arm training in five patients with chronic heart failure. An important recent study by Coats et al.[62] also examined exercise training in patients with chronic heart failure (LV ejection fraction 16% ± 8%). Patients demonstrated a significant improvement in peak VO_2, an improvement in symptoms, and a decrease in heart rate during submaximal exercise after training. Sympathetic nervous system activation at rest, as indicated by power spectral analyses of heart rate and radiolabeled norepinephrine spillover studies, was decreased after training, suggesting that long-term exercise may actually decrease afterload and thereby delay progressive LV dysfunction in this disorder.

Based on recent studies and the experience at our institution[40,56,59,60] and others,[55-58,61-69] it appears that medically stable patients with moderate heart failure and severe systolic LV dysfunction can benefit from participation in long-term aerobic exercise conditioning programs. Patients with persistent rales and uncontrolled edema on maximal medical therapy with digoxin, diuretics, and vasodilators have not been included in most previous studies and generally do not participate in exercise programs at the Duke Center for Living. However, a preliminary report by Kavanagh et al.[67] demonstrated that selected patients with functional class III to IV chronic heart failure can achieve important benefits, including improved peak VO_2, increased anaerobic threshold, and a decrease in symptoms from a progressive walking program. Patients with active ischemia and severe LV dysfunction should probably undergo angiography, and, if possible, myocardial revascularization before exercise training.[69] Previous studies have indicated that this group may accrue the largest absolute mortality reduction from surgical (or possibly angioplasty) intervention[70,71] but may not achieve a marked training benefit if they undergo training with

ongoing severe ischemia.[69] Analogous to the CABG experience,[70,71] it is possible that patients with severe LV systolic dysfunction may achieve the largest benefit in terms of morbidity or mortality from exercise training precisely because they are at highest risk. However, studies examining the long-term effects of exercise training on morbidity and mortality in patients with LV dysfunctions are currently unavailable and are needed. In light of recent studies,[55-69] it appears that patients with severe LV dysfunction and stable class I to III heart failure controlled by medical therapy achieve a clinically important improvement in exercise performance and symptoms, comparable with that achieved by vasodilator therapy, through exercise conditioning.[72-74]

MEDICAL THERAPY TO DELAY ATHEROSCLEROSIS PROGRESSION

Over the past 20 years important advances have paved the way for current research efforts aimed at inducing regression or delaying progression of atherosclerosis. A pioneering study by Keys et al.,[75,76] the Seven Countries Study, found that populations eating diets with lower saturated fat content tended to have lower blood cholesterol levels and less coronary artery disease than populations with high-fat intakes. By the 1980s further epidemiologic evidence had accumulated that provided strong evidence that elevated serum cholesterol levels play an important role in the pathophysiology of atherosclerosis.[77-83] Relationships have been established between coronary artery disease and lifestyle factors such as smoking,[84-87] obesity,[88-90] physical inactivity,[23-26,91,92] and psychosocial factors,[93-98] including social isolation[95,96] and lower socioeconomic status.[97,98] The discovery of the LDL receptor by Brown and Goldstein[99] and the elucidation of links between defects in LDL receptor activity, familial hypercholesterolemia, and early atherosclerosis served to focus research efforts on reducing serum cholesterol in this disorder. In concert with these breakthroughs, a number of effective cholesterol-lowering drugs were developed that could be used to test the cholesterol hypothesis pharmacologically.[100] Subsequent to these achievements, four primary prevention trials published in the early to mid-1980s, the Helsinki Heart Study,[101] the Oslo intervention trial,[102] the Lipid Research Clinics Coronary Primary Prevention Trial,[103] and the Coronary Drug Project,[104] were able to demonstrate that atherosclerosis-related mortality could be reduced by lowering plasma cholesterol levels, although total mortality was generally unchanged. A recent metaanalysis by Holme[105] that examined data from 19 studies of lipid-lowering therapy demonstrated that reducing serum LDL-C levels improves cardiovascular and possibly all-cause mortality in patients with established coronary artery disease.

Over the past 60 years, a large number of studies using

animal models have demonstrated that atherosclerosis can be experimentally induced by increasing fat and cholesterol in the diet over a period of months to years in a number of species.[106] Early studies by Armstrong et al.,[107,108] which were some of the first to demonstrate atherosclerosis regression unequivocally in nonhuman primates, have been followed by a host of investigations of atherosclerosis induction and regression in monkeys by several laboratories.[109-111] Although alterations in blood lipid levels have been believed to be the primary factor affecting the course of atherosclerosis in animal models, several studies have demonstrated that psychosocial stress and the degree of exercise conditioning may play important roles in the development of atherosclerosis independent of blood lipids. Kramsh et al.[112] examined the effect of aerobic exercise on coronary artery lesions in cynomolgus monkeys fed an atherogenic diet. When compared with sedentary animals on a similar atherogenic diet, animals who exercised had higher HDL-C levels, larger coronary arteries with less atheromatous obstruction due to lipid deposition (less intimal thickening), and less arterial fibrosis.

Investigators[113-116] at Bowman-Gray Medical Center have produced a series of elegant studies demonstrating that psychosocial stress may accelerate atherosclerosis induction in nonhuman primates. This group has demonstrated that cynomolgus monkeys subjected to social stressors in addition to a high-cholesterol diet developed more extensive lesions than those given the diet alone.[113,114] In a separate study, these investigators[115] demonstrated that introduction of β-blocker therapy to monkeys subjected to high levels of social stress blunted the increase in atherosclerosis. This group has also demonstrated that social isolation may lead to an increase in atherogenesis.[116] This finding is supported by the results of Nerem et al.,[117] who demonstrated that rabbits given atherogenic diets develop less plaque area if there is physical contact with supportive laboratory staff compared with animals who were isolated and were not handled by laboratory staff. These studies indicate that psychosocial factors and exercise conditioning are important in mediating the induction of atherosclerosis in animals and suggest the possibility that they may also play a role in the induction and possibly the reversal of atherosclerosis in humans.

In addition to reducing luminal diameter, atherosclerosis has been demonstrated to have important effects on coronary vasomotor function in animals[118-123] and humans.[124-126] Atherosclerosis leads to endothelial dysfunction and impairment of relaxation or a paradoxical vasoconstrictive response to a number of stimuli.[119-122,126] Harrison et al.[119] have demonstrated that in monkeys subjected to a high-fat diet, impaired coronary artery relaxation because of atherosclerosis may return almost to baseline after resuming a normal diet. These data suggest that alterations in coronary vasomotor tone, which may play an important role in the clinical course of coronary artery disease in humans, may be involved in the clinical response to intensive lipid-lowering interventions in patients with coronary artery disease.

Coronary artery atherosclerosis intervention trials in humans

Although early studies examining serial angiograms indicated that spontaneous regression of atherosclerosis was a rare event in humans,[127] there have now been almost a dozen studies that have demonstrated delayed progression or, in some patients, regression of atherosclerosis after intensive risk factor modification.[8-22] In interpreting the results of the coronary angiographic trials examining atherosclerosis regression in humans, one should keep in mind that a variety of angiographic methods were used and that the duration of the trials varied from 1 to 10 years. Tables 67-1 and 67-2 outline the procedures and results of these trials and the differences in angiographic definitions that were used to determine whether regression or progression occurred. Table 67-1 outlines the protocols and angiographic findings from these trials and includes information on patient selection and interventions. Table 67-2 describes the changes in lipids observed.

The *National Heart, Lung, and Blood Institute (NHLBI) Type II Coronary Intervention Study*[8,9] was the first double-blind, randomized controlled trial to demonstrate an alteration in coronary lesions using serial angiography after diet and cholestyramine therapy. Although the NHLBI Type II Coronary Intervention Study did not lower LDL-C to levels currently achieved by intensive lifestyle changes and drug therapy, it was the first to suggest that lowering LDL-C could retard the rate of progression of coronary heart disease in patients with type II hyperlipoproteinemia.

Blankenhorn et al.[10,11,128] conducted the *Cholesterol Lowering Atherosclerosis Study (CLAS)*, which randomized 188 nonsmoking white men who had undergone coronary artery bypass surgery. All patients successfully completed a 6-week run-in period on colestipol and niacin and had at least a 15% reduction in total blood cholesterol level. Patients were then randomized to a diet deriving 22% of calories from fat with 125 mg of cholesterol/day plus colestipol and niacin or to a less restricted diet of 26% fat (10% polyunsaturated, 5% saturated) and 250 mg of cholesterol/day with a placebo. Those in the drug treatment arm showed favorable changes in serum lipid values compared with the placebo subjects: total cholesterol levels decreased 26% vs. 4%, LDL-C levels decreased 43% vs. 4%, and HDL-C levels increased 37% vs. no change (all $P < 0.001$). After 2 years, visually estimated regression of coronary atherosclerosis assessed by lumen diameter was seen in 16% of

Table 67-1. Clinical angiographic coronary atherosclerosis regression trials, 1984-1992*

Yr of publication	Name of trial principal investigators	Profile of subjects	No.	Study duration (yr)	Intervention groups	Group no.	Angiographic outcome			Method
							Regression (%)	No change (%)	Progression (%)	
1984	NHLBI Type II Coronary Intervention Trial Brensike J, Levy R	Men and women with angiographically documented CAD and type II hyperlipoproteinemia (age 21-55)	116	5	1. Cholestyramine	59	15	53	32	Visual
					2. Placebo + usual care	57	9	42	49	
					Both groups on low-cholesterol (300 mg/day), low–saturated fat diet (polyunsaturated/saturated fat ratio >2:1)					
1985	Leiden Intervention Trial Arntzenius A	Men (35) and women (4) with stable angina and documented CAD (age 33-59)	39	2	1. Low-fat (polyunsaturated/to saturated fat ratio at least 2:1), low-cholesterol (<100 mg/day) vegetarian diet	39	0	46	54	Visual and computer assisted
1987	CLAS-I Blankenhorn D	Nonsmoking, white, married, employed, nonhypertensive men who had undergone bypass surgery and who had completed a 6-wk trial of colestipol and niacin with at least 15% reduction of serum cholesterol (age 40-59)	162	2	No control group					Visual
					1. Colestipol + niacin + diet (22% of total calories from fat, 125 mg of cholesterol/day)	80	16	5	39	
					2. Placebo + diet (26% of total calories from fat, 250 mg of cholesterol/day)	82	2	37	61	

*NHLBI, National Heart, Lung, and Blood Institute Type II Coronary Intervention Study; CAD, coronary artery disease; CLAS, Cholesterol Lowering Atherosclerosis Study; UCSF, University of California at San Francisco.

Continued.

Table 67-1. Clinical angiographic coronary atherosclerosis regression trials, 1984-1992—cont'd

Yr of publication	Name of trial principal investigators	Profile of subjects	No.	Study duration (yr)	Intervention groups	Group no.	Regression (%)	No change (%)	Progression (%)	Method
1990	CLAS-II Cashin-Hemphill L	Same subjects as CLAS-I	103	4	Same as CLAS-I	56	18	52	30	Visual
						47	6	15	79	
1990	Lifestyle Heart Trial Ornish D	Men (36) and women (5) with angiographically documented CAD (age 40-74)	41	1	1. Lifestyle change group	22	82	0	18	Computer assisted
					2. Usual care	19	42	5	53	
1990	Familial Atherosclerosis Treatment Study (FATS) Brown G	Men <62 yr old with documented CAD and apolipoprotein >125 mg/dL (mean age 47)	120	2.5	1. Lovastatin + colestipol	38	32	47	21	Computer assisted
					2. Niacin + colestipol	36	39	36	25	
					3. Placebo + usual care	46	11	43	46	
1990	UCSF Familial Hypercholesterolemia Study Kane J	Men and women with heterozygous familial hypercholesterolemia (ages 19-72)	72	2	1. Combined cholesterol-lowering drug treatment (colestipol, niacin and/or lovastatin)	32	33	47	20	Computer assisted
					2. Diet alone or diet + bile acid-binding resin	40	13	46	41	

Year	Study	Population	N		Treatment group					Method
1990	Program on Surgical Control of the Hyperlipidemias (POSCH) Buchwald H	Men and women who had survived a first myocardial infarction (mean age 51)	175	10	1. Ileal bypass surgery	95	19	26	55	Visual
					2. Usual care	80	8	7	85	
1992	Heidelberg Study II Schuler G	Employed men recruited after angiography for angina (mean age 51 ± 6 yr)	92	1	1. Physical exercise + low-fat diet	40	32	45	23	Computer assisted
					2. Usual care + some diet training	52	17	35	48	
1992	St. Thomas' Atherosclerosis Regression Study (STARS) Watts G	Men with angiographic proof of atherosclerosis and responsive to cholestyramine (mean age 51)	74	3	1. Diet	26	38	47	15	Computer assisted
					2. Diet + cholestyramine	24	33	55	12	
					3. Usual care	24	4	40	46	

Table 67-2. Lipid changes in clinical coronary atherosclerosis regression trials*

Trial name	Yr/angio	Interventions	No. of patients	Base total chol	Trial total chol	Change total (%)	Base LDL-C	Trial LDL-C	Change LDL (%)	Base HDL-C	Trial HDL-C	Change HDL (%)
NHLBI	5	1. Cholestyramine	59	331	256	−23	259	178	−31	38	39	2
		2. Placebo	57	315	289	−8	244	219	−10	40	41	2
LEIDEN	2	1. Diet	39	277	243	−12	NR	NR	NR	39	38	−3
CLAS	2	1. Colestipol, niacin, diet	80	246	180	−27	171	97	−43	45	61	36
		2. Placebo + diet	82	243	232	−5	169	160	−5	44	44	2
LHT	1	1. Diet, exercise, stress management	56	227	172	−24	152	95	−38	39	38	−3
		2. Usual care	47	245	232	−5	167	158	−5	52	51	−2
FATS	2.5	1. Lovastatin + colestipol	38	275	182	−34	197	107	−46	35	41	17
		2. Niacin + colestipol	36	270	209	−23	190	129	−32	39	55	41
		3. Placebo + some colestipol	46	263	253	−4	175	162	−7	38	40	5
SCOR	2.2	1. Colestipol, niacin, lovastatin	40	378	261	−31	283	172	−39	47	59	26
		2. Diet + some cholestyramine	32	367	335	−9	275	243	−12	51	51	0
POSCH	10	1. Ileal bypass surgery	95	251	196	−22	179	110	−39	40	41	3
		2. Usual care	80	251	241	−4	179	167	−7	41	39	−5
Heidelberg	1	1. Exercise + diet	40	234	210	−10	164	149	−8	36	36	2
		2. Usual care + diet training	52	236	236	0	164	168	2	35	35	0
STARS	3.3	1. Diet (no placebo)	26	278	239	−25	193	162	−16	44	44	0
		2. Diet + cholestyramine	24	288	215	−14	203	130	−36	48	46	−14
		3. Usual care	24	273	268	−2	186	180	−3	47	47	−2

*Chol, Cholesterol; LDL-C, low-density lipoprotein–cholesterol; HDL-C, high-density lipoprotein–cholesterol; NHLBI, National Heart, Lung, and Blood Institute Type II Coronary Intervention Study; Leiden, Leiden Intervention Trial; CLAS, Cholesterol Lowering Atherosclerosis Study; LHT, Lifestyle Heart Trial; FATS, Familial Atherosclerosis Treatment Study; SCOR, UCSF Arrtherosclerosis Specialized Center of Research Intervention Trial; POSCH, Program on Surgical Control of the Hyperlipidemias; Heidelberg, Heidelberg Study II; STARS, St. Thomas' Atherosclerosis Regression Study.

the treatment group vs. 2% in the placebo group. On average both groups progressed; however, in the drug group fewer patients showed progression (39%) when compared with placebo (61%) (P < 0.001).

At 4 years, 103 men participating in CLAS-II, the follow-up to CLAS, underwent a third angiogram that demonstrated continuing favorable results for the drug-treated group.[12] In addition to less angiographic progression (48% vs. 87%), patients in the treatment group also demonstrated a reduction in the formation of new lesions in both grafted and nongrafted native coronary arteries. However, the number of new arterial occlusions was not different, supporting the concept that progression of more severe lesions to occlusion may be "thrombosis-driven," whereas progression of new and less severe lesions may be "lipid driven."

The double-blind, randomized controlled *Familial Atherosclerosis Treatment Study (FATS)* by Brown et al.[13] examined changes in coronary anatomy in 146 men (120 completing the trial) treated with lipid-lowering drugs and followed for 2½ years. All were less than age 62 years, with apolipoprotein B levels greater than 125 mg/dL and documented coronary artery disease, including at least one lesion greater than 50%. Subjects were randomized into three groups: lovastatin and colestipol (N = 38), niacin and colestipol (N = 36), or conventional therapy with placebo and colestipol if the LDL level exceeded the 90th percentile for age (N = 46). All were instructed in a diet containing 30% of calories from fat and 200 to 300 mg of cholesterol/day. All patients underwent quantitative coronary angiography with analysis of lesions in multiple coronary artery segments before and after 2½ years of follow-up.

Total cholesterol and LDL-C levels dropped 32% and 45% in the lovastatin/colestipol group and 23% and 32% in the niacin/colestipol group, respectively, whereas HDL-C levels rose 16% and 41%, respectively. Lipids were essentially unchanged in controls. With regression or progression defined as a change of 10% or more in diameter in at least one proximal lesion with no comparable opposite change, quantitative arteriography demonstrated regression in 32% of the lovastatin/colestipol group, 39% of the niacin/colestipol group, and 11% of the control group, whereas progression occurred in 21%, 25%, and 46%, respectively.

An important finding of the FATS was that there was a reduction in adverse clinical events in treated patients when compared with controls (P < 0.05). To relate angiographic changes with clinical events, subjects were placed into three terciles based on percent increase in stenosis averaged from all lesions. Those in the lowest tercile (least progression) had one clinical event, the middle group had five clinical events, and the terciles with greatest overall increase in stenosis had nine clinical events. In a follow-up review of events, these investiga-

tors demonstrated that 1 of 683 insignificant lesions in the treatment groups and 8 of 414 insignificant lesions in the placebo group progressed to become symptomatic culprit lesions during the study.[129] These data provide evidence that intensive risk factor reduction stabilizes atheromatous plaques to prevent rupture during follow-up. Although the overall angiographic changes seen in this study were minor, they were linked to significant decreases in clinical events.

The UCSF Arteriosclerosis Specialized Center of Research Intervention Trial (SCOR) by Kane et al.[14] demonstrated delayed lesion progression in patients with documented coronary atherosclerosis and heterozygous familial hypercholesterolemia (average total cholesterol ≥ 373 mg/dL) using a combination of colestipol, niacin, and lovastatin. Using the same criteria as the FATS trial, 33% (13 of 40) of the pharmacologically-treated group demonstrated regression vs. 13% (4 of 32) of the control group. Progression occurred in 20% of the intervention group vs. 41% of controls.

Watts et al.[19] in the *St. Thomas' Atherosclerosis Regression Study (STARS)* examined the effects of dietary changes with or without cholestyramine in men with angina or previous MI. The St. Thomas diet limited total fat intake to 27% of calories, with no more than 10% of calories from saturated fat and at least 8% of calories coming from omega-6 and omega-3 polyunsaturated fats. In addition, fiber intake was increased and cholesterol level was limited to 100 mg for every 1000 kcal consumed.

Total cholesterol and LDL-C levels dropped 25% and 36% in the diet and cholestyramine group (N = 24) and 14% and 16% in the diet-alone group (N = 26), respectively. HDL-C levels dropped 4% in the diet and cholestyramine group but remained the same in the diet-alone group. Quantitative arteriography performed at baseline and after an average of 3.3 years revealed that almost half (46%) of those receiving usual care showed progression of coronary atherosclerosis vs. only 12% of those receiving diet and cholestyramine and 15% of those receiving diet alone. Regression was seen in 4% of the usual care group and in 33% and 38% of the diet plus cholestyramine and diet-alone groups, respectively. As in previous studies, lesions with greater than 50% stenosis demonstrated the most improvement. The large differences between the usual care and treatment groups (all intergroup P < 0.02) in the percent of patients exhibiting progression or regression indicate that diet alone can delay progression of coronary atherosclerosis. In addition to demonstrating anatomic effects of these diet-based therapies, the two treatment groups had fewer clinical cardiac events than the usual care group (P < 0.05) and had less angina compared with baseline (P < 0.05), whereas angina in controls did not change.

In the blinded, randomized controlled *Lifestyle Heart*

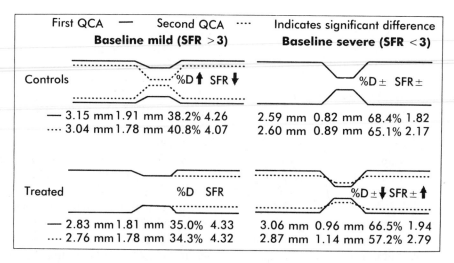

Fig. 67-4. Representation of average changes in lesion geometry for mild and severe lesions from both treated and untreated patients on the Lifestyle Heart Trial. (From Gould KL, Ornish D, Kirkeeide R, et al: Improved stenosis geometry by quantitative coronary arteriography after vigorous risk factor modification, *Am J Cardiol* 69:845-853, 1992. Used by permission.)

Trial, Ornish et al.[17] examined coronary anatomy before and after a comprehensive set of diet, exercise, and behavioral interventions. All participants in this 1-year study had significant coronary atherosclerosis and a left ventricular ejection fraction greater than 25% and were not taking lipid-lowering medications. Originally 48 men and women were randomized, and 41 completed the trial. The treatment group (N = 22) was assigned to a low-fat (10% of calories from fat) vegetarian diet, 1-hour/day of stress management, including stretching and progressive relaxation, and 3 hours or more of aerobic exercise/week. The trial began with 1 week-long retreat to introduce patients to the intervention. Throughout the year patients participated in two support group sessions/week, which were led by a clinical psychologist. These sessions focused on strategies for adhering to the program, improving communication skills, expression of emotions, and reducing hostility. Controls (N = 19) were given usual care and were counseled to follow a 30% fat diet and exercise.

Total cholesterol and LDL-C levels were reduced 24% and 37% in the intervention group vs. only 5% and 6% in controls, respectively. HDL-C levels did not change in either group. Treatment subjects also lost an average of 10 kg, whereas controls gained 1 kg. The incidence of angina dropped 91% in the treatment group with additional reductions in angina severity and duration, whereas controls experienced a 165% increase in angina incidence ($P < 0.01$). Quantitative angiography at 1 year revealed progression in 18% of the treatment group and 53% of controls and regression in 82% of treated patients and 42% of controls. It is important to note that progression and regression here were defined by a net directional change in global lesion severity. When more restrictive criteria (a minimum change in luminal diameter of 0.1 mm or a 10% change in lesion severity) were used to define progression or regression, 41% of the intervention group showed regression.[130]

Gould et al.[130] have carefully analyzed changes in lesions from angiograms of patients from this study. Using measures of lesion geometry, including entrance and exit angles, these investigators calculated coronary flow reserve in both groups before and after the study. As illustrated in Fig. 67-4, insignificant coronary artery lesions (<50% stenosis or flow reserve >3) tended to demonstrate overall progression in control patients (progression in segments proximal and distal to the lesion and lesion segments). Patients in the treatment group showed progression in the distal segment only. These changes led to a decrease in flow reserve in mild lesions in control patients over a 1-year follow-up interval. Lesions that at baseline were severe and had severely reduced flow reserve were not significantly different in the control group but demonstrated changes in all segments in treated patients. With intensive lifestyle changes, there was a decrease in luminal diameter in segments proximal and distal to the lesion with an increase in luminal diameter at the lesion. This remodeling improved minimal luminal diameter, reduced entrance and exit angles, and reduced percent stenosis from 66.5% to 57.5%, leading to a significant improvement in calculated coronary flow reserve. This analysis suggests that small to moderate changes in significant coronary stenosis as a result of intensive risk factor modification may be accomplished by physiologically significant improvements in coronary flow

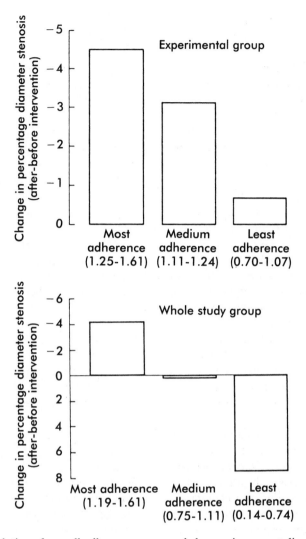

Fig. 67-5. Correlation of overall adherence score and changes in percent diameter stenosis in both treated and untreated patients from the Lifestyle Heart Trial. (From Ornish D, Brown SE, Scherwitz LW: Can lifestyle changes reverse coronary heart disease? The Lifestyle Heart Trial, *Lancet* 336:129-133, 1990. Used by permission.)

reserve. This is consistent with the finding that ischemia as measured by positron emission tomography after pharmacologic stress testing was reduced in patients in the treatment arm after this 1-year intervention. The LHT[17] was the first study to demonstrate that lesion progression could be slowed using dietary and lifestyle changes alone. Another important finding in this study was that the degree of adherence to the diet, exercise, and stress management regimen correlated with lesion changes in a dose-response fashion, as illustrated in Fig. 67-5. However, because all treated patients received multiple interventions simultaneously, the relative contribution of each facet of the intervention remains to be determined.

Schuler et al.[18,21] has published both a nonrandomized case control study and a randomized trial to examine the effects of exercise and a 20% fat diet in patients with coronary artery disease. The intervention groups in both studies received a 3-week in-hospital supervised initiation into a diet with less than 20% of calories from fat and less than 200 mg of cholesterol/day. In addition, they were asked to exercise at home on a bicycle ergometer for a minimum of 30 minutes daily and to participate in two intensive 60-minute group exercise sessions weekly. Controls received a 1-week in-hospital initiation into a prudent diet and were given instructions to exercise.

In the case-controlled study, quantitative angiographic analysis found regression of coronary atherosclerosis in 39% (7 of 18) of the treated patients vs. 6% (1 of 18) of case controls, whereas progression occurred in 28% (5 of 18) of the treatment group and 33% (6 to 18) of case controls.[18] Interestingly, treatment patients experiencing either regression or progression had very similar lipid profiles, and other risk factors could not account for the outcome differences. Controls, who had overall progression, had higher total cholesterol levels compared with controls who had no angiographic changes.

The larger randomized study by Schuler et al.[21] again found overall delayed lesion progression in the exercise and diet group vs. controls. Originally 111 men were randomized and began therapy, with 40 of 50 treatment subjects and 52 of 56 controls completing the study. In treated subjects total cholesterol levels dropped from 236 to 210 (11%), LDL-C levels dropped from 164 to 149 (9%), and HDL-C levels remained unchanged at 36, whereas controls had virtually no changes in lipid levels. Quantitative angiography demonstrated overall regression of coronary lesions in 32% of treated subjects and 17% of controls and overall progression in 23% and 48%, respectively. This group has also reviewed the effects of exercise intensity on coronary artery diameter in both treatment and control patients.[131] In both groups there was a modest relationship between weekly energy expenditure and increase in coronary artery luminal diameter. Patients with intensive exercise energy regimens (25 hours of aerobic exercise/week) tended to have the best angiographic outcomes. These data suggest that exercise influences coronary artery luminal diameter in humans. This trial also examined exercise-induced ischemia using exercise thallium scintigraphy before and after the intervention. Patients in the treatment group demonstrated less myocardial ischemia after the intervention, whereas there was no change in controls. This was accompanied by less exercise-induced angina in treated patients. This finding that inducible ischemia was reduced in treated patients is of potentially great importance because previous studies have not convincingly demonstrated that myocardial ischemia at a given rate-pressure product has been improved by exercise alone.[44,45]

Although the overall changes in minimal luminal areas were small in most treated patients in these trials, it appears that these minor changes were translated into a significant improvement in clinical outcome. This is supported by the finding that cardiovascular morbidity,[13,19] angina frequency,[17,19] and stress-induced myocardial ischemia[17,18,21] were reduced after intensive risk factor management. Several possible mechanisms may contribute to this reported clinical improvement, including (1) plaque stabilization, leading to a reduction in the incidence of plaque rupture[129]; (2) improved coronary vasomotor tone; and (3) increased coronary luminal diameter. These results,[18,21] when combined with the findings of the LHT,[17] suggest that intensive risk-factor intervention programs that can be applied through existing cardiac rehabilitation facilities may lead to improved coronary luminal diameter, improved myocardial blood flow, and reduced myocardial ischemia in patients with coronary artery disease.

COMPONENTS OF A COMPREHENSIVE CARDIAC REHABILITATION PROGRAM
Exercise program

The primary goals of an exercise program are to reduce cardiovascular morbidity,[5-7] increase the angina threshold,[43-51] and improve aerobic fitness, muscle strength, muscle endurance, and flexibility.[132] Most exercise programs are based on supervised outpatient activities, with the patient coming to the rehabilitation center three times weekly for 1 to 1.5 hours each session. Some hospitals use home-based exercise programs for low-risk patients.[133,134] The patient exercises at home on a stationary bike or by walking while using a portable heart rate monitor. To enhance compliance and review progress, a staff person telephones twice weekly, and the patient transmits his or her electrocardiogram during 1 minute of exercise and during 1 minute immediately after exercise. When home exercise was compared with supervised facility-based training with clinically uncomplicated MI patients, no difference was seen in the increase in functional capacity.[134,135] Although this approach has the advantage of being cost-effective and may reach patients from a wider geographic area, it may not meet the needs of high-risk patients.

The exercise prescription for cardiovascular fitness consists of the following four components: intensity, duration, frequency, and mode of activity. Usually exercise intensity is described as a percentage of individual functional capacity, using heart rate to calculate the appropriate level. The general recommendation for exercise intensity is 60% to 85% of maximal oxygen uptake,[132] although several studies suggest potential health benefits of regular exercise at lower intensity levels if combined with longer duration and higher frequency.[23,135] For totally sedentary individuals even a moderate level of activity such as walking may be beneficial in reducing cardiovascular events.[23] The most accurate way to calculate the prescribed intensity level, or training range (TR), is to obtain data from an exercise stress test and use the heart rate (HR) reserve method (Karvonen's formula) as follows:

Maximal HR (from exercise test) − Resting HR = HR reserve

HR reserve × (0.6 − 0.85) + Resting HR = TR

This will give a training intensity of approximately 60% to 85% of maximal oxygen uptake.[132] Higher-intensity exercise is often associated with increased risk of orthopedic injuries and lower compliance.[136-139] To optimize aerobic capacity, patients should exercise 20 to 45 minutes/day 3 to 5 days/week. Any activity that uses large-muscle groups in rhythmic, dynamic movements, such as walking, jogging, cycling, swimming, calisthenics, or cross-country skiing, will lead to aerobic conditioning. Aerobic exercise, as well as strength and flexibility training, should begin with an initial 5- to 10-minute warm-up period to adapt the cardiovascular system to the workout. It is equally important to allow 5 to 10 minutes at the end of the session for cooling down. Proper footwear should be emphasized when weight-bearing activities such as walking, jogging, or running are the aerobic exercise of choice. A properly-fitted running shoe, together with a gradually increased exercise prescription, is the best way to prevent foot, leg, and knee injuries. Exercise clothes should be made of breathable, sweat-absorbent material and worn in layers according to the air temperature, humidity, and wind-chill factor.

Many vocational tasks and activities of daily life include various types of lifting, carrying, or pushing. Therefore, it is important that the exercise program also improves muscle strength and endurance. Resistance exercise has been shown to be safe for patients with cardiovascular disease, even at a relatively high percentage of maximum voluntary contraction.[140,141] To avoid an excessive blood pressure response, rhythmic, dynamic movements during calisthenics or weightlifting should be used. Patients should emphasize the number of repetitions completed rather than the amount of weight lifted and should perform full range of motion in each exercise. Strengthening exercises should be performed two to three times weekly with a rest day in between. Stiffness and lack of normal range of motion in joints seen among the elderly is not entirely a function of age but rather, may result from a sedentary lifestyle. This condition may predispose the individual to exercise-related injuries; therefore, flexibility exercises designed to increase the extensibility of the muscles and ligaments by active or passive movements should be done three times weekly.

To translate the results of recent angiographic trials into clinical practice, cardiac rehabilitation programs will need to shift their focus from exercise alone to effective multifactorial risk-factor intervention programs. Facility-based programs like the Duke Center for Living have staffs composed of physicians, dietitians, exercise physiologists, psychologists, and physical therapists who provide all rehabilitation services in one setting. Patients with coronary artery disease are enrolled in a comprehensive risk-factor education program that includes exercise, nutritional education, cooking schools, patient support groups, and stress reduction classes. In this setting, patients can learn from both staff and each other in formal or informal support groups and maximize their ability to make important lifestyle changes.

Nutrition management of coronary artery disease

Nutrition intervention programs are a cornerstone of therapy in the prevention and treatment of coronary artery disease.[142-147] In many states nutrition education is required by law for cardiac rehabilitation patients and is provided by registered dietitians as part of the health care team. Although many individuals who have just experienced a heart attack or heart surgery are ready to change their eating patterns, they do not have the knowledge or behavioral skills to do this in a therapeutically appropriate manner. Questions and fears about diet are common among patients in a cardiac rehabilitation setting.

Three nutritional factors have been identified as atherogenic in humans: dietary saturated fatty acids (found in coconut and palm oil, animal fat and hydrogenated fat, shortening, and cocoa butter), which are the principal nutritional culprits in hyperlipidemia; excess caloric intake leading to obesity; and dietary cholesterol (found in meats, poultry, egg yolks, and dairy foods), which has an effect on lipids that is about half that of the effect of saturated fat intake.[142,146,148] Decreasing these three factors has been shown to significantly reduce plasma total cholesterol and LDL-C levels and is the main thrust of nutritional counseling in these patients. The National Cholesterol Education Program of the National Heart, Lung, and Blood Institute suggests the following algorithm for the dietary treatment of hyperlipidemia[145]: Step 1 dietary treatment calls for an intake of saturated fat of less than 10% of calories, total fat intake of less than 30% of calories, and dietary cholesterol intake of less than 300 mg/day. Step 2 calls for further reduction of saturated fat intake to less than 7% of calories and of dietary cholesterol to less than 200 mg/day.[145] Several dietary factors in addition to the amount of dietary saturated fats and cholesterol may alter serum lipid levels. First, the omega-6 class of polyunsaturated fats (corn oil, safflower oil, cottonseed oil) has been shown to reduce total and LDL-C levels. However, these oils may lower HDL-C levels and are linked with free-radical injury, a process that may be atherogenic because it is linked to oxidative modification of LDL-C.[149] Second, when substituted for saturated fatty acids, monounsaturated fatty acids (found in canola oil, olive oil, sesame oil, and peanut oil and the foods from which these oils are extracted) are known to lower total cholesterol and LDL-C levels yet do not lower the HDL-C levels.[142,145,148] Third, omega-3 fatty acids (found in cold-water fish such as mackerel, tuna, salmon, and bluefish), are hypotriglyceridemic and may be hypocholesterolemic.[143] Fourth, soluble fiber (found in barley, oats, legumes, pectin, gums, oranges, and apples), when added to a low-fat diet, can reduce plasma total cholesterol levels by 6% to 19%.[144] Fifth, when individuals are guided to lower the fat in their diets, a reciprocal relationship with dietary carbohydrate is invoked that has been shown to improve lipid levels and other cardiovascular risk factors. Most Americans consume approximately 45% of calories from carbohydrate and would benefit from increasing their carbohydrate intake to at least 55% to up to 70% of calories from carbohydrate. However, an increase in carbohydrate intake can raise triglyceride levels and lower the HDL level in some individuals[146]; therefore, gradual dietary changes and blood glucose monitoring for diabetics should be encouraged. Finally, a vegetarian pattern of eating, which usually incorporates the dietary guidelines for preventing and treating hyperlipidemia described earlier, has been shown to lower lipid levels.[142,144] Some studies also suggest that vegetarianism may favorably affect the lipid profile independent of the factors just listed.[150] Careful planning of a vegetarian diet is required to assure an adequate vitamin and nutrient intake and to avoid a high-fat, high–saturated fat intake, which often occurs when individuals omit meat.

Proceedings from a 1991 NHLBI Consensus Workshop on the role of antioxidants in the prevention of human atherosclerosis suggested that antioxidants may favorably affect the progression of atherosclerosis.[151] Several lines of evidence support the concept that antioxidants are beneficial in humans: First, increased vitamin E intake has been demonstrated to be associated with reduced rates of ischemic heart disease.[152-154] Second, some, but not all, studies suggest an association between vitamin C intake, overall mortality, and elevated HDL levels.[156] Finally, β-carotene supplementation may reduce the incidence of recurrent MI in men.[151] Although studies do not support the routine clinical use of antioxidants, the proceedings of the conference state, "It is doubtful that much is gained by increasing intake of vitamin E above 400-800 units/day; the intake of vitamin C above 1 g has little or no additional effect on plasma levels of vitamin C; and β-carotene, aside from causing skin pigmentation, has no known toxic side effects and therefore can be administered in maximum 'nonyellowing' doses."[151] In light of recent data indicating that high levels of plasma ferritin are linked to possible oxidation of LDL and to increased cardiovascular events, [156] large doses of vitamin C must be viewed with caution because ascorbic acid increases iron absorption. Although selenium, zinc, and copper have been implicated as having a role in oxidation and antioxidation,[151] more research is needed to make recommendations for these trace minerals other than the U.S. Recommended Dietary Allowances. Studies are currently underway to examine the role of antioxidants in altering atherosclerosis progression in humans.

It has become increasingly evident that acute thrombosis plays a major role in the development of an MI. Accordingly, the role of thrombosis and hemostatic factors and their interactions with nutrients have become the subject of intense research. Limited data suggest that excessive intake of saturated fatty acids is associated with an increased tendency for thrombosis. In contrast, high intake of omega-3 fatty acids has been shown to be antithrombogenic.[146] Although it is not possible to obtain these doses of omega-3 fatty acids from the diet, it is reasonable to suggest frequent consumption of seafood, which is rich in omega-3 fatty acids.

Obesity and an increased waist/hip ratio are possible risk factors for coronary heart disease. Although it has been demonstrated that being overweight is linked with the development of type II diabetes and hypertension, the effect on lipoprotein levels is mixed.[146] Excessive caloric intake raises triglyceride levels and lowers HDL-C levels. Dietary fat has been linked with the deposition of body fat and, as the most calorically dense nutrient, is targeted for reduction in the effort to reduce weight. Increased waist/hip ratios with excessive abdominal fat appears to be a cardiovascular risk factor. A moderate weight loss rate (½-2 lb/week) is optimal for maintaining muscle, bone mass, metabolic rate and for promoting long-term behavioral changes.

Type II, or adult-onset, diabetes mellitus is a risk factor for heart disease.[146] Among most persons with type II diabetes, the primary nutrition-related issue is being overweight or obese. Because 80% of type II diabetics are obese, weight reduction is the primary goal. Modification of dietary fat is the primary method for accomplishing weight loss; therefore, cardiovascular risk factors may be concurrently modified as well. The diabetic diet is essentially the same as the step 1 cardiovascular diet, so no conflicts arise with the nutritional needs of the diabetic with coronary artery disease.

Hypertension remains a risk factor for cardiovascular morbidity and mortality. Currently the Joint National Committee on Detection, Evaluation and Treatment of High Blood Pressure of the NHLBI, National Institutes of Health, recommends three nutrition interventions in the treatment of high blood pressure: caloric restriction for weight reduction, reduced consumption of alcohol, and sodium restriction. In addition to these widely established guidelines, epidemiologic, clinical, and animal data suggest that increasing dietary potassium and calcium levels may have beneficial effects on blood pressure.[157]

The American Heart Association, as well as many other health organizations, has long advised the public to reduce fat intake from the current U.S. consumption level of 37% to 40% of total calories to less than 30% of total calories.[145,146] The rationale for reducing fat intake is supported by the finding that such a decrease simultaneously promotes restricting the intake of saturated fat and cholesterol. In addition, dietary composition modification promotes weight reduction, which assists in blood pressure control and normalization of blood glucose levels among diabetics.

Table 67-3. Nutrition guidelines for heart health and weight control*

1. Reduce your intake of saturated fats as much as possible to lower your blood cholesterol level.
2. Stay within your fat gram budget to reach and maintain a healthy body weight. Weight loss should not exceed ½ to 2 lb/wk.
3. For at least half of your fat gram budget, choose mono- and unsaturated fats to lower your blood cholesterol level and maintain your HDL-C level.
4. Limit polyunsaturated fats to stay within your fat gram budget.
5. If you have high blood triglyceride levels, choose polyunsaturated fats rich in omega-3 fatty acids.
6. Limit your cholesterol intake to 200-300 mg/day.
7. Choose lean protein sources and limit your protein intake to 4-6 oz/day.
8. Increase your intake of complex carbohydrates (starches) to promote weight control and optimize blood cholesterol, blood pressure, and blood sugar.
9. Increase your intake of fruits, vegetables, and lowfat nonfat dairy foods for optimal blood pressure, bone health, and nutritional status.
10. If you drink alcohol, do so in moderation (<1-2 drinks each day).
11. Moderate your sodium intake to 1100-3300 mg sodium/day.
12. Gradually develop healthful eating and regular exercise habits for a balanced lifestyle.

*HDL, High-density lipoprotein.

The optimal dietary fat intake for patients with coronary artery disease has yet to be determined. It is important to note that patients in the usual care arms of the angiographic trials generally consumed a diet with 30% of calories from fat and had overall worsening of atherosclerosis on angiographic follow-up. In light of the recent recommendation that patients with coronary artery disease should have LDL-C levels less than 100 mg/dL and the findings of recent angiographic trials demonstrating improved stenosis severity in some patients treated with lower-fat diets (10%-27% of calories), it appears prudent for patients with coronary artery disease to lower fat intake to less than 25% of calories from fat. For patients who desire the best outcome from lifestyle changes in the management of coronary artery disease or those with advanced coronary artery disease, it may be advisable to reduce fat to 15% to 25% of total calories.

The nutrition and health research described earlier can be translated into the specific cardiac rehabilitation dietary guidelines found in Table 67-3. Within the cardiac rehabilitation program at the Duke Center for Living, the Sarah W. Stedman Nutrition Center has developed a nonjudgmental, positive approach to assist each client to develop nutritional knowledge, skills, and behaviors to promote his or her optimal health.

Clients participate in a cardiovascular and weight management peer-group program. The program provides individuals with the tools they need to begin assessing their eating patterns and developing their individual nutrition prescription. Table 67-4 is a food frequency questionnaire used for assessing dietary habits. It can provide a road map for practical ways to begin reducing fat intake. Because dietary fat is a major focus of this approach, patients are made aware of their fat gram budget for each day. Table 67-5 is an algorithm that allows patients to compute their caloric needs and develop their daily fat gram budget to reach their weight goal. At the Duke Center for Living, clients are guided to lower their fat intake to less than 25% of total calories while making changes at their own pace. Table 67-6 defines the fat gram amounts for various caloric requirements representing five different percentage fat levels. At the end of this initial program, clients design a personal nutrition plan that includes their goals for changing specific food patterns and identifies additional nutrition skills and behaviors they are required to implement to fulfill their nutrition prescription.

Patient compliance with diet

Perhaps the most difficult task a health professional has to deal with is that of patient compliance with a health care prescription, whether it be medication, nutrition, exercise, stress management, or other therapy. Several factors have been shown to dramatically enhance patient adherence in the area of nutrition. These include but are certainly not limited to the individual's readiness to change, a participatory mode of nutrition education with frequent follow-up, a focus on skill-building activities, social support, and an emphasis on a positive approach that allows the individual to move at his or her own pace and make personal decisions concerning nutritional patterns.[158-161] The process of dietary change is not an overnight one. Continuous support, reinforcement, and goal-setting is necessary for long-term dietary changes. At the Duke Center for Living, participatory nutrition programs are provided to effectively promote nutrition changes. We also combine nutrition education with patient support groups to emphasize the importance of lifestyle changes in these patients. Restaurant and supermarket programs and cooking schools are offered where new styles of food purchasing, cooking, and dining out are modeled and reinforced. A participatory style of assessment using a few simple questions to determine what changes the individual has already made may better facilitate nutrition behavior changes. The content of the education sessions varies so that it conforms to the patient's lifestyle. For example, if the patient never cooks, a session on how to select lean foods from a restaurant would provide a critical tool

Table 67-4. How does your diet measure up?

Circle the answer that best describes the way you have been eating recently.
  1. How much protein do you usually eat each day?*
     1. I mainly eat beans, grain, vegetables, and low-fat foods for protein.
     2. I eat 4 to 6 oz of seafood, poultry, or lean red meats per day.
     3. I eat 6 to 10 oz of meat, poultry, or seafood per day.
     4. I eat 10 or more oz of meat, poultry, or seafood per day.
  2. How much cheese do you eat per week?
     1. I avoid cheese altogether.
     2. I use only nonfat or low-fat cheese such as part skim ricotta, diet, or low-fat cottage cheese.
     3. I eat whole milk cheese once or twice per week (e.g., cheddar, Swiss, Monterey Jack).
     4. I eat whole milk cheese three or more times per week.
  3. What type of dairy foods do you use?
     1. I use only skim, ½% or 1% milk, nonfat or low-fat yogurt.
     2. I use skim milk but use regular yogurt.
     3. I use 2% milk, whole milk, or whole yogurt.
  4. How many egg yolks do you use per week?
     1. I eat 2 egg yolks or less per week.
     2. I eat 3 to 5 egg yolks per week.
     3. I eat 5 or more egg yolks per week.
  5. How often do you usually eat lunchmeat, hot dogs, corned beef, spareribs, sausage or bacon?
     1. I do not eat any of these meats.
     2. I eat them about once per week.
     3. I eat them about two to four times per week.
     4. I eat more than four servings per week.
  6. How many baked goods and how much ice cream do you usually eat (examples: cake, cookies, coffee cakes, sweet rolls, donuts)?
     1. I avoid commercial baked goods and ice cream or use the nonfat varieties.
     2. I eat commercial baked goods or ice cream once per week.
     3. I eat commercial baked goods or ice cream two to four times per week.
     4. I eat commercial baked goods or ice cream more than four times per week.
  7. What is the main type of fat you use in cooking?
     1. I use olive oil or canola oil.
     2. I use safflower, sunflower, corn, or soybean oil.
     3. I use shortening, fatback, or bacon drippings.
  8. How often do you eat snack foods such as chips, fries, or party crackers?
     1. I avoid these snack foods or choose nonfat or low-fat ones.
     2. I eat one serving of these snacks per week.
     3. I eat these snacks two to four times per week.
     4. I eat snack foods more than four times per week.
  9. What spread do you usually use on bread, vegetables, etc.?
     1. I don't use any spread.
     2. I use soft (tub) or diet margarine.
     3. I use stick margarine.
     4. I use butter.
 10. How often do you eat fresh or frozen fruits and vegetables?
     1. I eat at least four servings of both fruits and vegetables per day.
     2. I eat two or three servings of both fruits and vegetables each day.
     3. I eat less than two servings of both fruits and vegetables each day.
 11. How many servings of complex carbohydrates (starches) do you eat each day?
     1. I eat at least six to eleven servings per day.
     2. I eat three to five servings per day.
     3. I eat two or less servings per day.
Add up the numbers of your responses: _____
Higher scores indicate more fat and cholesterol. A score of 13 or 14 shows that you have a healthful, low-fat way of eating. A score of 19 or 20 shows that you have made some good choices but can still improve the balance of your foods. If you scored above 21, you have identified many fat sources in your foods. With a few changes you can dramatically improve your heart health.

*3 oz of meat, fish, or poultry is one of the following: one regular hamburger, one chicken breast, one chicken leg (thigh and drumstick), one pork chop, or three slices of presliced luncheon meat.

Table 67-5. Determine your daily fat gram budget

		Answer here
Step 1.	Write your current weight here.	_____ lb
Step 2.	Multiply your weight × 10 =	_____
Step 3.	If you want to improve your body composition (lose unwanted inches and tone up your body shape), maintain weight or lose less than 10 lb, **add 500** to **step 2** to get your daily calorie needs.	_____ calories
Step 4a.	If you want to lose 10, 15, 20, or 25 lb, use **step 2** as your daily calorie needs.	_____ calories
Step 4b.	If you want to lose between 25 and 75 lb, **subtract 500** from **step 2** to get your daily calorie needs.	_____ calories
Step 4c.	If you want to lose more than 75 lb, **subtract 1000** from **step 2** to get your daily calorie needs.	_____ calories
Step 5.	If you want to gain weight, **add 1000** to **step 2** to get your daily calorie needs.	_____ calories
Step 6.	We have assumed that you are exercising 3 to 5 times/wk in your prescribed training range. If you exercise more than 5 days/wk, ask your dietitian to adjust your calorie requirements.	
Step 7.	Use the chart below to determine your daily fat gram budget.	

Daily Fat Gram Budget Chart (25% of Calories from Fat)

Calorie needs	Maximum daily fat gram budget	Approximate fat grams per meal	Maximum daily saturated fat gram budget
1200	33	8	11
1400	39	9	13
1600	44	11	15
1800	50	12	17
2000	56	13	19
2200	61	15	20
2400	67	16	22
2600	72	18	24
2800	77	19	26
3000	83	20	28

Table 67-6. Daily fat gram amounts for various calorie requirements demonstrating five different percentage fat levels*

Calorie needs	10% calories from fat (g)	15% calories from fat (g)	20% calories from fat (g)	25% calories from fat (g)	30% calories from fat (g)
1200	13	20	27	33	40
1400	16	23	31	39	46
1600	18	27	36	44	53
1800	20	30	40	50	60
2000	22	33	44	56	66
2200	24	37	48	61	73
2400	27	40	54	67	80
2600	29	43	58	72	86
2800	31	47	62	77	93
3000	33	50	66	83	100

*The Duke Center for Living recommends no more than 25% fat, with particular emphasis on reducing saturated fats.

by which to live. If frozen dinners are a staple, a supermarket tour with a trip to the frozen food section can provide skills to improve behaviors and health. This style of education facilitates change and supports continued improvement of their nutritional patterns.

Social support for nutrition changes is enhanced when spouses or other family members attend the nutrition programs with the client. In a rehabilitation setting, additional contact can be made with clients during the 3 days/week exercise sessions where nutrition questions can be discussed with nutritionists, nurses, physicians, and exercise staff. Health behaviors are synergistic. If individuals improve their exercise patterns, they are more likely to begin and maintain the process of healthful eating. Programs at the Duke Center for Living that assist in the process of supporting behavior change include a weekly nutrition discussion group, a support group, and programs on changing and maintaining nutrition behaviors.

Table 67-7. Risk status based on the presence of coronary heart disease risk factors other than LDL-C

The patient is considered to have a high-risk status if he or she has one of the following:

Either:

Definite CHD*: the characteristic clinical picture and objective laboratory findings of:
- Definite prior myocardial infarction, or
- Definite myocardial ischemia, e.g., angina pectoris

Or:

Two other CHD risk factors:
- Male sex†
- Family history of premature CHD (definite myocardial infarction or sudden death before age 55 yr in a parent or sibling)
- Cigarette smoking (currently smokes >10 cigarettes/day)
- Hypertension
- Low HDL-C concentration (<35 mg/dL confirmed by repeat measurement)
- Diabetes mellitus
- History of definite cerebrovascular or occlusive peripheral vascular disease
- Severe obesity (≥30% overweight)

From *Report of the Expert Panel on detection, evaluation, and treatment of high blood cholesterol in adults*, NIH Publ No 89-2925, US Dept of Health and Human Services, Public Health Service, National Institutes of Health, January 1989, p. 23.
*CHD, Coronary heart disease.
†Male sex is considered a risk factor in this scheme because the rates of CHD are 3 to 4 times higher in men than in women in the middle decades of life and roughly 2 times higher in the elderly. Hence, a man with one other CHD risk factor is considered to have a high-risk status, whereas a woman is not so considered unless she has two other CHD risk factors.

Pharmacologic management of dyslipidemia

Recent angiographic trials have demonstrated that pharmacologic treatment of dyslipidemia combined with diet modification may lead to delayed progression of atherosclerosis[8-14] and reduced cardiac morbidity[13,17,19] in patients with coronary artery disease. The management of dyslipidemia is based on blood lipid levels with target values for LDL-C set by the National Cholesterol Education Program.[145] Although one can categorize these disorders by specific lipoprotein phenotype by measuring HDL-C, total-C (TC), and triglyceride (TG) levels and calculating LDL-C levels (LDL = TC − HDL − 1/5 TG), this classification may not give an accurate assessment of the underlying genetic defect. A given phenotype can result from several different genotypes, and, conversely, a given genotype can result in multiple, different phenotypes. To complicate the issue further, phenotypes can change over time. Therefore, it is reasonable to treat lipid disorders based solely on HDL-C, LDL-C, and triglyceride levels. In addition to the determination of the lipoprotein levels, one must make an accurate assessment of the patient's cardiovascular risk factors (Table 67-7), rule out secondary causes of dyslipidemia, and perform a careful physical examination to identify arcus cornea, vascular bruits, xanthelasma, cutaneous/tendinous xanthomas, or other signs associated with genetic disorders.

The initial classification and recommendations were made on the basis of total cholesterol and HDL-C levels and an assessment of nonlipid CHD risk factors. Adults 20 years old or older should have this screening test performed as part of their general medical care, and it should be repeated at least once every 5 years. If the total cholesterol level is 200 to 239 mg/dL, the HDL-C level is 35 mg/dL or more, and there are fewer than two risk factors present, one should provide information on dietary modification, physical activity, and risk factor reduction. The patient should be reevaluated in 1 to 2 years. If the HDL-C level is 35 mg/dL or less, if two or more risk factors are present, or if the total cholesterol level is 240 mg/dL or more, a lipoprotein analysis needs to be done. For primary prevention the goal is now a LDL-C level less than 130 mg/dL. If so, repeat in 5 years and provide general education in risk factor reduction. If the LDL-C level is borderline high, 130 to 159 mg/dL, and fewer than two risk factors are present, provide information on the step 1 diet and physical activity and provide annual reevaluation and education. Assignment of patients to diet or drug treatment should be based on the average of two LDL measurements. If the LDL-C level is more than 160 mg/dL, do a clinical examination, evaluate secondary causes, evaluate familial disorders, and consider other risk factors. In patients without CHD, after they have started the therapeutic step 1 diet, the serum cholesterol level should be measured and adherence to the diet assessed at 4 to 6 weeks and at 3 months. The monitoring goal for cholesterol is less than 240 mg/dL for patients with an LDL-C goal of less than 160 mg/dL or less than 200 mg/dL for patients with an LDL-C goal of less than 130 mg/dL. If the total cholesterol goal is met, the LDL-C level is measured and the patient seen quarterly for the first year and twice yearly thereafter. If the goals are not met, step 2 diet should be started, and if that fails, drug therapy may be considered. Drug therapy can often be delayed in young adult men (<35 years of age) and premenopausal women who have LDL-C levels less than 220 mg/dL.

According to the guidelines, the following risk factors are to be considered in the treatment of hypercholesterolemia: positive risk factors: age, men 45 years or more, women 55 years or more, family history of CHD, smoking, hypertension, HDL-C level less than 35 mg/dL, diabetes, inactivity, and overweight; negative risk factor: HDL-C level 60 mg/dL or more. For primary prevention, drug treatment can be considered for an adult patient who despite dietary therapy has an LDL-C level of 190 mg/dL or greater without two other risk factors or 160 mg/dL or greater with two other risk factors. *For secondary prevention in patients with coronary artery disease, the goal of therapy is an LDL-C level of 100 mg/dL or lower.* Drug therapy is indicated in patients with CHD if the LDL-C level is more than 130 mg/dL after maximal dietary therapy and lifestyle changes. The LDL-C levels achieved in treated patients in many angiographic regression trials have been less than 100 mg/dL,[13,17] suggesting that LDL-C levels lower than those currently achieved in most patients may confer an additional benefit in this disorder.

Decreased HDL-C levels play an important role in determining risk for morbidity in patients who have coronary artery disease.[101,162] Results of the Helsinki Heart Study suggest that increasing HDL-C levels through pharmacologic therapy decreases cardiovascular morbidity.[101] Patients with HDL-C levels less than 35 mg/dL are at high risk for development of atherosclerosis and for recurrent events after MI even if the LDL-C level is less than 160 mg/dL.[162] Studies have not examined pharmacologic or lifestyle interventions in this subgroup. However, some clinicians currently employ pharmacologic therapy for patients with isolated, very low HDL-C levels (<35 mg/dL) and desirable LDL-C levels (<130 mg/dL) who have significant coronary artery disease, especially in the setting of early disease onset (<45 years old) or a strong family history.

If, over a 6-month period, the desired blood lipid goal has not been achieved by intensive dietary modification and lifestyle changes and exercise, drug therapy may be initiated. The commonly used lipid-lowering agents are outlined in Table 67-8. Before drug therapy is initiated, levels of baseline liver enzymes, electrolytes, and blood glucose should be obtained. The bile acid–binding resins have the advantage of not being systemically absorbed. These agents can also be given after the evening meal in a once daily dose to enhance compliance. However, in cases where triglyceride levels are also elevated, the bile

acid–binding resins may cause an additional increase in triglyceride levels. In these instances, nicotinic acid is an alternative. Flushing is a major side effect of this medication, which can usually be ameliorated by taking aspirin 30 minutes before dosing, and nicotinic acid may also worsen diabetes. If patients have problems with side effects from these drugs, the 3-hydroxy-3-methylglutaryl coenzyme A (HMG CoA) reductase inhibitors are a suitable alternative with fewer side effects. After drug therapy is initiated, lipids and liver enzyme levels should be rechecked in 4 to 6 weeks and again at 3 months. If the LDL goals are met, lipids and liver enzyme levels should be rechecked every 3 to 4 months. In cases where the LDL goals are not met, combination therapy with two or three drugs may be necessary. Of note, nicotinic acid and the HMG CoA reductase inhibitors can be effectively combined, although the risk for myositis may be increased. The combination of an HMG CoA reductase inhibitor and a fibric acid derivative (Table 67-8) is not recommended for general use, because the risk of myositis is significant. In all cases of combination therapy, patients should be titrated to the lowest possible dose and followed very closely.

The indications for pharmacologic treatment of hypertriglyceridemia are somewhat controversial. Dietary changes, including lowering dietary fat, restricting calories to attempt weight loss when feasible, and reducing alcohol consumption are the first line of therapy. There is significant cardiovascular risk associated with hypertriglyceridemia in combination with low HDL levels.[162] Triglyceride levels greater than 1000 mg/dL are also associated with a significant risk for developing pancreatitis. If diabetes mellitus is also present, it should be aggressively managed to normalize blood glucose levels. When dietary therapy fails and triglyceride levels remain greater than 500 mg/dL, drug therapy may be instituted. Gemfibrozil and nicotinic acid are good choices for lowering triglyceride levels and for raising HDL-C levels. Again, baseline laboratory studies should be obtained before drug therapy is initiated. The lowest effective dose of medication should be used when this disorder is treated. Initially patients should be seen for follow-up lipid and liver enzyme analyses in 4 to 6 weeks and again at 3 months. If the triglyceride goal of less than 250 mg/dL is met, patients can be followed every 3 to 4 months. If goals are not met, combination therapy should be attempted and the patients followed closely.

It is important to note that patients in the "usual care" arms of angiographic trials were generally treated with diets similar to those recommended by the American Heart Association and the National Cholesterol Education Program (deriving 25%-30% of calories from fat), admonished to exercise and stop smoking, and given standard medical treatment usually without lipid-lowering drugs. These patients demonstrated a 40% to

Table 67-8. Lipid-lowering agents*

Drug	Effect on lipids (%)			Dose	Actions	Side effects
	TC + LDL	HDL	TG			
Bile acid–binding resins Cholestyramine Colestipol	↓ 20-25	(−)	(−) or ↑	1 scoop qd to 3 scoops bid	Binds bile acids in intestine and promotes excretion; bile acids synthesized in liver from cholesterol	Bloating Gas Constipation
Nicotinic acid	↓ 15-25	↑ 10-25	↓ 20-80	Sustained release: 250 mg qd to 750 mg tid Immediate release: 50 mg bid to 500 mg qid	Decreases VLDL synthesis	Flushing Itching Nausea Indigestion Diarrhea Increased liver enzymes Stomach ulcers Gout/arthritis, ↑ uric acid Glucose intolerance or worsening diabetes mellitus Skin rash Hypotension Liver inflammation
HMG CoA reductase inhibitors Lovastatin (Mevacor) Simvastatin (Zocor) Pravastatin (Pravachol)	↓ 15-40	↑ 5-10	↓ 10-15	20 mg qd to 40 mg bid 5 mg qd to 40 mg qd 10 mg qhs to 40 mg qhs	Inhibits cholesterol biosynthesis Induces LDL receptors, which promotes LDL uptake	Temporary ↑ liver enzymes Significant ↑ liver enzymes (>3 × normal) Stomach discomfort Muscle pains/unusual cramps/weakness Skin rash
Fibric acid derivatives Gemfibrozil (Lopid) Clofibrate (Atromid-S)	↓ 10-15	↑ 10-20	↓ 25-50	600 mg bid 500-1000 mg bid	Enhances breakdown of TG-rich lipids	Stomach discomfort/nausea Skin rash Abnormal liver enzymes Muscle pains Diarrhea Makes bile thicker ↑ risk of gallbladder problems Potentiate blood-thinning effect of (warfarin) (Coumadin)
Probucol (Lorelco)	↓ 10-15	↓ 15-30	(−)	500 mg bid	Decreases LDL-C levels by unclear mechanisms Decreases formation of HDL but enhances cholesterol removal from body tissues; antioxidant properties; can decrease cholesterol deposits in tendons	Gas Diarrhea Nausea Skin rash ECG changes

*TC, Total cholesterol; LDL, low-density lipoprotein; HDL, high-density lipoprotein; TG, triglyceride; VLDL, very low-density lipoprotein; HMG CoA, 3-hydroxy-3-methylglutaryl coenzyme A.

87% incidence of overall angiographic worsening, which was associated with increased angina.[13,17] These results indicate that "standard" risk factor management does not halt lesion progression in this disorder. Despite the increasing evidence that risk factor modification through diet, pharmacologic therapy, and lifestyle changes may have an impact on progression of atherosclerosis, at present only a minority of patients who have undergone angioplasty or coronary artery bypass receive comprehensive risk factor management. A recent study reviewed the records of outpatients who had been hospitalized for suspected coronary artery disease at a referral hospital.[163] Only a minority of patients were given appropriate risk factor counseling, and only 17% of those patients with significant hyperlipidemia were given appropriate antihyperlipidemic therapy. Although follow-up showed that these interventions had increased to 35% in 1990, the results demonstrated that, in general, efforts have not focused on risk factor reduction in patients with this disorder. This practice continues despite increasing evidence that patients who have coronary artery disease would benefit from intensive risk factor modification.

Psychosocial aspects of cardiac rehabilitation

Factors such as depression, low morale, and psychological distress are common in patients who have had an MI[164] and are significant predictors of mortality among post-MI patients.[165] Type A behavior patterns, including having a time urgency, being highly competitive, becoming frequently impatient with others, and becoming easily angered and hostile, have been identified as risk factors for coronary artery disease in some but not all studies.[166,169] Recent studies suggest that hostility and subsequent social isolation appear to be the most important factors in placing the type A personality at increased risk.[169] Orth-Gomer and Unden[170] found that socially integrated type A and B cardiac patients had significantly lower cumulative mortality rates (17.3% and 20.9%, respectively) than did socially isolated types A and B (68.9% and 43.8%, respectively). Although the relationship between social support and survival from cardiac-related mortality has been known for several decades,[169] these investigators[170] found that social activity predicted cardiac-related mortality as strongly as did serum lipid levels or arrhythmias in type A cardiac patients. This is supported by a recent study in which Williams et al.[98] demonstrated that social isolation and low socioeconomic status were independent predictors of survival in patients with coronary artery disease. It is hypothesized that psychological factors may increase the risk of coronary artery disease through heightened neuroendocrine arousal, which may increase blood pressure during stress and possibly affect vascular endothelium.[171] Thus, emotional problems contribute to both the increased risk of mortality and the psychological, social, and economic maladjustment in post-MI patients.

Several studies of cardiac outpatients have indicated that psychological treatment results in an enhanced sense of well-being and may lead to reductions in mortality and morbidity. In one of the earliest published reports, Adsett and Bruhn[172] noted that nondirective group therapy appeared to produce improved psychosocial adaptation in a group of six post-MI patients. A more extensive longitudinal study by Rahe et al.[173] demonstrated that group therapy did not alter traditional risk factors (e.g., obesity, smoking habits), although some coronary-prone behaviors (e.g., stressful work patterns and feelings of time urgency) were reduced. However, the group therapy patients had significantly lower morbidity and mortality rates than the control group. In another clinical trial of longer duration, Ibrahim et al.[174] found no significant differences in risk factors between a group therapy treatment and a control group. However, survival rates tended to be higher in the treated subjects, especially among the most severely ill patients. The largest study to examine a psychosocial intervention in patients was the Recurrent Coronary Prevention Project.[175] This study examined events in 862 patients randomized to risk-factor education groups or type A behavior modification and behavioral counseling, which were compared with a nonrandomized control group. There were fewer cardiac events in the behavior modification group, suggesting that biobehavioral interventions may improve outcome in this disorder. However, there was no effect on mortality, and patients who dropped out of the study had the lowest mortality. These data suggest that psychosocial interventions might improve outcome in this disorder.

Relaxation training and biofeedback are common aspects of cardiac rehabilitation programs[176,177] and may play a valuable role in treatment of chronic hyperreactivity to stress. Relaxation training and instruction in stress management appear to be effective in reducing blood pressure, serum lipid levels, and morbidity.[178,179] In a randomized study, patients who participated in both relaxation training and exercise training had a significantly lower recurrence rate of cardiac events than patients who participated in exercise only.[176] In addition to possibly altering outcome in patients with coronary artery disease, psychosocial interventions may greatly enhance patient compliance with risk-factor changes. The finding in the LHT[17] that patients were able to comply with a very low-fat, vegetarian diet and lower LDL-C levels by 36% over 1 to 4 years while reporting improved quality of life is likely due to the inclusion of relaxation training and patient support groups in the study. Thus, psychosocial interventions, including patient support groups, individual counseling, relaxation training, and behavior modification, may play an important role in cardiac rehabilitation.

CONCLUSION

In patients who have had an MI, cardiac rehabilitation has been demonstrated to reduce mortality and fatal reinfarction by 20%,[5-7] improve fitness,[34-38] reduce depression and anxiety,[32-33] increase the angina threshold,[43-51] and improve quality of life. Recent studies have demonstrated that exercise training leads to increased exercise tolerance, improved symptoms, and decreased neurohumoral activation in patients with chronic heart failure resulting from left ventricular systolic dysfunction.[55-69] Exercise training confers benefits that are of similar magnitude to those achieved with pharmacologic therapy in patients with this disorder. These findings, in conjunction with results from recent angiographic trials[8-21] showing delayed progression or regression of coronary atherosclerosis after intensive reductions in serum LDL-C levels and an associated reduction of cardiovascular morbidity,[17,19,22] suggest that combining standard cardiac rehabilitation practices with intensive risk-factor management in patients with established coronary artery disease may yield even greater reductions in morbidity and mortality than those achieved by exercise alone.

A recent editorial by LaFontaine and Roitman[180] suggests that cardiac rehabilitation programs should provide multidisciplinary intensive lifestyle intervention programs for patients with coronary artery disease. The results of recent angiographic trials suggest that these interventions may reduce health care expenditures for this disorder. Our current challenge is to design and implement cost-effective programs to meet these needs. At the Duke Center for Living we have integrated these findings into clinical practice with both long-term multidisciplinary risk-factor programs and an intensive 2-week retreat program for patients with coronary artery disease. The "Healing the Heart" retreat program combines dietary education, exercise, relaxation, patient support groups, and medical education for patients wishing to make significant lifestyle changes to delay progression of coronary artery disease and to improve prognosis. At present, cardiac rehabilitation efforts in many areas are expanding to provide these services. However, studies are needed to define the long-term cost benefits from this approach.

In addition to causing delayed progression of atherosclerosis, the combination of exercise with a diet containing less than 20% of calories from fat has been shown to reduce scintigraphic evidence of stress-induced ischemia and reduce angina.[17,19] Similar results from exercise alone have been difficult to demonstrate.

These studies begin a new era in the secondary prevention of coronary artery disease and indicate that medical therapy may halt the progression of atherosclerosis. New and more intensive risk-factor intervention strategies in patients with stable coronary artery disease offer the exciting possibility of reducing cardiovascular morbidity and mortality in patients while delaying disease progression. Although angiographic improvements have been small in treated patients in these studies, it is possible that future medical therapy may lead to significant regression of established arterial lesions.

REFERENCES

1. Health Technology Assessment Reports, US Department of Health and Human Services, Washington, DC, 1987, US Government Printing Office, vol 6, pp 1-89.
2. Thompson PD: The benefits and risks of exercise training in patients with chronic coronary artery disease, *JAMA* 259:1537-1540, 1988.
3. Wenger NK: Rehabilitation of the coronary patient in 1989, *Arch Intern Med* 149:1504-1506, 1989.
4. Van Camp SP, Peterson RA: Cardiovascular complications of outpatient cardiac rehabilitation programs, *JAMA* 256:1160-1163, 1986.
5. Collins R, Yusuf S, Peto R: Exercise after myocardial infarction reduces mortality: evidence from randomized controlled trials [abstract], *J Am Coll Cardiol* 3:622, 1984.
6. Oldridge NB, Guyatt GH, Fischer ME, et al: Cardiac rehabilitation after myocardial infarction: combined experience of randomized clinical trials, *JAMA* 260:945-950, 1988.
7. O'Connor GT, Buring JE, Yusuf S, et al. An overview of randomized trials of rehabilitation with exercise after myocardial infarction, *Circulation* 1989;80:235-244.
8. Brensike JF, Levy RI, Kelsey SF: Effects of therapy with cholestyramine on progression of coronary arteriosclerosis: results of the NHLBI Type II Coronary Intervention Study, *Circulation* 69:313-324, 1984.
9. Brensike JF, Kelsey SF, Passamani ER: National Heart, Lung, and Blood Institute Type II Coronary Intervention Study: design, methods, and baseline characteristics, *Contr Clin Trials* 3:91-111, 1982.
10. Blankenhorn DH, Nessim SA, et al: Beneficial effects of combined colestipol-niacin therapy on coronary atherosclerosis and coronary venous bypass grafts, *JAMA* 257:3233-3240, 1987.
11. Blankenhorn DH, Johnson RL, Nessim SA: The Cholesterol Lowering Atherosclerosis Study (CLAS): design, methods, and baseline results, *Contr Clin Trials* 8:354-387, 1987.
12. Cashin-Hemphill L, Mack WJ, Pogoda JM: Beneficial effects of colestipol-niacin on coronary atherosclerosis: a 4-year follow-up, *JAMA* 264:3013-3017, 1990.
13. Brown G, Albers JJ, Fisher LD: Regression of coronary artery disease as a result of intensive lipid-lowering therapy in men with high levels of apolipoprotein B, *N Engl J Med* 323:1289-1298, 1990.
14. Kane JP, Malloy MJ, Ports TA: Regression of coronary atherosclerosis during treatment of familial hypercholesterolemia with combined drug regimens, *JAMA* 264:3007-3012, 1990.
15. Buchwald H, Varco RL, Matts JP: Effect of partial ileal bypass surgery on mortality and morbidity from coronary heart disease in patients with hypercholesterolemia: report of the Program on the Surgical Control of the Hyperlipidemias (POSCH); *N Engl J Med* 323:946-955, 1990.
16. Buchwald H, Matts JP, Fitch LL: Program on the surgical control of the hyperlipidemias (POSCH): design and methodology, *J Clin Epidemiol* 42:1111-1127, 1989.

17. Ornish D, Brown SE, Scherwitz LW: Can lifestyle changes reverse coronary heart disease? The Lifestyle Heart Trial, *Lancet* 336:129-133, 1990.

18. Schuler G, Hambrecht R, Schlierf G: Myocardial perfusion and regression of coronary artery disease in patients on a regimen of intensive physical exercise and low fat diet, *J Am Coll Cardiol* 19:34-42, 1992.

19. Watts GF, Lewis B, Brunt JNH: Effects on coronary artery disease of lipid-lowering diet, or diet plus cholestyramine, in the St. Thomas' Atherosclerosis Regression Study (STARS), *Lancet* 339:563-569, 1992.

20. Arntzenius AC, Kromhout D, Barth JD: Diet, lipoproteins, and the progression of coronary atherosclerosis: the Leiden Intervention Trial, *N Engl J Med* 12:805-811, 1985.

21. Schuler G, Hambrecht R, Schlierf G, et al: Regular exercise and low-fat diet: effects on progression of coronary artery disease, *Circulation* 86:1-11, 1992.

22. Vogel RA: Comparative clinical consequences of aggressive lipid management, coronary angioplasty and bypass surgery in coronary artery disease, *Am J Cardiol* 69:1229-1233, 1992.

23. Blair SN, Kohl HW, Paffenbarger RS, et al: Physical fitness and all-cause mortality, *JAMA* 262:2395-2401, 1989.

24. Berlin HA, Colditz GA: A meta-analysis of physical activity in the prevention of coronary heart attacks, *Am J Epidemiol* 132:612-628, 1987.

25. Ekelund L-G, Haskell WL, Johnson SL, et al: Physical fitness as a predictor of cardiovascular mortality in asymptomatic North American men, *N Engl J Med* 319:1379-1384, 1988.

26. Ekelund L-G, Haskell WL, Troung YL, et al: Physical fitness as predictor of cardiovascular mortality in asymptomatic females [abstract], *Circulation* 78(supp II):110, 1988.

27. Astrand PO: From exercise physiology to preventive medicine, *Ann Clin Res* 20:10-17, 1988.

28. Brochier ML, Julian DG (eds): Physical training in patients with disease: training in coronary disease, 2nd workshop, *Eur Heart J* 9(suppl M):1-46, 1988.

29. Haskell WL: The influence of exercise training on plasma lipids and lipoproteins in health and disease, *Acta Med Scand* 711(suppl):25-37, 1986.

30. Thompson PD, Cullinane EM, Sady SP, et al: High density lipoprotein metabolism in endurance athletes and sedentary men, *Circulation* 84:140-152, 1991.

31. Holloszy JO, Shult J, Kusnierkiewicz A, et al: Effects of exercise on glucose tolerance and insulin resistance, *Acta Med Scand* 711(suppl):55-65, 1986.

32. Health and Public Policy Committee, American College of Physicians: Position stand on cardiac rehabilitation services, *Ann Intern Med* 109:671-673, 1988.

33. Taylor CB, Houston-Miller N, Ahn DK, et al: The effects of exercise training programs on psychosocial improvement in uncomplicated postmyocardial infarction patients, *J Psychosom Res* 30:581-587, 1986.

34. Clausen JP: Circulatory adjustments to dynamic exercise and effect of physical training in normal subjects and patients with coronary artery disease, *Prog Cardiovasc Dis* 18:459-495, 1976.

35. Varnauskas E, Bergman H, Houk P, et al: Hemodynamic effects of physical training in coronary patients, *Lancet* 2:8-12, 1986.

36. Detry JM, Rousseau M, Vandenbroucke G, et al: Increased arteriovenous oxygen difference after physical training in coronary heart disease, *Circulation* 44:109-118, 1971.

37. Clausen JP, Trap-Jensen J: Effects of training on the distribution of cardiac output in patients with coronary artery disease, *Circulation* 42:611-624, 1970.

38. Hagberg JM, Ehsani AA, Holloszy JO: Effect of 12 months of intense exercise training on stroke volume in patients with coronary artery disease, *Circulation* 67:1194-1199, 1983.

39. Letac B, Cribier A, Desplanches JF: A study of left ventricular function in coronary patients before and after physical training, *Circulation* 56:375-378, 1977.

40. Cobb FR, Williams RS, McEwan P, et al: Effects of exercise training on ventricular function in patients with recent myocardial infarction, *Circulation* 66:100-108, 1982.

41. Ferguson RJ, Taylor AW, Cote P, et al: Skeletal muscle and cardiac changes with training in patients with angina pectoris, *Am J Physiol* 243:H830-H836, 1982.

42. Williams MA, Maresh CM, Esterbrooks DJ, et al: Early exercise training in patients older than age 65 years compared with that in younger patients after acute myocardial infarction or coronary bypass grafting, *Am J Cardiol* 55:263-266, 1985.

43. Sim DN, Neill WA. Investigation of the physiological basis for increased exercise threshold for angina pectoris and physical conditioning, *J Clin Invest* 54:763-770, 1974.

44. Myers J, Ahnve S, Froelicher V, et al: A randomized trial of the effects of 1 year of exercise training on computer-measured ST segment displacement in patients with coronary artery disease, *J Am Coll Cardiol* 4:1094-1102, 1984.

45. Detry JMR, Bruce RA: Effects of physical training on exertional ST-segment depression in coronary artery disease, *Circulation* 44:390-398, 1971.

46. Nolewajka AJ, Kostuk WL, Rechnitzer PA, et al: Exercise and human collateralization: an angiographic and scintigraphic assessment, *Circulation* 60:114-121, 1979.

47. Hagberg JM: Physiologic adaptations to prolonged high-intensity exercise training in patients with coronary artery disease, *Med Sci Sport Exerc* 23(6):661-667, 1991.

48. Amsterdam EA, Laslett LJ, Dressendorfer RH, et al: Exercise training in coronary artery disease: is there a cardiac effect? *Am Heart J* 101:870-873, 1981.

49. Ehsani AA, Heath GW, Hagberg JM, et al: Effects of 12 months of intense exercise training on ischemic ST-segment depression in patients with coronary artery disease, *Circulation* 64:1116-1124, 1981.

50. Froelicher V, Jensen D, Genter F, et al: A randomized trial of exercise training in patients with coronary artery disease, *JAMA* 252:1291-1297, 1984.

51. Sebrechts CP, Klein JL, Ahnve S, et al: Myocardial perfusion changes following 1 year of exercise training assessed by thallium-201 circumferential count profiles, *Am Heart J* 112(6):1217-1225, 1986.

52. Ekelund LG, Ekelund CC: Cardiac rehabilitation today: programs, their effects and practical guidelines, *Scand J Med Sci Sports* 2:190-196, 1992.

53. Shephard RJ: The value of exercise in ischemic heart disease. A cumulative analysis, *J Cardiac Rehabil* 3:294-298, 1983.

54. P.R.E.COR Group: Comparison of a rehabilitation programme, a counseling programme and usual care after an acute myocardial infarction; results of a long-term randomized trial, *Eur Heart J* 12:612-616, 1991.

55. Lee AP, Ice R, Blessey R, et al: Long-term effects of physical training on coronary patients with impaired ventricular function, *Circulation* 60:1519-1526, 1979.

56. Conn EH, Williams RS, Wallace AG: Exercise responses before and after physical conditioning in patients with severely depressed left ventricular function, *Am J Cardiol* 49:296-300, 1982.

57. Jette M, Heller R, Landry F, et al: Randomized 4-week exercise program in patients with impaired left ventricular function, *Circulation* 84:1561-1567, 1991.

58. Hoffmann A, Duba J, Lengyel M, et al: The effect of training on the physical working capacity of MI patients with left ventricular dysfunction, *Eur Heart J* 8:43-49, 1987.

59. Sullivan MJ, Higginbotham MB, Cobb FR: Exercise training in

patients with severe left ventricular dysfunction: hemodynamic and metabolic effects, *Circulation* 78:506-515, 1988.

60. Sullivan MJ, Higginbotham MB, Cobb FR: Exercise training in patients with chronic heart failure delays ventilatory anaerobic threshold and improves submaximal exercise performance, *Circulation* 79:324-329, 1989.

61. Minotti JR, Johnson EC, Hudson TL, et al: Skeletal muscle response to exercise training in congestive heart failure, *J Clin Invest* 86:751-758, 1990.

62. Coats AJS, Adamopoulos S, Radaelli A: Controlled trial of physical training in chronic heart failure: exercise performance, hemodynamics, ventilation, and autonomic function, *Circulation* 85:2119-2131, 1992.

63. Giannuzzi P, Temporelli PL, Gattone M, et al: Exercise training in anterior myocardial infarction: ongoing multicenter study on ventricular function and topography, *Circulation* 84(suppl II):539, 1991.

64. Kellermann JJ, Ben-Ari E, Fisman E, et al: Physical training in patients with ventricular impairment, *Adv Cardiol* 34:131-147, 1986.

65. Coats AJS, Adamopoulos S, Meyer TE, et al: Effects of physical training in chronic heart failure, *Lancet* 335:63-66, 1990.

66. Shabetai R: Beneficial effects of exercise training in compensated heart failure [editorial], *Circulation* 78:775-776, 1988.

67. Kavanagh T, Myers MG, Baigrie RS, et al: Cardiorespiratory benefits of a walking training programme in chronic heart failure patients: a preliminary report. Paper presented at the Fifth World Congress of Cardiac Rehabilitation, Bordeaux, France, July 5-8, 1992.

68. Squires RW, Gau GT, Miller TD, et al: Cardiovascular rehabilitation: status, 1990, *Mayo Clin Proc* 65:731-755, 1990.

69. Arvan S: Exercise performance of the high risk acute myocardial infarction patient after cardiac rehabilitation, *Am J Cardiol* 62:197-201, 1988.

70. Alderman EL, Fisher LD, Litwin P, et al: Results of coronary artery surgery in patients with poor left ventricular function (CASS), *Circulation* 68:785-795, 1983.

71. Vigilante GJ, Weintraub WS, Klein LW, et al: Improved survival with coronary bypass surgery in patients with three-vessel coronary disease and abnormal left ventricular function: matched case-control study in patients with potentially operable disease, *Am J Med* 82:697, 1987.

72. Minotti J, Massie BM: Exercise training in heart failure patients, *Circulation* 85:2323-2325, 1992.

73. Drexler H, Banhardt U, Meinertz T, et al: Contrasting peripheral short-term and long-term effects of converting enzyme inhibition in patients with congestive heart failure, *Circulation* 79:491-502, 1989.

74. Captopril Multicenter Research Group: A placebo-controlled trial of captopril in refractory chronic congestive heart failure, *J Am Coll Cardiol* 2:755-763, 1983.

75. Keys A (ed): Coronary heart disease in seven countries, *Circulation* 41(4 suppl):I1-I198, 1970.

76. Keys A, Aravanis C, Van Buchem FSP, et al: The diet and all-causes death rate in the Seven Countries Study, *Lancet* 2:58-61, 1981.

77. Carlson LA, Bottiger LE: Ischaemic heart-disease in relation to fasting values of plasma triglycerides and cholesterol: Stockholm Prospective Study, *Lancet* 1:865-868, 1972.

78. Castelli WP, Doyle JT, Gordon T, et al: HDL cholesterol and other lipids in coronary heart disease: the Cooperative Lipoprotein Phenotyping Study, *Circulation* 55:767-772, 1977.

79. Dawber TR: *The Framingham Study: the epidemiology of atherosclerotic disease,* Cambridge, Mass, 1980, Harvard University Press.

80. Shekelle RB, Shryock AM, Paul O, et al: Diet, serum cholesterol, and death from coronary heart disease: the Western Electric Study, *N Engl J Med* 304:65-70, 1981.

81. Castelli WP, Garrison RJ, Wilson PWF, et al: Incidence of coronary heart disease and lipoprotein cholesterol levels: the Framingham Study, *JAMA* 256:2835-2838, 1986.

82. Martin MJ, Browner WS, Hulley SB, et al: Serum cholesterol, blood pressure and mortality: implications from a cohort of 361, 662 men, *Lancet* 1:933-936, 1986.

83. Shipley MJ, Pocock SJ, Marmot MG: Does plasma cholesterol concentration predict mortality from coronary heart disease in elderly people? 18 year follow up in Whitehall study, *Br Med J (Clin Res)* 303:89-92, 1991.

84. Rosenman RH, Brand RJ, Jenkins D, et al: Coronary heart disease in the Western Collaborative Group Study, *JAMA* 233:872-877, 1975.

85. Friedman GD, Petitti DB, Bawol RD, et al: Mortality in cigarette smokers and quitters: effect of base-line differences, *N Engl J Med* 304:1407-1410, 1981.

86. Neaton JD, Kuller LH, Wentworth D, et al: Total and cardiovascular mortality in relation to cigarette smoking, serum cholesterol concentration, and diastolic blood pressure among black and white males followed up for five years, *Am Heart J* 108:759-769, 1984.

87. Seltzer CC: Framingham study data and "established wisdom" about cigarette smoking and coronary heart disease, *J Clin Epidemiol* 42:743-750, 1989.

88. Hubert HB, Feinleib M, McNamara PM, et al: Obesity as an independent risk factor for cardiovascular disease: a 26-year follow-up of participants in the Framingham Heart Study, *Circulation* 67:968-977, 1983.

89. Bray AB: Complications of obesity, *Ann Intern Med* 103:1052-1062, 1985.

90. Reed D, Yano K: Predictors of arteriographically defined coronary stenosis in the Honolulu Heart Program. Comparisons of cohort and arteriography series analyses, *Am J Epidemiol* 134:111-122, 1991.

91. Fletcher GF, Blair SN, Blumenthal J, et al: Benefits and recommendations for physical activity programs for all Americans. A statement for health professionals by the committee on exercise and cardiac rehabilitation of the council on clinical cardiology, American Heart Association, *Circulation* 86:340-344, 1992.

92. Paffenbarger RS, Hyde RT, Wing AL, et al: A natural history of athleticism and cardiovascular health, *JAMA* 252:491-495, 1984.

93. Marmot MG, Syme SL, Kagan A, et al: Epidemiologic studies of coronary heart disease and stroke in Japanese men living in Japan, Hawaii and California: prevalence of coronary and hypertensive heart disease and associated risk factors, *Am J Epidemiol* 102:514-525, 1975.

94. Ruberman W, Weinblatt E, Goldberg JD, et al: Psychosocial influences on mortality after myocardial infarction, *N Engl J Med* 311:552-559, 1984.

95. Reed D, McGee D, Yano K, et al: Social networks and coronary heart disease among Japanese men in Hawaii, *Am J Epidemiol* 117:384-396, 1983.

96. Kaplan GA: Social contacts and ischaemic heart disease, *Ann Clin Res* 20:131-136, 1988.

97. Cassel J, Heyden S, Bartel AG: Incidence of coronary heart disease by ethnic group, social class, and sex, *Arch Intern Med* 128:901-906, 1971.

98. Williams RB, Barefoot JC, Califf RM, et al: Prognostic importance of social and economic resources among medically treated patients with angiographically documented coronary artery disease, *JAMA* 267:520-524, 1992.

99. Brown MS, Goldstein JL: A receptor-mediated pathway for cholesterol homeostasis, *Science* 232:34-47, 1986.

100. Grundy SM: Cholesterol and coronary heart disease: a new era, *JAMA* 256:2849-2858, 1986.
101. Frick MH, Elo O, Haapa K, et al: Helsinki Heart Study: primary-prevention trial with gemfibrozil in middle-aged men with dyslipidemia. Safety of treatment, changes in risk factors, and incidence of coronary heart disease, *N Engl J Med* 317:1237-1245, 1987.
102. Hjermann I, Holme I, Velve Byre K, et al: Effect of diet and smoking intervention of the incidence of coronary heart disease: report from the Oslo Study Group of a randomized trial in healthy men, *Lancet* 2:1303-1310, 1981.
103. Lipid Research Clinics Program: The Lipid Research Clinics Coronary Primary Prevention Trial results: I. Reduction in incidence of coronary heart disease, *JAMA* 251:351-364, 1984.
104. Canner PL, Berge KG, Wenger NK, et al: Fifteen year mortality in Coronary Drug Project patients: long-term benefit with niacin, *J Am Coll Cardiol* 8:1245-1255, 1986.
105. Holme I: An analysis of randomized trials evaluating the effect of cholesterol reduction on total mortality and coronary heart disease incidence, *Circulation* 82:1916-1924, 1990.
106. St.Clair RW: Atherosclerosis regression in animal models: current concepts of cellular and biochemical mechanisms, *Prog Cardiovasc Dis* 26:109-132, 1983.
107. Armstrong ML, Warner ED, Connor WE: Regression of coronary atheromatosis in rhesus monkeys, *Circ Res* 27:59-67, 1970.
108. Armstrong ML, Megan MB: Lipid depletion in atheromatous coronary arteries in rhesus monkeys after regression diets, *Circ Res* 30:675-680, 1972.
109. Clarkson TB, Lehner NDM, Bullock BC, et al: Atherosclerosis in New World monkeys, *Prim Med* 9:90-144, 1976.
110. Wissler RW, Vesselinovitch D: Atherosclerosis in nonhuman primates. In Brandly CA, Cornelius CE (eds): *Advances in veterinary science and comparative medicine,* Academic Press, 1977, New York, pp 351-420.
111. Malinow MR, McLaughlin P, Papworth L, et al: A model for therapeutic interventions on established coronary atherosclerosis in a nonhuman primate, *Adv Exp Med Biol* 67:3-31, 1976.
112. Kramsch DM, Aspen AJ, Abramowitz BM, et al: Reduction of coronary atherosclerosis by moderate conditioning exercise in monkeys on an atherogenic diet, *N Engl J Med* 305:1483-1489, 1981.
113. Manuck SB, Kaplan JR, Clarkson TB: Behaviorally induced heart rate reactivity and atherosclerosis in cynomolgus monkeys, *Psychosom Med* 45:95-108, 1983.
114. Kaplan JR, Manuck SB, Clarkson TB, et al: Social stress and atherosclerosis in normocholesterolemic monkeys, *Science* 220:733-735, 1983.
115. Kaplan JR, Manuck SB, Adams MR, et al: Inhibition of coronary atherosclerosis by propranolol in behaviorally predisposed monkeys fed an atherogenic diet, *Circulation* 76:1364-1372, 1987.
116. Shively CA, Clarkson TB, Kaplan JR: Social deprivation and coronary artery atherosclerosis in female cynomolgus monkeys, *Atherosclerosis* 77:69-76, 1989.
117. Nerem RM, Levesque MJ, Cornhill JF: Social environment as a factor in diet-induced atherosclerosis, *Science* 208:1475-1476, 1980.
118. Armstrong ML, Heistad DD, Marcus ML, et al: Structural and hemodynamic responses of peripheral arteries of macaque monkeys to atherogenic diet, *Arteriosclerosis* 5:336-346, 1985.
119. Harrison DG, Armstrong ML, Freiman PC, et al: Restoration of endothelium-dependent relaxation by dietary treatment of atherosclerosis, *J Clin Invest* 80:1808-1811, 1987.
120. Quillen JE, Selke FW, Armstrong ML, et al: Long-term cholesterol feeding alters the reactivity of primate coronary microvessels to platelet products, *Arterio Thromb* 11:639-644, 1991.
121. Lopez JAG, Armstrong ML, Piegors DJ, et al: Effect of early and advanced atherosclerosis on vascular responses to serotonin, thromboxane A2, and adenosine diphosphate (ADP), *Circulation* 79:698-705, 1989.
122. Williams JK, Armstrong ML, Heistad DD: Vasa vasorum in atherosclerotic coronary arteries: responses to vasoactive stimuli and regression of atherosclerosis, *Circ Res* 62:515-523, 1988.
123. Lopez JAG, Armstrong ML, Harrison DG, et al: Vascular responses to leukocyte products in atherosclerotic primates, *Circ Res* 65:1078-1086, 1989.
124. Zeiher AM, Drexler H, Wollschlaeger H, et al: Coronary vasomotion in response to sympathetic stimulation in humans: importance of the functional integrity of the endothelium, *J Am Coll Cardiol* 14:1181-1190, 1989.
125. Gordon JB, Ganz P, Nabel EG, et al: Atherosclerosis influences the vasomotor response of epicardial coronary arteries to exercise, *J Clin Invest* 83:1946-1952, 1989.
126. Golino P, Piscione F, Willerson JT, et al: Divergent effects of serotonin on coronary-artery dimensions and blood flow in patients with coronary atherosclerosis and control patients, *N Engl J Med* 324:641-648, 1991.
127. Bruschke AVG, Kramer Jr JR, Bal ET, et al: The dynamics of progression of coronary atheroclerosis studies in 168 medically treated patients who underwent coronary arteriography three times, *Am Heart J* 117:296-305, 1989.
128. Campeau L, Enjalbert M, Lespérance J, et al: The relation of risk factors to the development of atherosclerosis in saphenous-vein bypass grafts and the progression of disease in the native circulation: a study 10 years after aortocoronary bypass surgery, *N Engl J Med* 311:1329-1332, 1984.
129. Brown BG, Zhao Zue-Qiao, Sacco DE, et al: Lipid lowering and plaque regression. New insights into prevention of plaque disruption and clinical events in coronary disease, *Circulation* 87:1781-1791, 1993.
130. Gould KL, Ornish D, Kirkeeide R, et al: Improved stenosis geometry by quantitative coronary arteriography after vigorous risk factor modification, *Am J Cardiol* 69:845-853, 1992.
131. Hambrecht R, Niebauer J, Marburger C, et al: Various intensities of leisure time physical activity in patients with coronary artery disease: effects on cardiorespiratory fitness and progression of coronary atherosclerotic lesions, *J Am Coll Cardiol* 22:468-477, 1993.
132. American College of Sports Medicine: Position stand on the recommended quantity of exercise for developing and maintaining cardiorespiratory and muscular fitness in healthy adults, *Med Sci Sport Exerc* 22:265-274, 1990.
133. Kugler J, Dimsdale JE, Hartley H, et al: Hospital supervised vs home exercise in cardiac rehabilitation effects on aerobic fitness, anxiety, and depression, *Arch Phys Med Rehabil* 71:322-325, 1990.
134. Miller NH, Haskell WL, Berra K, et al: Home versus group exercise for increasing functional capacity after myocardial infarction, *Circulation* 70:645-649, 1984.
135. Haskell WL: Physical activity and health: need to define the required stimulus, *Am J Cardiol* 55:4D-9D, 1985.
136. Pollock ML: Prescribing exercise for fitness and adherence. In Dishman RK (ed): *Exercise adherence: its impact on public health.* Champaign, Ill, 1988, Human Kinetics Books, pp 259-277.
137. Pollock ML, Wilmore JH: *Exercise in health and disease: evaluation and prescription for prevention and rehabilitation,* ed 2, Philadelphia, 1990, WB Saunders.
138. Martin JE, Dubbert PM: Adherence to exercise. In Terjung RL (ed): *Exercise and sports sciences reviews.* New York, 1985, MacMillan, pp 137-167.
139. Dishman RK, Sallis J, Orenstein D: The determinants of physical activity and exercise, *Public Health Rep* 100:158-180, 1985.
140. Sparling PB, Cantwell JD, Dolan CM, et al: Strength training in

a cardiac rehabilitation program: a six-month follow-up, *Arch Phys Med Rehabil* 71:148-152, 1990.

141. Ghilarducci LE, Holly RG, Amsterdam EA: Effects of high resistance training in coronary artery disease, *Am J Cardiol* 64:866-870, 1989.

142. Grundy SM, Denke MA: Dietary influences on serum lipids and lipoproteins, *J Lipid Res* 1149-1172, 1990.

143. Connor WE, Connor SL: The dietary prevention and treatment of coronary heart disease. In Connor WE, Bristow JD (eds): *Coronary heart disease,* Philadelphia, 1984, JB Lippincott.

144. Kris-Etherton PM, Krummel D, Russel M, et al: The effect of diet on plasma lipids, lipoprotein, and coronary heart disease, *J Am Diet Assoc* 11:1373-1400, 1988.

145. Expert Panel on Detection, Evaluation, and Treatment of Blood Cholesterol in Adults: Summary of the second report of the National Cholesterol Education Program (NCEP) Expert Panel on Detection, Evaluation, and Treatment of High Blood Cholesterol in Adults (Adult Treatment Panel II), *JAMA* 269: 3015-3023, 1993.

146. Grundy SM, Brown WV, Dietschy JM, et al: Workshop III Basis for Dietary Treatment, *Circulation* 80:729-734, 1989.

147. Nutrition Committee, American Heart Association: Dietary guidelines for healthy American adults, *Circulation* 77:721A-724A, 1988.

148. Grundy SM, Barrett-Connor E, Rudel LL, et al: Workshop on the impact of dietary cholesterol on plasma lipoproteins and atherogenesis, *Arteriosclerosis* 8:95-101, 1988.

149. Steinberg D, Parthasarathy S, Carew TE, et al: Beyond cholesterol: modifications of low-density lipoprotein that increase its atherogenicity, *N Engl J Med* 320:915-924, 1989.

150. Sirtori CR, Gatti E, Mantero O, et al: Clinical experience with the soybean protein diet in the treatment of hypercholesterolemia, *Am J Clin Nutr* 32:1645-1658, 1979.

151. Steinberg D: Antioxidants in the prevention of human atherosclerosis. Summary of the proceedings of a National Heart, Lung and Blood Institute Workshop: Sept. 5-6, 1991, Bethesda, Maryland, *Circulation* 85:2338-2344, 1992.

152. Rimm EB, Stampfer MJ, Ascherio A, et al: Vitamin E consumption and the risk of coronary heart disease in men, *N Engl J Med* 328:1450-1456, 1993.

153. Stampfer MJ, Hennekens CH, Manson JE, et al: Vitamin E consumption and the risk of coronary artery disease in women, *N Engl J Med* 328:1444-1449, 1993.

154. De Keyser J, De Klippel N, Merkx H, et al: Serum concentrations of vitamin A and E and early outcome after ischemic stroke, *Lancet* 339:1562-1565, 1992.

155. Enstrom JE, Kanim LE, Klein MA: Vitamin C intake and mortality among a sample of the United States population, *Epidemiology* 3:194-202, 1992.

156. Salonen JT, Nyyssonen K, Korpela H, et al: High stored iron levels are associated with excess risk of myocardial infarction in Eastern Finnish men, *Circulation* 86:803-811, 1992.

157. Harlan WR, Harlan LC: Blood pressure and calcium and magnesium intake. In Laragh JH, Brenner BM (eds): *Hypertension: pathophysiology, diagnosis, and management,* New York, 1990, Raven Press.

158. Kristal RR, DeLett AC, Henry HJ, et al: Rapid assessment of dietary intake of fat, fiber and saturated fat. Validity of an instrument suitable for community intervention research and nutritional surveillance, *Am J Health Prom* 4:289-295, 1990.

159. DiMetteo MR: *Achieving patient compliance,* New York, 1982, Pergamon Press.

160. Save the Children: *Bridging the gap: a participatory approach to health and nutrition education,* Westport, Conn, 1982, Save the Children.

161. Shannon B, Bagby R, Want MQ, et al: Self-efficacy: a contributor to the explanation of eating behavior, *Health Educ Res* 5:395-407, 1990.

162. Miller M, Seidler A, Kwiterovich PO, et al: Long-term predictors of subsequent cardiovascular events with coronary artery disease and 'desirable' levels of plasma total cholesterol, *Circulation* 86:1165-1170, 1992.

163. Cohen MV, Byrne MJ, Levine B, et al: Low rate of treatment of hypercholesterolemia by cardiologists in patients with suspected and proven coronary artery disease, *Circulation* 83:1294-1304, 1991.

164. Schleifer SJ, Macari-Hinson MM, Coyle DA, et al: The nature and course of depression following myocardial infarction, *Arch Intern Med* 149:1785-1789, 1989.

165. Mumford E, Schlesinger H: The effects of psychological intervention on recovery from surgery and heart attacks: an analysis of the literature, *Am J Public Health* 72:141-151, 1982.

166. Nunes EV, Frank KA, Kornfeld DS: Psychological treatment for the type A behavior pattern and for coronary artery disease: a meta-analysis of the literature, *Psychosom Med* 48:159-173, 1987.

167. Mathews KA, Glass D, Rosenman R, et al: Competitive drive, pattern-A, and coronary artery disease: a further analysis of some data from the collaborative group study, *J Chronic Dis* 30:489-498, 1977.

168. Smith TW, Anderson NB: Models of personality and disease: an interactional approach to type A behavior and cardiovascular risk, *J Pers Soc Psychol* 6:1166-1173, 1986.

169. Williams R, Chesney M, Cohen S, Frasure-Smith N, Kaplan G, Krantz D, Manuck S, Muller J, Powell L, Schnall P, Wortman C: Behavior change and compliance: keys to improving cardiovascular health, *Circulation* 88(3):1406-1407, 1993.

170. Orth-Gomer K, Unden AL: Type A behavior, social support, and coronary risk: interaction and significance for mortality in cardiac patients, *Psychosom Med* 52(1):59-72, 1990.

171. Niaura R, Goldstein MG: Psychological factors affecting physical condition: cardiovascular disease literature review, *Psychosomatics,* 33:146-155, 1992.

172. Adsett CA, Bruhn JG: Short-term group psychotherapy for post-myocardial infarction patients and their wives, *Can Med Assoc J* 99:577-584, 1968.

173. Rahe RH, Ward HW, Hayes V: Brief group therapy in myocardial infarction rehabilitation: three to four year follow-up of a controlled trial, *Psychosom Med* 41:229-242, 1979.

174. Ibrahim MA, Feldman JG, Sultz HA, et al: Management after myocardial infarction: a controlled trial of the effect of group psychotherapy, *Int J Psychiatry Med* 5:253-268, 1974.

175. Friedman M, Thoresen C, Gill J, et al: Alteration of type A behavior and reduction in cardiac recurrences in post-myocardial infarction patients, *Am Heart J* 108:237-248, 1984.

176. Langosch W, Seer P, Brodner G, et al: Behavior therapy with coronary heart disease patients: results of a comparative study, *J Psychosom Res* 26:475-484, 1982.

177. Blumenthal JA, Emery CF: Rehabilitation of patients following myocardial infarction, *J Consult Clin Psychol* 56:374-381, 1988.

178. Mitsibounas DN, Tsouna-Hadjis ED, Rotas VR, et al: Effects of group psychosocial intervention on coronary risk factors, *Psychother Psychosom* 58:97-102, 1992.

179. Agras WS, Taylor CB, Kraemer HC, et al: Relaxation training for essential hypertension at the worksite: II. The poorly controlled hypertensive, *Psychosom Med* 49:264-273, 1987.

180. LaFontaine T, Roitman J: Life style changes can prevent or reverse the progression of atherosclerosis. Support for comprehensive cardiovascular rehabilitation, *J Cardiopulmonary Rehabil* 12:159-162, 1992.

Chapter 68

MEDICAL THERAPY OF HEART FAILURE FOLLOWING MYOCARDIAL INFARCTION

Michael B. Higginbotham

Whether it appears as an early or late complication of MI, heart failure represents a problem of major functional and prognostic significance.[1,2] Once heart failure develops, it is usually associated with marked left ventricular dysfunction and chamber dilation. The incidence of heart failure increases in the years following MI.[3] Numerous studies have shown that the extent of left ventricular dilation at the time of hospital discharge is the best predictor of late post-MI mortality.[4] Accordingly, effective prevention and management of left ventricular dilation in heart failure have been identified as major goals in the management of post-MI patients.

PATHOPHYSIOLOGY OF HEART FAILURE FOLLOWING MI

As a consequence of extensive research over the past 10 years it is now known that in the acute phase of MI, stroke volume and cardiac output are compromised if 20% or more of the myocardium is lost.[5] The subsequent development, perpetuation, and exacerbation of left ventricular dysfunction and heart failure is a complex and dynamic process involving the effects of hemodynamic and neurohumoral factors on the heart and blood vessels. Although these responses are initially adaptive, they later contribute to the development of clinical manifestations of heart failure and to the maintenance and progression of the heart failure state. An appreciation of

these pathophysiological processes is important to guiding our approach to therapeutic interventions (Table 68-1).

Cardiac changes

In a recent review Mitchell and Pfeffer[6] described three phases of left ventricular remodeling post-MI — early (hours to days), subacute (days to weeks), and late (months).

1. During *early* remodeling lengthening and thinning of the infarct zone is seen within 10 minutes. This is followed by infarct expansion, which is seen in 30% to 45% of infarcts, particularly when they are large, anterior, and first infarctions. The predilection of this process for anterior infarctions is related not only to a relatively large infarcted area but also to the loss of curvature of the apical region, so that wall stress (afterload) increases according to the law of LaPlace. This is described by the following formula:

$$\sigma \text{ (wall stress)} = PR/2h$$

where P = pressure, R = radius of curvature and h = wall thickness, and represents the interrelationship between increases in preload and afterload (Fig. 68-1).

Acute changes are also seen in the noninfarct zone, with "stunning" and abnormal regional

Table 68-1. Pathophysiologic mechanisms of progressive left ventricular dysfunction and heart failure following myocardial infarction

Pathologic change	Principal pathophysiologic mechanism(s)
Cardiac	
Early (infarct expansion)	Increased LV wall stress (law of LaPlace)
Subacute ⎤ Myocyte hyper- trophy & slip- page; matrix Late ⎦ hypertrophy	Increased LV wall stress "Trophic" effects of SNSA, catecholamines, angiotensin II
Peripheral	
Vasoconstriction (Increased SVR)	SNSA, catecholamines AVP RAS (AII) Endothelin
Sodium & water retention (Edema, increased vascular stiffness, hyponatremia)	RAS (Aldosterone) AVP Decreased GFR
Vascular remodeling (Increased vascular stiff- ness)	SNSA, catecholamines AVP RAS (AII) Endothelin
Skeletal muscle changes (Aerobic enzymes decrease, FT fibers increase)	Deconditioning ? Decreased blood flow ? Neurohumoral stimulation

loading in the border zone and distention as a result of increased wall stress and cell slippage in the remote zone.

2. *Subacute* remodeling is seen following early infarct expansion. This is a period of complex remodeling analogous to that following pressure overload hypertrophy. Within days, concentric and eccentric left ventricular hypertrophy are seen, resulting from an increase in myocyte diameter and length, in proportion to infarct size. The distribution of concentric vs. eccentric left ventricular hypertrophy is heterogeneous and depends on regional geometry and wall thickness. The net result of these subacute changes is that left ventricular end-diastolic pressure is maintained and volume increases. As already mentioned, subacute remodeling is not seen in all infarcts. Indeed, when early infarct expansion does not occur, left ventricular volumes may diminish during this phase.

3. *Late* remodeling begins 3 to 4 weeks after MI. Fibrous scarring reduces the area of the infarct zone. Continued increases in left ventricular wall stress result in a gradual but moderate and heterogeneous increase in left ventricular volume and a decrease in left ventricular ejection fraction. These changes have been seen in approximately

40% of subjects studied and are associated with large infarctions and early infarct expansion. Mitchell and Pfeffer[6] termed these subjects "enlargers," in contrast to the 60% of subjects who are "nonenlargers" and whose left ventricular size did not change over time. "Enlargers" tend to develop poor left ventricular function and congestive heart failure and have a poor prognosis.

The extent to which left ventricular dilation progresses during cardiac remodeling depends on two factors: the size of the MI and the patency of the infarct-related coronary artery. The latter finding has important implications for the benefits that may be derived from thrombolytic therapy. Remarkably, infarct vessel patency appears to reduce infarct expansion even when it does not achieve myocardial salvage. The mechanism by which these benefits are derived is unknown but may include improved border zone perfusion, "erectile" splinting of the infarct region, and preservation of the collagen and vascular framework. Whatever the mechanism, the end results are reduced infarct expansion, prevention of left ventricular aneurysm formation, less late remodeling, and improved survival.

The cellular basis of remodeling has not been completely characterized. Complex changes in structure[7,8] have been seen, with alterations in myocytes, vasculature, and interstitium analogous to hypertrophic remodeling seen in hypertension. Weber has expressed the opinion that the "origins of heart failure are rooted in the hypertrophic remodeling of the myocardium," noting that left ventricular hypertrophy is an important predictor of heart failure in hypertension and coronary artery disease.[9] Similarly, Katz[10] has suggested a "cardiomyopathy of overload," in which hypertrophy is initially compensatory but leads eventually to cell death from abnormal protein production and "energy starvation." From animal models of progressive cardiomyopathy, other investigators have suggested a role for ischemic necrosis resulting from microvascular spasm and myocardial cell damage from calcium overload.

Peripheral changes

Peripheral circulatory alterations in patients with heart failure post-MI arise largely, though not entirely, from compensatory neurohumoral activation involving the sympathetic nervous system and the renin-angiotensin system.[8,11,12] A defect in baroreceptor function may contribute to autonomic imbalance.[13] An increase in sympathetic nervous system activity results in augmented contractility and heart rate (beta receptors) and vasoconstriction (alpha receptors). An increase in the activity of the renin-angiotensin system causes potent vasoconstriction via an increase in angiotensin and sodium and water retention through stimulation of aldosterone.[14] In addition, angiotensin II directly

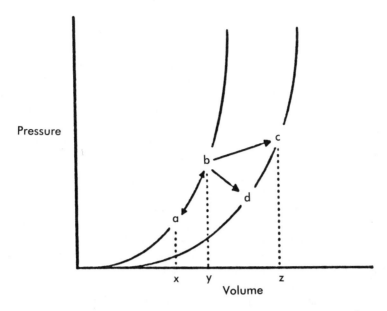

Fig. 68-1. LV Pressure-volume relationship following myocardial infarction.[6] During early remodeling (infarct expansion), increases in pressure and volume occur together (*a* to *b*). As remodeling progresses, the P-V curve shifts to the right, with higher volume associated with pressure that may be markedly elevated (*c*) or maintained near normal (*d*). (From Mitchell GF, Pfeffer MA: *Heart Failure* April/May:55-69, 1992.)

enhances sympathetic nervous system activity by stimulating presynaptic release of norepinephrine. The arginine-vasopressin system is also activated in heart failure[15] and may further contribute to peripheral vasoconstriction. In advanced heart failure stimulation of arginine vasopressin is responsible for hyponatremia; it reflects neurohumoral activation and predicts a poor prognosis.[16]

In addition to vasoconstriction the sympathetic, renin-angiotensin, and vasopressin systems, as well as endothelin, may contribute to alterations in vascular structure through chronic trophic effects.[8,17,18]

Activation of neurohumoral mechanisms is important from two perspectives: (1) the combined effects of vasoconstriction and of salt and water retention contribute to many of the symptoms and signs that characterize the heart failure state, such as peripheral edema, ascites, pulmonary congestion, fatigue, cold extremities, mental changes, oliguria, and poor exercise tolerance, and (2) although initially compensatory, these responses increase systolic and diastolic tension on the left ventricle, thereby producing excessive left ventricular wall stress according to the law of LaPlace, and they accelerate the process of remodeling. Thus alterations of the periphery in heart failure have therapeutic and prognostic implications far beyond improvement of the clinical manifestations of the condition.

A further peripheral change seen in patients with established heart failure is altered skeletal muscle function. Biochemical and histologic alterations have been demonstrated[19-22] that closely resemble those seen in deconditioning,[23] and can be at least partially reversed by training.[24] Although likely to represent an adaption to chronically limited blood flow rather than a primary limiting factor to exercise performance, skeletal muscle alterations may explain the inability to translate increases in cardiac output derived from therapy into immediate increases in exercise tolerance.

Neurohumoral activation and cardiac remodeling: a direct link

Although established concepts favor an indirect link between neurohumoral stimulation and cardiac remodeling (via mechanisms of increasing wall stress), a body of evidence has accumulated suggesting a direct interaction between neurohumoral activation and deterioration of left ventricular function.

Heart failure is known to cause a decline in norepinephrine stores and production, as well as a decrease in beta-adrenergic receptors.[25] In addition, high-dose catecholamine infusion can cause myocardial necrosis in experimental animals.[26] These effects could potentially contribute to myocardial dysfunction and to the remodeling process. Activation of both systemic and local renin-angiotensin systems has been implicated directly in the process of cardiac remodeling.[8,18] In experimental models of left ventricular hypertrophy, angiotensin II stimulates interstitial fibrosis, vascular hypertrophy and fibrosis; such changes have been prevented by pretreatment with the ACE inhibitor, captopril. The peptide endothelin is also activated in patients with heart failure and may play a role in remodeling through its actions as a vasoconstrictor and mitogenic growth factor.[8,18,27]

The combination of both direct and indirect effects on ventricular function by neurohumoral stimulation may explain its important and well-documented link to survival in heart failure.[16]

TREATMENT OF ESTABLISHED LEFT VENTRICULAR FAILURE POST-MI

The goals of therapy in heart failure have evolved as pathophysiological concepts have developed. Because current knowledge has established a clear link between left ventricular dysfunction, hemodynamics, neurohumoral function, heart failure symptoms, and mortality, we have come to expect a therapy to exert a positive impact on each of these areas. Thus, the current goals of therapy in heart failure are to relieve symptoms of edema, dyspnea, and fatigue; to improve functional capacity; to improve quality of life; to delay or prevent progression of the disease; and to prolong survival. Limiting neurohumoral activation and its consequences is implicit in achieving these goals.

General measures

Nonpharmacologic therapy is an important adjunct to managing the patient with heart failure. This includes (1) a *diagnostic workup* to rule out primary valvular heart disease, pericardial disease, heart failure due to diastolic dysfunction, or isolated right ventricular infarction. These conditions are often suspected clinically and are confirmed by echocardiography and/or cardiac catheterization, (2) *sodium and water restriction* commensurate with the severity of the heart failure, usually in the range of 1.5 to 2 liters of fluid and 2 to 3 grams of sodium daily, and (3) *selection of an appropriate level of physical activity*. It is now widely accepted that prolonged bed rest after MI is unnecessary and may be harmful. Exercise rehabilitation appears to improve long-term survival in the post-MI population as a whole.[28] The concept that physical activity may actually benefit post-MI patients with decreased left ventricular function has now developed, encouraged by the results of several small uncontrolled trials.[29-30] Jetté et al.[31] performed a controlled study of 4 weeks of intensive training in patients within 10 weeks following a large anterior MI. Although a training effect was reported in patients with ejection fractions less than 30%, 3 of 10 patients in this group suffered deterioration and were withdrawn. In the remaining patients exercise pulmonary artery wedge pressure was increased. More recently, Coats et al.[32] studied 19 patients with stable heart failure secondary to coronary artery disease in a controlled crossover trial of 8 weeks' exercise training. Although two patients dete-

riorated, the other 17 remained stable, with improved exercise tolerance and symptoms, increased exercise cardiac output, reduced minute ventilation, and partially normalized autonomic imbalance. The results of these small, short-term studies are insufficient to substantiate the safety or efficacy of exercise in patients with LV dysfunction post-MI; indeed, the high complication rate suggests that intensive training may have been detrimental in some patients. The issue of whether deterioration was related to neurohumoral stimulation during exercise and the significance of the results for long-term left ventricular function and for mortality are speculative. Until the results of long-term large controlled trials become available, it seems wise to permit exercise to comfortable levels, but to discourage unsupervised strenuous exertion in post-MI patients who have heart failure.

Drug therapy

Diuretics. Diuretics are widely regarded as appropriate first-line therapy in heart failure[33,34]; they rapidly remove excess salt and water and are well tolerated in the short term. Diuretics cannot be discontinued entirely once patients are on angiotensin-converting enzyme inhibitors[35] because sodium and water retention in heart failure results from low glomerular filtration as well as the actions of the renin angiotensin system.[36] In addition to its diuretic effect, intravenous furosemide may produce benefits from a venodilator action.[37]

Diuretic therapy can be initiated with a thiazide, but all but the patients with the mildest symptoms will require a loop diuretic such as furosemide. Metolazone is a very effective addition to the diuretic regimen of patients who do not respond well to furosemide alone.[38]

Despite their short-term efficacy, diuretics should be used as sparingly as is consistent with good symptom control. Diuretics are known to activate the sympathetic and renin-angiotensin systems,[39,40] which may have a detrimental long-term effect on hemodynamics[39] and ventricular arrhythmias.[41] The effect of diuretics on survival has not been studied, but there is a possibility that diuretics may enhance the progression of the disease.

Digitalis. The beneficial effects of digitalis glycosides were first described by William Withering in 1785. Since early in this century investigators both in the United Kingdom and the United States have noted that the main application of digitalis has been in the therapy of patients with heart failure complicated by atrial arrhythmias. The place of digitalis in patients with heart failure and sinus rhythm has been controversial, and recent trends have moved toward a reduced use of the drug.[42]

Experimental data have confirmed the significant inotropic effect from digitalis in both nonischemic and ischemic myocardium, which increases with the degree of left ventricular dysfunction.[43] Digitalis also has favorable effects on hemodynamics, improves baroreflex control, and attenuates neurohumoral activation.[44] Numerous clinical studies have confirmed digitalis' efficacy in patients with severe heart failure, characterized by a large heart, a third heart sound, a low ejection fraction, and severe congestion[45-48]; however, studies have produced evidence that digitalis has little or no effect in mild heart failure and mild left ventricular dysfunction.[45-47,49,50] Recent multicenter trials have demonstrated significant clinical deterioration following withdrawal of digoxin from patients with mild to moderate (functional Class II-III) heart failure, whether they were receiving ACE inhibitors[51] or not.[52] However, deterioration upon withdrawal of a drug cannot be equated with efficacy, and no prospective study to date has included this population. Furthermore, digitalis has been shown to be inferior to ACE inhibitors as first-line therapy.[53]

The ultimate role of digoxin will depend in large measure on its long-term effects on disease progression and survival. The fact that digitalis improves hemodynamics and decreases neurohumoral activation, at least acutely, is encouraging. On the other hand, there are good theoretical arguments against the use of an inotropic drug that increases rather than decreases myocardial oxygen and substrate utilization.[10] Experience with other inotropic agents has shown that possible detrimental effects on long-term LV remodeling and LV function must be considered.[10] Indeed, despite improving functional class and exercise tolerance to an extent similar to that of vasodilators in several studies, digitalis has not been demonstrated to improve survival. The long-term effects of the drug on neurohumoral activation are unknown. Digitalis has a low therapeutic-to-toxic ratio in the elderly, patients with renal impairment, patients with arrhythmia, and patients with chronic obstructive pulmonary disease and electrolyte disturbances.[54]

It is hoped that the appropriate clinical role of digitalis will be clarified with the results of a large prospective controlled mortality trial (the Digitalis Investigators Group or DIG study, being conducted by NHLBI) currently under way. Until these results become available (in 1995), it seems prudent to limit the use of digitalis to patients with severe (functional Class III and IV) heart failure and severe left ventricular dysfunction. These patients should be continued on the drug indefinitely because of the high incidence of deterioration after withdrawal seen in stable patients.[51,52] Alternative therapy should be selected for patients with mild left ventricular dysfunction and correspondingly mild symptoms.

Digitalis is commonly administered in doses of 0.125 to 0.25 mg daily as digoxin and adjusted appropriately in renal impairment and in the elderly. Digoxin levels are useful in obtaining a therapeutic benefit while avoiding toxicity; levels of .5 to 1.5 µg/mL are a common goal of therapy.[44] However, digitalis levels are no substitute for close clinical follow-up, and toxicity may develop even in the "therapeutic range."

Angiotensin-converting enzyme inhibitors. Given the importance of the renin-angiotensin system in heart failure, it is not surprising that we have seen the emergence of angiotensin-converting enzyme inhibitors as "a cornerstone of the therapy of heart failure."[55] Developed in the late 1970s because of their effects on the vasculature and kidney in hypertension, ACE inhibitors have now been shown to improve symptoms and exercise tolerance in severe, moderate, and mild heart failure.[56-58] In addition, ACE inhibitors have a favorable effect on survival during long-term therapy, reducing the likelihood of death from progressive heart failure[59,60] as well as sudden death[61-63] (Fig. 68-2). Although the effects of ACE inhibitors on preventing mortality in heart failure have been far from perfect, the quantitative importance has been at least equivalent to other interventions such as beta blockers and thrombolytic therapy post-MI.

The mechanism of action of ACE inhibitors in heart failure is complex and not completely understood. During chronic therapy a decrease in neurohumoral activation is seen, particularly for the renin-angiotensin system; thus the detrimental effects of neurohumoral activation on intravascular volume, hemodynamics, and long-term cardiovascular remodeling may be ameliorated. Although it is clear that long-term efficacy bears little relation to the initial hemodynamic effect of increasing stroke volume and cardiac output,[64] prolonged venodilation is seen, which may improve exercise tolerance by reducing left atrial and left ventricular diastolic pressures.[64,65] Besides having possible beneficial effects on pulmonary congestion, reduction of filling pressure also favors a decrease in left ventricular wall stress and improved left ventricular function; this corresponds to the small increase in ejection fraction seen in some studies.[57,58] Studies have demonstrated that a reduction in left ventricular filling pressures to normal levels is quite compatible with preserved stroke volume in ambulatory heart failure patients.[66] A decrease in pulmonary venous hypertension also results in a corresponding decrease in right ventricular diastolic pressure and wall stress, which may improve right ventricular function. The ability of ACE inhibitors to counter marked peripheral abnormalities caused by vasoconstriction and sodium and water retention may also play a role in their action.

Mancini et al.[67] have shown that even in the absence of an increase in cardiac output, enhanced limb blood flow is a prerequisite for improved exercise tolerance from ACE inhibitors in heart failure. Long-term benefits

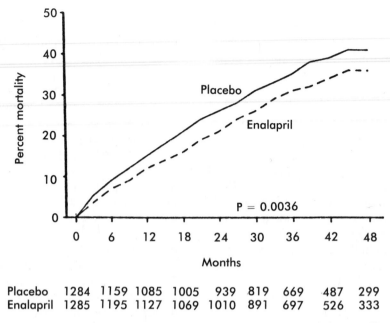

Fig. 68-2. Mortality curves for treatment and placebo groups in the SOLVD trial.[60] Mortality was reduced 16% by enalapril. (From The SOLVD Investigators: *New Engl J Med* 325(5):293-302, 1991.)

on mortality may result from peripheral hemodynamic improvements or reduction of the direct "trophic" effects of angiotensin II on the heart and blood vessels.[68] A favorable effect on electrolyte balance and arrhythmias has also been observed in several studies[41,69] and may contribute to the reduction in sudden death. Finally, recent evidence has demonstrated local synthesis of angiotensin II in the kidney, heart, and blood vessels, suggesting a possible dissociation between systemic ACE inhibition and the efficacy of these agents.[18,70] A recent study suggested that ultra–low-dose captopril, void of any systemic hemodynamic effect, may augment furosemide-induced natriuresis.[71]

Three ACE inhibitors—captopril,[56,57] enalapril,[53,58] and lisinopril[72]—are currently approved for use in heart failure, and preliminary studies with other agents have been promising.[73] Because of the early complications of hypotension and renal impairment,[74] ACE inhibitors usually are started at small doses (e.g., captopril 6.25 mg every 8 hours, enalapril 2.5 mg every 12 hours, or lisinopril 5 mg daily) and titrated up to "usual" doses of 25 mg every 8 hours for captopril, 10 mg every 12 hours for enalapril, or 20 mg daily for lisinopril.[75] It is important to realize, however, that the efficacy of ACE inhibitors in controlled trials has been generally confirmed at doses higher than the "usual" ones just described. Thus, an effort should probably be made to increase doses to 150 mg of captopril or 40 mg of enalapril, so long as severe hypotension can be avoided. The full effect of ACE inhibitors in improving symptoms and exercise tolerance typically is not seen for several

weeks after initiating therapy, possibly related to a slow reversal of the peripheral abnormalities discussed earlier. In patients at risk of hypotension and functional renal impairment (i.e., those with recent or severe heart failure, hyponatremia, renal artery stenosis, preexisting renal impairment, diabetic renal disease, preexisting hypotension, the elderly, or those on large doses of diuretics), only small doses of ACE inhibitor will be tolerated. Fortunately the phenomenon of hypotension and renal impairment is uncommon and usually mild, even with longer-acting agents.[59] The benefits of ACE inhibitors in small doses (in patients intolerant of higher doses) remains unproven, but their continued use appears justified at present. Initial hypotension or renal impairment with ACE inhibitors may be managed effectively by decreasing diuretics in most cases. ACE inhibitors rarely control the symptoms of heart failure in the absence of diuretics,[35] which appear to "sensitize" the circulation to the actions of ACE inhibitors[14] through neurohumoral stimulation.

Antiischemic effects of ACE inhibitors. A very interesting but generally unrecognized action of ACE inhibitors is their ability to reduce acute and chronic myocardial ischemia.[76] This effect may arise from indirect hemodynamic changes, such as a decrease in left ventricular filling pressure,[77] or from direct vasodilation of coronary arteries.[78] In addition, ACE inhibitors may have a profound effect on thrombosis and on the atherosclerotic process itself: via decreases in vascular angiotensin II and bradykinin, and increases in EDRF and prostaglandins, ACE inhibitors may significantly reduce vascular smooth muscle proliferation and migration, decrease matrix synthesis, decrease platelet aggregation, and increase tissue-plasminogen activator.[18,68] Finally, it is possible that captopril has a radical-free scavenging effect for preservation of ischemic myocardium by virtue of its sulfhydryl group.[79]

Activation of the renin-angiotensin system has been found to be an independent predictor of MI in patients with hypertension.[80] It appears also that the antiischemic actions of ACE inhibitors may have major clinical relevance to post-MI patients with heart failure. In the SOLVD trial[60] a reduction in recurrent MI and hospitalization for angina were observed during long-term follow-up.

Direct-acting vasodilators. Agents that have a direct dilatory action on the vasculature may primarily affect arteries (hydralazine and minoxidil), veins (nitrates), or both (alpha blockers and flosequinan). All have the potential of improving hemodynamics and left ventricular loading conditions. As discussed earlier, both arterial and venous vasodilation can have a beneficial effect on left ventricular wall stress (afterload).

Hydralazine. This direct-acting arteriolar vasodilator has marked hemodynamic benefits when given acutely and results in an increase in stroke volume and cardiac output and a decrease in systemic vascular resistance.[81] However, longer-term trials have demonstrated marked hemodynamic attenuation, poor long-term tolerance,[82] and a lack of benefit for symptoms or exercise tolerance.[83] Similar failure of long-term arterial vasodilation has been seen with minoxidil.[84]

Arterial vasodilation alone seems to be ineffective in the long-term management of heart failure. The combination of hydralazine and isosorbide dinitrate has been demonstrated to improve survival in heart failure[82]; however, the contribution of hydralazine to that effect is unproven and even somewhat doubtful given the ineffectiveness of hydralazine by itself. Not surprisingly, hydralazine given alone has not been shown to have effects on mortality comparable to ACE inhibitors.[63]

The use of hydralazine in chronic heart failure appears limited to patients with mitral regurgitation[85] and aortic regurgitation.[86] The effective dose of hydralazine is generally between 200 and 300 mg per day in divided doses every 6 hours.[33]

Nitrates. The nitrates are potent vasodilators with a predilection for epicardial coronary arteries, coronary collaterals, and systemic veins.[87] Initial administration of nitrates results in mixed arterial and venous vasodilation, with a decrease in blood pressure and systemic vascular resistance; an increase in stroke volume and cardiac output; and a decrease in right atrial, pulmonary artery, and pulmonary artery wedge pressures. Rapid attenuation of the arterial vasodilator effects follows during long-term therapy, but lower venous pressures persist.[88]

Some attenuation of venous pressure changes may occur[89] and can be prevented by the use of a nitrate-free period.

Long-term nitrates have not been demonstrated to be useful in achieving a benefit for heart failure patients in large placebo-controlled studies. However, smaller controlled trials have demonstrated that persistent decreases in filling pressure may be accompanied by an improvement in exercise tolerance and symptoms[88] during treatment with high doses of isosorbide dinitrate (120 to 160 mg daily). As for ACE inhibitors, the effect of nitrates on exercise tolerance was not seen immediately, which suggests a delayed redistribution of blood flow to skeletal muscle or a gradual process of reconditioning. Thus, as with ACE inhibitors, patients require a therapeutic trial of nitrates for at least several weeks.

The mechanism by which reduced filling pressure may improve symptoms in exercise tolerance in heart failure is unclear; possibilities include (1) relief of dyspnea by virtue of reduced pulmonary congestion, or (2) improved stroke volume and cardiac output reserve through decreases in left ventricular or right ventricular wall stress (afterload). It is of interest that improved exercise tolerance is not seen with arterial vasodilation; preservation of an adequate perfusion pressure may be important for the transfer of cardiac output to exercising skeletal muscle.[90]

It is also possible that nitrates may have a nonhemodynamic effect in chronic heart failure. By stimulating cyclic GMP, nitrates may inhibit vascular smooth muscle growth and reduce both peripheral and cardiac remodeling.[91]

Controlled trials have suggested that nitrates may alter the natural history of heart failure; combined with hydralazine, high-dose isosorbide dinitrate has been shown to improve prognosis in patients with moderate to severe heart failure,[82] though to a lesser extent than ACE inhibitors.[61] It is quite possible that such a benefit would be seen with nitrates alone, but this remains speculative. No study has demonstrated a benefit of the hydralazine/isosorbide dinitrate combination over nitrates alone.

Little support exists for the use of nitrates as first-line therapy in heart failure.[34] The clinical place of nitrates in heart failure appears to be as a replacement of (or supplement to) ACE inhibitors in patients with moderate to severe heart failure who are hypotensive and yet have persistently high filling pressures. The physician takes advantage of arterial tolerance, while hoping to maximize venodilation.

The usual dosage of nitrates starts at 10 mg every 8 hours for isosorbide dinitrate or 0.4 mg per hour of nitroglycerin in a transdermal preparation; the dose is then increased to the maximum level tolerated before the onset of intolerable headache or hypotension. Doses of 120 and 160 mg per day of isosorbide dinitrate[88] and 60 mg every 24 hours of transdermal nitroglycerin[89] appear to be desirable for maximal therapeutic effect. An effective nitrate-free interval can be achieved by administration of isosorbide dinitrate at 8-hour intervals[92] or by the temporary removal of nitroglycerin patches for 6 to 8 hours.[93]

Flosequinan. Approved in 1993 by the U.S. Food and Drug Administration for use in heart failure, flosequinan is a fluorinated quinolone compound with direct arterial and venous vasodilator effects comparable with nitroprusside.[94] A potent inotropic action has been demonstrated in animal models[95] but appears less pronounced in man.[96,97] Several placebo-controlled studies with orally administered flosequinan (100 mg) have demonstrated improvement in symptoms and exercise tolerance that are somewhat more pronounced than is seen with ACE inhibitors.[98-100] The drug also appears to be effective at this dose level when combined with commonly prescribed doses of ACE inhibitors.[101]

A potential disadvantage of flosequinan is that in high doses an increase in heart rate is observed; this heart rate increase is seen more during long-term than acute administration of flosequinan, suggesting a direct effect on the sinus node[94] rather than a reflex tachycardia. Doses of 100 mg are clinically effective and cause a modest increase in heart rate. Little increase in heart rate is seen at doses of 50 to 70 mg; however, efficacy has not been demonstrated for these dose levels.

A large survival trial (Prospective Randomized Flosequinan Longevity Evaluation or PROFILE) was initiated in 1991 to compare the effects in functional Class II to IV heart failure of placebo, 75 mg flosequinan, and 100 mg flosequinan. A disappointing early finding from this trial was that mortality was increased 51% with 100 mg flosequinan as compared with placebo in an interim analysis. A similar adverse trend was seen at the 75-mg dose level, and a decision was made to discontinue the trial.

The ultimate role of flosequinan in heart failure may depend on its efficacy in severe functional Class IV patients (in whom a clinical benefit may be considered more important than reduced survival) and in patients with mild to moderate heart failure at doses of 50 mg and 75 mg. No studies are currently underway to examine these issues.

Alpha-adrenergic blockers. Prazosin, the prototype alpha-adrenergic blocker, produces both arterial and venous dilation. However, there is marked early attenuation of its hemodynamic effects,[102] accompanied by an inconsistent improvement in symptoms and exercise tolerance.[103] Symptomatic improvement accompanies persistent venodilation in the face of attenuated arterial dilation[104] — a situation analogous to that achieved with long-term nitrates.

In one large controlled trial, prazosin had no effect on long-term mortality when compared with placebo.[82] It is notable that prazosin (like other arterial vasodilators) activates the renin-angiotensin system; this system is suppressed by ACE inhibitors, which have favorable effects on the natural history of heart failure.[105]

These observations indicate that alpha-adrenergic blockers have no role in the standard therapy of established heart failure. They may be used in the rare patient who is unable to tolerate the more effective regimens.

Calcium-channel antagonists. Because of their potent arteriolar dilating effects,[106] calcium-channel blockers have been evaluated for use in congestive heart failure. However, early experience with nifedipine was disappointing, with adverse hemodynamic effects and frequent clinical deterioration.[107,108] Effects with diltiazem were less unfavorable, but hemodynamics have tended to be preserved rather than improved.[109]

Unfortunately, despite a small reduction in reinfarction rates following non–Q-wave MI,[110] post-MI studies using nifedipine and diltiazem have indicated a trend toward increased complications and mortality in patients with heart failure.[111-113] Verapamil has demonstrated a reduction in cardiac events only in post-MI patients free of heart failure.[114]

Currently, newer vasoselective agents felodipine and amlodipine[115] are being investigated for early use in heart failure, based on animal data suggesting that verapamil may prevent experimental cardiomyopathy[116] by decreasing microvascular spasm and calcium overload. Two large trials are currently underway (V-HeFT III for felodipine and PRAISE (Prospective Randomized Amlodipine Survival Evaluation) for amlodipine). Although these agents may ultimately be shown to be helpful in limiting cardiac remodeling and in delaying the natural history of LV dysfunction, calcium-channel blockers are not currently indicated for the therapy of heart failure. In patients with significant left ventricular dysfunction and severe CAD with ischemia refractory to other agents, a careful trial of calcium-channel blockers may be necessary to relieve symptoms, but such patients should be monitored for development of worsening heart failure.

Beta-adrenergic blockers. As discussed earlier, sympathetic nervous system activation is seen early following MI and may contribute to many of the clinical manifestations of heart failure as well as to decreased left ventricular performance resulting from reduced beta receptor responsiveness, decreased norepinephrine production and release, increased left ventricular wall stress, coronary vasoconstriction, and even direct myocardial injury. Increased sympathetic nervous system activity is associated with poor survival in heart failure.[117,118] It is not surprising, then, that beta-adrenergic agonists have been shown to be ineffective heart failure therapy and may even lead to worsening of the condition and shortened survival.[119,120]

Interest in a possible role for beta-adrenergic blockers in the treatment of idiopathic cardiomyopathy developed from early studies by Waagstein et al.[121] Several subsequent reports primarily with the nonselective agents metoprolol and bucindolol appear to have confirmed improvement in ejection fraction and functional class following at least 2 months of therapy in patients with idiopathic cardiomyopathy.[122,123] Effects on exercise tolerance have been mixed, with an increase in some studies and a decrease in others. In a recent study (the Metoprolol in Dilated Cardiomyopathy [MDC] trial)[124] a strong trend was reported toward reduction in a combined endpoint, death or "need for transplantation," following beta-blocker therapy. However, no study to date has confirmed a significant improvement in survival with beta-blocker therapy in cardiomyopathy.

The beneficial results of beta blockers on functional class in patients with left ventricular dysfunction secondary to coronary disease has been studied very little. Woodly et al.[125] demonstrated a smaller (though significant) improvement in coronary vs. noncoronary patients treated with bucindolol. Andersson et al.,[126] in a non–placebo-controlled study, noted that apparent clinical benefits from metoprolol were seen only in idiopathic (nonischemic) cardiomyopathy.

The relative contribution of various mechanisms by which beta blockers may improve left ventricular function and symptoms in heart failure is unclear. However, recent studies have confirmed a decrease in neurohumoral activation, an increase in beta-receptor density, and improved hemodynamic response to catecholamine stimulation[127] following beta-blocker therapy.

Despite functional benefits and improvements in ventricular performance that may be achieved with long-term beta blockers in heart failure, initial deterioration of the heart failure state has been seen in 5% to 20% of subjects[128]; clearly it will be essential to establish guidelines for careful initiation of therapy if beta blockers are to be widely used for the treatment of heart failure.

Perhaps the greatest potential for beta blockers in heart failure post-MI may be through effects on the progression of heart failure, which may translate to important differences in survival. Preliminary studies have indicated that nonselective beta blockers may slow deterioration and prolong survival in patients with heart failure secondary to cardiomyopathy or MI[128,129] but that these results may not be applicable to beta blockers with intrinsic sympathomimetic activity.[129] Beta blockers may have the additional effect of preventing ventricular arrhythmias.[130] In the BHAT study[128] metoprolol sig-

nificantly decreased sudden death in patients with heart failure treated soon after MI.

It should be emphasized that the long-term effects of beta blockers on mortality in heart failure are unknown. Results of larger mortality studies currently in progress will be required before beta blockers are used for this purpose.

Newer inotropic agents. Myocardial contraction depends on effective intracellular calcium transport, and inotropic agents may facilitate this by various mechanisms[131]: digoxin acts by $Na+/K+$-dependent ATPase inhibition; beta agonists, glucagon, and histamine act on cardiac receptors to stimulate adenylate cyclase; phosphodiesterase inhibitors increase adenylate cyclase by reducing its breakdown. Other agents have been shown to have a direct action on calcium channels or sodium channels to increase calcium availability.

Triggered by the controversy surrounding the utility of digitalis in heart failure accompanied by normal sinus rhythm, early attempts to develop a nonglycoside, orally active inotropic agent for heart failure focused on beta-adrenergic agonists and phosphodiesterase inhibitors. The latter agents were reported to have an inotropic action with less adverse effects on myocardial energy requirement than beta agonists.[132] As mentioned earlier, beta-adrenergic agonists such as prenolterol, pirbuterol, and xamoterol, although having apparently beneficial hemodynamic effects, were demonstrated to be ineffective in the long term and to have possible detrimental effects on survival. Despite early encouraging results with L-dopa in heart failure, the oral dopamenergic agent ibopamine was not shown to be effective in U.S. studies.[133]

The phosphodiesterase inhibitors amrinone and enoximone, despite acute improvements in hemodynamics and exercise tolerance, also failed to show consistent beneficial effects on symptoms and hemodynamics.[134,135] In addition to rapid attenuation of their beneficial effects, cessation of these agents revealed deterioration from their baseline state. Also, an unexpectedly high mortality was noted in patients receiving these phosphodiesterase inhibitors. Several investigators concluded from this that inotropic stimulation may adversely affect the natural history of heart failure[136]; others have emphasized the possibility of calcium-dependent arrhythmias as a result of increased cyclic AMP production.[130]

Much of the recent development of phosphodiesterase inhibitors has focused on the potent agent milrinone, despite early indications of possible hemodynamic deterioration[137] and high mortality during follow-up,[138] as with the "first-generation" compounds. Encouraging initial results were obtained with this drug in clinical trials, including the demonstration of improved exercise tolerance and symptoms in a 3-month, double-

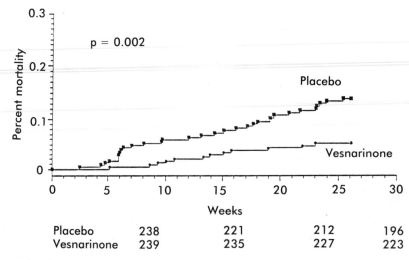

Fig. 68-3. Cumulative mortality observed with placebo and vesnarinone in patients with severe LV dysfunction (mean EF 20%) and functional Class II-IV congestive heart failure taking digoxin, diuretics, and ACE inhibitors. A 62% reduction in mortality was seen.[145] (From Feldman AM, Bristow MR, Parmley WW, et al. for the Vesnarinone Study Group: *New Engl J Med* 329:149-155, 1993.)

blind, placebo-controlled trial.[48] However, disappointing results were obtained when long-term survival was studied; milrinone was associated with a marked increase in mortality compared with placebo at 6 months.[139] These data do not support a role for oral phosphodiesterase inhibitors in heart failure.

Several "new-generation" inotropic agents are currently under development for heart failure. Pimobendan appears to owe its inotropic action to sensitization of the contractile proteins to intracellular calcium, as well as to phosphodiesterase inhibition. A recent multicenter trial has demonstrated beneficial effects of pimobendan on exercise tolerance and quality of life in heart failure patients.[140] Mortality data are not available for pimobendan. OPC-8212 or vesnarinone is an orally active agent that increases calcium availability by a complex array of direct actions on sodium, calcium, and potassium channels.[141] The agent does not appear to be proarrhythmic and may have an antiarrhythmic effect in low doses.[142] Early data on vesnarinone have been encouraging, with a decrease in symptoms and an increase in exercise tolerance, quality of life, and survival seen in double-blind, placebo-controlled trials.[143,144] Favorable trends seen in these small studies have been confirmed in a recent multicenter, placebo-controlled morbidity and mortality trial of 564 patients with advanced heart failure and ejection fractions less than 30%. In this trial, vesnarinone, given at a dose of 60 mg daily in addition to digoxin, diuretics, and ACE inhibitors, resulted in a highly significant improvement in quality of life, and a 62% decrease in mortality after 6 months of treatment[145] (Fig. 68-3). The major drug-related adverse effect was neutropenia, observed in 2.5% of patients within 16 weeks and reversible by

discontinuing the drug. An important aspect of this study was that, at a daily dosage of 120 mg, a trend toward increased mortality was observed; this suggests a dose-related alteration in the balance between vesnarinone's inotropic, vasodilator, and arrhythmic properties. Although further clarification of the drug's mode of action is necessary, it appears that vesnarinone will play an important role in the future treatment of severe heart failure.

Outpatient dobutamine therapy. Despite the clinical stability and improvement that can be obtained with diuretics, digitalis, ACE inhibitors, and direct vasodilating agents, many patients eventually develop refractory heart failure with severe symptoms, hypotension, and renal impairment. Such patients who are refractory to oral therapy may require hospital admission for inotropic support. Some patients are candidates for cardiac transplantation and may receive intravenous inotropic therapy on an inpatient basis; those who are not transplant candidates must be stabilized or face recurrent hospital admissions or early death from progressive heart failure.

The inotropic catecholamine dobutamine, developed in 1973 and tested in the United States soon afterward, has marked immediate hemodynamic effects, which can be maintained in the long term if appropriate dose levels are administered.[146] Beginning in 1980 several uncontrolled reports noted a sustained benefit from dobutamine that extended beyond the time of the dobutamine infusion.[147] Subsequently, sustained benefits were demonstrated from weekly 4-hour infusions of dobutamine in a controlled but unblinded study[148] and in a placebo-controlled trial following a single 72-hour infusion.[149] The observed benefits were attributed to a conditioning effect but may have resulted from alpha blockade or from a sustained improvement in sodium and water balance.

Unfortunately, in a multicenter trial of outpatient dobutamine vs. placebo no benefit was demonstrated, and there was an increase in sudden death in the dobutamine group.[150] The detrimental effect in that study has been ascribed to catecholamine-induced arrhythmia[151] and hypokalemia[152] but may have been caused by an adverse effect on cardiac function, induced by inotropic stimulation.

No recent studies of intermittent dobutamine therapy have been reported. It remains undetermined whether the benefits of hospitalization for inotropic therapy, which include close hemodynamic and electrocardiographic monitoring, careful adjustment of diuretics and vasodilators, and strict adherence to diet and relative rest, can be reproduced safely and effectively by administering dobutamine to outpatients.

The technology is now available to give patients continuous infusions of dobutamine at home, using portable pumps and permanent intravenous access via subcutaneously tunneled catheters.[153] Although still experimental in nature, this approach has shown promise and warrants further investigation.

Combination therapy. The use of drug combinations in heart failure follows the rationale, well established in the therapy of hypertension, that additive or even synergistic effects can be obtained while avoiding side effects of high-dose single-drug therapy. The approach has been successful in the management of acute heart failure, with hemodynamic benefits being derived from combinations of dobutamine and amrinone[154]; isosorbide and hydralazine,[155] and angiotensin-converting enzymes combined with hydralazine,[156] prazosin,[157] digoxin,[158] and milrinone.[159] However, the situation is far more complex in chronic heart failure. The exact mode of action of many drugs is unknown, and short-term hemodynamics may be irrelevant to the effects of therapy in the longer term. Finally, it is virtually impossible to study a drug combination across the dose range for each agent, so the question of whether two drugs in combination are better than one given at an adequate dosage is difficult to resolve.

Because of the methodological difficulties, very few long-term studies have been attempted to determine whether combining agents is better than using them alone. An excellent example of this problem is the combination of hydralazine and nitrates, which has been used effectively in two large multicenter mortality trials[61,82] but has never been demonstrated to provide more benefit than nitrates alone. In one of the rare combination studies that has been performed, milrinone and digoxin, both effective by themselves, had no additive value in combination.[48] In a recent study

flosequinan has been shown to be effective when added to long-term captopril therapy[101]; however, ACE inhibition was not administered at maximally tolerated levels, so the clinical role of this combination remains to be defined.

Most trials of drug therapy have in fact incorporated combination treatment into their study design: digoxin has been studied in addition to diuretics, and virtually all vasodilator studies have been conducted with "conventional therapy," including diuretics and usually digoxin, in both the treatment and placebo groups. Thus, we know that combination therapy is effective but are left to wonder about the relative benefit of combined vs. single-drug therapy.

Stevenson and co-workers[160] have proposed that combination therapy with digoxin, diuretics, and vasodilators be "tailored" to specific hemodynamic goals and that the short-term benefits can be maintained. However, these results, obtained in a uniform population of severely ill heart failure patients awaiting transplantation, may not apply to a broader heart failure population. In addition, measurements of hemodynamics in all patients with heart failure would be impractical.

It is clear then that few specific guidelines are available for combination therapy in heart failure. Unfortunately, one must attempt to use combined therapy based on pathophysiological considerations, as well as on the known effectiveness of each agent.

Recommendations. The selection of specific drug combinations will depend on the severity of heart failure. In patients who are severely ill (functional Class IV), relief of symptoms and correction of hemodynamic abnormalities are the highest priorities. Intensive sodium restriction and adequate rest are important. Initial therapy should include a combination of diuretics, digoxin, and an ACE inhibitor as tolerated. If the patient cannot tolerate ACE inhibition because of hypotension or other side effects, it is reasonable to add nitrates in an attempt to reduce filling pressures while maintaining systemic arterial pressure. The addition of nitrates in this situation seems preferable to increasing diuretics to high levels with attendant increases in neurohumoral activity. The precise role of flosequinan will remain unknown until further studies are available, whereas vesnarinone may be the most promising new agent for improving both symptoms and survival in severe heart failure.

For patients who are so ill as to require recurrent hospital admission for intravenous diuretics and inotropic agents, dobutamine at home may be attempted.

In patients with mild to moderate heart failure (functional Class II to III), the emphasis should be placed on early use of ACE inhibitors with the minimum diuretic therapy necessary to relieve edema. Digitalis should probably be reserved for patients with functional Class III heart failure and for functional Class II patients who have severe LV dysfunction and cardiac dilation. Despite encouraging results for the newer inotropic agent, vesnarinone, no role has yet been established for inotropic agents in patients with milder symptoms.

Treatment of ventricular arrhythmias

Approximately 40% of the deaths seen in heart failure patients are sudden[161] and quite unexpected, occurring in patients who are clinically stable. Some of these deaths may be caused by bradyarrhythmia or electromechanical dissociation,[162] but the majority arise from sustained ventricular tachycardia and ventricular fibrillation. Although ischemia, neurohumoral stimulation, and electrolyte imbalance have been implicated in triggering serious arrhythmias, the underlying mechanism in heart failure appears to be sustained reentry secondary to nonuniform ventricular conduction.[163]

It is not surprising that a close relationship exists between the extent of left ventricular dysfunction and the incidence of lethal arrhythmias. Left ventricular size and ejection fraction predict sudden death as well as they predict death caused by progressive heart failure.[164,165] The majority of patients with heart failure and left ventricular dysfunction have ventricular arrhythmias on Holter monitoring, and most have "complex" premature ventricular complexes or nonsustained ventricular tachycardia.[161] Although arrhythmias detected before hospital discharge for MI are associated with increased mortality, their independent predictive value is small,[161,166] after the degree of left ventricular dysfunction has been taken into account. This observation suggests that Holter arrhythmias and the arrhythmias that lead to sudden death are two largely independent consequences of severe left ventricular dysfunction. Similarly, sustained ventricular tachycardia inducible by electrophysiological study has been found in small studies to be predictive of subsequent mortality after MI,[167,168] but this observation has not been entirely uniform and has not been shown to be independently predictive once other variables such as left ventricular function are taken into account.[169] Signal-averaged electrocardiography has yielded similar early results,[170] but these are quite preliminary.

Although these observations do not strongly support the use of Holter monitoring or electrophysiological testing to select therapy, the incidence of lethal arrhythmias and sudden death in heart failure provides ample rationale for considering antiarrhythmic therapy in these patients. The use of antiarrhythmics is problematic because of frequent side effects, depression of left ventricular function,[171] and proarrhythmia, which is seen in 20% to 30% of patients with left ventricular dysfunction.[171-173] Furthermore, antiarrhythmics are relatively ineffective in heart failure patients.[174]

No trial has yet demonstrated reduction of mortality from antiarrhythmic therapy in either idiopathic or ischemic cardiomyopathy. In fact, recent studies have confirmed an increase in sudden death rate in patients treated with antiarrhythmics, despite apparently successful suppression of Holter arrhythmias.[175] Similar results have been observed in mixed populations treated with quinidine for atrial fibrillation.[176] Only two small uncontrolled studies—both using amiodarone—have suggested a benefit from antiarrhythmic therapy in heart failure. Simonton et al.[177] demonstrated a decrease in sudden death using amiodarone in patients receiving phosphodiesterase inhibitors, and Dargie et al.[178] observed a decrease in the sudden death rate in amiodarone-treated patients with heart failure caused by ischemic or idiopathic cardiomyopathy. A recent study by Pfisterer et al.[179] did not confirm a benefit from amiodarone in post-MI patients with impaired LV function. A Veterans' Affairs (VA) study is now evaluating the survival effects of amiodarone in a large multicenter heart failure trial.

The current approach toward preventing sudden death in patients with heart failure secondary to MI should be multifactorial and should not focus on the use of antiarrhythmic agents. Measures include (1) careful treatment of heart failure with early introduction of ACE inhibitors, which not only reduces ambient arrhythmias but has been demonstrated to decrease sudden death. ACE inhibitors may reduce ventricular arrhythmias by increasing serum potassium, decreasing wall stress, decreasing ischemia, or decreasing neurohumoral activation; (2) the avoidance of excessive diuretic use, which may lead to potassium and magnesium depletion, neurohumoral activation, and exacerbation of ventricular arrhythmias; (3) the reservation of drug treatment for symptomatic ventricular tachycardia, and perhaps prolonged nonsustained VT on Holter monitoring or sustained ventricular tachycardia on electrophysiological testing; (4) use of beta blockers in heart failure post-MI in patients able to tolerate such therapy; and (5) when antiarrhythmic therapy is to be used, it is probably best to avoid Class 1C agents and consider early introduction of amiodarone. Patients who do not tolerate amiodarone therapy should be considered for an implantable defibrillator.

Anticoagulation

Patients with severe nonischemic cardiomyopathy have a high incidence of systemic embolism regardless of whether an intraventricular thrombus is evident; long-term anticoagulants are recommended for them[180] unless specifically contraindicated. Milder cases of cardiomyopathy have a more favorable outlook, and the risk of anticoagulants does not appear to be warranted.[181]

Early after an anterior MI the incidence of left

ventricular thrombus is high,[182] and such patients are at considerable risk of embolism. Anticoagulation appears warranted, at least for the first 3 months post-MI, for prevention of reinfarction, systemic and venous thromboembolism, and death.[183-185] In contrast, chronic LV thrombi in the presence of an aneurysm have a low rate of embolism[186] and do not justify anticoagulation unless there is a history of previous embolism or the thrombus is seen to be mobile or protruding on echocardiography.[187] Additional consideration may be given to anticoagulation if the patient's heart failure is severe or complicated by atrial fibrillation.

The use of aspirin has not been investigated for the prevention of systemic embolism in heart failure. However, recent studies of patients with atrial fibrillation have yielded mixed results. In two large trials[188,189] aspirin appeared to have no advantage over placebo for the prevention of stroke or systemic embolism. In another trial[190] warfarin was more effective in preventing thromboembolism than aspirin, but aspirin (325 mg daily) was more effective than placebo. To the extent that left atrial and left ventricular thrombi are equivalent, these findings support a preference for warfarin in heart failure post-MI, and for the use of aspirin when warfarin is contraindicated.

MANAGEMENT OF THE PATIENT WITH ASYMPTOMATIC POSTINFARCTION LEFT VENTRICULAR DYSFUNCTION

Based on the known progression of left ventricular dilation and loss of left ventricular function through remodeling after MI and the prognostic implications of progressive left ventricular enlargement, there has been intense interest in developing interventions that limit infarct size, prevent early infarct expansion, and prevent associated late left ventricular remodeling before the patient becomes symptomatic from heart failure. Experimental data described earlier have led to the investigation of two approaches: (1) early revascularization, which may help reduce early infarct expansion and its sequelae even without myocardial salvage, and (2) drug therapy to reduce the harmful effects of neurohumorally mediated vasoconstriction and sodium retention on left ventricular wall stress, in addition to potential direct deleterious effects of sympathetic nervous system activation and renin-angiotensin system activation on the cardiovascular system.

Interest in drug therapy as a means of reducing post-MI left ventricular dysfunction became intense in 1985 with the studies of Pfeffer et al., who demonstrated a decrease in left ventricular dilation[191] and an increase in 1-year survival[192] in animals with moderately large MIs treated with an ACE inhibitor. Subsequent human studies appear to support these findings. Pfeffer et al.[193] found in a double-blind placebo-controlled trial that

subjects with anterior MIs and initial ejection fractions < 45% developed progressive ventricular enlargement. Administration of captopril in doses of up to 50 mg every 8 hours beginning 11 to 31 days post-MI reduced the progressive left ventricular enlargement and reduced left ventricular filling pressure in patients with at least 30% akinesis or dyskinesis of the left ventricle at 1-year follow-up; in addition, exercise tolerance was improved with captopril, suggesting the presence of subclinical heart failure in these apparently asymptomatic patients. Sharpe et al.[194] demonstrated comparable results from the administration of captopril beginning 8 to 9 days post-MI, preventing the progressive left ventricular dilation seen with placebo or furosemide. In 1991 Sharpe et al.[195] reported a similar effect in a 100-patient study in which captopril (50 mg bid) was administered beginning 24 to 48 hours post-MI. That a long-term effect on remodeling was achieved was supported by the observation that no clinical deterioration was seen when captopril was withdrawn for 48 hours 3 months after the initiation of therapy.

The mechanism by which ACE inhibitors favorably affect left ventricular remodeling is unknown. Effects on decreasing preload may be very important because it is known that most of the increase in wall stress in the post-MI ventricle is in diastole; venodilation is far more capable of reducing diastolic tension than arterial dilation is of reducing systolic tension.[196] In this context it is of interest that the venodilator nitroglycerin has been shown to limit infarct size and expansion,[197] but the arterial dilator hydralazine has not.[198] Although failure of hydralazine may have resulted from other mechanisms such as an unfavorable effect on pulsatile load[199] or stimulation of angiotensin II, lack of venodilation may have been responsible. ACE inhibitors have actions other than venodilation that may ameliorate the processes of infarct expansion and remodeling; these include a reduction of the trophic effects of angiotensin II on the cardiovascular system (as discussed earlier) and a reduction in direct cardiotoxic effects of the sympathetic nervous system. As detailed earlier, ACE inhibitors also have direct effects on the coronary arteries and reduce ischemic injury; this may well result in a decrease in MI size or ischemia-related remodeling.

The results of a large, 45-center survival trial of ACE inhibitors post-MI were reported recently. This study, the Survival and Ventricular Enlargement (SAVE) study,[200] enrolled 2231 patients who had an ejection fraction of 40% or less following AMI. The patients had an average age of 59.4 years and a mean ejection fraction of 31%. Thirty-five percent of the patients had had previous MIs, and 43% were hypertensive. Although none had heart failure requiring ACE inhibitors, 30% were on beta blockers and 40% were on calcium blockers for hypertension; 33% had received thrombolytics, and

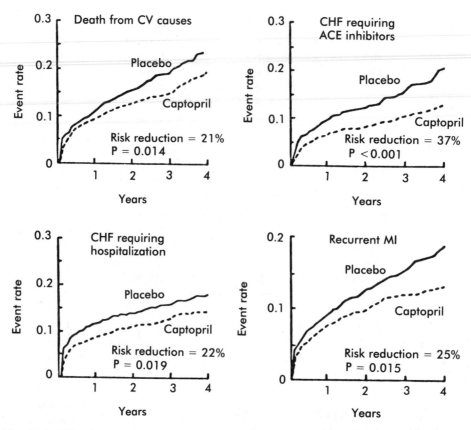

Fig. 68-4. Life tables for cumulative fatal and nonfatal cardiovascular events in the SAVE trial.[200] Significant reductions were seen in death from cardiovascular (CV) causes, congestive heart failure (CHF) requiring ACE inhibitors or hospitalization, and recurrent myocardial infarction (MI). (From Pfeffer MA, Braunwald E, Moye LA, et al. on behalf of the SAVE Investigators: *New Engl J Med* 327(10):669–677, 1992.)

12% had undergone percutaneous transluminal coronary angioplasty. Patients were randomized to captopril or placebo 3 to 16 days post-MI and were followed for 2 to 5 years; doses of captopril were relatively high, with 78% of patients taking 50 mg three times daily.

At a mean follow-up of 4 years 502 patients died, 274 from the placebo group (24.6%) and 228 from the captopril group (20.6%). Captopril was associated with a significant 17% decrease in total mortality and a similar 21% decrease in cardiac mortality (Fig. 68-4). The reduction in mortality was primarily caused by a decrease in death from pump failure, although a trend toward reduction of sudden death was also seen. The benefit of captopril for survival was seen independent of ejection fraction, Killip class, beta-blocker therapy, or thrombolytics. Interestingly, the trend for increased survival did not begin until 10 months postrandomization. In addition to its effects on mortality, captopril significantly reduced the onset of severe heart failure by 36%, hospitalization for heart failure by 19%, and recurrent MI by 24% (Fig. 68-4). In a subset of 419 patients studied with serial echocardiography, left ven-

tricular dilation was significantly reduced in the captopril-treated group.

It is important to note that in the SAVE trial, therapy was delayed 3 to 16 days. The question of whether greater benefit could be achieved with earlier therapy has not yet been answered. The rationale for early intervention is that infarct expansion provides the basis for later left ventricular remodeling. Experimentally it has been observed that the effects of ACE inhibitors in decreasing hypertrophy, necrosis, and fibrosis in left ventricular hypertrophy models are diminished after several days.[201] Unfortunately, there are potential dangers involved in the early use of ACE inhibitors post-MI as well. Because of early dependence on the compensatory role of the renin-angiotensin system, hypotension may occur with detrimental effects, as was seen in a study of intravenous nitroprusside administered less than 6 hours postinfarction.[202] Preliminary studies indicate that ACE inhibitors can be given 6 to 24 hours after the onset of MI without frequent hypotension.[203,204] Several large multicenter trials are currently underway, including ISIS-4, with randomization to captopril vs. placebo within 24 hours, and GISSI-3, with early randomization to lisinopril vs. placebo. Unfortunately, the design of these trials will not permit assessment of the relative benefit (or disadvantage) of early vs. late therapy, will not identify patient subgroups that may benefit especially (or not at all) from the intervention, and will not provide long-term follow-up data. One large study of early postinfarction administration of ACE inhibitors, CONSENSUS-II,[205] was terminated prematurely because of the lack of a beneficial effect of enalapril at 6 months; although these findings support the possibility that the benefits of ACE-inhibitor therapy early post-MI may be specific to captopril, failure of CONSENSUS-II may equally have resulted from early and sustained hypotension, or from the fact that the study was terminated too early for the benefits of therapy to become evident. Taken together, these results suggest that the theoretical benefits of very early ACE inhibition (within 24 hours post-MI) may not be clinically relevant, particularly given the possibility of a detrimental early fall in blood pressure.

The benefits of ACE inhibition in the early post-MI infarction period appear to extend to the asymptomatic patient with left ventricular dysfunction secondary to remote MI. In the "prevention" arm of the SOLVD trial[206] 4228 patients with ejection fractions 35% or less who were asymptomatic (67%) or minimally symptomatic (33%) were randomized to enalapril or placebo. The average age of the patients was 59 years and the average ejection fraction 28.3%, very similar to the population in the SAVE trial. Eighty-three percent had ischemic heart disease, and 80% had had a previous MI. Thirty percent were receiving nitrates, 24% beta blockers, 35% calcium channel blockers, 17% diuretics, and 12% digoxin for non–heart-failure indications. During a 4-year follow-up there were 329 deaths in the placebo group (15.5%) and 308 in the enalapril group (14.6%); the difference was insignificant ($P = 0.30$). Cardiovascular mortality was reduced significantly in the enalapril group (11.7%) compared with the placebo group (13.3%, $P = .048$) because of a difference in mortality from progressive heart failure. Although the effects on mortality were of borderline significance, enalapril markedly reduced hospitalization for congestive heart failure and reduced ischemic events such as MI (by 23%) and unstable angina (by 13%). It can be estimated from these results that for every 1000 patients treated for 3 years with enalapril, the drug would have prevented 15 deaths, 65 hospitalizations for heart failure, and 35 incidents of MI or unstable angina. A substudy confirmed neurohumoral activation, seen as an increase in plasma norepinephrine, renin, vasopressin, and atrial natriuretic factor levels in even asymptomatic patients.[207]

The evolving data on ACE inhibitors, in particular the results of the recent SAVE and SOLVD trials, appear to confirm the importance of neurohumoral activation in the natural history of heart failure and provide strong evidence that ACE inhibitors may be useful in any patient who has moderate to severe left ventricular dysfunction post-MI, whether or not they are symptomatic. ACE inhibitors are likely to become standard therapy in the post-MI patient.

FOLLOW-UP ASSESSMENT OF DRUG THERAPY

It is natural for both the physician and the patient to believe that once a drug is administered its effects should be followed in order to optimize its dosage, to add other drugs when necessary, and to withdraw it if it is ineffective.

However, the issue of follow-up is far from simple when applied to the individual patient. Two major obstacles must be confronted:

1. The first obstacle is the uncertainty about which is the best method of assessing improvement (or deterioration) on treatment.

In this regard one must choose among the patient's hemodynamics, LV function, functional class, quality of life, or submaximal or maximal exercise tolerance.

The optimal method of assessment will vary with the goals of therapy, and these have changed radically with increased understanding of pathophysiology and natural history to include not only improvement of symptoms and exercise tolerance but also prevention of progressive LV dysfunction and improved survival. Even these goals can be conflicting, as recent experience has shown with phosphodiesterase inhibitors and flosequinan.

- *In functional Class IV patients* the clinical consequences of abnormal hemodynamics are a primary target of therapy; therefore, serial evaluation of hemodynamics seems reasonable. However, it is far from established that achievement of "optimal" hemodynamics predicts long-term improvement and a better chance of survival.
- *In functional Class II-III patients* functional capacity is of great importance. In these patients New York Heart Association Class[208] or "quality of life" assessment[209] may reflect an individual's response to therapy.
  Exercise testing methods may also be useful, and measurement of peak O_2 consumption and of the anaerobic threshold are highly reproducible and sensitive to change with interventions.[210-212] The use of submaximal exercise testing, although functionally relevant, does not appear to have adequate reproducibility for following individuals.[213]
- *In asymptomatic patients with LV dysfunction*, symptoms and functional evaluations clearly cannot be used to evaluate the impact of therapy. However, the patient's progress over time can be followed with serial evaluations for signs of prognostically

important variables such as symptom development, deteriorating LV function, and worsening VO$_{2max}$.[214]

2. The second obstacle to be overcome is the complex and variable natural history of the individual heart failure patient, independent of drug therapy.

Over time the heart failure patient may change because of a variety of factors, including spontaneous improvement in condition, a placebo response, progressive LV deterioration, or events such as pulmonary embolism, recurrent infarction, infection, or other illness. Thus improvement or deterioration in symptoms or even exercise tolerance may not be drug-related; efficacy of therapy may be reflected by lack of deterioration rather than by measurable improvement. A series of drug withdrawals and "rechallenges" would be necessary to establish drug efficacy, and this clearly is impractical.

Thus although it is not possible to assess the response to *therapy* in an individual patient, in the current era of effective drug therapy and of alternatives such as myoplasty, transplantation, and defibrillators it remains essential to monitor *the patient* so that appropriate and timely management decisions can be made. This can be achieved with:

1. A complete baseline evaluation of hemodynamics, ejection fraction, and (in ambulatory patients) VO$_{2max}$
2. Selection of therapy based on known efficacy and application of pathophysiological concepts to the individual
3. Periodic assessment of EF, hemodynamics, and VO$_{2max}$

CONCLUSIONS

Much progress has been made over the last 10 years in the medical therapy of heart failure and LV dysfunction following MI. Two major developments have been responsible for this rapid progress: a rapid increase in our understanding of the pathophysiology and natural history of heart failure, and the discovery and development of effective new treatments.

We now see heart failure differently than we did 10 years ago. It is not a static hemodynamic problem but one in which dynamic forces must be contended with at an early stage in order to avoid progressive worsening of the heart's condition, increasing disability, and eventually death.

We have come to appreciate the role played by the *periphery,* in which activation of neurohumoral mechanisms, both systemic and local, appears to be of vital importance. Indeed, neurohumoral activation appears to trigger adverse chronic remodeling effects in the whole cardiovascular system. We have also learned that the *energy balance of the heart* itself must be respected and that "improvements" in cardiac performance cannot

be obtained at the expense of greatly increased energy utilization and decreased work efficiency; the ultimate price will be deterioration in cardiac function.

Development of effective therapies has combined the work of the basic researcher and the clinical researcher, often with the support of the pharmaceutical industry. ACE inhibitors, nonspecific vasodilators, beta blockers, and new inotropic vasodilators have all been shown to be useful, and proof of their effectiveness has depended in the final analysis upon large, multicenter, double-blind, placebo-controlled trials.

Future advances in heart failure therapy will continue to come from a coordinated effort from basic and clinical research. New drugs will evolve, and even the development and application of gene therapy that will alter cell function and growth in the cardiovascular system may not be far away. Patients with heart failure can only benefit from these future developments.

REFERENCES

1. McKee PA, Castelli WP, McNamara PM, et al: Kannel WB: The natural history of congestive heart failure: the Framingham Study, *New Engl J Med* 285:1441-1446, 1971.
2. Schocken DD, Arrieta MI, Leaverton PE, et al: Prevalence and mortality rate of congestive heart failure in the United States, *J Am Coll Cardiol* 20:301-306, 1992.
3. Kannel WB, Sorlie P, McNamara PM: Prognosis after initial myocardial infarction: the Framingham Study, *Am J Cardiol* 44:53-59, 1979.
4. Hammermeister KE, DeRouen TA, Dodge HT: Variables predictive of survival in patients with coronary disease: selection by univariate and multivariate analyses from the clinical, electrocardiographic, exercise, arteriographic, and quantitative angiographic evaluations, *Circulation* 59(3):421-430, 1979.
5. Herman MV, Gorlin R: Implications of left ventricular asynergy, *Am J Cardiol* 23:538-547, 1969.
6. Mitchell GF, Pfeffer MA: Left ventricular remodeling after myocardial infarction: progression toward heart failure, *Heart Failure* April/May:55-69, 1992.
7. Weber KT, Janicki JS: Pathogenesis of heart failure, *Cardiol Clin* 7(1):11-24, 1989.
8. Weber KT, Anversa P, Armstrong PW, et al: Remodeling and reparation of the cardiovascular system, *J Am Coll Cardiol* 20(1):3-16, 1992.
9. Kannel WB: Epidemiological aspects of heart failure, *Cardiol Clin* 7(1):1-9, 1989.
10. Katz AM: Changing strategies in the management of heart failure, *J Am Coll Cardiol* 13:513-523, 1989.
11. McAlpine HM, Morton JJ, Leckie B, et al: Neuroendocrine activation after acute myocardial infarction, *Br Heart J* 60:117-124, 1988.
12. Zelis R, Nellis SR, Longhurst J, et al: Abnormalities in the regional circulations accompanying congestive heart failure, *Prog Cardiovasc Dis* 18(3):181-199, 1975.
13. Creager MA: Baroreceptor reflex function in congestive heart failure, *Am J Cardiol* 69:10G-15G, 1992.
14. Cody RJ, Covit AB, Schaer GL, et al: Sodium and water balance in chronic congestive heart failure, *J Clin Invest* 77:1441-1452, 1986.
15. Goldsmith SR, Francis GS, Cowley AW Jr, et al: Increased plasma arginine vasopressin in patients with congestive heart failure, *J Am Coll Cardiol* 1(6):1385-1390, 1983.

16. Packer M, Lee WH, Kessler PD, et al: Role of neurohumoral mechanisms in determining survival in patients with severe chronic heart failure, *Circulation* 75(suppl IV):80-92, 1987.

17. Packer M: The neurohumoral hypothesis: a theory to explain the mechanism of disease progression in heart failure, *J Am Coll Cardiol* 20(1):248-254, 1992.

18. Dzau VJ: Autocrine and paracrine mechanisms in the pathophysiology of heart failure, *Am J Cardiol* 70:4C-11C, 1992.

19. Wiener DH, Fink LI, Maris J, et al: Abnormal skeletal muscle bioenergetics during exercise in patients with heart failure: role of reduced muscle blood flow, *Circulation* 73(6):1127-1136, 1986.

20. Massie B, Conway M, Yonge R, et al: Skeletal muscle metabolism in patients with congestive heart failure: relation to clinical severity and blood flow, *Circulation* 76(5):1009-1019, 1987.

21. Minotti JR, Christoph I, Oka R, et al: Impaired skeletal muscle function in patients with congestive heart failure: relationship to systemic exercise performance, *J Clin Invest* 88:2077-2082, 1991.

22. Drexler H: Skeletal muscle failure in heart failure, *Circulation* 85(4):1621-1623, 1992.

23. Holloszy JO, Booth FW: Biochemical adaptations to endurance exercise in muscle, *Ann Rev Physiol* 18:273-291, 1976.

24. Minotti JR, Johnson EC, Hudson TL, et al: Skeletal muscle response to exercise training in congestive heart failure, *J Clin Invest* 86:751-758, 1990.

25. Bristow MR, Ginsburg R, Minobe W, et al: Decreased catecholamine sensitivity and β-adrenergic receptor density in failing human hearts, *New Engl J Med* 307:205-211, 1982.

26. Rona G, Chappel CI, Balazs T, et al: An infarct-like myocardial lesion and other toxic manifestations produced by isoproterenol in the rat, *Arch Pathol* 67:443-455, 1959.

27. Lerman A, Hildebrand FL Jr, Aarhus L, et al: Endothelin has biologic actions at pathophysiological concentrations, *Circulation* 83:1808-1814, 1991.

28. O'Connor GT, Buring JE, Yusif S, et al: An overview of randomized trials of rehabilitation with exercise after myocardial infarction, *Circulation* 80:234-244, 1989.

29. Conn EH, Williams RS, Wallace AG: Exercise responses before and after physical conditioning in patients with severely depressed left ventricular function, *Am J Cardiol* 49:296-300, 1982.

30. Sullivan MJ, Higginbotham MB, Cobb FR: Exercise training in patients with severe left ventricular dysfunction: hemodynamic and metabolic effects, *Circulation* 78(3):506-515, 1988.

31. Jetté M, Heller R, Landry F, et al: Randomized 4-week exercise program in patients with impaired left ventricular function, *Circulation* 84:1561-1567, 1991.

32. Coats AJS, Adamopoulos S, Radaelli A, et al: Controlled trial of physical training in chronic heart failure: exercise performance, hemodynamics, ventilation, and autonomic function, *Circulation* 85:2119-2131, 1992.

33. Parmley WW: Pathophysiology and current therapy of congestive heart failure, *J Am Coll Cardiol* 13(4):771-785, 1989.

34. Packer M: Therapeutic options in the management of heart failure: is there a drug of first choice? *Circulation* 79(1):198-204, 1989.

35. Richardson A, Bayliss J, Seriven AJ, et al: Double-blind comparison of captopril alone against furosemide plus amiloride in mild heart failure, *Lancet* 2:709-711, 1987.

36. Hollenberg NK: The role of the kidney in heart failure. In Cohn J, (ed): *Drug treatment of heart failure,* Secaucus, NJ, 1988, Advanced Therapeutics Communications, pp 105-125.

37. Dikshit K, Vyden JK, Forrester JS, et al: Renal and extrarenal hemodynamic effects of furosemide in congestive heart failure after acute myocardial infarction, *New Engl J Med* 288:1087-1090, 1973.

38. Puschett JB: Physiologic basis for the use of new and older diuretics in congestive heart failure, *Cardiovasc Med* 2(2):119-134, 1977.

39. Ikram H, Chan W, Espiner EA, et al: Hemodynamic and hormone responses to acute and chronic furosemide therapy in congestive heart failure, *Clin Sci* 59:443-449, 1980.

40. Bayliss J, Norell M, Canepa-Anson R, et al: Untreated heart failure: clinical and neuroendocrine effects of introducing diuretics, *Br Heart J* 57:17-22, 1987.

41. Packer M, Gottlieb SS, Kessler PD: Hormone-electrolyte interactions in the pathogenesis of lethal cardiac arrhythmias in patients with congestive heart failure, *Am J Med* 80(4A):23-29, 1986.

42. Hlatky MA, Fleg JL, Hinton PC, et al: Physician practice in the management of congestive heart failure, *J Am Coll Cardiol* 8(4):966-970, 1986.

43. Braunwald E: Effects of digitalis on the normal and the failing heart, *J Am Coll Cardiol* 5(5):51A-59A, 1985.

44. Gheorghiade M (ed): A symposium: management of heart failure in the 1990s: a reassessment of the role of digoxin therapy, *Am J Cardiol* 69:1G-154G, 1992.

45. Arnold SB, Byrd RC, Meister W, et al: Long-term digitalis therapy improves left ventricular function in heart failure, *New Engl J Med* 303:1443-1448, 1980.

46. Lee DC, Johnson RA, Bingham JB, et al: Heart failure in outpatients. A randomized trial of digoxin versus placebo, *New Engl J Med* 306:699-705, 1982.

47. Gheorghiade M, St Clair J, St Clair C, et al: Hemodynamic effects of intravenous digoxin in patients with severe heart failure initially treated with diuretics and vasodilators, *J Am Coll Cardiol* 9(4):849-857, 1987.

48. DiBianco R, Shabetai R, Kostuk W, et al for the Milrinone Multicenter Trial Group: A comparison of oral milrinone, digoxin, and their combination in the treatment of patients with chronic heart failure, *New Engl J Med* 320:677-683, 1989.

49. Fleg JL, Gottlieb SH, Lakatta EG: Is digoxin really important in treatment of compensated heart failure? A placebo-controlled crossover study in patients with sinus rhythm, *Am J Med* 73:244-250, 1982.

50. Aronow WS, Starling L, Etienne F: Lack of efficacy of digoxin in treatment of compensated congestive heart failure with third heart sound and sinus rhythm in elderly patients receiving diuretic therapy, *Am J Cardiol* 58:168-169, 1986.

51. Packer M, Gheorghiade M, Young JB, et al for the RADIANCE Study: Withdrawal of digoxin from patients with chronic heart failure treated with angiotensin-converting-enzyme inhibitors, *New Engl J Med* 329(1):1-7, 1993.

52. Uretsky BF, Young JB, Shahidi FE, et al: Randomized study assessing the effect of digoxin withdrawal in patients with mild to moderate chronic congestive heart failure: results of the PROVED trial: PROVED Investigative Group, *J Am Coll Cardiol* 22:955-962, 1993.

53. Davies RF, Beanlands DS, Nadeau C, et al: Enalapril versus digoxin in patients with congestive heart failure: a multicenter study, *J Am Coll Cardiol* 18(7):1602-1609, 1991.

54. Surawicz B: Factors affecting tolerance to digitalis, *J Am Coll Cardiol* 5(5):69A-81A, 1985.

55. Braunwald E: ACE inhibitors—a cornerstone of the treatment of heart failure, *New Engl J Med* 325(5):351-353, 1991.

56. The Captopril-Digoxin Multicenter Research Group: Comparative effects of therapy with captopril and digoxin in patients with mild to moderate heart failure, *J Am Med Assoc* 259(4):539-544, 1988.

57. Captopril Multicenter Research Group: A placebo-controlled trial of captopril in refractory chronic congestive heart failure, *J Am Coll Cardiol* 2(4):755-763, 1983.

58. Sharpe DN, Murphy J, Coxon R, et al: Enalapril in patients with

chronic heart failure: a placebo-controlled, randomized, double-blind study, *Circulation* 70(2):271-278, 1984.

59. The CONSENSUS Trial Study Group: Effects of enalapril on mortality in severe congestive heart failure, *New Engl J Med* 316(23):1429-1435, 1987.

60. The SOLVD Investigators: Effect of enalapril on survival in patients with reduced left ventricular ejection fractions and congestive heart failure, *New Engl J Med* 325(5):293-302, 1991.

61. Cohn JN, Johnson G, Ziesche S, et al: A comparison of enalapril with hydralazine-isosorbide-dinitrate in the treatment of chronic congestive heart failure, *New Engl J Med* 325(5):303-310, 1991.

62. Newman TJ, Maskin CS, Dennick LG, et al: Effects of captopril on survival in patients with heart failure, *Am J Med* 84(3A):140-144, 1988.

63. Fonarow GC, Chelimsky-Fallick C, Stevenson LW, et al: Effect of direct vasodilation with hydralazine versus angiotensin converting enzyme inhibition with captopril on mortality in advanced heart failure: the Hy-C Trial, *J Am Coll Cardiol* 19(4):842-850, 1992.

64. Massie BM, Kramer BL, Topic N: Lack of relationship between the short-term hemodynamic effects of captopril and subsequent clinical responses, *Circulation* 69(6):1135-1141, 1984.

65. Ader R, Chatterjee K, Ports T, et al: Immediate and sustained hemodynamic and clinical improvement in chronic heart failure by an oral angiotensin-converting enzyme inhibitor, *Circulation* 61(5):931-937, 1980.

66. Stephenson LW, Tillisch JH: Maintenance of cardiac output with normal filling pressures in patients with dilated heart failure, *Circulation* 74(6):1303-1308, 1986.

67. Mancini DM, Davis L, Wexler JP, et al: Dependence of enhanced maximal exercise performance on increased peak skeletal muscle perfusion during long-term captopril therapy in heart failure, *J Am Coll Cardiol* 10(4):845-850, 1987.

68. Drexler H: Effect of angiotensin-converting enzyme inhibitors on the peripheral circulation in heart failure, *Am J Cardiol* 70:50C-54C, 1992.

69. Cleland JGF, Dargie HJ, Ball SG, et al: Effects of enalapril in heart failure: a double-blind study of effects on exercise performance, renal function, hormones, and metabolic state, *Br Heart J* 54:305-312, 1985.

70. Dzau VJ: Vascular wall renin-angiotensin pathway in control of the circulation: a hypothesis, *Am J Med* 77:31-36, 1984.

71. Motwani JG, Fenwick MK, Morton JJ, et al: Furosemide-induced natriuresis is augmented by ultra-low-dose captopril but not by standard doses of captopril in chronic heart failure, *Circulation* 86(2):439-445, 1992.

72. Chalmers JP, West MJ, Cyran J, et al: Placebo-controlled study of lisinopril in congestive heart failure: a multicenter study, *J Cardiovasc Pharmacol* 9(3):S89-S97, 1987.

73. Ribner HS, Colfer HT and the Benazepril Heart Failure Study Group: Improvement in exercise tolerance and clinical status with once-daily benazepril therapy in congestive heart failure: a double-blind, placebo-controlled trial (abstract), *Circulation* 82: III-323, 1990.

74. Packer M, Medina N, Yushak M: Relation between serum sodium concentration and the hemodynamic and clinical responses to converting enzyme inhibition with captopril in severe heart failure, *J Am Coll Cardiol* 3(4):1035-1043, 1984.

75. Parmley WW: Angiotensin converting enzyme inhibitors in the treatment of heart failure. In Cohn J(ed): *Drug treatment of heart failure*, Secaucus, NJ, 1988, Advanced Therapeutic Communications.

76. Sonnenblick EH, Zhao M, Eng C, et al: ACE inhibitors in acute and chronic ischemia: current status and future promise, *Br J Clin Pharmacol* 28:159S-165S, 1989.

77. DeMarco T, Daly PA, Liu M, et al: Enalaprilat, a new parenteral angiotensin-converting enzyme inhibitor: rapid changes in systemic and coronary hemodynamics and humoral profile in chronic heart failure, *J Am Coll Cardiol* 9:1131-1138, 1987.

78. Schunkert H, Dzau VJ, Tang SS, et al: Increased rate cardiac angiotensin converting enzyme activity and mRNA expression in pressure overload left ventricular hypertrophy: effects on coronary resistance, contractility, and relaxation, *J Clin Invest* 86:1913-1920, 1990.

79. Westlin W, Mullane K: Does captopril attenuate reperfusion-induced myocardial dysfunction by scavenging free radicals? *Circulation* 77(suppl I):I30-I39, 1988.

80. Alderman MH, Madhaven S, Ooi WL, et al: Association of the renin-sodium profile with the risk of myocardial infarction in patients with hypertension, *New Engl J Med* 324(16):1098-1104, 1991.

81. Chatterjee K, Ports TA, Brundage BH, et al: Oral hydralazine in chronic heart failure: sustained beneficial hemodynamic effects, *Ann Intern Med* 92(5):600-604, 1980.

82. Cohn JN, Archibald DG, Ziesche S, et al: Effect of vasodilator therapy on mortality in chronic congestive heart failure: results of a Veterans Administration Cooperative Study, *New Engl J Med* 314(24):1547-1552, 1986.

83. Franciosa JA, Weber KT, Levine TB, et al: Hydralazine in the long-term treatment of chronic heart failure: lack of difference from placebo, *Am Heart J* 104(3):587-594, 1982.

84. Franciosa JA, Jordan RA, Wilen MM, et al: Minoxidil in patients with chronic left heart failure: contrasting hemodynamic and clinical effects in a controlled trial, *Circulation* 70(1):63-68, 1984.

85. Greenberg BH, Massie BM, Brundage BH, et al: Beneficial effects of hydralazine in severe mitral regurgitation, *Circulation* 58(2):273-279, 1978.

86. Greenberg BH, DeMots H, Murphy E, et al: Beneficial effects of hydralazine on rest and exercise hemodynamics in patients with chronic severe aortic insufficiency, *Circulation* 62(1):49-54, 1980.

87. Abrams J: Pharmacology of nitroglycerin and long-acting nitrates, *Am J Cardiol* 56:12A-18A, 1985.

88. Leier CV, Huss P, Magorien RD, et al: Improved exercise capacity and differing arterial and venous tolerance during chronic isosorbide dinitrate therapy for congestive heart failure, *Circulation* 67(4):817-822, 1983.

89. Jordan RA, Seth L, Henry DA, et al: Dose requirements and hemodynamic effects of transdermal nitroglycerin compared with placebo in patients with congestive heart failure, *Circulation* 71(5):980-986, 1985.

90. Wilson JR, Falcone R, Ferraro N, et al: Mechanism of skeletal muscle underperfusion in a dog model of low-output heart failure, *Am J Physiol* 251(20):H227-H235, 1986.

91. Garg UC, Hassid A: Nitric oxide-generating vasodilators and 8-bromocyclic guanosine monophosphate inhibit mitogenesis and proliferation of cultured rat vascular smooth muscle cells, *J Clin Invest* 83:1774-1777, 1989.

92. Elkayam U, Roth A, Mehra A, et al: Randomized study to evaluate the relation between oral isosorbide dinitrate dosing interval and the development of early tolerance to its effect on left ventricular filling pressure in patients with chronic heart failure, *Circulation* 84(5):2040-2048, 1991.

93. Olivari MT, Cohn JN: Cutaneous administration of nitroglycerin: a review, *Pharmacotherapy* 3(3):149-157, 1983.

94. Kessler PD, Packer M, Medina N, et al: Cumulative hemodynamic response to short-term treatment with flosequinan (BTS 49465), a new direct-acting vasodilator drug, in severe chronic congestive heart failure, *J Cardiovasc Pharmacol* 12(1):6-11, 1988.

95. Greenberg S, Touhey B: Positive inotropy contributes to the hemodynamic mechanism of action of flosequinan (BTS 49465) in the intact dog, *J Cardiovasc Pharmacol* 15(6):900-910, 1990.

96. Yates DB: Pharmacology of flosequinan, *Am Heart J* 121: 974-983, 1991.

97. Corin WJ, Monrad ES, Strom JA, et al: Flosequinan: a vasodilator with positive inotropic activity, *Am Heart J* 121:537-540, 1991.

98. Elborn JS, Stanford CF, Nicholls DP: Effects of flosequinan on exercise capacity and symptoms in severe heart failure, *Br Heart J* 61:331-335, 1989.

99. Pitt B, Reflect II Study Group: A randomized, multicenter, double-blind placebo controlled study of the efficacy of flosequinan in patients with chronic heart failure (abstract), *Circulation* 84(suppl II):II-311, 1991.

100. Packer M, Narahara KA, Elkayam U, et al: Double-blind, placebo-controlled study of the efficacy of flosequinan in patients with chronic heart failure, *J Am Coll Cardiol* 22:65-72, 1993.

101. Massie BM, Berk MR, Brozena SC, et al: Can further benefit be achieved by adding flosequinan to patients with congestive heart failure who remain symtomatic on diuretic, digoxin, and an angiotensin converting enzyme inhibitor? Results of the flosequinan-ACE inhibitor trial (FACET), *Circulation* 88:492-501, 1993.

102. Arnold SB, Williams RL, Ports TA, et al: Attenuation of prazosin effect on cardiac output in chronic heart failure, *Ann Intern Med* 91(3):345-349, 1979.

103. Higginbotham MB, Morris KG, Bramlet DA, et al: Long-term ambulatory therapy with prazosin versus placebo for chronic heart failure: relation between clinical response and left ventricular function at rest and during exercise, *Am J Cardiol* 52:782-788, 1983.

104. Packer M, Medina N, Yushak M: Association of sustained drug-induced reduction in right and left ventricular filling pressures and subjective clinical response during long-term prazosin therapy in patients with severe chronic heart failure, *Heart Failure* 2:282-290, 1986.

105. Bayliss J, Norell MS, Canepa-Anson R, et al: Clinical importance of the renin-angiotensin system in chronic heart failure: double-blind comparison of captopril and prazosin, *Br Med J* 290:1861-1865, 1985.

106. Stone PH, Antman EM, Muller JE, et al: Calcium channel blocking agents in the treatment of cardiovascular disorders. Part II: Hemodynamic effects and clinical applications, *Ann Intern Med* 93(6):886-904, 1980.

107. Packer M, Lee WH, Medina N, et al: Prognostic importance of the immediate hemodynamic response to nifedipine in patients with severe left ventricular dysfunction, *J Am Coll Cardiol* 10(6):1303-1311, 1987.

108. Elkayam U, Amin J, Mehra A, et al: A prospective, randomized, double-blind, crossover study to compare the efficacy and safety of chronic nifedipine therapy with that of isosorbide dinitrate and their combination in the treatment of chronic congestive heart failure, *Circulation* 82(6):1954-1961, 1990.

109. Remme WJ, Krauss H, van Hoogenhuyze DCA, et al: Hemodynamic tolerability and antiischemic efficacy of high-dose intravenous diltiazem in patients with normal versus impaired ventricular function, *J Am Coll Cardiol* 21(3):709-720, 1993.

110. Gibson RS, Boden WE, Theroux P, et al: Diltiazem and reinfarction in patients with non-Q-wave myocardial infarction. Results of a double-blind, randomized, multicenter trial, *New Engl J Med* 315(7):423-429, 1986.

111. Wilcox RG, Hampton JR, Banks BC, et al: Trial of early nifedipine in acute myocardial infarction: the Trent Study, *Br Med J* 293:1204-1208, 1986.

112. The Multicenter Diltiazem Postinfarction Trial Research Group: The effect of diltiazem on mortality and reinfarction after myocardial infarction, *New Engl J Med* 319(7):385-392, 1988.

113. Goldstein RE, Boccuzzi SJ, Cruess D, et al., The Adverse Experience Committee, and the Multicenter Diltiazem Postinfarction Research Group: Diltiazem increases late-onset conges-tive heart failure in postinfarction patients with early reduction in ejection fraction, *Circulation* 83(1):52-60, 1991.

114. The Danish Study Group on Verapamil in Myocardial Infarction: Effect of verapamil on mortality and major events after acute myocardial infarction (The Danish Verapamil Infarction Trial II-DAVIT II), *Am J Cardiol* 66:779-785, 1990.

115. Packer M, Nicod P, Khandheria BR, et al: Randomized, multicenter, double-blind, placebo-controlled evaluation of amlodipine in patients with mild-to-moderate heart failure (abstract), *J Am Coll Cardiol* 17(2):274A, 1991.

116. Sonnenblick EH, Fein F, Capasso JM, et al: Microvascular spasm as a cause of cardiomyopathies and the calcium-blocking agent verapamil as potential primary therapy, *Am J Cardiol* 55:179B-184B, 1985.

117. Packer M, Lee WH, Kessler PD, et al: Role of neurohormonal mechanisms in determining survival in patients with severe chronic heart failure, *Circulation* 75(suppl IV):IV-80-IV-92, 1987.

118. Cohn JN, Levine TB, Olivari MT, et al: Plasma norepinephrine as a guide to prognosis in patients with chronic congestive heart failure, *New Engl J Med* 311(13):819-823, 1984.

119. Roubin GS, Choong YPC, Devenish-Meares S, et al: β-Adrenergic stimulation of the failing ventricle: a double-blind, randomized trial of sustained oral therapy with prenalterol, *Circulation* 69(5):955-962, 1984.

120. The Xamoterol in Severe Heart Failure Study Group: Xamoterol in severe heart failure, *Lancet* 336:1-6, 1990.

121. Waagstein F, Hjalmarson A, Varnauskas E, et al: Effect of chronic beta-adrenergic receptor blockade in congestive cardiomyopathy, *Br Heart J* 37:1022-1036, 1975.

122. Gilbert EM, Anderson JL, Deitchman D, et al: Long-term β-blocker vasodilator therapy improves cardiac function in idiopathic dilated cardiomyopathy: a double-blind, randomized study of bucindolol versus placebo, *Am J Med* 88:223-229, 1990.

123. Waagstein F, Caidahl K, Wallentin I, et al: Long-term β-blockade in dilated cardiomyopathy: effects of short- and long-term metoprolol treatment followed by withdrawal and readministration of metoprolol, *Circulation* 80:551-563, 1989.

124. Waagstein F, Bristow MR, Swedberg K, et al: Beneficial effects of metoprolol in idiopathic dilated cardiomyopathy, *Lancet* 342:1441-1446, 1993.

125. Woodley SL, Gilbert EM, Anderson JL, et al: β-Blockade with bucindolol in heart failure caused by ischemic versus idiopathic dilated cardiomyopathy, *Circulation* 84:2426-2441, 1991.

126. Andersson B, Blomström-Lundqvist C, Hedner T, et al: Exercise hemodynamics and myocardial metabolism during long-term beta-adrenergic blockade in severe heart failure, *J Am Coll Cardiol* 18(4):1059-1066, 1991.

127. Heilbrunn SM, Shah P, Bristow MR, et al: Increased β-receptor density and improved hemodynamic response to catecholamine stimulation during long-term metoprolol therapy in heart failure from dilated cardiomyopathy, *Circulation* 79(3):483-490, 1989.

128. Chadda K, Goldstein S, Byington R, et al: Effect of propranolol after acute myocardial infarction in patients with congestive heart failure, *Circulation* 73(3):503-510, 1986.

129. Yusuf S, Peto R, Lewis J, et al: Beta blockade during and after myocardial infarctions: an overview of the randomized trials, *Prog Cardiovasc Dis* 27(5):335-371, 1985.

130. Lubbe WF, Podzuweit T, Opie LH: Potential arrhythmogenic role of cyclic adenosine monophosphate (AMP) and cytosolic calcium overload: implications for prophylactic effects of beta-blockers in myocardial infarction and proarrhythmic effects of phosphodiesterase inhibitors, *J Am Coll Cardiol* 19(7):1622-1633, 1992.

131. Braunwald E, Ross J Jr, Sonnenblick EH: *Mechanisms of contraction of the normal and failing heart*, ed 2, Boston, 1976, Little, Brown.

132. Benotti JR, Grossman W, Braunwald E, et al: Effects of amrinone

on myocardial energy metabolism and hemodynamics in patients with severe congestive heart failure due to coronary artery disease, *Circulation* 62(1):28-34, 1980.

133. Rajfer SI, Rossen JD, Douglas FL, et al: Effects of long-term therapy with oral ibopamine on resting hemodynamics and exercise capacity in patients with heart failure: relationship to the generation of N-methyldopamine and to plasma norepinephrine levels, *Circulation* 73(4):740-748, 1986.

134. Massie B, Bourassa M, DiBianco R, et al. for the Amrinone Multicenter Trial Group: Long-term administration of amrinone for congestive heart failure: lack of efficacy in a multicenter controlled trial, *Circulation* 71(5):963-971, 1985.

135. Uretsky BF, Jessup M, Konstam MA, et al. for the Enoximone Multicenter Trial Group: Multicenter trial of oral enoximone in patients with moderate to moderately severe congestive heart failure: lack of benefit compared with placebo, *Circulation* 82(3):774-780, 1990.

136. Katz AM: Potential deleterious effects of inotropic agents in the therapy of chronic heart failure, *Circulation* 73(suppl III):III-184-III-188, 1986.

137. Sinoway LS, Maskin CS, Chadwick B, et al: Long-term therapy with a new cardiotonic agent, WIN 47203: drug-dependent improvement in cardiac performance and progression of the underlying disease, *J Am Coll Cardiol* 2(2):327-331, 1983.

138. Baim DS, Colucci WS, Monrad ES, et al: Survival of patients with severe congestive heart failure treated with oral milrinone, *J Am Coll Cardiol* 7(3):661-670, 1986.

139. Packer M, Carver JR, Rodeheffer RJ, et al. for the PROMISE Study Research Group: Effect of oral milrinone on mortality in severe chronic heart failure, *New Engl J Med* 325(21):1468-1475, 1991.

140. Kubo SH, Gollub S, Bourge R, et al. for the Pimobendan Multicenter Research Group: Beneficial effects of pimobendan on exercise tolerance and quality of life in patients with heart failure: results of a multicenter trial, *Circulation* 85(3):942-949, 1992.

141. Asanoi H, Sasayama S, Iuchi K, et al: Acute hemodynamic effects of a new inotropic agent (OPC-8212) in patients with congestive heart failure, *J Am Coll Cardiol* 9(4):865-871, 1987.

142. Lathrop DA, Varro A, Schwartz A: Rate-dependent electrophysiological effects of OPC-8212: comparison to sotalol, *Eur J Pharmacol* 164:487-496, 1989.

143. OPC-8212 Multicenter Research Group: A placebo-controlled, randomized, double-blind study of OPC-8212 in patients with mild chronic heart failure, *Cardiovasc Drug Ther* 4:419-426, 1990.

144. Feldman AM, Baughman KL, Lee WK, et al: Usefulness of OPC-8212, a quinolinone derivative, for chronic congestive heart failure in patients with ischemic heart disease or idiopathic dilated cardiomyopathy, *Am J Cardiol* 68:1203-1210, 1991.

145. Feldman AM, Bristow MR, Parmley WW, et al. for the Vesnarinone Study Group: Effects of vesnarinone on morbidity and mortality in patients with heart failure: results of a multicenter trial, *New Engl J Med* 329:149-155, 1993.

146. Unverferth DV, Blanford M, Kates RE, et al: Tolerance to dobutamine after a 72-hour continuous infusion, *Am J Med* 69:262-266, 1980.

147. Unverferth DV, Magorien RD, Lewis RP, et al: Long-term benefit of dobutamine in patients with congestive cardiomyopathy, *Am Heart J* 100(5):622-630, 1980.

148. Leier CV, Huss P, Lewis RP, et al: Drug-induced conditioning in congestive heart failure, *Circulation* 65(7):1382-1387, 1982.

149. Liang C-S, Sherman LG, Doherty JU, et al: Sustained improvement of cardiac function in patients with congestive heart failure after short-term infusion of dobutamine, *Circulation* 69(1):113-119, 1984.

150. Dres F: Intermittent dobutamine in ambulatory patients with chronic cardiac failure, *Br J Clin Proc* 40(suppl 45):37-39, 1986.

151. David S, Zaks JM: Arrhythmias associated with intermittent outpatient dobutamine infusion, *Angiology* 37:86-91, 1986.

152. Goldenberg IF, Olivari MT, Levine TB, et al: Effect of dobutamine on plasma potassium in congestive heart failure secondary to idiopathic or ischemic cardiomyopathy, *Am J Cardiol* 63:843-846, 1989.

153. Miller LW: Outpatient dobutamine for refractory congestive heart failure: advantages, techniques, and results, *J Heart Lung Transplant* 10(3):482-487, 1991.

154. Gage J, Rutman H, Lucido D, et al: Additive effects of dobutamine and amrinone on myocardial contractility and ventricular performance in severe heart failure, *Circulation* 74(2):367-373, 1986.

155. Massie B, Chatterjee K, Werner J, et al: Hemodynamic advantage of combined administration of hydralazine orally and nitrates nonparenterally in the vasodilator therapy of chronic heart failure, *Am J Cardiol* 40:794-801, 1977.

156. Massie BM, Packer M, Hanlon JT, et al: Hemodynamic responses to combined therapy with captopril and hydralazine in patients with severe heart failure, *J Am Coll Cardiol* 2(2):338-344, 1983.

157. Kugler J, Maskin CS, Frishman W, et al: Variable clinical response to long-term angiotensin inhibition in severe heart failure: demonstration of additive benefits of alpha-receptor blockade, *Am Heart J* 104:1154-1159, 1982.

158. Gheorghiade M, Hall V, Lakier JB, et al: Comparative hemodynamic and neurohumoral effects of intravenous captopril and digoxin and their combinations in patients with severe heart failure, *J Am Coll Cardiol* 13(1):134-142, 1989.

159. LeJemtel TH, Maskin CS, Mancini D, et al: Systemic and regional hemodynamic effects of captopril and milrinone administered alone and concomitantly in patients with heart failure, *Circulation* 72(2):364-369, 1985.

160. Stevenson LW: Tailored therapy before transplantation for treatment of advanced heart failure: effective use of vasodilators and diuretics, *J Heart Lung Transp* 10(3):468-476, 1991.

161. Francis GS: Development of arrhythmias in the patient with congestive heart failure: pathophysiology, prevalence and prognosis, *Am J Cardiol* 57:3B-7B, 1986.

162. Luu M, Stevenson WG, Stevenson LW, et al: Diverse mechanisms of unexpected cardiac arrest in advanced heart failure, *Circulation* 80(6):1675-1680, 1989.

163. El-Sherif N, Mehra R, Gough WB, et al: Reentrant ventricular arrhythmias in the late myocardial infarction period: interruption of reentrant circuits by cryothermal techniques, *Circulation* 68(3):644-656, 1983.

164. The Multicenter Postinfarction Research Group: Risk stratification and survival after myocardial infarction, *New Engl J Med* 309(6):331-336, 1983.

165. Mukharji J, Rude RE, Poole WK, et al. and the MILIS Study Group: Risk factors for sudden death after acute myocardial infarction: two-year follow-up, *Am J Cardiol* 54:31-36, 1984.

166. Bigger JT Jr, Fleiss JL, Kleiger R, et al: The Multicenter Post-Infarction Group: The relationships among ventricular arrhythmias, left ventricular dysfunction, and mortality in the 2 years after myocardial infarction, *Circulation* 69(2):250-258, 1984.

167. Hamer A, Vohra J, Hunt D, et al: Prediction of sudden death by electrophysiologic studies in high-risk patients surviving acute myocardial infarction, *Am J Cardiol* 50:223-229, 1982.

168. Richards DAB, Byth K, Ross DL, et al: What is the best predictor of spontaneous ventricular tachycardia and sudden death after myocardial infarction? *Circulation* 83:756-763, 1991.

169. Goldman L: Electrophysiological testing after myocardial infarction: a paradigm for assessing the incremental value of a diagnostic test, *Circulation* 83(3):1090-1092, 1991.

170. Kulakowski P, Dluzniewski M, Budaj A, et al: Relationship between signal-averaged electrocardiography and dangerous ventricular arrhythmias in patients with left ventricular aneurysm after myocardial infarction, *Eur Heart J* 12:1170-1175, 1991.

171. Wilson JR: Use of antiarrhythmic drugs in patients with heart failure: clinical efficacy, hemodynamic results, and relation to survival, *Circulation* 75(suppl IV):IV-64-IV-73, 1987.

172. Ruskin JN, McGovern B, Garan H, et al: Antiarrhythmic drugs: a possible cause of out-of-hospital cardiac arrest, *New Engl J Med* 309(21):1302-1306, 1983.

173. Parmley WW, Chatterjee K: Congestive heart failure and arrhythmias: an overview, *Am J Cardiol* 57(suppl B):34B-37B, 1986.

174. Hohnloser SH, Raeder EA, Podrid PJ, et al: Predictors of antiarrhythmic drug efficacy in patients with malignant ventricular tachyarrhythmias, *Am Heart J* 114(1):1-7, 1987.

175. Echt DS, Liebson PR, Mitchell LB, et al. and the CAST Investigators: Mortality and morbidity in patients receiving encainide, flecainide, or placebo, *New Engl J Med* 324(12):781-788, 1991.

176. Coplen SE, Antman EM, Berlin JA, et al: Efficacy and safety of quinidine therapy for maintenance of sinus rhythm after cardioversion: a meta-analysis of randomized control trials, *Circulation* 82(4):1106-1116, 1990.

177. Simonton CA, Daly PA, Kereiakes D, et al: Survival in severe left ventricular failure treated with the new nonglycosidic, nonsympathomimetic oral inotropic agents, *Chest* 92(1):118-123, 1987.

178. Dargie HJ, Cleland JGV, Leckie BJ, et al: Relation of arrhythmias and electrolyte abnormalities to survival in patients with severe chronic heart failure, *Circulation* 75(suppl IV):IV-98-IV-107, 1987.

179. Pfisterer M, Kiowski W, Burckhardt D, et al: Beneficial effect of amiodarone on cardiac mortality in patients with asymptomatic complex ventricular arrhythmias after acute myocardial infarction and preserved but not impaired left ventricular function, *Am J Cardiol* 69:1399-1402, 1992.

180. Fuster V, Gersh BJ, Giuliani ER, et al: The natural history of idiopathic dilated cardiomyopathy, *Am J Cardiol* 47(3):525-531, 1981.

181. Sugrue DD, Rodeheffer RJ, Codd MB, et al: The clinical course of idiopathic dilated cardiomyopathy: a population-based study, *Ann Intern Med* 117(2):117-123, 1992.

182. Keren A, Goldberg S, Gottlieb S, et al: Natural history of left ventricular thrombi: their appearance and resolution in the posthospitalization period of acute myocardial infarction, *J Am Coll Cardiol* 15(4):790-800, 1990.

183. Cregler LL: Antithrombotic therapy in left ventricular thrombosis and systemic embolism, *Am Heart J* 123:1110-1114, 1992.

184. Stein B, Fuster V: Antithrombotic therapy in acute myocardial infarction: prevention of venous, left ventricular and coronary artery thromboembolism, *Am J Cardiol* 64:33B-40B, 1989.

185. Smith P, Arnesen H, Holme I: The effect of warfarin on mortality and reinfarction after myocardial infarction, *New Engl J Med* 343(3):147-152, 1990.

186. Lapeyre AC III, Steele PM, Kazmier FJ, et al: Systemic embolism in chronic left ventricular aneurysm: incidence and the role of anticoagulation, *J Am Coll Cardiol* 6:534-540, 1985.

187. Jugdutt BI, Sivaran CA: Prospective two-dimensional echocardiographic evaluation of left ventricular thrombus and embolism after acute myocardial infarction, *J Am Coll Cardiol* 13(3):554-564, 1989.

188. Petersen P, Boysen G, Godtfredsen J, et al: Placebo-controlled, randomised trial of warfarin and aspirin for prevention of thromboembolic complications in chronic atrial fibrillation: The Copenhagen AFASAK Study, *Lancet* 1:175-179, 1989.

189. The Boston Area Anticoagulation Trial for Atrial Fibrillation Investigators: The effect of low-dose warfarin on the risk of stroke in patients with nonrheumatic atrial fibrillation, *New Engl J Med* 323(22):1505-1511, 1990.

190. Stroke Prevention in Atrial Fibrillation Investigators: Stroke Prevention in Atrial Fibrillation Study: final results, *Circulation* 84(2):527-539, 1991.

191. Pfeffer JM, Pfeffer MA, Braunwald E: Influence of chronic captopril therapy on the infarcted left ventricle of the rat, *Circ Res* 57:84-95, 1985.

192. Pfeffer MA, Pfeffer JM, Steinberg C, et al: Survival after an experimental myocardial infarction: beneficial effects of long-term therapy with captopril, *Circulation* 72(2):406-412, 1985.

193. Pfeffer MA, Lamas GA, Vaughan DE, et al: Effect of captopril on progressive ventricular dilatation after anterior myocardial infarction, *New Engl J Med* 319(2):80-86, 1988.

194. Sharpe N, Murphy J, Smith H, et al: Treatment of patients with symptomless left ventricular dysfunction after myocardial infarction, *Lancet* 1:255-259, 1988.

195. Sharpe N, Smith H, Murphy J, et al: Early prevention of left ventricular dysfunction after myocardial infarction with angiotensin-converting-enzyme inhibition, *Lancet* 337:872-876, 1991.

196. Sonnenblick EH, LeJemtel TH, Eng C, et al: The relationship of dynamic ischemia, ventricular wall remodeling, and reactive hypertrophy to the development of cardiomyopathies: pathophysiological and therapeutic considerations. In Sonnenblick EH, Laragh JH, Lesch M (eds): *New frontiers in cardiovascular therapy: focus on angiotensin converting enzyme inhibition,* New Jersey, 1989, Exerpta Medica.

197. Jugdutt BI, Warnica JW: Intravenous nitroglycerin therapy to limit myocardial infarct size, expansion, and complications: effect of timing, dosage, and infarct location, *Circulation* 78:906-918, 1988.

198. Raya TE, Gay RG, Aguirre M, et al: Importance of venodilation in prevention of left ventricular dilatation after chronic large myocardial infarction in rats: a comparison of captopril and hydralazine, *Circ Res* 64(2):330-337, 1989.

199. Mitchell GF, Pfeffer MA, Pfeffer JM: Equipotent antihypertensive agents variously affect pulsatile hemodynamics and regression of cardiac hypertrophy in spontaneously hypertensive rats (abstract), *Hypertension* 18:417, 1991.

200. Pfeffer MA, Braunwald E, Moye LA, et al. on behalf of the SAVE Investigators: Effect of captopril on mortality and morbidity in patients with left ventricular dysfunction after myocardial infarction: results of the Survival and Ventricular Enlargement Trial, *New Engl J Med* 327(10):669-677, 1992.

201. Jalil JE, Janicki JS, Shroff SG, et al: Captopril pretreatment and myocardial fibrosis and stiffness in renovascular hypertensive rats (abstract), *J Am Coll Cardiol* 13(2):82A, 1989.

202. Cohn JN, Franciosa JA, Francis GS, et al: Effect of short-term infusion of sodium nitroprusside on mortality rate in acute myocardial infarction complicated by left ventricular failure, *New Engl J Med* 306(19):1129-1135, 1982.

203. GISSI-3 Investigators: GISSI-3 Pilot Study: Safety of lisinopril and nitroglycerin in the first 72 hours after acute myocardial infarction (abstract), *Circulation* 84(4) (suppl II):II-366, 1991.

204. Flather M, Pipilis A, Foster C, et al. for the ISIS Pilot Study Collatorators' Group: Combination of oral captopril and oral isosorbide mononitrate is well tolerated in acute myocardial infarction (ISIS-4 Factorial Pilot Study) (abstract), *Circulation* 84:II-367, 1991.

205. Swedberg K, Held P, Kjekshus J, et al. on behalf of the CONSENSUS II Study Group: Effects of the early administration of enalapril on mortality in patients with acute myocardial infarction: results of the Cooperative New Scandinavian Enala-

pril Survival Study II (CONSENSUS II), *New Engl J Med* 327(10):678-684, 1992.

206. The SOLVD Investigators: Effect of enalapril on mortality and the development of heart failure in asymptomatic patients with reduced left ventricular ejection fractions, *New Engl J Med* 327(10):685-691, 1992.

207. Francis GS, Benedict C, Johnstone DE, et al: Comparison of neuroendocrine activation in patients with left ventricular dysfunction with and without congestive heart failure, *Circulation* 82:1724-1729, 1990.

208. Criteria Committee of the New York Heart Association: Nomenclature and criteria for diagnosis. In *Diseases of the heart and blood vessels,* ed 6, Boston, 1964, Little, Brown.

209. Rector TS, Cohn JN, with the Pimobendan Multicenter Research Group: Assessment of patient outcome with the Minnesota Living with Heart Failure questionnaire: reliability and validity during a randomized, double-blind, placebo-controlled trial of pimobendan, *Am Heart J* 124:1017-1025, 1992.

210. Simonton CA, Higginbotham MB, Cobb FR: The ventilatory threshold: quantitative analysis of reproducibility and relation to arterial lactate concentration in normal subjects and in patients with chronic congestive heart failure, *Am J Cardiol* 62:100-107, 1988.

211. Sullivan MJ, Higginbotham, MB, Cobb FR: Exercise training in patients with chronic heart failure delays ventilatory anaerobic threshold and improves submaximal exercise performance, *Circulation* 79(2):324-329, 1989.

212. Weber KT, Kinasewitz GT, Janicki JS, et al: Oxygen utilization and ventilation during exercise in patients with chronic cardiac failure, *Circulation* 65(6):1213-1223, 1982.

213. Lipkin DP, Scriven AJ, Crake T, et al: Six-minute walking test for assessing exercise capacity in chronic heart failure, *Br Med J* 292:653-655, 1986.

214. Mancini DM, Eisen H, Kussmaul W, et al: Value of peak exercise oxygen consumption for optimal timing of cardiac transplantation in ambulatory patients with heart failure, *Circulation* 83(3):778-786, 1991.

Part VI

OTHER ISSUES

Chapter 69

DEVELOPING A RATIONAL SYSTEM TO CONTAIN COSTS ON THE CARDIAC CARE UNIT

Robert M. Califf

Bradi Bartrug

Mark C. Rogers

Deborah Roth

Wanda Bride

Kevin Fitzpatrick

Daniel B. Mark

The practice of medicine in the United States is changing dramatically as both government and society attempt to cope with the generally accepted perception that we are spending too much on health care and getting too little in return. A significant proportion of the seemingly relentless growth in medical costs is driven by ongoing improvements in biotechnology,[1] much of which is focused around the use of intensive care. Simultaneously, improvements in medical information systems have yielded a new generation of tools that will allow clinical decisions to be related to subsequent outcomes. The capability to relate decision and outcome as never before in medicine will revolutionize our ability to discern which treatments are effective and to understand how those treatments affect the cost of medical care. We feel that as reliable outcome and cost information becomes more readily available to clinical personnel, its value in assessing and ensuring the quality of medical care while holding the line on costs will become clearly evident. The goal of this chapter is to describe our initial efforts to develop a rational, medically-sound plan for cost containment on the Duke Cardiac Care Unit that is centered around the ability to tie medical customs and the process of care to patient outcomes. The cornerstone of our approach is identification and use of clearly effective medical interventions and the abandonment of ineffective or marginally effective therapies, many of which are the product of medical folklore and individual physician habit.

Most cost-containment efforts have concentrated on reducing the volume of services provided to patients by introducing either administrative controls, such as preadmission certification, or caps on reimbursement.[2] Such efforts avoid directly addressing the fundamental underlying inefficiencies in our system of providing patient care; consequently they have not generally succeeded in controlling the nation's skyrocketing health care bill.[3] It is also clear that the societal demand for substantial controls on medical costs is not accompanied by a willingness on the part of patients and their families to forgo medical care. Patients expect to receive the most advanced "high-tech" medical care available and to have it provided in a service-oriented manner.[4] In addition, payors and regulators now expect providers to demonstrate that their services are high quality, appropriate, and cost-effective (all at once) and to reduce the rates at which their expenditures increase. The challenges facing medical practitioners and medical institutions are nothing less than revolutionary.

Medical institutions by their nature tend to be conservative, however, and revolutionizing "business as usual" comes very hard. At the hospital level, efforts to improve quality and contain costs have too often been developed and implemented in isolation, creating competing if not conflicting agendas among physicians, nurses, and administrators. If we are to ensure the continued general availability of quality medical care at a reasonable cost, we must aggressively pursue an understanding of the relationships among quality, efficiency, and cost so that an approach can be devised that harmonizes these objectives.

MEDICAL PRINCIPLES

The basic medical goal of an efficient, high-quality Cardiac Care Unit (CCU) is to provide care that will enable patients with heart disease to return to as normal a life, in terms of quantity and quality, as is possible, given the current state of medical science. To achieve this goal, the CCU team must identify and apply effective treatment strategies, measure the degree to which they are being used, assess the patient outcomes that are being achieved, and provide appropriate feedback to the unit personnel. Effective management strategies are identified principally from a thorough review of the relevant medical and nursing literature and an active group effort to stay abreast of new developments. In the CCU the number of basic diagnoses for which such a review must be conducted is limited predominantly to manifestations of ischemic heart disease (AMI and unstable angina), congestive heart failure, and arrhythmias. A number of other complex diagnostic categories or complications also require consideration, but these may be best managed by developing practice standards for particular situations, such as renal failure requiring dialysis or prolonged mechanical ventilation regardless of the precipitating cause. For example, patients with significantly impaired left ventricular function and ischemic heart disease should be placed on angiotensin-converting enzyme inhibitors except when directly contraindicated, whether they initially present with MI, congestive heart failure, or unstable angina. The presence of existing reviews and guidelines, such as those published by the AHA/ACC consensus groups and the Agency for Health Care Policy and Research, form a

valuable starting point in defining effective strategies and care plans.[5,6]

Once identified, the list of effective management strategies can be translated into a plan of care or CareMap™, which is a detailed specification of expected care over an established timeline for a typical patient with a specific diagnosis, such as an uncomplicated AMI (Fig. 69-1). This plan of care serves as a template, allowing actual practice to be compared with the "ideal." Although much has been written about CareMaps, and individual examples of successful implementation of plans of care can be found in the literature,[7-12] they have been most successful in managing the care process for elective procedures in which the vast majority of patients can be expected to have a "typical" course. In general they are more difficult to put into practice for acute medical conditions because of the multiple possible outcomes for a patient with a given diagnosis and the lack of adequate software and information systems to document the actual care and outcomes in a quantitative fashion. For example, the management of a patient with an AMI complicated by recurrent ischemia is quite different from the management of a patient whose course is complicated by ventricular tachycardia. Consideration of all of these possibilities can rapidly become complex and frustrating, often leading to failure to use the plan-of-care concept by medical practitioners. Nevertheless, the goal of reaching a consensus on the course of action for recurring medical problems remains a cornerstone of effective medical practice and control of costs.

From this perspective the plan of care can be based on a list of effective decisions, decisions of uncertain efficacy, and ineffective decisions. In the Duke CCU, categorization of "effective" decisions now includes all operational decisions on the unit, ranging from the obvious and critical issues of individual patient treatment decisions to less obvious management decisions about allocation of nursing staff or purchasing of equipment. In order to provide a "shorthand" method for discussing decisions, we have settled on an "ABCD" classification, modeled after the medical guidelines process. An "A" decision is one that is proven to be effective and should be routine practice with rare exceptions. A "B" decision is one that in the opinion of the staff is probably correct and should usually be routine, although definitive evidence supporting the decision or practice is not available. A "C" decision is one that is usually either unnecessary or not beneficial but may be worthwhile on occasion in the consensus of the staff and does not have definitive evidence to refute it as a reasonable practice. A "D" decision or practice has been proven ineffective in well-designed studies. "D" decisions should be discouraged whenever possible

Critical path	Arrival	30-60 Minutes	1 Hour	2 Hours	4 Hours
1. Consultants	Respiratory therapist Medical resident ED attending M.D.	CCU Fellow is consulted as needed			
2. Laboratory tests	Draw and send: ABC, PT, PTT, Total CK, CK-MB, OP7, Mg, Ca. Consider type and screen for 2 units of blood If on Digoxin, send level				Total CK, CK-MB
3. Diagnostic tests	Stat EKG Order old EKGs Order old chart Vital signs with BP in both arms	Stat portable CXR Repeat EKG with ↑ CP or s/p NTG	Repeat EKG Stat EKG if ↑ CP	Repeat EKG Stat EKG if ↑ CP	Repeat EKG Stat EKG if ↑ CP
4. Treatments	IV #1 saline lock Emergency cardiac drug box to bedside External pacer and defibrillator on standby	NS IV bolus for ↓ BP IV #2 and IV #3 if CP	Vital signs q 1 hour	Vital signs q 1 hour	Vital signs q 1 hour
5. Medications	No IM or SC injections Oxygen 21, per NC NTG 0.4 mg SL q 5 min prn x 3 if chest pain is present Chew four (4) baby ASA	Consider NTP 1-2" or NTG 50mg/in 250 ml NS to start at 10 mcg/min Consider MS 2-4 mg IV for pain or anxiety	Consider heparin IV bolus at 60 mg/kg then drip 25,000 units/in 500 at 15 units/kg/hour via plum	Continue chronic meds	
6. Monitoring	Continuous telemetry Pulse oximetry Continuous noninvasive BP/Pulse Apnea monitoring Estimate patient weight Rate each episode of CP 1-10 I & O q 1 hour Watch for complications: 1. Heart block, dysrhythmias 2. Hypotension 3. Evolving MI 4. Increased CP				
7. Diet	NPO	NPO	NPO	NPO	NPO
8. Activity	Bedrest	Bedrest	Bedrest	Bedrest	Bedrest
9. Teaching/discharge plan	Patient/family education of CP evaluation procedures Patient education of CP 1-10 scale				
10. Transfer planning			Transfer from ED stabilization area to ED CPEU		Prepare to assign to observation bed
11. Patient problem list	Knowledge deficit related to myocardial ischemia Anxiety and fear of the unknown Potential for chest pain and myocardial ischemia				
12. Referrals					

Fig. 69-1. A representative CareMap™ for use in patients presenting with AMI.

Critical path	8 Hours	12 Hours	18 Hours	23 Hours
1. Consultants	CCU fellow as needed			CCU Fellow for discharge
2. Laboratory tests	Total CK, CK-MB			
3. Diagnostic tests	Repeat ECG Stat ECG if ↑ CP	Repeat ECG Stat ECG if ↑ CP		
4. Treatments	Vital signs q 4 hours	Vital signs q 4 hours	Vital signs q 4 hours	
5. Medications	Continue cardiac meds as ordered Continue chronic meds			
6. Monitoring	Continuous telemetry Rate each episode of CP 1-10 I & O q 1 hour Watch for complications: 1. Heart block, dysrhythmias 2. Hypotension 3. Evolving MI 4. Increased CP			
7. Diet	NPO	AHA 1 as tolerated		
8. Activity	Bedrest	Bedrest	Bedrest with BRP	Ambulate as tolerated
9. Teaching/discharge plan				Chest pain evaluation patient/family ED information Discharge ECG
10. Transfer planning				
11. Patient problem list				
12. Referrals				Center for living: 1. GI services 2. Cardiologist ED resource nurse for follow-up call after discharge

Fig. 69-1. cont'd.

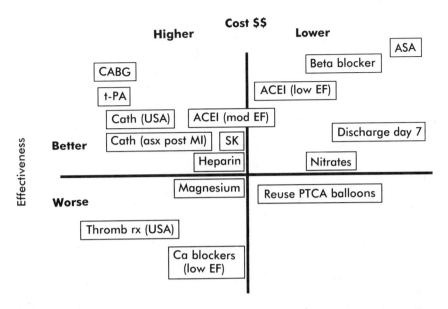

Fig. 69-2. A plot assessing the cost and effectiveness of several practices on the cardiac care unit. ASA, aspirin; CABG, coronary artery bypass graft surgery; ACEI, ACE inhibitors; EF, ejection fraction; Ca blockers, calcium blockers; Thromb rx, thrombolytic therapy; SK, streptokinase; t-PA, tissue-plasminogen activator; PTCA, percutaneous transluminal coronary angioplasty; asx, asymptomatic.

by the staff unless a very compelling justification can be made in a particular case.

This same strategy can be used to place decisions or practices on a four-quadrant chart to enable the unit staff to visualize costs vs. effectiveness. Several examples are provided in Figure 69-2.

An effective or "A" practice is one for which there is good evidence of improved survival or quality of life or a reduced incidence of an important adverse clinical outcome. Adequate evidence to consider a therapy effective consists of either an adequately powered randomized clinical trial or a carefully done observational study. In general, decisions supported by multiple high-quality studies, including at least one adequate randomized trial (e.g., thrombolysis for ST-elevation MI) are given more weight than therapies supported by only observational data (e.g., use of procainamide to treat atrial fibrillation). However, in many key areas of medical practice, observational data are the only kind that exist. Examples of "A" therapies for AMI patients with ST elevation include aspirin, thrombolysis, direct angioplasty, beta blockers, and angiotensin-converting enzyme (ACE) inhibitors (for ejection fraction < 40%); for acute ischemic heart disease patients without ST elevation, therapies include aspirin, heparin, beta blockers, and ACE inhibitors (for patients with ejection fraction < 40%) and discharge before day 7 in patients with uncomplicated infarctions.

A practice of uncertain efficacy is one that has not been shown to be effective but is nevertheless believed to be effective by a substantial portion of the medical staff based on observation, personal experience, extrapolation from pathophysiological data, or intuition. Examples include heparin and nitrates for patients with ST elevation and nitrates for patients without ST elevation. Routine administration of oxygen to patients with ischemic symptoms is an example of a "B" therapy, as is management of a patient with ECG changes but low suspicion for serious complications in a stepdown area rather than the CCU.

Many practices and therapies fall into the "C" category, and this category represents the area in which the most discussion should occur about cost reduction. For example, many patients with no lung disease and a normal physical exam are admitted with a suspicion of myocardial ischemia. Currently all of these patients are placed on oxygen at a charge of over $50 per day in most hospitals. In most cases this therapy is clearly unnecessary, but it is a time-honored tradition and has never been studied in a clinical trial. Similarly, cardiac rhythm monitoring is continued for many patients for several days after transfer from the CCU. The actual probability of an arrhythmic event and the cost effectiveness of continued monitoring have not been evaluated; yet if a patient were to arrest and die without receiving oxygen in the acute phase or without cardiac monitoring several days after CCU transfer, the legal risk might be considerable (see Chapter 70). Clinical practice guidelines provide the best approach to allow the clinical group to make rational choices, with a prospective defense against claims of inadequate care in the case of type C practices.

An ineffective or "D" therapy is one that has been shown either to have no effect on outcome or to actually increase the probability of a bad outcome, for example, calcium-channel blockers, prophylactic lidocaine, or magnesium for patients with ST elevation or, for patients without ST elevation, calcium-channel blockers (in the presence of ejection fraction < 40% or pulmonary edema) or magnesium therapy. "D" therapies should be eliminated from practice except in very carefully defined situations (e.g., diltiazem therapy in a low–ejection-fraction patient with rapid atrial fibrillation refractory to digoxin).

To provide efficient, high-quality patient care, physicians, nurses, and ancillary personnel must truly work together as a team. Members of this team must be able to challenge each other in a constructive way about what they do and how they do it. Particularly within the physician group and between the physicians and nurses, consensus standards must be established. In our experience this can be accomplished only by taking the time to meet and discuss new information about effective care so that the team can confront the difficulties and challenges in implementation away from the tense environment that often surrounds the critically ill patient.

To close the feedback loop, the CCU information system must be capable of providing regular reports about the extent to which the unit's idealized care plans are being followed. Significant deviations from expected care must be scrutinized to identify both deviations by the providers as well as inadequacies of the template being used to judge care. Additional reports must allow the CCU team to relate the major clinical decisions and care processes to subsequent hospital and short-term posthospital outcomes and costs. In our opinion, tracking costs and resource use with the goal of changing resource allocation provides an opportunity for serious mistakes unless outcomes are also tracked. Fortunately, in acute cardiac situations substantial data exist to allow stratification of risk upon entry into the hospital. Outcomes of patients cared for in a changing system can thus be compared over time, adjusting for differences in baseline characteristics to maximize the chances that the physicians, nurses, and administrators can distinguish whether different outcomes are the result of different types of patients or different medical care.

ECONOMIC ISSUES

Because there is strong societal pressure to constrain the growth in health costs and an equally strong sentiment against giving up the benefits of high-technology medicine, we must find a way to maximize the use of clearly effective therapies to maintain the benefits of high-technology medicine while eschewing approaches that are "not worthwhile." For illustrative

purposes, cost-containment measures can be considered in two categories: administrative and clinical. Administrative cost containment involves more efficient use of resources, such as personnel, operating systems, and materials, in the provision of a given medical service. Clinical cost containment encompasses any change in clinical decision-making relating to therapeutics, monitoring, or education of the patient. These are not totally distinct concepts, particularly because administrative decisions related to investment in systems to increase efficiency (such as staffing patterns and computer systems for decision support) have direct clinical ramifications.

There are three major obstacles to translating the desire to contain costs into practice in the CCU: (1) most hospitals do not know the true cost of producing specific cardiovascular (or other) services; (2) the fixed and variable components of the cost of various services and procedures are not known or cannot be separated, and clinicians therefore cannot know how changes in their practice will affect the cost; and (3) for many of the day-to-day details of medical practice there is virtually no information available to help judge the value of the activity in question or its relation to medical outcomes. A fourth issue that may come up in settings where medical practitioners are paid on a fee-for-service basis relates to the differing and occasionally conflicting economic self-interests of the physicians and the hospital administration.

The first obstacle, the lack of knowledge that most hospitals have about the true cost of their services, is surprising to those who have recently begun to pay serious attention to the problem of medical costs. The explanation for this state of affairs can be found in the way hospitals have been paid over the last 30 years.[2] The significant expansions of the role of the federal government as a payor for health care by President Lyndon Johnson in the mid-1960s, along with subsequent national campaigns to eradicate large classes of disease such as cancer, heart disease, and more recently AIDS, has had two effects on hospitals. First, until the era of prospective payment, hospitals were reimbursed based on their "reasonable" costs of providing care (which they largely defined themselves). Knowing they would be reimbursed for what they spent, they had no particular incentive to be thrifty or efficient. Second, until the institution of the current health care debate and the advent of managed competition, hospitals never faced serious price competition. Rather, they competed in a sort of technologic arms race—to have the biggest MRI, the most catheterization laboratories. As long as the national checkbook remained open, hospitals had no reason to be concerned with the costs of their services; in fact, because such information costs money to gather, there was actually a disincentive to obtain it.

Table 69-1. Costs and charges for typical procedures done on CCU patients*

Procedure	Total charge ($)	Total cost ($)	Fixed cost ($)	Variable cost ($)
Right heart catheterization	1383	789	352.80	436.10
Left heart catheterization, coronary angiogram and ventriculogram	2589	1240	618.10	621.60
Electrocardiogram	29	13.01	5.58	7.43
Chest x-ray (portable)	99	53.87	—	—
Automated blood count	14	5.74	4.02	1.72
Prothrombin time	18	7.55	3.98	3.01
Chemistry panel	15	6.78	4.56	2.22

*The dollar figures in this table are representative of those reported by several institutions participating in clinical trials.

Hospital administrators concentrated on keeping the overall budget "in the black." If one hospital department was losing money, raising prices in another, more profitable department was usually all that was required to cover the shortfall. In this fashion hospital charges or prices became a very distorted reflection of hospital costs.[2] The key point for current cost-containment efforts is that hospital charges provide a very inflated and inaccurate index of the true amount of cost savings available from changes in practice.

A second obstacle making it difficult for hospitals to relate practice patterns with their associated costs relates to the inability to distinguish between fixed and variable costs.[2] Every medical service has two cost components, one that changes with unit changes in service (variable cost) and one that does not change as additional units of service are provided (fixed cost). Reducing the number of laboratory tests or chest x-rays performed on the CCU will save the variable component of these costs but not the fixed cost. Fixed costs are typically saved only when capacity can be permanently reduced, such as by laying off employees, shutting down laboratories, or closing beds. If a fully staffed laboratory sits idle, the hospital must continue to pay the associated fixed costs of this excess capacity.

Distinguishing true costs from charges and fixed from variable components requires a sophisticated (and expensive) hospital cost-accounting information system. We believe that hospitals without such a system will be unable to compete in the currently evolving environment of health care. Table 69-1 demonstrates the abilities of such a system to explore hospital cost components. For example, the hospital charge for a right heart catheterization is $1383, whereas the true hospital cost is $789. However, neither of these figures reflects the amount saved if we reduce our use of this procedure. That latter figure is obtained by looking at the variable cost component, which in this case is $436.10. Note the large percentage of total true costs in Table 69-1 that are fixed. No matter how efficient the clinician becomes, these costs (which include the allocated expenses of adminis-

tration, laundry, housekeeping, medical records, etc.) will continue to accrue. Thus, cost-efficient medical care clearly requires shared responsibility for fat-trimming and efficiency between practitioners and administration.

The third major obstacle to cost containment is uncertainty about the relationship between accepted patterns of practice and outcome. In the 1940s and 1950s hospitalization after AMI usually involved 3 or more weeks of bed rest.[13] By the early 1970s a 1-week stay was considered as safe as a longer hospitalization for uncomplicated patients.[14] Most recently a 3-day stay has been proposed for selected low-risk patients with successful early revascularization.[15] The current 7- to 9-day average length of stay after AMI may be excessive for a significant minority of patients, but it is impossible to judge from current data the extent to which this practice can be safely altered. One major impediment is that there is no consensus in the medical community about how low the risk of adverse events must be to be acceptable.[16] To take another example, we know that not every patient in the CCU needs a chest x-ray and routine blood work every day, but we are uncertain about the safe minimum use of these tests. This is one area where the risk-benefit judgment of the physician favors more testing, a practice sometimes referred to as "defensive medicine." Because malpractice cases are always judged with the end result known, it is difficult, for example, to defend not ordering a routine hematocrit that may have provided early warning of an unsuspected catastrophic retroperitoneal bleed, even if that event occurs only once in 1000 patients. Thus, uncertainty about relationships between practice and outcome and the absence of clear practice standards tend to push the physician to a more costly style of practice.

The final major obstacles to cost containment are the differing financial motivations of hospitals and physicians. Under prospective payment, hospitals are rewarded for spending as little as possible per hospital admission. In many practice environments, however, physicians still get paid for doing more, not less. Where no professional fee is involved, such as in routine blood work, there is no direct conflict between physician and hospital. Areas where conflict might arise in the CCU include the use of pulmonary artery catheters, temporary pacemakers, and intraaortic balloon pumps. Additional conflicts may arise because the physician wishes to provide the best possible care for the patient, regardless of cost, whereas the hospital must keep in mind what is likely to be reimbursed. Use of t-PA over streptokinase and use of nonionic vs. ionic contrast are two contemporary examples of this type of conflict in many hospitals.

ADMINISTRATIVE COST CONTAINMENT

In this section we will review the main options for administrative cost constraints in the CCU in three categories: labor, supplies, and operations/systems.

Labor

One of the key strategies for effective control of labor costs is to convert fixed costs to variable costs wherever possible. Typically, once a staffing pattern is established for a patient unit, it is only adjusted during the annual hospital budgetary review process. Accordingly, most units are not able to adjust staffing levels (and, consequently, labor expenses) to account for daily variations in census and patient acuity. By treating labor as a variable expense, however, staffing patterns may be increased or decreased in concert with fluctuations in the census. In this model, which we currently use in our unit, a specified nurse-to-patient ratio is established; when the census decreases, the number of nurses used to staff the unit is decreased proportionally. Operationally this may be achieved by reassigning staff members to other units or allowing the use of vacation time or educational time. One strategy to decrease reassignment to multiple units is to develop a reciprocal relationship with a sister unit, "trading" nurses back and forth to meet changing census needs. A less desirable but sometimes necessary option for meeting decreased patient census needs is mandated time off, (i.e., sending nurses home without pay), which causes loss of income and frustration with the system. We believe that this option should be exercised only as a last resort because of its negative impact on staff morale. Nurses should be involved in decisions regarding variable staffing in response to fluctuating census in order to decrease the negative repercussions of reassignment or time off without pay. By playing an integral part in the decision-making process, staff nurses develop a sense of control and take pride in their role, the unit, and the institution.

In order to provide coverage when the census increases, additional staffing resources must be available on a timely basis. This may be accomplished through the use of a central staffing pool that provides nurses with training in specific clinical service areas (such as critical care). In order to establish the pool without adding new positions, each unit in the hospital is expected to relinquish a predetermined number of budgeted positions and in return will receive additional help on an as-needed basis. Another option is to recruit unit-specific per-diem nurses for times of high acuity or volume, an approach that allows flexibility in patient coverage while decreasing costs to the institution. A third option is to establish a group of nurses who are willing to work flexible hours and on an as-needed basis. Their time can be scheduled directly with the unit, and their performance can be evaluated by that unit's leadership.

Supplies

There are two main ways to reduce supply costs at the unit level: reducing the use of unnecessary supplies and paying less per supply item by substituting less expensive supplies or negotiating better pricing. The following strategies may be useful in achieving these objectives:

1. Track supply costs and use on an ongoing basis, including the total expenditures for supplies on a monthly basis as well as expenditures within specific categories (office supplies, IV solutions and supplies, sterile supplies, etc.). An effective information monitoring system allows problems in supply use to be quickly identified and interventions to be implemented before a major financial impact occurs. It also ensures that any errors in the amount billed for the supplies may be identified and corrected on a timely basis. Actual expenditures should then be compared with budgeted expenditures, and variances may be calculated and analyzed. The major disadvantage of this approach is that comparing actual expenditures with a fixed monthly budget does not take into account fluctuations in patient volume and acuity and therefore cannot be used to interpret variances. Accordingly, it is helpful to track expenditures in relation to actual activity, such as calculating the supply cost per patient day in each major supply category. The ideal method would incorporate a measure of acuity into the calculation. Finally, a flexible budgeting approach may be used, in which each month's budgeted expense is adjusted to reflect volume and/or acuity and then compared with the actual expense.

2. Assign the responsibility for monitoring supply use and expenses to a head nurse, assistant head nurse, or unit clerk, depending on the size of the unit. If nursing staff members are to be held accountable

for the use of unit resources such as supplies, this expectation should be included in the orientation of all new staff as well as in performance standards and evaluations. Approaches to this problem might include programs for minimizing waste, using the most appropriate supply item for a particular task and ensuring that items used are properly recorded for accounting and billing purposes. Ultimately, the head nurse and medical director must assume responsibility for monitoring supply utilization and expenditures.

3. Identify lower-cost alternatives to commonly used supplies by comparing and evaluating items. During the evaluation consider a variety of factors in addition to cost such as time savings, reduced waste, etc. Ensure that decisions to choose a high-cost item over a low-cost item are based on an improvement in some aspect of patient care (outcome, infection control, safety, etc.) or the demonstrated offsetting of other costs rather than on anecdotal information or personal preference. Some examples include using traditional vs. tympanic thermometers, using a higher-priced oximeter pulmonary artery catheter for specific cases rather than for all patients, drawing up normal saline flushes vs. using prefilled syringes, and using sandbags vs. groin site occlusive devices. It is intriguing that despite the multimillion-dollar implications of the systematic choice of one supply item over another in routine practice, little is known about the true incremental value of more expensive medical supplies.

4. Reduce inventory expense by minimizing the number and types of particular items that are routinely stocked on the unit and reviewing the use of each item regularly. Seek consensus from the personnel involved regarding the most acceptable item and eliminate the others from the unit stock. This strategy requires collaboration within the hospital to ensure the availability of "second-line" items that are rarely needed in an individual unit, but that may be frequently used among units. Additionally, items needed by an individual hospital only several times per year should ideally be shared between hospitals.

5. Evaluate the cost differential between reusable and disposable items, including cloth underpads instead of disposable underpads, scissors, hemostats, suction cannisters, 12-lead ECG electrodes, blood pressure cuffs, urinals, bedpans, and thermometers. In the near future the issue of reusing diagnostic and therapeutic catheters will need to be addressed. Preliminary data from Canada supported the safety of this approach with angioplasty balloons,[17] although there was a significantly increased incidence of both abrupt closure and adverse clinical events in the center that reused the catheters.[18]

6. Ensure appropriate accessibility to supplies. Care must be taken to avoid restricting supplies too much. Efficiency can be reduced in other areas of care when clinicians and nurses do not have rapid and easy access to necessary supplies, thereby increasing personnel cost. At its extreme, restriction of supplies can lead to impairment of patient outcome.

In many cases these strategies will require changes in established practices and may consequently generate resistance from the staff. In order to achieve such change it is vital to recognize the extent to which staff members must be involved in the process. Before initiating cost-reduction efforts, we have found it helpful to review with staff members the key issues relating to health care costs nationally as well as at institutional and unit levels. Although health care workers and the general public are being bombarded continuously with information regarding the "health care cost crisis," staff members are not generally familiar with cost issues at a unit level and consequently may not fully appreciate the significant role they can play by supporting and participating in cost-reduction efforts. Estimating the amount of money that could be saved annually simply by reducing the personnel budget of each department by as little as 10% (through more flexible staffing patterns) may make a considerable impression on staff members who do not believe that they are in a position to make an impact. Such an educational effort might begin by introducing staff members to the size of the unit's annual budget, as well as the proportion of the budget allotted for personnel, supplies, equipment, maintenance, and other expenses (Fig. 69-3). In the area of supplies it will be critical to educate staff about the actual cost of individual supply items in order to raise their consciousness about the economic impact of these items on the unit budget and the patient's bill. This could be accomplished by making cost (and charge) information readily accessible to staff members, perhaps by highlighting the cost and charge of a few individual items each month. Key items to focus on might include both the most expensive items as well as several low-cost, high-volume items.

After education, the second key step in the implementation of a successful unit-based cost-reduction effort is involving staff in a meaningful and substantive way. Involving staff in research-based product evaluation (at the unit level) enhances staff ownership of cost issues, teaches the evaluation research process, pro-

Total FTE's-67.9

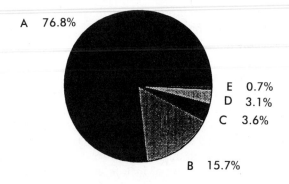

A 76.8%

E 0.7%
D 3.1%
C 3.6%

B 15.7%

A-Nursing payroll   D-Clerical support payroll
B-Fringe benefits   E-Maintenance and other
C-Supplies

Fig. 69-3. This pie chart demonstrates a breakdown of the Duke Cardiac Care Unit annual expense budget for fiscal year 1993-1994.

motes independent thinking and creativity, and encourages interdisciplinary and intradisciplinary respect. Such exercises have been shown to increase job satisfaction and retention among staff nurses.[19,20]

A model was developed by nurses in our CCU to answer clinical, cost, and product-evaluation questions in a systematic and research-based manner. Questions are recorded by the staff at the patient's bedside on note pads (Post-it™ notes). These questions include anything about patient care or product evaluation, implementation, substitution, or discontinuation. The notes are posted on a central STICK (So This is Investigating Clinical Knowledge) board in the conference room for general staff observation and review. Each month the research committee (staff nurses, nurse clinician, clinical nurse specialist, and director of the center for nursing research) meets to review all questions and concerns on the STICK notes. The questions are answered based on a review of the current literature (via Medline search) using a unit-based personal computer. Answers are posted monthly on a central bulletin board in the CCU. Questions not answered conclusively in the literature are then considered for unit research projects. Staff interested in various issues form a team, which formulates a clinical research question and carries out a study either alone or in collaboration with other units or hospitals (Fig. 69-4).

One example of the STICK board process involved tympanic thermometers. A staff member posted a question requesting a substitution of our traditional digital oral/rectal thermometer for the newer, faster tympanic thermometer. The research committee pro-

duced conclusive data from the literature to support the reliability and validity of tympanic temperature correlation with core temperature. Average time for temperature readout was 3 seconds with the tympanic thermometer as compared with 30 seconds orally. In addition, the data revealed a significantly decreased rate of nosocomial infection when using a tympanic as compared with a traditional oral/rectal device. A unit-based trial of the tympanic thermometers was conducted for 1 month, with similar supporting results. A cost comparison of the two devices revealed a 125% greater cost for the tympanic thermometer. A risk-to-benefit analysis was done that included a review of nosocomial device–related infections in the CCU over the past 2 years. No cases of thermometer-mediated *E. coli* transmission were identified (these had been most prevalent in an immunosuppressed pediatric population). As a result of these data the research committee recommended that the unit not purchase the new thermometers because the time savings was not significant enough to outweigh the cost, and our patient population is not at unusual risk for thermometer-transmitted infection.

DEVELOPING EFFICIENT SYSTEMS AND OPERATIONS

Another important administrative aspect of ensuring high-quality patient care while controlling costs is to create and maintain highly efficient operating systems that facilitate and streamline patient flow. First, the care delivery process must recognize the patient's needs as the focus around which the hospital revolves, rather than subjecting the patient to less efficient care for the

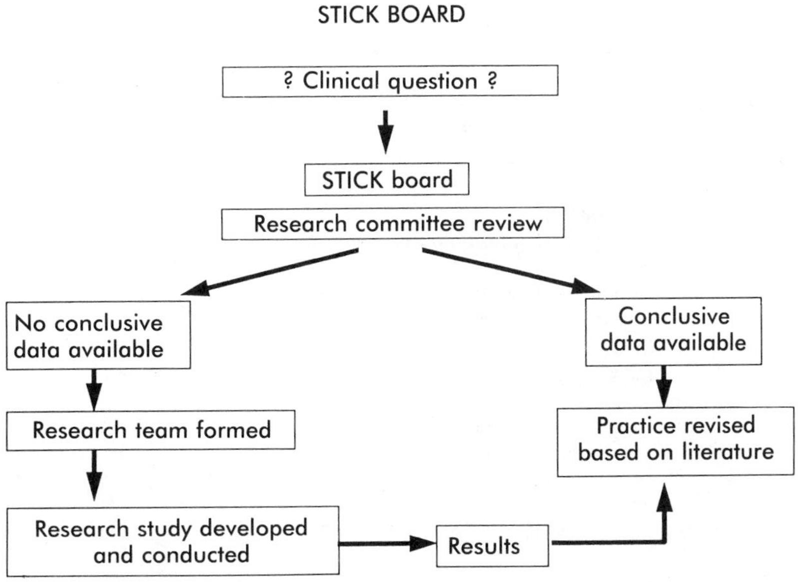

STICK BOARD

Fig. 69-4. The STICK (So This is Investigating Clinical Knowledge) board method of clinical research uses the method illustrated in this figure.

convenience of staff or departments. For example, if a patient's discharge is contingent on the results of a diagnostic test, the test should be scheduled early in the day to facilitate the discharge decision and the availability of that bed for another patient. This may entail developing flexible working hours for personnel in diagnostic areas (e.g., cath lab, nuclear radiology) to meet patient needs. The sequence of physician rounds on an inpatient unit should be structured so that patients with the potential to be discharged that day are seen first. Finally, if it is likely that a patient will be discharged the following day, necessary paper work should be completed the night before in order to ensure that all personnel and departments involved in the discharge process are able to anticipate the patient's needs and plan accordingly. Although this is less of an issue for CCU patients directly, many hospitals repeatedly encounter problems where the lack of available floor beds unnecessarily prolongs a patient's CCU stay, resulting in significant overuse of resources and increase in costs.

The scheduling of diagnostic tests and ancillary services may present a particular challenge throughout the patient's stay and during preparation for discharge. Often the patient's care is dependent on when a particular laboratory can perform the given test. If the patient needs multiple tests, coordination problems and delays are likely to occur. These obstacles to efficient patient flow may be decreased by designating the ICU bedside nurse as coordinator of all tests and ancillary services. Generally, the care nurse is in the best position to determine the appropriate sequence of these services

and to schedule them to meet the patient's needs best. Another key area to address is the admission, transfer, and discharge process. A system of communication between referral hospitals, the admissions department, bed control, housekeeping, patient transport staff, and nurses and physicians on the unit is essential in order to facilitate timely patient admission and treatment. An efficient system will also help minimize turnover time on the unit when patients are transferred within the hospital or discharged. The smooth flow of patients through the hospital will not only facilitate high-quality care and timely access to treatment but will also enhance satisfaction among patients, families, and referring physicians and help reduce lengths of stay and hospital costs.

CLINICAL-ADMINISTRATIVE INFORMATION DISSOCIATION

It is important for both clinicians and administrators to understand the differences between administrative/financial data systems and clinical data systems. Currently, most administrative and financial data systems include minimal clinical data, primarily the diagnosis-related group (DRG), a system of classification-by-discharge diagnoses that determines hospital payment for Medicare patients. Importantly, the assigned DRG category does not have to agree with the clinical admitting diagnosis, and substantial inaccuracies have been found in the diagnostic ICD-9 codes on insurance forms that are used to determine the DRG.[21] Despite the seemingly homogeneous nature of the CCU patient

Table 69-2. Top 20 DRGs in 1581 consecutive CCU admissions*

DRG	DRG: Description	N	LOS	Mean LOS
112	Percutaneous cardiovascular procedure	338	2,824	8.4
106	Coronary bypass with cardiac catheterization	211	3,143	14.9
124	Circulatory disorders except AMI	134	1,044	7.8
110	Major cardiovascular procedure	130	1,567	12.1
121	Circulatory disorders with AMI and complication	125	1,348	10.8
127	Heart failure and shock	74	921	12.4
122	Circulatory disorders with AMI without complication	60	436	7.3
107	Coronary bypass without cardiac catheterization	38	432	11.4
125	Circulatory disorders except AMI with cardiac catheterization without complex diagnosis	31	123	4.0
475	Respiratory system diagnosis with ventilator support	29	341	11.8
116	Permanent cardiac pacemaker implant	29	329	11.3
138	Cardiac arrhythmia and conduction	29	291	10.0
104	Cardiac valve procedures with cardiac catheterization	29	676	23.3
483	Tracheostomy except for mouth	28	1,942	69.4
123	Circulatory disorders with AMI, expired	27	220	8.1
470	Ungroupable	19	245	12.9
478	Other vascular procedures with cardiac catheterization	18	286	15.9
144	Other circulatory system diagnosis	16	149	9.3
140	Angina pectoris	13	89	6.8
143	Chest pain	12	34	2.8
Other	N/A	191	3,052	16.0
Grand total		1581	19,492	12.3

*CCU, cardiac care unit; DRG, diagnosis-related group; MI, myocardial infarction; CABG, coronary artery bypass graft; CHF, congestive heart failure; LOS, length of stay

population, during a 1-year period (July 1992 to June 1993) on the Duke CCU 1581 patients received treatments that ranged across 20 different DRGs (Table 69-2).

When a patient is admitted to the hospital with an AMI and then has an angioplasty, that patient is classified by the hospital administrative database into the percutaneous cardiovascular procedures DRG. In contrast, a clinical information system would classify the patient as presenting with an MI with certain baseline characteristics and complications. By the time a patient is in the percutaneous cardiovascular procedures DRG, the most expensive decision of the inpatient stay has already been made: to do the angioplasty. One critical aspect of cost containment is therefore to judge, prospectively if possible, whether such high-cost decisions are appropriate.

In order to resolve the clinical-administrative dissociation problem, the clinical staff and administrators should have access to both an adequate clinical database and a functional financial database. The clinical database should capture the baseline characteristics and admitting diagnoses of the patients, as well as the key therapies they received and the important complications that were encountered. Without this information aggregate data cannot be used to review appropriateness of therapy. The financial database should allow the user to

determine the actual cost to the institution of performing a particular service or procedure. Total costs should be broken down into variable-vs.-fixed costs so that the actual savings that could be realized by reducing the volume of services can be calculated. In a similar manner, this information allows the determination of the cost of additional resources that would be required to institute an incrementally effective treatment approach.

We have become convinced that the most effective approach to cost containment will occur when the clinical and administrative databases are effectively linked. Such a linkage will allow examination of the cost and resource use profiles of patients who are grouped in clinically meaningful ways. For example, the resources used to care for patients with MI in general and for patients with particular complications can be examined. Without a clinical system such an analysis is hampered by the fact that when a complication affects DRG assignment, patients with widely diverse intensity of illness and resource utilization may all be classified to the same DRG. DRG 121, for example, includes patients with a single complication, whether that complication is nonsustained ventricular tachycardia or cardiogenic shock. Additionally, proper risk stratification can occur only with clinical databases[22] because administrative databases do not reflect quality control adequate for clinical purposes.

Table 69-3. Costs, charges, and reimbursements for selected cardiology DRGs*

DRG: Description	N	Mean LOS (days)	Charge ($)	Cost ($)	Reimbursement ($)
121 : Complicated MI	125	10.8	17,830	11,659	12,028
122 : Uncomplicated MI	60	7.3	11,981	8294	11,481
123 : MI with death	28	7.9	19,100	12,185	10,947
112 : Percutaneous procedure	338	8.4	19,580	12,608	16,886
127 : Heart failure and shock	74	12.4	19,831	11,540	10,018
106 : CABG with catheterization	211	14.9	37,668	23,426	34,171
107 : CABG without catheterization	38	11.4	28,032	18,001	26,295
999 : Other	769	14.0	32,495	20,262	22,038

*The dollar figures in this table are representative of those reported by several institutions participating in clinical trials.
DRG, diagnosis-related group; MI, myocardial infarction; CABG, coronary artery bypass graft; LOS, length of stay.

CLINICAL COST CONTAINMENT: THE DUKE CCU COST REDUCTION PROGRAM

With the foregoing principles in mind we have developed a six-step approach to clinically responsible cost control on the CCU. This approach represents an ideal, which we continue to refine as we gain more experience; coming as close as possible to the ideal remains a challenging goal.

Understanding the patient population

The first step in cost control is to understand the patient population, in both clinical and administrative terms, that is being cared for on the CCU. Reports addressing this issue should include the DRG categories, admitting clinical diagnoses, and lengths of stay of the patients treated on the CCU. An example of such a report from the Duke CCU is displayed in Table 69-3. The mix of patients with complicated AMI, "rule-out" infarction, or unstable angina can vary considerably, depending on whether the institution is a tertiary referral center or a community hospital and upon the practice patterns and availability of "step-down" or monitored beds.

Understanding patient outcome

The next step toward ensuring that the quality of patient care is not sacrificed in the process of reducing costs is to understand the outcomes of patients treated in the intensive care unit by developing a mechanism for collecting and analyzing relevant outcome data. At a minimum the report from this effort should include mortality rates. As the system becomes more detailed, major nonfatal complications, quality of life, and patient satisfaction should also be recorded. To provide these data, an on-line clinical data collection system is required.

Many such systems have now been developed to allow comparative assessment of outcomes across institutions. Regression models have been developed to relate patient characteristics at the time of admission to

mortality.[22-24] In this manner a hospital can keep track of its "scorecard." Difficult issues must be addressed in the analysis and reporting of individual physician- and institution-specific "scorecards."[25]

Understanding resources used in treating patients

Until recently, physicians and nurses had little knowledge of or interest in the costs of medical care and the budgets of hospital inpatient units. Because of the issues just discussed, however, the future clinical and financial success of physicians and nurses will be critically dependent upon an in-depth understanding of the influence of clinical decision-making on cost. The problem is complex because of the traditional dissociation between the "budget" for the individual hospital unit and the cost of providing services as influenced by the mix of patients and determination of appropriate medical care. In the past, budgets have generally reflected the cost of running the unit the previous year, with an adjustment factor for changes in policy on the unit.

Sophisticated new cost-accounting systems now allow analyses of inpatient budgets to be constructed using both the "top-down" approach and the "bottom-up" approach.[2] The "top-down" approach evaluates the cost of providing the array of services needed to operate an intensive care unit; the "bottom-up" approach constructs a cost profile from the individual patients composing a (homogeneous) diagnostic category. Theoretically these two estimates should lead to similar conclusions about the total resources needed to operate the intensive care unit, although little empirical data are available on this issue. Available data indicate that the costs of treating a patient with AMI are driven in large part by patient-related characteristics (the demographics of the patient and the presenting features of the disease), disease-related characteristics (particularly the occurrence of complications), and treatment-related characteristics (the therapies chosen and resulting events).[2] The accompanying box demonstrates the independent factors related to increased costs obtained from studies of AMI involving thrombolytic treatment (TAMI 5)[26] and direct angioplasty (PAR).[26,27] Figures 69-5 to 69-11 demonstrate the distribution of costs as a function of these risk factors. The different personnel and resource intensity required to treat patients with different clinical characteristics can now be quantified.

Independent factors for increased cost in patients with AMI

Age
Anterior MI
Initial Killip Class
Number of diseased arteries
Recurrent ischemia
New heart failure
Revascularization

Comparing costs with national and regional norms to identify differences

Without a frame of reference all of the preceding steps are simply exercises that raise interesting issues. Only by comparison with other institutions can a sense be gained of whether the clinical and financial practices are reasonable compared with national or regional norms. We believe that comparing data institution-to-institution is the best method for reaching a consensus on reasonable costs for cardiovascular services. When local costs are above the norm they must be scrutinized to assess whether the difference represents cost shifting to offset imbalances in other parts of the medical center or a difference in medical practice, nursing practice, or administrative practice. A difference in any of these areas could be either good (because the difference results in better outcome and is worth the extra cost) or bad (because the difference results in the same or

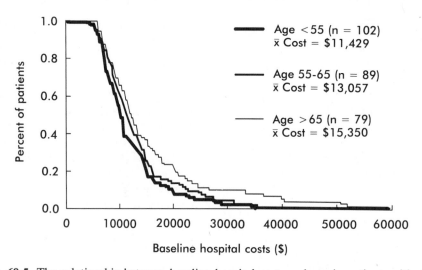

Fig. 69-5. The relationship between baseline hospital costs and age in patients with AMI.

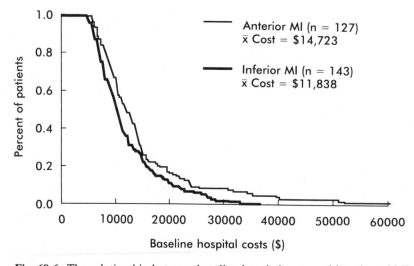

Fig. 69-6. The relationship between baseline hospital costs and location of MI.

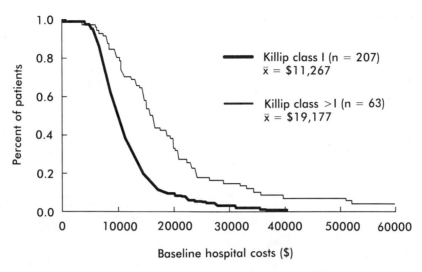

Fig. 69-7. The relationship between baseline hospital costs of Killip Class at presentation.

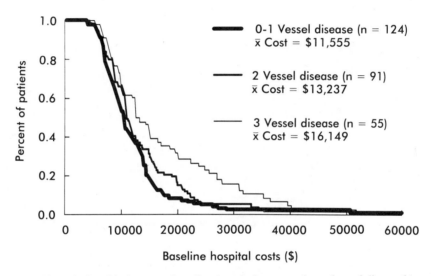

Fig. 69-8. The relationship between baseline hospital costs and number of diseased arteries.

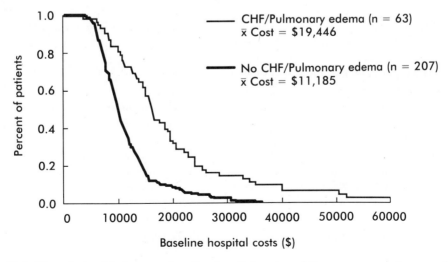

Fig. 69-9. The relationship between baseline hospital costs and the presence or absence of recurrent ischemia.

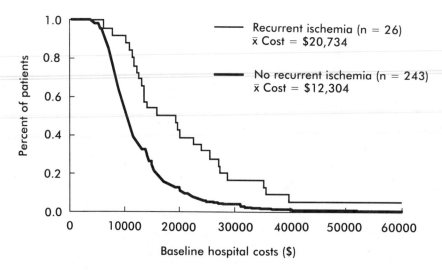

Fig. 69-10. The relationship between baseline hospital costs and congestive heart failure or pulmonary edema.

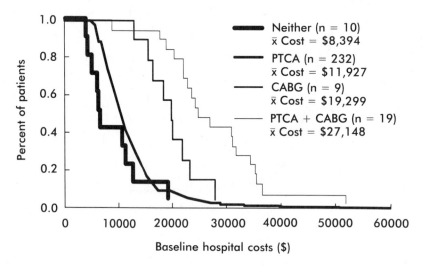

Fig. 69-11. The relationship between baseline hospital costs and revascularization procedures.

worse outcome at higher cost). Only through careful analysis can such a conclusion be reached. Although adjustment of the cost data for severity of illness in different institutions cannot currently be accomplished accurately, this approach will be possible in the near future. In the Primary Angioplasty Registry both charges and costs varied as a function of hospital, even after using a sophisticated adjustment procedure for severity of illness.[27,28]

We believe that this information should be made available to the physicians and nurses caring for patients on the CCU. In this manner, assumptions of the cost accounting system can be challenged and the most effective course of action can be planned.

Developing a cost reduction plan

The administrative team, nurses, physicians, and other personnel involved in the care of patients on the

unit should review the clinical, outcome, and cost data and develop a plan for cost reduction. Wherever possible the costs of supplies and unnecessary equipment should be reduced through efficient buying practices as just outlined.

When economic and clinical variances from norms do not result in better patient outcome, a plan for change should be instituted. Such a plan can be most conveniently packaged and tracked through a set of rules implemented in a tracking database. An example of such a rule is that uncomplicated AMI patients (no heart failure, recurrent ischemia, ventricular tachycardia, or atrioventricular block) should be transferred to the less intensive stepdown unit 24 hours after admission. At first glance this rule seems easy to track, but it actually requires a system that simultaneously records the circumstances and time of admission, major complications, and time of transfer on every patient. Although these rules should be configured into a Care Map™ for coherent presentation, existing hospital databases are not adequate for collecting and tracking the array of data needed for care maps.

An understanding of the potential for a simple rule to have an effect on global costs can be gained by evaluating the length of hospitalization per facility in the GUSTO-I trial.[29] For this example we have chosen patients with first infarction and no heart failure, recurrent ischemia, heart block, or serious ventricular arrhythmia during the hospitalization. The length of stay for the 20,000 patients meeting these criteria ranged from 1 to 20 days, with 25% of patients hospitalized for less than 8 days and 25% hospitalized for more than 11 days (Table 69-4). Within the United States substantial variability existed, although it was much greater outside the United States.

Outcomes should be tracked not in terms of whether the agreed-upon strategy is being followed (e.g., is the uncomplicated patient transferred out within 24 hours?) but to ensure that the pieces combine to have an effect on the whole; the costs should also be tracked in terms of the global CCU budget and DRG per-patient costs. Reports on these aspects of the administration of the unit should be tracked on a monthly or quarterly basis. Of course none of this can be placed effectively in context without knowledge of patient outcomes.

Developing a system of adequate incentives that will not compromise care

We believe that some fraction of savings from efficiency must be reflected in benefits for employees in the area that realized the savings. Several issues need to be considered before implementation of an incentive program, such as group vs. individual incentives, tangible vs. intangible incentives, the incorporation of cost containment into job expectations, and the use of performance appraisals with merit-based salary increases. All members of the unit and the health care team must participate in the development of cost-containment efforts if success is to be achieved. A successful plan will encourage local leadership to be exerted without concern that success will lead only to shifting of resources to other hospital areas that are not as successful.

The role of the physician in the reward structure for cost containment is a volatile but crucial concern. One potential conflict may arise when the physician is reimbursed for procedures done, but the hospital is attempting to reduce costs. We believe that some mix of direct financial rewards for practicing cost-effective medicine and incentives to provide better information should be combined with an emphasis on the latter. Careful safeguards, predominantly involving peer collaboration and review, must be in place to prevent incentives that encourage substandard care as a way to

Table 69-4. Length of stay (days) for uncomplicated MI (GUSTO-I trial—1991-93)

	Hospital			Intensive care unit		
	25%	Median	75%	25%	Median	75%
Overall	7	9	11	2.5	3.5	5
US	6	8	10	2.5	3.5	5
Non-US	7	10	13	3	4	5

reduce cost. A continuous effort involving both the physician and nursing staffs will have the best chance to responsibly identify practices that can be eliminated without compromising patient outcome.

Group incentives could include payment for unit activities such as annual staff meetings; computers with educational, data analysis, and word processing programs; financial support for unit-based educational offerings; a personnel lounge that is private and restful; or family facilities that are attractive, comfortable, and easily accessible to the health care team. Individual incentives could focus on professional development, including a nominal budget for each staff member for educational development, presentation of posters, and speaking engagements; recognition of professional certifications such as CCRN; and the use of "class days" for learning and preparation of unit-based educational offerings.

Cost-containment standards for resource utilization should be incorporated into job expectations, and compliance with these standards should be reflected in the performance appraisal. One approach could be the use of a merit-based salary increase system. In order to implement such a system, objective and measurable criteria need to be established. The amount of salary increase would then be directly proportional to the level of overall job performance, which would *include* cost-conscious practice.

In order to be involved in and supportive of cost containment, the entire unit staff must feel that their status on the health care team is recognized and appreciated. Respect and recognition of the valuable roles both nurses and physicians play are essential to promote involvement and professional behavior. Because nurses in particular coordinate the delivery of patient care, they are in an excellent position to identify cost-containment issues at the unit level. A concerted and cohesive effort by a collaborative health care team would provide optimal cost containment without a loss of quality.

REFERENCES

1. Newhouse JP, (ed): *Measuring medical prices and understanding their effects,* Santa Monica, Calif, 1988, Rand.
2. Mark DB: Medical economics and health policy issues for interventional cardiology. In Topol EJ, (ed): *Textbook of interventional cardiology,* ed 2, Philadelphia, 1994, WB Saunders.

3. Rice DP, Hodgson TA, Kopstein AN: The economic cost of illness: a replication and update, *Health Care Financ Rev* 7:61-80, 1985.

4. Ginzberg E: High-tech medicine and rising health care costs, *JAMA* 263:1820-1822, 1990.

5. Braunwald E, Mark DB, Jones RH, et al: Unstable angina: diagnosis and management, Clinical Practice Guideline No. 10, AHCPR Publication No. 94-0602. Rockville, Md; Agency for Health Care Policy and Research and the National Heart, Lung, and Blood Institute, Public Health Service, U.S. Department of Health and Human Services, March 1994.

6. Ryan TJ, Bauman WB, Kennedy JW, et al: Guidelines for percutaneous transluminal coronary angioplasty: a report of the American College of Cardiology/American Heart Association Task Force on Assessment of Diagnostic and Therapeutic Cardiovascular Procedures (Committee on Percutaneous Transluminal Coronary Angioplasty), *J Am Coll Cardiol* 22:2033-2054, 1993.

7. Barnsteiner JH, Mohan A, Milberger P: Implementing managed care in a pediatric setting, *AACN Clin Iss Crit Care Nurs* 3:777-787, 1992.

8. Strong AG, Sneed NV: Clinical evaluation of a critical path for coronary artery bypass surgery patients, *Prog Cardiovasc Nurs* 6:29-37, 1991.

9. Guiliano KK, Poirier CE: Nursing care management: critical pathways to desirable outcomes, *Nurs Manage* 22:52-55, 1991.

10. McElroy MJ, Campbell S: Case management with the nurse manager in a role of case manager in an interventional cardiology unit, *AACN Clin Iss Crit Care Nurs* 3:749-760, 1992.

11. Collard AF, Bergman A, Henderson M: Two approaches to measuring quality in medical case management programs, *QRB* 16:3-8, 1990.

12. Thompson KS, Caddick K, Mathie J, et al: Building a critical path for ventilator dependency, *Am J Nurs* 91:28-31, 1991.

13. Pryor DB, Hindman MC, Wagner GS, et al: Early discharge after acute myocardial infarction, *Ann Intern Med* 99:528-538, 1983.

14. McNeer JF, Wallace AG, Wagner GS, et al: The course of acute myocardial infarction: feasibility of early discharge of the uncomplicated patient, *Circulation* 51:410-413, 1975.

15. Bates ER, Topol EJ: Early hospital discharge in the myocardial reperfusion era, *Clin Cardiol* 12(suppl III):III-65-III-70, 1989.

16. Mark DB, Sigmon K, Topol EJ, et al: Identification of acute myocardial infarction patients suitable for early hospital discharge after aggressive interventional therapy: results from the Thrombolysis and Angioplasty in Acute Myocardial Infarction Registry, *Circulation* 83:1186-1193, 1991.

17. Goulet G, Plante S, Strauss BH, et al: Preliminary report on the safety and performance of reused PTCA catheters, *Circulation* 88(suppl I):I-479, 1993.

18. Plante S: Personal communication, March 31, 1994.

19. Kacuba A: Turning tradition upside down: staff nurses in research, *Am J Nurs* (suppl) 5-10, 1993.

20. Campbell G, Chulay M: Establishing a clinical nursing research program in a service setting. In Spicer J, Robinson M, (eds): *Environmental management in critical care,* Baltimore, Md, 1990, Williams and Wilkins.

21. Jollis JG, Ancukiewicz M, DeLong ER, et al: Discordance of databases designed for claims payment versus clinical information systems: implications for outcomes research, *Ann Intern Med* 119:844-850, 1993.

22. Selker HP, Griffith JL, Beshansky JR, et al: The thrombolytic predictive instrument project: combining clinical study data bases to take medical effectiveness research to the streets. In Grady ML, Schwartz HA, (eds): Summary report: medical effectiveness research data methods, Rockville, Md, 1992, Agency for Health Care Policy and Research.

23. Goldman L, Weinberg M, Weisberg M, et al: A computer-driven protocol to aid in the diagnosis of emergency room patients with acute chest pain, *N Engl J Med* 307:588-596, 1982.

24. Goldman L, Cook EF, Brand DA, et al: A computer protocol to predict myocardial infarction in emergency department patients with chest pain, *N Engl J Med* 318:797-803, 1988.

25. Topol EJ, Califf RM: Scorecard cardovascular medicine: its impact and future directions, *Ann Intern Med* 120:65-70, 1994.

26. Califf RM, Topol EJ, Stack RS, et al: Evaluation of combination thrombolytic therapy and timing of cardiac catheterization in acute myocardial infarction: results of thrombolysis and angioplasty in myocardial infarction—phase 5 randomized trial. TAMI Study Group, *Circulation* 83:1543-1556, 1991.

27. O'Neill WW, Brodie BR, Ivanhoe R, et al: Primary coronary angioplasty for acute myocardial infarction (The Primary Angioplasty Registry), *Am J Cardiol* 73:627-634, 1994.

28. Mark DB, Brodie B, Ivanhoe R, et al: Effects of direct angioplasty on hospital costs in acute myocardial infarction: results from the multicenter PAR study (abstract), *Circulation* 83(suppl I):I-237, 1991.

29. The GUSTO Investigators: An international randomized trial comparing four thrombolytic strategies for acute myocardial infarction, *N Engl J Med* 329:673-682, 1993.

Chapter 70

MEDICOLEGAL ISSUES

M. Lee Cheney
Daniel B. Mark

In legal parlance medical malpractice is a type of *tort,* which is a private or civil wrong/injury, other than breach of contract, for which the court will provide a remedy. Tort law is based upon the recognition in this country that one who is harmed either intentionally or unintentionally by another is entitled to recover compensation for the resulting loss, detriment, or injury. Torts can be *intentional,* in which one deliberately does that which the law has declared wrong, such as assault, battery, or libel, or *unintentional,* the result of negligence, in which one fails to exercise the requisite degree of care in doing what is otherwise permissible. Another category of tort law involves *strict liability,* in which the question of intent or fault is irrelevant. For example, activities deemed inherently dangerous no matter how much care is exercised, such as dynamite blasting, can give rise to strict liability for all injuries proximately caused by the activity. By contrast with intentional and strict liability torts, *negligence,* or *fault,* is central to most unintentional tort actions, including medical malpractice.

Whether one is rendering diagnosis and treatment or driving a car, all persons are required to adhere to certain duties of care in carrying out their professional and personal activities. *Negligence* is the failure to exercise the degree of care ordinarily exercised by a "reasonably prudent person" under the same or similar circumstances. One whose conduct falls below that standard may be liable in damages for any resulting injuries or losses. Thus, one who operates a motor vehicle in a manner inconsistent with a reasonably prudent person (e.g., runs a red light) may be deemed negligent and liable to persons injured as a result. In the context of medical malpractice, a physician is required to exercise the average degree of care, skill, and diligence

ordinarily exercised by members of the same profession under similar circumstances. This measure is referred to as *the standard of care.* In arguments to juries, plaintiff lawyers frequently suggest that the failure to comply with the applicable standard of care is the medical analogue of running a red light. The applicable standard of care must be proved in each case.

ESSENTIAL ELEMENTS OF A MEDICAL MALPRACTICE CASE

Not every act of medical negligence gives rise to malpractice liability. In order to establish a case that is legally sufficient to be submitted to a jury, a plaintiff must meet a number of technical and substantive requirements. The technicalities include filing suit within the relevant state's statutory time limit for bringing suit after the right to do so accrued (known as the *statute of limitations*), suing and properly effecting timely service of suit papers (*summons* and *complaint*) on the right defendants, properly stating a claim for relief in the complaint, and complying with other technical rules. Substantively, a malpractice plaintiff must be able to show four essential elements in order to file a suit:

1. A duty on the part of the physician to comply with an applicable standard of care, and
2. a breach of that duty of care, or failure to comply with the applicable standard of care, which is
3. a proximate cause of
4. damage to the patient.

If the plaintiff fails to present sufficient evidence of each of these four essential elements, the defendant may be entitled to ask the court for a summary judgment or a dismissal of the case as a matter of law without the necessity of a trial.

Duty and breach of duty

The existence of a doctor-patient relationship at the time of the alleged negligence has long been a threshold requirement for any medical malpractice case. This is because the duty of a physician to a patient arises out of that relationship. Historically, the doctor-patient relationship has been considered a contractual relationship, subject to the legal doctrine of "freedom of contract." That is, physicians and patients are deemed free to decide whether and with whom to contract. Absent a doctor-patient relationship, we formerly believed that no duty runs from the doctor to a patient that is capable of being breached and serving as the basis for a malpractice case. This is still pretty much the rule, although, as discussed below, the recently recognized exceptions to the rule may signal a trend toward its erosion.

A duty is an obligation, to which the law gives recognition and effect, to conform to a particular standard of conduct toward another. Once a doctor-patient relationship has been established, or some other basis for a duty exists, a physician owes the patient a duty to comply with the applicable standard of care in rendering diagnosis, care, and treatment. In a general theoretical sense the standard of care to which a doctor owing a duty must comply is that degree of care, skill, and diligence ordinarily exercised by the average practitioner of the defendant's specialty under similar circumstances. In practice, the standard of care applicable to a given situation is established by expert witness testimony. Ironically, expert witnesses are usually required to educate lay juries on standards of care because such matters are not within the common knowledge and experience of most jurors. Yet almost every malpractice case that goes to the jury presents one set of opinions from expert witnesses for the plaintiff, promoting one view of the standard of care and the defendant's breach thereof, and another generally contradictory set of opinions from expert witnesses for the defendant, articulating a different standard of care and opinion of the defendant's conduct. Alternatively, the experts for both sides may agree on the standard of care issue, but may disagree concerning causation. Ultimately, then, lay jurors are still often expected to decide between competing technical, scientific, or medical theories.

The only time a plaintiff is not required to come forward with an expert witness to testify concerning the standard of care is when the alleged negligence fits within the "common knowledge exception." The exception refers to matters that are within the common knowledge and experience of the average juror, such that expert testimony would be unnecessary. For example, no expert testimony is needed to help a jury understand that putting an intraaortic balloon pump in the wrong patient is a deviation from standards of care.[1] Expert testimony would be necessary, however, to establish that the physician's technique in implanting the intraaortic balloon pump was incorrect.

Proximate cause

Before a defendant physician can be liable for medical negligence, the patient must have suffered some injury or damage as a result of the physician's negligence. The physician's negligence need not be the sole cause of the plaintiff's injuries, but it must be one of the causes without which the injury would not have occurred. For example, if the physician orders a medication to which the patient is allergic or which is otherwise contraindicated, but the patient suffers no harm as a result, then the element of proximate cause cannot be established. On the other hand, if one physician orders the wrong medication, and another physician improperly treats the patient's consequent anaphylaxis, both acts of negligence may be causes of the patient's resulting injuries and both physicians may therefore be jointly and separately liable.

Physicians often have difficulty with the legal definition of causation, which is not as rigorous as a scientific notion of causation. In most cases, the physician's negligence need only be *more likely than not* a cause of the plaintiff's injuries. Expert testimony is usually required to establish, by a probability of 51% or greater, that the physician's negligence was a cause of the plaintiff's injuries.

Damages

Clever, new theories of harm are continually being advanced by plaintiffs and their attorneys and recognized by the courts, thus adding to the ever-increasing size of malpractice settlements and jury awards. In our civil litigation system, physical, mental, emotional, and financial injuries to a plaintiff are all compensable damages. In general in this context the law recognizes three types of damages: economic, noneconomic, and punitive damages. Economic damages involve compensation for past and future economic losses, such as medical expenses; funeral expenses; lost wages, including lost benefits; pharmaceutical and special equipment costs; and expenses related to transportation, rehabilitation, and home health care. Noneconomic losses include past and future pain and suffering, scarring and disfigurement, emotional distress, loss of enjoyment of life, as well as the loss of a chance for cure, and loss of ability to be gainfully employed. Punitive damages are monetary awards to the plaintiff that are unrelated to issues of compensation for losses sustained. Punitive damages are awarded to punish physicians who are found to have been grossly negligent, or who have acted willfully, maliciously, or fraudulently. A defendant physician who commits a simple act of negligence is not ordinarily subject to punitive damages.

THEORY VS. PRACTICE

As the federal and legislative branches of government grapple with complex proposals to legislate containment of the exponential growth of health care costs, the judicial arm of that same government seems bent on continuing to expand the potential exposure of health care providers to malpractice liability. For example, some courts have recently been willing to find a physician's breach of duty even in the *absence* of a doctor-patient relationship.[2] Other courts have recently decided that plaintiffs need not necessarily establish proximate causation, which has always been accepted as a crucial element of a plaintiff's case.[3] Courts continue to recognize new theories of damages, constructed by creative plaintiff attorneys to inflate amounts that may be recovered by successful malpractice plaintiffs (and thus their lawyers). Some of the emerging damage theories include recent cases allowing recovery for negligent infliction of severe emotional distress by persons other than the injured patient,[4] for so-called hedonic damages, which speak to an assumed loss of enjoyment of life,[5] and for a patient's fear of certain consequences (e.g., contracting AIDS) that have not actually occurred.[6]

The increasing pressure on individual physicians to reduce medical resource use for the explicit purpose of reducing costs may well increase their risks of being sued successfully in a malpractice case. Consider, for example, the prevalent drive to discharge patients from the hospital as early as possible. In uncomplicated AMI patients enrolled in the GUSTO-I trial, one quarter of the U.S. patients were discharged from the hospital on or before the sixth hospital day whereas the median length of stay for such patients was 8 days. If an uncomplicated AMI patient who was sent home on day 6 or on day 7 had a cardiac arrest and died (a rare event that does happen), there would undoubtedly be physician expert witnesses willing to testify for a plaintiff that (for reasons only evident in retrospect) it was inappropriate and a violation of the standard of care to send this patient home early. In a malpractice case defense attorneys are reluctant to raise the issue of cost savings because of the general perception that juries will not accept such justification in the setting of a bad outcome. (Plaintiff attorney: "Doctor, do you mean to tell the jury that you were not willing to spend $300 to keep Mr. Jones in the hospital one day longer so that his fatal arrhythmia could have been successfully treated, and his children would still have a father...") We believe that the lack of adequate malpractice reform clashes directly with desires for cost containment. The only protection that doctors currently have in this area comes from professional group consensus. In particular, practice guidelines may help establish the boundaries of safe and acceptable medical practice without specific reference to cost containment.

APPLICATIONS TO CARDIOLOGY

The cardiologist's primary exposure to malpractice liability arises from diagnostic errors.[7] Other important issues include informed consent, withdrawing and withholding treatment, documentation, complications and adverse outcomes, drug-related events, and patient abandonment. To the extent possible, each of these issues is discussed with specific reference to the specialty of cardiovascular medicine and will be accompanied by some suggestions for risk minimization. The reader must appreciate that the details of various malpractice cases may vary according to patient diagnosis, physician specialty, other factual distinctions, and state law. Ultimately, however, all cases generally adhere to the framework outlined in the preceding section.

Diagnosis-related issues

Diagnostic errors are the leading cause of loss in malpractice suits against cardiologists.[7] A delayed diagnosis, or failure to recognize a diagnosis altogether, can result not only in costly delays in providing necessary treatment but also in consequent mistreatment. Cases involving diagnostic errors are among the most susceptible to evaluation through the "retrospectoscope." For this reason, these cases are often difficult to defend. Frequently, when the patient's entire medical record, including knowledge of the outcome, is available for plaintiff experts to study in great detail, the damning clues to the patient's (by then known) diagnosis can be located and made to appear to the jury as obvious evidence of the defendant physician's negligence.

Failure to diagnose AMI in the emergency department or outpatient clinic is one of the most common allegations in cardiology malpractice cases. In one such case an emergency department physician failed to recognize hyperacute T-wave changes in a patient with prolonged chest pain and sent the patient home. After expert review of this case by the defense attorney, it became clear that the major debate with the plaintiffs would not be about negligence (since the negligence was obvious) but rather about damages—how much the plaintiff was entitled to recover.

Some of the most difficult failure-to-diagnose-AMI cases involve a patient who presents with some form of discomfort that might be ischemic and a normal or ambiguous ECG. We have seen several such situations where the physician's note is inadequately detailed to support the decision not to admit the patient, while the description by the ED nurse on the chief complaint line is quite graphic: "Patient feels like an elephant is sitting on his chest..." A careful, well-documented history, physical exam, and 12-lead ECG interpretation can provide powerful justification for a decision not to admit even if that decision is shown *in retrospect* to be wrong. However, the doctor must provide a convincing argument in her note that the patient's symptoms do not represent acute ischemic heart disease (i.e., "I considered the possibility of acute ischemic heart disease but do not feel this to be the correct diagnosis for the following reasons. . ."). One mistake that we see too often is for the clinician to focus on ruling out the less serious (but perhaps more likely) diagnoses in the differential before doing an adequate evaluation of the possibility of unstable CAD. Statements such as "I will get an upper GI series and if this is negative will consider an exercise thallium. . ." are of little help when the patient dies the day after his normal GI study and before any subsequent work-up has been initiated.

Another type of failure-to-diagnose case involved failure to diagnose intracranial hemorrhage following t-PA therapy. The patient, a 35-year-old man, was hospitalized for AMI and treated promptly with IV t-PA. Over the next 2 days the medical record showed increasing headaches, nausea, vomiting, and vertigo. The patient subsequently became comatose and died shortly thereafter. The defendant doctor admitted that he had considered the possibility of intracranial hemorrhage but had rejected it in favor of alternative explanations for the patient's symptoms. The plaintiffs convincingly argued that an early CT scan would have revealed the hemorrhage at a treatable stage before the development of herniation. The result was a jury verdict in favor of the plaintiff for $1.15 million.

The importance of a patient's medical history cannot be overemphasized. Too often plaintiff experts criticize defendant physicians for failure to elicit or to appreciate certain aspects of a patient's medical history. Often the aspect of the medical history allegedly overlooked by the defendant appears in a history obtained by someone else (e.g., nurse, consultant). It probably will not be a good enough excuse that the defendant did not read that section of the chart or that the patient failed to give that particular information to the defendant personally. Plaintiff experts will testify that the defendant had an obligation to ask the questions that would elicit the information and to read the medical histories obtained by others, including nurses. A single symptom or occurrence reported by the patient to just one health care provider making entries in the patient's chart can constitute a critical piece of evidence in a failure to diagnose or delayed diagnosis case.

The process of arriving at and ruling out differential diagnoses has become an important weapon in the arsenal of malpractice plaintiff attorneys and their expert witnesses. Ignoring the role of clinical judgment, plaintiff lawyers portray inclusion of a diagnosis in the differential as a matter of scientific requirement. This then supports a conclusion that failure to rule out the possible diagnosis definitively was medical negligence. An experienced plaintiff attorney, writing on this subject

for other plaintiff attorneys, has counseled: ". . . the differential diagnosis is not a theoretical exercise. The possible causes of illness, in order of severity and . . . [acuity] . . . must actually be ruled out. And if you can't rule it out, you better check it out."[8]

Health care reform is expected to curtail the practice of defensive medicine, which has developed at least in part as a response to the cookbook approach taken by plaintiff attorneys. Although this may be a positive step in the effort to control costs, it is not clear what protection, if any, will be offered to the physician who gets sued for failure to order a costly diagnostic test to rule out that unlikely but theoretically possible diagnosis suggested by the plaintiff's signs and symptoms. Medical practice guidelines being developed by professional organizations and research groups may help to eliminate some of this uncertainty; however, practice guidelines are usually not so comprehensive and rigorous as to preclude the need for clinical judgment. Guidelines may actually have the effect of increasing the number of malpractice claims if they are too rigidly written because failure to follow them in every case (for whatever reason) will become persuasive evidence of negligence. Since 1992 the state of Maine has been conducting the Maine Medical Liability Demonstration Project, which allows some specialists to use compliance with practice guidelines as an affirmative defense in malpractice cases. State-approved practice guidelines for 20 conditions in four specialties judged at particularly high risk (obstetrics, radiology, emergency medicine, and anesthesiology) were developed for the program. This project is scheduled to conclude in 1996.

Informed consent

Informed consent is first a *doctrine* predicated upon fundamental rights of privacy, bodily integrity, and self-determination recognized by our Constitution and court case law.[9] To safeguard the rights each individual has not to be touched without authorization, the *process* of informed consent has emerged. The process of informed consent ensures that patients give permission before submitting to medical procedures and certain therapies. Because most patients lack the medical knowledge needed to make meaningful choices, health care providers have been charged with the duty of providing sufficient information to allow the patient to decide whether to undergo the proposed procedure.

Informed consent is one of the rare situations in which a physician may be exposed to *intentional* tort liability. If a physician obtains *no consent* to a procedure, a lawsuit alleging battery can be brought by the patient, whether or not the patient sustained any damages. In the context of a battery, defined as an unconsented to, offensive touching of one person by another, damage is presumed and need not be proven. Negligent performance of the procedure is not an element of an action for battery. That is, a physician may be liable for performing an unconsented-to procedure even if the procedure was performed flawlessly and the patient actually benefited from it.

Most informed consent cases today arise not because the patient's consent was entirely lacking but because the patient claims that inadequate information was provided to truly inform the patient's decision. Cases involving the *quality* of the disclosure underlying a patient's consent are *unintentional* torts, or negligence actions. These cases arise after a patient has experienced a complication, and the lawsuit alleges that the physician failed to inform the patient that the particular complication was an inherent risk of the procedure. Multiple studies have documented patients' inability to recall information given during the informed consent process, and patients invariably fail to recall having been informed of a risk once it has actually occurred.[10]

In order to satisfy informed consent requirements, physicians must advise their patients of the most frequent and serious risks and hazards inherent in a proposed procedure. Although extremely remote risks or those with only slight injury potential ordinarily need not be disclosed, some states may require, and the best practice involves, disclosure of even remote risks that involve serious complications. Disclosure should also include the patient's diagnosis, the nature and a description of the recommended procedure, its expected benefits, any available alternatives (whether or not recommended by the physician), including nontreatment, and the expected benefits and potential risks of the alternatives, including the potential consequences of refusing the recommended procedure.

State laws usually establish either a professional or a lay standard against which a physician's disclosure is to be measured. The majority of states apply the professional standard, which is based upon the standard of practice among members of the same health care profession under similar circumstances.[11] In states that apply the lay standard, the test is an objective one, that is, whether the physician disclosed all the information a reasonably prudent person would have considered material in making a treatment decision.[12] Expert testimony is usually required to establish the professional standard for informed consent but is not necessary to establish the lay standard. Under the lay standard, however, expert testimony is still required to prove the existence and magnitude of the inherent risks.

Once a physician's breach of the relevant (professional or lay) standard has been established, the plaintiff must then demonstrate proximate causation. That is, the plaintiff must show that consent would not have been given had the risk of the complication that occurred been disclosed before the procedure.[13] Again,

the inquiry in most states is objective, requiring the jury to consider whether a reasonable person in the plaintiff's position would have consented to the procedure had the risk been disclosed. In this context a subjective test is no test at all. This is because plaintiffs generally maintain and undoubtedly believe, in retrospect, that they would not have consented to the procedure if they had been told about a particular risk, which in fact occurred (even though they acknowledge having consented with knowledge of other risks, including death).

Although consent may validly be expressed orally or in other nonwritten forms, and may even be implied in some instances, the medical record should contain documentation of the patient's consent. A patient's signature on a preprinted form is the bare minimum documentation that must be obtained. Such forms are usually general enough to apply to any and all risks of any and all procedures, stating that "all the risks and benefits have been explained to me by my physician." Because almost half of patients have no subsequent recall of risks disclosed to them by their physicians before undergoing procedures,[10] separate documentation should memorialize the specific risks of which the patient was informed. The record should also document that the patient was informed of the diagnosis or differential diagnoses, the nature and a description of the proposed procedure, its expected benefits, any alternatives to the proposed procedure, including nontreatment, as well as the expected benefits and potential risks of these alternatives, including the consequences of nontreatment. In addition, the physician's rationale for recommending one procedure over the alternative procedures should be explained to the patient, and the record should reflect that the patient appeared to understand the disclosure and voluntarily consented to the procedure.

Exceptions to informed consent requirements include emergencies and incompetent patients. The requirements of informed consent are suspended in emergency situations, unless the physician has reason to know that the patient would have withheld authorization or the patient's life or health is not in immediate jeopardy.[11] Incompetent patients are those who are unconscious, senile, retarded, psychotic, intoxicated, unemancipated minors, or those who have been adjudicated by the courts to be incompetent to make their own health care decisions. It is sometimes difficult to measure a patient's competence. Although rare cases may require formal legal proceedings, the President's Committee for the Study of Ethical Problems in Medicine and Biomedical and Behavioral Research recommends that the attending physician make these determinations with institutional regulation and review.[14]

The President's Commission identified the following

five factors for an attending physician to consider when assessing patient competence: (1) patient capacity to understand relevant information; (2) patient capacity to communicate decisions to caregivers; (3) patient capacity to reason about reasonable alternatives against a background of sound, stable, personal values and life goals; and, in some instances, (4) a psychiatric assessment.[14]

Intermittent incompetence can result from such things as medication, intoxication, and depression. A patient's competence or capacity to make health care decisions should not be confused with the ability to communicate those decisions. For example, a competent patient may be prevented from voicing preferences by such mechanisms as intubation. As long as a patient is competent for purposes of consenting to treatment, notwithstanding inability to easily communicate that consent, consent should be obtained from the patient. Consent by an incompetent patient, by contrast, is invalid. A physician may be held liable for rendering treatment based upon an incompetent patient's consent or for failing to render treatment based upon an incompetent patient's refusal to consent. Consent for an incompetent patient must be obtained from a parent, guardian, or some other person with legal authority to make health care decisions for the patient. In the absence of a legal surrogate, the incompetency exception permits health care providers to render necessary treatment without consent.[11]

The fact that all patients have a right to full disclosure before giving consent does not mean that they must submit to this process. Patients also have the right to consent without a detailed discussion of the possible risks of treatment. Patient waiver constitutes a third exception to informed consent requirements. The patient's chart must document that the physician attempted to make the requisite disclosure and that the patient declined to receive the information.

In a malpractice case the test for whether a particular procedure requires obtaining informed consent is a standard-of-care one. In other words, if the majority of individuals in a particular specialty get informed consent to do a given procedure or to administer a particular therapy, then failure to do so provides grounds for a malpractice suit. In emergencies, however, the emergency exception, described just above, may apply.

Withdrawing and withholding treatment

Just as patients have a right to consent to medical treatment, they also have a right to withhold that consent. A competent patient has a legal right to refuse any form of medical intervention, including life-saving treatment such as a blood transfusion, cardiopulmonary resuscitation, and even artificial hydration, nutrition, and respiration.[15] An incompetent patient has the same right to refuse treatment through the patient's legal surrogate for making health care decisions.[16]

State legislation usually designates a hierarchy of appropriate health care decision-makers for incompetent patients, and physicians should familiarize themselves with the relevant laws of the states in which they practice. Many state laws now recognize the right of a patient to prepare an advance directive, or "living will," at a time when the patient is competent to give directions to health care providers in the event of the patient's future incompetence. States are also enacting "Natural Death Legislation" to assist physicians in caring for incompetent patients who are not known to have previously executed living wills. In general, extraordinary means of keeping the patient alive may be withheld or discontinued in patients who are comatose with no reasonable probability of returning to a cognitive sapient state, or who are otherwise mentally incapacitated, with a condition their physician has determined is terminal, incurable, and irreversible. The statutes typically establish a hierarchy of appropriate decision-makers on this question, including the patient's attending physician in concurrence with the patient's spouse, guardian, a majority of the patient's relatives in the first degree, or an institutional committee.[17]

Documentation

The primary evidence available to plaintiff attorneys and their expert witnesses concerning a patient's care and treatment is the patient's medical record. Of considerable concern to malpractice defense attorneys is the susceptibility of the record to interpretation by looking through the "retrospectoscope," a perspective that was unavailable to the defendant physician when treating the patient. Although the primary purpose of medical records is to ensure continuity and quality of patient care by recording an accurate chronology of the patient's presentation, diagnostic work-up, treatment, and results, health care providers who enter information in a patient's chart should always be alert to the fact that they are creating a legal document that could one day end up in court. By being mindful of both purposes for creating and maintaining a record, health care providers should be able to avoid most documentation pitfalls. Too many physicians, however, still regard documentation requirements as something extraneous to patient care and resent the time and effort involved in record keeping. In the setting of a bad medical outcome and a malpractice suit, the defendant physician's assertion that he or she is too busy taking care of patients to waste time on the medical record usually comes across very poorly.

Medical liability experts estimate that 35% to 40% of all medical malpractice suits are rendered indefensible by problems with the medical record.[18] Poorly maintained records reflect adversely on the quality of the record keeper's practice, and a bad result combined with a bad record can result in a jury verdict of liability, notwithstanding a lack of any real negligence on the part of the health care provider.

A proper medical record should memorialize a factual and objective chronology of the patient's course of treatment. It should legibly and understandably document the patient's medical history and presenting complaints; physical examination and findings (including negative findings); laboratory or other diagnostic testing and the results; differential diagnoses and the ultimate diagnosis, including an explanation of how it was arrived at and the other diagnoses excluded. In addition, all important conversations with the patient and the patient's family should be summarized, including all informed consent discussions, patient refusals, noncompliance, and failure to keep appointments. Finally, the physician's treatment of and instructions to the patient should be recorded, including directives concerning follow-up, medication, and life-style changes.

Entries in medical records should be sequential, and each health care provider who makes entries in a medical record should date and sign that entry, noting the time of day a patient visit occurred, a particular observation or patient complaint was made, and test or consult was ordered. Once made, entries should not be modified. If additional information needs to be recorded, a separately dated, timed, and signed entry should be made. Alterations to medical records look suspicious, and can render an otherwise defensible case indefensible.

A medicolegal reviewer has recently noted a disturbing increase in the proportion of cases that involve altered medical records.[19] One such case implicated an attending physician in an emergency department who failed to document a physical examination of a 55-year-old woman who presented with complaints of acute left-sided chest pain and history of a recent fall resulting in a chest contusion. Twelve hours later the patient returned in cardiac arrest, and a description of "normal cardiac exam" was added to the initial emergency department note.[19] Although a cardiac examination may well have been normal on the patient's initial presentation, such an alteration will be portrayed by a plaintiff attorney as dishonest. As a result the physician's credibility will be compromised and the case may be rendered indefensible.

In addition to reviewing information obtained by other health care providers from the patient, or those accompanying the patient, it is recommended that all available prior medical records, including previous electrocardiogram strips, radiographs, and the like, be reviewed for any information that may be pertinent to the patient's present condition. If previous electrocardiograms, for example, are not readily available but would be useful or necessary for comparison purposes,

they should be requested and efforts made to obtain them as soon as possible. Toward this end technologic advances such as facsimile transmission are very useful.

Finally, it is equally important to know what not to write in a patient's medical record. For example, a disgruntled consultant should discuss any differences of opinion orally with the attending physician who requested the consultation. Airing differences in a patient's medical record neither contributes to quality care for the patient nor helps the consultant's position in the event of a subsequent malpractice suit, given that most juries expect physicians to direct their time and efforts to treating patients rather than scribbling childish notes in the medical record. In addition, a patient's medical record is not the place for creative writing, editorializing, or making personal observations or comments about the patient or the patient's family. Moreover, a medical record should never contain criticisms of care rendered by other health care providers.

Complications and adverse outcomes

Medical maloccurrence and medical malpractice are not synonyms. In the event of a recognized complication or adverse outcome, a physician should be able to defeat a subsequent medical malpractice case with adequate informed consent and documentation. The law recognizes that certain risks are inherent in all medical procedures. Cardiac catheterizations, for example, carry risks of bleeding, infection, vascular complications, thrombosis, anaphylactoid reactions, and dysrhythmias. Although these complications certainly can occur as a result of negligence, the mere occurrence of a complication that is a recognized risk of the procedure does not establish negligence. In other words, the existence of the proximate cause and damage elements of a particular case does not automatically create liability because the plaintiff must also prove medical negligence or a deviation from the applicable standard of care by the defendant physician. Although a physician would not be liable for an allergic reaction to contrast, physicians have been found liable for patient deaths resulting from perforation of a patient's pulmonary artery by a Swan-Ganz catheter[20] and from the improper insertion of a chest tube causing a bilateral pneumothorax.[21]

Medical negligence, or fault, in connection with the performance of a procedure must ordinarily be proved by expert testimony. Naively trusting their colleagues to exercise intellectual fairness and honesty, physicians tend to feel reassured by the knowledge that plaintiffs will have to come forward with an expert to testify that there was a violation of a standard of care. Increasingly, however, as expert witness referral services proliferate and courts continue to approve large expert witness fees, any reassurance physicians feel from the expert witness requirement for plaintiffs may be misplaced. Thus, physicians must be prepared to defend their decisions and their practices in court by demonstrating a thorough knowledge of the procedure or device involved, its indicated uses, that the physician's decision to use and the performance of the procedure complied with accepted standards of practice, that the benefits outweighed the potential risks, and that the patient's informed consent was obtained.

Lawsuits related to procedures can also arise from the failure to use an indicated technology. For example, a Connecticut physician was sued for failure to use a Swan-Ganz catheter in a patient who subsequently died. The plaintiff's expert witness testified that the Swan-Ganz catheter would have helped to diagnose hypovolemia; however, the patient did not die from problems related to hypovolemia. Inasmuch as there was no evidence that the physician's failure to use the Swan-Ganz catheter caused or contributed to the patient's death, (i.e., the essential element of proximate causation was lacking), the court decided the case in favor of the defendant physician as a matter of law without the necessity of a trial.[22]

Physicians are charged with a duty to keep abreast of evolving technologies, new information, and changes in medical practice, but not every physician must or should offer the latest technology. The strong association that exists between volume rates and outcome suggests that many physicians should refer patients for certain types of treatment. For example, the ACP/ACC/AHA Task Force on Clinical Privileges in Cardiology has established the minimum number of angioplasty procedures an individual should perform or an institution should offer on an annual basis in order to provide rather than refer angioplasty procedures.[23] For individual physicians the estimate is 75 PTCA procedures per year as the primary operator, and for institutions the estimate is 200 PTCA procedures annually. Cardiac catheterization and coronary bypass procedures give rise to the same analysis.[24]

Drug-related claims

Errors in prescribing medication account for 6% to 10% of all medical malpractice claims.[25] These figures may suggest that the single semester of pharmacology offered in medical schools is inadequate. Because approximately 75% of the pharmacologic agents available today were not available 15 years ago,[30] the more important factor may be the lack of continuing pharmacologic education offered to physicians, who instead must rely on the information provided by detail men and women whose sole interest is in promoting their employer's products.

Drug-related claims against physicians involve prescribing the wrong drug, the wrong dose, inadequate or excessive duration of drug treatment, failure to prescribe an indicated drug, failure to advise of and monitor for side effects, failure to consider drug allergies, interactions with other drugs being taken, teratogenic effects in pregnant women, and causing or allowing patient addiction. Physicians not only must be knowledgeable about the toxic potential of each drug they prescribe but also must know about the cumulative and synergistic effects of the various combinations of medications their patients may be receiving. In teaching hospitals the average patient is estimated to receive more than six medications either simultaneously or consecutively.[25] Patients receiving six drugs are 64 times more likely to experience the effects of drug interactions than patients receiving only two drugs.[25]

Physicians must not only be familiar with the drugs they are prescribing, the recommended dosages and durations of therapy, and the other drugs being taken by the patient and their interactions with the new drug being prescribed, but they must also advise the patient of and perform adequate monitoring for side effects, including signs of patient addiction. In addition, prescriptions and medication orders must be legible, complete, and unambiguous, leaving no room for misinterpretation by pharmacists filling prescriptions and nurses taking off medication orders. Finally, any instructions to the patient concerning administration, monitoring, and refilling the prescribed medication should be documented.

A drug-related claim that has become more frequent in the last few years relates to failure to administer thrombolytic therapy to an AMI patient. For patients who meet the usual eligibility criteria (see Chapter 18) and who do not have any contraindications, some form of reperfusion therapy (thrombolysis, direct PTCA) is now clearly the standard of care. As discussed in other sections of this book, direct PTCA is a viable alternative to thrombolytic therapy at experienced centers but is not an option at many sites. Thus, most often the clinician's decision about reperfusion therapy centers around whether to give a thrombolytic agent. If a decision is made not to administer such therapy, the reasons for this should be clearly documented in the patient's medical record. It is quite useful in this regard for hospitals to have a thrombolytic therapy checklist and drug administration protocol. This allows the doctor to state that "at my hospital, we do not give thrombolytic therapy in the situation where..." rather than having to state "I thought the risks of therapy were too high..." or "I didn't think thrombolytics were helpful in this type of patient." Such protocols must be revised periodically to keep up with new knowledge and developing consensus in the field.

Although we are not currently aware of any cases, it is possible that an enterprising plaintiff lawyer might allege that an MI patient with a bad outcome should have received a different thrombolytic regimen than was actually given (e.g., t-PA vs. SK). However, the distinctions among different regimens are still a matter of ongoing scientific debate and should not be viewed as standard-of-care issues.

Abandonment

Claims of patient abandonment can arise when a physician unilaterally and unjustifiably terminates the doctor-patient relationship, refuses to continue treating a patient, withdraws from the care of a patient without the consent or knowledge of the patient, or fails to come to the hospital to treat a patient. In addition, failure to provide competent coverage during periods of physician unavailability also constitutes abandonment. In contrast to most other issues of medical negligence, the question of abandonment may be decided by a lay jury without the necessity of expert testimony.

For example, if a physician admits a patient to the hospital, then goes on vacation and fails to arrange competent coverage, a lay jury would be permitted to decide whether the defendant physician had abandoned the patient. By contrast a physician may cease medical treatment based upon a decision that medical treatment is no longer required. Whether the physician is liable for abandonment will depend upon whether the decision that treatment was no longer necessary was correct or incorrect, a question for which expert testimony is required. Issues of abandonment can arise in the context of *consults* and *referrals*, two words that are erroneously used interchangeably. A physician who refers a patient to another physician should document that the patient will be managed by that physician. By contrast, a consultant should make sure the record clearly limits his or her role in the management of another physician's patient. In either situation, clear communications between the physicians are essential and should be confirmed in writing.

IDENTIFICATION OF POTENTIAL MALPRACTICE PLAINTIFFS

One of the most contentious debates in the area of medical malpractice centers around whether there are too many suits or too few. Advocates of the former position cite the many frivolous lawsuits that are filed each year and the sense that many plaintiffs (and their attorneys) view bad medical outcomes as a potential financial bonanza. Those supporting the latter position bring up statistics from the Harvard Medical Practice Study and other sources showing that up to 1% of hospitalizations result in adverse events caused by medical provider negligence and the vast majority of such cases do not result in malpractice suits.[26,27] A recent study from the University of Oklahoma prospectively examined all calls to six plaintiff attorneys' offices with claims relating to medical negligence during a 10-day period.[28] An average of 12 such calls were

received by each office. Of the factors motivating the call, among the most prevalent were poor relationship with the physicians and/or nurses before the injury (53%), television advertising by the law firm (73%), explicit recommendations by another health care provider to seek legal counsel (27%), and advice from a family member or friend (14%). Eighteen percent of callers had previously filed a lawsuit of some kind. The five physician specialties most often named by these callers were obstetrics, family practice, orthopedic surgery, emergency medicine, and general surgery. The acts of negligence most frequently claimed were failure to diagnose (25%) and failure to perform a procedure properly (23%). Economic issues were important to many callers. A significant percentage had medical bills that exceeded 50% of their annual income. In addition, the unemployment rate for these potential plaintiffs was over three times that of the general population in the area.

Only 1 call in 30 led to the filing of a lawsuit. Small recoverable damages and an expired statute of limitations were the two most common reasons attorneys gave for declining to pursue a case. Medical records and expert reviews were obtained in about 15% of cases; of these, over 40% were subsequently judged to have insufficient damages and in one quarter there was no negligence found on the part of the provider.

Thus this study shows that the stereotypic litigious patient is not the major source of malpractice actions. Poor rapport is clearly a risk factor, but good rapport does not guarantee a career free from suits. Perceived lack of adequate information provided and perceived low availability of the practitioner were other major complaints cited by potential plaintiffs.

NATIONAL PRACTITIONERS' DATA BANK

Created by the Health Care Quality Improvement Act of 1986 to improve the ability of the health care profession to police itself, the National Practitioners' Data Bank (NPDB) began on September 1, 1990 to collect data on adverse actions against, and malpractice payments made on behalf of, individual physicians.[29] Medical malpractice insurers, state medical and dental boards, and professional societies involved in peer review are required to report to the NPDB the following four categories of actions taking place on or after September 1, 1990: (1) medical malpractice indemnity payments; (2) adverse licensure actions taken by state medical and dental boards; (3) adverse actions taken on clinical privileges; and (4) adverse actions taken on membership in professional societies. These data are subsequently made available to entities authorized by the Act to receive a report.

Medical malpractice indemnity payments made by any insurer or entity on behalf of an individual practitioner must be reported to the NPDB regardless of amount; that is, nuisance value settlements are not excluded from reporting requirements. When a report is made to the NPDB, state licensing and disciplinary boards also receive a copy of the report, and many undertake a separate investigation. Having settled or concluded the trial of a malpractice case, a physician may subsequently find himself or herself being called before the state licensing or disciplinary board to answer questions about the case.

The reporting form on which information about malpractice indemnity payments is submitted to the NPDB requests a "brief description of the acts or omissions and injuries or illnesses on which the action or claim was based." The form is not designed to reflect denials of liability, or to summarize the defenses to the claims that were made. There is a procedure for dispute resolution whereby the subject practitioner can request a modification of the report. The process is cumbersome, but ultimately either the report will be modified or the physician will be permitted to include a brief statement concerning the dispute in the file so that all entities that receive the report will also receive the dissenting statement.

CONCLUSION

For the foreseeable future, medical malpractice litigation is likely to continue with little or no meaningful reforms. As jury awards and settlement amounts continue to increase and state appellate courts continue to expand theories of physician liability and damages, health care providers must protect themselves by becoming informed about the grounds for malpractice liability and the ways to avoid it. This chapter is not intended to serve as and should not be construed as legal advice; it is designed to provide a general understanding of medical malpractice law. Answers to particular questions depend upon applicable state law.

REFERENCES

1. *Totten v Adongay,* 337 SE 2d, W Va., 1985.
2. *Mozingo v Pitt Co Memorial Hospital,* 331 NC 182, 1992; *McNeil v Bradley, Guilford County Superior Court,* 91 CVS 5594; *Schendel v Hennepin County Medical Center,* 484 NW2d 803, Minn. App. 1992; *Daly v United States,* 946 F2d 1467, 1991.
3. *Gouse v Cassel,* 1 MD 1990, Pa. Sup. Ct., Oct. 8, 1992.
4. *Johnson v Ruark Obstetrics,* 395 SE2d 85, NC, 1991.
5. Havrilesky T: *Valuing life in the courts: an overview, J Foren Econ* 3:71-74, 1990.
6. *Faya v. Almarez,* 620 A 2d 327, Md, 1993; *Carroll v Sisters of St Francis Health Services, Inc,* No 9110-CV-00121, Oct 12, 1992.
7. Kuehm SL, Abraham E: Medical malpractice claims in cardiology, *NJ Med* 87:393-398, 1990.
8. Shrager DS: Strategy for negligent diagnosis cases, *Trial* May: 20-25, 1991.
9. *Schloendorff v. The Society of NY Hospital,* 105 NE 92, NY 1914.
10. Cassileth BR, Zupkis RV, Suton-Smith K, et al: Informed consent—why are its goals imperfectly realized? *N Engl J Med* 302:896-900, 1980.
11. Nyman DJ, Sprung CL: Ensuring informed consent: essentials and specific exceptions, *J Crit Illness* 6:891-906, 1991.
12. *Goodreau v State,* 514 NYS2d 291, 1985.
13. NC Gen Stat 90-321, Cum Supp, 1991.
14. President's Commission for the Study of Ethical Problems in Medicine and Biomedical and Behavioral Research: Making health care decisions: the ethical and legal implications of informed consent in the patient-practitioner relationship, vol. 2, Washington, DC, 1982, US Government Printing Office, pp. 17-410.
15. *Clark,* 510 A2d 136, 1986.
16. Brock DW, Wartman SA: When competent patients make irrational choices, *N Engl J Med* 322:1595-1599, 1990.
17. NC Gen Stat 90-321, Cum Supp, 1991.
18. Curran WJ: Medical malpractice claims since the crisis of 1975: some good news and some bad, *New Engl J Med* 309:1107, 1983.
19. Prosser RL: Alteration of medical records submitted for medicolegal review, *JAMA* 267:2630-2631, 1992.
20. *Taylor v Security Industrial Insurance Co,* 454 So2d 1260, 1984.
21. *Jones v City of New York,* 395 NYS2d 429, 1977.
22. *Sochard v St Vincent's Medical Center,* 510 A2d 1367, 1986.
23. ACP/ACC/AHA Task Force on Clinical Privileges in Cardiology: Clinical competence in percutaneous transluminal coronary angioplasty, *J Am Coll Cardiol* 15:1469-1474, 1990.
24. American College of Cardiology/American Heart Association Ad Hoc Task Force on Cardiac Catheterization: ACC/AHA guidelines for cardiac catheterization and cardiac catheterization laboratories, *J Am Coll Cardiol* 18:1149-1182, 1991.
25. Medication-related claims on the rise, *Malpractice Digest* Fall 1985.
26. Brennan TA, Leape LL, Laird NM, et al: Incidence of adverse events and negligence in hospitalized patients. Results of the Harvard Medical Practice Study I. *N Engl J Med* 324(6):370-376, 1991.
27. Brennan TA, Localio AR, Leape LL, et al: Identification of adverse events occurring during hospitalization. A cross-sectional study of litigation, quality assurance, and medical records at two teaching hospitals, *Ann Intern Med* 112(3):221-226, 1990.
28. Huycke LI, Huycke MM: Characteristics of potential plaintiffs in malpractice litigation, *Ann Intern Med* 120:792-798, 1994.
29. Robb J: National Practitioner Data Bank, *NY State J Med* 92:12-13, 1992.

Chapter 71

HEALTH POLICY IMPLICATIONS OF THROMBOLYTIC THERAPY FOR ACUTE MYOCARDIAL INFARCTION

C. David Naylor

When medical historians appraise this century's advances in the treatment of acute ischemic syndromes, few will rank alongside intravenous thrombolysis and related strategies for coronary reperfusion during and after AMI. This closing chapter reviews some health policy implications of the reperfusion revolution, focusing on three interrelated points: (1) the diffusion and utilization of thrombolytic therapy; (2) the resource implications of reperfusion therapy, particularly in reference to use of revascularization procedures; and (3) the cost-effectiveness of thrombolytic therapy.

ADOPTION AND UTILIZATION OF THROMBOLYTIC AGENTS
Clinical efficiency

The effectiveness of therapies is commonly summarized as the percent reduction in relative risk of death during some defined follow-up period. Pooled trial data[1] show that thrombolysis for younger patients reduces MI mortality from 9.4% in controls to 7.3% among treated subjects—a 22% relative risk reduction (0.094-0.073/ 0.094). A more salient number is the absolute risk difference, which is 2.1%, or its reciprocal −48 (derived from 1/0.021), which indicates the number of persons who must be treated to prevent one death.[2,3] Such

measures relate clinical efforts to therapeutic yields in a way that is relevant for physicians and patients alike.[4]

In thrombolysis trials the focus on relative risk reductions has probably generated some confusion about the merits of therapy for high-risk groups. For example, pooled data from elderly trial subjects show mortality rates of 22.1% among controls and 17.9% in treated patients. This 4.2% absolute difference is about twice as great among elderly as opposed to nonelderly subjects,[1] but the corresponding relative risk reduction is only 19% (derived from 0.221-0.179/0.221), which is actually lower than that seen in younger persons. Use of relative risk reductions therefore fails to convey the excellent clinical efficiency inherent in treating patients with high baseline mortality rates. These statistical framing or data format effects, along with exclusion criteria in many early trials, may have contributed to the underuse of thrombolysis in high-risk patients such as the elderly.

The same arithmetic considerations dictate that treatment effects with thrombolysis will seem to diminish over time if relative summary measures are used because the baseline mortality rate is necessarily rising.[5] However, the absolute difference in mortality between treatment and controls at the end of one or more years is generally similar to that seen in the first few weeks of follow-up.[5]

Development and diffusion

Earlier chapters have documented the historical development of clot-lysing therapy for AMI. Clearly no therapy in medical history has been subject to such exhaustive investigation, with over 100,000 patients randomized in placebo-controlled and drug-drug comparative trials. Enormous trials, starting with GISSI-1 (1986),[6,7] unequivocally established the safety and effectiveness of intravenous thrombolysis as compared with conventional therapy. ISIS-2 (1988),[8] with an elegant factorial design, showed that aspirin had a synergistic effect when added to streptokinase.[9,10] Such simple but powerful "tombstone trials," with mortality as their endpoint, were inherently more persuasive than trials using proxy measures such as left ventricular function or angiographic reperfusion of the infarct-related artery. They had the additional advantage of involving scores of smaller hospitals. By taking therapy out of highly specialized centers with aggressive interventional strategies, they proved that intravenous thrombolysis was feasible in a variety of community hospital settings. Indeed, the trials provided a "technological inoculation": large numbers of community practitioners learned to use these drugs because so many centers participated.

A concurrent boost to the profile of thrombolytic therapy came with the media coverage of t-PA. As one of the first products of recombinant DNA technology to be used in human medicine, the drug enjoyed enormous publicity and was cleverly promoted by its manufacturers. Its demonstrably superior clot-lysing performance[11,12] and excellent side-effect profile led to strong endorsements from the American cardiology establishment, which helped catalyze the rapid diffusion of thrombolytic therapy in the U.S.A.

A survey of a sample of 1065 American practitioners in early 1987 offers insight into this diffusion pattern.[13] Whereas in 1980 only 2% of respondents used these drugs for MI, the number rose to 50% by 1985 and 66% by 1987. However, 58% of respondents gave thrombolytic drugs to one quarter or less of their patients. Factors independently affecting acceptance of thrombolytic therapy were medical specialty, number of patients with MI treated in the preceding year, physician age, and availability of a cardiac catheterization laboratory in the hospital.[13]

In contrast to the stratified random sample used in the American survey, a British survey[14] attempted to capture all consultants in the United Kingdom and Northern Ireland who might be involved in treatment of AMI. Response rates in 1987 and again in 1989 exceeded 75%. Changes were dramatic, in that routine use of thrombolytics rose from 2% in 1987 to 68% in 1989, with 96%

administering these drugs "sometimes." Antiplatelet therapy was routinely given by 9% and 84% of respondents in 1987 and 1989 respectively—a remarkable change catalyzed by ISIS-2.[14,8] The experience of ISIS-2 and reported overviews of patient experience from 7 to 12[15] hours after symptom onset also altered views of the appropriate time frame from symptom onset within which the agents remained effective. Only 18% of consultants were willing to use these drugs more than 6 hours from symptoms onset in 1987, but by 1989 the figure had risen to 46%, with a minority using the drugs out to 24 hours from symptom onset.[14]

All such surveys must be interpreted with caution, however, because they represent self-reported practices. Research in other fields of practice has shown that self-reported compliance with changing standards of practice may not be reflected in actual practice.[16] The question therefore arises: is thrombolytic therapy underused? If so, are some groups denied therapy more often than others?

Age bias in drug utilization

In their survey Collins and Julian[14] found that the age of the patient was a factor in use of thrombolysis for 69% of British consultants in 1987 and 54% in 1989. Many of those influenced by age indicated arbitrary thresholds (e.g. refusing to treat patients over age 70 or 75). Similarly, Hlatky et al.[13] found that most of their physician respondents viewed age as very (40%) or somewhat (45%) important in any decision about use of a thrombolytic drug. As reviewed by Gurwitz et al.,[17] reluctance to treat the elderly is partly explicable by clinical features of their presentation and the increased risks of reperfusion therapy in this age group. For example, in GISSI-2[18] and the companion International streptokinase/t-PA Mortality Trial, of 38,086 patients admitted to CCUs, 25,596 or 67.2% were excluded.[19] However, the exclusion rates were 80% vs. 61% for those over and under 70 years of age respectively. The higher rate of exclusion among the elderly reflected more late arrivals, more atypical presentations (e.g. unconvincing symptoms and/or equivocal ECGs), and more contraindications to therapy. Also, once thrombolysis is given, the elderly have a higher rate of bleeding complications, including hemorrhagic stroke.[17] They are similarly subject to more complications with coronary arteriography, coronary bypass surgery, and PTCA.[17]

Nonetheless, any element of age bias is worrisome because of the high in-hospital case fatality rate for first AMI among the very elderly. Recent data from the Worcester Heart Attack Study[20] show the case fatality rate to be 5% among those less than 55 years of age and 32% in those over 75. There was a 94% 1-year survival among survivors to discharge under age 55, but only a 77% 1-year survival for those 75 years of age and older.[20]

Table 71-1. Proportion of patients (%) treated by various means in each of the age strata

	Age (years)			
	< 55	55-64	65-74	≥ 75
Thrombolytic Rx	39	29	22	5
Angiogram in-hospital	76	65	54	22
PTCA	29	25	19	7
CABG	11	12	14	5
Aspirin	82	76	72	57
Heparin	78	69	61	35
Beta blocker	25	26	19	11

All *P*-values are for Chi-square tests on 3 df: uniformly < 0.0001 (From Weaver WD, Litwin PE, Martin JS, et al: Effect of age on use of thrombolytic therapy and mortality in acute myocardial infarction, *J Am Coll Cardiol* 18:657-662, 1991.)

Thus, although physicians may be chagrined by treatment-induced side effects in the elderly, the risk-to-benefit ratio will almost always be favorable.

Unfortunately, age biases may be formalized in treatment protocols. Burrell et al.[21] surveyed English districts and found that of 55 districts with established policies or draft guidelines for thrombolysis, 25 districts stated an upper age limit; the limits ranged from 65 to 80 years of age. Moreover, practice data corroborate that younger persons are more likely to receive thrombolytic drugs. In data from the SAVE trial, multivariate analysis showed age to be a strong independent predictor of nonuse of thrombolytic drugs.[22] The Myocardial Infarction, Triage and Intervention [MITI] project in Metropolitan Seattle logged 3256 consecutive patients hospitalized in 19 hospitals during 1989 with AMI.[23] The majority of the patients with presumed MI were elderly: 28% were 65 to 74 years of age, and another 28% were aged 75 or over. About 39% of persons under 55 years of age received thrombolysis, with an in-hospital case fatality rate of 2%. Among persons over 75 years of age, only 5% received thrombolytic drugs, and the in-hospital case fatality rate was 17.8%. Weaver et al.[23] attribute the low use of these drugs to comorbidity, a greater prevalence of nondiagnostic ECG abnormalities, higher frequency of silent infarction or atypical symptoms, and "physicians' concerns about the benefit/risk ratio in this group." Remarkably, MITI data show that even aspirin was used significantly less often in persons over age 75 (see Table 71-1).

Similar results have been seen in utilization studies from a variety of jurisdictions. In a Canadian teaching hospital, Montague et al.[24] reviewed 402 consecutive patients seen between July 1, 1988 and June 30, 1989. They found that thrombolytic drugs, invasive and noninvasive tests, beta blockers, and aspirin were all used less frequently in the elderly subgroup of patients. In Israel[25]

a multicenter registry study of 413 consecutive patients presenting in early 1990 showed that patients were significantly less likely to receive thrombolytic drugs if they were over 75 years old.

Improvements in these treatment patterns are readily achievable. A before-after study from a coronary care unit in Plymouth, England[26] found that only 12% of patients over age 65 received thrombolysis in the baseline period. Forty-six percent received drugs in the second period after a simple intervention involving feedback of the low utilization rate to physicians and instructions that nurses should question house officers in the event of failure to use lytic agents in any elderly patient. The usual trade-offs between specificity and sensitivity were evident, in that all treated patients had confirmed MI in the baseline period, whereas 16% did not in the second. Although mortality did not differ significantly in the two periods, there was a positive trend (26.4% vs. 19.2%).[26]

Other factors leading to reduced usage or effectiveness

Other factors adversely affecting utilization are reviewed elsewhere in this volume. They include excessively stringent exclusion criteria based on fears of hemorrhagic complications. Many earlier contraindications carry much less weight today, including recent CPR, remote or questionable upper gastrointestinal bleeds, and remote cerebrovascular events. However, no reports document whether practice patterns have shifted in response to this gradual relaxation of eligibility criteria. Also, evidence from Israel[25] and the United States[22] suggests that drugs are given more often to patients with first MIs and less often to those with recurrent MIs. Although ECG interpretation may be a factor, the reluctance to treat recurrent MIs is difficult to explain and may represent an unfortunate byproduct of a misleading subgroup analysis in GISSI-1.[6,7] (For example, in ISIS-2[8] there was a strongly significant treatment effect for patients with previous MI, as would indeed be expected because such persons have more limited ventricular reserve.)

One key issue is the continuing controversy about the effectiveness of lytic agents when given 6 to 12 hours after symptom onset. The survey by Collins and Julian[14] clearly documents the shift in self-reported practice patterns that occurred in the United Kingdom after the ISIS-2 report.[8] In the absence of recent and comparable survey data from North America, practitioners' views on eligibility periods are uncertain. Anecdotally there appears to be continuing reticence about late treatment unless the patient has ongoing pain or a stuttering onset. This uncertainty has been reinforced by the lack of statistical benefit in EMERAS, a major South American study of late treatment with streptokinase.[27] The preliminary results of LATE, a recently completed mortality trial examining t-PA vs. placebo more than 6 hours from symptom onset, show unequivocal benefit for patients treated within 6 to 12 hours from symptom onset. Specifically, 35-day mortality was reduced by 27% (95% confidence interval: 8%-46%). The final publication of the LATE results should resolve this issue, especially when those data are combined with results of previous studies.

Regardless of the chosen time window of therapy, any needless delay between the patient's symptom onset and initiation of therapy should be avoided. Patients themselves are vital here; some still present several hours from onset of pain, and there is little evidence that public education campaigns shift the time of presentation.[28-31] On the other hand, one reason for the lack of an incremental effect of specific public education campaigns may be a secular trend for patients to present earlier after symptom onset—a phenomenon that led to unexpectedly slow recruitment in the LATE trial mentioned above. In any case, it is particularly important that the medical care system not exacerbate the problem of patient-related delays.

A logical way to minimize delay is prehospital therapy, (e.g., paramedic administration of thrombolysis at home or in the ambulance). Early studies of prehospital therapy suggested that it was safe and feasible and saved time in initiating therapy but did not clearly lead to better patient outcomes.[32-36] The trials were small, and questions of statistical power led to larger trials (see Chapter 20). In both the MITI trial and the EMIP trial, prehospital treatment saved about an hour.[37,38] However, preliminary analyses of both trials have shown no difference in clinical outcomes with prehospital therapy—a finding probably attributable to very rapid treatment in the emergency room and also possibly related to any broad trends for patients to seek attention earlier after symptom onset. In consequence, prehospital initiation will probably see limited use and attention will focus on the many reversible factors[39,40] that delay the use of thrombolysis in the emergency room. Not the least of these is the need for a paradigm shift on the part of all staff, so that an AMI is understood as being myocardium that is acutely infarcting. One obvious starting point is for every emergency room to log the time from entry to initiation of thrombolysis for its AMI patients and then seek to identify and address the points at which time is lost.

Finally, adjuvant therapies of all kinds have been given rather superficial consideration in utilization studies. The evidence is very strong in support of concurrent and continued use of aspirin, along with early and continued treatment with beta blockers for most patients and ACE inhibitors for all who have impaired left ventricular function. There are limited data showing that these drugs are underused,[23-24] whereas calcium-channel antagonists continue to enjoy a popularity post-MI out of all proportion to the trial evidence that has accumulated for them.[41]

Magnitude of the problem

It should be emphasized that the uptake of thrombolytic therapy has been very rapid by the usual standards of medical history, and there is continued diffusion. For example, the SAVE trial found that the proportion of MI patients receiving thrombolytic drugs in 112 American and Canadian coronary care units rose from 26.5% during 1987 to 39.9% during 1989.[22]

On the other hand, the continuing underuse of thrombolytic drugs is illustrated by an informal survey of English health districts[21] carried out in January 1989. The authors concluded that up to 20,000 eligible patients in England were not receiving thrombolytic therapy in any given year. Utilization rates of streptokinase based on drug expenditures indicated that the treatment rates were not higher in districts with guidelines, or even in those where there were teaching hospitals or local cardiologists.[21]

A similar large-scale analysis by Muller and Topol[42] estimated that there were 675,000 patients hospitalized annually in the United States with AMI. At least 33% should be eligible for thrombolytic therapy (i.e., about 225,000 persons). Yet, based on manufacturers' sales figures, only 124,000 (17%) were treated.[42] This estimate is corroborated exactly by a national survey of 164 hospital pharmacies carried out in late 1988.[43]

In sum, there is a clear role for quality management techniques aimed at improving the process and outcomes of care so as to ensure that thrombolytic therapy and appropriate adjuvant and postlysis interventions are used rapidly in the widest possible range of eligible patients. These quality improvement techniques must themselves be assessed rigorously. As we move from establishment of efficacy to assurance of effectiveness, the most important trials may well test methods to optimize utilization of proven therapies, rather than continuing to focus on minor refinements of the therapies themselves.

Gender bias in treating AMI

From 1987 to 1988 in the Seattle-Tacoma metropolitan area Maynard et al.[44] found that eligible women were less likely to receive thrombolysis. However, age and gender are confounded because women are more likely to be older with first and subsequent infarcts. Other analyses have not shown gender bias in the use of thrombolytic therapy once age was taken into account.[22,24,45] Nonetheless, several groups report that practitioners are less willing to perform invasive procedures in women with CHD,[46-50] and this phenomenon has been demonstrated on MI admissions specifically. Ayanian and Epstein[50] used administrative datasets with information on over 80,000 admissions for coronary heart disease to hospitals in Massachusetts and Maryland and found that men were significantly more likely to undergo either coronary angiography or revascularization. The difference persisted after controlling for principal diagnosis, age, congestive heart failure or diabetes mellitus, race, and insurance status. It was replicated in a subset analysis limited to persons hospitalized with MI. Results from the SAVE study[48] showed that men and women had similar rates of procedures during the index hospitalization for MI. In post-MI care, however, about twice as many men as women underwent coronary angiography (503/1842 or 27.3% vs. 60/389 or 15.4%) or CABG (234/1842 or 12.7% vs. 23/389 or 5.9%). Gender was an independent predictor of the likelihood of intervention.[48] Krumholz et al. studied patients hospitalized with definite AMI at Boston's Beth Israel Hospital between 1984 and 1990.[47] There were 1350 men and 1123 women. Although women apparently underwent coronary angiography less often on the index admission (22% vs. 34%), the difference was abolished by controlling for age. PTCA rates were similar between sexes, but bypass surgery rates were higher in men. This was of borderline significance after controlling simultaneously for age and anatomic severity of coronary disease.[47] One Canadian study has analyzed gender bias in procedure use after MI, drawing on linked administrative data to review 4462 men and 2487 women discharged during fiscal 1990 in Ontario. In-hospital mortality was 14.5% among men and 23.5% among women, a difference that remained significant after controlling for age and comorbidity. Over a follow-up ranging from 6 to 12 months, 18.4% of men vs. 9.9% of women underwent angiography. Angioplasty and/or CABG were performed in 12.1% of men and 6.4% of women. Procedure rates were far lower than seen in the United States, but gender differences remained significant after adjustment for age, comorbidity, and mortality.[51]

What has remained uncertain is whether the bias is towards too little intervention in women, too much in men, or both. There is evidence that women have higher rates of complications and less benefit from CABG and perhaps PTCA as well, but these factors must be weighed against the unequivocally higher mortality of females after MI. If procedures are underused in women, errors would have to be rooted in clinical misperceptions of risk-to-benefit ratios of procedures around the time of MI or in less benign influences such as overt sexism.

RESOURCE IMPLICATIONS OF REPERFUSION THERAPY: USE OF INVASIVE PROCEDURES
Rate variations: general observations

International and interregional variations in rates of cardiovascular procedure utilization are striking.[52] For example, throughout the early 1980s the American

CABG rate remained about twice the Canadian national rate. In 1989 to 1990 the California bypass rate was 112.5 per 100,000 adults, whereas Ontario had a rate of 66.2 per 100,000 adults; (i.e., little had changed). Despite the lower rate of utilization and strict regionalization[53] of CABG services under national health insurance in Canada, there are moderate regional and municipal variations in CABG use.[54,55] Taking the entire population rather than adults alone, CABG rates in major census metropolitan areas from 1986 to 1987 ranged from 19.5 to 46.9 per 100,000.[54] In 1989 provincial rates varied from a low of 27.2 in Alberta to a high of 49.3 in Quebec.[56] The Canadian PTCA rate tripled between 1986 and 1989, but like CABG it remains less than half the American rate.

Researchers with the Rand Corporation have used delphi processes with scenario ratings to develop criteria for the appropriate use of CABG.[57] Application of these criteria to a sample of 386 patients undergoing CABG at three hospitals in a western American state in 1979, 1980, and 1982 showed that only 14% of procedures were deemed inappropriate. Appropriate indications were present in 56%, but 30% of CABG were for uncertain indications.[58] A parallel panel process was run in the Trent region of the United Kingdom.[59] As expected, British clinicians were more conservative. When applied to the same group of 386 American patients, British criteria suggested that 35% of cases were inappropriate (vs. 14% with American ratings).[59] A second British panel was run to update the criteria for application in the Trent region.[60] An audit of 319 patients' charts from 1987 to 1988 showed 58% of cases to be appropriate, 26% equivocal, and 16% inappropriate. These results are of particular interest because the rate of CABG in the Trent region was low by even British standards (11 per 100,000 in 1985).[60] These findings underscore the fact that low CABG rates do not necessarily mean more appropriate utilization. Previous analyses for other medical and surgical procedures have similarly failed to show a consistent or strong relationship between the proportion of appropriate procedures and the rate of use.[61-63]

Rate variations in reperfusion therapy of AMI

No published data directly address the extent of variation in, and appropriateness of, practice patterns for reperfusion therapy. The area is ripe for investigation because of the pace and, above all, the direction of movement. Historically in medicine, invasive procedures are first used in a limited sphere and then indications broaden over time. In contrast the movement in reperfusion therapy of MI has been away from routine use of invasive procedures and towards a more conservative approach. Intravenous administration of thrombolysis-supplanted intracoronary therapy, and as discussed earlier in this text, routine use of angiography and revascularization after intravenous thrombolysis were set aside as unnecessary in the wake of several randomized trials. Fox[5] has recently confirmed that at 1 year, mortality rates for the "conservative strategies" validated by TIMI–II-B, SWIFT, and the six TAMI studies are essentially identical to those seen with aggressive regimens.

Canadian centers never adopted an aggressive approach to mechanical revascularization for MI,[64,65] but many American centers did so. The open-ended multipayer system supported the proliferation of invasive facilities in smaller community hospitals—a policy stringently curbed in Canada's state-administered system.[53,66,67] Thus in the late 1980s there arose an interesting situation wherein fee-for-service invasive cardiologists in scores of American for-profit hospitals confronted strong evidence,[68-76] suggesting that reduced use of angiography, PTCA, and CABG might be appropriate. Examination of the responses to this evidence is overdue.

Analyses of all these practice patterns should be strengthened by the availability of clear guidelines promulgated by various groups concerning the management of the MI patient. One such set of guidelines was recently developed by Canadian and American expert panels. The panels completed a Rand-style group process, rating case scenarios to derive explicit criteria for the appropriate use of coronary angiography and revascularization in general. These indications included responses to various postthrombolysis and post-MI scenarios. A detailed comparison of use between two Canadian provinces and New York state should be available by early 1993. As well as helping to clarify how different countries use revascularization services, such explicit criteria have the advantage of facilitating comparative analyses across smaller regions and could be applied specifically to the post-MI postlysis subpopulation.

Does thrombolysis necessitate an increase in invasive procedures?

Many conservative practitioners would now recommend perilysis and postlysis coronary angiography only for three situations: hemodynamic deterioration despite treatment, suggesting both failure to reperfuse and an extensive infarct; early postinfarction angina or sudden deterioration suggestive of reocclusion; and unequivocally positive noninvasive tests in the first few days to weeks after use of clot-lysing agents. The first of these indications remains fluid and contentious; whether a randomized trial of "salvage angioplasty" will ever be ethically acceptable is still unclear. Better markers of either failed lysis or early reocclusion (e.g., continuous computerized ST-segment monitoring)[77] could well catalyze a major growth in acute mechanical interventions. However, in general the second and third indica-

tions are not clearly dissimilar to practice patterns in the prethrombolytic era. Thus one question that arises is whether a conservative approach to reperfusion therapy necessarily leads to a short-term increase in invasive procedures beyond that which would have resulted, given already established trends to more aggressive risk stratification following MI.

To address this issue we performed a metaanalysis[78] of seven controlled trials performed in Europe,[79,80] North America,[81,82] and Australia and New Zealand.[83-85] These data allowed a direct randomized comparison of how patients fared with thrombolysis as opposed to conventional care. All trials used a "conservative" approach to mechanical revascularization, with follow-up ranging from 14 to 30 days; six of the seven trials were blinded. We found that streptokinase and t-PA were associated with an 80% increase in mechanical revascularization procedures (95% CI: 33%-144%, $2P = 0.0003$).[78] Although study-related angiography was a potential confounder, the absolute rates of revascularization in the first few weeks postthrombolysis were all lower in these trials than in TIMI–II-B,[68] where 33% of patients in the "conservative" arm underwent angiography in the first 2 weeks after randomization. Assuming then that clot lysis truly shifts practice patterns, the question remains: what is the optimum rate of intervention in a "conservative" approach to this patient population?

Variable procedure use in "conservative" clinical trials

In the conservative arm of the TIMI–II-B study, treatment with t-PA, heparin, and aspirin was followed by cardiac catheterization only in response to symptoms of recurrent ischemia or a positive exercise test before discharge.[68] Both tertiary and community hospitals participated; the latter had access to invasive procedures at a regional hospital. Six-week procedure rates were much higher if the index admission was to a tertiary hospital—for catheterization 48% vs. 32%, for PTCA 18% vs. 11%, and for CABG 12% vs. 8%. Yet outcomes at community hospitals were identical to those in tertiary centers with respect to mortality, reinfarction, recurrence of angina, and various noninvasive markers of residual ischemia and left ventricular function.[71] Geltman has extrapolated that nationwide differences in these two strategies could increase costs "between $550 and $600 million per year."[70]

Note, however, that the total revascularization rate over 6 weeks was almost 20% even in community hospitals. In the trials included in our metaanalysis[78] this was the high end of observed rates in the first few weeks after thrombolysis, with some trials reporting rates as low as 5%. The difference may be a function of when the trials were performed and/or the effectiveness of the clot-dissolving and patency-maintaining regimens used.

Table 71-2. Longer-term data on revascularization after thrombolysis: data from controlled trials

Trial	Follow-up	Treated (%)	Controls (%)	Difference (%)
ASSET[87]	6 mos	2.3	2.8	− 0.5
GISSI-1[7]	6 mos	3.3	3.0	+ 0.3
France[88]	1 yr	9.5	9.5	0.0
ISAM[89]	7 mos	13.3	9.3	+ 4.0
Netherlands[90,91]	1 yr	24.9	17.0	+ 7.9
Western Washington[81]	1 yr	27.2	18.6	+ 8.5
TICO[92]	1 yr	35.1	15.5	+ 19.6

It is also likely to be influenced by three other factors. First, there is continuing uncertainty and interpretive variability as to the patterns of results of noninvasive tests that signal the need for intervention. Second, there are international variations in overall use of PTCA and CABG. One might postulate similar variations in the specific case of postlysis intervention, with lower procedure use outside the United States. A third factor is timing. Because waiting lists for revascularization procedures are the norm in Canada and various European countries,[56,66,48] it could be that procedures tend to be "front-loaded" in the United States. That is, in the USA, they occur on the index admission for MI. If so, one would expect convergence in revascularization rates among countries, as patients are followed postthrombolysis over the course of months or years.

Table 71-2 shows some longer-term data from various controlled trials of thrombolytic therapy, in which an aggressive postlysis strategy was not prespecified. Using the Mantel-Haenszel method,[86] the aggregate relative increase in the odds of revascularization is smaller than was found in the short-term metaanalysis, at about 24% (95% CI: 10%-41%, $2P = 0.001$). This is partly a function of the rising base rate, but absolute differences are also narrower. ASSET[87] and GISSI-1[7] drive this phenomenon, as both were large, were characterized by low procedure rates, and showed minimal differences between placebo and thrombolysis arms. As the ASSET investigators commented,[87] these findings in ASSET and GISSI-1 "may reflect either a relative underprovision of facilities for such treatments in the European countries which took part in these studies, or a genuine lack of need." Aggregating the other five trials leads to a relative increase of 49% (95% CI: 25%-77%, $2P = 0.000007$). However, while the relative differences between thrombolysis and conventional therapy are attenuated, the international and interstudy variations in rates of revascularization are enormous.

Thus, many questions persist about the use of mechanical revascularization in conjunction with lytic therapy for AMI. Some increase relative to conventional therapy seems inevitable and appropriate, but we do not know how much mechanical revascularization is really

necessary to consolidate or extend the initial gains achieved with intravenous thrombolysis. Similarly, the choice of procedure itself is moot, with limited evidence suggesting that CABG may be superior to PTCA in improving left ventricular function following thrombolysis.[93] Albeit fraught with confounders, international outcomes research using observational databases may be the only way to clarify the extent to which differing rates and modes of postlysis intervention alter long-term morbidity and mortality.

COSTS AND COST-EFFECTIVENESS OF THROMBOLYTIC THERAPIES
t-PA vs. streptokinase: Canada vs. the United States

The choice of agents for thrombolysis has been colored by differing side-effect profiles, convenience of administration, and above all by early emphasis on proxy measures such as recanalization rather than by harder endpoints such as left ventricular function or, better yet, mortality. Indeed the ultimate endpoint for policymakers and patients alike must surely be some composite of all-cause mortality and overall morbidity or functional status.

In Canada, insistence on the latter type of evidence was primarily responsible for what evolved into a national movement away from routine use of t-PA. t-PA received American Food and Drug Administration approval in November 1987, and Canadian federal approval came the same week. By early 1988 Genentech Canada reported steady sales of the new drug. However, in Ontario, the largest of Canada's 10 provinces, leaders of organized medicine were struck by t-PA's price— C$2900 per 100 mg dose. This cost meant that special per-case funding might be needed to supplement the prospective annual budgets for acute care hospitals using t-PA. An expert panel was therefore convened. The panel's guidelines not only rejected the trend toward aggressive investigation and revascularization of patients receiving thrombolytics[64] but also offered cautionary advice about the choice of drug:

As yet no definitive evidence has been marshalled to prove the superior efficacy of t-PA or streptokinase in terms of

Table 71-3. Thrombolytic preferences of a sample of Ontario internists and cardiologists in November 1988

Question: Which agent would you prefer to receive if you suffered an AMI and were an appropriate candidate for thrombolytic treatment with either streptokinase or t-PA?

	Any respondent (N = 388)	Respondents using thrombolytics in previous 12 months (N = 268)
Strongly prefer t-PA	38.3	45.4
Mildly prefer t-PA	22.8	23.0
Indifferent	26.9	23.0
Mildly prefer streptokinase	3.6	3.7
Strongly prefer streptokinase	3.4	3.7
No response	5.6	2.2

(From Naylor CD, et al: Coronary thrombolysis, clinical guidelines, and public policy: results of an Ontario practitioner survey, *Can Med Assoc J* 142:1069-1080, 1990.

mortality (short- or long-term) or myocardial preservation . . . Both thrombolytic agents appear to carry a similar, small risk of producing serious bleeding complications in patients who are not subjected to invasive procedures. t-PA has a shorter half-life and reduced systemic fibrinolytic activity, both of which may be helpful in the event that bleeding develops or urgent intervention is needed. t-PA also appears to be more efficient in initial clot lysis . . . Other side effects, including hypotension and anaphylaxis, are more common with streptokinase. These latter concerns must be weighed against the longer experience with streptokinase, the more complete database on its efficacy (particularly with respect to mortality), and its lower cost. Currently, streptokinase is less than one tenth the price of a comparable dose of t-PA. A verdict on the agent of choice must therefore be deferred pending additional evidence as to comparative efficacy, side effects, and cost effectiveness.[64]

This cautionary view led the provincial government to reject the concept of special funding for t-PA, and severely limited the adoption of t-PA in Ontario hospitals.[94] Intense controversy arose, and specialists and governments in other provinces were openly critical at first. Indeed, a 1988 survey of Ontario cardiologists and internists in about 150 hospitals showed that the majority would themselves prefer to receive t-PA in the event of an MI[94,95] (Table 71-3). Over time, however, all provinces followed Ontario's lead. Thus even before the results of GISSI-2, the International SK/t-PA Mortality Trial, and ISIS-3, streptokinase dominated the Canadian market; about 75% of all cases were treated with SK rather than t-PA—the exact opposite of the American situation. The response to the results of the GUSTO-I trial (Global Utilization of Streptokinase and Tissue plasminogen activator in Occluded coronary arteries) will therefore be fascinating for policy analysts and students of the sociology of medicine and science. GUSTO-I has various objectives, but foremost among them is a comparison of the mortality benefits with conventional intravenous streptokinase accompanied by full-dose intravenous heparin vs. a "front-loaded" regimen of t-PA and an arm using a combination of t-PA and streptokinase. Should t-PA win the race, those who have favoured this drug will be tallying the lives lost in Canada and other jurisdictions where a skeptical approach was taken. Should t-PA lose, the dollars wasted in America are likely to lead to a brief flurry of recrimination against the medical-industrial establishment. In either case, however, the unresolved issue is how much evidence we need to support therapeutic policies with major funding and clinical implications.[95]

Cost-effectiveness of thrombolytic therapy

In tallying the relationship of expenditures and outcomes, the standard paradigm is cost-effectiveness analysis. Various authors have analyzed the cost-effectiveness of reperfusion therapy. In these analyses, as is generally true, the economic impact of any approach stems from the balance of its absolute or incremental costs and absolute or incremental economic benefits relative to previous patterns of practice. Chapter 15 covered the key cost variables in relation to reperfusion therapy. To recapitulate, the primary incremental costs associated with thrombolytic therapy are payments for the drugs themselves and any associated invasive procedure costs over and above those incurred with conventional therapy. Procedure costs will be greatest, obviously, if there is major reliance on direct and salvage angioplasty or if an aggressive strategy of angiography and follow-up CABG or PTCA is pursued. Other incremental costs are either small or, if larger on a per-occurrence basis, greatly reduced on average because they are rarely incurred. Examples respectively are additional tests used routinely to monitor coagulation status (common but inexpensive), and hemorrhagic stroke (very costly but offset economically in part by reduced rates of nonhemorrhagic stroke, and also rare). Potential economic benefits come in several categories, including the reduction in length of stay on the index MI admission because of improved left ventricular function, fewer downstream hospitalizations for congestive heart failure, and, depending on the analytic perspective, some allowance for wages and salaries of individuals who would otherwise be disabled or dead. Once costs and benefits are tallied, the net incremental cost is then compared with the incremental effects in clinical terms, usually expressed as additional survivors or potential life-years gained, with or without some adjustment for expected quality of life.

Laffel et al.[96] have published a cost-effectiveness model for reperfusion therapy that explored subgroups according to time to treatment and other risk factors for in-hospital death. However, the model included assumptions about a continuous and graded relationship between time to treatment from symptom onset and both extent of left ventricular damage and in-hospital mortality. Treatment effects were assumed to disappear by 6 hours from symptom onset. In the absence of a pricing structure, t-PA was priced at $1500 per dose. Although this model is now outdated, its strength was the explicit consideration of time from symptom onset.

Silberberg and McGregor[97] examined cost-effectiveness calculated as the incremental cost per 1-year survivor with various strategies for intravenous streptokinase. They assumed no increase in invasive procedures compared with conventional therapy, an assumption that will underestimate the incremental costs of the reperfusion strategy. Cost-effectiveness ratios were only a few thousand dollars per additional survivor.

Steinberg et al.[98] used trial evidence and a delphi process to generate inputs for a detailed model of the cost-effectiveness ratios for a conservative revascularization strategy after thrombolysis. Major increases in the use of invasive procedures were projected for both streptokinase and t-PA, as compared with placebo. The incremental cost per additional life saved in their model was based on a 1.3% absolute mortality advantage over placebo for streptokinase and a further 0.7% advantage for t-PA. Unfortunately, the model was built using Medicare charges and payments, and neither t-PA (at $2200) nor streptokinase (at $190) was specifically reimbursed under Medicare. Thus, the incremental costs were $52,796 per life saved for streptokinase vs. conventional treatment, $56,900 for t-PA vs. conventional treatment, and only $64,571 for t-PA vs. streptokinase.

Simoons et al.[91] have provided a particularly useful analysis of the cost-effectiveness of thrombolytic therapy, based on 3- to 5-year follow-up data from the Netherlands Inter-University Trial of streptokinase. The generalizability of this model is limited by the fact that all the patients presented less than 4 hours from symptom onset, aspirin was not used, and the intracoronary lysis regimen was atypical. The strength of the model is that survival, hospital days, reinfarction, procedure and medication use, and morbidity were all empirically derived. Long-term survival was projected based on appropriately matched subjects in published life tables. With appropriate discounting of deferred benefits and costs, the cost per year of life gained was only $2690, rising to $2940 after adjustment for quality of life. For anterior MI the cost per year of life gained was $2000, whereas for inferior MI it was $7030. Thus, from a cost-effectiveness standpoint it is hard to defend the continuing bias of some practitioners against treating modest inferior MIs with thrombolytic drugs, unless

there are other relative contraindications that put the patient at increased risk from treatment.

Krumholz et al.[99] recently addressed the specific question of the cost-effectiveness of treating elderly patients. Pooled data from elderly subgroups in large randomized controlled trials were used to generate a baseline estimate that intravenous streptokinase within 6 hours would lead to a relative reduction in mortality of 13%. In keeping with our earlier caveats about relative risk reductions, this figure translates to a substantial absolute risk difference because the baseline case fatality rate for MI among elderly patients is high—29% in the data reviewed by Krumholz et al.[99] The authors used a simulation model to estimate post-MI life expectancy of older persons and factored in the costs of complications of treatment. They estimated the incremental cost per year of life saved for an 80-year-old patient with suspected AMI to be $21,200 in current American dollars and found that over "a wide range of assumptions about risks, benefits, and costs, the cost per year of life saved remained less than $55,000".[99]

Given the fact that the cost of streptokinase is one sixth that of t-PA in Canada (and up to one twentieth in the United States, depending on whether charge or cost data are used), it seems useful to anticipate what cost-effectiveness ratios would be associated with various results of the GUSTO-I trial. Informal projections would suggest a very high cost-effectiveness ratio. For example, with an overall 8% case fatality rate for MI patients given streptokinase and aspirin, and a 7% rate for t-PA, one would have to treat 100 patients to save one life. On the basis of Canadian differences in drug costs, this alone would amount to ($2430 × 100) $243,000 per survivor. However, potential costs per life-year saved are acceptable. For example, even assuming only an extra 5 years of survival for each person "saved" by t-PA, the cost-effectiveness ratio is under $50,000 per life-year gained. Continuing this simple example, another long-term consideration is whether hypothetical benefits accrue not just to the 1 extra survivor out 100 persons treated with t-PA instead of streptokinase but also to the other 99 persons who would have survived with either drug. This situation could occur if t-PA results in superior left ventricular preservation because of greater early reperfusion rates, or if a higher rate of infarct-artery patency leads to better left ventricular healing and/or reduced arrhythmogenesis.

We have recently published a formal economic evaluation of the potential incremental benefits of intravenous t-PA vs. streptokinase for treatment of AMI.[100] The analysis used a third-party payer perspective, with short-term costs and charges in 1988 Canadian dollars. Cost differentials included drug costs (which were then $2900 for t-PA and $300 for streptokinase) and those resulting from an assumed higher rate of

Table 71-4. Incremental cost per life year gained in 1988 Canadian dollars for treatment with t-PA vs. streptokinase for different combinations of the effect of t-PA on short- and long-term mortality

		Annual difference in hazard rate		
		0%	0.1%	0.5%
Absolute	0	∞	$188,400	$37,400
Short-term				
mortality	1%	$58,600	$ 44,600	$22,700
Advantage	2%	$29,300	$ 25,300	$16,300

NOTE: An absolute short-term mortality difference of 1% could occur with any pairing, (e.g., streptokinase mortality of 8% vs. t-PA mortality of 7%, or 12% vs. 11% etc.) An annual difference in hazard rates of 0 presumes no further benefits except the long-term survival of persons saved from death on the index admission by use of t-PA (1 or 2 per 100 here). A hazard difference of 0.1% or 0.5% means that the persons treated with t-PA die at a slightly or moderately reduced rate over ensuing years.
(From Goel V, Naylor CD: Potential cost effectiveness of intravenous tissue plasminogen activator versus streptokinase for acute myocardial infarction, *Can J Cardiol* 8:31-38, 1992.)

Table 71-5. Comparative cost/effectiveness ratios of some interventions to reduce mortality from coronary heart disease in middle-aged males (1988 Canadian dollars)

Intervention	Approximate MCE
Beta blockers post-MI in 55-year-old male at medium risk	$ 5,000
CABG for left mainstem disease	$ 9,000
CABG for three-vessel disease	$ 20,000
Treatment of severe hypertension (diastolic blood pressure ≥ 105 mm)	$ 20,000
Treatment of moderate hypertension (diastolic blood pressure 95-104 mm)	$ 45,000
CABG for two-vessel disease	$120,000
Lifelong cholestyramine, serum cholesterol = 6.85 mmol/L after diet, average risk profile	> $250,000

NOTE: Adapted from references 101 to 103. Exact cost-effectiveness ratios will vary according to methodology of analysis, hence ratios are rounded for ease of comparison. None of these studies made allowance for indirect benefits in the form of wages and salaries.

procedures among patients receiving t-PA. In the latter case we took the position that if t-PA is to attain mortality advantages over streptokinase, there would also be superior arterial patency in association with viable myocardium; hence, the proportion of patients with post-MI angina and positive exercise tests would also be somewhat increased. The target group was nonelderly patients with uncomplicated MI. Impact of treatment-associated morbidity was not considered because of more or less offsetting differences for stroke and major bleeding, (i.e. an additional 3 per 1000 with t-PA and streptokinase respectively in GISSI-2[18] and the International t-PA/Streptokinase Mortality Trial[19]). Costs for the increased reinfarction rate seen among streptokinase patients were explicitly included. Lastly, we modeled potential life-years gained only out to 5 years from treatment, applied a 5% discount rate to these deferred clinical benefits, but assumed that all other clinical benefits were lost thereafter.

Key results are summarized in Table 71-4. If t-PA achieves a 1% short-term mortality advantage over streptokinase, with no other advantages, cost per life year gained was comparable with other cardiovascular interventions (Table 71-5) at $58,600. In the absence of immediate survival advantages, but assuming greater left ventricular preservation, the constant annual hazard rate advantage must be about 0.5% per year for competitive cost-effectiveness ratios. Results were more or less insensitive to changes in any factors apart from the short-term and longer-term mortality rates with t-PA, major changes in cost differential between t-PA

and streptokinase, and, to a small extent, the relative procedural volume ratio for t-PA vs. streptokinase. An update of the model using 1991 costs, including the increased price of streptokinase ($470 vs. $300 in 1988), has yielded very similar results. Nonfatal long-term outcomes, such as quality of life, could also be incorporated into the model as these are obtained in GUSTO-I substudies. It is possible, for example, that functional status may differ between drugs if left ventricular preservation is superior for one. Analyses of this nature can be used to assist policymakers in determining whether or not additional funds should be provided for new thrombolytic treatment strategies or if further investment in investigations on existing agents would be efficient.

A more general conclusion is that as the short-term mortality from AMI is driven lower, immediate benefits from new therapies will be not only more difficult to prove in clinical trials but also more difficult to justify on economic grounds, given the phenomenon of diminishing marginal returns. Data collection in trials must be oriented to both short- and longer-term outcomes and costs, including quality-of-life benefits, if the eventual worth of in-hospital treatments for MI is to be fairly appraised.

Effectiveness research: from trials to practice and treatment to outcomes

The benefits from thrombolytic therapy of AMI appear to be enduring when compared with placebo or conventional care. For example, aggregated anistreplase data[5] show that the 1-year mortality was 10.1% for APSAC vs. 17.8% for placebo, a 7.7% absolute difference. Much longer-term follow-up data from the Netherlands Inter-University Trial of intracoronary streptokinase show 5-year survival to be 81% in treated patients vs. 71% in controls—a remarkable 10% absolute difference.[90] The biggest advantage was seen for patients presenting with anterior MI (81% vs. 64% alive after 5 years).[90] In several large trials most of the gains have occurred in the immediate post-MI period, with parallel tracking of survival curves thereafter (e.g. GISSI-1, ASSET, and ISIS-2). However, follow-up of the Netherlands Inter-University Trial included an intriguing analysis counting only those persons alive at 1 year: their 5-year survivals were 87% and 81% among treated and control patients respectively, suggesting that there are indeed incremental benefits, perhaps related to left ventricular function, that accrue to treated patients well beyond the immediate periinfarct period. Unfortunately, the generalizability of these results is unclear for reasons noted above. No long-term data are available comparing one agent to another with adequate heparinization.

Apart from thrombolysis, further survival advantages would be expected with validated post-MI interventions such as aspirin and beta blockers, with revascularization procedures for various patterns of coronary stenosis, and with angiotensin-converting enzyme inhibitors for patients with impaired left ventricular function. One might therefore reasonably expect to see dramatic declines in the in-hospital MI case fatality rates and longer-term mortality rates from incident cases of MI surviving after hospitalization.

A metaanalysis of all observational studies published between 1960 and 1988 has been undertaken by de Vreede et al.[104] to assess in-hospital mortality from MI. Mean case fatality rates indeed decreased from 29% during the 1960s to 21% during the 1970s and further to 16% during the 1980s. However, there was little evidence for a change in 5-year prognosis during this period. A subsequent report from the Minnesota Heart Survey showed an improvement in 28-day mortality as well as 4-year survival for 1980 vs. 1970, but no further improvements when 1985 was compared with 1980.[105] Here, as in other reports, data are largely confined to the prethrombolytic era. Thrombolysis trial data are limited by severe selection bias because many more patients are excluded than are treated. We urgently need contemporary community-based studies to indicate what has happened since the widespread adoption of reperfusion therapy.

One of the few such studies, the Worcester Heart Attack Study, examined treatment and outcomes of patients with confirmed MI in a network of 16 community and tertiary hospitals.[106] The report showed virtually no change in incidence and outcome of cardiogenic shock. However, the use of thrombolytic therapy did rise

from 9.3% of cases in 1986 to 20.2% in 1988, even though the latter is still much lower than ideal. More important, the in-hospital mortality for all AMI patients was 17.9%—a contrast with the single-digit case fatality rates reported in the treatment or even placebo arms of many modern thrombolysis trials. Not only did the majority of subjects not receive thrombolytic drugs, but also those with most to gain were least likely to receive treatment.[106,107] Clearly more attention needs to be paid to how advances in treatment of acute coronary disease are being translated into practice and what the outcomes are for all our patients, as opposed to the reassuring results in the fortunate minority deemed eligible for reperfusion therapy.[107]

Lastly, some studies have shown that patients have a more favorable outcome in hospitals with higher MI caseloads. This is presumably related to physician and/or hospital experience.[108-111] A recent analysis by Farley and Ozminkowski[112] is particularly helpful, showing that increases in volumes within a hospital lead to better patient outcomes for that institution. On the other hand, one planning epiphenomenon of the advent of thrombolytic therapy is the need to temper enthusiasm for regionalized MI care in high-volume centers, since patients will suffer needless delays in receiving lytic drugs if they wait for transfer to a regional center. Moreover, the TIMI–II-B data quoted above suggest that the high-volume centers may be more aggressive in the use of invasive procedures without any resulting benefits.[70,71]

This type of research—looking beyond the randomized trials and therapeutic efficacy toward real-world effectiveness—is generally known as *effectiveness* or *outcomes research*. Patient Outcomes Research Teams (PORTs) are now working in the United States to examine treatment of AMI and management of the patient with chronic manifestations of ischemic heart disease. There is a logical connection between the types of utilization management research outlined above, with its focus on process of care, and the newer wave of research into patient outcomes. Both will be more prominent in the 1990s, as health service researchers and managers attempt to link evidence from research to practices, and in turn, evidence from practice to an agenda of applied research.

CONCLUSIONS

The reperfusion revolution in the care of patients with MI is still in progress. The small marginal returns of very aggressive intervention with angiography and CABG or PTCA, combined with the feasibility of using thrombolytic drugs in a variety of settings, has made it possible to offer enormous numbers of patients the benefits of this important therapeutic advance. Although data show that practitioners have rapidly accepted thrombolytic therapy, this technology has not diffused optimally. There is incontrovertible evidence that thrombolytic drugs are underused, particularly in the elderly. Yet indices of clinical efficiency, such as the numbers of patients who must be treated to avert one in-hospital death, reveal that it is highly appropriate to treat the elderly and other groups that have high case fatality rates. Assuming that thrombolytic therapy is generally underused among persons at the greatest risk of dying from MI, it is understandable that registry studies show only a modest decline in in-hospital MI case–fatality rates.

There is accordingly a pressing need for research into, and dissemination of, quality improvement methods that will facilitate the most effective use of thrombolytic therapy. Pivotal points include broadening the eligibility criteria to provide treatment to persons of all ages with ST-segment elevation or bundle branch block on the presenting ECG, ignoring spurious contraindications based on unproven bleeding risks, consideration of treatment in the period from 6 to 12 hours from symptom onset, and ensuring expeditious use of these drugs in the emergency department setting.

Metaanalyses of randomized controlled trials confirm that the diffusion of thrombolytic therapy will almost certainly lead to some increased caseloads on catheterization laboratories and revascularization services, even with very conservative approaches to postlysis investigation and intervention. However, rates of procedure utilization vary dramatically in randomized trials, and the optimum intervention strategy has yet to be determined. Minimal procedure use, with trivial increases among thrombolysis-treated patients, has not led to a loss of the initial survival advantages seen with streptokinase or t-PA. But it remains possible that larger advantages, with divergence in survival curves and/or improved quality of life and functional status, might be attainable with more liberal use of revascularization. Randomized trials, as well as observational research comparing patient outcomes across different levels of intervention, should help set effective and efficient benchmarks for revascularization practices in the post-MI context. Utilization analyses of postlysis practice patterns are particularly pertinent in the United States, where aggressive use of PTCA and CABG in MI patients was widely accepted from the mid- through the late 1980s.

Despite the increased use of invasive procedures associated with intravenous thrombolytic therapy and the costs of the drugs themselves, this innovation is highly cost-effective. Cost-effectiveness ratios for intravenous streptokinase typically run only a few thousand dollars per life-year gained—far less than many other cardiovascular interventions that are routinely funded. Although t-PA is also cost-effective relative to conventional therapy, the more appropriate comparison is with streptokinase. The relative effectiveness and hence the cost-effectiveness of t-PA vs. streptokinase is unclear at this time. Based on GISSI-2, the International Streptokinase/t-PA Mortality Trial, and ISIS-3, the cost-effectiveness ratio for t-PA vs. streptokinase is infinite because no clinical advantages have been shown. However, absolute mortality advantages over streptokinase as small as 1% render t-PA reasonably cost-effective in comparison with other routinely funded therapies. Even negligible short-term differences do not preclude the possibility that t-PA will prove cost-effective if there are longer-term advantages that lead to lower mortality rates for t-PA patients.

In Canada the lack of evidence to support the putative superiority of t-PA, along with its cost of $2900 per dose, led to considerable debate about whether special funding should be provided to help hospitals purchase it for routine use. From 1988 onwards no Canadian government has proved willing to offer such special per-case funding for the drug. Thus, in contrast to the United States the overwhelming majority of Canadian patients have received streptokinase. Practitioners across North America and indeed around the world now eagerly await the results of the GUSTO-I trial, which will have important practical and pathophysiologic implications.

REFERENCES

1. Grines CL, DeMaria AN: Optimal utilization of thrombolytic therapy for acute myocardial infarction: concepts and controversies, *J Am Coll Cardiol* 16:223-231, 1990.
2. Laupacis A, Sackett DL, Roberts RS: An assessment of clinically useful measures of the consequences of treatment, *N Engl J Med* 318:1728-1733, 1988.
3. Laupacis A, Naylor CD, Sackett DL: How should results of clinical trials be interpreted? *ACP Journal Club/Ann Int Med* 116(suppl 3):A12-A14, 1992.
4. Naylor CD, Chen E, Strauss B: Measured enthusiasm: does the method of reporting trial results alter perceptions of therapeutic effectiveness? *Ann Intern Med* 117(11):916-921, 1992.
5. Fox KAA: Comparative analysis of long-term mortality after thrombolytic therapy, *Am J Cardiol* 67:38E-44E, 1991.
6. GISSI Collaborative Group: Effectiveness of intravenous thrombolytic treatment in acute myocardial infarction, *Lancet* 1:397-401, 1986.
7. Gruppo Italiano per lo Studio della Streptochinasi nell'Infarto Miocardico: Long-term effects of intravenous thrombolysis in acute myocardial infarction: final report of the GISSI study, *Lancet* 2:871-874, 1987.
8. ISIS-2 (Second International Study of Infarct Survival) Collaborative Group: Randomised trial of intravenous streptokinase, oral aspirin, both, or neither among 17,187 cases of suspected acute myocardial infarction: ISIS-2, *Lancet* 2:349-360, 1988.
9. Basinski A, Naylor CD: Aspirin and fibrinolysis (C), *Lancet* 2:1188-1189, 1988.
10. Basinski A, Naylor CD: Aspirin and fibrinolysis in acute myocardial infarction. Meta-analytic evidence for synergy, *J Clin Epidemiol* 44(10):1085-1096, 1991.
11. The TIMI Study Group: The thrombolysis in myocardial infarction (TIMI) trial. Phase I findings, *N Engl J Med* 312:932-936, 1985.

12. Verstraete M, Bernard R, Bory M, et al: Randomised trial of intravenous recombinant tissue-type plasminogen activator versus intravenous streptokinase in acute myocardial infarction: report from the European Cooperative Study Group for Recombinant Tissue-type Plasminogen Activator, *Lancet* 1:842-847, 1985.

13. Hlatky MA, Cotugno H, O'Connor C, et al: Adoption of thrombolytic therapy in the management of acute myocardial infarction, *Am J Cardiol* 61:510-514, 1988.

14. Collins R, Julian D: British Heart Foundation surveys (1987 and 1989) of United Kingdom treatment policies for acute myocardial infarction, *Br Heart J* 66:250-255, 1991.

15. Collins R, Peto R, Sleight P: Significant reduction in mortality with streptokinase given 7-24 hours after pain onset, *Lancet* 2:1187-1188, 1988.

16. Lomas J, Anderson GM, Domnick-Pierre K, et al: Do practice guidelines guide practice? The effect of a consensus statement on the practice of physicians, *N Engl J Med* 321:1306-1311, 1989.

17. Gurwitz JH, Goldberg RJ, Gore JM: Coronary thrombolysis for the elderly? *JAMA* 265:1720-1723, 1991.

18. Gruppo Italiano per lo Studio della Sopravvivenza nell'Infarto Miocardico: GISSI-2: a factorial randomised trial of alteplase versus streptokinase and heparin versus no heparin among 12,490 patients with acute myocardial infarction, *Lancet* 336:65-71, 1990.

19. The International Study Group: In-hospital mortality and clinical course of 20,891 patients with suspected acute myocardial infarction randomised between alteplase and streptokinase with or without heparin, *Lancet* 336:71-75, 1990.

20. Goldberg RJ, Gore JM, Gurwitz JH, et al: The impact of age on the incidence and prognosis of initial acute myocardial infarction: the Worcester Heart Attack Study, *Am Heart J* 117:543-549, 1989.

21. Burrell CJ, Skehan JD, Cowley ML, et al: Districts' use of thrombolytic agents, *Br Med J* 300:237-238, 1990.

22. Pfeffer MA, Moye LA, Braunwald E, et al: Selection bias in the use of thrombolytic therapy in acute myocardial infarction, *JAMA* 266:528-532, 1991.

23. Weaver WD, Litwin PE, Martin JS, et al: Effect of age on use of thrombolytic therapy and mortality in acute myocardial infarction, *J Am Coll Cardiol* 18:657-662, 1991.

24. Montague TJ, Ikuta RM, Wong RY, et al: Comparison of risk and patterns of practice in patients older and younger than 70 years with acute myocardial infarction in a two-year period (1987-1989), *Am J Cardiol* 68:843-847, 1991.

25. Behar S, Abinader E, Caspi A, et al: Frequency of use of thrombolytic therapy in acute myocardial infarction in Israel, *Am J Cardiol* 68:1291-1294, 1991.

26. Hendra TJ, Marshall AJ: Increased prescription of thrombolytic treatment to elderly patients with suspected acute myocardial infarction associated with audit, *Br Med J* 304:439-441, 1992.

27. Paolasso E: Randomized trial of late thrombolysis in Acute Myocardial Infarction: Estudia Multicentrico Estreptoquinasa Republicas de America del Sur (EMERAS). In Sleight P, Tavassi L, (eds): *The major clinical trials on thrombolysis for acute myocardial infarction,* New York, 1992, Raven Press.

28. Ho MT, Eisenberg MS, Litwin PE, et al: Delay between onset of chest pain and seeking medical care: the effect of public education, *Ann Emerg Med* 18:727-731, 1989.

29. Herlitz J, Hartford M, Blohm M, et al: Effect of a media campaign on delay times and ambulance use in suspected acute myocardial infarction, *Am J Cardiol* 64:90-93, 1989.

30. Moses HW, Engelking N, Taylor GJ, et al: Effect of a two-year public education campaign on reducing response time of patients with symptoms of acute myocardial infarction, *Am J Cardiol* 68:249-251, 1991.

31. Mitic WR, Perkins J: The effect of a media campaign on heart attack delay and decision times, *Can J Public Health* 75:415-418, 1984.

32. Castaigne AD, Herve C, Duval-Moulin AM, et al: Prehospital use of APSAC: results of a placebo-controlled study, *Am J Cardiol* 64:30A-33A, 1989.

33. Herve C, Gaillard M, Castaigne AD, et al: Thrombolysis at home, *Lancet* 2:1278, 1987.

34. Kereiakes DJ, Weaver WD, Anderson JL, et al: Time delays in the diagnosis and treatment of acute myocardial infarction: a tale of eight cities. Report from the Pre-hospital Study Group and the Cincinnati Heart Project, *Am Heart J* 120:773-779, 1990.

35. Koren C, Weiss AT, Hasin Y, et al: Prevention of myocardial damage in acute myocardial ischemia by early treatment with intravenous streptokinase, *N Engl J Med* 313:1384, 1985.

36. Roth A, Barbash GI, Hod H, et al: Should thrombolytic therapy be administered in the mobile intensive care unit in patients with evolving myocardial infarction? A pilot study, *J Am Coll Cardiol* 15:932-936, 1990.

37. Report of the European Myocardial Infarction Project (EMIP) subcommittee: Potential time-saving with pre-hospital intervention in acute myocardial infarction, *Eur Heart J* 9:118-124, 1988.

38. Weaver WD, Eisenberg MS, Martin JS, et al: Myocardial infarction triage and intervention Project Phase I: patient characteristics and feasibility of prehospital initiation of thrombolytic therapy, *J Am Coll Cardiol* 15:925-931, 1990.

39. Moses HW, Bartolozzi JJ, Koester DL, et al: Reducing delay in the emergency room in administration of thrombolytic therapy for myocardial infarction associated with ST elevation, *Am J Cardiol* 68:251-253, 1991.

40. Sharkey SW, Brunette DD, Ruiz E, et al: An analysis of time delays preceding thrombolysis for acute myocardial infarction, *JAMA* 262:3171-3174, 1989.

41. Yusuf S, Wittes J, Friedman L: Overview of results of randomized clinical trials in heart disease. I: Treatments following myocardial infarction, *JAMA* 260:2088-2093, 1988.

42. Muller DWM, Topol EJ: Selection of patients with acute myocardial infarction for thrombolytic therapy, *Ann Intern Med* 113:949-960, 1990.

43. Grasela TH, Green JA: A nationwide survey of prescribing patterns for thrombolytic drugs in acute myocardial infarction, *Pharmacotherapy* 10:35-41, 1990.

44. Maynard C, Althouse R, Cerqueira MD, et al: Underutilization of thrombolytic therapy in eligible women with acute myocardial infarction, *Am J Cardiol* 68:529-530, 1991.

45. Cragg DR, Friedman HZ, Bonema JD, et al: Outcome of patients with acute myocardial infarction who are ineligible for thrombolytic therapy, *Ann Intern Med* 115:173-177, 1991.

46. Tobin JN, Wassertheil-Smoller S, Wexler JP, et al: Sex bias in considering coronary bypass surgery, *Ann Intern Med* 107:19-25, 1987.

47. Krumholz HM, Douglas PS, Lauer MS, Pasternak RC: Selection of patients for coronary angiography and coronary revascularization early after myocardial infarction: is there evidence for a gender bias? *Ann Intern Med* 116:785-790, 1992.

48. Naylor CD, Baigrie RS, Goldman BS, et al: Revascularization Panel Consensus Methods Group. Assessment of priority for coronary revascularization procedures, *Lancet* 335:1070-1073, 1990.

49. Khan SS, Nessim S, Gray R, et al: Increased mortality of women in coronary artery bypass surgery: evidence for referral bias, *Ann Intern Med* 112:561-567, 1990.

50. Ayanian JZ, Epstein AM: Differences in the use of procedures between women and men hospitalized for coronary heart disease, *N Engl J Med* 325(4):221-225, 1991.

51. Jaglal SB, Naylor CD, Goel V: Gender differences in the use of invasive procedures after acute myocardial infarction in Ontario,

1990: a population-based analysis, ICES Working Paper Series no. 6, 1993.

52. Naylor CD, Ugnat AM, Weinkauf D, et al: Coronary artery bypass graft surgery in Canada: what is its rate of use? Which rate is right? *Can Med Assoc J* 146(6):851-858, 1992.

53. Anderson GM, Lomas J: Regionalization of coronary artery bypass surgery. Effects on access, *Med Care* 27:288-296, 1989.

54. Peters S, Chagani K, Paddon P, et al: Coronary artery bypass surgery in Canada, *Health Reports* 2(1):9-26, 1990.

55. Roos LL, Sharp SM: Innovation, centralization, and growth: coronary artery bypass graft surgery in Manitoba, *Med Care* 27:441-452, 1989.

56. Higginson LAJ, Cairns JA, Keon WJ, et al: Rates of cardiac catheterization, coronary angioplasty and open-heart surgery in adults in Canada, *Can Med Assoc J* 146:921-925, 1992.

57. Chassin MR, Park RE, Fink A, et al: Indications for selected medical and surgical procedures—a literature review and ratings of appropriateness: coronary artery bypass graft surgery (RAND R-3204/2CWF/HF/PMT/RWJ), Santa Monica, 1986, Rand Corporation.

58. Winslow CM, Kosecoff JB, Chassin MR, et al: The appropriateness of performing coronary artery bypass surgery, *JAMA* 260:505-509, 1988.

59. Brook RH, Kosecoff JB, Park RE, et al: Diagnosis and treatment of coronary artery disease: comparison of doctors' attitudes in the USA and the UK, *Lancet* 1:750-753, 1988.

60. Gray D, Hampton JR, Bernstein SJ, et al: Audit of coronary angiography and bypass surgery, *Lancet* 335:1317-1320, 1990.

61. Roos NP, Roos LL, Henteleff PD: Elective surgical rates: do high rates mean lower standards? *N Engl J Med* 297:360-365, 1977.

62. Chassin MR, Kosecoff JB, Park RE, et al: Does inappropriate use explain geographic variations in the use of health care services? A study of three procedures, *JAMA* 258:2533-2537, 1987.

63. Leape LL, Park RE, Solomon DH, et al: Does inappropriate use explain small-area variations in the use of health care services? *JAMA* 263:669-672, 1990.

64. Naylor CD, Armstrong PW: Guidelines for the use of thrombolytic therapy in acute myocardial infarction, *Can Med Assoc J* 137:1289-1299, 1989.

65. Floras JS, Naylor CD, Armstrong PW: Coronary revascularization after thrombolytic therapy for myocardial infarction: what caseloads could Canadian centres face? *Can Med Assoc J* 141:783-790, 1989.

66. Naylor CD: A different view of queues in Ontario, *Health Aff (Millwood)* 10(3):110-128, 1991.

67. Anderson GM, Lomas J: Monitoring the diffusion of a technology: coronary artery bypass surgery in Ontario, *Am J Public Health* 78:251-254, 1988.

68. The TIMI Study Group: Comparison of invasive and conservative strategies after treatment with intravenous tissue plasminogen activator in acute myocardial infarction: results of the thrombolysis in myocardial infarction (TIMI) Phase II trial, *N Engl J Med* 320:618-627, 1989.

69. The TIMI Study Group: Immediate vs delayed catheterization and angioplasty following thrombolytic therapy for acute myocardial infarction. TIMI IIa results, *JAMA* 260:2849-2858, 1988.

70. Geltman EM: Conservative management after thrombolysis: the strategy of choice, *J Am Coll Cardiol* 16:1535-1537, 1990.

71. Feit F, Mueller HS, Braunwald E, et al: Thrombolysis in myocardial infarction (TIMI) Phase II trial: outcome comparison of a "conservative" strategy in community versus tertiary hospitals, *J Am Coll Cardiol* 16:1529-1534, 1990.

72. Simoons ML, Arnold AER, Betriu A, et al: Thrombolysis with tissue plasminogen activator in acute myocardial infarction: no additional benefit from immediate percutaneous coronary angioplasty, *Lancet* 1:197-202, 1988.

73. Guerci AD, Gerstenblith G, Brinker JA, et al: A randomized trial of intravenous tissue plasminogen activator for acute myocardial infarction with subsequent randomization to elective coronary angioplasty, *N Engl J Med* 317:1613-1618, 1987.

74. Guerci AD, Ross RS: TIMI II and the role of angioplasty in acute myocardial infarction, *N Engl J Med* 320:663-665, 1989.

75. Topol EJ, Califf RM, George BS, et al: A randomized trial of immediate versus delayed elective angioplasty after intravenous tissue plasminogen activator in acute myocardial infarction, *N Engl J Med* 317:581-588, 1987.

76. Topol EJ: Coronary angioplasty for acute myocardial infarction, *Ann Intern Med* 109:970-980, 1988.

77. Krucoff MW, Green CE, Satler LF, et al: Noninvasive detection of coronary artery patency using continuous ST-segment monitoring, *Am J Cardiol* 57:916-922, 1986.

78. Naylor CD, Jaglal SB: Impact of intravenous thrombolysis on short-term coronary revascularization rates: a meta-analysis, *JAMA* 264:697-702, 1990.

79. The ISAM Study Group: A prospective trial of intravenous streptokinase in acute myocardial infarction (ISAM), *N Engl J Med* 314:1465-1471, 1986.

80. Van de Werf F, Arnold AER: Intravenous tissue plasminogen activator and size of infarct, left ventricular function and survival in acute myocardial infarction, *Br Med J* 297:1374-1379, 1988.

81. Kennedy JW, Martin GV, Davis KB, et al: The Western Washington intravenous streptokinase in acute myocardial infarction randomized trial, *Circulation* 77:345-352, 1988.

82. Armstrong PW, Baigrie RS, Daly PA, et al: Tissue plasminogen activator: Toronto (TPAT). Randomized trial in myocardial infarction, *J Am Coll Cardiol* 13:1469-1476, 1989.

83. O'Rourke M, Baron D, Keogh A, et al: Limitation of myocardial infarction by early infusion of recombinant tissue-type plasminogen activator, *Circulation* 77:1311-1315, 1988.

84. White HD, Norris RM, Brown MA, et al: Effect of intravenous streptokinase on left ventricular function and early survival after acute myocardial infarction, *N Engl J Med* 317:850-855, 1987.

85. National Heart Foundation of Australia Coronary Thrombolysis Group: Coronary thrombolysis and myocardial salvage by tissue plasminogen activator given up to 4 hours after onset of myocardial infarction, *Lancet* 1:203-207, 1988.

86. Mantel N, Haenszel W: Statistical aspects of the analysis of data from retrospective studies of disease, *J Natl Cancer Inst* 22:719-748, 1959.

87. Wilcox RG, von der Lippe G, Olsson CG, et al: Effects of alteplase in acute myocardial infarction: 6-month results from the ASSET study, *Lancet* 335:1175-1178, 1990.

88. Lardoux H, Louvard Y, de Vernejoul D, et al: French multicenter trial of anistreplase versus heparin in acute myocardial infarction, *Cardiovasc Drug Ther* 4:1337-1344, 1990.

89. Schroder R, Neuhaus KL, Leizorovicz A, et al: A prospective placebo-controlled double-blind multicenter trial of intravenous streptokinase in acute myocardial infarction (ISAM): long-term mortality and morbidity, *J Am Coll Cardiol* 9:197-203, 1987.

90. Simoons ML, Vos J, Tijssen JGP, et al: Long-term benefit of early thrombolytic therapy in patients with acute myocardial infarction: 5-year follow-up of a trial conducted by the Inter-University Cardiology Institute of the Netherlands, *J Am Coll Cardiol* 14:1609-1615, 1989.

91. Simoons ML, Vos J, Martens LL: Cost-utility analysis of thrombolytic therapy, *Eur Heart J* 12:696-699, 1991.

92. Wilkes NPF, Jones MP, O'Rourke MF, et al: Determinants of recurrent ischaemia and revascularization procedures after thrombolysis with recombinant tissue plasminogen activator in primary coronary occlusion, *Int J Cardiol* 30:69-76, 1991.

93. Kereiakes DJ, Califf RM, George BS, et al: Coronary bypass surgery improves global and regional left ventricular function

following thrombolytic therapy for acute myocardial infarction, *Am Heart J* 122:390-399, 1991.

94. Naylor CD, Hollenberg AA: Practice guidelines and professional autonomy in a universal health insurance system: the case of tissue plasminogen activator in Ontario, *Soc Sci Med* 31:1327-1336, 1990.
95. Naylor CD, Hollenberg AA, Ugnat AM, et al: Coronary thrombolysis, clinical guidelines, and public policy: results of an Ontario practitioner survey, *Can Med Assoc J* 142:1069-1080, 1990.
96. Laffel GL, Fineberg HV, Braunwald E: A cost-effectiveness model for coronary thrombolysis/reperfusion therapy, *J Am Coll Cardiol* 10:79B-90B, 1987.
97. Silberberg JS, McGregor M: Restoration of flow in acute coronary obstructive syndromes: consequences of different management strategies, *Can J Cardiol* 5:129-135, 1989.
98. Steinberg EP, Topol EJ, Sakin JW, et al: Cost and procedure implications of thrombolytic therapy for acute myocardial infarction, *J Am Coll Cardiol* 12:58A-68A, 1988.
99. Krumholz HM, Pasternak RC, Weinstein MC, et al: Cost effectiveness of thrombolytic therapy with streptokinase in elderly patients with suspected acute myocardial infarction, *N Engl J Med* 327:7-13, 1992.
100. Goel V, Naylor CD: Potential cost effectiveness of intravenous tissue plasminogen activator versus streptokinase for acute myocardial infarction, *Can J Cardiol* 8:31-38, 1992.
101. Goldman L, Cook EF, Hashimoto B, et al: Evidence that hospital care for acute myocardial infarction has not contributed to the decline in coronary mortality between 1973-74 and 1978-79, *Circulation* 65:936-942, 1982.
102. Naylor CD, Basinski A, Frank JW, et al: Asymptomatic hypercholesterolemia: a clinical policy review, *J Clin Epidemiol* 43:1029-1121, 1990.
103. Toronto Working Group on Cholesterol Policy: *Detection and management of asymptomatic hypercholesterolemia,* Toronto, 1989, Task Force on the Use and Provision of Medical Services.
104. de Vreede JJM, Gorgels APM, Verstraaten GMP, et al: Did prognosis after acute myocardial infarction change during the past 20 years? A meta-analysis, *J Am Coll Cardiol* 18:698-706, 1991.
105. McGovern PG, Folsom AR, Sprafka JM, et al: Trends in the survival of hospitalized myocardial infarction patients between 1970 and 1985. The Minnesota Heart Survey, *Circulation* 85:172-179, 1992.
106. Goldberg RJ, Gore JM, Alpert JS, et al: Cardiogenic shock after acute myocardial infarction. Incidence and mortality from a community-wide prespective, 1975 to 1988, *N Engl J Med* 325:1117-1122, 1991.
107. Naylor CD, Armstrong PW: Cardiogenic shock after acute myocardial infarction, *Ann Int Med* 116(2):58, 1992.
108. Kelly JV, Hellinger FJ: Heart disease and hospital deaths: an empirical study, *Health Serv Res* 22(3):369-395, 1987.
109. Luft HS, Hunt SS, Maerki SC: The volume-outcome relationship: practice makes perfect or selective-referral patterns? *Health Serv Res* 22(2):157-182, 1987.
110. Maerki SC, Luft HS, Hunt SS: Selecting categories of patients for regionalization: implications of the relationship between volume and outcome, *Med Care* 24(2):148-158, 1986.
111. Shortell SM, LoGerfo JP: Hospital medical staff organization and quality of care: results for myocardial infarction and appendectomy, *Med Care* 19(10):1041-1055, 1981.
112. Farley DE, Ozminkowski RJ: Volume-outcome relationships and inhospital mortality: the effect of changes in volumes over time, *Med Care* 30:77-94, 1992.

INDEX

Prostacyclin
  aspirin and, 327-328
  reperfusion injury and, 383
Prostacyclin analogue, 343-344
Prostaglandin, 679
Prostaglandin E$_1$, 343-344
Protein, plasmin and, 30-31
Protein C, 29
  age and, 39
  as antithrombotic agent, 332
  deficiency, 36
Protein C antigen, 38
Prourokinase; *see also* Single-chain urokinase-type
    plasminogen activator
Proximate cause, 916
Pseudoaneurysm, femoral artery catheterization and,
    689-690
Psychiatric symptoms, delirium as, 757; *see also*
    Delirium
Psychological factors
  of cardiac rehabilitation, 865-866
  exercise testing and, 775
Psychological support for patient, 818
Psychosocial factors, 49-55
  depression as, 51
  hostility and, 49-54
  social isolation as, 51, 52
  type A behavior and, 49-54
Pulmonary capillary wedge pressure, 724
Pulmonary edema, 724
Pulse pressure, 642
Pump, intraaortic balloon; *see* Intraaortic balloon
    pump
Purkinje system, 232-234

Q

Q wave
  myocardial infarction, 241
  reperfusion and, 457
Q wave myocardial infarction
  exercise testing and, 773-774
  stress perfusion imaging for, 792
QRS complex
  exercise testing and, 773-774
  myocardial infarction and, 235-236, 604
Quality of care, 146
Quality of life assessment, 183-199
  in acute ischemic disease, 193-196
  background of, 183-184
  measurements for, 185-193
  reasons for, 184-185
Questionnaire, hostility assessment, 54
Quinidine
  dosage of, 486
  monitoring levels of, 486-487
  for ventricular tachycardia and, 620
Q-wave infarction, 525

R

Race
  emergency room evaluation and, 257

Race—cont'd
  stroke risk and, 639
Radiation therapy, streptokinase versus, 298-299
Radiography, in renal failure, 677-678
Radionuclide imaging
  angiographic, 797-813
    assessment of prognosis with, 801-807
    congestive heart failure and, 799-801
    as endpoint in trial, 153-154
    in experimental infarction, 797-799
    thrombolytic therapy and, 807-811
  clinical applications of, 786-793
  in right ventricular myocardial infarction, 745
  techniques of, 786-790
  thallium for, 781-786
  of ventricular function, 446
Randomized Evaluation of Salvage Angioplasty With
    Combined Utilization of Endpoints trial, 392-393
Ratio scale, 189
Receptor, platelet membrane, 99, 101
Recombinant antistatin, 332
Recombinant tick anticoagulant peptide, 102
Recombinant tissue-type plasminogen activator
  angioplasty versus, 410
  antibody treatment and, 101-102
  antithrombotic therapy and, 329
  streptokinase vs, 91-92
Recurrent ischemia, as endpoint in trial, 162; *see also*
    Reperfusion, failure of
Recurrent stenosis, unstable angina and, 552-553
Reflex, Bezold-Jarisch, 610
Reform, malpractice, 917
Refusal to treat, 923
Registry
  of myocardial infarction patients, 248
  primary angioplasty, 307-309
Regression of atherosclerosis, 537-538; *see also*
    Atherosclerosis, control of progression of
Regurgitation
  aortic, 727-732
  mitral, 732-735
    ischemic, 651-655
  tricuspid, 737-738
    in right ventricular myocardial infarction, 746
Rehabilitation, 843-870
  early, 815-819
  exercise and, 844-847, 856-857
  medical therapy in, 847-856
  nutrition and, 857-861
  pharmacologic therapy in, 862-865
  psychosocial aspects of, 865-866
  stroke and, 646-647
Reinfarction
  after reperfusion, 584-598; *see also* Reperfusion,
    failure of
  as endpoint in trial, 160-161
Relaxation, myocardial, 711
Relaxation training, 865
Remodeling of left ventricle, 119-126
  heart failure and, 871-874
  radionuclide angiography and, 801